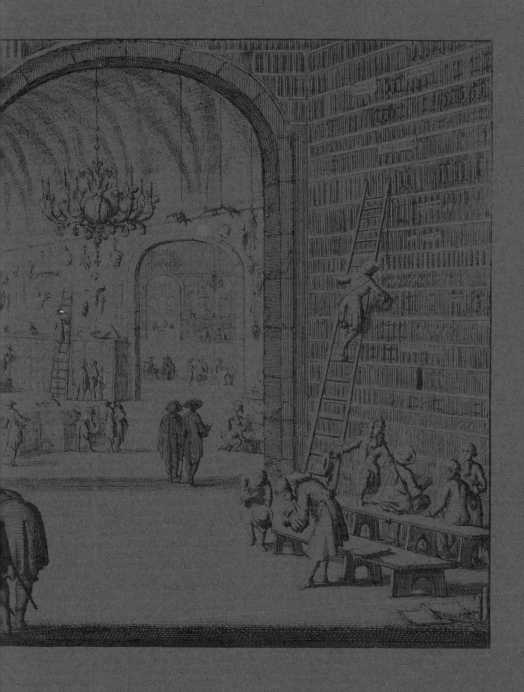

HISTORY OF THE LIFE SCIENCES

An annotated bibliography

by

PIETER SMIT

Catholic University of Nijmegen

With a foreword

by

FRANS VERDOORN

HAFNER PRESS
A Division of Macmillan Publishing Co., Inc.
New York
Collier Macmillan Canada Ltd.

HAFNER PRESS

A Division of Macmillan Publishing Co., Inc.

866 Third Avenue, New York, N.Y. 10022

Collier Macmillan Canada Ltd.

Library of Congress Cataloging in Publication Data:

Smit, Pieter, Dr.
   History of the Life Sciences: An annotated bibliography

    1. Life sciences - History - Bibliography.   I. Title.
Z5320.S55   016.57'09   74-12091

ISBN 0-02-852510-8

FOREWORD

In the early 1940's, after moving Chronica Botanica and related activities to the U.S.A., I started building up - in conjunction with the gathering of documentation towards our 'Index Botanicorum' project (a biographical encyclopaedia of plant scientists) - a number of card indices of the world literature relating to various historical and not mainly biographical aspects of the life, particularly the plant sciences.

In 1958, all this documentation, together with the former Chronica Botanica Library, was repatriated to the Netherlands where I was enabled to start building up the Utrecht University Biohistorical Institute. Owing to the pressure of various new duties and to broadening the scope of what I started in the New World, according to the gradual development of our biohistorical ideology, not too much was added to our documentation apparatus, our 'Index Ultrajectinus', for some time.

When Dr. Smit, already widely known, *i.a.*, for his research, editorial and bibliographic work at the Leiden University Institute for Theoretical Biology, joined our staff in 1963, he started materially adding to various indices of the 'Index Ultrajectinus', thoroughly covering the entire biological field.

A few years later, we made tentative plans for a vademecum type short-title, selective, and only incidentally briefly annotated guide to cover the entire biohistorical spectrum. It became, however, soon clear that we did not, as yet, have enough data on hand for this extensive subject matter and that a couple of guides of a more limited scope, with proper annotations, might well be preferable.

Since then, Dr. Smit has been compiling his annotated bibliography, mainly of the history of the life sciences. After combing the books, serials, card indices, *etc.* available at our Institute, he proceeded to consult the relevant holdings of many Netherlands libraries. Much additional material was gathered by him on several trips abroad (for a number of which we are under obligation to Z.W.O., the Netherlands Organisation for the Advancement of Pure Research).

I think that Dr. Smit, tirelessly labouring for several years on his 'Annotated Bibliography', succeeded in elucidating by a proper selection, as well as by appropriate and informative annotations, the history of the life sciences in its manifold ramifications. On the one hand, his guide includes also much of interest to workers in medical history as well as various branches of the humanities. On the other hand, much relating to the role of life sciences and their subject matter through cultural history has been covered.

I am happy that the results of Dr. Smit's careful preparatory work and sound judgment are now being presented in a most fitting manner, and I hope - or rather feel certain - that it will stimulate and be of considerable aid to research and related activities in the history of the life and allied sciences, as well as in various related aspects of biohistory.

FRANS VERDOORN

INTRODUCTION

This 'History of the Life Sciences: an annotated Bibliography' originated as a plan to produce an extension of those parts of Sarton's 'Guide to the History of Science' that deal with the life sciences. The growing interest in the history of the life sciences on the part of scientists, philosophers and historians of all sorts, made the creation of a useful instrument advisable for an easy retrieve of some basic information concerning a certain subject or period. Like Sarton's book, this annotated bibliography primarily will serve the historian of science, but at the same time it will attract the scientific and scholarly biologist and medical man and may be of value to the librarian.

The text is composed of more than 4,000 entries; each of them gives full bibliographical information - such as: author, title, edition where applicable, collation, series, imprint, etc. - followed by a summary review of an average length of 90 words about the selected literature regarding a certain subject on account of its importance to the history of the life sciences. These reviews are in English; the composition, however, varies greatly. Journal articles have been considered only exceptionally. Unfortunately it has not been possible to standardize in the entries the method of transliteration from the Russian, Arabic, etc. There also may be discrepancies in the spelling of names. The form of the names chosen is the English version in the case of famous men; otherwise I have given preference to the vernacular or Latin version.

The contents have been based in the first place on the rich collections of the Biohistorical Institute of Utrecht University, but in order to attain a higher level of completeness, several libraries were visited, in the Netherlands as well as abroad, such as: the university libraries of Leiden and Utrecht, the library of the Wellcome Medical Historical Institute, the British Museum of Natural History, the University of Cambridge, the Senckenberg Institute for the history of Medicine, the Medical Historical Institute of the University of Bonn, and the Bibliothèque Nationale of Paris.

Most of the books included have been consulted by the editor personally, but a number of journals containing critical bibliographies have been considered as well, like: Isis, Sudhoffs Archiv, Archives Internationales d'Histoire des Sciences, Bulletin of the History of Medicine, Journal of the History of Medicine and Allied Sciences, Bri h Journal for the History of Science, Medical History, Janus, Science, Nature (Lond.), and some others. In spite of these efforts, however, I must have missed many relevant entries. Except for a few cases, the deadline for listing new works and new editions was the middle of the year 1971.

The present text is composed of four parts. The first chapter deals with general references and methods used with historical research. Separate sections deal with general works on the philosophy and methodology of history; with comprehensive works on the history of science and civilization; with comprehensive standard bibliographies, dealing with such subjects as: the pure and applied plant sciences, animal sciences, incl. veterinary science, the medical sciences, incl. therapy and pharmacy, gastronomy, hunting, psychology, occult sciences, etc.; with biographical dictionaries, dealing with men and women who were active in the fields of biology, medicine, and pharmacy; and with some recommended encyclopaedias, chronologies, historical atlases, dictionaries, explanatory glossaries, taxonomic indexes, etc. in the fields of biology s.l., pure and applied plant sciences, animal sciences, incl. apiculture and veterinary science, medicine, incl. dentistry, therapy, and pharmacy, geographical dictionaries, guides to literature on travel, etc.

The second chapter deals with the historiography of the life and medical sciences during the ancient and mediaeval periods, and is arranged in chronological and ethnographical order. It is composed of the following sections: antiquity in general, the life and medical sciences in prehistoric times, in Egypt, Mesopotamia, India, the Far East, the life and medical sciences of the Hebrews, in Classical Antiquity, in the Near East (Byzantium, Syria, Persia, Arabs) and in the Latin West in the Middle Ages. Each of these sections has been subdivided into three or four sub-sections as follows: History of science and culture in general; History of the plant and animal sciences; History of the medical sciences; Some individual scientists. In this last sub-section biographical studies or modern reissues of publications are assembled - as a rule in the form of an annotated translation in one of the modern languages - of some of the authors from the periods considered. The identification of personalities appeared to be a time-consuming task. Often the original sources gave no decisive clue as to the identity of personality and the fact that the references were in many different languages, some involving problems of transliteration, often made matters complicated.

The third part dealing with the historiography of the life and medical sciences during the Renaissance and later periods, has been divided according to the subjects into four sections. First, the section History of the life sciences in general, with the sub-sections: history of general biology, human biology and anthropology, human and animal behaviour, anatomy and cytology, embryology, physiology, microbiology, genetics and evolution theory, palaeontology, the domestication of animals and plants, and the history of plant and animal geography and ecology. Second, the section History of the animal sciences, with the sub-sections: history of zoology in general, entomology, ornithology, and veterinary science. Third, the section History of the plant sciences with sub-sections: history of the pure plant sciences, agriculture, horticulture, forestry, phytopathology and mycology. The fourth section deals with the history of the medical sciences; the first part of this section deals, *inter alia,* with the histories of some specialties of a more general importance, incl. the histories of some diseases, the history of some social aspects of medicine, of medical education and the care of the sick, the history of public health, industrial hygiene, occupational diseases, epidemiology, medical geography, preventive medicine, immunization, military-, naval-, and aviation hygiene and medicine, *etc.* The second part of this fourth section deals with the history of therapy, incl. the history of pharmaco-therapy, pharmacy, pharmacognosy and the apothecary, pharmacology and toxicology, and the history of chemo-therapy. Throughout this whole third part, special attention has been paid to histories of only a regional importance; special subsections deal with them in the sections on the history of the pure and applied plant sciences, the medical sciences and therapy.

The fourth and last part of the text consists of a selected list of biographies, bibliographies, *etc.* of famous biologists, medical men, *etc.,* including some modern reissues of their publications.

Cross-references facilitate searching; throughout the book a moderate number of cross-references call attention to closely allied headings and to individual works listed under other subjects. An extensive index of authors listed and of names included in the text completes this volume.

Without the generous help of many colleagues this bibliography could not have been compiled. The first name to be mentioned is that of Frans Verdoorn, director of the Biohistorical Institute, Utrecht University, who suggested to me some eight years ago to start this work and who always remained interested in it ever since. I am also much indebted to the directors and staff members of institutes who allowed me to consult their libraries. Of course, I can not hope to mention each one of the many helpers separately, but I would like to name in particular Dr. C. H. Talbot of the Wellcome Medical Historical Institute for his valuable suggestions for and his examination of the section 'Life and medical sciences in the Latin West in the Middle Ages'; Dr. R. Y. Ebied of the Department of Semitic Studies, University of Leeds, who was so kind to go through the section 'Life and medical sciences in the Near East in the Middle Ages'; Dr. G. Preiser of the Senckenberg Institute for the History of Medicine, Frankfurt a. M., who made some valuable suggestions concerning the section 'Life and medical sciences in Classical Antiquity'; Dr. H. H. Eulner, Department of the History of Medicine, University of Göttingen, with whom I had a fruitful discussion about the arrangement of the section 'History of the medical sciences'; Dr. J. Needham, Master of Gonville and Caius' College, Cambridge University, who enabled me to explore the rich collections of the Cambridge University Library, where I composed the greater part of the sections dealing with the Middle Ages; Dr. J. G. M. van der Poel of the Department of Agricultural History of the Agricultural College, Wageningen, for his help in completing the sections on agrarian history; and Drs. A. G. Mathijsen, Librarian of the Veterinary Faculty, Utrecht University, for his information concerning the sections dealing with veterinarian science. I also would like to mention Dr. Jerry Stannard of Kansas University both for his interest in this bibliographic project and for his additions to the section 'Life and medical sciences in Classical Antiquity'. Furthermore I am indebted to my former colleagues of the Biohistorical Institute, Utrecht University, in particular to Miss A. J. M. Koenheim (now Mrs. Heniger) and to Miss P. H. van der Linden (now Mrs. Blans) for checking many of the references and for the preparation of the index. Then I will not fail to express my thanks to the publishers, A. Asher & Co., for their valuable assistance with the final completion of the book.

Last but not least I would like to express my deep appreciation to the late Dr. Hugh Nicol, Shoreham-by-Sea, England, who was so instrumental in correcting and standardizing the text, in supplying additional bibliographical information, in correcting the proofs, in teaching the English language, and in stimulating the whole project, that here I want to call him my closest co-worker during the preparation of this book.

Despite all this help and advices, responsibility for the accuracy and completeness of the information given in this book rests solely with its editor. No one but myself knows better the deficiencies of this work. The decision to publish it in its present form, rests on my hope that it will in some measure fulfil its object of assisting those who are interested in the history of the life and medical sciences. Although every effort has been made to check the accuracy of the references and other data, it has not been possible to be successful in every case. I also am fully aware of the fact that some books included may have been superseded, that much has been omitted which might have been included, but also that much is included which better had been omitted. It appeared to be too extensive a task for one single scientist to review the steadily growing field of the history of the life and medical sciences, but I still believe that it is necessary to have a starting point. In the future this starting point may perhaps be considered worthy of serving as a basis for further improvement. Opportunities will certainly arise to close some of the gaps to bring the book more into line with the existing situation. Anyway, the editor will gratefully accept any suggestion regarding errors, inclusions or omissions.

TABLE OF CONTENTS

XIV

CHAPTER I: GENERAL REFERENCES AND TOOLS

1. SOME WORKS ON THE PHILOSOPHY AND METHODOLOGY OF HISTORY
(incl. some bibliographical guides)

AGASSI, J., 1963: Towards a historiography of science, 117 p. (History and theory: studies in the philosophy of history, Beiheft 2) ('s-Gravenhage: Mouton).—

> According to the author, two defects are responsible for the lamentable state in which the study of the history of science finds itself, *viz.,* the application of the inductive philosophy (according to which scientific theories emerge from facts) and the conventionalist philosophy (according to which scientific theories are mathematical pigeonholes for classifying facts). Both methods are thoroughly criticized, and as an alternative Popper's critical philosophy of science should provide a possible remedy. *(Cf.* POPPER, K.R., 1959: The logic of scientific discovery, 479 p., London: Hutchinson; and POPPER, K.R., 1963: Conjectures and refutations: the growth of scientific knowlegde, 412 p., London: Routledge & Kegan Paul). Although the author does not concern himself with biological problems, the book is (due to its provocative character) of interest to everyone concerned with historical problems, whether or not he can agree with the author's statement that "historical explanation of any value is rare in the annals of the history of science, mainly because of a naive acceptance of untenable philosophical principles."

ARTELT, W., 1949: Einführung in die Medizinhistorik. Ihr Wesen, ihre Arbeitsweise und ihre Hilfsmittel, 240 p. (Stuttgart: Enke).—

> A manual of historical research and publication, in which the author adapts the rules, methods, *etc.,* as they are described by BERNHEIM *(vide infra)* to the special needs of the medical historian. Separate chapters deal with the understanding of sources, the finding of material, criticism and interpretation, and with the presentation of the results.

BERNHEIM, E., 1908: Lehrbuch der historischen Methode und der Geschichtsphilosophie. Mit Nachweis der wichtigsten Quellen und Hilfsmittel zum Studium der Geschichte, 2 vols., ed. 6, 852 p. (Leipzig: Duncker & Humblot).—

> The contents of the book are divided into six parts: 1. Concept and essence of historiography (p. 1-178) (the concept of the science of history and its evolution, limitations, relations to other sciences, *etc.);* 2. Methodology (p. 179-251) (the specific character of the historical method, objectivity *vs.* subjectivity, evolution and classification of methodology); 3. Knowledge of sources (p. 252-323) (heuristic: classification of sources, supplementary sciences, *e.g.,* philology, palaeography, heraldry, numismatics, *etc.);* 4. Criticism (p. 324-561) (authenticity and falsification, tradition, influence of place and time, reliability of the sources, critical evaluation of sources, multiple control of sources, *etc.);* 5. Interpretation (p. 562-776) (interpretation of tradition, language, time of origin, combination of interpretations, the role of phantasy, *etc);* 6. Representation (p. 777-798). Author- and subject-indexes. The first edition appeared in 1889. The sixth edition has been reprinted quite recently (undated) by Franklin (New York, N.Y.).

CABANÈS, A., 1921: L'histoire éclairée par la clinique, 320 p. (Paris: Michel).—

> To demonstrate the contents of this book the chapter headings are stated: La médecine, science auxiliaire de l'histoire: Du rôle de l'individualité dans l'histoire; Qu'entend-on par dégénérescence? Il n'y a pas de logiques (Michelet, Taine); La méthode scientifique: Littré et son école; Origine du psychopathologie historique; Les rapports de la médecine d'une part et de la sociologie, de la philosophie, de l'histoire d'autre part; Application des notions médicales à l'interprétation de l'histoire.

COLLINGWOOD, R. G., 1956: The idea of history, 339 p. (New York, N.Y.: Oxford U.P.).—

> A reprint of the posthumously published work of a famous English historian. The introduction deals with such subjects as: the philosophy of history, its nature, object, method, and value. The rest of the text has been divided into 5 parts. 1. Graeco-Roman historiography; 2. The influence of Christianity; 3. The threshold of scientific history; 4. Scientific history (in England, France, Germany and Italy); 5. Epilegomena (dealing with such subjects as: human nature and human history, the historical imagination, historical evidence, history as re-enactment of past experience, the subject-

matter of history, history and freedom, progress as created by historical thinking. The original ed. appeared in 1946 (Oxford: Clarendon Press).

DANTO, A. C., 1968: Analytical philosophy of history, 318 p. (Cambridge: U.P.).—

First published in 1965. The best way to make clear the contents of this book seems to be to give the table of contents: Substantive and analytical philosophy of history; A minimal characterization of history; Three objections against the possibility of historical knowledge; Verification, verifiability, and tensed sentences; Temporal language and temporal scepticism; Evidence and historical relativism; History and chronicle; Narrative sentences; Future and past: contingencies; Historical explanation: the rôle of narratives; Methodological individualism and methodological socialism. "This book is an analysis of historical thought and language, presented as a systematic network of arguments and clarifications, the conclusions of which compose a descriptive metaphysic of historical existence." (From the preface).

DUTCHER, G. M., et al., 1931: Guide to historical literature, 1222 p. (New York, N.Y.: Macmillan).—

Contains a review of the larger publications of source-material and a selection of standard works. Its subject-matter is arranged under subjects and under countries. Each section is annotated by a specialist. Reprinted 1949 (New York, N.Y.: National Bibliophile Service). A German equivalent is: FRANZ, G., 1956: Bücherkunde zur Weltgeschichte, 279 p. (Munich: Oldenbourg). Particularly valuable for French material is: LANGLOIS, 1901-1904, *vide infra.*

GARDINER, P., ed., 1959: Theories of history, 549 p. (Glencoe, Ill.: Free Press).—

A collection of some outstanding writings on the philosophy of history, starting with Vico (1668-1744). The first part of the book (p. 1-262) contains selections from thinkers who have constructed "systems" concerning the nature of the historical process (Vico, Condorcet, Kant, Herder, Hegel, Marx, Comte, Spengler, Croce, Toynbee), together with some "classical" philosophers of history like Mill or Tolstoy. The second part contains contemporary contributions with critiques of classical theories of history (*e.g.,* Popper, B. Russell, P. Geyl, A. Toynbee). Both parts are preceded by introductions, and each selection

included contains a prefatory comment, prepared by the editor.

GARRAGHAN, G. J., 1946: A guide to historical method, 482 + 30 p. (New York, N.Y.: Fordham U.P.).—

A partial translation of A. FEDER's "Lehrbuch der geschichtlichen Methode" (Regensburg, 1924). A comprehensive manual, mainly to be used by the expert scholar. The first section (p. 3-99) deals with the meaning and methods of history, certainty in history, and with auxiliary sciences; the second section (p. 103-140) deals with nature and classification of historical sources and with mechanical aids to research; the third part (p. 143-317) deals with the logical processes in history (*viz.,* analogy, generalizations, statistics, hypothesis, conjecture, the argument from silence, the argument *a priori),* the authenticity, analysis, integrity and credibility of sources; the fourth part (p. 321-426) deals with the presentation of the results of the researches. Included are a selected bibliography of historical method (p. 427-431), an index of authors (p. 433-457), and an index of subjects (p. 458-482).

GEYL, P., 1954: Use and abuse of history, 97 p. (New Haven, Conn.: Yale U.P.).—

This booklet is the result of the Terry lectures held by the author at Yale University in October, 1954. It is a very provocative book, discussing many general problems of history. To mention some of them: the different ways in which history is and has been used (and even abused) in the course of time; the organismic conception and the role of "Historismus" in the 19th century application of the methods of (natural) science in history (Comte); the influence of Hegelianism; the relativity of truth in history; fact, cause and effect in history; *etc.* A Dutch translation exists: Gebruik en misbruik der geschiedenis, 1956, 76 p. (Groningen: Wolters).

LANGLOIS, C. V., 1901-1904: Manuel de bibliographie historique, 2 vols. Vol. I: Instruments bibliographiques; Vol. II: Histoire et organisation des études historiques, 634 p. (Paris: Hachette).—

The first part was published in 1896 and deals with bibliographical tools. A second ed. of this part appeared in 1901. The second part deals with the history and organisation of historical studies in various countries from the Renaissance to the end of the nineteenth century. A reprint edition appeared in 1968 (Graz: Akad. Druck- und Verlagsanstalt).

—— & C. SEIGNOBOS, 1932: Introduction to the study of history, 350 p. (London: Duckworth).—

> Originally published in French: Introduction aux études historiques, [ed. 5, 1913] (Paris: Hachette). English translation first published in 1889 (London) and has been reprinted many times. The work is divided into three books: I. Preliminary studies (search for documents, auxiliary sciences); II. Analytical operations (external and internal criticism); III. Synthetic operations (construction, exposition). Two appendixes concerning the teaching of history in the French high schools and universities.

ROTENSTREICH, N., 1958: Between past and present: an essay on history, 329 p. (New Haven, Conn.: Yale U.P.).—

> The table of contents includes: Res gestae and their narration; objectivity; historical time; history and social science; causality and laws. Detailed analytical table of contents.

SARTON, G., 1948: The life of science: essays in the history of civilization, 197 p. (New York, N.Y.: Schuman).—

According to an editorial note, the present essays "have been selected from the author's writings over a period of some thirty years with the aim of giving both the general reader and the student a better understanding of the history of science, its scope, purpose and methods." The essays deal with: the scope of the history of science; how to write short interpretative biographies; the fundamentals of science in eastern and western civilizations; the organization and aim of the history of science.

VERDOORN, F., 1944: On the aims and methods of biological history, 27 p. (Chronica Botanica 8: 427-448).—

> With the aid of some concrete examples the author illustrates the preparation of biographies, especially as they should be written in the field of the biological sciences.

WALSH, W. H., 1951: An introduction to philosophy of history, 173 p. (London: Hutchinson; New York, N.Y.: Longmans).—

> An interpretation of the nature of historical thinking as diverging from other kinds of thinking and a discussion of the traditional metaphysical problems raised by the philosophy of history.

2. COMPREHENSIVE WORKS ON THE HISTORY OF SCIENCE AND CIVILIZATION

ANTHONY, H. D., 1948: Science and its background, 304 p. (London: Macmillan).—

> A rather popular introduction into the history of science, taking account of human development and the evolution of social institutions. The subject-matter has largely been grouped around individual men of science, selected because of the value of their work today. The author clearly elucidates how human action, knowledge and vision together helped man to reach his present state. The subject has been dealt with under the following headings: The beginning of science in the "Rivers Period", the Mediterranean period (Classical and Mediaeval), the Atlantic period (Renaissance to modern), the World period (international conflict and world co-operation).

BARKER, E., G. CLARK & P. VAUCHER, eds., 1954: The European inheritance, 3 vols. Vol. I: Prehistory; Greece and Rome; the Jews and the beginnings of the Christian Church; the Middle Ages, 543 p.; Vol. II: The early modern period; political, economic and social development in the 18th century;

the development of literature and culture in the 18th century, 391 p.; Vol. III: The nineteenth century (1815-1914), 1914-1950; review and epilogue, 406 p. (Oxford: Clarendon Press).—

> "This work originated during the War at a conference of the ministers of education of eight allied governments then resident and active in London. It is divided into seven chronological parts (from the beginnings of prehistory to the middle of the twentieth century), each accompanied by maps, illustrations, and primary historical documents. Each section is written by a specialist." (From Isis 47 : 256).

BERNAL, J. D., 1953: Science and industry in the nineteenth century, 230 p. (London: Routledge & Kegan Paul).—

> Starting from the emergence of the energy concept, the controversy between Pasteur and Liebig about the nature of ferments, the birth and early history of the steel industry, and the introduction of electric light, Bernal demonstrates "the close and necessary connections between

technical developments and the advancement of scientific knowledge".

—— 1965: Science in history, ed. 3, 1039 p. (London: Watts).—

This book is intended for a wide public and deals with the vital problem: what has science meant in history from earliest time to present day? Stress has been laid on the interrelations between science and society. In the first 490 pages, an analysis has been given of the manner in which scientific facts and theories are created in close connection with current social circumstances. The later pages deal with science in our time, including the development of science in the socialist part of the world and the new orientation of the emergent peoples of Asia and Africa. First published in 1954. A fourth ed. appeared in 1969, 1325 p.

BLAKE, R. M., et al., 1960: Theories of scientific method: the Renaissance through the nineteenth century, 346 p. (Seattle, Wash.: Univ. Washington Press).—

The contents of this book consist of 13 studies of historical and philosophical investigations of the theories of scientific method held by some leading thinkers from the Renaissance through the 19th century. The titles of the studies are: Natural science in the Renaissance; Theory and hypothesis among the Renaissance astronomers; Francis Bacon's philosophy of science; The role of experience in Descartes' theory of method; T. Hobbes and the rationalistic ideal; Isaac Newton and the hypothetico-deductive method; David Hume on causation; J. F. W. Herschel's methods of experimental inquiry; W. Whewell's philosophy of scientific discovery; J. Stuart Mill's system of logic; W. S. Jevons on induction and probability; C. S. Peirce's search for a method; and Chauncey Wright and the American functionalists. With notes and index.

BOAS, M., 1962: The scientific renaissance, 1450-1630, 380 p. (New York, N.Y.: Harper; London: Collins).—

This is the second volume of a planned series of eight on "The rise of modern science", edited by A. R. HALL. Although it mainly deals with 16th- and early 17th-century science, it also points on many occasions to the development of science during the Middle Ages. The text deals inter alia with such subjects as: science and learning, navigational instruments, popular knowledge, experiment and magic, the organization of science, science in the

universities, the conflict of Galileo and the Church. Separate chapters deal with Harvey, Kepler, and Galileo. The terminal date of the period considered is characterized by the publication of Galileo's "Dialogue on the two chief systems of the world", appearing two years after Harvey's "De motu cordis", both works marking "at once the culmination of the work of a preceding century and the beginning of a new age". Also in German translation: Die Renaissance der Naturwissenschaften, 1450-1630. Das Zeitalter des Kopernicus, 1965, 407 p. (Gütersloh: Mohn).

BÖHM, W., 1961: Die Naturwissenschaftler und ihre Philosophie, 316 p. (Freiburg i.B.: Herder).—

According to the author, the history of the separate scientific disciplines is greatly influenced by the history of philosophy, and not vice versa. Thus many parallels should exist between the history of philosophy and the history of these disciplines. The author believes that the history of chemistry is not a chain of fortuitously successful experiments, but that, on the contrary, the experiments should be directed by speculative ideas arising from philosophy which are practised upon a certain class of phenomena. This book is an attempt to study the history of chemistry from this point of view.

BOYNTON, H., ed., 1948: The beginnings of modern science: scientific writings of the 16th, 17th and 18th centuries, 634 p. (New York, N.Y.: Black).—

The subject-matter has been divided into 9 parts, viz.: 1. Matter and motion; 2. Light, heat and fire; 3. The study of air and of chemistry (e.g., Paracelsus); 4. Electricity; 5. The earth and its waters (e.g., da Vinci, Agricola, Buffon, Hutton); 6. How plants grow (v. Helmont, Grew, Hales, Linnaeus, Priestley, Ingenhousz); 7. The structure of the human body (Vesalius, Servetus, Fabricius, Harvey, Leeuwenhoek, Spallanzani); 8. The science of healing (Fracastorius, Paré, Sydenham, Montagu, Auenbrugger, Cook, Jenner); 9. Scientists think about science (e.g., Agricola, Bacon, Descartes). The whole book consists of 85 excerpts, each being preceded by a brief descriptive passage by the editor, explaining its contents and meaning.

BRÉHIER, E., 1926-1932: Histoire de la philosophie, 2 vols.+2 supplementary vols., 1938 and 1949. (Paris: Alcan).—

A clearly-written text, supplemented

by useful bibliographical information. The two vols. are issued in seven parts. Vol. I deals with classical antiquity and the Middle-Ages and consists of the following parts: Période hellénique, Période hellénistique et romaine; Moyen Âge et Renaissance. Vol. 2 deals with modern philosophy and consists of the following parts: Le XVIIe siècle; Le XVIIIe siècle; Le XIXe siècle-période des systèmes (1800-1850); Le XIXe siècle après 1850; Le XXe siècle. Bibliographies at the end of each chapter. The first supplement has been written by MASSON-OURSEL, P., 1938: La philosophie en Orient, 188 p.; the second supplement has been written by TATAKIS, B., 1949: La philosophie byzantine, 324 p.

BRINTON, C., J. B. CHRISTOFER & R. L. WOLFF, 1955: A history of civilization, 2 vols. Vol. I: Prehistory to 1715, 686 p.; Vol. II: 1715 to the present, 722 p. (New York, N.Y.: Prentice Hall).—

A well-written political, social, economic and intellectual history of the world from prehistory up to the 1950's. Many beautiful illustrations.

BRYK, O., 1967: Entwicklungsgeschichte der reinen und angewandten Naturwissenschaft im XIX. Jahrhundert. Vol. I: Die Naturphilosophie und ihre Ueberwindung durch die erfahrungsgemässe Denkweise (1800-1850), 654 p. (Leipzig: Zentral-Antiquariat der D.D.R.).—

Originally published in 1909 (Leipzig: Barth). Separate sections deal with the history of physics (p. 1-116), chemistry (p. 117-199), technique (p. 200-260), mineralogy (p. 261-290), geology, incl. palaeontology (p. 291-339), mathematics (p. 340-369), astronomy (p. 370-431), zoology (p. 432-494), botany (p. 495-542), and medicine (p. 543-629). As to the life sciences, special attention has been paid to the concept of "Naturphilosophie" and the influence of the cell theory.

BURY, J. B., 1955: The idea of progress: an inquiry into its origins and growth, 40+357 p. (New York, N.Y.: Dover).—

The author shows how the idea of progress is intimately connected with the growth of modern science, the growth of rationalism and the struggle for political and religious liberty. The book was first printed in 1920; this is a reprint. According to G. Sarton it is an excellent book.

BUTTERFIELD, H., 1957: The origins of modern science, 1300-1800, ed. 3, 242 p. (London: Bell).—

This is a history of science written by a historian. His main thesis is that great advances in science do not depend on a new discovery of facts, but that they depend rather on someone having the genius to look at the old material in a new way. The innovator must also have the political and dialectical skill to force people to give attention to his new point of view. This thesis has been illustrated by many examples. The author considers the 17th century as the culminating point of the scientific revolution in which the foundations of the evolution theory already were being laid which in its turn originated in the 14th century when the Aristotelian explanations of motion were being challenged. In a review of this book I.B. Cohen writes that this is one of the most stimulating and fascinating books. (Isis 41 : 231-233).

CLAGETT, M., ed., 1959: Critical problems in the history of science: proceedings of the Institute for the History of Science at the University of Wisconsin, September 1-11, 1957, 555 p. (Madison, Wisc.: Wisconsin U.P.).—

The book contains papers in the following 6 main areas of study: 1. The scientific revolution; 2. Teaching the history of science; 3. Science and the French revolution; 4. Conservation of energy; 5. Evolution; 6. The structure of matter and chemical and physical theory. The following chapters are of a special biohistorical interest: A.C. CROMBIE: The significance of medieval discussions of scientific method for the scientific revolution (p. 79-101); J.W. WILSON: Biology attains maturity in the nineteenth century (p. 401-418); J. C. GREENE: Biology and social theory in the nineteenth century: Auguste Comte and Herbert Spencer (p. 419-446), and the commentaries on the two last-mentioned chapters by R. H. SHRYOCK (p. 447-453) and C. ZIRKLE (p. 454-466).

COLLINGWOOD, R. G., 1945: The idea of nature, 183 p. (Oxford: Clarendon Press).—

The last and posthumously published work of the famous English archaeologist, historian, and philosopher, a book of which the reviewer in Isis 40, p. 395 writes: "The present volume is an historical study of the idea of nature, from the Ionians to Whitehead, from the standpoint of the philosopher. As such the work is of distinct interest to the historian of science, even though the approach is purely philosophical."

COPLESTON, F. C., 1947 →: A history of philosophy, 6 vols. (London: Burns, Oates & Washbourne; Westminster, Md.: Neuman).—

The only recent extensive history of philosophy in English. It has been written from "the standpoint of the scholastic philosopher". The following volumes have appeared: Vol. 1 (1947): Greece and Rome; vol. 2 (1950): Augustine to Scotus; vol. 3 (1953): Ockham to Suárez. Up to now vols. 4-6 seem not to have appeared.

CROMBIE, A. C., 1953: Robert Grosseteste and the origin of experimental science 1100-1700, 369 p. (Oxford: Clarendon Press).—

The author attempts to prove that the origin of the experimental method is to be found in the Middle Ages. In order to set the stage, he discusses extensively the position of 12th-century science, and against this background he examines Grosseteste's writings, for, as Crombie states, Grosseteste embodies "the two twelfth-century traditions of technology and logic". The distinction between experimental fact and theoretical (or rational) knowledge of the cause of the fact came to the West with Aristotle's logic and Galen's medicine, and so Crombie shows how Grosseteste's opinions are related to those of Aristotle and Galen, and how they on the other hand influenced such men as Roger Bacon, Albertus Magnus and William of Ockham. The book contains much material for the study of mediaeval scientific methodology and a very complete bibliography has been included.

——— 1959: Medieval and early modern science. Vol. I: Science in the Middle Ages: V-XIII centuries, 296 p.; Vol. II: Science in the later Middle Ages and early modern times: XIII-XVII centuries, 380 p. (Garden City, N.Y.: Doubleday).—

This is the second edition of CROMBIE's "Augustine to Galileo: the history of science A. D. 450-1650" (London, 1952; Cambridge, Mass., 1953). Vol. I deals with science in Western Christendom until the 12th-century renaissance, with the reception of Graeco-Arabic science in Western Christendom, with what Crombie calls the system of systematic thought in the 13th century and with mediaeval technology, incl. agricultural techniques and medicine. Vol. II deals with scientific methods and developments in physics in the later Middle Ages,

and with the revolution of scientific thought in the 16th and 17th centuries. At the end of each chapter very complete bibliographies have been added. A fascinating analysis of the history and methodology of science in the mediaeval and early modern periods.

CUVIER, G., 1834-1836: Histoire des progrès des sciences naturelles depuis 1789 jusqu'à 1831, 5 pts., 376, 419, 493, 381, 507 p. (Paris: Librairie encyclopédique de Roret).—

This work is of a great biohistorical value, because large parts are devoted to the history of biology (including physiology and anatomy), agriculture, and medicine. The first part deals with the period 1789-1808, the second, third, and fourth parts with the period 1809-1827, and the fifth part with the period 1827-1831.

DAMPIER, W. C., 1943: A history of science and its relations with philosophy and religion, 574 p. (Cambridge: U.P.; New York, N.Y.: Macmillan).—

A classic, especially valuable for those scholars who wish to have a bird's eye view of any given period in the history of science. Good index and bibliography. (1st ed., 1929). A fourth edition appeared in 1949. Also in French translation: Histoire de la science et de ses rapports avec la philosophie et la religion, 1951, 608 p. (Paris: Payot). A paperback edition appeared in 1966 (London: Cambridge U.P.). The same author also wrote a condensation of this book: A shorter history of science, 1944, 189 p. (Cambridge: U.P.). Of this work a German translation exists: Kurze Geschichte der Wissenschaft in ihren Beziehungen zur Philosophie und Religion, 1946, 228p. (Zurich: Rascher).

DANNEMANN, F., 1920-1923: Die Naturwissenschaften in ihrer Entwicklung und in ihrem Zusammenhange, ed. 2, 4 vols. Vol. I: 486 p.; vol. II: 508 p.; vol. III: 434 p.; vol. IV: 628 p. (Leipzig: Engelmann).—

Subtitles of vol. I: "Von den Anfängen bis zum Wiederaufleben der Wissenschaften"; of vol. II: "Von Galilei bis zur Mitte des 18. Jahrhunderts"; of vol. III: "Das Emporblühen der modernen Natur-Wissenschaften bis zur Aufstellung des Energieprinzipes"; of vol. IV: "Das Emporblühen der modernen Naturwissenschaften seit der Entdeckung des Energieprinzipes". The work as a whole is mainly concerned with European circumstances. There also exists a condensation of this work: Vom Werden der naturwissenschaftlichen Probleme. Grundriss einer Geschichte der Naturwissenschaften, 1928, 376 p. (Leipzig: Engelmann).

DAUMAS, M., ed., 1957: Encyclopédie de la pléiade. Histoire de la science, 48+1904 p. (Paris: Gallimard).—

> A comprehensive survey of the history of science. An introductory essay (by DAUMAS) discusses the changing conditions under which scientists have worked. Subsequent chapters deal with science in antiquity, the Middle Ages, the 17th century, histories of the separate sciences, and the science of man (incl. anthropology, sociology, demography, and psychology). Included are a synchronous table, an analytical table of contents and a bibliography.

DE CANDOLLE, A., 1885: Histoire des sciences et des savants depuis deux siècles précédée et suivie d'autres études sur des sujets scientifiques en particulier sur l'hérédité et la sélection dans l'espèce humaine, ed. 2, 594 p. (Geneva-Basle: Georg).—

> De Candolle was especially interested in the way in which human genetic characters are mutable under the influence of the (educational and social) environment, and the role played by selection. In order to outweigh this role, the author makes use of the life-histories of excellent scientists, living in 17th- and 18th-century Europe; and as criterion of excellency is chosen the (corresponding) membership of a native or foreign learned society, starting from the assumption that these self-supporting societies select only leading scientists. In this way the author tries to discover in what country and under which conditions science can reach its maximum expansion. This also in connection with problems of civilization and the future of the human race. First ed. 1873. The book is somewhat complementary to F. GALTON's English men of science: their nature and nurture, 1874 (London: Macmillan), in which the nature-nurture controversy is the central problem. Also in German translation: Zur Geschichte der Wissenschaften und Gelehrten seit zwei Jahrhunderten, 1911, 466 p. (Leipzig). A modern book concerned with the explosion in numbers of scientists and scientific publications since about 1600 is: DE SOLLA PRICE, D. J., 1963: Little science, big science, 119 p. (New York, N. Y. & London: Columbia U. P.). Mainly based on American circumstances; some mathematical treatment is given.

DE MORSIER, G., 1965: Essai sur la genèse de la civilisation scientifique actuelle avec une histoire du cerveau, 243 p. (Geneva: Georg).—

> This volume has been composed of two books, of which the second book contains a sketchy history of brain anatomy from the days of the ancient Greek physicians to the 17th century. Starting from this historical introduction, the author develops a theory, illustrating the genesis of present-day scientific civilization. In doing so the author has chosen two groups of scientific pioneers, born between 1450 and 1800. The first group comprises 174 mathematicians, astronomers, physicists, chemists, geologists, and geographers; the second group comprises 127 biologists, botanists, zoologists, anatomists, physiologists, and physicians. For each of these men the author analyses his place of birth, social origin, religion, and biological data. From these data he arrived at some very interesting conclusions.

DEVAUX, P., 1955: De Thalès à Bergson. Introduction historique à la philosophie européenne, 607 p. (Liège: Sciences et Lettres).—

> A history of philosophy designed for students. Of the philosophers discussed, biographical accounts have been given concerning their relationships to the scientific, religious and political movements of their era. The book starts from the basic assumption that European thought is based upon the Graeco-Roman and the Judaic-Christian traditions. According to the author, modern European thought is principally founded on what he calls continental rationalism (originated by Descartes and further developed by Malebranche, Spinoza and Leibniz) and British empiricism (Hobbes, Locke, Berkeley, and Hume). Kant was thought to have united both streams; he sought to reconcile natural science and Christian faith. A last chapter has been devoted to evolutionism and pragmatism, discussing among others Darwin, Nietzsche, Poincaré, Jaurès, and Bergson.

DINGLER, H., 1932: Geschichte der Naturphilosophie, 174 p. (Berlin: Junker & Dünnhaupt).—

> A compact survey of the history of the principles of (natural) science, together with a correlated history of philosophy in so far as it relates to nature. Thus the author discusses, *e.g.,* the animistic natural philosophy of primitive people, natural philosophy of the classical Greeks and its decline, the Alexandrian period, early Chris-

tianity, the Arabs, scholasticism, and science in modern times.

DRACHMAN, J. M., 1936: Studies in the literature of natural science, 487 p. (New York, N.Y.: Macmillan).—

In criticizing scientific writings as literature, the author limits himself to 19th-century English works on (natural) science. The central theme is the history of the evolutionary theory, and among the authors considered are: C. Darwin, Hutton, Wells, E. Darwin, H. Miller, Buffon, Spencer, Wallace, and T. Huxley. The authors have been divided into the following groups; the great synthesists, the popularizers of science, essayists and journalists, and astronomists, i.e., writers who raised the question of life on other planets.

DUBOS, R., 1961: The dreams of reason: science and utopias, 167 p. (New York, N.Y. & London: Columbia U.P.).—

A series of lectures discussing the social and humanistic implications of the development of science. The central theme of the book is a critical discussion and evaluation of certain concepts of Francis Bacon. The author also critically examines the machine theory of life.

FEHL, N. E., 1965: Science and culture. Vol. I: Time, space and motion, 417 p. (Chung Chi College Philosophy of Life Series, No. 7) (Hong Kong: Chung Chi College, Chinese Univ. Hong Kong).—

This book deals with the history of science from the beginnings up to 1700. In the text Eastern science (ca. 10 per cent of its contents) is integrated in the discussion of the development of science in the West. Many passages from the "classics of science", helpful bibliography, index.

GILLISPIE, C. C., 1959: Genesis and geology: the impact of scientific discoveries upon religious beliefs in the decades before Darwin, ed. 2, 306 p. (New York, N.Y.: Harper).—

The main topic of this work is the growth of geology as a scientific discipline between 1790 and 1850. In the meantime the author illuminates the basic difficulty between science and religion of those days, which he sees as a problem of religion within science, rather than one of religion versus science. It is his aim to give an account of the immediate background of the

pattern of scientific disagreement which culminated in disputes about Darwin's book on the origin of species and to attempt to analyse the causes of that disagreement. The book is divided into 8 chapters: 1. Introduction to the evolutionary thought of the early 19th century; 2. Neptune and the flood; 3. From vulcanism to palaeontology; 4. Catastrophist geology; 5. The uniformity of nature; 6. The vestiges of creation; 7. How useful is thy dwelling place; 8. The place of providence in nature. The first edition appeared in 1951 under the title: Genesis and geology: a study in the relations of scientific thought, natural theology, and social opinion in Great Britain, 1790-1850, 315 p. (Harvard Historical Studies, 58) (Cambridge, Mass.: Harvard U.P.).

—— 1960: The edge of objectivity: an essay in the history of scientific ideas, 562 p. (Princeton, N.J.: U.P.).—

The author tries to give a history of the "objectivation" of science, in which objectivation appears to be closely related to mathematization. It is his aim to free science from anthropocentric elements, and, as he states in his own words: "This book is no attempt to recount in summary the whole history of science from Galileo to Maxwell and Mendel. Instead, its purpose is to set out in narrative form what I take to be the structure of classic science. This I find in the route which the advancing edge of objectivity has in fact taken through the story of nature from one science to another."

GODE VON AESCH, A., 1941: Natural science in German romanticism, 302 p. (New York, N.Y.: Columbia U.P.).—

This book deals with philosophy of Romanticism, rather than with natural science. Romanticism is the prevailing mode of thought which dominated German cultural life during the period between the last decades of the 18th century and the first four decades of the 19th century. The speculative ideas dominating Romanticism were largely taken over from ancient and mediaeval philosophy and theology, and as a consequence many scientific terms, such as: magnetism, galvanism, gravitation, etc., are often associated with non-scientific speculations. In the present volume the philosophical speculations of many more or less romantic authors are described, illustrated and analysed, and it has been made clear how science on the one hand, and literature and philosophy on the other hand, were closely interconnected during Romanticism; and the book is illuminated by showing the ways in which prevailing scientific ideas found literary expression.

GORCE, M. & R. MORTIER, eds., 1944-1951: Histoire générale des religions, 5 vols. (Paris: Quillet).—

A profusely illustrated history of religions. The titles of the separate vols. are respectively: 1. (1948) Introduction générale. Magie et religion. Les primitifs. L'ancien Orient. Les Indo-européens; 2. (1944) Grèce. Rome; 3. (1945) Indo-Iraniens. Judaïsme. Origines chrétiennes. Christianismes orientaux; 4. (1947) Christianisme médiéval. Réforme protestante. Islam. Extrême-Orient. With suppl.: Panorama des religions vivantes, 1949; 5. (1951) Folklore et religion. Magie et religion. Tableaux chronologiques de l'histoire des religions.

GUERLAC, H., 1952: Science in Western civilization: a syllabus, 198 p. (New York, N.Y.: Ronald Press).—

This syllabus gives a "selection from the voluminous available material... (that)... should be an indispensable core of materials for a course on science in Western civilization." It is composed of 91 topics (21 dealing with the period from prehistory through the time of the Romans, 12 with the Middle Ages, 10 with the Renaissance, 14 with the 17th-, 10 with the 18th-, and 20 with the 19th and the 20th century, and 3 with science in the U.S.A.). Each topic may serve as material for a single lecture (for an undergraduate course) and is introduced by a brief general outline (throwing light on the main ideas, events, individuals, institutions, *etc.,* of the period considered) and is accompanied by a short bibliography (of books in the English language) of readings on that topic. At the end of the book sections of general references have been added.

HALL, A. R., 1954: The scientific revolution, 1500-1800: the formation of the modern scientific attitude, 390 p. (London, New York & Toronto: Longmans, Green).—

A well-written book dealing with the development of (positive) science from 1500 to 1800. The author treats his work in a new way, by trying to give an insight into the nature of science in general and into 17th-century scientific developments in particular, thereby underlining the methodology and philosophy of the scientific achievements of the scientific pioneers of those times. Separate chapters have been devoted to the development of biology in the first half of the 17th century, to the biological thoughts of Descartes, and to descriptive biology in the late 17th and early 18th century.

——— & M. B., 1964: A brief history of science, 352 p. (New York, N.Y.: New American Library).—

The first two divisions (entitled "Philosophy and physics in the ancient world" and "Philosophy and physics in medieval Europe") trace astronomical and mechanical concepts and theories from the Greeks to the precursors of Copernicus. A short section ("Biological knowledge before the microscope", 42 p.) deals with biological and medical theories and practices up to Paracelsus and van Helmont. The last third of the book ("The scientific revolution" and "The establishment of science in the West") is devoted to the accomplishments of modern science, and deals with a small number of topics of high interest, such as: the role of science in the growth of technology and society; evolution and heredity; cell theory; wave theory of light; atomic theory in chemistry; electrodynamics; quantum theory and relativity.

HARVEY-GIBSON, R. J., 1929: Two thousand years of science, 362 p. (New York, N.Y.: Macmillan).—

"The 4 sections of this work deal respectively with the birth of science, science in the middle ages, advances in the 18th and early 19th centuries, and science today. All phases of science are briefly discussed and their progress interrelated. Brief accounts are given of the major discoveries and hypotheses in botany, zoology, physiology, genetics, and evolution, with some data of the instruments used." (Biol. Abstracts 4: 2495).

JONES, H. M. & I. B. COHEN, eds., 1963: Science before Darwin: a nineteenth-century anthology, 372 p. (London: Deutsch).—

This book brings "a collection of scientific prose whose literary quality is outstanding" in order to re-create the scientific climate reigning in educated Britain during the period immediately preceding the publication of Wallace's and Darwin's revolutionizing ideas. Thus, the situation in astronomy (Chalmers, Herschel), the physical sciences (Dalton, Davy, Faraday, Joule), geology (Lyell, Playfair), and biology (R. Brown, R. Chambers, C. Bell) has been considered. One chapter is devoted to the organization of science. The philosophical climate of those days can be characterized by Paley's "Natural theology", and accordingly the book starts with a discussion of this work.

KROEBER, A. L., 1944: Configuration of

culture growth, 882 p. (Berkeley, Calif.: Univ. Calif. Press).—

An approach to an analysis of our culture from a historical and psychological point of view, written by one of the greatest anthropologists of our century.

LEWIS, J., 1954: Introduction to philosophy, 236 p. (London: Watts).—

A well-written introduction for the general reader without training in philosophy. The text has been built up historically: its begins with Plato and Aristotle, and ends with Bergson, James, Russell, and Whitehead.

LILLEY, S., ed., 1953: Essays on the social history of science, 182 p. (Centaurus Vol. 3).—

A collection of papers treating the development of science as a social phenomenon, starting from the assumption that up till now enough facts have been accumulated for the historian of science to try to discover the general laws of cause and effect operating within the various fields of learning.

LINDSAY, R. B., 1963: The role of science in civilization, 318 p. (New York, N.Y.: Harper).—

A discussion of science in its relation to the humanities, philosophy, history, communication, technology, the state and human behaviour. (From Isis 55: 495).

MASON, S. F., 1953: Main currents of scientific thought: a history of the sciences, 520 p. (New York, N.Y.: Schuman; London: Routledge & Kegan Paul).—

A well-written, informative and instructive short history of science which may prove to be a valuable textbook for students. It is an attempt to integrate the history of science with general history. It consists of 48 chapters. There also exists a French translation: Histoire des sciences, 1956, 476 p. (Paris: Colin) and a German translation: Geschichte der Naturwissenschaft in der Entwicklung ihrer Denkweisen, 1961, 724 p. (Stuttgart: Kroner).

PLEDGE, H. T., 1939: Science since 1500: a short history of mathematics, physics, chemistry, biology, 357 p. (London: H.M. Stationery Office).—

One of the best short surveys of modern science available. Chapters especially dealing with biological subjects are: 2. Biology before the microscope; 7. Microscopy, classification, geology; 11. Evolution and the microscope; 14. Cytology and genetics; 17 en 18. Growth and unity of the individual I and II; 19.Ecology.Subject- and name-index. There also exists an American edition, 1947 (New York, N.Y.: Philos. Library) and a reprint edition, 1959 (New York, N.Y.: Harper). A second edition appeared in 1966, 357 p. (London: H.M.S.O.).

RITCHIE, A. D., 1958: Studies in the history and methods of the sciences, 230 p. (Edinburgh: U.P.).—

"It covers in a remarkably short space the origin of geometry, astronomy, chemistry via alchemy, biology in many aspects, 'human order' and cosmologies: and it leaves no doubt of its author's conclusion that all these sciences, including mathematics, were derived originally from observation and experience, from the practical arts. That does not mean, as he insists, that an even greater part in their development was not played by intellectual curiosity, by bold and critical thought, by trying to find order amid disorder: but the order to be found was among real things, thrown up by measurement, by construction, by working metals, by observing the sky and the seasons, by breeding plants and animals and by medicine." (From Nature 184: 4). Reprinted in 1960, 1963, and 1965.

RUSSELL, B., 1952: The impact of science on society, 64 p. (London: Allen & Unwin).—

The contents of this booklet consist of a series of three lectures held at Columbia University in 1950. They are entitled Science and tradition, Effects of scientific technique, and Science and values.

RUSSO, F., 1951: Histoire de la pensée scientifique, 125 p. (Paris: Ed. du Vieux Colombier).—

A rather popular introduction to the history of the great thoughts which guided the course of science from antiquity up to recent times.

SARTON, G., 1927-1948: Introduction to the history of science, 3 vols. Vol. I (1927): From Homer to Omar Khayyam, 839 p.; vol. II (1931): From Rabbi ben Ezra to Roger Bacon, 2 parts, 1251 p.; vol. III (1947-

1948): Science and learning in the fourteenth century, 2 parts, 2155 p. (Carnegie Publ., No. 376) (Baltimore, Md.: Williams & Wilkins).—

As to the purpose of this work, Sarton states that it is its aim to explain briefly, yet as completely as possible, the development of one essential phase of human civilization which has not yet received sufficient attention — the development of science, that is of systematized positive knowledge. Virtually every branch of science (incl. historiography, law, sociology, and philology) has been included and virtually all peoples, all religions, and all languages receive attention. The material has been arranged chronologically; each chapter contains an introduction, surveying briefly the material which is to follow. This is followed by notes on the lives and works, criticism and bibliographical history of the principal persons concerned. This work is indispensable as a reference work. Photographic reprints of vols. I and II were published in 1950. Addenda and errata are included in the "Critical bibliography of the history and philosophy of science", appearing in ISIS (cf. section Bibliographies, sub-section a).

—— 1936: The study of the history of science, 75 p. (Cambridge, Mass.: Harvard U.P.).—

This booklet tries to explain the meaning of the history of science. Nearly half of the book consists of bibliographical information which may serve as a starting-point for further research. Moreover, the book contains selected lists with information on catalogues of scientific literature, scientific periodicals and journals, handbooks and guides, encyclopaedias, societies and congresses. Reprinted in 1957 (New York, N.Y.: Dover).

—— 1955: The appreciation of ancient and medieval science during the Renaissance (1450-1600), 233 p. (Philadelphia, Pa.: Pennsylvania U.P.).—

This book gives the text of the lectures of Sarton as Rosenbach Fellow in Bibliography at the Univ. of Pennsylvania. Its main problem is a study of the means by which knowledge of the science of classical antiquity and of the Middle Ages has been transmitted to the scientists of the Renaissance. The crucial point in this transmission was the discovery of printing which made the production and multiplication of scientific works easier. The first two lectures are of special interest to biohistorians:

the first deals with the survival and revival of the medical works of Hippocrates, Celsus, Soranos, Galen, and Avicenna, the second deals with the discovery and dissemination of the works on natural history of Aristotle, Theophrastos, Dioscorides, and Pliny the Elder, contains a discussion about herbals, e.g., of Dodonaeus, and considers some encyclopaedists, such as Gesner and Aldrovandi. In an epilogue Sarton shows how the Renaissance became a turning point in the close association between Eastern and Western cultures, and that from here both cultures go their own way, the West exploiting the experimental science, foreshadowing the gigantic development of science in the 17th and later centuries, the East remaining isolated in scholasticism and orthodoxy.

—— 1957: Six wings: men of science in the Renaissance, 318 p. (Bloomington, Ind.: Indiana U.P.).—

This book is the result of the Patten lectures delivered in 1955 and it can be seen as a supplement of Sarton's "The appreciation of ancient and medieval science during the Renaissance" (vide supra). Renaissance science is shown as a part of Renaissance living and thinking, and the book gives an integrative view of the subject, showing how early scientists in the fields of mathematics and astronomy; physics, chemistry and technology; natural history; anatomy and medicine, had to struggle in order to emerge from mediaeval dogma and superstition. A final chapter on Leonardo da Vinci, his art and science, has been included (as the sixth wing), embodying Sarton's ideals of beauty and scientific truth.

SCHWARTZ, G. & P. W. BISHOP, eds., 1958: Moments of discovery, 2 vols. Vol. I: The origins of science, 500 p.; Vol. II: The development of modern science, 510 p. (New York, N.Y.: Basic Bks.).—

An anthology containing numerous brief selections from scientific writers, accompanied by an editorial commentary. According to a review in Science 129: 460-461, it is "unfortunate that such interesting selections and illustrations should be so badly edited", for, according to this reviewer, the editorial commentary is "incredibly inaccurate in its history and sophomorically naive in its conception of science."

SEDGWICK, W. T., H. W. TYLER & R. P. BIGELOW, 1939: A short history of science, 512 p. (New York, N.Y.: Macmillan).—

This is a complete revision of a book originally published in 1917 by SEDGWICK & TYLER. It is an attempt "to trace briefly the history of the foundations upon which recent, as well as earlier, advances were based; to correlate the steps of progress with the spirit of the time; and to increase the emphasis on the evolution of scientific methods." The book is well-illustrated. Lists of references for further reading follow each chapter. Excellent index. According to a review in Isis (32: 465) it is an admirable book, highly recommended as a text both for the undergraduate and the general reader. Also in Spanish translation: Breve historia de la ciencia, 1950, 508 p. (Buenos Aires: Argos).

SIEGEL, C., 1913: Geschichte der deutschen Naturphilosophie, 390 p. (Leipzig: Akad. Verlagsges.).—

The author defines "Naturphilosophie" as follows: "eine wissenschaftliche Disziplin, die bewusst neben und nach der Naturwissenschaft auftritt, ... gefordert von ihr als unentbehrliche Ergänzung". Deals more particularly with the following philosophers: Kepler, Leibniz, Kant, Fries, Herder, Goethe, Schelling, Schopenhauer, Herbart, Feuerbach, Lotze, Fechner.

SINGER, C., 1928: From magic to science: essays on the scientific twilight, 253 p. (London: Benn).—

This volume consists of 7 essays: 1. Science under the Roman Empire (a study of Greek science in decay); 2. The Dark Ages and the dawn of science (deterioration and recovery of scientific thought, infiltration of Arabian culture); 3. The Lorica of Gildas the Briton (a magical formulary illustrating the attitude of men of the Dark Ages to nature); 4. Anglo-Saxon magic (the inheritance of Anglo-Saxon culture from Teutonic saga, Celtic magic, classical myths, and Christian tradition); 5. The visions of St. Hildegard of Bingen (illustrating the mystico-magical point of view); 6. The history of the herbal (from Theophrastos to the 16th century A.D.); 7. The School of Salerno and its legends (the rise of the first university in Europe). Paperback reprint, 1958 (New York, N.Y.: Dover).

—— 1959: A short history of scientific ideas to 1900, 525 p. (New York, N.Y. & London: Oxford U.P.).—

In his preface Singer states that he wants to give an elementary idea of how science came to occupy its distinctive position in the life of our time. Separate chapters deal with: 1. The nature of the scientific process; 2. The rise and foundations of mental coherence; 3. The unitary system of thought: Athens; 4. Alexandria; 5. Imperial Rome; 6. The Middle Ages: theology; 7. The rise of humanism: attempted return to antiquity, 1250-1600; 8. Downfall of Aristotle, 1600-1700: new attempts of synthesis; 9. The mechanical world: enthronement of determinism (1700-1850); 10. Culmination of the mechanical view of the world (1850-1900).

STÖRIG, H. J., 1954: Kleine Weltgeschichte der Wissenschaft, ed. 2, 794 p. (Stuttgart: Kohlhammer).—

A book primarily written for the scientist having no historical training and for the interested layman. In his first chapter the author tackles the problem of why a history of science should be useful. The second chapter deals with methodological problems, such as science and society, science and religion, science and art, science and technique, and science and philosophy. Other chapters deal with the origin of science in Greece, science and Hellenism, Rome, science and Islam, science in the Latin West, the beginnings of modern science (Leonardo da Vinci, Francis Bacon, Cardano, Paracelsus, Paré, Vesalius, etc.), science in the 17th century (Hooke, Leeuwenhoek, Swammerdam, Harvey, etc), science in the 18th century (e.g., Linnaeus, Buffon, E. Darwin, Goethe, Haller, Bichat, Jenner, etc.); science in the 19th century (dealing with e.g., the theory of evolution, A. von Humboldt, C. Darwin, Lyell, Weismann, Morgan, Pasteur, Koch, Mendel, etc.).

STRUIK, D. J., 1962: Yankee science in the making, 544 p. (New York, N.Y.: Collier).—

Revised version of the 1948 edition. The text is in three parts, viz., 1. Beginnings: the colonial setting (with sections on emigration to New England, agriculture, urban centers, interest in science, British influence on science, religion and science, and medical study); 2. The federalist period (with sections on John Adams and the American Academy, the Massachusetts medical society, science in the coastal towns, the earliest canals, early inventions, Whitney and the cotton gin, the beginning of textile industry, early textbooks, chemistry and geology, medicine, botany and chemistry at Harvard, Bigelow's botany); 3. The Jacksonian period (with sections on: the origin of the A.A.A.S., the new type of scientist, the lyceums, school reform, the physicians, the dentists, anaesthesia, the public health report, the great naturalists: Nuttall, Rafinesque, Audubon, Lyell, Agassiz, Gray, Dana, *etc.*, science and religion, the beginnings of Darwinism, primitive laboratories, *etc.*). Useful bibliography and index.

TATON, R., ed., 1957-1964: Histoire générale des sciences, 3 vols. Vol. I (1957): La science antique et médiévale (dès origines à 1450), 627 p.; Vol. II (1958): La science moderne (de 1450 à 1800), 800 p.; Vol. III: La science contemporaine, part 1 (1961): Le XIXᵉ siècle, 775 p.; part 2 (1964): Le XXᵉ siècle, 1080 p. (Paris: Presses Univ. de France).—

> This series intends to give a synthetic presentation of the entire history of science and the contribution of science to civilization, and is addressed to the general reader. It is written co-operatively by a (rather large: Vol. I: 21, Vol. II: 25) number of specialists. Vol. 1 spans the period from the first scientific achievements of prehistoric man up to 1450 and deals with ancient science in the Orient (Egypt, Mesopotamia, Phoenicia and Israel, India, China), with science in the Graeco-Roman world (mathematics, physics, astronomy, biology and medicine) and with science in the Middle Ages (America before Columbus, India, China, Byzantium, Arabic and Jewish science, and mediaeval science in the Christian West). Vol. II is divided into 4 parts (Renaissance, 17th century, 18th century, science outside Europe); each part is preceded by a general introduction. Within each part the subjects are grouped as exact sciences (mathematics, physics, astronomy) and descriptive sciences (geology, chemistry, biology). Vol. III concentrates on Western contributions in the various fields of natural science during the 19th and 20th centuries. Also in English translation: Vol. I (1963): Ancient and medieval science from the beginnings to 1450, 551 p.; Vol. II (1964): The beginnings of modern science from 1450 to 1800, 665 p.; Vol. III, part 1 (1965): Science in the nineteenth century, 623 p.; Vol. III, part 2(1966): Science in the twentieth century, 638 p. (New York, N.Y.: Basic Bks.; London: Thames & Hudson).

TAYLOR, F. S., 1949: Science, past and present, new ed., 368 p. (London: Heinemann).—

> First published in 1945. A popular, yet scientific historical review of the growth of science. It deals with the histories of mechanics, physics, chemistry, biology, geology, *etc.*, but, besides, it also deals with such studies as the history of public health,

and the problem of the limitations of science. Good bibliography, illustrations, and diagrams. Reprinted 1962. An American edition, adapted to the American public by having the French and German abstracts presented in English and by the addition of some new material, appeared under the title: A short history of science and scientific thought, with readings from the great scientists from the Babylonians to Einstein, 1949, 368 p. (New York, N.Y.: Norton).

THORNDIKE, L., 1958-1960: A history of magic and experimental science, 8 vols., 6429 p. (New York, N.Y.: Columbia U.P.).—

> After a general introduction, vol. I contains Book I: the Roman Empire (Pliny, Seneca, Galen, Aelian, *etc.*); Bk. II: Early Christian thought (Christianity and natural science, Augustine, fusion of pagan and Christian thought); Bk. III: The early Middle Ages (post-classical medicine, Boethius, Isidore, Bede, Gregory, Const. Africanus, Marbod, Anglo-Saxon, Salernitan, and other Latin medicine, *etc.*). Vol. II contains Bk. IV: The twelfth century (Abelard, Adelard of Bath, Hildegard, Alexander Neckam, Maimonides, ancient and mediaeval dream books, *etc.*); Bk. V: The thirteenth century (M. Scot, T. Cantimpré, Bartholomew Anglicus, R. Grosseteste, Vincent of Beauvais, Petrus Hispanus, Albertus Magnus, Thomas Acquinas, Roger Bacon, medical and biological experiments and secrets, Arnald of Villanova, *etc.*). Vol. III deals with *e.g.*, alchemy, old pest tractates, Gentile de Foligno and 14th-century medicine, the Pope and the calendar, astrology and medicine, Oresme on marvels of nature, Guy de Chauliac and his contemporaries, works on poisons, encyclopaedias of the 14th century. Vol. IV deals with *e.g.*, the alchemical collection of Raymond Lull, astrology in the 15th century, astrological surgery and medicine, Michael Savonarola and his "Practica medica", Ant. Guaineri, Conrad Heingarter, humanism in relation to natural and occult science, Ant. Benivieni, the attack on Pliny. Vol. V discusses such topics as: Leonardo da Vinci, Achillini as Aristotelian and anatomist, astrology and astronomy, the Copernican theory, German medicine, Brasavola and pharmacy, poisons, fascination, and hydrophobia, Fracastoro, anatomy from Carpi to Vesalius, Cardan, Gratarolo, the Paracelsan revival, T. Erastus. Vol. VI contains *inter alia* chapters on: medicine after 1550, the 16th-century naturalists, Cesalpino's view on nature, efforts towards a Christian philosophy of nature, for and against Aristotle, natural philosophy and natural magic, witchcraft and magic after Johannes Wier. Vol. VII

contains chapters dealing with *e.g.,* Francis Bacon, alchemy and iatro-chemistry to 1650, v. Helmont, natural magic, Harvey and Patin, Descartes. Vol. VIII deals with *e.g.,* natural history, esp. of animals, with botany, pharmacy, medicine and physiology, physiognomy, divination, mental disease and magic. General and bibliographical indexes, and index of mss. Very valuable work.

UEBERWEG, F., 1923-1928: Grundriss der Geschichte der Philosophie, ed. 11 and 12, 5 vols. (Berlin: Mittler).—

This work has many times been reprinted. It is indispensable to any student of the history of philosophy by reason of its invaluable bibliographical information. Vol. 1: Die Philosophie des Altertums (ed. 12, 1926, by K. PRAECHTER); vol. 2: Die patristische und scholastische Philosophie (ed. 11, 1928, by B. GEYER); vol. 3: Die Philosophie der Neuzeit bis zum Ende des 18. Jahrhunderts (ed. 12, 1924, by M. FRISCHEISEN-KÖHLER & W. MOOG); vol. 4: Die deutsche Philosophie des 19. Jahrhunderts und der Gegenwart (ed. 12, 1923, by T. K. OESTERREICH); vol. 5: Die Philosophie des Auslandes vom Beginn des 19. Jahrhunderts bis auf die Gegenwart (ed. 12, 1928, by T. K. OESTERREICH).

WHITE, A. D., 1960: A history of the warfare of science with theology in Christendom, 2 vols. Vol. I: 415 p.; Vol. II: 474 p. (New York, N.Y.: Dover).—

A reprint of the 1896 edition. Chapters of special value from our point of view are: ch. 1. From creation to evolution (ancient and mediaeval views regarding the manner, the matter, the time and the date of creation, theological teachings regarding the animals and Man, theological and scientific theories of an evolution in animate nature; attacks on Darwin and his theories in England, in France, in Germany, and in America; final victory of evolution); ch. 5: From Genesis to geology; ch. 6: The antiquity of Man, Egyptology and Assyriology; ch. 7: The antiquity of Man, and prehistoric archaeology (considering, *e.g.,* flint weapons and implements); ch. 8: The "fall of Man" and anthropology; ch. 9: *Idem* and technology; ch. 10. *Idem* and history; ch. 13: From miracles to medicine (the early and sacred theories of disease; growth of legends of healing; the mediaeval miracles of healing: the attribution of disease to satanic influences; theological opposition to anatomical studies; new beginnings of medical science: Galen; theological discouragements of medicine: the doctrine of signatures, theological opposition to surgery, fashion in pious cures, *etc.;* fetich cures

under Protestantism; theological opposition to inoculation and vaccination, *etc.);* ch. 14: From fetich to hygiene (the theological view of epidemics and sanitation, *etc.);* ch. 15: From "demoniacal possession" to insanity; ch. 16: From diabolism to hysteria.

WIGHTMAN, W. P. D., 1950: The growth of scientific ideas, 495 p. (London & Edinburgh: Oliver & Boyd).—

An analysis of the historical development of thought and the origin of certain basic ideas or concepts. This has largely been done by extensive quotations from original writings in order to bring the reader into closer contact with the minds of great discoverers.

—— 1962: Science and the Renaissance, 2 vols. Vol. I: An introduction to the study of the emergence of the sciences in the sixteenth century, 327 p.; Vol. II: An annotated bibliography of the sixteenth-century books relating to the sciences in the library of the University of Aberdeen, 293 p. (London & Edinburgh: Oliver & Boyd).—

The first volume discusses the emergence of the sciences during the 16th century; roughly speaking, its first half is occupied with the cultural and general background and its second half is almost fully devoted to the development of the biological and medical sciences. The author tries to distinguish the mainstream of advance during that period and evaluates the separate contributions of the different scientists in the light of this criterion. The second volume contains an informative and richly-annotated catalogue of the early printed books in the Aberdeen library (to which belong several famous collections).

WINTER, H. J. J., 1952: Eastern science: an outline of its scope and contribution, 114 p. (London: Murray).—

An attempt to outline the value of Eastern science to the West. The account is divided as follows: 1. Antiquity (Babylonia, Egypt, India, China); 2. Mediaeval China; 3. Mediaeval India; 4. The scope of Arabic science; a) The Arabic period and the diffusion of science; b) Some great Arabic thinkers and experimenters; c) The scientific legacy of Islam to Latin Christendom; 5. Modern times: what Asian science teaches us. Useful bibliography.

WOLF, A., 1951: A history of science, technology, and philosophy in the 16th and 17th centuries, new ed., 692 p. (London: Allen & Unwin; New York, N.Y.: Macmillan).—

A history of the various branches of science, *viz.*, of astronomy, mathematics, mechanics, light, sound, botany, zoology, medicine, *etc.* Many illustrations. Originally published in 1935. A reprint edition was published in 1959, in 2 vols., 686 p. (New York, N.Y.: Harper).

—— 1952: A history of science, technology, and philosophy in the eighteenth century, ed.

2, 814 p. (London: Allen & Unwin; New York, N.Y.: Macmillan).—

An introduction to science of the 18th century. The text is divided as follows: mathematics, 16 p.; mechanics, 35 p.; physics, 113 p.; astronomy, 65 p.; chemistry, 45 p.; meteorology, 68 p.; geology, 23 p.; geography, 16 p.; botany, 34 p.; zoology, 18 p.; medicine, 20 p.; technology, 170 p.; psychology, 27 p.; social sciences, 51 p.; philosophy, 153 p. Originally published in 1939. A reprint edition was published in 1959 (New York, N.Y.: Harper).

3. COMPREHENSIVE STANDARD BIBLIOGRAPHIES AND BIOGRAPHICAL DICTIONARIES

α. BIBLIOGRAPHIES
(incl. some bibliographical periodicals and some library catalogues)

a. *General* (incl. some bibliographies of bibliographies, bibliographies dealing with gastronomy, geography, alchemy and chemistry, hunting, psychology, occult sciences, *etc.*)

ARTELT, W., ed., 1953: Index zur Geschichte der Medizin, Naturwissenschaft und Technik, Vol. I: 398 p. (Unter Mitwirkung von J. STEUDEL, W. HARTNER & O. MAHR) (Munich & Berlin: Urban & Schwarzenberger).—

A bibliography containing the literature pertaining to the history of medicine, dentistry, pharmacy, exact sciences, technology, and biology for the years 1945-1948. It contains 7,022 medical, 182 dental, 374 pharmaceutical, and 751 biological items. This "Index" can be considered as a continuation of the "Mitteilungen zur Geschichte der Medizin, der Naturwissenschaften und der Technik" *(vide infra).* Reprinted 1967 (Würzburg: Journalfranz). A second volume of this "Index" has been published under the editorship of STEUDEL, J., 1966, *vide infra.* It deals with the literature published in the years 1949-1952.

BESTERMAN, T., ed., 1965-1966: A world bibliography of bibliographies and of bibliographical catalogues, calendars, abstracts, digests, indexes, and the like, ed. 4, revised and greatly enlarged throughout, 5 vols. (Lausanne: Societas Bibliographica).—

A very extensive bibliography of bibliographies in which the material is arranged by subjects. This bibliography is limited to separate published bibliographies. It includes, however, bibliographies of every sort of written matter, including letters, documents, broadsides, periodicals, as well as the more substantial types of manuscript material and collections of abstracts. Excluded are booksellers' and sale catalogues, lists of works of art, library catalogues and general handbooks. Vol. 5 contains the index.

BIBLIOGRAPHIC INDEX, 1938 → (New York, N.Y.: Wilson).—

A cumulative bibliography of bibliographies, covering material published in books, pamphlets, and periodicals since 1937, mostly in English. For this purpose more than 1,500 periodicals are examined. Vol. 1 covers the period 1937-1942, 1780 p.; vol. 2: 1943-1946, 831 p.; vol. 3: 1947-1950, 796 p.; vol. 4: 1951-1955, 709 p.; vol. 5: 1956-1959, 801 p. A sixth vol. (1960-1962) appeared in 1963, and a seventh vol. (1963-1965) in 1966. Appears twice a year, with annual and other cumulations. German bibliographies are listed in the BIBLIOGRAPHIE DER VERSTECKTEN BIBLIOGRAPHIEN aus deutschsprachigen Büchern und Zeitschriften der Jahre 1930-1953 (1956) (Leipzig: Deutsche Bücherei), continued by the annual BIBLIOGRAPHIE DER DEUTSCHEN BIBLIOGRAPHIEN (Leipzig: Deutsche Bücherei). *Cf.* also: BOHATTA, H. & F. HODES, eds., 1950: Internationale Bibliographie der Bibliographien, 652 p. (Frankfurt a.M.: Klostermann), a systematically arranged bibliography of bibliographies, covering universal and national bibliography, and subject bibliography with detailed subarrangement.

BITTING, K. G., ed., 1939: Gastronomic bibliography, 718 p. (San Francisco, Calif.: A. W. Bitting).—

A collection of more than 3,000 books upon foods, cookery and dining. It includes many American cookery books published by societies, lodges, churches, and similar organizations. Government and official publications have not been included. The description of the books is very complete. A bibliography dealing with the same topic is: SIMON, A. L., 1953: Bibliotheca gastronomica: a catalogue of books and documents on gastronomy, 196 p. (London: Wine and Food Society). This is a catalogue of the author's own library, now housed at the Wine and Food Society. The catalogue extends back as far as 1861, and contains 1,644 entries; there are many books published since 1861 in the library which will be published in another catalogue at a later date. The entries contain valuable information on the authors and the contents of the books; numerous quotations from the works included are given. Excellent subject-index divided under 51 headings. (cf. also VICAIRE, G., 1954, vide infra).

BULLETIN SIGNALÉTIQUE du C.N.R.S., 1954 → (Paris: Centre National de la Recherche Scientifique).—

The whole work consists of some 32 sections, of which only those dealing with the sciences of biology, of medicine, and of man are of interest to the present bibliography. Subscriptions can be obtained for the following combinations: Sciences biologiques et médicales (comprising the sections: biophysics, biochemistry, analytical biological chemistry; pharmacology, toxicology; microbiology, virology, immunology; general and experimental pathology; biology and physiology of animals; endocrinology, reproduction, genetics; biology and physiology of plants; agricultural sciences, zootechnics, phytopharmacology, food industries; psychology and psychopathology); and Sciences humaines (comprising the sections: philosophy, religion; pedagogy; sociology, ethnology, prehistory, archaeology; history of science and technique; history and science of literature and art; sciences of language). Annual indexes of authors and subjects.

CAILLET, A. L., ed., 1964: Manuel bibliographique des sciences psychiques ou occultes, 3 vols. Vol. I: 67+531 p.; Vol. II: 533 p.; Vol. III: 767 p. (Nieuwkoop, the Netherlands: de Graaf).—

A reprint of the 1912 edition (Paris: Dorbon). Its subject matter may be illustrated by the sub-title: "Sciences des mages-hermétique-astrologie-kabbale-francmaçon-nerie-médecine ancienne-mesmérisme-sor-cellerie-singularités-aberrations de tout ordre-curiosités. Sources bibliographiques et documentaires sur ces sujets." Cf. GRAESSE, J. G. T., 1968: Bibliotheca psychologica oder Verzeichnis der wichtigsten über das Wesen der Menschen- & Thierseelen und die Unsterblichkeitslehre handelnden Schriftsteller älterer und neuerer Zeit, 60 p. (Amsterdam: Bonset). A reprint.

CHOULANT, L., ed., 1924: Graphische Incunabeln für Naturgeschichte und Medicin. Enthaltend Geschichte und Bibliographie der ersten naturhistorischen und medicinischen Drucke des XV. und XVI. Jahrhunderts, welche met illustrirenden Abbildungen versehen sind, 168 p. (Munich: Verlag der Münchner Drucke).—

A source book for illustrated medical incunabula, in which stress has been laid on the significance of the illustration for a better understanding of history in general and of medical history in particular.

DUVEEN, D., ed., 1949: Bibliotheca alchemica et chemica: an annotated catalogue of printed books on alchemy, chemistry and cognate subjects in the library of Denis I. Duveen, 669 p. (London: Weil).—

This catalogue of what is probably by now the largest collection in this field contains a great number of early English and French alchemical works. It consists of about 3,000 items, each being well described. The arrangement is in alphabetical order of authors' names (or of titles for anonymous books) and for each author his works are listed chronologically. No biographical information concerning the authors mentioned is given. (Cf. also: FERGUSON, vide infra).

ENGELMANN, W., ed., 1858: Bibliotheca geographica. Verzeichnis der seit der Mitte des vorigen Jahrhunderts bis zu Ende des Jahres 1856 in Deutschland erschienenen Werke über Geographie und Reisen, mit Einschluss der Landkarten, Pläne und Ansichten, 1225 p. (Leipzig: Engelmann).—

A comprehensive list arranged for the most part by geographical location. Subject-index (p. 1149-1225). Reprinted in 1965 in 2 vols. (New York, N.Y.: Meridian).

FERGUSON, J., ed., 1954: Bibliotheca chemica: a catalogue of the alchemical, chemical and pharmaceutical books in the collection of the late James Young of Kelly and Durris, 2 vols. Vol. I: 487 p.; Vol. II: 598 p. (London: Holland Press).—

> A photo-lithographic reprint of the original 1906 edition. This bibliography consists of about 1,400 accurately-described items and includes many copious biographical notes and extensive references pertaining to the sources. The arrangement is in alphabetical order of authors' names or of titles for anonymous books. (Cf. also DUVEEN, vide supra).

GRÄSZE, J. G. T., ed., 1960: Bibliotheca magica et pneumatica oder wissenschaftlich geordnete Bibliographie der wichtigsten in das Gebiet des Zauber-, Wunder-, Geister- und sonstigen Aberglaubens, vorzüglich älterer Zeit, einschlagenden Werke, 179 p. (Hildesheim: Olms).—

> A reprint of the original edition of 1843 (Leipzig). Separate sections deal with the literature of such subjects as: superstition in general, wonderful things in nature, the devil, hell, angels, were-wolf, vampires, fairies, magic-books, trials for witchcraft, amulets, talismans, somnambulism, magnetism, sorceries, demoniac possession, apparition of spirits, dreams, fortune-telling, visions, natural magic. This bibliography also contains the catalogues of two libraries specialized in these fields, viz., those of HAUBER and of HORST.

ISIS, critical bibliography of the history of science and its cultural influences, 1913 → (Washington, D.C.: Smithsonian Instn.).—

> This critical bibliography is part of the journal Isis, "an international review devoted to the history of science and its cultural influences", founded in 1912 by George Sarton. Up to 1968, 92 of these bibliographies have been published. They are each ca. 125-150 pages in length, and they include a list of periodicals and serials examined systematically and an index of personal names. Its subject matter has been divided into 4 main sections, viz., A. History of science: general references and tools; B. Science and its history from special points of view (scientific instruments, institutions, etc., scientific education, social and humanistic relations); C. Histories of special sciences (in which special sections deal with the history of the biological sciences, the sciences of Man, and with medicine and the medical sciences, incl. pharmacy); D. Chronological classifications. This is the most useful bibliography of current literature in the field of the history of biology.

KLEBS, A. C., ed., 1938: Incunabula scientifica et medica: short title list, 359 p. (Osiris IV) (Bruges: St. Catherine Press).—

> A carefully-selected list of some 3,000 editions of some 1,000 incunabula; as such it is one of the most valuable tools for the historian of mediaeval science. The author has brought together the material of the most important libraries of America and Western Europe. Most of the incunabula mentioned were examined by the author. This bibliography of Klebs is supplemented by a long review by G. SARTON (1938): The scientific literature transmitted through the incunabula, 204 p. (Osiris V: 41-245). For more extensive bibliographical information, cf. HAIN, L., ed., 1948: Repertorium bibliographicum ad annum MD, 4 vols. (Milan: Gorlich). Originally published 1826-1838. It is an authors' list, containing 16,229 items, with short bibliographical descriptions. These volumes are supplemented by: COPINGER, W. A., 1926: Supplement to Hain's "Repertorium bibliographicum"; or, collections towards a new edition of that work, 3 vols. (London: Sotheran). Originally published 1895-1902. Contains some 6,000 items not listed by Hain, together with corrections to Hain. This work is supplemented by: REICHLING, D., 1905-1911: Appendices ad Hainii-Copingeri Repertorium bibliographicum: additiones et emendationes, 7 vols. (Monaco: Rosenthal) + supplement, 1914. Also very valuable in this respect is the GESAMTKATALOG DER WIEGEDRUCKE (1925-1940) of which 7 volumes have appeared thus far (A-EIG) and of vol. 8, part 1 (Eike-Federicis). These published parts contain some 10,000 items; locations of the incunabula included are given for European and American libraries. Many references to Hain's "Repertorium". These 7 vols. will be reprinted, and the publication of this "Gesamtkatalog" will be continued, by Hiersemann (Leipzig).

MALCLÈS, L. N., ed., 1950-1958: Les sources du travail bibliographique, 3 vols. Vol. I (1950): Bibliographies générales, 364 p.; Vol. II (1952): Bibliographies spécialisées: sciences humaines, 960 p.; Vol. III (1958): Bibliographies specialisées: sciences exactes et techniques, 575 p. (Geneva: Droz; Paris: Minard).—

> A very useful guide to reference-material of all kinds. The general pattern is to consider material in chapter form, beginning with a survey and then listing material, with analysis of contents or addition of annotations. Vol. I includes chap-

ters on: bibliographies of bibliographies; universal bibliographies; 15th- and 16th-century books; printed library catalogues; union catalogues; national bibliographies; encyclopaedias; biographical dictionaries; periodicals; publications of learned societies; indexes to periodicals; included are sections on the Slav and Balkan countries, and on arts of books. Vol. II includes chapters on: prehistory, anthropology, ethnology, sociology; linguistics; history; language and literature; religion; geography; archaeology and art; music; law; political and social sciences; philosophy; the Near-, Middle-, and Far East. Vol. III is an introductory guide to the literature of the various aspects of the natural) sciences. Separate chapters deal with: the history of science, general and animal biology, zoology, botany and plant physiology, the medical sciences, and pharmacy.

MITTEILUNGEN zur GESCHICHTE der MEDIZIN und der NATURWISSEN-SCHAFTEN, 1902 → (Leipzig: Voss).—

The first vol. appeared in 1902, ed. by G. W. A. KAHLBAUM, M. NEUBURGER, and K. SUDHOFF. The last vol. published was vol. 40, 1941-'42, 372 p., ed. by R. ZAUNICK. This journal was almost exclusively bibliographical; practically all the German publications dealing with the history of science and medicine have been considered, but a good many foreign publications are included as well. Recently reprinted (1967) (Leipzig: Zentral-Antiquariat D.D.R.).

MOORAT, S. A. J., ed., 1962: Catalogue of Western manuscripts on medicine and science in the Wellcome Historical Medical Library. Vol. I: Manuscripts written before 1650 A.D., 679 p. (London: Wellcome Historical Medical Library).—

This bibliography lists 800 mss., arranged in alphabetical order of names. Each item gives a description of the ms., details of collation, script, *etc.*, and supplies much information on authorship and subject matter of the text. Indexes have been added, allowing orientation concerning the age, bindings, illustrations, bookplates, owners of the mss., the libraries of their provenience, the language in which the texts were written, and the subjects they deal with.

PEDDIE, R. A., ed., 1933-1948: Subject index of books published before 1880. 1st ser., 1933, 745 p.; 2nd ser., 1935, 857 p.; 3rd ser., 1939, 945 p.; new ser., 1948, 872 p. (London: Grafton).—

Each series contains an alphabetical subject-list of some 50,000 books in various languages published before 1880, the date from which the British Museum subject-indexes continue the subject record. The third series includes in its alphabetical arrangement every subject-heading used in the first two series (with cross-references to the first and second series). This record is not continued in the "new series".

PETZHOLDT, J., ed., 1961: Bibliotheca bibliographica. Kritisches Verzeichnis der das Gesammtgebiet der Bibliographie betreffenden Literatur des In- und Auslandes in systematischer Ordnung, 939 p. (Nieuwkoop, the Netherlands: de Graaf).—

First published in 1866 (Leipzig). A very good bibliography of those days, extending to about 5,500 entries. The classification is relatively simple, but, of course, somewhat obsolete. *Cf.* also BESTERMAN, *vide supra.*

RAND, B., ed., 1940-1949: Bibliography of philosophy, psychology, and cognate subjects, 2 vols. (New York, N.Y.: Smith).—

This is the third volume of BALDWIN's Dictionary of philosophy and psychology, *vide* section Some recommended encyclopaedias *etc.*, subsection a. It is the most comprehensive systematical bibliography of its kind, for both books and periodical articles. It contains: 1. Bibliographical information (general bibliographies, dictionaries, periodicals); 2. Literary information (histories of philosophy, individual philosophers, systematic philosophy, logic, aesthetics, philosophy of religion, ethics, psychology). No author-index, but sub-arrangement is alphabetical. *Cf.* also: SCHÜLING, H., 1964: Bibliographisches Handbuch zur Geschichte der Psychologie, 292 p. (Giessen: Universitätsbibliothek), und: SCHÜLING, H., 1967: Bibliographie der psychologischen Literatur des 16.Jahrhunderts, 301 p. (Hildesheim: Olms).

REUSS, J. D., ed., 1801-1821: Repertorium commentationum a societatibus litterariis editarum, 16 vols. (Göttingen: Dieterich).—

A classified index to the publications of learned societies from their inception to 1800. For the present purpose the following volumes are of major importance: 1. Historia naturalis, generalis et zoologia; 2. Botanica et mineralogia; 8. Historia; 10-16. Scientia et ars medica et chirurgica. A continuation of this work is provided by the

ROYAL SOCIETY of London catalogue of scientific papers, 1800-1900, *infra*.

ROYAL SOCIETY of London. Catalogue of scientific papers, 1800-1900, 19 vols. (London: H.M. Stationery Office; Cambridge: U.P.).—

The standard index to 19th-century scientific papers and author-index to 1,555 periodicals, including transactions of European academies and other learned societies. A continuation of REUSS, J. D., *vide supra*. Vols. 1-6: first series, 1800-1863; vols. 7-8: second series, 1864-1873; vols. 9-11: third series, 1874-1883; vol. 12: supplementary vol., 1800-1883; vols. 13-19: 4th series, 1884-1900. It gives for each article entered: author's name in full when it can be found, full title of periodical, volume, date and inclusive paging. There are to be published separate index-volumes for each of the seventeen sciences of the International Catalogue (among which: palaeonthology, biology, botany, zoology, anatomy, anthropology, physiology, and bacteriology). Up to now the following subject-index volumes have appeared: Pure mathematics, Mechanics and Physics (partly). These subject-indexes can be used independently of the author vols.

RUSSO, F., ed., 1954: Histoire des sciences et des techniques: bibliographie. Ouvrage publié avec le concours du Centre National de la Recherche Scientifique et de l'Union Internationale de l'Histoire des Sciences, 186 p. (Actualités Scientifiques et Industrielles, 1204) (Paris: Hermann).—

A select bibliography, listing general and special bibliographies, important standard works, dictionaries, encyclopaedias, periodicals, and transactions. Arranged by subject. Brief indications as to character, value, *etc.*, of the works included.

SARTON, G., 1952: Horus: a guide to the history of science, 316 p. (Waltham, Mass.: Chronica Botanica).—

The first part of this book contains three introductory essays, entitled: Science and tradition; The tradition of ancient and mediaeval science; Is it possible to teach the history of science? In these essays the author elucidates the problem of the transmission of scientific achievements and the reasons for studying the history of science. The second part (p. 66-304) "gives the means of implementing the purpose which they advocate" and is primarily an extensive bibliog-

raphy of the history of science, divided into four chapters with 26 sections. A) History: 1. Historical methods, 2. Historical tables and summaries, 3. Historical atlases, 4. Gazetteers, 5. Encyclopaedias, 6. Biographical collections. B) Science: 7. Scientific methods and philosophy of science, 8. Science and society, 9. Catalogues of scientific literature, 10. Union lists of scientific periodicals, 11. General scientific journals, 12. Abstracting and review journals, 13. National academies and scientific societies. C) History of science: 14. Chief reference books on the history of science, 15. Treatises and handbooks on the history of science, 16. Scientific instruments, 17. History of science in special countries, 18. History of science in special cultural groups, 19. History of special sciences, 20. Journals and serials concerning the history and philosophy of science. D) Organizations of the study and teaching of the history of science: 21. National societies devoted to the history of science, 22. *Idem* international, 23. The teaching of the history of science, 24. Institutes, museums, libraries, 25. International congresses, 26. Prizes.

SOUHART, R., ed., 1886: Bibliographie générale des ouvrages sur la chasse, la vénerie et la fauconnerie publiés ou composés depuis le XV siècle jusqu'à ce jour, en français, latin, allemand, anglais, espagnol, italien, etc., avec des notes critiques et l'indication de leur prix et de leur valeur dans les différentes ventes, 750 p. (Paris: Rouquette).—

The text is in two parts. The first part (p. 1-507) deals with books; it is arranged alphabetically according to the name of the authors. It includes many books in such related fields as biology, forestry, or legislation, and also many works which are of importance to the literary-historical aspects of biohistory (*e.g.*, poems, theatre, *etc.*). The second part (p. 510-738) lists anonymous publications, serials, reviews, collections, *etc.* Cf. also THIÉBAUD, *vide infra*.

STEUDEL, J., ed., 1966: Index zur Geschichte der Medizin, Naturwissenschaft und Technik, Vol. 2: 312 p. (Unter Mitwirkung von W. RICKER & C. NISSEN) (Munich & Berlin: Urban & Schwarzenberger).—

This volume contains the literature pertaining to the history of medicine, dentistry, pharmacy, exact sciences, technology, and biology for the years 1949-1952. It contains 5,037 medical, 172 dental, 380 pharmaceutical, and 822 biological items. Reprinted 1967 (Würzburg: Journalfranz). The first vol. of this index was published in 1953 by W. ARTELT, *vide supra.*

THIÉBAUD, J., ed., 1934: Bibliographie des ouvrages français sur la chasse, 1039 p. (Paris: Nourry).—

This alphabetically arranged bibliography contains books on hunting published in or translated into the French language, published in France or in other parts of the world since the 15th century. It includes works by French authors that are written in Latin or other languages, Greek, Latin, and Byzantine authors of Antiquity and the Middle Ages. *Cf.* also SOUHART, *vide supra.*

TOTOK, W., R. WEITZEL & K. H. WEIMANN, eds., 1966: Handbuch der bibliographischen Nachschlagewerke, ed. 3, 362 p. (Frankfurt a.M.: Klostermann).—

A manual of bibliographical science. The first part deals with general bibliographies, incl. bibliographies of bibliographies, encyclopaedias, library catalogues, national biographies (chronological and geographical), bibliographies of translations, of dissertations, and of publications of learned societies, *etc.* The second part deals with special bibliographies, *e.g.,* on psychology, linguistics, archaeology, history (chronological and geographical), geology, palaeontology, biology, botany, zoology, anthropology, medicine, agriculture, forestry, *etc.* Table of contents in German, English, and French.

VAN DE VELDE, A. J. J., ed., 1933-1936: Bromatologicon of bibliographie der geschriften over de levensmiddelen tot 1800, 6 parts, 300 p. (Gent: Vanderpoorten).—

A bibliography of publications dealing with foodstuffs, published before 1800. It is in 6 parts, published in the "Verslagen en Mededeelingen van de Kon. Vlaamse Academie voor Taal- en Letterkunde". It contains 1,315 items, dealing with such subjects as: water, feeding, beer, wine, coffee, tea, fish, cookery, tobacco, bread, honey, *etc.* Of many of the entries included, supplementary information has been given as to illustrations, rarity, *etc.;* sometimes short biographies of the authors are included.

—— 1937-1941: Zuid- en Noord-Nederlandse bibliographie over Natuur- en Geneeskunde tot 1800, 12 parts, 895 p. (Lede-

berg/Gent: Erasmus).—

A bibliography consisting of 3,233 items, dealing with books published in the Netherlands (South and North) before 1800 on science and medicine. This bibliography is published in the "Verslagen en Mededeelingen van de Kon. Vlaamse Academie voor Taal- en Letterkunde". A supplement appeared in 1947 in the "Verslagen en Mededeelingen", 1947, p. 47-64.

VICAIRE, G., ed., 1954: Bibliographie gastronomique, ed. 2, 971 p. (London: Derek Verschoyle Academic and Bibliographical Publications).—

This bibliography lists many thousands of works on gastronomy, based on exhaustive researches in the Bibliothèque Nationale and many other libraries, both public and private. It is a bibliography of books appertaining to food and drink and related subects from the beginning of printing up to 1890. This is a reissue of the original edition of 1890. *(cf.* also BITTING, K. G., 1939, *vide supra).*

WILDHABER, R., ed., 1966: Internationale volkskundliche Bibliographie/International folklore bibliography/Bibliographie intl. des arts et traditions populaires/für die Jahre 1963 und 1964 mit Nachträgen für die vorausgehenden Jahre, 634 p. (Bonn: Habelt).—

This bibliography is published by the International Society for Ethnology and Folklore. Some sections are of a certain biohistorical interest, *viz.,* those on: folklore in general, relations between folklore and psychology, theories and methods, principles and methodology, bibliography, magic and countermagic, folk medicine, plant- and animal lore.

b. *General biology* (incl. anatomy, genetics, *etc.*)

ANATOMISCHER ANZEIGER, Centralblatt für die gesamte wissenschaftliche Anatomie, 1886 →

A record of current anatomical literature appears in each volume from 1886. This periodical is published semi-monthly, two volumes a year. Each issue contains a section of about 15 pages of current bibliography on anatomy arranged under headings; the combined bibliography of each volume totals *ca.* 125 pages.

ANNÉE BIOLOGIQUE, comptes rendus annuels des travaux de biologie générale, 1895 → (Paris: Masson).—

Abstracts, bibliographical reviews and critical reports.

BERICHT ÜBER DIE GESAMTE BIOLOGIE. Abt. A. Bericht über die wissenschaftliche Biologie. Referierendes Organ der deutschen botanischen Gesellschaft und der deutschen zoologischen Gesellschaft, 1926 → (Berlin, Heidelberg & New York, N.Y.: Springer).—

Includes abstracts and also lengthy reviews of books and periodical articles. Author- and subject-indexes in each volume. The abstracts are prepared and signed by someone other than the author. Abstracts are mainly from European publications. Appears irregularly. In 1966 13 vols. appeared, together consisting of nearly 8,000 pages of abstracts and of approximately 1,500 pages of author- and subject-indexes. In 1956 these numbers were *ca.* 3,100 and 500 pages resp.

BIOLOGICAL ABSTRACTS: a comprehensive abstracting and indexing journal of the world's literature in theoretical and applied biology, exclusive of clinical medicine, 1926 → (Philadelphia, Pa.: Univ. of Pennsylvania Press).—

This journal is now published by the trustees of "Biological abstracts", with the co-operation of international biologists, biological institutions, and biological journals. There are many subsections, each with its own editor. The abstracts are signed. Author- and subject-indexes. Five sections are also sold separately, *viz.,* A: General biology; B: Basic medical sciences; C: Microbiology, immunology, and parasitology; D: Plant sciences; E: Animal sciences. Vol. 30(1956) carried 33,355 signed indicative abstracts; vol. 36 (1961) 87,022, and vol. 48 (1967) 125,027 signed indicative abstracts. Before 1926 it was published under the titles: "Botanical abstracts" and "Abstracts of bacteriology".

BIOLOGICAL AND AGRICULTURAL INDEX: a cumulative subject index to periodicals in the fields of biology, agriculture, and related sciences, *vide* subsection c2, AGRICULTURAL INDEX.

BIOLOGICAL SCIENCES SERIAL PUB-LICATIONS: a world list, 1950-1954, prepared under the sponsorship of the Natural Science Foundation, 1955, 269 p. (Philadelphia, Pa.: Biological Abstracts).—

The 1954 list of journals abstracted by "Biological Abstracts" was used as the starting-point of this bibliography. It contains some 3,500 titles, grouped under the following headings: general biology; botany; zoology; science of Man; general science. Each entry usually includes title, issuing agency and publisher, date of first issue, frequency, bibliographical and descriptive notes, and contents. It also includes an index of titles and subjects and an index of societies and institutions arranged according to the 85 countries covered.

BOURLIÈRE, F., ed., 1941: Eléments d'un guide bibliographique du naturaliste, 302 p., with two supplements by P. LECHEVALIER, 1941, p. 303-368. (Mâcon: Protat).—

"Pour la biologie, la zoologie, la botanique, la géologie et l'ethnographie, ce répertoire fait connaître: 1) les travaux historiques, bibliographiques, méthodologiques, les vocabulaires et les traités, 2) les études régionales intéressant les cinq continents; au total 6357 notices de signalement, très complètes." (Cited after MALCLÈS, p. 301, *vide* subsection a). No index. General sections are followed by regional sections, covering all parts of the world.

BRITISH MUSEUM (Natl. Hist.), 1903-1940: Catalogue of the books, manuscripts, maps and drawings in the British Museum (Natural History), 8 vols. (London: Brit. Mus. Natl. Hist.).—

An author catalogue; if the author's name is absent, the book is catalogued under the principal word or words of the title. Societies and corporate bodies are considered to be authors of their publications. Vol. I (1903): A-D; Vol. II (1904): E-K; Vol. III (1910): L-O; Vol. IV (1913): P-Sn; Vol. V (1915): So-Z. Together these 5 vols. comprise 4202 pages. Vol. VI (1922): Suppl. A-I; Vol. VII (1933): suppl. J-O; Vol. VIII (1940): Suppl. P-Z. Together these 3 supplementary vols. comprise 1480 pages. One of the most valuable bibliographies in the field of biology.

HOLMES, S. J., ed., 1924: Bibliography of eugenics, 514 p. (Univ. California Publ. in Zoology, Vol. 25) (Berkeley, Calif.: Univ. Calif. Press).—

References under about 40 headings.

ISIS, Critical bibliography of the history of science and its cultural influences, 1913 → (Washington, D.C.: Smithsonian Instn.).—

> This is the most useful bibliography of current literature in the field of the history of biology. For more detailed information *vide supra,* subsection a.

KROGMAN, W. M., ed., 1941: A bibliography of human morphology, 1914-1939, 385 p. (Chicago, Ill.: U.P.).—

> A comprehensive, classified bibliography of human morphology, dealing with the period 1914-1939, including some titles of earlier years (on race, prehistory, osteology). It contains some 13,000 references classified under the following headings: osteology, races, prehistory, craniology, teeth, heredity, nervous system, myology, blood, hair, dermatoglyphics, phylogeny, soft parts, body-type, and growth. Reviews are cited. Author-index and extensive table of contents.

MEISEL, M., ed., 1924-1929: A bibliography of American natural history: the pioneer century, 1769-1865. The rôle played by the scientific societies; scientific journals; natural history museums and botanic gardens; state geological and natural history surveys; federal exploring expeditions in the rise and progress of American botany, geology, mineralogy, palaeontology and zoology, 3 vols. Vol. I: An annotated bibliography of the publications relating to the history, biography and bibliography of American natural history and its institutions, during colonial times and the pioneer century, which have been published up to 1924; with a classified subject and geographic index; and a bibliography of bibliographies, 244 p.; Vol. II: The institutions which have contributed to the rise and progress of American natural history, which were founded or organized between 1769 and 1844, 741 p.; Vol. III: The institutions founded or organized between 1845 and 1865. Bibliography of books. Chronological tables. Index of authors and institutions. Addenda to Vol. I, 749 p. (Brooklyn: Premier Publ. Comp.).—

> In the preface we read: "This work aims to trace bibliographically the rise and progress of natural history in the U.S.A. from the formation of an active American Philosophical Society at Philadelphia in 1769 to the close of the Civil War in 1865 ... The bibliography aims to recover the natural history contents of the publications of nearly ninety societies; of twenty-five journals; of thirty-six state geological and natural history surveys; of fifteen natural history museums and botanic gardens, and of over seventy Federal exploring expeditions and surveys." The contents of vol. I are fairly well described in its sub-title. The classified subject-index (p. 104-140) makes searching easy; the geographical index (p. 141-155) makes it easy to prepare an account of scientific work done in a particular state, section or locality. A long list of biographies and bibliographies of pioneer American scientists closes vol. I. The second volume contains a series of (chronologically arranged) articles devoted to American societies and other institutions (journals) founded or organized between 1769 and 1844. For each of them the author gives a historical outline, including lists of the main officers, a list of their publications and a special list of their papers on natural history. The first part of vol. III (p. 1-329) is a continuation of Vol. II and deals with the institutions, journals, expeditions, *etc.,* founded between 1845 and 1865. The second part of this volume (p. 329-495) is a bibliography of books, pamphlets, and miscellaneous articles on American natural history from 1590-1865. The period 1590-1768 occupies 20 pages; the period 1769-1865 occupies 45 pages. The rest of this volume contains chronological tables of the publications considered, and very elaborate indexes of authors, naturalists, and institutions. Reprinted 1967 (New York, N.Y.: Hafner).

REFERATIVNYI ZHURNAL, 1954 → (Moscow: Akad. Nauk. SSSR).—

> The Russian abstracting journal, ed. by A. S. BUCHINSKI, appearing semimonthly in eight series, one of which covers biology. The abstracts are in Russian, the titles are in the language of the published paper. Table of contents and author-index. Names in author-index are first arranged according to script (Cyrillic, West European, Armenian, Georgian, and Chinese), then the names are arranged alphabetically within each script printed. All entries, most of them carrying abstracts, include the author's name, title of publication, title of the source publication.

RESUMPTIO GENETICA, 1924-1953. ('s-Gravenhage: Nijhoff).—

> Abstract journal, international in

scope. Abstracts in English, French or German. Each volume contains a list of current literature (paged separately), the greater part consists of abstracts of books and journal articles. It includes literature on: general works, zoology, botany, anthropology, medicine, agriculture, eugenics, floriculture, *etc*. The last vol. appeared in 1953(vol. 19).

c. *Plant sciences* (excl. bibliographies of a regional importance; for these bibliographies *vide* section History of the plant sciences, subsection Regional histories).

c1. *Pure plant sciences*

BAY, J. C., ed., 1910: Bibliographies of botany: a contribution toward a bibliotheca bibliographica, 125 p. (Progressus Rei Botanicae III: 331-456) (Jena: Fischer).—

>Separate sections of this valuable bibliography deal with: 1. Methodology; 2. Periodicals and collective indexes to periodicals; 3. General, national, and comprehensive bibliographies; 4. Morphology, anatomy, microtechnique, and teratology; 5. Plant geography, systematic botany, ecology, and nomenclature; 6. Plant physiology, phenology, and biology; 7. Palaeobotany; 8. Economic botany; 9. Bibliographies of individual works; 10. Libraries and lists of publications of institutions; 11. Auction and sales catalogues; 12. Bookseller's catalogues.

BOTANY SUBJECT INDEX, compiled by the U.S. Department of Agriculture library, 1958, 15 vols. (Boston, Mass.: Hall).—

>The Botany subject index (or "Plant science subject catalog") is a semi-classed catalogue arranged alphabetically by subjects, names of countries, scientific names, and some vernacular names, with appropriate divisions and subdivisions under these. The catalogue is world-wide in scope and contains references to botanical literature from earliest times as published in books and scientific serials. In addition to the more strictly botanical publications on such subjects as: taxonomy, useful and injurious plants, phyto-geography, ecology, physiology, anatomy, and plant introduction, it includes also collateral subjects such as: voyages and travels, biographies, and textbooks. Names of genera are under the name of the family, the family names appear in their regular alphabetical sequence. *Ca.* 315,000 cards reproduced.

EXCERPTA BOTANICA. Sectio A: Taxonomica et chorologica, 1959 → (Stuttgart: Fischer).—

Contains abstracts of books and periodical articles. The abstracts are prepared and signed by someone other than the author. The abstracts are arranged under the following headings: Taxonomia et phylogenia (nomenclature, terminology, morphology, anatomy, embryology, palynology, cytotaxonomy, phytochemistry, pharmacognosy, systematics); Chorologia (subdivision geographical); Palaeobotanica; varia (herbals, botanical gardens, museums, biographical papers, bibliographies, ethnobotany, *etc.*). Published in co-operation with the International Association for Plant Taxonomy.

JACKSON, B. D., ed., 1881: Guide to the literature of botany: being a classified selection of botanical works, including nearly 6000 titles not given in Pritzel's "Thesaurus", 40 + 626 p. (London: Longmans, Green).—

>A classified subject-index of short titles mainly based on PRITZEL's "Thesaurus" *(vide infra)*. Introductory works in foreign (= non-English) language, theses, lectures, inaugural dissertations, works of more medical than botanical interest, and works on foreign local floras are excluded. The main sections into which the work has been divided are: Bibliography; History; Biography (consists entirely of works not given by Pritzel); Indexes (of terminology and of plant names); Encyclopaedias; Nomenclators; Systems; Pre-Linnaean botany (*i.e.*, biblical, classical, and early modern botany); Physiological and morphological botany (divided into many subsections according to functions and organs); Descriptive botany (divided into the main systematic groups); Palaeobotany; Economic botany; Emblematic works (poems, calendars, mythology, emblems); Practical botany (plant collection, plant-drawing, *etc.*); Local works (incl. directories, voyages); Local floras (geographically arranged); Botanical gardens (geographically arranged); Serial publications (transactions and journals). Extensive index (p. 513-623). Reprinted, 1964 (New York, N.Y.: Harper). Another valuable source is: JUNK, W., 1909: Bibliographia Botanica, 228 p., with suppl. (1916), p. 229-1052. (Berlin: Junk). Together these two volumes contain a mine of information.

LINDAU, G. & P. SYDOW, eds., 1908-1917: Thesaurus litteraturae mycologicae et lichenologicae, 5 vols. (Leipzig: Borntraeger).—

>The first two vols. consist of an alphabetical list of publications in the fields

of mycology and lichenology, published up to 1907. Vol. III (1913) considers the literature in these fields published between 1907 and 1910. Together they contain *ca.* 42,000 items. Vols. IV and V (1915-1917) contain an important subject-index. These volumes have quite recently been reprinted by Johnson (New York, N.Y.). No publication-date is given. In 1959, R. CIFERRI published a supplement containing the literature between 1911 and 1930 (Papia: Cortina).

PRITZEL, G. A., 1851: Thesaurus literaturae botanicae omnium gentium, inde a rerum botanicorum initiis ad nostra usque tempora Quindecim millia operum recensens, 547 p.; editio nova reformata, 1872-1877, 576 p. (Leipzig: Brockhaus).—

The book is in two parts. The first part gives an alphabetically arranged bibliography of botany from ancient times up to the end of 1871 (Editio nova), containing 10,675 items, together with a list of anonyma, periodicals and herbals (*ca.* 200 items). The first edition contains more information concerning botanical medicine, gardening, chemistry and philology; the Editio nova contains much biographical information, while horticultural literature has been excluded. (For further information concerning the differences between the original edition and the Editio nova, *cf.* JACKSON, B. D., 1880: Remarks on botanical bibliography, in: J. Bot., N.S., 9: 167-177). The second part of both editions is systematical and contains the following chapters: I. General botany (incl. sections on historical botany, pamphlets and collected works, botanical iconography and iconology, popular works arranged in geographical order); II. Systematic botany (incl. a section on Horti botanici); III. Geographical botany (incl. fossil plants); IV. Physiological botany (incl. morphology, general anatomy and physiology, and physico-chemical aspects). The second part of the Editio nova reformata was, after the author's death, edited by K. JESSEN. This Editio nova was reprinted in 1924 and 1950. (Milan: Görlich). *Cf.* also JACKSON, B. D., ed., 1881, *vide supra*.

QUINBY, J. & A. STEVENSON, eds., 1958-1961: Catalogue of botanical books in the collection of Rachel McMasters Miller Hunt, 2 vols. Vol. I (1958): Printed books 1477-1700, with several manuscripts of the 12th, 15th, 16th and 17th centuries, 84+517 p.; Vol. II, pt. 1 (1961): Introduction to printed books 1701-1800, 254 p.; Vol. II, pt. 2 (1961): Printed books 1701-1800, 655 p. (Pittsburgh, Pa.: Hunt Bot. Library).—

The introduction of vol. 1 contains the following essays: Botany from 840-1700 (by H. W. RICKETT); Medical aspects of early botanical books (by J. F. FULTON); The dawn-time of modern husbandry (by P. B. SEARS); The illustration of early botanical works (by W. BLUNT); Printing in the 15th and 16th centuries as represented in the Hunt Collection (by M. B. STILLWELL). Then follows the chronological catalogue of 405 books printed between 1477 and 1700 and of mss., with extensive descriptions of the items included. Appendix dealing with facsimiles, transcripts and reprints. Vol. II, pt. 1 contains the following essays: 18th-century botanical prints in color (by G. DUNTHORNE); Gardening books of the 18th century (by J. S. L. GILMOUR); Botanical gardens and botanical literature in the 18th century (by W. T. STEARN); A bibliographical method for the description of botanical books (by A. STEVENSON). The second pt. contains a chronological index of books printed in the 18th century and present in the library (764 in all) with extensive descriptions, an index to scientific names (p. 557-579) and a general index (p. 581-655), compiled by A. STEVENSON.

STAFLEU, F. A., 1967: Taxonomic literature: a selective guide to botanical publications with dates, commentaries and types, 556 p. (Regnum Vegetabile, Vol. 52) (Utrecht, Neth.: Int. Bureau for Plant Taxonomy and Nomenclature).—

The main purpose of the present book is to bring together the available information on dates of publication, references, commentaries and other publications which have a certain importance for present-day taxonomy. The main entries consist of paragraphs on *ca.* 650 authors (p. 1-513), giving information on their herbaria and types and references to bibliographical and biographical literature, followed by information as to their publications (*e.g.,* dates of publication, bibliographical or nomenclatural details, artists and illustrations, *etc.*). Index to personal names and index to titles of books.

WARNER, M. F., M. A. SHERMAN & E. M. COLVIN, eds., 1934: A bibliography of plant genetics, 552 p. (U.S. Dept. of Agriculture, Miscellaneous Publ., No. 164) (Washington, D.C.: U.S. Dept. Agriculture).—

A comprehensive bibliography of the literature up to 1930 bearing on plant genetics. It is mainly based on the catalogue of the Bureau of Plant Industry and it has been supplemented by articles from other sources. Japanese and Russian works have been listed only when accompanied by summaries in other languages; these and other summaries of non-English-language articles are carefully noted. Author-index; the subject-index contains all the names of plants and crops, with many features of interest to the breeder.

c2. *Applied plant sciences* (*i.e.*, agriculture, forestry, and horticulture)

AGRICULTURAL INDEX: ... subject index to a selected list of agricultural periodicals, books and bulletins, 1916 → (New N.Y.: Wilson).—

A detailed alphabetical subject-index to a selected list of agricultural periodicals, books and bulletins, issued in 11 parts per annum. From 1955 onwards (= vol. 14), cumulated volumes appear at two-yearly intervals instead of three years as formerly. Mainly English-language publications are listed, incl. some in entomology and applied zoology. The arrangement is alphabetical under subject, states, and major and minor topics. Since Vol. 50, No. 1 (October 1964): BIOLOGICAL AND AGRICULTURAL INDEX: a cumulative subject index to periodicals in the fields of biology, agriculture, and related sciences. (Published monthly except September). *Cf.* BIBLIOGRAPHY OF AGRICULTURE, *vide infra.*

ANDERSON, A., ed., 1961: Catalogue of the Walter Frank Perkins Agricultural Library, the University Library of Southampton, 291 p. (Southampton: University Library).—

After a preface (by M. J. HENDERSON), and a memoir by Perkin's daughter, Mary HOPKIRK, the alphabetically arranged catalogue follows (2,009 items). Appendixes deal with: books printed in England and Scotland up to 1700; periodicals; Board of Agriculture county reports (England [1793-1815], Scotland [1793-1815], and Wales [1794-1815]).

ASLIN, M. S., ed., 1940: Library catalogue of printed books and pamphlets on agriculture published between 1471 and 1840, ed. 2, 293 p. (Harpenden, Herts.: Rothamsted Experimental Station Library).—

This bibliography contains an alphabetical list of English authors and translations (p. 9-164), a list of reprints and later editions, an alphabetical list of foreign authors and translations (p. 169-226), a historical and geographical list of foreign authors and translations (p. 227-278), a list of books in Latin printed in different parts of Europe, a list of incunabula, of farm accounts, of portraits and of cattle prints, and a list of illustrations of agricultural operations. First ed. 1926.

BIBLIOGRAPHIA HISTORIAE RERUM RUSTICARUM INTERNATIONALIS, 1964 → (Budapest: Museum rerum rusticarum hungariae).—
Cf. GUNST, P., ed., *vide infra.*

BIBLIOGRAPHIE DES FORST- UND HOLZWIRTSCHAFTLICHEN SCHRIFTTUMS, 1955 → (Reinbek bei Hamburg: Bundesforschungsanstalt für Forst- und Holzwirtschaft).—

The contents represent a selection of titles important to forest research and practice, being gathered and analysed by the Documentation Centre of the Federal Research Station for Forestry and Forest Products, Reinbek near Hamburg. The titles have been arranged under the subheadings of number 634.0 of the U.D.C.; Oxford-system classification numbers have been published above the titles of the publications. One vol. comprises *ca.* 7,000 to 8,000 titles.

BIBLIOGRAPHY OF AGRICULTURE, 1942 → (Washington, D.C.: Govt. Print. Office).—

A large bibliography of agriculture prepared by a special staff in the library of the Dept. of Agriculture of the U.S.A. It is published monthly and there are two volumes a year. It contains the following major headings: Plant science (incl. phytopathology), Soils and fertilizers, Forestry, Animal industry (incl. veterinary medicine), Entomology, Agricultural engineering, Agricultural products, Agricultural economics and rural sociology, and Miscellanea (incl. biographies, history, *etc.*). Each issue carries an author-index, and the December-issue contains author- and subject-indexes. (*Cf.* also AGRICULTURAL INDEX, *vide supra.*

BLANCHARD, J. R. & H. OSTVOLD, eds., 1958: Literature of agricultural research,

231 p. (Berkeley, Calif.: Univ. California Press).—

A bibliographic guide to the literature of agriculture in its broadest meaning, listing bibliographies, indexes and abstracting services under the following section headings: A. Agriculture in general (23 p); B. Plant sciences (incl. horticulture, agronomy, plant breeding, plant pathology, forestry and forest products, 39 p.); C. Animal sciences (incl. economic zoology, animal husbandry, poultry, veterinary medicine, economic entomology, apiculture, pest control, fisheries, 62 p.); D. Physical sciences (incl. agricultural chemistry, soils and fertilizers, irrigation, meteorology, 14 p.); E. Food and nutrition (18 p.); F. Social sciences (incl. agricultural economics, statistics, rural sociology, agricultural education, 19 p.); G. Additional recent references.

DICTIONARY CATALOG of the library of the MASSACHUSETTS HORTICULTURAL SOCIETY, 1962, 3 vols. (Boston, Mass.: Hall).—

This catalog lists more than 31,000 entries of books and serial publications in the possession of the largest and most comprehensive library in this field.

DICTIONARY CATALOGUE of the YALE FORESTRY LIBRARY, 1962, 12 vols. (Boston, Mass.: Hall).—

This dictionary catalogue presents an accumulation of references to forestry literature from the early 18th century to the present. Yale Forestry Library possesses some 90,000 volumes (in 1962), included in this dictionary catalogue, together with some 38,000 cards representing periodical articles.

GUNST, P., ed., 1969: Bibliographia historiae rerum rusticarum internationalis, 1966, 274 p. (Budapest: Museum rerum rusticarum hungariae).—

This comprehensive international bibliography is published by the Hungarian Museum for Agriculture and deals with the literature on nearly every aspect of agriculture, *inter alia,* with: bibliographies relating to the history of agriculture; methods of agricultural history; the history of agricultural historiography; general works on agriculture; agricultural production and technology; plant gathering, hunting, fishing, and fishery; forestry, seed-growing; plant

growing in general; field crops; horticulture, plantation; viticulture and viniculture; animal husbandry. Regular publication of succeeding annual volumes is planned, with titles in English, except those in German, French, Italian, or Spanish. The following vols. have appeared: Vol. I (listing publications appearing in 1960 and 1961) was issued in 1964, 208 p.; Vol. 2 (1962-1963), 1965, 272 p.; Vol. 3 (1964), 1967, 267 p.; Vol. 4 (1965), 1968, 344 p.

JACKSON, B. D., ed., 1882: Vegetable technology: a contribution towards a bibliography of economic botany, with a comprehensive subject-index (founded upon the collections of G. J. SYMONS), 355 p. (London: Longmans, Green).—

This index is designed as a help in finding the books on a given subject which are distributed under the authors' names. Excluded are books and papers on horticulture, therapeutic, chemical, commercial, or manufacturing interest, unless they contain a sufficient account of the raw product and/or its cultivation. Part I consists of a catalogue of authors (p. 1-215); a list of serials (p. 217-219) and a list of anonymous publications (p. 221-239). Part II contains an extensive subject-index (p. 259-354) which facilitates searching.

LAUCHE, R., ed., 1957: Internationales Handbuch der Bibliographien des Landbaues, 411 p. (Munich: Bayerischer Landwirtschaftsverlag).—

An annotated list of 4,157 entries, of which 300 are current bibliographies and periodicals carrying bibliographical sections. 58 countries are dealt with. Subject-index.

LIBRARY CATALOGUE OF PRINTED BOOKS AND PAMPHLETS ON AGRICULTURE published between 1471 and 1840, ed. 2, 1940, 293 p. (Harpenden, Herts.: Rothamsted Experimental Station).—

An author-catalogue with indexes of authors, translations, and a historical and geographical list of foreign authors and translations. In 1949 a supplement was published, listing the additions since 1940 (15 p.). Another bibliography of agriculture, listing about 2,500 items is: A SELECTED AND CLASSIFIED LIST OF BOOKS RELATING TO AGRICULTURE, HORTICULTURE, *etc.,* in the library of the Ministry of Agriculture, Fisheries and Food of Great Britain, ed. 3, 1954, 87 p. (Bulletin

No. 78) (London: H. M. Stationery Office).
With subject-index. In 1958 a fourth edition
appeared, 95 p.

NAFTALIN, M. L., ed., 1967: Historic
books and manuscripts concerning general
agriculture in the collection of the National
Agricultural Library, 94 p. (Library List, No.
86, Febr. 1967, of the USDA Nat. Agric.
Library) (Washington, D.C.: USDA Nat.
Agric. Library).—

> "For more than a hundred years the
> United States Department of Agriculture
> Library has accumulated a rare collection
> of agricultural history materials. Included
> in this listing are all the Library's materials
> published in Europe prior to 1800 and those
> published in America before 1830. The items
> listed may be purchased in photocopy."
> (From: Agricult. Hist. 42(1): 74-75).

SPRINGER, L. A., ed., 1936: Bibliographisch overzicht van geschriften, boek- en
plaatwerken op het gebied der tuinkunst
(Bibliography of works relating to the art of
gardening), 166 p. (Fonds Landbouw Export
Bureau 1916-1918, Publicatie No. 15) (Wageningen: Veenman).—

> An international bibliography chiefly
> concerned with landscape gardening, but
> including many related subjects. Frequent
> annotations. Particularly useful for the
> Dutch references. The number between
> brackets, given after several titles, refers to
> the author's collection which has been de-
> posited in the main library of the College of
> Agriculture at Wageningen, The Nether-
> lands.

d. *Animal sciences* (incl. veterinary science)

DEAN, B., ed., 1962: A bibliography of
fishes, 3 vols. Vol. I: Publications grouped
under the names of authors A-K, 718 p.;
Vol. II: Author's titles L-Z, 702 p.; Vol.
III: Indices, *etc.,* 707 p. (New York, N.Y.:
Russell & Russell).—

> A reissue of the 1916-1923 edition.
> A very useful and complete bibliography.
> The first two volumes contain a list of about
> 50,000 papers and books which appeared
> between 1758 and 1914. Vol. III has mainly
> been prepared with the combined efforts of
> EASTMEN, GUDGER, and HENN. This
> volume contains: Addenda to vols. I and II
> (203 p.); Titles of pre-Linnean ichthyologic-
> al publications (p. 204-338, a section of ut-

most interest to the historian of biology);
General bibliographies which include references to fishes (incl. fisheries, pisciculture,
and angling); Voyages and expeditions which
relate to fishes; Periodicals relating to fish
and fish culture; and a subject-index of an
encyclopaedic nature (p. 361-707, including
a morphological section, a systematic section and a finding index). *Cf.* WESTWOOD
& SATCHELL, *vide infra.*

DERKSEN, W. & U. SCHEIDING, eds.,
1963 →: Index literaturae entomologiae. Serie II: Die Weltliteratur über die gesamte
Entomologie von 1864 bis 1900. (Berlin:
Deutsche Akad. der Wissenschaften).—

> The whole work will consist of 5
> vols., dealing with entomological literature
> published between 1864 and 1900. Up to
> now vol. I has been published (A-E); the
> whole work will contain some 90,000 en-
> tries. For older literature on entomology
> *cf.* HAGEN, 1862-1863, *vide infra.*

EALES, N. B., 1969: The Cole library of
early medicine and zoology, 425 p. (Oxford:
Alden).—

> This is the first part of a chronologi-
> cal catalogue prepared from the book col-
> lection (of about 8,000 vols.) of the late
> F. J. Cole, formerly professor of zoology,
> Univ. of Reading. The collection is now in
> the library of the university of Reading. The
> major sections of this collection are those
> dealing with sexual generation and with
> comparative anatomy; books included as
> "medical" deal with anatomical subjects.

ENGELMANN, W., ed., 1960: Bibliotheca
historico-naturalis. Verzeichnis der Bücher
über Naturgeschichte welche in Deutschland, Skandinavien, Holland, England,
Frankreich, Italien und Spanien in den
Jahren 1700-1846 erschienen sind, 786 p.
(Hildesheim: Olms).—

> A reissue of a general classified bib-
> liography concerning all zoological litera-
> ture from 1700-1846, first published in 1846
> (Leipzig: Engelmann). The literature cover-
> ing the years 1846-1860 can be found in:
> CARUS, J. V. & W. ENGELMANN, 1861:
> Bibliotheca Zoologica, 2 vols. (Leipzig: En-
> gelmann), and the literature published be-
> tween 1861 and 1880 in: TASCHENBERG,
> O., 1887-1913: Bibliotheca Zoologica II, in
> 7 vols. Engelmann's work is supplemented
> by: AGASSIZ, J. L. R., 1968: Bibliographia
> zoologiae et geologiae, 4 vols., 506 + 492
> + 658 + 684 p. (New York, N.Y.: Johnson).

Originally published 1848-1854 in London for the Ray Society.

HAGEN, H. A., ed., 1862-1863: Bibliotheca entomologica. Die Litteratur über das ganze Gebiet der Entomologie bis zum Jahre 1862, 2 vols. Vol. I: A-M, 566 p.; Vol. II: N-Z, 512 p. (Leipzig: Engelmann).—

This bibliography covers the literature from the beginning of entomological literature down to the year 1862. It includes both separate works and articles in serial literature. The arrangement is by authors. Author- and subject-index, and index of taxonomic groups. A revision of this bibliography, containing some more than 8,000 titles is: HORN, W & S. SCHENKLING, 1928-1929: Index literaturae entomologicae. Die Weltliteratur der gesammten Entomologie bis inklusive 1863, 4 vols., 1426 p. (Berlin: Dahlem). This work covers the literature on entomology up to the appearance of the Zoological Record. It has no index. For literature on entomology published between 1864 and 1900, *cf.* DERKSEN, W. & U. SCHEIDING, 1963, *vide supra.*

HARTING, J. E., ed., 1964: Bibliotheca accipitraria: a catalogue of books ancient and modern relating to falconry. With notes, glossary and vocabulary, 28+289 p. (London: Holland Press).—

This work is the only bibliography in English relating to falconry. Books in over 20 languages are catalogued, all with extensive and illuminating notes. First published in 1891; this is a photomechanical reprint.

INDEX-CATALOGUE of medical and veterinary zoology, 1902 → (Washington, D.C.: Govt. Print. Office). —

An author-bibliography which has appeared in 3 series of bulletin-sized publications issued by the U.S. Government Printing Office. It is a world bibliography with a broad interpretation of the field. It is fairly complete in the cestodes, nematodes, trematodes, and thorn-headed worms. The rather complex structure of this index is explained *in extenso* by SMITH, R. C., 1962: Guide to the literature of zoological sciences, ed. 6, *vide* section Some recommended encyclopaedias, *etc.*

INDEX VETERINARIUS, 1933 → (*Cf.* SCHÜTZLER, G., A. ZANDER & K. BARESAL, *vide infra*).—

KLEE, R., ed., 1901: Bibliotheca veterinaria oder Verzeichnis sämtlicher bis zur Gegenwart im deutschen Buchhandel erschienenen Bücher und Zeitschriften auf dem Gebiete der Veterinärwissenschaften, 247 p. (Leipzig: Seeman).—

This is mainly a compilation of the following catalogues: ENSLIN, T. C. F., 1825: Bibliotheca veterinaria, oder Verzeichniss aller brauchbaren... in Deutschland erschienenen Bücher über alle Theile der Thierheilkunde, 34 p. (Berlin: Enslin); ENGELMANN, W., 1843: Bibliotheca veterinaria oder Verzeichniss der in älterer und neuerer Zeit bis zur Mitte des Jahres 1842 in Deutschland erschienenen Bücher über alle Theile der Thierarzneikunde, ed. 2, 75 p. (Zuerst hrsg. von T.C.F. ENSLIN) (Leipzig: Engelmann); BÜCHTING, A., 1867: Bibliotheca veterinaria oder Verzeichniss der 1842-1866 im deutschen Buchhandel erschienenen Bücher und Zeitschriften über alle Theile der Thierarzneikunde. Im genauen Anschluss an die W. Engelmann'sche Bibliotheca veterinaria bis... 1842, 68 p. (Nordhausen: Büchting), continued as: VERZEICHNISS DER GESAMTEN LITERATUR ÜBER VETERINÄRWISSENSCHAFT und populäre Thierheilkunde... von 1866-1883 im deutschen Buchhandel erschienen, 69 p. (Leipzig: Gracklauer). For the period 1841-1865 one may also consult the JAHRESBERICHT über die FORTSCHRITTE der THIERHEILKUNDE, 1842-1865. (1842-1850: Erlangen: Enke; 1851-1865: Würzburg: Stahel). (This journal appeared from 1850 onwards under the title: C. CANSTATT's JAHRESBERICHT, *etc.*). For the literature of 1841, *cf.* HERTWIG, 1843: Jahresbericht über die Fortschritte der gesamten Thierarzneikunde in In- und Auslande. Leistungen des Jahres 1841, 35 p. (Erlangen). For the period 1889-1907, *cf.* SCHOETZ, R., 1902: Die Literatur der Veterinär-Wissenschaft und verwandten Gebiete von 1889-1. Dez. 1901, 112 p. (Berlin: Schoetz). From 1881 onwards the JAHRESBERICHT über die LEISTUNGEN auf dem Gebiete der VETERINÄRMEDIZIN appeared, *cf.* SCHÜTZLER, G., *et al.*, 1965; and WINDISCH, W., 1958, *vide infra. Cf.* also GRMEK, M. D., 1955, *vide* section History of the medical sciences, subsection b (Croatia).

MENNESSIER DE LA LANCE, 1915-1917: Essai de bibliographie hippique, donnant la description détaillée des ouvrages publiés ou traduits en latin et en français sur le cheval et la cavalerie avec de nombreuses biographies d'auteurs hippiques, 2 vols. Vol. I (1915): A à K, 760 p.; Vol. II (1917): L à Z et supplément, 736 p. (Paris: Dorbon).—

The publications are arranged in alphabetical order of names of authors. Contains much that is of importance to the history of agriculture; publications of iconographical importance also are included.

NISSEN, C., 1966: Die zoologische Buchillustration. Ihre Bibliographie und Geschichte. (Stuttgart: Hiersemann).—

For more details, *vide* section History of the animal sciences, subsection a.

RONSIL, R., ed., 1948-1949: Bibliographie ornithologique française, 2 vols. Vol. I: 534 p.; Vol. II: 84 p. (Encyclopédie ornithologique VIII and IX) (Paris: Lechevalier).—

Vol. I contains an alphabetically arranged bibliography (3,496 authors; 11,607 publications) of ornithological literature, published in the French or Latin language, and published in France or in one of the French colonies between 1473 and 1944. The second vol. consists of indexes of abbreviations of periodical publications incorporated in the bibliography, ornithological terms, geographical terms, bird names (French and Latin), ornithological monographs, the history of ornithology, and ornithological applications.

SAWYER, F. C., ed., 1955: Books of reference in zoology, chiefly bibliographical, 19 p. (J. Soc. Bibliogr. nat. Hist. 3 (2): 72-91).—

This publication lists 212 titles, including the leading periodicals. The aim of the author has been to compile a concise and briefly annotated list of books which experience has shown to be of service in assisting students to track down a paper from an incomplete or incorrect citation; also to list specialized bibliographies and some other reference-works relating to the various sub-divisions of the animal kingdom. The full titles are listed under authors. First come general bibliographical works, followed by special works under the various phyla and classes. Included is a topographical index of works restricted to specific regions.

SCHÜTZLER, G., A. ZANDER & K. BARESEL, eds., 1965: Bibliographie der Veterinärmedizin und ihrer Grenzgebiete, 1943-1947. Monographien, Hochschulschriften und Zeitschriftenaufsätze aus Deutschland, Oesterreich und der Schweiz, 855 p. (Berlin: Trenkel).—

This bibliography includes the literature on veterinary medicine published between 1943 (when the last vol. of the "Jahresbericht der Veterinärmedizin" appeared, *cf.* KLEE, R., *vide supra)* and 1948 (when the publication of "Die Veterinärmedizin" started). It is restricted to the German speaking countries, and it contains some 10,000 items, including literature dealing with such related fields as: some aspects of human medicine, agriculture, pure and applied biology, and technology. The items are arranged according to subject. Biographical index. *Cf.* also: WINDISCH, W., 1958, *vide infra.* For literature of the English speaking countries, *cf.* INDEX VETERINARIUS, published by the Imperial (Commonwealth) Bureau of Animal Health, Weybridge, 1933 → (Still in progress).

SMITH, R. C., 1966: Guide to the literature of the zoological sciences, ed. 7, 238 p. (Minneapolis, Minn.: Burgess).—

For more details, *vide* section Some recommended encyclopaedias, *etc.,* subsection Zoology.

STRONG, R. M., ed., 1939-1946: A bibliography of birds, 3 vols. Vol. I (1939): Author catalogue A to J, 464 p.; Vol. II (1939): Author catalogue K to Z, p. 469-937; Vol. III (1946): Subject index, 528 p. (Field Museum of Natural History, Vol. 25, parts 1-3) (Chicago, Ill.: Field Museum of Natural History).—

According to the subtitle this bibliography emphasizes anatomy, behaviour, biochemistry, embryology, pathology, physiology, genetics, ecology, aviculture, economic ornithology, poultry culture, evolution and related subjects up to 1939. Contains some 25,000 entries. Some other bibliographies on birds are: GIEBEL, C. G., ed., 1872-1877: Thesaurus ornithologiae. Repertorium der gesammten ornithologischen Literatur und Nomenclator sämmtlicher Gattungen und Arten der Vögel nebst Synonymen und geographischer Verbreitung, 3 vols. Vol. I (1872): 868 p.; Vol. II (1875): 787 p.; Vol. III (1877): 861 p. (Leipzig: Brockhaus), and IRWIN, R., ed., 1951: British bird books: an index to British ornithology A.D. 1481 to A.D. 1948, 398 p. (London: Grafton). *Cf.* also ZIMMER, J. T., 1926, *vide infra,* and RONSIL, R., 1948-1949, *vide supra.*

WESTWOOD, T. & T. SATCHELL, eds., 1966: Bibliotheca piscatoria: a catalogue of books on angling, the fisheries and fish-culture, with bibliographical notes and an appendix of citations touching on angling and fishing from old English authors, 397 p. (London: Dawson).—

A reprint of the 1883 edition (London: Satchell), to which is added a supplement, ed. by A. B. MARSTON. In this work 3,158 editions and reprints of 2,148 distinct works are registered. The subject matter has been divided into the following sections: Books on angling (p. 1-245); Books on fisheries (p. 247-330); Books on fish-culture (p. 331-354). There are two appendixes, the first contains a "Collection of citations touching on angling and fishing, from old English authors, dramatists, and poets" (p. 355-368), the second contains "A skeleton chronicle of dated, redated, and undated editions and reprints, with dissimilar imprints, of Izaak Walton's 'Compleat Angler', enumerated in this work" (p. 369-370). Extensive index (p. 371-397). A comparable work is: MULDER BOSGOED, D., 1873: Bibliotheca ichthyologica et piscatoria. Catalogus van boeken en geschriften over de natuurlijke geschiedenis van de visschen en walvisschen, de kunstmatige vischteelt, de visscherijen, de wetgeving op de visscherijen, enz., 474 p. (Haarlem, Neth.: Loosjes). Cf. DEAN, vide supra.

WINDISCH, W., 1958: Titelbibliographie der deutschsprachigen Veterinärhistorik 1900-1957, 144 p. (Munich: Inst. Staatsveterinärmed. und Gesch. Tiermed. Tierärztl. Fakult. der Universität).—

A list of titles on veterinary medicine, extracted from journals and reference works. The titles are listed according to subject, and then alphabetically. The section dealing with historical matters has been arranged according to cultural epochs and to disciplines.

WOOD, C. A., ed., 1931: An introduction to the literature of vertebrate zoology, 643 p. (London: Oxford U.P.).—

A classified bibliography based chiefly on the titles in the Blacker library of zoology, the Emma Shearer Wood Library of ornithology, the Bibliotheca Osleriana and other libraries of McGill University, Montreal, Canada. The volume consists of three parts: A. Introduction to the literature of vertebrate zoology consisting of 19 chapters with very good guides and references to the 19th century and earlier literature. B. Student's and librarian's ready index to short author-titles on vertebrate zoology, arranged geographically and in chronological order. C. A partially annotated catalogue of the titles on vertebrate zoology in the libraries of the McGill University. A photomechanical reprint was published in 1967 (Hildesheim: Olms). Later on a more complete bibliography of this book collection was published: A DICTIONARY CATALOGUE of the BLACKER-WOOD LIBRARY of zoology and ornithology, 1966, 9 vols. (Boston, Mass.: Hall). In J. Soc. Bibliogr. nat. Hist. 4: 320, F. C. Sawyer writes that Dr. Casey A. Wood's "Introduction" has proved to be a most valuable book of reference during the past three decades; and he adds that this new "Dictionary catalogue, recording the vast store of knowledge contained in these 60,000 volumes, should be of even more use for easy and quick reference". Author-, title-, and subject-entries are interfiled in a single alphabetical sequence. Estimated 135,000 cards are reproduced. A classified bibliography of mammalogy can be found in: WALKER, E.P., et al., 1964: Mammals of the world, Vol. III, 769 p. (London: Oxford U.P.; Baltimore, Md.: Johns Hopkins Press).

ZIMMER, J. T., ed., 1962: Catalogue of the Edward E. Ayer ornithological library, 2 vols., 706 p. (Chicago, Ill.: Field Museum of Natural History).—

Mr. E. E. Ayer is a successful business man who collected many books on ornithology. The present volume is the very elaborate catalogue of his ornithological library and it gives a rather complete bibliography on ornithology. The collection is particularly full with regard to books containing bird illustrations. Each book is completely described and many a description is accompanied by a critical note discussing many technical details and referring to reviews in scientific periodicals. Cf. also STRONG, R. M., 1939-1946, and RONSIL, R., 1948-1949, vide supra.

ZOOLOGISCHER ANZEIGER, 1878 → (Leipzig: Geest & Portig).—

From the commencement of this periodical in 1878, records of current literature, arranged systematically, appeared in each part. From 1896 onwards the records of literature were issued separately under the title "Bibliographia Zoologia". Comprehensive indexes are issued at varying intervals. No issues appeared between 1945 and 1950. From 1950 onwards it is published by Geest & Portig (Leipzig); it appears irregularly in issues of ca. 80 pages in connection with the "Verhandlungen der deutschen Zool. Gesellschaft".

ZOOLOGISCHER BERICHT, 1922-1944:
55 vols. (Jena: Fischer).—

> Issued in parts, in which short ab-
> stracts of current papers are arranged sys-
> tematically. Two to three vols. were issued
> yearly, each containing an author- and sub-
> ject-index; an overall-index covering the
> first twenty vols. was issued in 1931.

e. *Medical sciences* (incl. therapy, pharmacy, *etc.,* excl. bibliographies of a
regional importance; for these works,
vide section History of medicine, subsection Regional histories).

BIBLIOGRAPHY of the HISTORY of
MEDICINE, 1965 → (U.S. Dept. Health,
Education and Welfare: Public Health Ser-
vice Publ., No. 1540) (Washington, D.C.:
Govt. Print. Office).—

> A by-product of the Index Medicus
> *(vide infra),* produced in the National Li-
> brary of Medicine's Historical Division.
> This "Bibliography" will appear annually
> and then in quinquennial cumulations. It
> can be considered as a complement to the
> Wellcome Institute's CURRENT WORK in
> the HISTORY of MEDICINE *(vide infra).*

BISHOP, W. J., ed., 1958: Bibliography of
international congresses of medical sciences,
238 p. (Oxford: Blackwell).—

> This work has been prepared under
> the auspices of the "Council for Internation-
> al Organizations of Medical Sciences". The
> purpose of the present list is described by
> the editor as follows: "it is a guide for
> congress organisers, librarians, editors and
> others who wish to trace the published pro-
> ceedings of medical congresses". It gives a
> list of the more important publications
> arising from international congresses in the
> medical field. The information provided:
> the subject of the congress, the members
> of the congress, the place of meeting, the
> precise date of the congress, a bibliogra-
> phical description (title, numbers of vols.,
> number of pages, note of illustrations, place
> of publication, publisher, and date of publi-
> cation), the languages represented in the
> congress, *etc.* The present bibliography
> gives particulars of 1,427 congress meetings
> devoted to some 362 different aspects of
> medicine.

BLACK, A. D., ed., 1921-1939: Index of
the periodical dental literature published in
the English language, 1839-1936/'38, 15
vols. (Buffalo, N.Y.: Dental Index Bureau;
Chicago, Ill.: Amer. Dental Assn.).—

> Each volume is in two parts: 1. a clas-
> sified subject-index arranged following the
> Dewey decimal classification, and 2. an
> author-index. Vol. 1 (1923): 1839-1875; vol.
> 2 (1925): 1876-1885; vol. 3 (1926): 1886-
> 1890; vol. 4 (1927): 1891-1895; vol. 5 (1930):
> 1896-1900; vol. 6 (1931): 1901-1905; vol.
> 7 (1934): 1906-1910; vol. 8 (1921): 1911-
> 1915; vol. 9 (1922): 1916-1920; vol. 10
> (1928): 1921-1923; vol. 11 (1929): 1924-
> 1926; vol. 12 (1932): 1927-1929; vol. 13
> (1936): 1930-1932; vol. 14 (1938): 1933-1935;
> vol. 15 (1939): 1936-1938. This work is con-
> tinued as INDEX TO DENTAL LITERA-
> TURE in the English language (Chicago,
> Ill.: Amer. Dental Assn.). Separate vols.
> appeared in 1943, 1946, 1949, and 1951 resp.,
> dealing with the literature of the periods
> 1939-1941, 1942-1944, 1945-1947, and 1948-
> 1949. From 1951 onwards it appears yearly,
> each vol. considering the literature published
> during the previous years, thus, *e.g.,* in
> 1968 appeared a vol. dealing with the liter-
> ature of 1967, *etc.* The bibliography is pre-
> pared by the Bureau of Library and Indexing
> Service of the Amer. Dental Assn. *Cf.* also:
> WEINBERGER, B. W., ed., 1929-1932:
> Dental bibliography: index to the literature
> of dental science and art as found in the
> libraries of the New York Academy of Med-
> icine, and Bernhard Wolf Weinberger, ed.
> 2, 2 vols. (New York, N.Y.: First Dental
> District Dental Soc., State of New York).
> Contains a reference-index, a subject-index,
> and an additional reference-index. For den-
> tal literature in the German and French
> languages, *cf.* PORT, G., ed., *vide infra.*
> *Cf.* also: STRÖMGREN, N. W., ed., 1957;
> and CAMPBELL, J. M., ed., 1949, *vide
> infra.*

BLAKE, J. B. & C. ROOS, eds., 1967: Medical reference works, 1679-1966: a selected
bibliography, 343 p. (Chicago, Ill.: Medical
Library Assn.).—

> This book essentially is a new and
> completely revised version of the "Bibliog-
> raphy of the reference works and histories
> in medicine and the allied sciences", the
> appendix to DOE, J. & M. L. MARSHALL's
> Handbook of medical library practice, *vide
> infra.* Compared with this original version
> over a thousand items have been excluded,
> but 1,800 wholly new titles have been in-
> cluded; the new ed. contains 2,703 entries,
> divided as follows: 1. General medicine (413
> entries); 2. History of medicine (419 entries,
> of which 226 are national histories); 3.
> Special subjects (1,871 entries; of particular
> interest to the historian of biology are the

categories dealing with: general biology, anatomy, botany, genetics, microbiology, parasitology, physiology, zoology, and science). Authors, subjects and titles are arranged in one alphabet. Complete bibliographical details; each entry being accompanied by an annotation.

BLOOMFIELD, A. L., ed., 1960: A bibliography of internal medicine, selected diseases, 312 p. (Chicago, Ill.: U.P.).—

This is a guide to selected medical writings of the recent past (*i.e.,* from the beginnings of the 19th century onwards), intended for those students and physicians who have no special historical training. The text is divided into sections, each dealing with one of 21 selected non-communicable diseases. Each section comprises *ca.* 20 principal references, and each reference is the subject of a short description or résumé, usually including a number of extracts. The author tries to bring continuity into his book and to bring documentation up to date. A comparable book of the same scope is: BLOOMFIELD, A. L., ed., 1958: A bibliography of internal medicine: communicable diseases, 560 p. (Chicago, Ill.: U.P.).

BRITTAIN, R. P., ed., 1962: Bibliography of medico-legal works in English, 252 p. (London: Sweet & Maxwell).—

A bibliography of publications on forensic medicine written in English.

CAMPBELL, J. M., ed., 1949: A dental bibliography, British and American, 1682-1880, with an index of authors, 63 p. (London: Low).—

A bibliography of British and American dental books and pamphlets printed between 1682 and 1880. It comprises 417 dental books and pamphlets published in Great Britain and Ireland and 306 items published in the U.S.A. between 1801 and 1880. Title, number of pages, *etc.,* are not very complete.

CHATTON, M. J. & P. J. SANAZARO, eds., 1967: Current medical references, ed. 5, 595 p. (Los Angeles, Calif.: Lange Med. Publ.).—

An annotated compilation of representative references in the English-language literature, divided into some 34 sections corresponding with the existing specialities and subspecialities.

CHOULANT, L., ed., 1924: Graphische Incunabeln für Naturgeschichte und Medicin, *vide supra,* subsection a.

—— ed., 1956: Handbuch der Bücherkunde für die ältere Medicin. Zur Kenntniss der griechischen, lateinischen und arabischen Schriften im ärztlichen Fache und zur bibliographischen Unterscheidung ihrer verschiedenen Ausgaben, Uebersetzungen und Erläuterungen, 434 p. (Graz: Akad. Druck- und Verlagsanstalt).—

This is one of the best check lists of printed works of the older medical writers. The present edition is a reissue of the second edition of 1841. It contains biographical and historical notes as well as lists of editions of the works of the early Greek, Latin and Arabian writers.

CURRENT WORK in the HISTORY of MEDICINE 1954 →: An international bibliography. (London: Wellcome Hist. Med. Libr.).—

This is a quarterly index of articles on the history of medicine and the allied sciences appearing in a wide range of periodicals, published by the Wellcome Historical Medical Library. From 1965 onwards it is compiled with the co-operation of the National Library of Medicine at Bethesda (Md.). *Cf.* BIBLIOGRAPHY of the HISTORY of MEDICINE, *vide supra).* Each issue contains a subject- and author-index as well as a list of addresses of authors. New books on the history of medicine and science are listed alphabetically by author's names at the end of each number.

DOE, J. & M. L. MARSHALL, eds., 1956: Medical Library Association handbook of medical library practice, with a bibliography of the reference works in the history of medicine and the allied sciences, ed. 2, 601 p. (Chicago, Ill.: Amer. Library Assn.).—

Individual chapters discuss such subjects as: medical libraries, the Medical Library Association, the medical librarian, administration, acquisition and preservation, classification, cataloguing, non-book materials, photoduplication, public relations, reference and bibliographic services. Of particular bibliographical interest is the chapter on: Rare books and the history of medicine, supplemented by a bibliography of the reference works on the history of medicine and allied sciences. This check list, taking up almost half of the volume, is classified by subject and has a special table of contents to make it easier to use. *Cf.* **BLAKE & ROOS**, *vide supra.*

DURLIN, R. J., ed., 1967: A catalogue of sixteenth century printed books in the national library of medicine, 698 p. (Bethesda, Md.: U.S. Dept. Health, Education and Welfare, Public Health Service, Natl. Libr. Med.).—

This catalogue describes 4,818 books and broadsides, most of them related to the healing arts. The order of entries under each heading is alphabetical. There are four indexes: a geographical index of printers and publishers (p. 621-636); a name index of printers and publishers (p. 637-692); a concordance of STC items and serial numbers used in this catalogue (p. 693); and an index of vernacular imprints (p. 695-698). Many Renaissance eds. of Greek, Roman, Byzantine, and Arabic writers. In conjunction with the items included in Vol. I of the Wellcome Catalogue, Durlin's book provides the basis for a comprehensive survey of medical publishing in the 16th century. *Cf.* **POYNTER, F. N. L.**, ed., *vide infra.*

EMMERSON, J. S., ed., 1965: Translations of medical classics: a list, 82 p. (Newcastle-upon-Tyne: Univ. Libr. Publ.).—

A list, arranged alphabetically by authors, of translations of medical works of classical interest and importance, published before 1900.

EXCERPTA MEDICA 1947 → (Amsterdam: Excerpta Medica Foundation).—

The most comprehensive medical abstracting journal, containing abstracts in English from every available medical journal published throughout the world. It consists of 17 sections which are issued monthly, with author- and subject-indexes to each volume. The sections are: 1. Anatomy, anthropology, embryology and histology (1947 →); 2. Physiology (1948 →); 3. Endocrinology (1947 →); 4. Microbiology: bacteriology, virology, mycology, and parasitology (1948 →); 5. General pathology and pathological anatomy (1948 →); 6. Internal medicine (1947 →); 7. Pediatrics/ (1947 →); 8. Neurology and neurosurgery (1947 →); 9. Surgery (1947 →); 10. Obstetrics and gynaecology (1948 →); 11. Otorhinolaryngology (1948 →); 12. Ophthalmology (1947 →); 13. Dermatology and venereology (1947 →); 14. Radiology (1947

→); 15. Chest diseases, thoracic surgery, and tuberculosis (1948 →); 16. Cancer (1953 →); 17. Public health, social medicine and hygiene (1955 →); 18. Cardiovascular diseases and cardiovascular surgery (1957 →); 19. Rehabilitation and physical medicine (1958 →); 20. Gerontology and geriatrics (1958 →); 21. Developmental biology and teratology (1961 →); 22. Human genetics (1963 →); 23. Nuclear medicine (1964 →); 24. Anesthesiology (1966 →); 25. Hematology (1967 →); 26. Immunology, seriology and transplantation (1967 →); 27. Biophysics, bio-engineering and medical instrumentation (1967 →); 28. Urology and nephrology (1967 →); 29. Biochemistry (1948 →); 30. Pharmacology and toxicology (1948 →); 31. Arthritis and rheumatism (1965 →); 32. Psychiatry (1948 →); 33. Orthopedic surgery (1956 →); 34. Plastic surgery (1970 →); 35. Occupational health and industrial medicine (1971 →); 36. Health economics (1971 →).

GARRISON, F. H. & L. T. MORTON, eds., 1954: A medical bibliography: a check-list of texts illustrating the history of the medical sciences, ed. 2, 655 p. (London: Grafton).—

This is the most widely-used standard guide to the classic books and papers which mark the development of knowledge in the medical sciences; it is meant for research workers, librarians, biographers, and students of the history of medicine. The first edition appeared in 1943 (5,506 items); this greatly expanded 2nd. ed. contains over 6,000 items. A revised edition appeared in 1965; and a third ed. in 1970, under the editorship of L. T. MORTON (6,804 items). The subject-headings are in accordance with the International Decimal Classification, and under each subject-heading the titles are arranged in chronological order. Very useful author- and subject-indexes have been added. A valuable supplement to this volume is: ASH, L., 1961: Serial publications containing medical classics: an index to citations in Garrison-Morton, 147 p. (New Haven, Conn.: Antiquarium). In this book the author indexes the titles of journals containing the individual papers cited in Garrison & Morton's "Medical Bibliography". Each title is followed by details of the issues containing Garrison-Morton items. The book is preceded by an introduction of L. T. MORTON, entitled "The story of the Garrison-Morton Bibliography". The book is of importance to librarians and bibliographers, and also to students of the history of medicine. A much older bibliography is: ENSLIN, T. C. F., ed., 1838: Bibliotheca medico-chirurgica et pharmaceutico-chemica oder Verzeichniss derjenigen

medizinischen, chirurgischen, geburtshilfli-
chen und pharmazeutisch-chemischen Bücher, welche vom Jahre 1750 bis zur Mitte
des Jahres 1837 in Deutschland erschienen
sind. Von neuem gänzlich umgearbeitet von
W. ENGELMANN, ed. 5, 1838-1841, 588
p. (Leipzig: Engelmann). *Cf.* also: GIL-
BERT, J. B., 1962: Disease and destiny: a
bibliography of medical references to the
famous, 535 p. (London: Dawsons). For
more details, *vide* section History of the
medical sciences, subsection a (General).

GUITARD, E. H., ed., 1968: Index des travaux d'histoire de la pharmacie de 1913 à
1963, 80 + 103 p. (Paris: Soc. d'Histoire de
la Pharmacie).—

The contents of this index may become clear from its sub-title: Répertoire
des auteurs et des sujets d'articles et d'ouvrages soit publiés soit analysés dans les
revues ou éditions des 51 premières années
de la "Société d'Histoire de la Pharmacie".
This bibliography is preceded by a rather
long introduction, in which the author tries
to give the historical development of the
concepts pharmacon, pharmacist, apothecary, and druggist. *Cf.* also FERCHL-MIT-
TENWALD, F., ed., 1937, *vide* subsection
Biographical dictionaries.

INDEX-CATALOGUE of the LIBRARY
of the SURGEON-GENERAL's OFFICE,
United States Army, 1880 → Series 1 (1880-
1895), 16 vols.; series 2 (1896-1916), 21
vols.; series 3 (1918-1932), 10 vols.; series 4
(1936 →) Washington, D.C.: Govt. Print.
Office).—

A dictionary catalogue, listing books
and periodical articles belonging to one of
the largest medical libraries of the world.
Includes many biographical entries.

INDEX MEDICUS, New Series, 1960 →
(Washington, D.C.: U.S. Dept. Health).—

This current index to medical literature has appeared under the following series
titles: Current list of medical literature
(1959-1960); Quarterly Cumulative Index
Medicus (1927-1959). This journal originated
as a junction of the Quarterly cumulative
index to current literature (1916-1926, vols.
1-12) and the Index medicus (1879-1926).
It is published monthly. More than 5,000
journals are indexed. There is a list of major
subheadings in each issue, but the references
are listed alphabetically by author under
secondary or minor subheadings. Author
index. The older vols. have been reprinted
by Johnson (New York, N.Y.). An annual

catalogue, in appearance and arrangement
resembling the Index medicus is: CATA-
LOG of books in the LIBRARY of the
WASHINGTON UNIVERSITY SCHOOL
of MEDICINE, published by the Univ. of
Washington School of Medicine (St. Louis,
Mo.). A list of new accessions of the li-
brary, published from 1969 onwards.

LIBRARY of the ROYAL COLLEGE of
OBSTETRICIANS and GYNAECOLO-
GISTS: short title catalogue of books printed
before 1851, ed. 2, 1968, 85 p. (London:
Roy. Coll. Obstet. Gynaec.).—

Nearly 1,200 titles have been listed
under the names of some 600 different
authors. First ed. 1956.

MANN, G., ed., 1970: Internationale Bibliographie zur Geschichte der Medizin 1875-
1901, 591 p. (Hildesheim & New York,
N.Y.: Olms).—

A collection of reprints of medico-
historical bibliographies, *viz.*, those of: J.
PAGEL: Historisch-Medicinische Bibliographie für die Jahre 1875-1896 (from: Geschichte der Medicin, II, 1898, p. 575-960);
T. PUSCHMANN & R. v. TÖPLY: Geschichte der Medicin und der Krankheiten
(from: Jahrb. über die Leistungen und Fort-
schr. in der Ges. Medicin 22, vol. 1, 1898,
p. 293-329); J. PAGEL, *Idem*, 23, 1899, p.
307-341; 24, 1900, p. 300-341; 25, 1901, p.
297-344; 26, 1902, p. 348-396.

MILLER, G., ed., 1964: Bibliography of the
history of medicine of the United States and
Canada (1939-1960), 428 p. (Baltimore,
Md.: Johns Hopkins U.P.).—

This work is a reissue in consolidated
form of the "Bibliography of the History
of Medicine of the United States and Canada" which was published annually in the
"Bulletin of the History of Medicine" after
1939, and it includes the literature published
between 1939 and 1960. The main subjects
which constitute separate sections are: biography, dentistry, diseases, general, hospitals, journals, libraries, museums, local history and societies, medical education, medical science and specialties, military medicine, nursing, pharmacy, primitive medicine,
professional history, public health, and
social medicine.

MORTON, L. T., ed., 1970: A medical
bibliography: an annotated check-list of
texts illustrating the history of medicine, ed.
3, 872 p. (London: Deutsch).—

For details, *vide* GARRISON, F. H. & L. T. MORTON, *supra*.

Osler, W.-FRANCIS, W. W., R. H. HILL & A. MALLOCH, eds., 1929: Bibliotheca Osleriana: a catalogue of books illustrating the history of medicine and science, collected, arranged, and annotated by Sir William Osler, Bt., and bequeathed to McGill University, 36+758 p. (Oxford: Clarendon Press).—

From the editor's preface: The library here catalogued consists of literature illustrating the history of medicine and science, collected with a definite educational purpose by the late Sir William Osler, and bequeathed by him to the Medical Faculty of McGill University, Montreal. The arrangement of this catalogue is mainly chronological. It contains sections named: Bibliotheca litteraria, -historica, -biographica, -bibliographica, Incunabula, Manuscripts.

PASZTOR, M. & J. HOPKINS, eds., 1968: Bibliography of pharmaceutical reference literature, 167 p. (London: Pharmaceutical Press).—

A review of the most important reference works in the field of pharmacy. The table of contents lists the following subjects: pharmacopoeias, catalogues of medicaments (general and regional), abstracting journals, bibliographies, encyclopaedias, yearbooks, nomenclature, dictionaries, and a list of chemical and pharmaceutical organizations of Great Britain.

PAULY, A., ed., 1954: Bibliographie des sciences médicales, 1758 cols. + 74 p. index. (London: Verschoyle).—

A reprint of the 1874 edition (Paris: Tross). This bibliography was begun by C. V. DAREMBERG. After his death in 1872, the compilation was continued by A. PAULY. The contents of this bibliography covers the following fields of medicine: bibliography, history of medicine, professional history, history of schools and societies, controversies, medical philosophy and literature, history of the different branches of medicine, including the history of diseases, hospitals, epidemics and endemics. Its chapters are subdivided into countries, and subsections give the history of each period. Titles are listed in chronological order of printing and all titles found in VON HALLER (Bibliotheca chirurgia, 1774-1775; and Bibliotheca medicinae practicae, 1776),

CHOULANT *(vide supra)*, and CALLISEN *(vide* section Biographical dictionaries, subsection c) are included.

PAZZINI, A., 1948: Bio-bibliographia di storia della chirurgia, 525 p. (Rome: Cosmopolita).—

For more details, *vide* section Biographical dictionaries, subsection c.

PORT, G., ed., 1922: Index der deutschen zahnärztlichen Literatur und zahnärztlichen Bibliographie, umfassend die Literatur von 1847 bis 1902, 2 vols. (Berlin: Meusser).—

This bibliography has been compiled under the auspices of the Zentralverein deutscher Zahnärzte. A compilation of the German dental literature published in 1903 was published in 1904 by the Heidelberger Verlagsanstalt, and compilations of this literature of the years 1904, 1905, 1906-1907, 1908-1912, 1913, and 1914 appeared in 1922, 1922, 1909, 1922, 1914, and 1916 resp. (Published by Meusser, Leipzig). In 1934 appeared the INDEX DER DEUTSCHEN UND AUSLÄNDISCHEN ZAHNÄRZTLICHEN LITERATUR, considering the literature published between 1915 and 1918. This publication was succeeded by the following series: in 1936 2 vols. dealing with the literature published between 1919 and 1928, in 1934 with 1929, in 1933 with 1930, in 1933 with 1931, in 1934 with 1932, in 1935 with 1933, and in 1936 with 1934 (published by Lehmann, Munich). From 1936-1945 the dental bibliography is included in the ZENTRALBLATT FÜR DIE GESAMTE ZAHN-, MUND-, UND KIEFERHEILKUNDE, edited under the auspices of the Deutsche Gesellschaft für Zahn-, Mund-, und Kieferheilkunde, and published by Meusser (Leipzig). (Included is the literature up to 1943/'44). From 1948 onwards the bibliography is published in: DEUTSCHE ZAHN-, MUND-, UND KIEFERHEILKUNDE. Mit: Zentralblatt für die gesamte Zahn-, Mund-, und Kieferheilkunde, 1948 → (Leipzig: Barth). For the French dental literature, *cf.*: NOTICES SIGNALÉTIQUES DES TRAVAUX ORIGINAUX D'ODONTO-STOMATOLOGIE DE LANGUE FRANÇAISE, 1960 → (Paris: Centre français de documentation odontostomatologique). Appears irregularly (vol. 7 in 1968). As to the dental literature in the English language, *Cf.* BLACK, *vide supra*.

POYNTER, F. N. L., ed., 1962-1966: Catalogue of the Wellcome Historical Medical Library. Vol. I (1962): Books printed before 1641, 407 p.; Vol. II (1966): Books printed between 1641 and 1850, A-E, 540 p. (London: Wellcome Hist. Med. Library).—

Vol. I of this catalogue contains 6,959 items, including a supplement of 131 items (containing great rarities). In each item are given biographical dates of the authors, a brief collation of pages, the presence of plates, woodcuts, portraits and tables. Brief references are given to the incunabula, of which a detailed catalogue was published in 1954, *viz.*, POYNTER, F. N. L., ed., 1954: A catalogue of incunabula in the Wellcome Historical Medical Library, 159 p. (Publ. of the Wellcome Hist. Med. Museum, N.S., No. 5) (London: Wellcome Hist. Med. Library). The year 1641 has been chosen because it coincides approximately with the decline of classical and mediaeval ideas and the beginning of modern scientific medicine. Vol. II contains, as the title indicates, the entries of books printed in the years 1641 to 1850 in the possession of the Wellcome Historical Medical Library. (Vol. III: F-L, in press). *Cf.* DURLIN, R. J., 1967, *vide supra.*

RUCH, T. C., ed., 1941: Bibliographia primatologica, 241 p. (Yale Medical Library, Hist. Libr. Publ., No. 4) (Springfield, Ill.: Thomas).—

A classified bibliographie of "primates other than Man". No works are included which were published after 1939. Excellent index. The volume contains some 4,630 entries. The author promised to publish a second volume, devoted to the literature on diseases of the primates that, up to now (1969), seems not to have been published.

SHOCK, N. W., ed., 1957: A classified bibliography of gerontology and geriatrics, 1900-1948, 599 p. Suppl. I, 1949-1955, 38+525 p. (Stanford, Calif.: U.P.).—

In the first volume the historical references were relegated to the Miscellaneous section; in the suppl., however, a section "Historical references" has been included, in which section some 50 papers are listed (partly published even before 1900).

STRÖMGREN, H. L., ed., 1955: Index of dental and adjacent topics in medical and surgical works before 1800, 255 p. (Library res. monogr., No. 4) (Copenhagen: Munksgaard).—

The author has gone through many works on medicine and surgery before 1800 for references to dental subjects, the references being specified under each entry.

THORNTON, J. L., 1966: Medical books, libraries and collectors: a study of bibliography and the book trade in relation to the medical sciences, 445 p. (Rev. ed.; introd. by G. KEYNES) (London: Deutsch).—

Originally published 1949. The first half of the book is devoted to medical literature from the earliest times up to and including the 19th century, including biographical sketches of prominent medical writers and comments on selected titles *(e.g.,* on variant, spurious and facsimile editions, translations, contents, plagiarisms, locations of copies, *etc.).* Other chapters deal, *inter alia,* with: medical societies, periodical literature, and medical libraries.

VESTER, H., 1953: Deutsche pharmazie-historische Bibliographie. 1. Deutsche pharmazeutische Zeitschriftenliteratur 1945-1951, 32 p. (Stuttgart: Int. Gesell. Gesch. Pharmazie).—

Includes articles on general and foreign pharmacy printed in the German periodicals indexed. Author- and catchword indexes.

——, 1956-1961: Topographische Literatursammlung zur Geschichte der deutschen Apotheken, 474 p. (Int. Gesell. Gesch. Pharm. Veröffentl., N.S., vols. 9, 14, 17 and 19) (Stuttgart: Int. Gesell. Gesch. Pharm.).—

This work is in 3 sections, *viz.,* 1. Deutsche Städte und Ortschaften, A-Z (p. 1-411); Deutsche Länder, Provinzen, *etc.* (p. 413-464); 3. Deutsches Reichsgebiet (p. 467-474). Under each local entry are lists of dispensatories, pharmacopoeias, registries, ordinances, tariffs, *etc.,* chronologically subarranged; general works, and works on individual pharmacists or apothecaries. Included are publications from the 15th century up to 1950.

Waller, E.-SALLANDER, H., ed., 1955: Bibliotheca Walleriana: a catalogue of the Erik Waller collection, 2 vols. Vol. I: 471 p.; Vol. II: 494 p. (Uppsala: Almqvist & Wiksells).—

A catalogue of books collected by the late Dr. Erik Waller and bequeathed to the library of the Royal University of Uppsala. The volumes contain 20,428 entries, together illustrating the history of medicine and science. Extensive index of names.

WARING, E. J., 1878-1879: Bibliotheca therapeutica, or bibliography of therapeutics, chiefly in reference to articles of the materia medica, with numerous critical, historical, and therapeutical annotations, and an appendix containing the bibliography of British mineral waters, 2 vols., 934 p. (London: New Sydenham Soc.).—

"Vol. 1 has sections on general and special therapeutics, arranged according to method of use, classes of medicines, then sections devoted to the individual articles of materia medica. Vol. 2 continues the latter section and contains in addition the appendix on mineral waters and the indexes to both vols. There is much incidental information, including lists of relevant journals, techniques of prescribing drugs, *etc.* The indexes, incidentally, are divided according to diseases, authors, and subjects. Altogether an extremely valuable reference book which we have found most useful. So far as I know it has not been reprinted." (From a letter by Mr. E. J. Freeman of the Wellcome Inst. of the Hist. of Medicine). *Cf.* also: GUITARD, E. H., ed., 1968; PASZTOR, M. & J. HOPKINS, eds., 1968; and VESTER, H., 1953 and 1956-1961; *vide supra.*

β. BIOGRAPHICAL DICTIONARIES
(incl. some cumulative biographies)

a. *General* (incl. some dictionaries of national biography and some dictionaries of scientists)

BINET, L., 1954: Médecins, biologistes et chirurgiens, 285 p. (Paris: S.E.G.E.P.).—

A series of rather popular biographies (with supplementary bibliographical information) of some biologists and physiologists, including: Leonardo da Vinci, Descartes, Lavoisier, Laënnec, Orfila, A. Boyer, E. Woillez, C. Bernard, Brown-Séquard, L. Pasteur, C. Richet, A. d'Arsonval, C. Vincent, H. Roger, Quénie, Duval, Gosset, M. Arthus, J. A. Sicard, G. Roussy, L. Portes.

DEBUS, A. G., ed., 1968: World Who's Who in science: a biographical dictionary of notable scientists from antiquity to the present, 1855 p. (Marquis Biographical Library) (Chicago, Ill.: Marquis Who's Who).—

This book lists "notable scientists from antiquity to the present", including

distinguished alchemists, astrologers, and mystics. It includes some 30,000 entries.

The DICTIONARY of NATIONAL BIOGRAPHY, 1885-1900. With many supplements. (Oxford: U.P.).—

This biographical dictionary contains biographies of people born in Great Britain, Ireland, the British Commonwealth and colonies, and of Englishmen born abroad. It was begun in 1885 and later on was reprinted in 22 vols. Various supplements cover the period 1900-1950. The last volume appeared in 1959 and deals with the period 1941-1950, and contains an index covering the years 1901-1950 in one alphabetical series. Of each of the persons included rather extensive biographical and bibliographical information has been given. In 1966 appeared a list of "Corrections and additions to the Dictionary of National Biography", cumulated from the Bulletin of the Institute of Historical Research, Univ. of London, covering the years 1923-1963, 212 p. (Boston, Mass.: Hall). There also appeared a one-volume edition: The dictionary of national biography. The concise dictionary, from the beginning to 1930. Being an epitome of the main work and its supplement, to which is added an epitome of the twentieth century volumes, covering 1901-1930, 1456 p. (Earliest times to 1900) + 183 p. (Epitome of the 20th-century) (London: Oxford U.P.).

DICTIONNAIRE de BIOGRAPHIE FRANÇAISE, 1935 → (Paris: Letouzey & Ané).—

Of this biography vol. 12 (Dugueyt - Espigat-sieurac) appeared in 1970.

FIGUIER, L., 1868-1883: Vies des savants illustres depuis l'antiquité jusqu'au dix-neuvième siècle avec l'appréciation sommaire de leurs travaux. Vol. I (1872): Savants de l'antiquité, ed. 2, 468 p.; Vol. II (1883): Savants du Moyen Age, ed. 3, 503 p.; Vol. III (1868): Savants de la Renaissance, ed. 1, 474 p.; Vol. IV (1876): Savants du XVIIe siècle, ed. 2, 528 p.; Vol. V (1874): Savants du XVIIIe siècle, ed. 2, 496 p. (Paris: Hachette).—

Vol. I discusses *inter alia:* Thales, Pythagoras, Plato, Aristotle, Hippocrates, Theophrastos, Pliny, Dioscorides, Galen; Vol. II: Avicenna, Averroës, Roger Bacon, St. Thomas Aquinas, Arnald of Villanova; Vol. III: Paracelsus, Agricola, Gessner, Cardan, Vesalius, A. Paré, Van Helmont,

Palissy; Vol. IV: F. Bacon, Descartes, Boyle, Harvey, Huygens; Vol. V: Leibniz, Boerhaave, Linnaeus, Fontenelle, Maupertuis, d'Alembert, von Haller, de Buffon, de Jussieu, and Spallanzani.

FREUND, H. & A. BERG, eds., 1963-1964: Geschichte der Mikroskopie. Leben und Werk grosser Forscher, 2 vols. Vol. I: Biologie, 376 p.; Vol. II: Medizin, 506 p. (Frankfurt a.M.: Umschau).—

   A collection of short biographies of scientists who have used the microscope as a tool and of those men who made any contribution to microscopy as such. Of each of them a photograph or portrait has been included. Many references concerning the persons mentioned.

HOWARD, A. V., ed., 1951: Chambers's dictionary of scientists, 499 p. (Edinburgh: Chambers).—

   This work contains biographies of ca. 1,300 individual scientists, mainly of the 19th and 20th centuries. The entries contain information about nationality, place of birth and death, education, research, etc. Reprinted, 1956.

HYAMSON, A. M., ed., 1951: A dictionary of universal biography of all ages and of all peoples, ed. 2, 680 p. (London: Routledge & Kegan Paul).—

   This book "is a guide to the biographies of ... every man or woman, not still alive, who has achieved eminence, or prominence, from the dawn of history until this day ..." Entries, usually single-line, include name, nationality, country of adoption, profession, dates (where known) and references to work(s) from which fuller biographical information can be obtained.

JOHNSON, A. & D. MALONE, eds., 1946: Dictionary of American biography, 20 vols. +Suppl. I (1946) and II (1958). (Centenary edition) (New York, N.Y.: Scribner).—

   The dictionary is published under the auspices of the American Council of Learned Societies, with the cooperation of an Advisory Committee. The first 20 vols. contain 13,633 biographical articles, by 2,243 contributors, on "persons who have made significant contributions to American life". Suppl. I contains 652 articles on persons who died within the period 1928-1935, and Suppl. II contains 585 biographies of persons who died during the period 1935-1940. Each biographical article gives a summary review of the life of the person considered, and contains a critical appraisal of his accomplishments. A bibliography has been added to each of these descriptions, containing sources of information concerning the subject considered. The American Naturalist 72 (1938), p. 534-546, contains a handlist of American naturalists, based on this dictionary, compiled by P. H. OEHSER.

LINDROTH, S., 1952: Swedish men of science 1650-1950, 295 p. (Stockholm: Almqvist & Wiksell).—

   This book contains a group of brief biographies of some 29 scientists, including such men as: O. Rudbeck (1630-1702); U. Hiärne (1641-1724); E. Swedenborg (1688-1772); A. Celsius (1701-1744); C. von Linné (1707-1787); C. de Geer (1720-1778); C. W. Scheele (1742-1786); C. P. Thunberg (1743-1828); E. Fries (1794-1878); S. Hedin (1865-1952); H. Nilsson-Ehle (1873-1949); The Svedberg (1884- —).

MURCHISON, C. A., ed., 1929-1932: Psychological register, 2 vols. Vol. II: 580 p.; Vol. III: 1269 p. (Worcester, Mass.: Clark U.P.; London: Oxford U.P.).—

   Contains brief biographies with very full bibliographies of psychologists throughout the world, arranged by country; vol. 2. includes 1,250 psychologists from 29 countries, and vol. 3, a revision and expansion of the 1929 vol., includes 2,400 psychologists from 40 countries. Vol. 1 never appeared; it was announced to include psychologists deceased before the initiation of this series and to extend back to the time of the early Greek psychologists.

NEUE DEUTSCHE BIOGRAPHIE, 1953 →: (Berlin: Duncker & Humblot).—
   A biographical dictionary, published by the historical commission of the Bavarian Academy of Science. In 1966 vol. 7 appeared (Grassauer-Hartmann). This work succeeds the "Allgemeine deutsche Biographie" (55 vols., Leipzig, 1871-1910), and is completely rewritten. Cf. also: Deutsche Forscher aus sechs Jahrhunderten. Lebensbilder von Aerzten, Naturwissenschaftlern und Technikern, 1965, 440 p. (Leipzig: Bibliographisches Institut).

NOBEL FOUNDATION, 1964-1967: Nobel lectures. Physiology or medicine, including presentation speeches and laureates' biographies, 3 vols. Vol. I (1967): 1901-1921, 564 p.; Vol. II (1965): 1922-1941, 548 p.; Vol. III (1964): 1942-1962, 839 p. (Amsterdam, London & New York, N.Y.: Elsevier).—

The Nobel Foundation has arranged for the Nobel lectures to be published in the English language, arranged in chronological order and according to the various prizefields. They represent an effort to present a semi-popular but very accurate review of the events leading up to whatever accomplishment was rewarded by the prize. The present vols. contain the lectures in physiology and medicine for 1901-1962. The lectures are preceded by the presentation addresses to the prize-winners and followed by a biography. The first vol. contains biographies of, *inter alia,* von Behring, Carrell, Ehrlich, Golgi, Koch, Krogh, Metchnikoff, Pavlov, Ramón y Cajal, and Ross. The second vol. contains biographies of, *inter alia,* E. D. Adrian, Banting, Dale, Domagk, Eykman, Einthoven, A. V. Hill, Landsteiner, Meyerhof, T. H. Morgan, Sherrington, Spemann, Szent-Györgyi, O. H. Warburg, and G. H. Whipple. The third vol. contains biographies of, *inter alia,* G. W. Beadle, G. von Békésy, F. M. Burnet, Crick, A. Fleming, Florey, H. A. Krebs, J. Lederberg, P. B. Medawar, H. J. Muller, S. Ochoa, E. L. Tatum, H. Theorell, S. A. Waksman, and J. D. Watson. *Cf.* also STEVENSON, L. G., ed., 1953, *vide infra.*

SCHWERTE, H. & W. SPENGLER, eds., 1955: Forscher und Wissenschaftler im heutigen Europa, Vol. 2. Erforscher des Lebens. Mediziner, Biologen, Anthropologen, 339 p. (Oldenburg: Stalling).—

A series of biographies of 31 20th-century scientists, written by some 25 authors. There are three sections, *viz.,* a. Medicine (considering A. Carrel, Sauerbruch, L. Aschoff, V. von Weizsäcker, Pavlov, Ramón y Cajal, O. Foerster, W. R. Hess, E. Bleuler, J. H. Schultz, O. H. Warburg, Szent-Györgyi, G. Domagk, A. Fleming); b. Biology (Boveri, Correns, Michurin, Nilsson-Ehle, Driesch, Spemann, M. Hartmann, O. Meyerhof, Frey-Wyssling, von Frisch); c. Anthropology (Boule, Fischer, Schwalbe, Klaatsch, Mollison, von Eickstedt, Biasutti). There are 27 portraits.

STEVENSON, L. G., ed., 1953: Nobel prize winners in medicine and physiology, 1901-1950, 291 p. (New York, N.Y.: Schuman).—

The book deals with 59 Nobel Prize winners between 1901 and 1950. Of each of them a biographical sketch has been given together with a description of the prize-winning work and a selection from the writings in which that work was presented. Most data concerning the description of the work have been derived from the Nobel Address delivered at the Presentation Ceremony; those not delivered in English have been translated by the editor. A new ed. seems to have appeared in 1968: STEVENSON, L. G., 1968: Nobel prize winners in medicine and physiology, 1901-1965, 464 p. (New York, N.Y. & London: Abelard-Schuman). *Cf.* also NOBEL FOUNDATION, *vide supra.*

TURKEVICH, J. & L. B., 1968: Prominent scientists of continental Europe, 204 p. (New York, N.Y.: Elsevier).—

A collection of 3,154 short biographies of some of the leading European scientists. The selection has been limited to members of national academies and to professors at leading universities. This biographical collection is especially valuable for its information concerning East European scientists (it contains, *e.g.,* 149 scientists of Czechoslovakia, 68 of Hungary, 160 of Poland, 170 of Rumania, 486 of the Sovjet Union, and 107 of Yugoslavia). The closing date for information was July 1, 1966. The arrangement is geographical.

UNGHERINI, A., 1967: Manuel de bibliographie biographique et d'iconographie des femmes célèbres, 2 vols., 896 cols. Suppl. I (1968): 638 cols.; Suppl. II (1968): 760 cols. (Naarden, The Neth.: Bekhoven).—

Reprint of the 1892-1905 edition. The contents of this book may become clear from its subtitle: "Contenant: un dictionnaire des femmes qui se sont fait remarquer à un titre quelconque dans tous les siècles et dans tous les pays: les dates de leur naissance et de leur mort; la liste de toutes les monographies biographiques relatives à chaque femme, avec la mention des traductions; l'indication des portraits joints aux ouvrages cités et de ceux gravés séparément, avec les noms des graveurs; les prix auxquels les livres, les portraits et les autographes ont été portés dans les ventes ou dans les catalogues; suivi d'un répertoire de biographies générales, nationales et locales et d'ouvrages concernant les portraits et les autographes." *Cf.* LIPINSKA, M., 1930: Les femmes et le progrès des sciences médicales, *vide* section History of the medical sciences, sub-section a.

WEBSTER'S BIOGRAPHICAL DICTIO-

NARY: a dictionary of names of noteworthy persons, with pronunciations and concise biographies, 1953, 1697 p. (Springfield, Mass.: Merriam).—

> In this volume American and British names have been included on a more generous scale than those of non-English speaking people. Included are about 40,000 persons. New edition, 1967, 1736 p.

WILLIAMS, T. I., ed., 1968: A biographical dictionary of scientists, 592 p. (With assistance of S. WITHERS) (London: Black).—

> Authoritative accounts of the lives of over 1,000 eminent scientists and technologists from early times to the present; each written by a specialist, with additional bibliographical, iconographical and other reference information.

WILLIAMSON, G. C., ed., 1921-1925: Bryan's dictionary of printers and engravers, new ed., 5 vols., each *ca.* 400 pages. (London: Bell).—

> First published 1816, revised 1849. The names are alphabetically arranged. Vol. I: A-C; Vol. II: D-G; Vol. III: H-M; Vol. IV: N-R; Vol. V: S-Z.

ZISCHKA, G. A., ed., 1961: Allgemeines Gelehrten-Lexikon. Biographisches Handwörterbuch zur Geschichte der Wissenschaften, 710 p. (Stuttgart: Kröner).—

> A selective list of 7,000 biographies of scientists of all times. Much bibliographical information (*ca.* 50,000 items).

b. *Biology* (incl. veterinary science).

ADAMS, A. B., 1969: Eternal quest: the story of the great naturalists, 512 p. (New York, N.Y.: Putnam).—

> This book consists of a series of biographies of the major contributors to systematic biology, *viz.*, Linnaeus, Buffon, Lamarck, Cuvier, A. von Humboldt, C. Darwin, Wallace, A. Wilson, Audubon, Lyell, Agassiz, and Mendel. Each of the subjects considered has been placed within the framework of his time; his character, education, intentions, successes, *etc.*, have been elucidated.

BARNHART, J. H., ed., 1965: Biographical notes upon botanists, 3 vols. (44,700 cards).

Compiled by John Hendley BARNHART, bibliographer, 1903-1941 and maintained in the New York Botanical Garden Library. (Boston, Mass.: Hall).—

> This biographical file contains information about 44,700 botanists from early times to the present. The entry for each name includes the botanist's dates, education, and professional activities; sources of information are also indicated.

BRITTEN, J., G. S. BOULGER, & A. B. RENDLE, eds., 1931: A biographical index of deceased British and Irish botanists, ed. 2, 342 p. (London: Taylor & Francis).—

> Over 2,000 concise standardized biographical sketches which include an enormous amount of information (*e.g.,* concerning main publications, biographical articles, location of mss., herbaria, *etc.*). A revised edition is being prepared by R. DESMOND. This new ed. will be increased in scope to include horticulturists, plant collectors and naturalists with interests on the margins of formal botany. Pp. vii-xii: list of sources. For more detailed data about principal botanists *vide* The DICTIONARY of NATIONAL BIOGRAPHY, *supra*, subsection a. *Cf.* also PRAEGER, R. L., 1941: Some Irish naturalists, *vide infra.*

CARPENTER, M. M., ed., 1945: Bibliography of biographies of entomologists, 116 p. (Amer. Midl. Nat. 33: 1-116).—

> This publication can be considered as a second edition of WADE's "Bibliography of entomologists" (Ann. Ent. Soc. Amer. 21: 489-520, 1928); it covers the literature up to 1943. The references include not only obituaries, but also birthdays, portraits, anniversaries, biographies, and disposition of collections. As regards the last-named item, information concerning the disposal and location of collections up to 1937 can be found in a series of papers by HORN, W. & J. KAHLE, 1935-1937: Ueber entomologische Sammlungen, Entomologen und Entomo-museologie. Ein Beitrag zur Geschichte der Entomologie, 388 p. (Unter Mitarbeit von R. KORSCHEFSKY) (Entomologische Beihefte aus Berlin-Dahlem II (1935): 1-160; III (1936): 161-296; IV (1937): 297-388), *vide* section History of the animal sciences, subsection entomology.

CATTELL, J., ed., 1965-1967: American men of science in the physical and biological sciences: a biographical directory, ed. 11, 6 vols. (New York, N.Y.: Bowker).—

The authoritative biographical directory of American scientists, containing biographies of more than 150,000 living American and Canadian scientists actively engaged in the physical or biological sciences. The details given for each include the name, position, address, field, birthplace, degrees, positions held, memberships and research specialities. The first vol. (A-E) appeared in 1965, the others in sequence at six-month intervals.

EYCLESHYMER, A. C. & D. M. SCHOEMAKER, 1917: Anatomical names ... with biographical sketches, 744 p. (New York, N.Y.: Wood).—

For more details, *vide* section Some recommended encyclopaedias, *etc.*, subsection b.

GEBHARDT, L., ed., 1964: Die Ornithologen Mittel-Europas, 404 p. (Giessen: Brühlscher).—

A very useful biographical dictionary because many of the 1,250 names included had interests beyond ornithology. Of the persons included references have been given to published biographies or obituaries. Included are such men who studied birds in museums, or on expeditions, field ornithologists, students of birds in zoos, *etc.* Living ornithologists are not included.

INDEX des ZOOLOGISTES, 1953, 431 p. +Suppl., 1959, 429 p. (Paris: Secrétariat de l'Union int. des Sciences Biologiques).—

A directory of zoologists, arranged alphabetically. Date of birth and specializations are given. International coverage.

MIALL, L. C., 1912: The early naturalists: their lives and work (1530-1789), 396 p. (London: Macmillan).—

Much biographical information on, *e.g.*, O. Brunfels, H. Bock, L. Fuchs, V. Cordus, C. Gesner, l'Obel, Cesalpino, P. Belon, Rondelet, Turner, J. Gerard, J. Caius, C. Butler, O. de Serres, J. Ray, F. Willughby, R. Hooke, Malpighi, N. Grew, J. Swammerdam, A. van Leeuwenhoek, F. Redi, C. Perrault, Réaumur, Trembley, Bonnet, Lyonet, Roesel von Rosenhof, Linnaeus, B. and A. L. de Jussieu, and de Buffon.

The NATURALISTS' DIRECTORY, 1961, ed. 39, 176 p. (Phillipsburg, N.J.: Anthony).—

This is an bi-annual publication which lists the names, addresses, and biological interests particularly of amateur and professional plant and animal taxonomists in the Western Hemisphere. The arrangement of the names is alphabetical by states or countries. The name of the groups of plants or animals collected, identified, exchanged or sold, is printed in bold-faced type. Included are lists of scientific societies and periodicals with headquarters, addresses and the subscription rate and a list of natural history museums. (From SMITH, R. C., *vide* section Some recommended encyclopaedias, *etc.*, subsection d).

PRAEGER, R. L., 1941: Some Irish naturalists: a biographical notebook, 208 p. (Dundalk: Tempest).—

Contains brief biographical descriptions of about 300 zoologists, botanists, and geologists from the 12th to the 20th century. It also contains a section dealing with societies and institutions.

RATZEBURG, J. T. C., ed., 1872: Forstwissenschaftliches Schriftsteller-Lexikon, 516 p. (Berlin: Nicolai).—

Unfortunately I am not able to give any details about this book.

SCHRADER, G. W. & E. HERING, eds., 1863: Biographisch-literarisches Lexicon der Thierärzte aller Zeiten und Länder, sowie der Naturforscher, Aerzte, Landwirthe, Stallmeister u.s.w., welche sich um die Thierheilkunde verdient gemacht haben, 490 p. (Stuttgart: Ebner & Seubert).—

A biographical dictionary, indispensable for any study of the history of veterinary medicine. It is alphabetically arranged, according to the names of the persons included. It also contains much biographical information. Included are the names of those anatomists, zoologists, botanists, agriculturists, *etc.*, who made any contribution to the field of veterinary medicine. Reprinted 1967 (Leipzig: Zentralantiquariat der DDR).

STEENIS-KRUSEMAN, M. J. v., 1950: Malaysian plant collectors and collections: being a cyclopedia of botanical exploration in Malaysia and a guide to the concerned literature up to the year 1950, 152+639 p. (Flora Malesiana, Vol. I)+supplement, 1957, 108 p. (Groningen/Djakarta: Noordhoff-Kolff).—

For more details, *vide* section Some recommended encyclopaedias, *etc.*, subsection C1.

c. *Medical sciences* (incl. therapy, pharmacy, *etc.*; excl. biographical dictionaries of a regional importance; for these works, *vide* section History of medicine, subsection Regional histories)

ALEXANDER, F., S. EISENSTEIN & M. GROTJAHN, eds., 1966: Psychoanalytic pioneers, 616 p. (New York, N.Y.: Basic Bks.).—

A collection of 41 biographies of individuals who "having recognized the truth and importance of Freud's teachings, devoted [their lives] to the advance and spread of our knowledge through research and teaching". Each of these essays provides an outline of the subject's life, a brief description of his contributions to psychoanalysis and a brief bibliography of his works.

ANNAN, G. L., ed., 1960: Catalog of biographies in the library of the New York Academy of Medicine, 165 p. (Boston, Mass.: Hall).—

This book contains photographic reproductions of the 3,450 cards representing the shelf list of that section in the library of the New York Academy of Medicine which contains single biographies of physicians and scientists, with a few autobiographies, family histories and occasional biographies written by physicians. The entries, arranged under the names of the subjects, are chiefly for books. Volumes of collected biographies are not included. Excluded are also biographies of less than 100 pages, unless bound in hard covers.

——— ed., 1960-1965: Portrait catalog of the library of the New York Academy of Medicine, 5 vols., 4564 p.; First suppl., 1959-1965 (1965), 842 p. (Boston, Mass.: Hall).—

A photographic reproduction of index cards representing 10,784 separate portraits (paintings, woodcuts, engravings, photographs), on hand in the Academy, and 151,792 entries of portraits which appeared in books and journals. Special signs indicate whether the portrait is accompanied by biographical information. The supplement contains 1,073 separate portraits in possession of the Academy, and 35,976 entries of portraits from books and journals. *Cf.* LEFANU, W., 1960, *vide infra*.

BAILEY, H. & W. J. BISHOP, eds., 1959: Notable names in medicine and surgery, ed. 3, 216 p. (London: Lewis).—

For more details, *cf.* section Some recommended reference works, subsection e.

BAUDOUIN, M., 1906: Femmes médecins d'autrefois. Étude de psychologie sociale internationale, 263 p. (Paris: Rousset).—

Short biographies of some 200 women who were active in the field of medicine as healer or as nurse, obstetrician, *etc.* Separate sections deal with women physicians in Portugal, Spain, Byzantium, Syria, and with military women physicians. *Cf.* SCHÖNFELD, W., 1947: Frauen in der abendländischen Heilkunde; and LIPINSKA, M., 1930: Les femmes et le progrès des sciences médicales, *vide* section History of the medical sciences, subsection a.

BAYLE, A. L. J. & A. J. THILLAYE, eds., 1967: Biographie médicale par ordre chronologique, 2 vols. Vol. I: 560 p.; Vol. II: 950 p. (Amsterdam: Israel).—

A chronologically arranged biographical dictionary of physicians. *Ca.* 2,000 names are included. Originally published in 1855 (Paris).

BRAUCHLE, A., 1944: Grosse Naturaerzte, 368 p. (Leipzig: Reclam).—

A summary of the author's "Die Geschichte der Naturheilkunde in Lebensbildern" *(vide* section History of Therapy, subsection a1).

CALLISEN, A. C. P., ed., 1962-1965: Medicinisches Schriftsteller-Lexikon der jetzt lebenden Aerzte, Wundärzte, Geburtshelfer, Apotheker, und Naturforscher aller gebildeten Völker, ed. 2, 33 vols. (Nieuwkoop: de Graaf).—

Unchanged photomechanical reprint of the 1830-1845 ed. (Copenhagen). An author-catalogue of 99,001 numbered items. Vols. 1-21 A → Z.; Vol. 22 anonymous and miscellaneous works; Vols. 23-25 periodicals; Vols. 26-33 A → Z. Covers for the greater part 19th-century references, and some from the 18th century. According to Garrison: "Of well-nigh infallible accuracy as to names, dates, numerical data and cross-references; ... (contains) collateral biographic and historic data. Vols. 23-25 contain a definitive catalogue not only of the medical periodicals of 1780-1833, but also of secular and scientific journals of the period containing matter of medical interest." *(Cf.* HIRSCH, A., ed., 1962, *infra).*

DUMESNIL, R. & F. BONNET-ROY, eds., 1947: Les médecins célèbres, 371 p. (Geneva: Mazenod).—

A collection of 92 medical biographies contributed by 72 different authors, covering the period from Hippocrates up to Sauerbruch. The purpose of this book is popular rather than scholarly. Many illustrations of portraits, title-pages, letters, anatomical drawings, medical instruments, *etc.,* some of which are very beautiful reproductions. Also in German translation: DUMESNIL, R. & H. SCHADEWALD, eds., 1967: Die berühmten Aerzte, ed. 2, 420 p., 179 illus. (Köln: Aulis). Some other books containing many portraits of physicians are: JONAS, S., 1960: Cent portraits de médecins illustres, 350 p. (Paris: Masson); and STRIKER, C., ed., 1963: Medical portraits, 279 p. (Cincinnati, Ohio: Acad. of Medicine of Cincinnati).

FERCHL-MITTENWALD, F., ed., 1937: Chemisch-pharmazeutisches Bio- und Bibliographicon, 603 p. (Hrsg. im Auftrage der Gesellschaft für Geschichte der Pharmazie) (Mittenwald: Nemayer).—

This book consists of short biographies of chemists and pharmacists who lived between *ca.* 1500 and *ca.* 1850. Their most important achievements and publications have been given, together with existing biographical literature.

GIBSON, W. C., 1958: Young endeavour: contributions to science by medical students of the past four centuries, 292 p. (Springfield, Ill.: Thomas; Oxford: Blackwell).—

This book is a collection of 66 examples of outstanding medical practitioners who, during their study, were able to carry out notable research and even to conduct fundamental discoveries. The persons considered are grouped according to subject: a biographical sketch is included. A somewhat comparable book is DIEPGEN, P., 1960: Unvollendete. Vom Leben und Wirken frühverstorbener Forscher und Aerzte aus anderthalb Jahrhunderten, 223 p. (Stuttgart: Thieme). This book contains a series of biographies of medical men and other scientists who died young, but who, during their short life, made valuable contributions to medicine and science.

GROSS, S. D., 1967: Lives of eminent physicians and surgeons of the nineteenth century, 838 p. (New York, N.Y.: Da Capo).—

A reprint of the 1861 edition (Philadelphia, Pa.: Lindsay & Blakiston). Still a useful book, although limited by its restriction to 32 individuals who achieved considerable fame in American medicine.

HAYMAKER, W., ed., 1953: The founders of neurology, 479 p. (Springfield, Ill.: Thomas).—

Biographical sketches of 133 neurologists: each biographical sketch is provided with a portrait.

HIRSCH, A., ed., 1962: Biographisches Lexikon der hervorragenden Aerzte aller Zeiten und Völkern, ed. 3, 5 vols. + supplement. Vol. I: 40 + 898 p.; Vol. II: 926 p.; Vol. III: 873 p.; Vol. IV: 964 p.; Vol. V: 1058 p.; Suppl.: 426 p. This work is continued as: FISCHER, I., ed., 1962: Biographisches Lexikon der hervorragenden Aerzte der letzten fünfzig Jahre, ed. 2 and 3, 2 vols., 1741 p. (Berlin: Urban & Schwarzenberg).—

The first edition of Hirsch's work appeared in 1884-1888; a second ed. in 1929-1935. The first edition of Fischer's work appeared in 1932-1933. Together these volumes are the standard work of medical biography. The volume edited by Fischer replaces J. PAGEL's Biographisches Lexikon hervorragender Aerzte des 19. Jahrhunderts. Mit einer historischen Einleitung, 1901, 1983 p. (Berlin: Urban & Schwarzenberg).

KAGAN, S. R., 1941: Leaders of medicine: biographical sketches of outstanding American and European physicians, 176 p. (Boston, Mass.: Medico-Historical Press).—

Contains biographical sketches of: Jacob Henle (1809-1885), Rudolf Virchow (1821-1902), Silas Weir Mitchell (1829-1914), Abraham Jacobi (1830-1919), Thomas Clifford Allbutt (1836-1925), Jacob da Silva Solis-Cohen (1838-1927), John Shaw Billings (1838-1913), Julius Cohnheim (1838-1884), Carl Weigert (1849-1904), William Osler (1849-1919), William Henry Welch (1850-1934), and Paul Ehrlich (1854-1915).

KELLY, E. C., ed., 1948: Encyclopedia of medical sources, 476 p. (Baltimore, Md.: Williams & Wilkins).—

For more details, *cf.* section Some recommended reference works, subsection e.

KOLLE, K., ed., 1956-1963: Grosse Nervenärzte, 3 vols. Vol. I (1956): 21 Lebensbilder, 284 p.; Vol. II (1959): 22 Lebensbilder, 251 p.; Vol. III (1963): 22 Lebensbilder, 228 p. (Stuttgart: Thieme).—

In its totality the work can be considered as a biographical history of neuropsychiatry from the end of the 18th century to the present. The first volume especially deals with the creators of neuro-psychiatry; the chapters are arranged alphabetically. Of vol. I a second ed. appeared in 1970 (309 p.); same publisher. In the second volume the biographies are grouped into sections, *viz.,* basic investigators, inventors, clinicians-psychiatrists, neurologists, therapist-surgeons, and psychotherapists. It also contains a chapter written by E. H. ACKERKNECHT on the history of psychiatric and neurological teaching and research institutions in France, Great Britain, Italy, Russia, Switzerland, Belgium, Holland, and the Scandinavian countries. Vol. III deals with anatomists, physiologists, neurologists, neuro-surgeons, psychiatrists, and psychologists. A more complete biographical reference work is: KIRCHHOFF, T., 1921: Deutsche Irrenärzte. Einzelbilder ihres Lebens und Wirkens, 274 p. (Berlin: Springer).

LEFANU, W., ed., 1960: A catalogue of the portraits and other paintings, drawings and sculpture in the Royal College of Surgeons of England, 119 p. (Edinburgh: Livingstone).—

The book consists of two parts. The first part contains 359 items in all, 244 of which are portraits. The second part includes paintings of racial types, historical material, drawings of human skulls, animals and birds. The book is very important from the iconographical point of view; it gives useful details of the works of art included. There are 145 illustrations, 4 in color. Indexes to artists and subjects. (*Cf.* ANNAN, G. L., ed., 1960-1965, *vide supra*).

MONDOR, H., 1949: Anatomistes et chirurgiens, 531 p. (Paris: Fragrance).—

A series of biographies of Guy de Chauliac (p. 3-52); Ambroise Paré (p. 53-122); Andreas Vesalius (p. 123-164); Jean-Louis Petit (p. 165-218); J. Desault (p. 219-260); Guillaume Dupuytren (p. 261-322); François Malgaigne (p. 323-370); Paul

Lecène (p. 371-424); Charles Lenormant (p. 425-472); Clovis Vincent (p. 473-530). *Cf.* BINET, L., *vide supra,* subsection a.

MUNK, W., ed., 1878: The roll of the Royal College of Physicians of London; comprising biographical sketches, ed. 2, 3 vols. (London: Royal College of Physicians).—

These first three volumes cover the period from 1518 to 1825. A fourth volume appeared in 1955 under the editorship of G. H. BROWN. This volume of 637 p. contains short biographies of Fellows elected between 1826 and 1925 and who died before 1st January 1954. A still later vol. appeared in 1965 under the editorship of R. R. TRAIL: Royal College of Physicians, London. Lives of the Fellows, continued to 1965, 476 p. (Munk's Roll, vol. 5) (London: Royal College of Physicians).

PAZZINI, A., 1948: Bio-bibliografia di storia della chirurgia, 525 p. (Rome: Cosmopolita).—

This book consists of two parts. The first part deals with biographies of surgeons and contains the following sections: surgery of primitive peoples, Greek and Hellenistic surgeons, surgeons of the Middle Ages (Byzantine, Arabic, Italian, French, Flemish, English), surgeons of the Renaissance (Italian, French, Spanish, German, Swiss, Dutch, and English), and surgery in the 17th, 18th, and 19th centuries respectively (Italian, French, German, Swiss, Dutch, Belgian, English, Scandinavian, and American). The second part consists of the same sections and deals with the relevant surgical literature.

PLARR, V. G., ed., 1930: Plarr's lives of the Fellows of the Royal College of Surgeons of England, 2 vols. Vol. I: 752 p.; Vol. II: 596 p. (Thelwall Thomas memorial) (Rev. by Sir D'Arcy POWER) (Bristol: Wright).—

Contains biographies of Fellows who died before 1930. A continuation of this work is: POWER, D'Arcy & W. R. LEFANU, 1953: Lives of the Fellows of the Royal College of Surgeons of England: 1930-1951, 889 p. (London: Royal College of Surgeons). These volumes contain accurate descriptions of the lives of the Fellows; this information is derived from obituary notices, relatives and friends. References to publications, portraits, and other sources of additional information are included. Inasmuch as Fellows of this College come from, and go to, all parts of the world and whereas leading surgeons of many countries are elected Honorary Fellow of the Royal College of Surgeons, these volumes are of great value for medical biography.

THORNTON, J. L., A. J. MONK & E. S. BROOKS, eds., 1961: A select bibliography of medical biography, 112 p. (Library Assn. Bibliographies, No. 3) (London: Library Assn.).—

> There are two sections. The first deals with collective biographies and contains 57 entries. The second section contains over 700 individual biographies dealing with *ca.* 350 individual physicians. The selection is limited to works in English published in the 19th and 20th centuries. The arrangement is alphabetically, by author in the first sec-

tion, by subject of the biography in the second section.

ZEKERT, O., ed., 1955-1962: Berühmte Apotheker, 2 vols. Vol. I: 160 p.; Vol. II: 95 p. (Stuttgart: Deutscher Apotheker Verlag).—

> Short biographies of famous pharmacists almost restricted to the German-speaking countries. The first volume considers those pharmacists living in the 15th-18th centuries (67), the second volume those of the 19th and 20th centuries (55). Of each of the persons considered short biographical sketches have been given together with a portrait (when available).

4. SOME RECOMMENDED ENCYCLOPAEDIAS, CHRONOLOGIES, HISTORICAL ATLASES, DICTIONARIES, EXPLANATORY GLOSSARIES, TAXONOMIC INDEXES, AND OTHER AUXILIARY REFERENCE WORKS

a. *Some general works of reference* (guides to reference books, chronologies and encyclopaedias of science and history, explanatory glossaries of scientific terms, philosophical, psychological, and geographical dictionaries, guides to literature on travel, *etc.*)

BALDWIN, J. M., 1940-1949: Dictionary of philosophy and psychology, 3 vols. Vol. I: 644 p.; Vol. II: 892 p. (New York, N.Y.: Smith).—

> Originally published 1901-1905 (New York, N.Y.: Macmillan), a new ed. with corrections appeared in 1925, of which edition this is a reprint. Its coverage may become clear from its full title: Dictionary of philosophy and psychology, including many of the principal conceptions of ethics, logic, aesthetics, philosophy of religion, mental pathology, anthropology, biology, neurology, physiology, economics, political and social philosophy, philology, physical science and education, and giving a terminology in English, French, German and Italian. Appended to vol. 2 are indexes of Greek, Latin, German, French and Italian terms. Vol. 3, edited by B. RAND, is entitled: Bibliography of philosophy, psychology, and cognate subjects. It is the most comprehensive bibliography of its kind; *vide* section Bibliographies, subsection a. Reprinted 1966. (Magnolia, Mass.: Smith). *Cf.* EISLER, R., ed., 1927-1930; and WARREN, H. C., 1935, *vide infra.*

BARTHOLOMEW, J. G., 1952: The citizen's atlas of the world, ed. 10. (Edinburgh: Bartholomew).—

> This atlas contains 200 pages of maps designed primarily to show settlement and boundaries, both national and international. The first 16 pages contain world maps showing climate, land use, population, air routes, and time zones. Index with *ca.* 95,000 names. An atlas of physical geography is: BARTHOLOMEW, J. G., 1954: The Columbus atlas; or, regional atlas of the world. (Edinburgh: Bartholomew). It contains 160 pages of maps, 137 pages of text, and a gazetteer of some 50,000 names.

BERTHIER, J. & C. LAUVERNIER, 1930: Tableaux d'histoire générale. Présentation synchronique des principaux événements contemporains à travers les siècles. Politiques, religions, philosophies, lettres, arts, sciences, découvertes, inventions, institutions, 7 p. +43 tables. (Paris: Société Mercasia).—

> This volume consists of 43 double-page folio tables presenting the events of history from the 6th century B.C. to 1900 A.D. There are *ca.* 2,300 entries, classified by subject in similar sequences in successive tables. Much biographical information.

BRITISH UNION-CATALOGUE of periodicals, *vide* STEWART, *infra.*

BROWN, R. W., 1956: Composition of scientific words: a manual of methods and a lexicon of materials for the practice of logotechnics, rev. ed., 882 p. (Washington, D.C.: R. W. Brown, U.S. Natl. Museum).—

> After a general discussion of the methods for creating words, especially of terms used in the sciences, the author gives a cross-reference lexicon, in which the English key-words receive their appropriate Latin, Greek and other synonyms. Many of the words considered are of bio-medical importance. First published 1927: Materials for word study. *Cf.* FLOOD, W. E., 1960, *vide infra.*

COLLOCOTT, T. C. & J. O. THORNE, eds., 1954: Chambers's world gazetteer and geographic dictionary, 792 p. (Edinburgh & London: Chambers).—

> Chambers' world gazetteer and geographic dictionary is essentially an alphabetically arranged list of places, describing these places with respect to location, importance, interest, and size. The normal layout of articles is: heading (in heavy type), pronunciation, location, description, population, historical notes. In a supplementary index are gathered cross-references in the form of variant names of alternative spellings. This work has been published in the U.S.A. as The Macmillan world gazetteer and geographical dictionary (New York, N.Y.: Macmillan). The emphasis is primarily on Great Britain. It contains about 12,000 entries. *Cf.* WEBSTER's Geographical dictionary, *vide infra.*

COX, E. G., ed., 1935-1949: A reference guide to the literature of travel, including voyages, geographical descriptions, adventures, shipwrecks, and expeditions, 3 vols. Vol. I (1935): 402 p.; Vol. II (1938): 591 p.; Vol. III (1949): 732 p. (Univ. Wash. Publ. in language and literature, vols. 9, 10, 12) (Seattle, Wash.: Univ. of Washington).—

> Source material is covered up to 1800; entries are arranged chronologically under area or subject. Vol. 1 deals with the Old World; vol. 2 with the New World and includes an index of personal names; vol. 3 deals with Great Britain and includes chapters on maps and charts, general reference books and bibliographies.

DARMSTAEDTER, L., 1908: Handbuch zur Geschichte der Naturwissenschaften und der Technik in chronologischer Darstellung,

ed. 2, 1262 p. (Berlin: Springer).—

> A chronological list of about 12,000 scientific discoveries and inventions arranged year by year, giving for each its date, name of discoverer or inventor and other brief data. Indexes of personal names and of subjects. Sarton wrote about this book: valuable; but to be used with caution.

DELORME, J., 1956: Chronologie des civilisations, 453 p. (Paris: Presses Univ. de France).—

> This book mainly consists of tables, containing an analytic chronology of world history from 3000 B.C. to 1945 A.D. Within the tables, different columns deal with different civilizations occurring synchronously in different parts of the world.

DESCHAMPS, P. C. E., ed., 1870: Dictionnaire de géographie ancienne et moderne à l'usage du libraire et de l'amateur des livres, 796 p. (Paris: Didot).—

> The contents of the book are explained in its sub-title: "Contenant: 1° Les noms anciens, grecs et latins, de la décadence latine et la renaissance, des principales divisions de l'Europe, provinces, villes, bourgs, abbayes, etc. avec leur signification actuelle en langues vulgaires; 2° Les recherches les plus étendues et les plus consciencieuses sur les origines de la typographie dans toutes les villes, bourgs, abbayes d'Europe, jusqu'au XIXe siècle exclusivement; 3° Un dictionnaire français-latin des noms de lieux, destiné à servir de table." Reprinted 1965 (Hildesheim: Olms). A comparable book is: GRAESSE, J. G. T., 1922: Orbis latinus oder Verzeichnis der wichtigsten lateinischen Orts- und Ländernamen, ed. 3, 348 p. (Berlin). Contains only the Latin names with German equivalents and brief identification.

DITLER, R., G. JOOS, *et al.*, 1931-1935: Handwörterbuch der Naturwissenschaften, ed. 2, 10 vols. + Sachregister, 1935, 242 p. (Jena: Fischer).—

> An authoritative work, covering all the natural sciences, botany, zoology, physiology, mineralogy, geology, physics, and chemistry. Contains much biographical and bibliographical information. No separate articles on small subjects, such as species of plants or animals. No definitions or derivations of terms.

DUDEN-Wörterbuch geographischer Namen, 1966: Europa (ohne Sowjetunion), 40

+740 p. (Mannheim: Bibliographisches Institut).—

A geographical dictionary, comprising names of towns, mountains, hills, lakes, rivers, counties, *etc.*, in Eastern Europe, excluding the Soviet Union. A useful tool, because of the many changes which have occurred in that part of the world during the last 50 years.

EISLER, R., 1927-1930: Wörterbuch der philosophischen Begriffe, ed. 4, 3 vols. Vol. I: 893 p.; Vol. II: 780 p.; Vol. III: 906 p. (Berlin: Mittler).—

Contains very full definitions of philosophical terms, with detailed documentation of their use by philosophers. Many bibliographical references (bibliography vol. 3, p. 695-906). A condensation and popularization of this "Wörterbuch" is EISLER's Handwörterbuch der Philosophie, ed. 2, 785 p. (Berlin: Mittler). A (German) one-volume philosophical dictionary is: SCHMIDT, H., 1951: Philosophisches Wörterbuch, ed. 12, 658 p. (Stuttgart: Kröner). Includes many biographies. For an English dictionary of philosophy, *vide* BALDWIN, *supra*.

ELLIS, J. C., ed., 1949: Nature and its applications: over 200,000 selected references to nature forms and illustrations of nature, as used in every way, 861 p. (Boston, Mass.: Foxon).—

The purpose of the book is "to lead its enquirer to a picture of some nature object, in some particular form or design, for the purpose of a lesson, lecture, or artistic work." It indexes some 130 books (including some encyclopaedias) and journals.

ELSEVIER Wereldatlas, 1959. (Amsterdam: Elsevier).—

An unpretentious school atlas which will answer the average questions.

FLOOD, W. E., 1960: Scientific words: their structure and meaning, 220 p. (London: Oldbourne).—

An explanatory glossary listing about 1,150 word-elements (roots, prefixes, suffixes) which enter into the formation of scientific terms. Very common elements, *e.g.*, un-, -ation-, -able, are not included. The meaning of each element is given and its origin is explained. *Cf.* BROWN, R. W., 1956, *vide supra*.

GOODALL, G., 1947: Philip's historical atlas, ancient, medieval and modern, ed. 7, 68 pl.+32 p. (London: Philip).—

Coverage is 1500 B.C. to date. It is a revised and enlarged edition of an atlas issued in 1927, and consists of a combination of Philip's "Historical atlas, medieval and modern" (ed. 6, 1927) and Philip's "Atlas of ancient and classical history" (1938).

GREGORY, W., ed., 1943: Union list of serials in the libraries of the United States and Canada, ed. 2, 3065 p. (New York, N.Y.: Wilson).—

With supplements covering the years 1941-1953. A new edition is in preparation. It contains a list of the 225 libraries which cooperated in this compilation and a list of some 75,000 serial publications in the U.S.A. in the possession of these libraries, and lists of those volumes which each of them has. An excellent source of information about the correct name, place of publication, cumulative indexes, *etc. Cf.* also: STEWART, J. D., ed., 1955-1958, *vide infra*.

HARRIMAN, P. L., ed., 1946: The encyclopaedia of psychology, 897 p. (New York, N.Y.: The Philosophical Library).—

A most ably edited and valuable reference work. One of the most useful volumes published during this century in the field of psychology. (From Isis 39: 125). *Cf.* also: PIÉRON, H., 1968, and WARREN, H. C., 1935, *vide infra*.

LANA, G., L. IASBEZ & L. MEAK, eds., 1968: Glossary of geographical names: in six languages, English, French, Italian, Spanish, German, and Dutch, 184 p. (Amsterdam & New York, N.Y.: Elsevier).—

A multilingual glossary of nearly 6,000 geographical names in English, French, Italian, Spanish, Dutch, and German. The names are cross-indexed in such a way that one can quickly find the names of places, using any of the given languages as a basis. Besides place names, such items as countries, counties, regions, waterways and rivers, are also included.

LANGER, W. L., 1940: An encyclopaedia of world history: a revised and modernized version of Ploetz's "Epitome", 28+1155+66 p. (Boston, Mass.: Houghton Mifflin; London: Harrap).—

A chronologically-arranged encyclopaedia of world history, ancient, mediaeval, and modern, with emphasis on the 18th and 19th centuries. M. F. Ashley Montague writes in Isis 33, p. 164 about this book: "The factual data, the maps, the tables and index (which contains about 15,000 entries) comprise so useful an integrated unit that the word 'indispensable' automatically comes to mind." A fourth ed. appeared in 1968, 1504 p.; this ed. has been completely revised. Main additions to the sections prehistory and recent history up to 1964.

LITTLE, C. E., ed., 1900: Cyclopedia of classified dates, with exhaustive index, 1454 p. (New York, N.Y.: Funk & Wagnalls).—

Primary arrangement is alphabetically by countries, then by period, then by subject (*e.g.,* art, science, nature, deaths, society, *etc.),* each subject being finally arranged by date. Coverage is up to 31st December 1894. Index p. 1163-1454. A comparable work: KELLER, H. R., 1934: Dictionary of dates, 2 vols. (New York, N.Y.: Macmillan).

MALCLÈS, L. N., ed., 1950: Les sources du travail bibliographique, Vol. I. (*vide* section Bibliographies, subsection a).

MAYERHÖFER, J., *et al.,* 1959 →: Lexikon der Geschichte der Naturwissenschaften. Biographien, Sachwörter und Bibliographien, Pt. 1 (1959): Einführung; Aachen-Achard, 128 p.; Pt. 2 (1961): Achard-Aryabhata, p. 129-288; Pt. 3 (1962): Arzachel-Bewegung, p. 289-448; Pts. 4 and 5 (1965): Bewegung-Daniel von Morley, p. 449-704; Pt. 6 (1970): Daniel von Morley - Arnold Dodel, p. 705-847. (To be continued) (Vienna: Hollinek).—

An elaborate lexicon of personal names, subjects, and geographical terms, used in the field of the (natural) sciences. Contains much biographical and bibliographical information that is of interest to the historian of biology and medicine.

NELSON's dictionary of dates, n.d., 1253 p. (London & Edinburgh: Nelson).—
"The object of this dictionary of dates is to provide a clear, systematic, and accurate record of the most important events in the world's history-political, social, ecclesiastical, legal, scientific, geographical, educational, and commercial". A compa-

rable booklet of the same scope (and partly dealing with the same subjects) is: A dictionary of dates, n.d., 346 p. (London: Dent; New York: Dutton): *Cf.* also PASCOE, L. C., 1968, *vide infra.*

NEWMAN, J. R., ed., 1965: The international encyclopedia of science, 4 vols., 1379 p. (Edinburgh & London: Nelson).—

This work was first published in the U.S.A. as "The Harper Encyclopedia of Science" in 1963. A second edition appeared in 1967, 1379 p. (New York, N.Y.: Harper & Row). 450 scientists have contributed nearly 4,000 articles. It includes both pure and applied sciences. Many tables, valuable bibliographies, and a useful index.

PASCOE, L. C., ed., 1968: Encyclopaedia of dates and events, 776 p. (London: English Universities Press).—

In four parallel columns for each year outstanding events in political history, literature, the arts, economics, exploration and science have been recorded. *Cf.* PUTNAM, *infra;* and NELSON's dictionary of dates, *vide supra.*

PIÉRON, H., 1968: Vocabulaire de la psychologie, ed. 4, 575 p. (Paris: Presses Univ. de France).—

Special attention has been paid to the definition of the terms included. A number of English terms are included and there are some German and English equivalents mentioned. Appendixes deal with such subjects as: abbreviations, symbols, *etc.* A more recent French dictionary of psychology is: AMAR, A., ed., 1967: La psychologie moderne de A à Z, 544 p. (Paris: Denoël). *Cf.* also WARREN, H. C., 1935, *vide infra;* HARRIMAN, P. L., 1946, *vide supra;* and BALDWIN, J. M., ed., 1940-1949, *vide supra.*

PUTNAM, G. P. & G. H., 1936: Dictionary of events: a handbook of universal history, 565 p. (New York, N.Y.: Grosset & Dunlap).—

Its contents become clear from its subtitle: A series of chronological tables presenting, in parallel columns, a record of the noteworthy events of history from the earliest times to the present day, together with an index of subjects and genealogical tables. *Cf.* PASCOE, *supra.*

ROBERTS, A. D., ed., 1958: Introduction to reference books, ed. 3, 237 p. (London: Library Assn.).—

> The majority of the chapters of this book are devoted to descriptions of the various kinds of reference books that exist; this book does not deal in detail with the literature of special subject fields. Chapters deal with encyclopaedias, dictionaries, newspapers and other records of events, yearbooks, directories and other business publications, bibliographies, serials, indexing and abstracting services, current national bibliographies and bibliographies of books in print, bibliographies of older British books, directories of societies, institutions, *etc.*, bibliographies, government publications, biographical works of reference, atlases and maps, and the literature of special subjects.

SMITH, B. E., ed., 1905: The century cyclopedia of names, 1085 p. (London: The Times; New York, N.Y.: The Century Co.).—

> A pronouncing and etymological dictionary of names in geography, biography, mythology, history, ethnology, art, archaeology, fiction, *etc.* A very useful work for biographical details. The biographical entries are reasonably full; the work seems to be biographically quite comprehensive. It gives exact date (day, month, year) of birth and death for all entries wherever ascertainable. The work states that it was an outcome of the Century Dictionary.

STEIN, W., 1954: Kulturfahrplan. Die wichtigsten Daten der Kulturgeschichte von Anbeginn bis Heute, 1311 p. (Berlin-Grunewald: Herbig).—

> A chronological table of discoveries arranged year by year in 7 parallel columns, representing respectively politics; theatre; religion, philosophy, education; plastic arts, architecture, film; music; science and technics; economics, daily life.

STEWART, J. D., ed., 1955-1958: British union-catalogue of periodicals: a record of the periodicals of the world, from the seventeenth century to the present day, in British libraries, 4 vols.+suppl. (1962) (London: Butterworth).—

> The fullest list of periodicals, containing more than 140,000 titles, permanently filed in 441 libraries of the United King-

dom. *Cf.* also GREGORY, W., ed., 1943, *vide supra;* ULRICH's periodicals directory, *vide infra* and WORLD LIST of scientific periodicals, *vide infra.*

STIELER, A., 1930: Stieler's Hand-atlas, ed. 10, 336 p. + 108 plates. (Gotha: Perthes).—

> Contains 108 plates of maps on which 263 maps are printed. Extremely detailed name plates. Index of about 300,000 entries.

STOKVIS, A. M. H. J., 1888-1893: Manuel d'histoire, de généalogie et de chronologie de tous les états du globe, 3 vols. (Leiden: Brill).—

> According to Sarton (Isis 39: 237), "one of the most valuable tools used by historians everywhere... one of those indispensable books which everyone uses but seldom quotes."

ULRICH's periodicals directory: a classified guide to a selected list of current periodicals, foreign and domestic, ed. 12, 1967, 540 p. (New York, N.Y.: Bowker).—

> A classified guide to selected world periodicals, giving titles, supplements, date of origin, frequency, price, size, publisher, place of publication, how and where indexed, whether books are reviewed, *etc.* Indexes to subjects and titles. *Cf.* also: STEWART, J. D., ed., 1955-1958: British union-catalogue of periodicals, *vide supra;* GREGORY, N., ed., 1943, *vide supra:* and WORLD LIST of scientific periodicals, *vide infra.*

VAN NOSTRAND's Scientific Encyclopaedia, ed. 4, 1968, 2010 p. (Princeton, N.J. & London: Van Nostrand).—

> Included are about 15,000 articles, covering mathematics, engineering, medicine, and the physical and biological sciences. Alphabetical arrangement of subjects, with frequent cross-references.

WALDEN, P., 1952: Chronologische Uebersichtstabellen zur Geschichte der Chemie von den ältesten Zeiten bis zur Gegenwart, 118 p. (Berlin, Göttingen & Heidelberg: Springer).—

> A chronological list of discoveries, major publications, *etc.*, from 1600 onwards,

arranged year by year. Index of personal names.

WALFORD, A. J., ed., 1963: Guide to reference material, 543 p. (London: The Library Assn.).—

> This book "provides an annotated list of the leading reference books and bibliographies, with emphasis on current publications, and particularly on material published in Britain." It contains about 3,000 items, each being annotated; the annotations often contain references to other material. Separate sections deal with: generalities, philosophy, religion, social sciences, languages, science and technology, mathematics and natural sciences, applied sciences, the arts, literature, geography, biography, exploration and travel, and history.

WALTHER, E., 1949: Geschichte der Philosophie in Tabellen, 119 p. (Geschichte der Wissenschaften in Tabellen, vol. 1) (Kevelaer: Butzon & Bercker).—

> The subject matter has been divided into 5 parts, viz., 1. Greek philosophy; 2. Middle Ages; 3. Humanism and Renaissance; 4. Modern philosophy (Baroque, Enlightenment, French encyclopaedists, philosophy of the previous century in Germany, France, Great Britain); 5. Contemporary philosophy. Glossary and index of personal names.

WARREN, H. C., 1935: Dictionary of psychology, 372 p. (London: Allen & Unwin).—

> The scope of this book is to explain the meaning of technical terms which the reader will meet in psychological literature or which the psychologist may wish to use in his writings. Appendix (p. 303-339) with tables on: Colour vision tests; Fundamental types of complexes; Dextrality; Errors occurring in experimental investigation; Glands treated in psychological literature; Logical fallacies; Musical intervals; Phobias, common types; Prefixes and suffixes; Reflexes treated in human psychology; Retinal layers in the human eye; Sensory illusions; Spectral lines and range of colours; Statistical formulae; Symbols and technical abbreviations; Topographical reference terms; Topographical terms relating to the human body; Topography of the human central nervous system. Then follows a list of technical dictionaries and vocabularies, and glossaries of French and German terms. More recent psychological dictionaries are: DREVER, J., 1952: A dictionary of psychology, 316 p. (Harmondsworth, Middlesex: Penguin Bks.), a concise English psychological dictionary; DORSCH, F., 1963: Psychologisches Wörterbuch, ed. 7, 552 p. (Hamburg: Meiner; Bern: Huber); and the LAROUSSE dictionnaire de la psychologie, 1965, 319 p., edited by SILLAMY, N. *Cf.* also: HARRIMAN, P. L., 1946; PIÉRON, H., 1957; and BALDWIN, J. M., 1940-1949, *vide supra.*

WEBSTER's geographical dictionary, 1955: A dictionary of names of places with geographical and historical information and pronunciation, 1293 p. (Springfield, Mass.: Merriam; London: Bell).—

> Includes *ca.* 40,000 entries and 177 maps. Sarton remarks about this volume: "This is truly an excellent work, the best of its size at present (1952) available." Ancient and mediaeval place-names are included. Tables of geographical terms in various languages. Designed primarily for the North American user. In 1966 a new ed. appeared. *Cf.* COLLOCOTT, T. C. & J. O. THORNE, eds., 1954, *vide supra.*

WINCHELL, C. M., ed., 1951: Guide to reference books, ed. 7, 645 p. + suppl., 1950-1952 (1953), 117 p. + second suppl., 1953-1955 (1956), 134 p. (Chicago, Ill.: American Library Assn.).—

> This guide was first published in 1902. It contains some 7,500 reference works dealing with *e.g.*, libraries, societies, encyclopaedias, mythology, popular customs, folklore, language dictionaries, science (special sections deal with ethnology, biology, botany, zoology, bacteriology, genetics, entomology, natural history, agriculture, forestry, and medicine); symbolism, numismatics, biography, bibliography, geography, and history. Very useful! This work is kept up to date by the half-yearly supplements appearing in the January- and July-issues of College and Research Libraries, to begin with vol. 18, no. 1, Jan. 1957, p. 28-35.

WORLD LIST of scientific periodicals, 1963-1965, ed. 4, 3 vols. (London: Butterworth).—

> This fourth edition of the "World List" is edited by P. BROWN & G. B. STRATTON, and deals with the periodicals published in the years 1900-1960. It lists 59,404 periodicals, arranged alphabetically under the name. It gives the place of publication and other names by which the serial has been known. Much care has been given to abbreviations for titles of the pe-

riodicals issued. Location of sets in the British Islands has been given. This is followed by a list of published reports of periodic international scientific congresses (556 items). The first edition of this work appeared in 1925-1927, in 2 vols. The "World List" is now edited by K. PORTER and is being incorporated with British Union Catalogue (*vide* STEWART, *supra*). *Cf.* also ULRICH's periodicals directory, *vide supra*. In 1953 UNESCO published a list of "World medical periodicals", 237 p. (Paris: Unesco), an international list of 3,908 medico-biological periodicals, arranged according to the code of rules introduced by this "World List" and according to the World List's abbreviations. Subject-index and index of journals by countries are included. In 1957 a second edition appeared, 340 p. (New York, N.Y.: World Medical Assn.). This 2nd ed. contains 4,841 entries. Included are veterinary medicine (items 4773-4841) and the principal international medical abstracting and indexing journals. In 1961 a third ed. appeared, supplemented by: FLEURENT, C. H. A., 1968: World medical periodicals: supplement to the 3rd edition, 68 p. (New York, N.Y.: World Med. Assn.). About 700 new and changed titles have appeared since 1961.

WRIGHT, J. K. & E. T. PLATT, eds., 1947: Aids to geographical research: bibliographies, periodicals, atlases, gazetteers and other reference books, ed. 2, 331 p. (New York, N.Y.: Columbia U.P.).—

    This valuable book contains lists of bibliographies of general reference works and bibliographies, of geographical bibliographies, geographical institutions, periodicals, serials, manuals, gazetteers and related works, travellers' manuals, maps, atlases, historico-geographical studies, physical geography, biogeography, human geography, and a list of regional aids and general geographic periodicals.

b. *Biology* (incl. anatomy, embryology, anthropology, genetics, physiology, bacteriology, *etc.;* excl. botany and zoology)

ABERCROMBIE, M., C. J. HICKMAN & M. L. JOHNSON, eds., 1957: A dictionary of biology, 254 p. (Harmondsworth, Middx.: Penguin Bks.).—

    "Every biological technical term used in a definition is ... itself defined elsewhere in the dictionary; though some semitechnical terms, which can be found in any

English dictionary ... are omitted"(from the preface). It contains about 2,500 definitions. Reprinted 1967 (Chicago, Ill.: Aldine). *Cf.* SAYERS, 1951; GRAY, P., ed., 1967; and HENDERSON, I. F. & W. D., 1963, *vide infra*.

ALTSHELER, B., ed., 1940: Natural history index guide: an index to 3,365 books and periodicals in libraries. A guide to things natural in the field, ed. 2, 583 p. (New York, N.Y.: Wilson).—

    An index to 3,365 books and periodicals of places, animals, flora, insects, birds, tribes, and the like in outstanding travel records. The first section (p. 1-79) contains the general index, being an alphabetical list of all the subject-headings which are grouped in the various sections and divisions in which they are classed. There are 9,447 place-names and natural objects in botany, zoology, *etc.*, including the corresponding scientific names in Latin of about 4,200 of them. The subject-matter has been grouped in some 14 sections (geography, microscopy, palaeontology, botany, zoology, anthropology, food and drink, *etc.),* then the bibliography follows (p. 455-584), containing a complete list of titles indexed.

ARTSCHWAGER, E. F., ed., 1930: Dictionary of biological equivalents, German-English, 239 p. (London: Baillière, Tindall).—

    Contains about 12,000 entries, and a list of 16 important reference-books and dictionaries.

BIASS-DUCROUX, F., *et al.,* 1969: Glossary of genetics, 350 p. (Glossarium Interpretum, G. 16) (Amsterdam: Elsevier).—

    "This glossary has been compiled to provide the user with a rapid and adequate translation of the terms in current use in the field of genetics. Much care has been taken to avoid a mere transposition of words from one language into the other." It contains 2,930 entries in English, French, German, Russian, Italian, and Spanish. *Cf.* KING, R. C., 1968; KNIGHT, R. L., 1948; and RIEGER, R. & A. MICHAELIS, 1958, *vide infra*.

BOTTLE, R. T. & H. V. WYATT, eds., 1966: The use of biological literature, 286 p. (London: Butterworth).—

    An attempt at a complete coverage of the literature on the biological sciences to be used by both librarians and scientists.

Separate sections deal with: libraries and classification; the primary sources of information; abstracts, reviews and bibliographies as keys to the literature; foreign serials and translations; quick reference sources of data, techniques and background information; taxonomy, treatises, museums; zoology; biochemistry and biophysics; anatomy, physiology and pathology; microbiology; the use of patent literature; government publications and trade literature; the literature of applied biology (pharmacy, food and agriculture); some general and interdisciplinary aspects; history and biography of biology.

CARPENTER, J. R., ed., 1938: An ecological glossary, 306 p. (Norman, Okla.: Oklahoma U.P.).—

In this volume the author tries to bring together and to make available the more technical and restricted usages of some 3,000 terms which have been and are used in ecological literature. After each term included a reference has been added to the first use of the term or to a more available work or standard text in which the term is used or discussed.

DE VRIES, L., ed., 1946: German-English science dictionary for students in chemistry, physics, biology, agriculture, and related sciences, ed. 2, 558 p. (New York, N.Y.: McGraw-Hill).—

Contains some 48,000 entries. The same author also published: French-English science dictionary for students in agricultural, biological and physical sciences, 1940, 546 p. (New York, N.Y.: McGraw-Hill).

DOBSON, J., 1962: Anatomical eponyms: being a biographical dictionary of those anatomists whose names have become incorporated into anatomical nomenclature, with definitions of the structures to which their names have been attached and references to the works in which they are described, 235 p. (Edinburgh & London: Livingstone).—

The book is a biographical dictionary of anatomists associated with eponymously-named structures in the human body, and with descriptions of the structures named after them. Besides this function its aim is to preserve a terminology, for, as WOOD JONES writes in his foreword: "The policy of eliminating all eponyms from anatomical nomenclature has deprived the student of his main incentive to learn of the history and of the great masters of his subject."

Whereas no new anatomical eponyms are now likely to be introduced, this reference work may be considered as the definitive authority on this subject. Cf. TERRA, P. DE, 1913, vide infra.

DUMBLETON, C. W., ed., 1964: Russian-English biological dictionary, 512 p. (Edinburgh & London: Oliver & Boyd).—

"The terms included in this dictionary have been taken from numerous Russian textbooks and monographs, of which the most important are listed in the appendix, and from a multitude of research papers and journal articles ... Some obsolete terms have been included, particularly those connected with discarded biological theories, since they may be encountered in review articles as well as in the less recent literature. Terms connected with pathology have not been included." A comparable dictionary seems to be: CARPOVICH, E. A., 1958: Russian-English biological and medical dictionary, 400 p. (New York, N.Y.: Technical Dictionaries).

EYCLESHYMER, A. C. & D. M. SCHOEMAKER, eds., 1917: Anatomical names, especially the Basle Nomina Anatomica ("BNA"), ... with biographical sketches by R. L. MOODIE, 744 p. (New York, N.Y.: Wood).—

A classified list of ca. 5,000 Latin terms used in anatomy as determined at the Basle Conference (1895), with an index for the English equivalents, and a translation of the report of the Commission on Nomenclature. It also contains biographies of some 800 anatomists. Cf. also: KOPSCH, F., 1956; TRIEPEL, H., 1957; and TERRA, P. DE, 1913, vide infra.

FIELD, E. J. & R. J. HARRISON, 1947: Anatomical terms: their origin and derivation, 165 p. (Cambridge: Heffer).—

The editors describe this booklet as an attempt to explain to the student having little or no knowledge of Latin or Greek the origin of terms commonly used in the description of familiar structures of the body. Notes are added on their historical and literary associations. Cf. JAEGER, E. C., 1955; and MELANDER, A. L., 1940, vide infra.

FITTER, R. & M., 1967: The Penguin dictionary of British natural history, 348 p. (Harmondsworth, Middx.: Penguin Bks.).—

A little dictionary dealing with "all living things and natural phenomena of the earth and its atmosphere" which occur in the British Isles and Ireland. Internal organs have been, in the main, excluded. Comprehensive scientific index of species with their popular equivalents, together with cross-references. Some well-annotated line drawings.

FRAUENDORFER, S. v., ed., 1969: Survey of abstracting services and current bibliographical tools in agriculture, forestry, fisheries, nutrition, veterinary medicine and related subjects, 192 p. (Munich: BLV Verlagsges.).—

This publication consists of two main parts. The first part comprises a discussion of the possibilities of digesting the increasing amount of literature, considering abstracting and indexing services, methods of presenting documentation material, managing and organizing abstracting and indexing services, *etc.* The second part contains an international list of abstracting and indexing services, mainly periodicals, in an alphabetical order (692 items), with short descriptions. Subject- and country-indexes are added.

GRAY, P., ed., 1961: The encyclopedia of the biological sciences, 1119 p. (New York, N.Y.: Reinhold; London: Chapman & Hall).—

This is a relatively complete encyclopaedia, containing numerous shorter or longer articles (most being more than 500 words in length on many subjects of a general biological importance. Most articles are written by specialists of international repute. For historians the greatest merit of this reference work lies in its numerous biographies.

—— 1967: The dictionary of the biological sciences, 612 p. (New York, N.Y.: Reinhold).—

The dust jacket informs us that this book contains about 40,000 definitions, including botanical and zoological taxa down to families, mutant genes and their symbols, and organic compounds of biological importance. The entries incorporated are listed by roots (as far as possible). *Cf.* ABERCROMBIE *et al.,* 1957, *vide supra.*

HENDERSON, I. F. & W. D., 1963: A dictionary of biological terms: pronunciation,

derivation, and definition of terms in biology, botany, zoology, anatomy, cytology, genetics, embryology, physiology, ed. 8, 640 p. (Edinburgh & London: Oliver & Boyd).—

The first edition of this book appeared in 1920 under the title: A dictionary of scientific terms; this eighth edition has been edited by J. H. KENNETH, and appeared under a new title. Specific, generic, ordinal and other taxonomic names of plants and animals are omitted. The total number of terms is *ca.* 16,500. *Cf.* ABERCROMBIE *et al.,* 1957, *vide supra.*

HIRSCH, G. C., ed., 1928: Index biologorum: investigatores, laboratoria, periodica, 545 p. (Berlin: Springer).—

The first part (p. 1-335) contains a list of biologists with brief biographical and professional notes. The second part (p. 336-539) contains a list of laboratories and biological institutions, arranged by subject and then by city. Of each institute personnel and main objects of study are given. The third part (p. 540-545) contains a list of biological journals. *Cf.* also: LIST of SERIAL PUBLICATIONS in the British Museum (Natural History) library, 1164 p. (London: Brit. Mus. N.H.).

JACOBS, M. B., M. J. GERSTEIN & W. G. WALTER, 1957: Dictionary of microbiology, 276 p. (Princeton, N.J.: Van Nostrand).—

A dictionary of some 4,000 terms commonly used in microbiology and the related fields of bacteriology, mycology, virology, cytology, immunology and immunochemistry, serology, and microscopy. The authors have followed, as far as possible, the system of nomenclature and classification of bacteria used in BERGEY's "Manual of determinative bacteriology".

JAEGER, E. C., 1955: A source-book of the biological names and terms, ed. 3, 34 + 317 p. (Springfield, Ill.: Thomas).—

An alphabetically arranged list of 12,000 elements from which scientific biological names and terms are made. With them are given their Greek, Latin, or other origins and their concise meaning, together with examples of their use in scientific nomenclature. In an appendix a considerable number (more than 280) of short biographies are added of persons commemorated in botanical and zoological generic names. (First ed. 1944 - here, however, no appendix). A book set up along the same lines is: WERNER, C. F., 1956: Wortelemente lateinisch-griechischer Fachausdrücke in der Biologie, Zoologie, und vergleichende Anatomie, 397 p. (Leipzig: Akad. Verlagsgesellschaft). *Ca.* 1,700 terms; explanation of prefixes and suffixes, *etc. Cf.* MELANDER, A. L., 1940, *vide infra.*

KING, R. C., 1968: A dictionary of genetics, 300 p., 250 illus. (New York, N.Y. & London: Oxford U.P.).—

> Thoroughly up-to-date in its coverage, this concise volume defines some 4,300 terms which the student or researcher in biology, genetics, and related sciences is likely to encounter. Also included are structural formulas and molecular weights for biological materials, and selected tables. *Cf.* KNIGHT, R. L., 1948; and RIEGER & MICHAELIS, *vide infra.*

KNIGHT, R. L., 1948: Dictionary of genetics: including terms used in cytology, animal breeding and evolution, 183 p. (Waltham, Mass.: Chronica Botanica).—

> An attempt to define and standardize genetic terms. Separate appendixes deal with: useful formulae; coefficients of the terms in the expansion of $(1 + x)^n$ for values of n from 1 to 20; 2^n and 4^n for values of n from 3 to 20; distribution of x^2; genotypes expected in backcrosses and in F_2's; percentage of homozygotes in each generation following a cross the whole progeny of which is continuously selfed; rate of elimination of donor genotype by backcrossing; international rules for symbolizing genes and chromosome aberrations; planting distances recommended to avoid seed contamination. *Cf.* KING, 1968, *vide supra;* and RIEGER & MICHAELIS, *vide infra.*

KOPSCH, F., ed., 1957: Nomina anatomica, ed. 5. Vergleichende Uebersicht der Basler, Jenaer und Pariser Nomenklatur. Bearb. von K. H. KNESE, 155 p. (Stuttgart: Thieme).—

> An alphabetical list of anatomical terms as they have been proposed at the anatomical congresses in Basle (1895), Jena (1935), and Paris (1955) respectively. *Cf.* EYCLESHYMER & SCHOEMAKER, *vide supra,* and TRIEPEL, *vide infra.*

MELANDER, A. L., 1940: Source book of biological terms, 157 p. (New York, N.Y.: City College, Dept. of Botany).—

> Nearly half of the book deals with matters as: biological nomenclature, clas-

sical sources for names, word homologies, word phylogeny, the origin of words, derivations of words, early anatomical conceptions, unnatural history, colour terms, acceptuation, pronunciation, suffixes and prefixes, plurals, *etc.* The other part of the book (p. 62-157) consists of an alphabetical list of the components of biological vocabulary. *Cf.* JAEGER, E. C., 1955, *vide supra.*

NAUMANN, E., 1931: Limnologische Terminologie, 776 p. (Berlin & Vienna: Urban & Schwarzenberg).—

> A dictionary of technical terms used in limnology with often very elaborate explanations. Included are many ecological and geographical terms, excluded are names of plant and animal species and morphological terms.

PARTRIDGE, W., ed., 1927: Dictionary of bacteriological equivalents, 141 p. (London: Ballière, Tindall & Cox; Baltimore, Md.: Williams & Wilkins).—

> This dictionary contains French-English, German-English, Italian-English, and Spanish-English lists of words having a specific and special bacteriological significance in any of the given languages. The numbers of words dealt with are: French about 2,400; German about 2,600; Italian about 1,200; Spanish about 1,600.

RIEGER, R. & A. MICHAELIS, 1958: Genetisches und cytogenetisches Wörterbuch, ed. 2, 648 p. (Berlin, Göttingen & Heidelberg: Springer).—

> An alphabetical list of *ca.* 4,000 genetical and cyto-genetical terms. The first edition appeared as a supplement of the journal "Züchter". The second edition also includes many terms used in the fields of reproduction, developmental physiology, evolution, and statistics. Anglo-American terms have often been accompanied by a German equivalent and *vice versa.* The third ed. is in English (based on the third German ed.), ed. by RIEGER, R., A. MICHAELIS & M. M. GREEN, 1968: A glossary of genetics and cytogenetics: classical and molecular, 507 p. (London: Allen & Unwin; Heidelberg & New York, N.Y.: Springer). *Cf.* also: BIASS-DUCROUX, F., *et al.*, 1969, *vide supra.*

ROTHSCHUH, K. E., 1952: Entwicklungsgeschichte physiologischer Probleme in Tabellenform, 122 p. (Munich & Berlin: Urban & Schwarzenberg).—

A chronological survey of physiological discovery in synoptic tables arranged according to physiological subjects. The period covered extends from the 16th century till about 1920. Each entry included is preceded by a running number (which is used in the index of names at the end of the book), and gives the year, names, short description, and place of publication of the discovery and the discoverer respectively. This book is a useful supplement to ROTHSCHUH's "Geschichte der Physiologie" *(vide* section History of Physiology).

SAYERS, N. F., 1951: A biological glossary, 168 p. (London: London U.P.).—

In the preface the author writes that this glossary is intended to assist the student to understand and use the various scientific terms associated with botany and zoology in the senior forms of schools and the first year of the university course. Words in general use in the standard text-books have been arranged in groups according to their derivation. *Cf.* ABERCROMBIE *et al.,* 1957, *vide supra.*

SHARAF, M., 1928: An English-Arabic dictionary of medicine, biology, and allied sciences (based upon recent scientific literature), ed. 2, 971 + 12 + 42 p. (Egyptian Ministry of Education Publication) (Cairo: Govt. Press).—

"This is a very elaborate dictionary which will facilitate the translation of most technical treatises from English (and indirectly from other languages) into Arabic. The author has taken into account the very rich scientific literature already available in Arabic and adapted its terminology to modern needs. There is a long Arabic preface (42 p.) and 12 p. of errata and addenda." (Sarton in Isis 14: 537-538).

SHAW, H. K. A., ed., 1948: Directory of natural history societies, 155 p. + suppl. (1949) (London: Amateur Entomologists' Soc.).—

A geographically arranged list of societies with detailed index. A new directory of natural history societies seems to be in preparation by the British Association for the Advancement of Science.

SHERBORN, C. D., ed., 1940: Where is the . . . collection? An account of the various natural history collections which have come under the notice of the compiler . . . between

1880 and 1939, 149 p. (Cambridge: U.P.).—

Under the name of the collection is given its location and supplementary information, including journal references, *etc.*

TERRA, P. DE, 1913: Vademecum anatomicum. Kritisch-etymologisches Wörterbuch der systematischen Anatomie; mit besonderer Berücksichtigung der Synonymen. Nebst einem Anhang: Die anatomischen Schriftsteller des Altertums bis zur Neuzeit, 647 p. (Jena: Fischer).—

Contains *ca.* 14,000 anatomical terms and their synonyms. p. 601-647 contain a list of anatomical writers and of those anatomists whose name is connected with the name of some anatomical term, together with short biographical and bibliographical information. *Cf.* DOBSON, J., 1962, *vide supra.*

TRIEPEL, H., 1957: Die anatomischen Namen, ihre Ableitung und Aussprache, ed. 25. Völlig neu bearbeitet und entsprechend den neuen anatomischen Namen (Pariser N.A.) ergänzt von R. HERRLINGER, 82 p. (Munich: Bergmann).—

A comprehensive and almost entirely etymological glossary, first published in 1905. It covers the etymology of all terms used in the Basle (1895) and Jena (1935) nomenclatures, as well as the additions made in the Nomina Anatomica (Paris, 1955). *Cf.* EYCLESHYMER & SCHOEMAKER, 1917; and KOPSCH, 1957, *vide supra..*

WINICK, C., 1958: Dictionary of anthropology, 579 p. (London: Owen; Totowa, N.J.: Littlefield & Adams).—

A vocabulary covering the various fields of anthropology, such as: archaeology, cultural- and physical anthropology, and linguistics. Included are *ca.* 10,000 entries.

WOODS, R. S., 1966: An English-classical dictionary for the use of taxonomists, 345 p. (Claremont, Calif.: Pomona College).—

This book contains all words occurring in Latin and Greek which are or could be used in taxonomic nomenclature, together with their Latin and Greek equivalents. Its main purpose is to help botanists and zoologists in the selection and construction of suitable epithets for new taxa. Greek words are transliterated into Roman characters.

c. *Plant sciences*

c₁ Pure plant sciences

AINSWORTH, G. C. & G. R. BISBY, 1954: A dictionary of the fungi, ed. 4, 475 p. (Kew: Commonwealth Mycological Institute).—

This book contains an alphabetical list of orders, families, and genera, together with a list of mycological terms, short biographies of mycologists, common fungal diseases, and formulae for the preparation of culture media. *Cf.* SNELL & DICK, *vide infra.*

ANDRÉ, J., 1956: Lexique des termes de botanique en latin, 343 p. (Paris: Klincksieck).—

An alphabetically arranged list of Latin botanical terms setting forth their meaning and etymologies. It lists generic plant terms, names of species, and terms for parts of plants with their meanings.

ARTSCHWAGER, E. & E. M. SMILEY, eds., 1925: Dictionary of botanical equivalents, 124 p. (Baltimore, Md.: Williams & Wilkins).—

A dictionary of botanical technical terms, containing German- English, Dutch-English, Italian-English, and French-English lists of terms.

ASHBY, H., H. RICHTER, E. ASHBY & J. BÄRNER ,1938: German-English botanical dictionary, 195 p. (London: Murby).—

This booklet is an introduction to German and English terms used in botany, including plant physiology, ecology, genetics, and plant pathology. This has been done in the form of a brief survey of botanical science, printed in English and in German on opposite pages. Many technical terms are included in the text. Appendixes contain the names of common, wild, and cultivated European plants in English, German, and Latin, a list of the most important common names of plant diseases, and a list of abbreviations frequently used in botanical literature. English and German indexes.

BEDEVIAN, A. K., 1936: Illustrated polyglottic dictionary of plant names in Latin, Arabic, Armenian, English, French, German, Italian and Turkish languages, 614+466 p. (Cairo: Argus & Papazian Presses).—

This volume includes all the cultivated crops, fruit trees, and vegetables, the industrial, medicinal and poisonous plants, most ornamental plants used in public gardens, and the most common weeds. The book consists of two parts. The first part contains a dictionary and appendixes (concerning the Arabic transliteration system, the Armenian and Turkish alphabets, and a bibliography) and the second part consists of a list of common names of plants in English, French, German, Italian, Turkish, Armenian and Arabic. *Cf.* ISSA BEY, *vide infra.*

BRITTEN, J. & R. HOLLAND, 1886: Dictionary of English plant-names, 618 p. (London: Trübner).—

Originally published as Publications nos. 22, 26, and 45 of the English Dialect Society (1878-1884). An authoritative work on the subject. Each entry consists of the common name and the scientific name of the plants included, together with explanations of origin, and references to uses in literature. An index of country names of (English) plants can be found in: GRIEVE, M., 1931: A modern herbal: the medicinal culinary, cosmetic and economic properties, cultivation, folk-lore of herbs, grasses, fungi, shrubs and trees, with all their modern scientific uses, 2 vols., 888 p. (London: Cape). Vol. 2 includes an index of country names of plants covered. Reprinted 1959 (New York, N.Y.: Hafner). *Cf.* FISHER, R., 1932-1934; and MACLEOD, R. D., 1952, *vide infra.*

CLUTE, W. N., 1942: The common names of plants and their meanings, ed. 2, 164 p. (Indianapolis, Ind.: W. N. Clute).—

In this book the author tries to unravel a few of the terms applied to some common American plants of fields and wood. Its contents can be explained by giving the chapter headings: 1. Whence came our plant names; 2. Technical names; 3. Our first plant names; 4. Indian names; 5. Pioneer names; 6. The contribution of ignorance; 7. Manufactured names; 8. Transferred names; 9. Saints and heroes; 10. Plants named for demons; 11. *Idem* for animals; 12. *Idem* for serpents; 13. The banes; 14. Medicinal plants; 15. Hyphenated names; 16. Imported names.

—— 1939: A second book of plant names and their meaning, 164 p. (Indianapolis, Ind.: W. N. Clute).—

A booklet of the same character as the preceding one. Chapter headings are as follows: 1. Origin of the common names; 2. The technical names; 3. Puzzling technical terms; 4. Evolution in plant names; 5. Associated names; 6. Duplicate plant names; 7. Mistakes of typist and printer; 8. Names in series; 9. Sunflowers and frost-weeds; 10. Milk-weeds and wartworts; 11. Madworts and rattleweeds; 12. Burs and sticktights; 13. Odoriferous plants; 14. Dye-plants; 15. Forget-me-nots; 16. Plants named for bugs; 17. Curious and unusual.

—— 1940: American plant names, 285 p. (Indianapolis, Ind.: W. N. Clute).—

This volume brings together all the vernacular names by which the plants of Northern America are known. The genera in each family and the species in each genus are arranged alphabetically. The book has been divided into two parts; the first part contains the vernacular names arranged under their proper genus and species, the second part is a cross-referenced index to the first list.

DAVUIDOV, N. N., 1960: Botanicheskii slovar: Russko-Anghliisko-Nemetzko-Frantzuszko-Latininskii, 334 p. (Moskva: Red. Inostr. Nauchno-Tekhn. Slovarei Fizmatghiza).—

Botanical dictionary. Russian-English-German-French-Latin. It contains ca. 6,000 botanical terms of which approximately 30 percent are names of plants with references to the families to which they belong. Russian is the basic language of this dictionary.

FISHER, R., 1932-1934: The English names of our commonest wild flowers, 2 vols. Vol. I (1932): 249 p.; Vol. II (1934): 344 p. (Arbroath: Buncle).—

This work is intended to meet difficulties by giving to each plant a standard name. Therefore, each name included is referred to this standard name, and all the other names of the plants are given under this standard name. By this plan a plant known by any particular or local name can be identified by reference to its standard name, and all its other names known also. The meaning of the names is also added. The first volume contains those plants which are common in all districts of Britain; the

second volume also includes many plants of a more restricted distribution. A somewhat comparable work is that of BRITTEN, J. & R. HOLLAND, 1886, vide supra. A study especially dealing with Irish and Scottish plant names is: HOGAN, E. & J. & J. C. MACERLEAN, 1900: Irish and Scottish Gaelic names of herbs, plants, trees, etc., 137 p. (London).

FOURNIER, P., 1947-1948: Le livre des plantes médicinales et vénéneuses de France. 1500 espèces par le texte et par l'image d'après l'ensemble de nos connaissances actuelles. Vol. I (1947): Abricot à Coloquinte, 78 + 448 p.; Vol. II (1948): Consoude à Melon, 504 p.; Vol. III (1948): Menthe à Zacinthe, 637 p. (Paris: Lechevalier).—

The first volume contains a brief historical review of phytotherapy, a review of French medicinal plants and their modes of action. The work as a whole is a flora giving a key leading to the species included. Of each species included is a systematic description, a very interesting history of their use in former days, a summing-up of their medical, chemical, etc., properties and a description of their present use, preparation, etc. This work contains much that is of interest to the biohistorian.

GATIN, C. L., 1965: Dictionnaire aide-mémoire de botanique, 848 p. (Vaduz: Kraus).—

A reprint of the 1924 edition (Paris: Lechevalier). A comparable French dictionary seems to be: GUINOCHET, M., 1965: Notions fondamentales de botanique générale, 446 p. (Paris: Masson).

GERTH VAN WIJK, H. L., 1909-1916: A dictionary of plant-names, 4 vols. Vol. I (1909): p. 1-710; Vol. II (1909): p. 711-1444; Vol. III (1916): Index A-K, 34 p. + p. 1-880); Vol. IV (1916): Index L-Z, p. 881-1696. (The Hague: Nijhoff).—

"The work is so planned, that it will enable one to find the name, by which a plant is known in four modern languages, if one knows the Latin name, but also to find the Latin name, if only the name in one of these four languages is known. To make this possible the first two parts are alphabetically arranged to the Latin names, while the last two parts ... form a large index, arranged alphabetically according to the names of the plants in the modern languages." The modern languages are: English, French, German, and Dutch. Reprinted 1962-1963 (Amsterdam: Asher).

ISSA BEY, A., 1930: Dictionnaire des noms des plantes en latin, français, anglais et arabe, ed. 1, 16+223+64 p. (Cairo: Imprimerie Nationale).—

"J'ai transcrit les noms des plantes tels que je les ai découverts, en respectant l'orthographe des termes purement arabes aussi bien que celle des mots arabisés ou métis. De plus, je me suis efforcé de ne commettre aucune omission, répondant ainsi aux buts suivants qui sont actuellement poursuivis par tous les écrivains et les savants du siècle: (1) Que le dictionnaire contienne tous les noms des plantes cités dans les ouvrages arabes, quelle que soit l'origine de ces noms. (2) Qu'il ne serve pas seulement de référence pour connaître les noms des plantes, mais qu'il puisse être également utile à identifier l'origine des mots étrangers cités dans les ouvrages arabes. Il sera donc en quelque sorte, un supplément aux autres dictionnaires arabes, supplément auquel on se reportera pour reconnaître les origines des mots." This is derived from a quotation by Sarton in Isis 20, p. 586, to which quotation he adds: "L'ordre principal est celui des mots latins, mais la valeur pratique de l'ouvrage est augmentée par la présence d'index français, anglais, et arabe. Ce dernier sera surtout précieux; il remplit 64 p. de 3 colonnes chacune." *Cf.* BEDEVIAN, *supra.*

JACKSON, B. D., 1928: A glossary of botanic terms with their derivation and accent, ed. 4, 481 p. (London: Duckworth).—

A very good glossary, including nearly 25,000 botanical terms. Words drawn from the same leading word have been grouped into paragraphs. Derivations have been given and pronunciation of the words has been indicated. Offset reprints were issued by Hafner, New York, 1950, and by Duckworth, London, 1965. The first ed. appeared in 1900.

LANJOUW, J. & F. A. STAFLEU, 1954-1964: Index herbariorum. Part I: The herbaria of the world, ed. 5 (1964), 249 p., Part II: Collectors. First instalment A-D (1954), 174 p.; second instalment: E-H (1957), p. 175-295. (Utrecht: Intern. Bureau for Plant Taxonomy).—

The "Index Herbariorum" will consist of 4 parts. Part I deals with the herbaria of the world, arranged topographically in alphabetical order. It gives information with regard to the herbaria (date of foundation, details of staff and publications, *etc.)* with detailed indexes; it may also serve as an address book of taxonomists; large index to personal names). Part II contains a list of all collectors of any importance with indication of the herbaria in which their collections are preserved. Two instalments have been published (A-H), and a third one (I-K) is in course of preparation. Part III will contain a geographical index of collections and Part IV will contain an alphabetical list of authors of types.

LINSBAUER, K., ed., 1917: C. K. SCHNEIDERs illustriertes Handwörterbuch der Botanik, ed. 2, 824 p. (Leipzig: Engelmann).—

A botanical dictionary containing about 7,000 botanical terms. Many illuminating illustrations. Etymological review of Greek and Latin word stems used in botany. The first edition was published in 1905. *Cf.* also: WITTSTEIN, G. C., 1967: Etymologisch-botanisches Handwörterbuch, ed. 2, 952 p. (Wiesbaden: Sändig). A reprint of the 1852 edition. Two somewhat shorter and more modern dictionaries are: BOROS, G., 1958: Lexikon der Botanik, 276 p. (Stuttgart: Ulmer); and SCHUBERT, R. & G. WAGNER, eds., 1962: Botanische Pflanzennamen und Fachwörter, 327 p. (Radebeul: Neumann), a pocket dictionary containing some 5,000 terms. An elaborate botanical dictionary in the French language is: BAILLON, M. H., 1876-1892: Dictionnaire de botanique, 4 vols., 788 + 776 + 756 + 340 p. (Paris: Hachette).

MACLEOD, R. D., 1952: Key to the names of British plants, 94 p. (London: Pitman).—

A dictionary explaining the origin and meaning of the scientific and common names of British wild flowers and trees. There is a large introduction explaining such matters as: the form of scientific names, their pronuncation and origin, basic forms of Latin and Greek nouns and verbs, the form of common names, origin and analysis of popular names, *etc. Cf.* BRITTEN & HOLLAND, 1886; and FISHER, R., 1932-1934, *vide supra.*

MARZELL, H., 1937 →: Wörterbuch der deutschen Pflanzennamen. Vol. I (1937-1943): Anfangsbuchstaben A, B und C, 1412 p.; Vol. II (1951-1960): Daboecia-Knautia, 1119 p.; Vol. III (1963 →): Macleya-Nigella, 319 p. Vol. V (1958): Registerband, 651 p. (Leipzig: Hirzel).—

From the preface: "Das vorliegende Wörterbuch macht den Versuch, die deutschen Pflanzennamen aus allen Zeiten und aus allen Mundartgebieten zu sammeln, sie mit den Pflanzennamen anderer europäischer Sprachen zu vergleichen und sie nach Benennungsgründen geordnet vorzuführen. Dabei wird im Gegensatz zu allen früheren derartigen Sammlungen jeder Pflanzennamen genau quellenmässig belegt werden." As far as I am aware Vols. III and IV are still to be completed. An older and more comprehensive dictionary of German plant names is: VOSS, A., 1922: Wörterbuch der deutschen Pflanzennamen, ed. 3, 488 p. (Stuttgart).

PLOWDEN, C. C., 1968: A manual of plant names, 260 p. (London: Allen & Unwin).—

> This book explains botanical terminology, gives a simplified classificatory system of flowering plants, and gives the meaning and derivation of generic names and their English translation, together with the separate translation of specific epithets. Included are plants grown for a variety of reasons, such as: ornament, food, or science. It aims to be of interest for both amateur and professional botanists and gardeners.

SNELL, W. H. & E. A. DICK, 1957: A glossary of mycology, 32 + 169 p. (Cambridge, Mass.: Harvard U.P.).—

> A dictionary containing nearly 7,000 terms as used in mycological literature or in general literature of interest to mycologists, e.g., technical terms and their derivations; common or popular, vernacular, and obsolete terms; terms used in the fields of medical mycology and antibiotics; names of the originators of the terms; folk-lore terms; and colour terms. Cf. AINSWORTH & BISBY, vide supra.

STEARN, W. T., 1966: Botanical Latin: history, grammar, syntax, terminology and vocabulary, 566 p. (London & Edinburgh: Nelson).—

> This book is meant to supply a working tool to enable those botanists who are not classical scholars to prepare a diagnosis or description in Latin which should accompany new names of taxa according to the standards set by the International Code of Botanical Nomenclature. This book also is of high value for anyone interested in botanical historiography because, up to a century ago, nearly all botanical texts were written in Latin. The book contains a historical review of botanical Latin terminology, a condensed outline of the grammar and syntax, standard descriptions in Latin of representatives of various plant groups, and a comprehensive vocabulary, containing all the terms commonly used in botanical Latin, with exact definitions.

STEENIS-KRUSEMAN, M. J. v., 1950: Malaysian plant collectors and collections: being a cyclopedia of botanical exploration in Malaysia and a guide to the concerned literature up to the year 1950, 152 + 639 p. (Flora Malesiana, Vol. I) + supplement, 1957, 108 p. (Groningen/Djakarta: Noordhoff-Kolff).—

> The text has been divided into a general and a special part. The special part (p. 1-639) consists of an alphabetical list of collectors giving information of their lives, expeditions, collections, main publications, etc. The general part contains information on such topics as, e.g., private collections of Malaysian plants; lists of works principally containing illustrations of Malaysian plants, and of collections of drawings or photographs; an annotated list of literature for the use of botanists and explorers; the technique of plant collecting and preservation in the tropics; the chronology of collections; desiderata for future collection, etc. The supplement has been arranged in the same way.

WILLIS, J. C., 1966: A dictionary of the flowering plants and ferns, ed. 7, 1214 + 53 p. (Cambridge: U.P.).—

> The first edition appeared in 1897, the sixth edition in 1931; that edition has been completely rewritten by H. K. A. SHAW. The ca. 40,000 entries in this new edition are confined by generic (1,753) and family (1,789) names; botanical terms, common and vernacular names, and economic products are omitted. The generic names contain many variant spellings and intergeneric hybrids. Brief characters of subfamilies are usually given. In an appendix (53 p.), the synopses of the Bentham-Hooker and Engler-Prantl systems have been retained.

ZANDER, R., 1964: Handwörterbuch der Pflanzennamen und ihre Erklärungen. Entsprechend den Beschlüssen der letzten internationalen Nomenklatur — Tagungen in Stockholm (1950), London (1951 und 1952) und Paris (1954) gänzlich neu bearbeitet, ed. 9, 623 p. (Stuttgart: Ulmer).—

> The first ed. was published in 1927. This volume contains: a general introduction to the rules of botanical nomenclature;

a systematic review of the plant kingdom; an alphabetical list of names of families, genera and species of plants (p. 46-375); an alphabetical list of German plant names; an alphabetical list of Latin plant names with an explanation of their composition and a translation of their meaning; and a list of the names of those authors who used the names first (together with some biographical notes).

ZIMMER, G. F., 1949: A popular dictionary of botanical names and terms with their English equivalents, 122 p. (London: Routledge & Kegan Paul).—

This little dictionary is intended for the use of botanists and horticulturists, as well as for lovers of the flowers of garden, field and wood, as the author states in the subtitle.

c2 *Applied plant sciences (i.e., agriculture, viticulture, forestry, and horticulture)*

ANONYMOUS, 1965: Dicţionar forestier poliglot, 2 vols. Vol. I: 760 p.; Vol. II: 408 p. (Bucarest: Minsterul economici forestiere).—

Vol. I consists of a forest dictionary in Rumanian, Russian, French, German, English, and Hungarian. Vol. II contains an index of the names used in the above-mentioned languages and in Latin. *Cf.* BOERHAAVE BEEKMAN, 1964-1966, *vide infra.*

BAILEY, L. H., 1943: The standard cyclopedia of horticulture, 3 vols., 3639 p. + 4056 figs. (New York, N.Y.: Macmillan).—

A classic, reprinted many times since 1900 when the first edition appeared. Its contents are very well described in its subtitle: a discussion, for the amateur, and the professional and commercial grower, of the kinds, characteristics and methods of cultivation of the species of plants grown in the regions of the United States and Canada for ornament, for fancy, for fruit and for vegetables; with keys to the natural families and genera, descriptions of the horticultural capabilities of the states and provinces and dependent islands, and sketches of eminent horticulturists.

BEZEMER, T. J., ed., 1934: Dictionary of terms relating to agriculture, horticulture, forestry, cattle-breeding, dairy industry in English, French, German and Dutch, 1061 p. (London: Allen & Unwin).—

The work is paged separately for each language-sequence (English-German, Dutch, French; German-Dutch, French, English; Dutch-French, English, German; French-English, German, Dutch) and equivalents in each subsidiary language are given.

BOALCH, D. H., ed., 1960: World directory of agricultural libraries and documentation centres, 280 p. (Harpenden, Herts: Rothamsted Exp. Statn.).—

This book records nearly 2,600 libraries in more than 20 countries, concerned with agriculture and related subjects, including such fields as: agricultural engineering, veterinary medicine, forestry, fisheries, food and nutrition. Of the libraries included, it gives such information as: date of foundation, number of volumes held, current serials received, size of staff, system of classification, *etc.* The arrangement is geographical. Indexes of places, of names, and of subjects.

——, 1965-1968: Current agricultural serials, 2 vols. Vol. I (1965): 351 p.; Vol. II (1968): 95 p. (Oxford: Intl. Assn. Agricult. Librarians and Documentalists).—

A world list of serials in agriculture and related subjects, excl. forestry and fisheries, current in 1964. It includes such details as: place of publication, starting-year, frequency of issue, name of the publisher. Many indexes.

BOERHAVE-BEEKMAN, W., ed., 1964-1966: Wood dictionary, 3 vols. Vol. I (1964): 479 p.; Vol. II (1966): 642 p.; Vol. III (1968): 460 p. (New York, N.Y. & Amsterdam: Elsevier).—

The first volume was primarily concerned with commercial and botanical nomenclature of world-timbers and with sources of supply. The second vol. presents tables of production, transportation, and trade in seven languages, *viz.,* English/American, French, Spanish, Italian, Swedish, German, and Dutch. The third vol. deals with matters of research, manufacture and utilization. This dictionary is a useful tool for explorers, timber experts, merchants, and institutions involved with world forests and forestry. *Cf.* CORKHILL, 1948, *infra,* and ANONYMOUS, 1965, *supra.*

CHITTENDEN, F. J., ed., 1956: Dictionary of gardening: a practical and scientific encyclopaedia of horticulture, ed. 2, 4 vols.,

2316 p.+suppl., 1968 (ed. by J. SYNGE), 555 p. (Oxford: Clarendon Press).—

This work aims at describing every plant suitable for cultivation in the British Isles both outdoors and under glass, thereby also covering almost all plants suitable for cultivation in temperate climates. Whereas additional notes on many tropical and subtropical plants are included, the dictionary should prove valuable to gardeners all over het world. Each genus has a general account, followed by descriptions of individual species and such hybrids as are long established and widely grown. Many species are illustrated by drawings. The supplement contains lists of recommended varieties of flowers, fruits and vegetables. The whole work has been prepared under the auspices of the Royal Horticultural Society. The suppl. vol. consists of alphabetical sections on flowers, fruit and vegetables, and of additions and corrections to the main vols.; this supplement will be revised periodically.

CHOUARD, P. & E. LAUMONNIER, eds., 1947: Le bon jardinier, nouvelle encyclopédie horticole, ed. 151, 1842 p. (Paris: Librairie agricole, horticole, forestière et ménagère).—

The whole work has been divided into 6 parts. The first part deals with general questions such as: What is horticulture?, garden calendars, lexicon of terms used in horticulture, horticultural and botanical nomenclature, etc. The second part deals with the scientific aspects of horticulture (botanical morphology, physiology, genetics, variation, selection, environment and amelioration of plants, etc.). The third part deals with horticultural techniques, the fourth with horticultural products, the fifth with economical aspects of horticulture, and the sixth part deals with the aesthetic aspects of horticulture (garden design, public gardens, etc.). Index (p. 1195-1839). The first edition appeared in 1755.

CORKHILL, T., 1948: A glossary of wood, 656 p. (London: Nema Press).—

This glossary contains explanations of about 10,000 terms and expressions used in forestry, lumbering, marketing, woodworking trades and in all other forms of application of wood. More than 1,000 of these terms are also illustrated by line diagrams. *Cf.* BOERHAVE BEEKMAN, *supra.*

ELSEVIER's DICTIONARY OF HORTICULTURE, 1970, 561 p. (Amsterdam, London & New York, N.Y.: Elsevier).—

"This dictionary in nine languages, compiled under the auspices of the Netherlands Ministry of Agriculture and Fisheries, has been prepared with the help and cooperation of many international experts in the field of horticulture. The basic table is in English, with terms arranged alphabetically and numbered in that order. The English terms are followed by their equivalents in the eight other languages. Separate alphabetical indexes are supplied for each of these languages; these lead the user to the appropriate numbered entry in the basic table."

FAES, H., 1940: Lexique viti-vinicole international, 278 p. (Paris: Office international du Vin).—

This volume consists of separate lists of terms in French, Italian, Spanish, and German, used in viticulture, together with their explanation.

GREEN, C. E. & D. YOUNG, eds., 1907-1909: Encyclopaedia of agriculture. By the most eminent authorities, 4 vols. (Edinburgh & London: W. Green).—

The whole work consists of four 600-page volumes, dealing with nearly every aspect of agriculture and husbandry. Many illustrations. *Cf.* HUNTER, H., 1931, *vide infra.*

HAENSCH, G. & G. HABERKAMP, eds., 1966: Dictionary of agriculture, ed. 3, 744 p. (Munich: Bayrischer Landwirtschaftsverl.).—

"Contents: In this third edition, the number of entries has been extended to 10,057. The first part of the dictionary is a systematic basic table in which each term is numbered and is given column-wise in German, English, French and Spanish. The second part comprises alphabetical indexes for each language, which permit the reader to trace each numbered term back to the basic table, where its translation into the three other languages will then be found. The compilers have been careful to distinguish English from American usage, to differentiate between European and Latin American Spanish and to account for differences in linguistic usage in the German- and French-speaking communities of Europe." (After a publisher's announcement in Nature 220: xv, Dec. 21, 1968). Originally published in 1963; Russian and Italian supplements. *Cf.* also RIES, L. W., ed., 1957, *vide infra.*

HALE, P. H., 1915: Hale's history of agriculture by dates: a simple record of historical events and victories of peaceful industries, ed. 5, 95 p. (St. Louis, Mo.: Hale).—

Citation of events in agriculture from 4241 B.C. to 1910 A.D.

HAWLEY, R. C., ed., 1950: Forestry terminology: a glossary of technical terms used in forestry, new ed., 93 p. (Washington, D.C.: Society of American Foresters).—

This glossary is restricted to "terms used in a special sense by foresters and to terms from other sciences and industries the meaning of which a forester should know" and which may not be defined in other glossaries normally available to foresters. Included is a list of 23 glossaries in allied sciences. A third edition appeared in 1958. *Cf.* WECK, 1966, *infra.*

HUNTER, H., ed., 1931: Baillière's encyclopaedia of scientific agriculture, 2 vols. (London: Baillière, Tindall & Cox).—

"Although the subject-matter is largely concerned with British agriculture, it is applicable ... to ... other countries characterized by a temperate climate" (from the preface). A much older agricultural encyclopaedia is: GREEN, C. E. & D. YOUNG, *vide supra.* A more recent agricultural dictionary, of which I - unfortunately - cannot give further details is: WINBURNE, J. N., 1962: A dictionary of agriculture and allied terminology, 905 p. (Michigan, Wisc.: Michigan State U.P.).

JACKS, G. V., ed., 1955: Multilingual vocabulary of soil science, 439 p. (Rome: Agricultural Division F.A.O., United Nations).—

Separate sections deal with physics, texture, structure, chemistry, biology, ecology, cultivation, geology, mineralogy, *etc.,* of the soil, with soil water, -humus, soil formation, -classification, -irrigation, -erosion, *etc.,* and with organic-, peat-, podsolic-, meadow-, arid-, saline-, *etc.* soils. Indexes in English, French, German, Spanish, Portuguese, Italian, Dutch, and Swedish.

JOHNSON, A. T. & H. A. SMITH, 1947: Plant names simplified, rev. ed., 120 p. (London: Collingridge).—

In this book the authors have set out to explain the names of mainly garden and greenhouse plants and to indicate their correct pronunciation. *Cf.* SMITH, A. W., 1963, *vide infra.*

KELSEY, H. P. & W. A. DAYTON, eds., 1942: Standardized plant names, ed. 2, 675 p. (Harrisburg, Pa.: McFarland).—

This work has been prepared under the auspices of the American joint Committee on Horticultural Nomenclature in accordance with the international rules of botanical nomenclature. It is described in its sub-title as a revised and enlarged listing of approved scientific and common names of plants and plant products in American commerce and use.

LANDWIRTSCHAFTLICHES WÖRTERBUCH in acht Sprachen, 1970, 2 vols. Vol. I: 1045 p.; Vol. II: 676 p. (Berlin: Deutscher Landwirtschaftsverlag).—

An extensive agricultural dictionary (ed. by I. I. SINJAGIN) in eight languages, *viz.,* Russian, Bulgarian, Czech, Polish, Hungarian, Rumanian, German, and English, containing 25,780 terms in the field of crop production, agricultural economy, agricultural technique, forestry, hunting, farming, animal production, and veterinary medicine. *Cf.* also: POSHARSKI, W. K., 1968: Wörterbuch der Landwirtschaft Russisch-Deutsch, 454 p. (Leipzig: Enzyklopädie), containing some 29,000 terms; and HORATSCHEK, E., K. FREYSE & E. HASSENRÜCK, 1967: Wörterbuch der Landwirtschaft. Deutsch-Tschechisch-Russisch-Polnisch, 652 p. (Leipzig: Enzyklopädie), containing some 6,500 terms.

LEXIKON DES LANDWIRTES, hrsg. von einer Arbeitsgemeinschaft von Fachwissenschaftlern und Praktikern, 1948, 448 p. (Vienna: Leinmüller).—

An alphabetical lexicon, containing "Antworten auf Tausende von Fragen aus allen Gebieten der Landwirtschaft, wie Acker- und Pflanzenbau, Pflanzenschutz, Düngerlehre, Tierzucht, Tierheilkunde, Fütterung, Milchwirtschaft, Bauwesen, Maschinenkunde, Wetterkunde, Rechtsleben, usw. Bei der Wahl der Stichworte war der Grundsatz massgebend, alles Wesentliche zu erfassen und so darzustellen, dass der praktische Landwirt daraus unmittelbaren Nutzen ziehen kann." Many illustrations. *Cf.* RIES, L. W., ed., 1957, *vide infra.*

LINNARD, W., 1966: Russian-English forestry and wood dictionary, 109 p. (Commonwealth Agricultural Bureau, Forestry Dept.) (Farnham Royal, Bucks.: Commonwealth Agricult. Bureau).—

A bilingual dictionary of forestry, containing *ca.* 7,000 terms or expressions, most of them accompanied by explanatory commentaries. It covers the whole field of sylviculture and deals, *e.g.*, with utilisation and composition of woods, animals and plants of the forest, *etc.*

MERINO-RODRÍGUEZ, M., 1966: Lexicon of plant pests and diseases, 351 p. (Amsterdam, London & New York, N.Y.: Elsevier).—

>A compilation of vernacular names in English, French, Spanish, Italian, German, and Latin. Latin has been adopted as the basic language. The text consists of a systematic and an alphabetical part. The systematic part contains two sections dealing with zooparasites and phytoparasites respectively. There are three appendixes: 1. Symptoms of diseases; 2. Non-parasitic diseases; 3. Unclassified virus diseases. 2,396 entries.

NIJDAM, J., 1961: Horticultural dictionary (Dutch, English, French, German, Danish, Swedish, Spanish and Latin), 504 p. (The Hague: Staatsdrukkerij; London & New York, N.Y.: Interscience).—

>Nearly all of the *ca.* 4,000 words and expressions included in this dictionary are related to the practice of horticulture, which, in the Netherlands, is interpreted to include the production of vegetables, fruit, flowers, bulbs, trees and shrubs, herbs and seeds as well as apiculture. The words have been arranged alphabetically on the basis of their Dutch spelling. Alphabetical lists of English, French, German, Danish, Swedish, Spanish and Latin words are included; of each word the reference-letter and number under which the equivalents in the other languages will be found in the main list, are given. A fifth ed. is published under the following title: Elsevier's dictionary of horticulture, 1970, 561 p. (ed. by J. NIJDAM & A. DE JONG) (Amsterdam: Elsevier). Another horticultural dictionary is: ZANDER, R. & M. HECKEL, 1938: Wörterbuch der gärtnerischen Fachausdrücke in vier Sprachen (German, English, French, Italian), 419 p. (Berlin: 12. Int. Gartenbau Kongress).

RIES, L. W., ed., 1957: Pareys Landwirtschaftslexikon, ed. 7, 2 vols., 805 p. (Unter Mitwirkung von E. KLAPP & F. HARING) (Hamburg & Berlin: Parey).—

>A lexicon of over 8,000 terms appertaining to agriculture, including many terms belonging to related fields, such as: botany, zoology, genetics, husbandry, soil science, viticulture, apiculture, fruit-growing, forestry, phytopathology, pisciculture, *etc.* Many illustrations. *Cf.* also: HAENSCH, G. & G. HABERKAMP, eds., 1966; and LEXIKON DES LANDWIRTES, 1948, *vide supra.*

SELTENSPERGER, C., 1922: Dictionnaire d'agriculture et de viticulture, 1064 p. (Paris: Baillière).—

>A (somewhat obsolete) encyclopaedia of scientific and technical terminology used in agriculture, husbandry, apiculture, viticulture, *etc.*, and related industries, incl. some terms from the fields of biology, chemistry and other related sciences. Many illustrations. *Cf.* RIES, L. W., ed., 1957, *vide supra.*

SMITH, A. W., 1963: A gardener's book of plant names: a handbook of the meaning and origin of plant names, 428 p. (New York, N.Y. & London: Harper & Row).—

>After a list of some botanical definitions, explaining the botanical terms most often used, an alphabetical list of plant names follows with short explanations of the meaning of these names. Therefore it contains much that is of importance to the biohistorian.

STÄHLIN, A., 1967: Die landwirtschaftlichen Kulturpflanzen Mitteleuropas in den europäischen Sprachen, 174 p. (Unter Mitarbeit von A. STÄHLIN) (Frankfurt a.M.: DLG).—

>A list of 105 economically useful Central-European plants (food plants, esp. graminaea and leguminous plants, wheat, oil plants, *etc.*), in 23 languages (Albanian, Bulgarian, Danish, English and American, Finnish, French and Canadian French, Greek, Irish, Icelandic, Italian, Dutch, Norwegian, Polish, Portuguese, Rumanian, Russian, Swedish, Serbo-Croat, Spanish, Czech, Turkish and Hungarian).

TAYLOR, N., ed., 1948: Taylor's encyclopedia of gardening, horticulture and landscape design, ed. 2, 1225 p. (Boston, Mass.: Houghton Mifflin).—

>An elaborate, alphabetically arranged, encyclopaedia. The main articles, however, have been rearranged according to the main divisions of gardening, in order to give a more simultaneous view of the whole field of gardening. They are: 1. Green-

houses, conservatories, cold frames, and hot beds; 2. Climate and hardiness; 3. Soils and soil operations; 4. Specialized gardens; 5. Garden planning and design; 6. Propagation; 7. Plant breeding; 8. Pests; 9. Miscellaneous horticultural operations, special types of gardening, and miscellaneous articles; 10. Special cultural articles on the best varieties and how to grow them. A smaller and handsome encyclopaedia of gardening is: WRIGHT, W. P., 1941: An illustrated encyclopaedia of gardening, 494 p. (London: Dent).

UPHOF, J. C. T., 1968: Dictionary of economic plants, ed. 2, 591 p. (Lehre: Cramer; Hitchin, Herts.: Wheldon & Wesley).—

The first ed. was published in 1959. It lists in alphabetical order some 6,000 species of economic plants and gives brief descriptions of each of them. Cross-indexes of synonyms and vernacular names. The term economic plants comprises all crops "of importance to agriculture, forestry, fruit and vegetable growing, pharmacognosy, (and) also those that are of importance to the world trades as well as plants that are strictly of local value." Ornamental plants are excluded.

WECK, J., ed., 1966: Wörterbuch der Forstwissenschaft. Dictionary of forestry, in five languages: German-English-French-Spanish-Russian, compiled and arranged on a German alphabetical basis, 573 p. (Amsterdam: Elsevier; Munich: Bayrischer Landwirtschaftsverlag).—

Contains *ca.* 10,000 scientific terms arranged alphabetically according to the German language. Indexes in English, French, Spanish, and Russian. Some other dictionaries of forest terminology are: RABER, O., 1939: German-English dictionary for foresters, 346 p. (Washington, D. C.: Forest Service, Dept. of Agriculture); SIMONEN, M. E., 1955: Forestry dictionary: Swedish-English-German-French, 284 p. (Stockholm: Swedish Forestry Assn.). *Cf.* HAWLEY, *supra.*

WELTFORSTATLAS, published by the Bundesanstalt für Forst- und Holzwirtschaft, Reinbek, in collaboration with F.A.O., 1951. (Berlin: Haller).—

Each map covers one country or area, showing distribution of forest types and wood species, location of wood-working industries, *etc.* In 1956, Ronald Press (New York, N.Y.) published "A world geog-

raphy of forest resources", 736 p., consisting of a series of contributions by specialists. The treatment is regional.

WOLFE, L. S., 1949: Farm glossary, 360 p. (Orangeburg, S. C.: L. S. Wolfe).—

In his preface, the author writes that his book is not offered as an exhaustive or technical presentation concerning agriculture and its allied sciences, but is thought to be comprehensive enough to be of real value to farmers, ranchers, salesmen catering to farmers, students of agriculture, rural preachers and teachers, farm editors, farm radio program directors, beginners in professional agriculture and to the many others who seek the broadening influence of reading agricultural literature.

ZANDER, R., 1952: Geschichte des Gärtnertums mit Zeittabellen vom Jahre 30-1935, 120 p. (Stuttgart: Ulmer).—

The greater part of this booklet consists of a concise history of horticulture (p. 1-97); it is more or less restricted to the German-speaking peoples. This history is supplemented by a table (p. 97-112), illustrating the text.

d. *Animal sciences* (incl. apiculture and veterinary science)

BARTHOLOMEW, J. G., 1911: Atlas of zoogeography: a series of maps illustrating the distribution of over seven hundred families, genera and species of existing animals, 6+67+11 p. (Edinburgh: Bartholomew).—

Consists of about 200 maps, "illustrating the present distribution of the higher animals over the surface of the earth". Covers all the families of mammals, birds, reptiles, amphibians, most of the families of fishes, and a selection of families and genera of molluscs and insects. The text deals with such subjects as: general principles of distribution, the history of the geographical distribution, and the explanation of the plates (36 double plates in all). Bibliography of about 1,000 items, arranged by regions and then by animals. Index.

CRANE, E. E., ed., 1951: Dictionary of beekeeping terms with allied scientific terms, 74 p. (London: Bee Research Assn.).—

The main section lists a thousand of English terms used in beekeeping, with

French, German, and Dutch translations. There are separate (alphabetical) indexes of French, German, Dutch, and Latin terms. *Cf.* ROOT, A. I., ed., 1954, *vide infra.*

DALLING, T., ed., 1966: International encyclopaedia of veterinary medicine, 5 vols., 3168 p. (Edinburgh: W. Green; London: Sweet & Maxwell).—

This is by far the most complete existing veterinary encyclopaedia, supplying accurate information. Poultry and other birds and laboratory animals are dealt with in specific articles. Emphasis has been placed on such aspects as diagnosis, differential diagnosis, control, prevention, treatment, and, where appropriate, economic importance. The subjects are arranged in alphabetical order. Many cross-references. Generally, references to the literature on a subject are not included. A one-volume veterinary dictionary is: MILLER, W. C. & G. P. WEST, eds., 1967: Black's veterinary dictionary, ed. 8, 1051 p. (London: Black). This dictionary has been modelled upon the plan and general design of Black's medical dictionary, *vide infra.* A German veterinary dictionary: WIRTH, D., ed., 1956-1958: Lexikon der Therapie und Prophylaxe für Tierärzte, ed. 2, 2 vols., 1588 p. (Munich, Berlin & Vienna: Urban & Schwarzenberg). *Cf.* also: WAMBERG, K. & E. A. MCPHERSON, eds., 1968, *vide infra.*

HUSSON, R., 1964: Glossaire de biologie animale, 280 p. (Paris: Gauthier-Villars).—

A dictionary of terms used in modern biology, "un glossaire des termes spéciaux les plus couramment utilisés, glossaire auquel le non-spécialiste aussi bien que l'étudiant pourra se reporter pour avoir non seulement une orthographe exacte, mais aussi une définition et une explication précise, ainsi que la racine étymologique qui bien souvent éclaire la signification du vocabulaire et en justifie l'emploi." Pure descriptive zoological terms are excluded, as far as possible. This glossary is intended for students of biology, medicine, and agriculture.

JAEGER, E. C., 1931: A dictionary of Greek and Latin combining forms used in zoological names, 157 p. (Springfield, Ill.: Thomas).—

The author writes in his preface: "Over two thousand of the most commonly used Greek and Latin forms that enter into the make-up of zoölogical terms and classificatory names have been catalogued, con-

cisely defined, and illustrated by thousands of familiar examples taken from the standard text books and manuals of zoölogy of the leading British and American publishers. It is especially rich in its explanation of generic names, and of ecological and morphological terms... Each definition has been designed to show if possible the application of the stem forms employed..."

KÉLER, S. von, 1963: Entomologisches Wörterbuch mit besonderer Berücksichtigung der morphologischen Terminologie, ed. 3, 774 p. (Berlin: Akademie Verlag).—

A valuable dictionary of terms used in the fields of insect morphology and systematics and in the field of applied entomology. In this third edition many references to supplementary literature have been included. Many illustrations. The dictionary also contains bibliographies of entomological dictionaries, zoological dictionaries, nomenclators, dictionaries of (natural) science, manuals of entomology, forest- and agricultural entomology, medical and veterinary entomology. A French entomological dictionary is: SEGUY, E., 1967: Dictionnaire des termes techniques d'entomologie élémentaire, 465 p. (Paris: Lechevalier). For an English entomological dictionary, *vide* TORRE-BUENO, *infra.*

KOLLER, G., 1949: Daten zur Geschichte der Zoologie. Zeittafel, Forscherliste, Artentafel, 64 p. (Bonn: Athenäum).—

The greater part of this booklet consists of a time scale summing up the most important zoological discoveries and achievements during the period between 1551 and 1915. It also contains information concerning the foundation of important zoological institutes, societies, gardens, *etc.,* improvements in laboratory techniques, *etc.* There also is a list of birth and death dates of prominent zoologists, and a review of the number of animals known since Linnaeus's time.

LAROUSSE, P., 1967: The Larousse encyclopedia of animal life, 640 p. (New York, N.Y.: McGraw-Hill).—

Of this encyclopaedia 200 pages are devoted to the invertebrates, 130 pages to the fishes, amphibians, and reptiles, and 300 pages to birds and mammals. The book contains some 1,000 illustrations (including some 50 colour-plates). The French original (La vie des animaux, ed. by the late L. BERTIN) is strongly revised by a staff of British authors, and many North American examples and North American common names have been introduced. The work is arranged in a strictly taxonomic order; at the end of the book, a guide to the classification used in the text is included.

LEFTWICH, A. W., 1967: A dictionary of zoology, 319 p. (London: Constable).—

This book includes definitions of all the principal phyla and classes of animals as well as a large number of orders, suborders and families. *Ca.* 4,500 words are defined. There is an appendix on classification and nomenclature. First published 1963 as: A student's dictionary of zoology (290 p.). *Cf.* also: ZIEGLER, H. E. & E. BRESSLAU, 1927, *vide infra.*

MILLER, W. C. & G. P. WEST, eds., 1967: Black's veterinary dictionary, ed. 8, 1017 p. (London: Black).—

The first edition appeared in 1928. A useful and illustrated dictionary of veterinary science, including some aspects of anatomy, physiology, veterinary medicine, animal husbandry, public health matters, and techniques of interest to farmers. *Cf.* DALLING, T., 1966, *vide supra;* and MOULÉ, L., 1913, *vide* section Middle Ages in the West, subsection b.

NEAVE, S. A., ed., 1939-1950: Nomenclator zoologicus: a list of names of genera and subgenera in zoology from the tenth edition of Linnaeus 1758, to the end of 1945, 5 vols. Vol. 1: A-C, 957 p.; vol. 2: D-L, 1025 p.; vol. 3: M-P, 1065 p.; vol. 4: Q-Z, 758 p.; vol. 5: years 1936-1945, 308 p. (London: Zoological Soc. of London).—

About 250,000 entries consisting of name, namer, date, source (journal reference, *etc.),* and genus.

ROOT, A. I., ed., 1954: The ABC and XYZ of bee culture: an encyclopedia pertaining to scientific and practical culture of bees, 703 p. (Medina, Ohio: A. I. Root).—

The first ed. appeared in 1877. An encyclopaedia on bee-keeping. Many of the entries included have been written by various specialists.

SMITH, R. C., 1962: Guide to the literature of the zoological sciences, ed. 6, 232 p. (Minneapolis, Minn.: Burgess).—

A valuable guide. Separate chapters deal with: The literature problems of the scientist (methods of obtaining information); The mechanics of the library and book classifications (libraries and their organization); Bibliographies of the zoological sciences (p. 39-87); Abstract journals; The form of bibliographies; The forms of literature; The preparation of a scientific paper; Taxonomic indexes and literature; Library assignments. The scope of the book makes it useful to a wide range of biologists. A seventh ed. appeared in 1966, ed. by R. C. SMITH & R. H. PAINTER, 238 p.

THOMSON, A. L., ed., 1964: A new dictionary of birds, 928 p. (London & Edinburgh: Nelson).—

An encyclopaedic work dealing with birds in all their aspects, such as: migration, singing, skeleton, falconry, domestication, ringing, photography, folk-lore, heraldry, poetry, music, *etc.,* terms used in ornithology, English names of birds, *etc.* Many illustrations and explanatory diagrams. Many references to other languages, *i.c.* South Italian dialects and Egyptian.

TORRE-BUENO, J. R. de la, 1937: A glossary of entomology. Smith's "An explanation of terms used in entomology", completely revised and rewritten, 336 p. (Brooklyn, N.Y.: Brooklyn Entomological Soc.).—

HAVE

A vocabulary or dictionary of technical terms, furnishing information as to their contents and use. For a German or French entomological dictionary, *cf.* KÉLER, S. von, 1963, *vide supra.*

WAMBERG, K. & E. A. MCPHERSON, eds., 1968: Veterinary encyclopaedia. Diagnosis and treatment: small and large animals. Loose-leaf volumes written entirely for the practitioner, 4 vols., *ca.* 2,700 pages. (Copenhagen: Medical Book Comp.).—

This encyclopaedia covers the whole field of veterinary and surgical science, containing *ca.* 1,000 informative pictures. Recognizing that the last word is never written in any veterinary, surgical or medical subject, the Veterinary Encyclopaedia is bound on the loose-leaf plan. As progress is made or material becomes obsolete or as new discoveries or developments take place, new pages are furnished. The revisions are sent automatically on approval without any obligation. *Cf.* DALLING, 1966, and MILLER & WEST, 1967, *vide supra.*

ZIEGLER, H. E. & E. BRESSLAU, 1927: Zoologisches Wörterbuch. Erklärung der zoologischen Fachausdrücke, ed. 3, 786 p. (Jena: Fischer).—

> A well-known German dictionary of zoological, anatomical, and embryological terminology. Many illustrations. Another useful German zoological dictionary is: HIRSCH-SCHWEIGGER, E., 1925: Zoologisches Wörterbuch, 628 p. (Berlin: de Gruyter). *Cf.* also: LEFTWICH, A. W., 1967, *vide supra*.

e. *Medical sciences* (incl. dentistry, therapy, pharmacy, *etc.*)

ABDERHALDEN, R., 1948: Medizinische Terminologie. Wörterbuch der gesamten Medizin und der verwandten Wissenschaften, 1213 p. (Basel: Schwabe).—

> Besides medical terminology, it includes many chemical, physical, botanical, and zoological terms. *Cf.* DUDEN Wörterbuch medizinischer Fachausdrücke, 1968; and ZETKIN, M., *et al.*, 1964, *vide infra*.

AGARD, W. R. & C. H. BUNTING, 1937: Medical Greek and Latin at a glance, 87 p. (New York, N.Y.: Hoeber).—

> This brief compendium is offered... not as a substitute for a medical dictionary, but to lighten the difficulties of the student with Greek and Latin terms by familiarizing him with the commonly used roots of words, with prefixes and suffixes, and with the compounding of these stems. (From the introduction.) A seemingly comparable book is: MCCULLOCH, J. A., 1962: A medical Greek and Latin workbook, 154 p. (Springfield, Ill.: Thomas). (Not seen). *Cf.* also: ROBERTS, F., 1959, *vide infra*.

ALTSCHUL, E., 1864: Real-Lexicon für homöopatische Arzneimittellehre, Therapie und Arzneibereitungskunde, 450 p. (Lübeck: Bolhoevener).—

> Before describing the properties of each herb, plant or drug, there is a historical note about its discovery and early history and literature.

ANDREWS, E., 1947: A history of scientific English: the story of its evolution based on a study of biomedical terminology, 342 p. (New York, N.Y.: R. R. Smith).—

> So far medical history has been confined to the history of Man and his ideas. This book, however, shows in a very profound manner how a careful philologic dissection of words used to express ideas may serve to elucidate obscure problems, and how medical English has undergone influences of foreign languages. Reference work for the cultured of the professions of biology and medicine. Very complete index.

ARENDS, G., 1948: Volkstümliche Namen der Arzneimittel, Drogen, Heilkräuter und Chemikalien. Eine Sammlung der im Volksmunde gebräuchlichen Benennungen und Handelsbezeichnungen, ed. 13, 262 p. (Berlin, Göttingen & Heidelberg: Springer).—

> Originally written by J. HOLFERT. It consists of a list of names of drugs, herbs, chemicals, *etc.*, used by apothecaries. Included are many folk-names of plants as they are used in Germany, the Netherlands, Luxemburg, Austria, Switzerland, and some parts of Czechoslovakia. A more extensive and somewhat more elaborate work of the same purpose is: BERGER, F., 1954/1955: Synonyma-Lexikon der Heil- und Nutzpflanzen, 1221 p. (Vienna: Oesterreichische Apotheker-Verlags Ges.). A dictionary, more especially dealing with more or less modern therapeutic materials is: BERNOULLI, E. & H. LEHMANN, 1955: Uebersicht der gebräuchlichen und neueren Arzneimittel für Aerzte, Apotheker und Zahnaerzte, 508 p. (Basle: Schwabe). *Cf.* also: HUNNIUS, C., 1966, *vide infra*.

ASCHOFF, L., P. DIEPGEN & H. GOERKE, 1960: Kurze Uebersichtstabelle zur Geschichte der Medizin, ed. 7, 85 p. (Heidelberg, Göttingen & Berlin: Springer).—

> This is the 7th edition of a handy little reference work. It is a guide to the chronology of the advances and discoveries in medicine from the earliest times to the present day. The first 20 pages deal with primitive medicine and with early civilizations, a period during which no exact dates can be given. Extensive indexes of names and subjects have been included. *Cf.* LEIBBRAND, W., 1963; POWER, D'Arcy S. & C. J. S. THOMPSON, 1923; SCHMIDT, J. E., 1959; and VEILLON, E., 1950, *vide infra*.

BAILEY, H. & W. J. BISHOP, 1959: Notable names in medicine and surgery, ed. 3, 216 p. (London: Lewis).—

> This book is especially devoted to students and nurses who want to know who

the people were whose names are connected to eponyms used in general medical practice, in the chemical laboratory, in the factory, in the nursing profession, *etc.* It consists of 83 short biographies, each illustrated with a portrait. Often a picture of the hospital in which they worked and a diagram of what they described have been included. In the third edition many more names are included than in the second edition (1946), but some others have been omitted. For a more thorough discussion of these matters, *vide:* LEIBER, B. & T. OLBERT, *et al.,* 1968: Die klinischen Eponyme. Medizinische Eigennamenbegriffe in Klinik und Praxis, 456 p. (Munich: Urban & Schwarzenberg). *Cf.* also FISCHER, I., 1931; and KELLY, E. C., 1948, *vide infra.*

CLARK, P. F. & A. S., 1942: Memorable days in medicine: a calendar of biology and medicine, 305 p. (Madison, Wisc.: Univ. Wisconsin Press).—

Like a true calendar, this book gives information from day to day about birth and death days of famous medical men (including many biologists), about the foundation of learned societies, colleges, and hospitals, and about dates of the first publication of famous books, *etc. Cf.* SCHMIDT, J. E., 1959, *vide infra.*

DORLAND's illustrated medical dictionary, ed. 24, 1965, 1724 p. (Philadelphia, Pa.: Saunders).—

The contents of this volume are explained in its subtitle: a complete dictionary of the terms used in medicine, surgery, dentistry, pharmacy, chemistry, nursing, veterinary science, biology, medical biography, *etc.*, with the pronunciation, derivation, and definition. There are some 942 illustrations, including 283 portraits. Reprinted 1968. A concise but fairly comprehensive English dictionary is: WAKELEY, C., ed., 1953: The Faber medical dictionary, 471 p. (London: Faber & Faber). This dictionary gives the Anglicized spelling and is as such a useful complement to Dorland's dictionary. *Cf.* also: HOERR, N. L. & A. OSOL, eds., 1956; THOMSON, W. A. R., ed., 1968; and STEDMAN's medical dictionary, *vide infra.*

DUDEN Wörterbuch medizinischer Fachausdrücke, 1968, 56+639 p. (Ed. by K. AHLHEIM, auf Grund einer Materialsammlung von H. LICHTENSTERN) (Mannheim: Bibliographisches Inst.; Stuttgart: Thieme).—

Contains: "Etwa 30,000 Stichwörter aus der Medizin und ihren Randgebieten:

Rechtschreibung, Aussprache, Herkunft, Bedeutung, Verwendungsweise." (From: Deutsche Bibliographie. Das deutsche Buch, 1968: 692-693). *Cf.* ABDERHALDEN, R., 1948, *vide supra.*

DUNNING, W. B. & S. E. DAVENPORT, eds., 1936: A dictionary of dental science and art, comprising the words and phrases proper to dental literature, with their pronunciation and derivation, 635 p. (Philadelphia, Pa.: Blakiston).—

This dictionary gives pronunciation, derivation and definition of dental terms. Reprinted 1947 (London: Churchill). A German, English, French, Spanish dental vocabulary is: HOLZAPFEL, A., 1939: Dental lexicon, 640 p. (Mainz: Medizinische Verlagsanstalt).

EIDELBERG, L., ed., 1968: Encyclopedia of psychoanalysis, 37+571 p. (New York, N.Y.: Hafner).—

"This work establishes a standard for understanding and judging the value of those concepts that are an inherent part of classical psychoanalysis and provides a basis for further changes and additions . . ." (From a publisher's announcement). *Cf.* also: MOORE, B. E., *et al.,* 1967: A glossary of psychoanalytic terms and concepts, 96 p. (New York, N.Y.: Amer. Psychoanalytic Soc.); LAPLANCHE, J. & J. B. PONTALIS, 1967: Vocabulaire de la psychanalyse, 520 p. (Paris: Presses Univ. de France); and: RYCROFT, C., 1968: A critical dictionary of psychoanalysis, 189 p. (London: Nelson).

FISCHER, I., 1931: Die Eigennamen in der Krankheitsterminologie, 143 p. (Vienna & Leipzig: Perles).—

According to Garrison-Morton: the best dictionary of medical eponyms so far produced. It gives references to the original papers and books concerned, and records wherever possible the first use of the eponym. *Cf.* also: BAILEY, H. & W. J. BISHOP, 1959, *vide supra.*

GALTIER-BOISSIÈRE, E., 1923: Larousse médical illustré, 1294 p. (Paris: Larousse).—

A French medical encyclopaedia, containing 2,242 illustrations and 78 synoptic tables. New ed., 1967 (Paris). An extensive French medical encyclopaedia is DECHAMBRE, A., 1864-1889: Dictionnaire encyclopédique des sciences médicales, 100 vols. (Paris: Asselin & Masson).

GARNIER, M. & V. DELAMARE, 1945: Dictionnaire des termes techniques de médecine, ed. 14, 909 p. (Paris: Maloine).—

The scope and contents of this French dictionary can best be described by giving its full title: Dictionnaire des termes techniques de médecine, contenant: les étymologies grecques et latines, les noms des maladies, des opérations chirurgicales et obstétricales, les symptômes cliniques, des lésions anatomiques, les termes de laboratoire, *etc.*

HOCKING, G. M., 1955: A dictionary of terms in pharmacognosy and other divisions of economic botany, 284 p. (Springfield, Ill.: Thomas).—

The book gives definitions of terms used in pharmacognosy arranged in an alphabetical order. According to the author himself the term pharmacognosy is "now generally restricted to the science of crude drugs, that branch of pharmacy relating to medicinal substances from the plant, animal, and mineral kingdoms in their natural, crude, or unprepared state, or in the form of such primary derivatives as oils, waxes, gums, and resins." The dictionary is designed to meet the special needs of students and practitioners in the various health professions and of people in trade and industry.

HÖFLER, M., 1899: Deutsches Krankheitsnamen-Buch, 922 p. (Munich: Piloty & Löhle).—

"Verfasser spricht die Hoffnung aus, dass sein Buch dem praktischen Aerzte, dem Mediziner überhaupt, dem Freunde der Medizin und Kulturgeschichte, dem Germanisten, Mythologen, Folkloristen, sogar dem Botaniker etwas Brauchbares bieten wird." (From a book review in Janus 4: 314).

HOERR, N. L. & A. OSOL, eds., 1956: Blakiston's new Gould Medical Dictionary: a modern comprehensive dictionary of the terms used in all branches of medicine and allied sciences, ed. 2, 1463 p. (New York, N.Y.: McGraw-Hill).—

A very extensive medical lexicon, containing nearly 100,000 brief entries, indicating pronunciation and including much biographical information. An appendix covering more than 100 pages consists of tabulated data on anatomy, blood constituents, enzymes, hormones, isotopes, *etc. Cf.* also DORLAND's illustrated medical dictionary, *vide supra,* and STEDMAN's medical dictionary, *vide infra.*

HUNNIUS, C., 1966: Pharmazeutisches Wörterbuch, ed. 4, 858 p. (Berlin: de Gruyter).—

An up-to-date standard dictionary of pharmacy. *Cf.* ARENDS, G., 1948, *vide supra;* and MARLER, E. E. J., 1961, *vide infra.*

JAEGER, E. C., 1953: A source-book of medical terms, 145 p. (Springfield, Ill.: Thomas).—

In this book are assembled in alphabetical sequence the word-elements, combining forms, prefixes and suffixes from which modern medical terms have been coined. Included are the Greek, Latin, French or other words from which they were derived, together with their original meaning. A separate section deals with the basic principles and formal rules used in the construction or synthesis of words. *Cf.* ROBERTS, F., 1959, *vide infra.*

KELLY, E. C., 1948: Encyclopedia of medical sources, 476 p. (Baltimore, Md.: Williams & Wilkins).—

This encyclopaedia lists more than 70,000 items, most of which are names of physicians. Each personal name is followed by a concise statement of the subject's nationality, field of work, and dates. Principal contributions are listed, each of which is supplemented by one or more bibliographical citations. The purpose of the book is to provide the reader with key references to source material. *Cf.* BAILEY, H. & W. J. BISHOP, 1959, *vide supra.*

LEIBBRAND, W., 1963: Kompendium der Medizingeschichte, 242 p. (Munich: Banaschewski).—

As the title indicates, this is a compendium, giving the most essential events of the history of medicine in a few lines *(e.g.,* medicine in Egypt, p. 16-21; China, p. 30-31; Byzantine medicine, p. 60-64; surgery in the 18th century, p. 129-132; history of plague, p. 187-189; dental surgery, p. 223-224). Few bibliographical references, but extensive index of personal names. *Cf.* ASCHOFF, L., *et al.,* 1960, *vide supra.*

LEIBER, B. & G. OLBRICH, 1966: Wörterbuch der klinischen Syndrome, ed. 4, 1133 p. Vol. I: Syndrome; Vol. II: Symptomenregister. (Munich & Berlin: Urban & Schwarzenberg).—

About 440 syndromes (for the greater part eponyms) are described with their synonyms, definitions, biographical data about the authors concerned (with year of first description), symptoms, aetiology and pathogenesis, differential diagnosis, literature references, and classification (according to the decimal and WHO classification). P. 653-966: "Symptomenregister". The data about authors, first descriptions and literature references have been prepared in such a careful and critical way that this is an invaluable work for all concerned with the history of clinical medicine. A fourth edition appeared in 1966 in 2 vols. A book of the same scope is: DURHAM, R. H., 1960: Encyclopedia of medical syndromes, 628 p. (New York, N.Y.: Hoeber). The book contains some 1,000 entries in alphabetical order, each syndrome is described, its synonyms listed; historical information and references are included. *Cf.* also: PSCHYREMBEL, W., 1969: Klinisches Wörterbuch mit klinischen Syndromen, new ed., 1348 p. + 2275 illus. (Founded by O. DORNBLÜTH) (Berlin: de Gruyter).

LINDNER, J., 1957: Zeittafeln zur Geschichte der pharmakologischen Institute des deutschen Sprachgebietes, 167 p. (Aulendorf: Cantor).—

> The first part contains a review of pharmacological institutions in the German-speaking countries with a chronological review of their teachers. The second part consists of short biographical reviews of the persons mentioned in the first part, and a third part contains a review of pharmacological laboratories of the industry. Bibliography and index.

LOUROS, N. C., 1964: Glossaire des termes obstétricaux et gynécologiques, 444 p. (Amsterdam, London & New York, N.Y.: Elsevier).—

> This dictionary contains 2,576 entries in French, Latin, English, Russian, German, Spanish, Italian, and Greek of terms currently used in obstetrics and gynaecology and authorized by the Fédération Internationale de Gynécologie et d'Obstétrique, Geneva.

MARLER, E. E. J., ed., 1961: Pharmacological and chemical synonyms, ed. 3, 267 p. (Amsterdam, London & New York, N.Y.: Excerpta Medica Foundation).—

> A collection of more than 13,000 names of drugs and other compounds drawn from the medical literature of the world;

it is meant as a guide to the identification of substances which appear under a variety of names.

MAYRHOFER, B., 1937: Kurzes Wörterbuch zur Geschichte der Medizin, 224 p. (Jena: Fischer).—

> "An index of medical men and discoveries containing very brief biographic sketches and useful notes giving dates of first descriptions of diseases, operations, *etc.* A useful volume for quick reference." (After Doe & Marshall, p. 388).

The NOMENCLATURE OF DISEASES, drawn up by a Joint Committee appointed by the Royal College of Physicians of London, ed. 8, 1961, 398 p. (London: H.M. Stationery Office).—

> This book provides a list of "approved terms for describing and recording abnormal and pathological observations". Included are synonyms and lists of eponyms. This 1961 edition has since been reprinted (last reprint 1968).

PARR, J. A. & R. A. YOUNG, 1965: Parr's concise medical encyclopaedia, 514 p. (Amsterdam, London & New York, N.Y.: Elsevier).—

> Medical concepts and expressions have been defined and explained in clear, concise and non-technical language. This down-to-earth treatment of the subject makes it suitable for the many non-medical people who frequently have to deal with medical terminology. 11,000 entries. (From a publisher's announcement).

PEPPER, O. H. P., 1949: Medical etymology: the history and derivation of medical terms for students of medicine, dentistry and nursing, 263 p. (Philadelphia, Pa.: Saunders).—

> A history of medical terms for students of medicine, dentistry and nursing. The terms are grouped under subjects beginning with anatomy; the vocabularies of the clinical subjects are last. *Cf.* ROBERTS, F., 1959, *vide infra*.

PODOLSKY, E., ed., 1953: Encyclopaedia of aberrations: a psychiatric handbook, 550 p. (London: Arco).—

> An alphabetically arranged dictionary of psychopathology, offering brief defi-

nitions of unfamiliar terms and, in other instances, short articles representing summaries of various psychiatric subjects. It includes such subjects as: mental disturbances related to organic diseases of the brain, juvenile delinquency, alcoholism, hallucinations, delusions, *etc.* A large French dictionary considering the same kind of topics is CHOISY, M., ed., 1949: Dictionnaire de psycho-analyse et psychotechnique, 1200 p. (Paris: Psyché). *Cf.* POROT, A., 1960, *infra.*

POROT, A., 1960: Manuel alphabétique de psychiatrie clinique et thérapeutique, ed. 2, 560 p. (Paris: Presses Univ. de France).—

    An alphabetically arranged dictionary of psychiatry, psychoanalysis, and the pathogenesis of mental disorders. *Cf.* PODOLSKY, E., 1953, *supra.*

POWER, D'Arcy, S. & C. J. S. THOMPSON, 1923: Chronologia medica: a handlist of persons, periods and events in the history of medicine, 278 p. (London: Bale).—

    A chronology of the chief persons in the history of the healing art from traditional times up to the present. Some interesting details concerning each person, epoch, or event, have been added. *Cf.* ASCHOFF, L., *et al.,* 1960, *vide supra.*

PRINZ, H., 1945: Dental chronology: a record of the more important historic events in the evolution of dentistry, 189 p. (Philadelphia, Pa.: Lea & Febiger).—

    A concise chronological survey of the history of dentistry with valuable references for further reading. The appendix contains tables on such subjects as: important dates relating to the introduction of general anaesthesia; important dates related to the introduction of local anaesthesia; the evolution of the extracting instruments; and chronological data on the invention of porcelain teeth.

ROACH, L. K. & E. S., 1951: A dictionary of antibiosis, 373 p. (New York, N.Y.: Columbia U.P.).—

    An alphabetical list of antibiotic substances, plants from which they are derived, and test organisms, together with technical data. Bibliography included.

ROBERTS, F., 1959: Medical terms: their origin and construction, ed. 3, 92 p. (London: Heinemann).—

    The book explains in an easy way the origin of many medical terms and it sets out to make easier and more interesting the studies of those medical students who were deprived of knowledge of the classics. *Cf.* SKINNER, H. A., 1961; VOLKMANN, H., 1948; WAIN, H., 1958; *vide infra;* and AGARD, W. R. & C. H. BUNTING, 1937; JAEGER, E. C., 1953; PEPPER, O. H. P., 1949,*vide supra.*

SCHMIDT, J. E., 1959: Medical discoveries: who and when, 555 p. (Springfield, Ill.: Thomas).—

    Its contents are fairly well described by its subtitle: "A dictionary listing thousands of medical and related scientific discoveries in alphabetical order, giving in each case the name of the discoverer, his profession, nationality, and floruit, and the date of the discovery." The "first" or presumed first description of a disease, operation, procedure, instrument, invention, *etc.* is described and annotated. Included are many references to dentistry, pharmacy, and some other related fields of medicine. *Cf.* ASCHOFF, L., *et al.,* 1960; and also: CLARK, P. F. & A. S., 1942, *vide supra.*

SCHNEIDER, W., ed., 1962: Lexikon alchemistisch-pharmazeutischer Symbole, 140 p. (Weinheim: Verlag Chemie).—

    A useful dictionary of alchemical symbols and terms. The text has been divided into three parts. The first part consists of a facsimile reprint of the anonymously published "Medicinisch-Chymisch- und Alchemistisch Oraculum" (Ulm, 1755), a dictionary of alchemical symbols and terms as they were used by physicians, apothecaries, chemists and alchemists during the Middle Ages. A second part contains information supplementary to the terms included and the third part consists of an index and a list of synonyms.

——, 1968: Lexikon zur Arzneimittelgeschichte. Sachwörterbuch zur Geschichte der pharmazeutischen Botanik, Chemie, Mineralogie, Pharmakologie, Zoologie, 4 vols. Vol. I (1968): Tierische Drogen. Sachwörterbuch zur Geschichte der pharmazeutischen Zoologie, 92 p.; Vol. II (1968): Pharmakologische Arzneimittelgruppen. Sachwörterbuch zu ihrer Geschichte, 92 p.; Vol. III (1968): Pharmazeutische Chemikalien und Mineralien. Sachwörterbuch zur Geschichte der pharmazeutischen Chemie und Mineralogie, 412 p.; Vol. IV (1969): Geheimmittel und

Spezialitäten. Sachwörterbuch zu ihrer Geschichte bis um 1900, 307 p. (Frankfurt a. M.: Govi).—

> These are the first four vols. of a greater lexicon (consisting of *ca.* 7 vols.), dealing with the history of medicaments. In the first vol. the author discusses the role animal medicaments have played in the course of time and for which purposes they have been used; in the second vol. medicaments with a similar function (such as: splanchnica, splenetica, stimulantia, stomachica, aphrodisiaca, *etc.*) are considered; in the third vol. those chemical and mineral substances which have been used as medicaments are enumerated and their chemical composition explained; and in the fourth volume attention has been paid to medicaments of a vegetable origin.

SCHUURMANS STEKHOVEN, W., 1955: Geneeskundig woordenboek. Engels-Nederlands. Nederlands-Engels, ed. 2, 284 p. (Amsterdam: de Bussy).—

> An English-Dutch and Dutch-English medical dictionary written primarily for students and nurses.

SKINNER, H. A., 1961: The origin of medical terms, ed. 2, 437 p. (Baltimore, Md.: Williams & Wilkins).—

> A general reference work of medical terms particularly directed toward the basic medical sciences: anatomy, physiology and pathology. It explains the origin and history of the words used; these words are arranged alphabetically. Many terms incorporate the personal name of the discoverer, and in these cases brief biographies of these discoverers have been included. *Cf.* ROBERTS, F., 1959, *vide supra.*

SLIOSBERG, A., ed., 1964: Elsevier's medical dictionary in five languages, English/American, French, Italian, Spanish and German, 1588 p. (Amsterdam, London & New York, N.Y.: Elsevier).—

> This volume comprises some 35,000 terms taken from all branches of medical science, and covering in the most practical way the standard terminology of the languages mentioned in the title. A separate list of the most commonly encountered English synonyms is included. Columnwise translations and cross-keyed indexes for each of the languages represented. *Cf.* VEILLON, E., ed., 1950, *vide infra,* especially CLAIRVILLE's polyglot dictionary.

—— ed., 1968: Dictionary of pharmaceutical science and techniques in five languages: English, French, Italian, Spanish, German. Vol. I: Pharmaceutical technology, compiled and arranged on an English alphabetical basis, 686 p. (Amsterdam, London & New York, N.Y.: Elsevier).—

> "Contents: This dictionary contains the equivalents of 7,507 technical terms used in pharmaceutical technology. The work comprises a basic table of the English terms and their synonyms arranged alphabetically, followed by their translation in French, Italian, Spanish and German. The section part includes indexes of each of these languages with a reference to the number in the basic table where corresponding translations into the other languages can be found." (After a publisher's announcement in Nature 220: xv, Dec. 21, 1968). A second vol., dealing with materia medica is in preparation. It will contain approximately 6,000 entries in English, French, Italian, Spanish, German, and Latin. *Ca.* 650 pages.

STEDMAN's medical dictionary: a vocabulary of medicine and its allied sciences, with pronunciations and derivations, ed. 21, 1966, 49+1836 p. (Baltimore, Md.: Williams & Wilkins; Edinburgh & London: Livingstone).—

> A very useful medical dictionary comparable to DORLAND's *(vide supra).* Since the 20th edition (1961), 9,183 new words have been included. No etymological explanations; the book has been compiled primarily for practical purposes.

STEEN, E. B., 1968: Dictionary of abbreviations in medicine and the related sciences, ed. 2, 102 p. (London: Cassell).—

> A source of reference and an attempt at standardization of abbreviations used in medical and related literature. Another little volume of the same scope is: PEYSER, A., 1950: Pars pro toto: breviarium medicum internationale, 196 p. (Stockholm: Almqvist & Wiksell). A polyglot repertory of abbreviations has been edited by LEREBOULLET, J., W. TRUMMERT & G. D. KRASSNOFF (n.d.): Abréviations utilisées en médecine et en biologie médicale (published by the Union internationale de la presse médicale). The following languages are included: French, German, English, Italian, Spanish, and Portuguese.

STEINBICHLER, E., 1963: Lexikon für die Apothekenpraxis in sieben Sprachen mit fünf selbständigen Alphabeten und einer pharmazeutischen Phraseologie, 488 p. (Frankfurt a.M.: Govi).—

Contains *ca.* 2,500 equivalents in German, English, French, Spanish, Italian, Greece, Russian of all terms used in pharmacy. *Cf.* also: Glossario europeo dei termini farmaceutici, 114 p. (Milan: Library A.E.I.O.U.).

TCHERNICHOWSKY, S., ed., 1934: Dictionary of medecine and allied sciences: Latin-English-Hebrew, 790 p. (Jerusalem).—

"Very elaborate dictionary, containing the Hebrew equivalents of some sixty-three thousand medical and scientific terms." (G. Sarton in Isis 33: 390).

THOMSON, W. A. R., ed., 1968: Black's medical dictionary, ed. 28, 1014 p.+400 illus. (London: Black).—

A popular encyclopaedia devoted to domestic medicine. *Cf.* DORLAND's illustrated medical dictionary, *vide supra*.

UNESCO list of world medical periodicals, 237 p. (Paris: Unesco).—

For more details, *vide* subsection a, WORLD LIST. *Cf.* also the UNION CATALOG of Medical Periodicals I and II, published by the Medical Library Center of New York (New York, N.Y.).

UNSELD, D. W., 1968: Medizinisches Wörterbuch der deutschen und englischen Sprache, ed. 5, 511 p. (Stuttgart: Wissenschaftliche Verlagsgesell.).—

Standard dictionary (English-German and German-English). Included are many terms used in veterinary medicine, pharmacy, chemistry, and physics. *Cf.* VEILLON, E., ed., 1950, *vide infra*.

VALENTIN, H., 1950: Geschichte der Pharmazie und Chemie in Form von Zeittafeln. Unter besonderer Berücksichtigung der Verhältnisse in Deutschland, ed. 3, 126 p. (Stuttgart: Wissenschaftliche Verlagsgesell.).—

A chronology of pharmaceutical history. Many points of contact with cultural history are indicated. The subject-matter has been divided into 3 main sections, *viz.*, antiquity (Mesopotamia, Egypt, Persia, the Semites, India, China, Greece, Rome), the Middle Ages (incl. the Arabs), and modern developments (from the 16th century onwards, p. 27 ff.).

VEILLON, E., ed., 1950: Medizinisches Wörterbuch, 476+496+435 p. (Bern: Huber).—

With the contributions of many specialists, this work consists of three distinct alphabetical vocabularies, *viz.*, German-English-French; French-German-English; English-French-German, each arranged in three synoptic columns. The book is primarily intended for the research worker and general practitioner. The largest polyglot dictionary of medical terms is CLAIR-VILLE, A. L., 1950 →: Dictionnaire polyglotte des termes médicaux. Vol. I (ed. 2, 1955): Français-anglais-allemand-latin; Vol. II (1952): Portuguese supplement; Vol. III (1952): Version española; Vol. IV (1955): Italian supplement. (Paris: S.I.P.U.C.O.). Arabic, Dutch, and other supplements are in preparation.

VIERORDT, H., 1916: Medizin-geschichtliches Hilfsbuch mit besonderer Berücksichtigung der Entdeckungsgeschichte und der Biographie, 469 p. (Tübingen: Laupp).—

This book is in two parts, the first part containing a list by authors of remarkable medical books and writings (p. 1-326), the second part containing a list of authors with short biographical information. Elaborate subject-index. *Cf.* ASCHOFF, L., *et al.*, 1960, *vide supra*.

VOLKMANN, H., 1948: Medizinische Terminologie. Ableitung und Erklärung der gebräuchlichsten Fachausdrücke aller Zweige der Medizin und ihrer Hilfswissenschaften, ed. 34, 522 p. (Berlin & Munich: Urban & Schwarzenberg).—

A medical dictionary with many illustrations. Included are many terms from the fields of chemistry, physics, botany and zoology. Explanations of the Latin and Greek stems. The first edition appeared in 1902. *Cf.* ROBERTS, F., 1959, *vide supra*.

WAIN, H., 1958: The story behind the word: some interesting origins of medical terms, 342 p. (Springfield, Ill.: Thomas; Oxford: Blackwell).—

A medical lexicography containing over 5,700 medical terms, including the principal eponyms and many recently-coined words. The words are arranged alphabetically. *Cf.* ROBERTS, F., 1959, *vide supra.*

ZETKIN, M., E. H. KÜHTZ & K. FICHTEL, 1964: Wörterbuch der Medizin, ed. 2, 1087 p. (Berlin: Volk und Gesundheit).—

"Das Wörterbuch der Medizin" ist eine Terminologie für Aerzte aller Fachgebiete und Wirkungskreise, für Studenten und für das mittlere medizinische Personal und bringt die notwendigen Ausdrücke aller Fachgebiete der Medizin in sorgfältig erwogener Auswahl." (From the preface). *Cf.* ABDERHALDEN, R., 1948, *vide supra.*

1. PHILOSOPHY OF THE LIFE SCIENCES AND THEIR HISTORICAL ASPECTS

ANDRÉ, H., 1931: Urbild und Ursache in der Biologie, 371 p. (Munich: Oldenbourg).—

"After the historical introduction, this work discusses from a philosophical point of view the struggle of the mathematical with the biological and anthropomorphic interpretation during the last century, giving in detail the contributions of Driesch, Scheler, Buytendijk, Plessner, Friedmann and Hartmann; it then applies these theories to present-day botanical problems, discussing morphogenesis, death and rejuvenescence in the individual and in the larger groups, and phylogeny from the aspect of metabolism, convergence, divergence, *etc.*" (after Biol. Abstr. 7: 764).

ARBER, A., 1950: The natural philosophy of plant form, 247 p. (Cambridge: U.P.).—

The book contains elements of science, philosophy, and history, and the whole is dominated by a teleological viewpoint. Some chapters are of a historical character: chapter 2 deals particularly with Aristotelian morphology and Theophrastos's theories. In chapter 3 these theories are traced into the Middle Ages (Albertus Magnus and Cesalpino) and chapter 4 bears the title "Plant morphology from Joachim Jung to Goethe and de Candolle". This historical approach serves as an introduction to a new theory of form.

BAVINCK, B., 1924: Ergebnisse und Probleme der Naturwissenschaft. Eine Einführung in die moderne Naturphilosophie, ed. 3, 470 p. (Leipzig: Hirzel).—

Deals largely with the problems of biology and evolution in the 19th century.

BERNAL, J. D., 1967: The origin of life, 345 p. (London: Weidenfeld & Nicolson; Cleveland, O.: World).—

In his preface the author writes: "We are here trying to settle a question of a different character from those of the rest of science; it is not merely a description ... but an attempt to carry out an intellectual reconstruction based on assumptions of inner logic themselves drawn from experimental science here and now". The book contains much that is of interest from the historical point of view.

BERTALANFFY, L. v., 1933: Modern theories of development: an introduction to theoretical biology, 204 p. (London: Oxford U.P.).—

This book is an annotated translation (by J. H. WOODGER) of von Bertalanffy's "Kritische Theorie der Formbildung", 1928, 243 p. (Berlin: Borntraeger). It is a discussion and evaluation of theories current around the thirties, in which biological development is considered from the organismic point of view; at the same time it is an attempt to overthrow the old contradiction between mechanism and vitalism.

BLOCH, K., 1956: Zur Theorie der naturwissenschaftlichen Systematik. Unter besonderer Berücksichtigung der Biologie, 138 p. (Acta Biotheoretica, Suppl. I) (Leiden: Brill).—

This book is in two parts. The first 50 pages contain a discussion of some basic concepts, such as: principle, abstraction, reality, general and individual, *etc.* The second part consists of a theory of systematics in general (p. 52-79) and a discussion of the fundamental principles on which biological systematics rest, their specific character, the various ways in which biological systems may be and have been interpreted, the reality of biological systems and their ultimate goals and results.

BLUM, H. F., 1951: Time's arrow and evolution, 222 p. (Princeton, N.J.: Princeton U.P.).—

By time's arrow is essentially meant the Second Law of thermodynamics, as a key concept in his thesis to show how the nature and evolution of the non-living world place limits upon the nature and evolution of life. *Cf.* NICOL, H., 1967, The limits of Man, *infra,* which also relies on entropy and the Second Law.

BREWSTER, E. T., 1927: Creation: a history of non-evolutionary theories, 295 p. (Indianapolis, Ind.: Bobbs-Merrill).—

This book essentially contains a history of creationist theories, *i.e.,* such theories as those of spontaneous generation, primitive special creationism, catastrophic special creationism, uniformitarian special creationism, and evolutionism.

BUNGE, M., 1959: Causality: the place of the causal principle in modern science, 380 p. (Cambridge, Mass.: Harvard U.P.).—

A very provocative book in which the author tries to analyse the concept of causality. Some interesting aspects of the author's point of view are 1) that not everything that exists needs to be explained and 2) that there are other forms of determinism besides causal determinism. Both notions - causality as well as determinism - are crucial notions in biology and they were that also in the past. Because the author combines a vast range of the knowledge of science with a thorough knowledge of the history both of science and of philosophy, this book contains many points of interest for the historically-minded biologist.

BUTLER, J. A. V., 1951: Man is a microcosm, 159 p. (New York, N.Y.: Macmillan).—

A survey of our knowledge of the nature and basis of life, with particular reference to man.

CHILDE, V. G., 1951: Man makes himself, 192 p. (A Mentor book) (New York, N.Y.: New American Library).—

A very readable introduction dealing with such subjects as: human and natural history, organic evolution and cultural progress, time scales, food gatherers, the Neolithic revolution, prelude to the second revolution, the urban revolution, the revolution in human knowledge, and the acceleration and retardation of progress. With index. Originally published in 1936, 275 p. (London: Watts). Reissued 1939, rev. ed., 1941. *Cf.* also: CHILDE, V. G., 1963: Social evolution, 191 p. (Toronto: S. J. R. Saunders), a reprint of the book first published by Watts (London), 1951. It contains the text of the Josiah Mason lectures on anthropology 1947-'48.

DARLINGTON, C. D., 1955: The facts of life, 467 p. (New York, N.Y.: Macmillan).—

The author tries to give an answer to the fundamental problems of biology: What is life, Where did it come from, What

"forces" operate upon it, and Can Man influence his own evolution? In order to come nearer to a solution of these problems, the first part of the book develops the history of evolution and genetics, especially during the period after the publication of the "Origin of Species", in which part the author tries to discover the underlying factors which caused science to develop as it did. A chapter describing the rise and fall of Lysenkoism follows, and the latter part of the book covers topics such as: Man as an individual and as a member of society, sex and temperament, marriage and fertility, irrational elements in human behaviour, the biological interpretation of history. *Cf.* HARDIN, G., 1959, *vide infra.*

DOBZHANSKY, T., 1956: The biological basis of human freedom, 139 p. (New York, N.Y.: Columbia U.P.).—

Whereas man is a part of nature, he is a subject for biological investigation, whatever may be his additional qualities. From this point of view Dobzhansky discusses heredity as a basis for human culture. According to this view, present men are the result of the interaction of our biological and cultural evolution and we have to understand the basic principles of both kinds of evolution in order to understand how our species came to be as it is. The text consists of the Page-Barbour lectures for 1954 at the University of Virginia.

DRIESCH, H., 1905: Der Vitalismus als Geschichte und als Lehre, 246 p. (Leipzig: Barth).—

The first part of this book (p. 1-167) deals with the history of vitalism in a rather elaborate way, and as such is of great biohistorical value. Among the older vitalists are discussed: Aristotle, Harvey, Stahl, K. F. Wolff, and some nature philosophers; among the neovitalists, *inter alia.* E. von Hartmann and E. Montgomery. Special attention is paid to Kant's "Critique of judgment". The book deals also shortly with the materialistic reaction of the preceding century, culminating in the Darwinian theory. The second part of the book is devoted to the learning of vitalism and is of less biohistorical value. Also in English: The history and theory of vitalism, 1914, 239 p. (London: Macmillan). Second edition entitled: Geschichte des Vitalismus, 1922, 213 p. (Leipzig: Barth). *Cf.* WHEELER, L. R., 1939, *vide infra.*

GEDDA, L., 1961: Twins in history and science, 240 p. (Springfield, Ill.: Thomas).—

Besides the genetic, embryological, and anatomical aspects of twin-studies, the author deals with many aspects of biohistorical importance, *e.g.,* superstition and folk practices, legends about twins in Persian, India, Greek, Roman, and North American mythology, twins in the arts, the historical development of the scientific study of twins *(e.g.,* Hippocrates, Empedocles, Democritos, Aristotle, Galen, Cicero, *etc.).* Very beautiful illustrations.

GRENE, M., 1968: Approaches to a philosophical biology, 295 p. (New York, N.Y.: Basic Bks.).—

The text consists essentially of a summary of the works and thoughts of Adolf Portmann, Helmuth Plessner, F. J. J. Buytendijk, Erwin W. Strauss, and Kurt Goldstein, who are all representatives of the holistic approach to biology.

HARDIN, G., 1959: Nature and Man's fate, 375 p. (New York, N.Y.: Rinehart).—

This book deals with the essential biological questions: What is life? From where did it come? How did it reach its present stage? and What about its future?, questions which are directly relevant to our own existence. In connection the author briefly reviews Darwinian evolution theory. The book is intended for all interested in human life, but not quite for the professional biologist. *Cf.* DARLINGTON, C. D., 1955, *vide supra.*

HARTMANN, M., 1956: Einführung in die allgemeine Biologie und ihre philosophischen Grund- und Grenzfragen, 132 p. (Sammlung Göschen, Vol. 96) (Berlin: de Gruyter).—

A very readable semi-popular introduction into the methodology of biology. A first chapter deals with the contents of the science of biology. According to the author, the phenomena of assimilation and dissimilation, sensitiveness, and inconsistency of form are the main criteria of the living organism; the science of genetics ought to be considered as the central science of biology. In a second chapter the author deals with the philosophical foundation of biology; the author appears to belong to the neo-Kantian school of philosophy. In a third chapter some of these principles are applied to some problems of biology, *viz.,* the difference between organic and inorganic nature, the origin of life, causality *vs.* finality, the mind-body problem, and the controversy between mechanism and vitalism.

LIPPMANN, O. von, 1933: Urzeugung und Lebenskraft. Zur Geschichte dieser Probleme von den ältesten Zeiten an bis zu den Anfängen des 20. Jahrhunderts, 136 p. (Berlin: Springer).—

The book contains much material concerning the history of opinions about the origin of life and the nature of the vital force. The author gives the opinions of men of science as well as of speculative philosophers from antiquity up to the beginning of the 20th century. He concludes that not much has altered during these 25 centuries of thought on these problems, which, according to the author, do not belong to natural (physical) science, but are problems belonging to the realm of metaphysics. Reprint announced (Wiesbaden: Sändig).

MEYER-ABICH, A., 1963: Geistesgeschichtliche Grundlagen der Biologie, 322 p. (Stuttgart: Fischer).—

In this book the author tries to analyse the historical and cultural background from which the various biological disciplines originate. Thus, *e.g.,* morphology finds its origin in the works of Aristotle, Plato, *etc.* (which still finds its expression in idealistic morphology); physiology finds its origin in the causal and mechanistic principles of Cartesianism and Kantianism; phylogeny typically is a child of the 19th century, when the historical point of view stood in the centre of interest. An introductory chapter deals with probiology (considering the definition, logic, and classification of biology), and a last chapter deals with metabiology.

——, 1964: The historico-philosophical background of the modern evolution-biology, 170 p. (Acta Biotheoretica, Vol. 13, Suppl. secundum) (Leiden: Brill).—

This book consists of a series of 9 lectures delivered at the Dept. of Zoology, Univ. of Texas in Austin, Texas, U.S.A. The first lecture deals with problems of probiology, historico-philosophical definition, and classification of biology; the second lecture contains some introductory remarks about phenomenology, metaphysics and logic of biological knowledge; the third and fourth lectures treat of the historico-philosophical background of taxonomy and morphology in their relationship to evolution; the fifth and sixth lectures deal with the historico-philosophical background of physiology and ecology in their relationship to evolution; the seventh and eight lectures deal with the historico-philosophical background of phylogeny in its relationship to evolution; and the ninth lecture considers problems of metabiology.

MITTERER, A., 1947: Die Zeugung der Organismen, insbesondere des Menschen. Nach dem Weltbild des Hl. Thomas von Aquin und dem der Gegenwart, 240 p. (Vienna: Herder).—

In Isis 41: 339, G. Sarton writes about this book: "A study of procreation, especially in man, with continuous and abundant references to the Latin text of St. Thomas, the other half by Professor Mitterer. This is enough to prove the uptodateness of St. Thomas' teaching in Catholic circles. A good part of his wisdom applies to all men, whether Catholic or not. Latin and German indices."

NEUBURGER, M., 1930: The doctrine of the healing power of nature throughout the course of time, 184 p. (New York, N.Y.: Author).—

The original title was "Die Lehre von der Heilkraft der Natur im Wandel der Zeiten", 1926, 212 p. (Stuttgart: Enke). It is the standard work in this field. In it the author traces the role of the "vis naturae medicatrix", the healing force of Hippocrates, through the history of medicine. The author makes clear how new discoveries and a better understanding of the mechanism of normal and pathological reactions led to a gradual enrichment of this originally mystical concept.

NICOL, H., 1967: The limits of Man: an enquiry into the scientific bases of human population, 283 p. (London: Constable).—

In this book the author discusses population from the strictly scientific standpoint. "The book is founded on the absolute unity of nature in giving 'nothing for nothing' in every chemical, biological and thermodynamic respect, and thus controlling the recent rise in population through adoption of fossil fuel (oxidisable substances) for food-production, notably since about 1880 - a factor which historians, sociologists, etc. have overlooked in its chemical i.e., population, connotations. Equally confidently, a decline in human population (and cultural achievement) back to the level of approximately mediaeval times is foreseeable within a few centuries." (Summary by H. Nicol).

ROTHSCHUH, K. E., 1959: Theorie des Organismus. Bios, Psyche, Pathos, 330 p.

155

(Munich & Berlin: Urban & Schwarzenberger).—

An attempt to construct an organismic theory based upon the result of the experimental sciences, such as: physics, chemistry, biology, physiology, pathology, and psychology, written by an outstanding physiologist and theoretical biologist. Cf. ROTHSCHUH, K. E., 1936: Theoretische Biologie und Medizin, 203 p. (Berlin: Junker & Dünnhaupt).

——, 1965: Prinzipien der Medizin. Ein Wegweiser durch die Medizin, 298 p. (Munich & Berlin: Urban & Schwarzenberger).—

The text is in two parts. The first part (p. 1-126) is of a more or less general character, considering such matters as: concept, self-evidence, and subjects of medicine; grouping, structure and classification of medicine; Principia medica normativa (incl. a section on rights and duties of the physician); methodology of medical knowledge; Man in the light of a medico-scientifically-founded anthropology. The special part deals with such aspects as: Man and disease, principles of somatopathology; psychopathology and psychosomatics; sickness, health, and care of health; diagnostics, prognosis, and therapy. Bibliography and index.

SCHAXEL, J., 1922: Grundzüge der Theorienbildung in der Biologie, ed. 2, 367 p. (Jena: Fischer).—

In this book the author tries to make an inventory of all elements composing biological theories. The first part: "Der Theoriengehalt der Biologie", contains examples from the various theories and disciplines together composing the science of biology, e.g., from Darwinism, phylogeny, developmental physiology, genetics, physiology, mechanism, vitalism, etc. The second part contains an analysis of these elements, which are reduced to some basic principles, viz., the energetic, the historic, and the organismic principles. In the third part the author tries to set up order in these matters, and to formulate the main problems of general biology in a new and logical way.

TSCHULOK, S., 1910: Das System der Biologie in Forschung und Lehre. Eine historisch-kritische Studie, 409 p. (Jena: Fischer).—

Essentially, this book is a historico-critical study of biological concepts. The first part deals with the evolution of the ideas concerning the distinction and inter-

156

relation of the various disciplines into a system of biology. Especially the systems of A. P. de Candolle, M. J. Schleiden, and E. Haeckel have been considered. The second part contains an attempt to construct a new system of biological disciplines and the various possible ways to construct such a system. The third part contains a critical review of contemporary biological systems as they are expounded in some current biological textbooks.

WHEELER, L. R., 1939: Vitalism: its history and validity, 275 p. (Diss. Univ. London) (London: Witherby).—

The book has been written from the vitalistic point of view; by the term vitalism the author means to describe "living things as actuated by some power or principle additional to those of mechanics and chemistry"; this definition implicates autonomy in living things generally, consciousness or something of that sort in animals, and independence of mind in Man. According to the author, in the course of time there has been some kind of alternation between vitalistic and mechanistic conceptions in the development of the life sciences. Thus ancient biology was vitalistic (Aristotle, Ga-

len). The 17th century offered mechanistic hypotheses, and this in its turn led to a reaction in the early 19th century. The development of physics, of chemistry, and the hypothesis of natural selection again caused a revival of mechanistic principles, and, according to the author, in more recent times, vitalism is again in the ascendent. Cf. DRIESCH, H., 1905, vide supra.

WHITROW, G. J., 1961: The natural philosophy of time, 324 p. (London & Edinburgh: Nelson).—

In quite recent years the concept of time becomes more and more a subject of natural science both in the inorganic (e.g., in the theory of relativity, in far-distant astronomical observations, in time-reversible processes in thermodynamics) and in the organic (e.g., in rhythmic phenomena both in physiology and ecology, in time-interval mechanisms, in psychological problems, such as time-sense and memory) natural sciences. These and many other topics are discussed in Whitrow's book, which has also historical value, albeit (not least) for its many adequate citations of historical sources.

A. HISTORIOGRAPHY OF THE LIFE AND MEDICAL SCIENCES DURING THE ANCIENT AND MEDIAEVAL PERIODS: CHRONOLOGICAL AND ETHNOGRAPHICAL

1. ANTIQUITY IN GENERAL (i.e., WORKS DEALING WITH VARIOUS CULTURES)

a. *History of science and culture in general*

BRUNET, P. & A. MIELI, 1935: Histoire des sciences. Antiquité, 1224 p. (Paris: Payot).—

A very good, mainly chronologically-arranged, review of the history of ancient science from prehistory up to the 8th century. The separate historical reviews are followed by selected abstracts from the authors considered, and these abstracts are accompanied by numerous annotations. The book is divided into the following sections: I. Introduction. Primitive science: Prehistory, Egypt, Babylon (90 p.); II. Hellenistic science (100 p.); III. Aristotle and his School (100 p.); IV. Alexandrian period (258 p.); V. Beginnings of Graeco-Roman science (182 p.); VI. The last great scholars of Graeco-Roman antiquity: from Ptolemy to Pappus (186 p.); VII. Decline of the science of antiquity (158 p.).

BUCHWALD, W., A. HOHLWEG & O. PRINZ, 1963: Tusculum-Lexikon griechischer und lateinischer Autoren des Altertums und des Mittelalters, 544 p. (Munich: Heimeran).—

A very valuable biographical dictionary of authors living during classical antiquity, during the Middle Ages in the Latin West, and during the Byzantine Age. Of each of the authors included, the most important writings are given, together with some essential biographical details. Cf. CHEVALIER, U., 1905-1907, *vide infra*.

The CAMBRIDGE ANCIENT HISTORY, 1923-1939, 12 vols. + 5 vols. of plates. (Cambridge: U.P.).—

A standard work, in which each chapter has been written by a specialist. Vol. 1: Egypt and Babylonia, to 1580 B.C.; vol. 2: The Egyptian and Hittite Empires, to ca. 1000 B.C.; vol. 3: The Assyrian Empire;

vol. 4: The Persian Empire and the West; vol. 5: Athens, 478-401 B.C.; vol. 6: Macedon, 401-301 B.C.; vol. 7: The Hellenistic monarchies and the rise of Rome; vol. 8: Rome and the Mediterranean, 218-133 B.C.; vol. 9: The Roman Republic, 133-44 B.C.; vol. 10: The Augustan Empire, 44 B.C.-A.D. 70; vol. 11: The Imperial peace, A.D. 70-192; vol. 12: The Imperial crisis and recovery, A.D. 193-324. Very valuable volumes of plates, illustrating the arts and cultures of the ancient peoples. Maps are included in the text-volumes. Extensive bibliographies. *Cf.* also The CAMBRIDGE MEDIEVAL HISTORY, *vide infra.*

The CAMBRIDGE MEDIEVAL HISTORY, 1911-1936, 8 vols. (Cambridge: U.P.).—

A standard work of reference for the history of the Middle Ages. Vol. 1: The Christian Roman Empire and the foundation of the Teutonic kingdoms; vol. 2: The rise of the Saracens and the foundation of the Western Empire; vol. 3: Germany and the Western Empire; vol. 4: The Eastern Roman Empire, 717-1453; vol. 5: Contest of Empire and Papacy; vol. 6: Victory of the Papacy; vol. 7: Decline of Empire and Papacy; vol. 8: The close of the Middle Ages. *Cf.* also The CAMBRIDGE ANCIENT HISTORY, *vide supra,* and PREVITÉ-ORTON, C. W., 1952, *vide infra.*

CASSON, L., 1960: The ancient mariners: seafarers and sea fighters of the Mediterranean in ancient times, 285 p. (London: Gollancz).—

The book deals with the first men (the Egyptians) who went down to the sea in ships to explore the surroundings and to carry on trade (*ca.* 4000 B.C.). Vase and tomb paintings, as well as written records (2700 B.C.) make reconstruction possible. Crete was the first nation to establish a sea empire and accordingly Cretan pottery can be found over a large part of the old Mediterranean world. Mercantile fleets were built, and to protect these, war ships had to be built, which also played a role in the settlement of trading posts; and by 550 B.C. the Greek colonization of the Mediterranean was virtually complete: Greece became a leading sea power from the Homeric age down to the 5th century. After the Greeks came the supremacy of Rhodes and then of Rome. Tables with dates, a select bibliography, and a glossary of Greek and Latin nautical terms have been added. *Cf.* KORNEMANN, E., 1948, *vide* section Classical Antiquity X., subsection a.

CHEVALIER, U., 1894-1903: Répertoire des sources historiques du Moyen Âge. To-

po-bibliographie, 3383 p. (Montbéliard: Soc. anon. d'Imp. Montbéliardaise).—

Very useful list of names of towns, cloisters, castles, *etc.*, together with biographical information. Reprinted 1959-1960 (New York, N.Y.: Kraus).

——, 1905-1907: Répertoire des sources historiques du Moyen Âge, 2 vols. Bio-bibliographie. Vol. I (A-I); Vol. II (J-Z), 2436 p. (Paris: Picard).—

Very useful list of names, together with bibliographical information. Indispensable to anyone working on mediaeval history. Reprinted 1959-1960. (New York, N.Y.: Kraus). *Cf.* BUCHWALD, W., *et al.*, 1963, *vide supra.*

CLAGETT, M., 1955: Greek science in antiquity, 217 p. (New York, N.Y.: Abelard-Schuman).—

A well-written introduction to the study of ancient Greek science, including medicine. The book starts with a good survey of science in Egypt and Mesopotamia. The fourth chapter deals with Greek medicine and biology; many fragments and excerpts from ancient authors have been given. The author does not restrict his researches to ancient Greece, for in Ch. 8 he discusses Roman science (Lucretius, Celsus, Seneca, Pliny) and Ch. 9-14 are devoted to science in late antiquity (church fathers, the Physiologus, Boethius, Isidore of Seville, Bede, and others).

DURANT, W., 1950: The age of faith. A history of medieval civilization - Christian, Islamic, and Judaic - from Constantine to Dante: A. D. 325-1300, 1196 p. (New York, N.Y.: Simon & Schuster).—

" 'The Age of Faith' describes the activities inspired by the three religions which dominated the medieval scene in the Western World, but it refers to much else, politics and government, wars and rebellions, philosophy, arts and letters, education, manners and customs... It is an admirable panorama of the Middle Ages, very well documented, pleasantly written, good descriptions being spiced with epigrams and humor; its outstanding merit is to be informed throughout with a generous spirit." (Sarton in Isis 42: 349-350). *Cf.* WEINBURG, J., 1964, *vide infra.*

FARRINGTON, B., 1936: Science in antiquity, 257 p. (The Home Univ. Library of

Modern Knowledge) (London: Butterworth).—

A popular introduction. There are chapters on Egypt and Mesopotamia, the Ionian schools, the Italian schools, the atomic theory, Greek medicine, Socrates and Plato, Aristotle, the Alexandrian age, and the Graeco-Roman world.

FRANKFORT, H. & H. A., J. A. WILSON, T. JACOBSEN & W. A. IRWIN, 1946: The intellectual adventure of ancient Man: an essay on speculative thought in the ancient Near East, 401 p. (Chicago, Ill.: Chicago U.P.).—

The text of the book consists of the contents of a series of introductory lectures. After an introduction discussing the connection between myth and reality, three chapters follow, the first of which deals with Egypt (the nature of the universe, the function of the state, the values of life), the second with Mesopotamia (the cosmos as a state, the function of the state, the good life), and the third with the Hebrews (God, Man, and World, nation, society, and politics). A concluding chapter is entitled: The emancipation of thought from myth.

GRANT, R. M., 1952: Miracle and natural law in Graeco-Roman and early Christian thought, 293 p. (Amsterdam: North-Holland Publ. Co.).—

The book opens with a chapter on the various meanings of the term "nature" in antiquity. Then the author shows that, whereas the Greeks did not believe in a personal God who transformed non-being into being, they searched for an immutable law of physical nature. In this world view there was no room for miracles. Early Christianity, however, was indifferent to natural science and they had no *a priori* objections to miracles, for these were considered as signs of their God, and many parallels with paganism exist. The concluding section discusses the meaning and value of the miracle story.

HAUSSIG, H. W., ed., 1965: Götter und Mythen im vorderen Orient, In: Wörterbuch der Mythologie, Abt. I: Die alten Kulturvölker, Vol. I, 601 p. (Stuttgart: Klett).—

A dictionary of mythology of Mesopotamia (Sumerians, Accadians), Asia Minor (Hittites and Hurrites), Syria (Ungarites, Phoenicians), Egypt, the people of north and central Arabia during the pre-Islamic era, South Arabia (Saba', Qatāban, *etc.*) and of the Semites in Ethiopia. Extensive index of subjects and names.

MAS-LATRIE, L., 1889: Trésor de chronologie, d'histoire et de géographie, pour l'étude et l'emploi des documents du Moyen Âge, 2300 cols. (Paris: Palme).—

Contains chapters on and tables of the various periods, lists of saints and fathers of the church, of popes, cardinals, councils and emperors, rulers and ecclesiastics, for the countries of Europe, Asia, and Africa, with emphasis on France. A reprint seems to be in preparation.

PEATOW, L. J., 1964: A guide to the study of medieval history, 643 p. (New York, N.Y.: Kraus).—

An attempt to assemble the historical literature concerning the Middle Ages compiled between *ca.* 1815 and 1915. The first part of this bibliographical review (p. 3-138) comprises the most important general books useful in a study of mediaeval history (bibliographical works, books of reference, and some other auxiliaries to the study of mediaeval history, a review of modern historical works and a review of large collections of original sources). The second part (p. 139-358) contains a general history of the Middle Ages and has been divided into 35 sections. The third part (p. 359-546) considers mediaeval culture and has been divided into 28 sections; each section is divided into three parts: A. An outline, aiming to present the subject matter of the section in an orderly fashion, including the principal names and dates; B. Special recommendations for reading; and C. A bibliography. The book was first published in 1917.

POUCHET, F. A., 1853: Histoire des sciences naturelles au Moyen Âge, ou Albert le Grand et son époque, considérés comme point de départ de l'école expérimentale, 656 p. (Paris: Baillière).—

This book consists of 5 chapters, each dealing with one of the several schools to be distinguished. Ch. 1 deals with the Scandinavian School (p. 1-36), its natural history, zoology of the sagas, medicine; ch. 2 deals with the French-Gothic School (p. 37-110), the encyclopaedists: Isidore of Seville, Theodoric, Boethius, Cassiodorus, Alcuin, Charlemagne, *etc.*, alchemy (Geber), agriculture (Strabo), Frederick II and cynegetic zoology, bestiaries, medicine (Hildegard of

Bingen, Salerno, Montpellier); ch. 3 deals with the Byzantine School (p. 109-138), medicine (Alexander of Tralles, Paulos Aegineta, Aëtios of Amida), natural history (George Pisides), and with agriculture (Cassianos Bassos); ch. 4 deals with the Arabian School (p. 138-202), medicine (Avicenna, Rhazes, al-Kindi, Averroës, Albucasis, *etc.*), natural history (al-Kazwīnī, al-Demiri, Abdallah-Tif, Ibn Baiṭār, Serapion, Mesuë the Elder, Alfarabi), and with alchemy (Geber); ch. 5 deals with the Experimental School (p. 203-614), *e.g.*, with Albert the Great (p. 203-319), esp. with his zoology and botany), Thomas Aquinas, Roger Bacon, R. Lull, Duns Scotus, *etc.*, the natural history of Vincent of Beauvais, Adelard of Bath, Bartholomaeus Anglicus, the zoology of Richard de Furnival, and Agricola, the botany of Joh. Platearius, Gilbertus Anglicus, Simon de Corda, Jean de Dondis, Nicholas Leoniceno, the medicine of Arnald of Villanova, Pietro d'Albano, Lanfranc, Guy de Chauliac, Jean de Vigo, Henri de Mondeville, John of Arderne, Paracelsus, the anatomy of Mundinus, Berengarius, Vesalius, Achillini, and the agriculture of Pietro dei Crescentii.

PREVITÉ-ORTON, C. W., ed., 1952: The shorter Cambridge Medieval History, 2 vols., 1202 p. (New York, N.Y.: Cambridge U.P.).—

This is a digest of the great Cambridge Medieval History in eight volumes, *q.v.* This shorter edition is supplied with a large number of illuminating illustrations.

REY, A., 1930-1948: La science dans l'antiquité, 5 vols. Vol. I (1930): La science orientale avant les Grecs, 495 p.; Vol. II (1933): La jeunesse de la science grecque, 537 p.; Vol. III (1939): La maturité de la pensée scientifique en Grèce, 574 p.; Vol. IV (1946): L'apogée de la science technique grecque. Les sciences de la nature et de l'homme, les mathématiques d'Hippocrate à Platon, 313 p.; Vol. V (1948): L'apogée de la science technique. L'essor de la mathématique, 322 p. (Paris: Michel).—

Vol. I deals with Chaldeo-Assyrian, Egyptian, Chinese and Hindu science (esp. astronomy and mathematics). Short sections deal with Chaldeo-Assyrian speculations on alchemy (p. 190-196) and medicine (p. 196-197), with Egyptian medicine (p. 305-329), with Chinese cosmology (p. 398-404), and with Hindu medicine (p. 426-428). Vol. II deals with Greek science down to the middle of the 5th century. According to the author, during this period physics ceased to be mythical, because of the awakening of experimental science and the strong development of inductive mathematics and the method of logical deduction. Of this vol., the following parts are of more particular importance: Beginnings of Greek science, the School of Miletos (75 p.); Evolution of Greek thought around Pythagorism (79 p.); the School of Pythagoras: Xenophanes, Parmenides; a section on medicine and biological theories (17 p.); and a section on geography, geology and history (8 p.). Vol. III largely deals with Plato and Aristotle, a period during which scientific thought was preoccupied with subjective abstractions. A relatively large section is devoted to the interrelation between Greek medicine and Greek science in general (esp. p. 420-458). Other sections deal with the medical or/and other scientific achievements of Anaxagoras (p. 69-93), Empedocles (p. 94-136), Leucippos and Democritos (p. 393-419). Vol. IV deals *inter alia* with acoustics and optics, with medicine (p. 117-146), natural sciences (p. 147-170) and the science of Man (p. 171-185). Vol. V is of no special importance for this Guide. In their totality the books give a clear picture of the history of ancient science.

ROBINSON, C. A., 1951: Ancient history, 738 p. (New York, N.Y.: Macmillan).—

This volume deals with the essential points of the history of Man from his earliest beginnings to the death of Justinian in 565 A. D. Good bibliography. Index. M. F. A. Montague writes about this book (in Isis 42: 346) that it is a magisterially-written volume which will long hold the leading place in its field.

SANDYS, J. E., 1921: A history of classical scholarship. Vol. I: From the VIth century B.C. to the end of the Middle Ages, ed. 3, 702 p. (Cambridge: U.P.).—

The first ed. of this volume appeared in 1903 (2nd ed. 1906) and vols. II and III were published in 1908. There also exists a summary of the whole work: A short history of classical scholarship from the sixth century B.C. to the present day, 1915, 455 p. (Cambridge: U. P.). The volume under discussion consists of 6 sections: 1. The Athenian age (600-300 B.C.); 2. The Alexandrian age (300 B.C. - beginning of Christian Era); 3. The Roman age of Latin scholarship (168 B.C. - 530 A.D.); 4. The Roman age of Greek scholarship (beginning of Christian era - 530 A. D.); 5. The Byzantine age (530-1350 A.D.); 6. The Middle Ages in the West (530-1350 A. D.).

STAHL, W. H., 1962: Roman science: origins, development, and influence to the later Middle Ages, 308 p. (Madison, Wisc.: Univ. Wisconsin Press).—

This book covers 600 years of antiquity (from Cato to Martianus Cappella) and 800 years of the Middle Ages (from Balthius to the School of Chartres), an epoch characterized by an abundance of textbook-literature, compendia, and uncritical compilations. The subject-matter has been divided into three parts. The first part deals with the Greek origins of Roman science (p. 3-64), in which the early Hellenistic handbook-tradition is discussed. The second part (p. 65-192) deals with the period between 200 B.C. and 450 A.D., and discusses at length such authors as: Lucretius, Virgil, Horace, Varro, Cicero, Mela, Vitruvius, Celsus, Seneca. A special chapter has been devoted to Pliny's theoretical science. The third part deals with Roman science in the Middle Ages, e.g., with classical learning under the Ostrogoths, with encyclopaedic science in the borderlands and with Roman survivals in the later Middle Ages. Much information has been given of encyclopaedic science in such borderlands as Spain (Isidore of Seville) and England (Bede). According to the author, the disinterest of the Romans in the original writings of the Greek scientists, must be held responsible for much of the detiorated state of scientific knowledge in Western Europe during the first millennium of the Christian era. This view is also supported by H. BUTTERFIELD, 1957: The origins of modern science, 1300-1800, ed. 3, 242 p., vide section Comprehensive works on the history of science.

STRUNZ, F., 1904: Naturbetrachtung und Naturkenntnis im Altertum. Eine Entwicklungsgeschichte der antiken Naturwissenschaften, 168 p. (Hamburg & Leipzig: Voss).—

An attempt to show that observation and reflection of nature ultimately lead to science. The author pursues this argument into the ancient Near- and Far East and in Classical Antiquity.

WEINBURG, J., 1964: A short history of medieval philosophy, 304 p. (Princeton, N.J.: Princeton U.P.).—

According to its author this book is a sketchy history of the various philosophers and philosophical schools from Augustine to Nicholas of Autrecourt, intended for the non-specialist. The author starts with

the view that practically all philosophy in the Middle Ages developed in association with one or the other of three major religions: Judaism, Christianity, or Mohammedanism. According to a review in Speculum 40: 373, this book offers a better than usual survey of both Arabic and Jewish philosophy. Cf. DURANT, W., 1950, vide supra.

b. *History of the plant and animal sciences*

BODENHEIMER, F. S., 1960: Animal and man in Bible lands, 232 p. (Coll. de travaux de l'Acad. Intl. d'Hist. des Sciences, Nr. 10) (Leiden: Brill).—

In an introductory part (p. 1-38) the author sets out his scope, methods and sources, faunal history, hunting, agriculture and husbandry in the Natufian age. The second part (p. 39-148) deals with ancient zoology in the Middle East (e.g., animals in the life of ancient Mesopotamia and Egypt, Graeco-Roman zoology) and the third part (p. 149-220) deals with the period between the Neolithic and the end of the Iron Age (e.g., animals in the excavations of the Bronze and Iron Ages in Palestine, the Old Testament and its animals, animal sacrifices in the Bible, the zoology of the Bible in the light of Frazer's analysis of comparative folklore). Indexes of Latin names of animals and of quotations.

BUDGE, E. A. W., 1928: The divine origin of the craft of the herbalist, 96 p. (London: Society of Herbalists).—

The book starts with a brief description of the attributes and works of the earliest gods of medicine in Mesopotamia and Egypt, who were considered as herbalists by having knowledge of divine medicines. They made this knowledge available to the priests, and the author shows how the Sumerian, Egyptian, Babylonian and Assyrian Herbals formed the foundation of the Greek Herbals (e.g., of Diocles of Carystos, Theophrastos, Dioscorides, Galen) and how the contents of these herbals (especially via the School of Alexandria) were translated into Syriac and Arabic (and even Coptic and Ethiopian), and so became known throughout Western Asia. From there it spread to Europe and even to Turkestan and China. Cf. SINGER, C., 1927: vide infra.

CLAPHAM, J. H. & E. POWER, eds., 1941: The Cambridge economic history of Europe from the decline of the Roman Empire. Vol. I: The agrarian life of the Middle Ages, 650 p. (Cambridge: U.P.).—

A very profound study of medieval economic life, based as it was on the soil, the crops, the peasant and his cattle, his toil, and his agricultural implements. It describes social life and the way in which villages and fields were occupied and laid out. Some chapters describe the great "sweeping movements" which affected all Europe, such as the settlement and colonization of Europe (Ch. I), the evolution of agricultural technique (Ch. III), the rise of manory. (Ch. VI), and the factors deeply affecting rural life of late mediaeval times (Ch. VIII). Ch. II deals with agriculture and rural life in the later Roman Empire; Ch. IV with agrarian institutions of the Germanic kingdoms from the fifth to the ninth century; Ch. VII deals with the situation in separate countries or regions at what we call the height of the Middle Ages (11-14th century); and Ch. V is devoted to mediaeval agrarian conditions in the Byzantine Empire.

DOUGLAS, N., 1928: Birds and beasts of the Greek anthology, 215 p. (London: Chapman & Hall).—

A natural history of the fauna of the Greek anthology. After a short introduction, chapters follow on: mammals; birds; reptiles and batrachians; sea-beasts; creeping things. Domestic animals are not included.

DÜRST, J. U., 1899: Die Rinder von Babylonien, Assyrien und Ägypten und ihr Zusammenhang mit den Rindern der alten Welt, 94 p. (Diss. Univ. Zurich) (Berlin: Reimer).—

Unfortunately, I am unable to give further details.

GOTHEIN, M. L., 1928: A history of garden art from the earliest times to the present day, vol. I (London: Dent).—

For more details, *vide* section History of the applied plant sciences, subsection History of horticulture.

GRADMANN, R., 1909: Der Getreidebau im deutschen und römischen Altertum, 111 p. (Jena: Costenoble).—

According to the author, the Germanics borrowed from the Romans the pear, cherry, peach, quince, walnut, vine, cabbage, caper, parsley, onions, black radish, fennel,

anise, cummin, lettuce, asparagus, mustard, pumpkin, rose, lily, but no cereal. Before the arrival of the Romans, the Germanics already cultivated bald wheat, barley, rye, *Triticum spelta, Tr. monococcum*, lentils, *Pisum sativum, Faba vulgaris, Daucus carota, Linum nsitatissimum, Cannabis sativa, Isatis tinctoria, Papaver somniferum, Pyrus malus* and an *Allium*-species.

HOPF, L., 1904: Die Anfänge der Anatomie bei den alten Kulturvölkern, 126 p. (Abh. Gesch. Med. IX) (Breslau/Wrocław: Kern).—

Unfortunately I am unable to give further details as to the contents of this publication.

JORET, C., 1892: La rose dans l'Antiquité et au Moyen-Âge. Histoire, légendes et symbolisme, 483 p. (Paris: Bouillon).—

The first part treats of the rose in antiquity, dealing with such subjects as: the species of roses known in antiquity, its culture; the rose in Graeco-Roman literature and pharmacology; the rose in the ancient Orient. The second part treats of the rose in the Middle Ages, dealing with such subjects as: its culture in East and West; its role in literature, in art and in cults; the rose as pharmaceutic and gastronomic object. *Cf.* WATKINS, G. M., 1896, *vide infra*.

———, 1897-1904: Les plantes dans l'Antiquité et au Moyen-Âge. Histoire, usages et symbolisme, 2 vols. Vol. I (1897): Les plantes dans l'orient classique I: Egypte, Chaldée, Assyrie, Judée, Phénice, 504 p.; Vol. II (1904): Les plantes dans l'orient classique II: L'Iran et l'Inde, 657 p. (Paris: Bouillon).—

The first part of vol. I (p. 1-326) entirely deals with the plants in Egypt, *e.g.*, with the Pharaonic flora, with agriculture, horticulture, fruit trees, ornamental trees, vegetables, plants used in industry, plants in arts and literature, in myths and cults, and the medical use of plants. The second part of vol. I (p. 327-501) deals with the role of plants with Semitic people, *e.g.*, with the flora of Asia Minor, Syria, Mesopotamia, Arabia, the vegetables used, plants used in industry, agriculture, horticulture, plants in art and literature, *etc.* Vol. II, part 1 deals with the plants of the Iranians (p. 1-182); part 2 with the plants of the Hindoos (p. 183-654), considering the same topics as those discussed above.

KELLER, O., 1963: Die antike Tierwelt, 2 vols. Vol. I: 434 p.; Vol. II: 617+46 p. (Hildesheim: Olms).—

A photographic reprint of the 1909-1913 edition. The volumes contain a summing-up of all animals known by the ancients (Egyptians, Greeks, Romans), as it becomes clear from literary- and art-historical sources. The first volume deals with mammals, the second volume with birds, reptiles, fishes, insects, Arachnidea, Myriapoda, Crustacea, Vermes, Mollusca, Echinodermata, and Coelenterata.

LANGKAVEL, B., 1964: Botanik der spaeteren Griechen. Vom dritten bis dreizehnten Jahrhunderte, 207 p. (Amsterdam: Hakkert).—

Reprint of the 1866 edition (Berlin: Berggold). During the period between the 3rd and 13th century, many botanical synonyms took their origin in the many translations made during this period. Langkavel prepared an index of the plant names which are to be found in the writings issued during that period and, "Aus dem so entstandenen zahlreichen Verzeichnissen stellte ich dann für jedes Wort die verschiedenen Stellen zusammen, sichtete sie, je nachdem sie selbständig oder nur entlehnt waren, prüfte die etwa gegebenen oft sehr vagen Pflanzendiagnosen an den lebenden Pflanzen... verglich sodann die medicinische Anwendung und Wirkung der so bezeichneten Pflanze mit den früheren Ueberlieferungen und den Resultaten neuer pharmacologischen Werke, und gelangte so endlich zu einer gewissen Ordnung in diesem wüsten Felde der bunten Synonymen." The main part of the book consists of an alphabetical list of plants, according to the family names (p. 1-133), a list of Latin plant names (p. 134-144) and an elaborate index (p. 145-207). Among the authors considered are: Theodorus Priscianus, Marcellus Empíricus, Isidore of Seville, Oribasios, Aëtios, Alexander of Tralles, Psellos, Nonnos, Joannes Actuarios, Nicolaus Damascenos, Paulos Aegineta, Hildegard of Bingen, Albert the Great, Simon Genuensis, Matthaeus Sylvaticus, and Dioscorides.

LEY, W., 1968: Dawn of zoology, 280 p. (Englewood Cliffs, N.J.: Prentice Hall).—

A valuable study of the beginnings of zoology in Classical Antiquity and during the Middle Ages. Especially valuable sections deal with allegorical and clerical attitudes to zoology.

MEYER, E. H. F., 1854-1857: Geschichte der Botanik, 4 vols. (Königsberg: Borntraeger).—

For more details, *vide* section History of the pure plant sciences, subsection a.

SAVASTANO, L., 1890/'91: La patologia vegetale dei Greci, Latini ed Arabi, 75 p. (Ann. Scuo. Sup. Agric. Portici, Vol. 5).—

A collection of those passages in the works of Theophrastos, Pliny and Ibn al-Awam which deal with phytopathology. The author attempts to show that most contemporary plant diseases were also known to the ancient writers, especially to the Arabs.

SEIDENSTICKER, A., 1886: Waldgeschichte des Altertums. Ein Handbuch für akademische Vorlesungen, 2 vols. Vol. I: Vor Caesar, 403 p.; Vol. II: Nach Caesar, 460 p. (Frankfurt a.O.: Trowitzsch).—

Contains information concerning such subjects as: the various trees in the forests, the names of the various types of forests, sacred forests and sacred trees, their usage, protection, upkeep, *etc.*

SINGER, C., 1927: The herbal in antiquity and its transmission to later ages, 52 p. (J. Hellenic Studies 47: 1-52).—

A very clear survey of the history of herbals from antiquity to the Middle Ages, down to the incunabula. It contains many very fine illustrations and, therefore, is especially valuable from the iconographical point of view. Herbals considered in more or less detail are those of Diocles of Carystos (the earliest herbal of which we know, *ca.* 350 B.C.); Theophrastos (the earliest herbal which has survived, *ca.* 250 B.C.); Nicander (*ca.* 200 B.C.); Crateuas (*ca.* 75 B.C.), the first herbarium with illustrations drawn from the object); Pamphilos; Damocrates; Andromachos; Menecrates; Dioscorides (whose work has survived entire; the most influential herbal ever written, including a list of synonyms derived from languages many of which are now unknown); Galen; Oribasios; Apuleius; Pliny. *Cf.* BUDGE, E. A. W., 1928, *vide supra. Cf.* also SINGER, C., 1921, *vide* section History of Biology in general, subsection a.

WATKINS, G. M., 1896: The natural history of the ancients, 274 p. (London: Stock).—

In this book the term "ancient" comprises the period between Homer and *ca.*

1800. The text deals with such subjects as: the gardens of Homer, the Romans, Pliny, Chaucer, and Bacon; the Romans in Britain as acclimatizers; roses in Greece and Rome, roses of Chaucer and Shakespeare; the connection between our present wild and domesticated animals and those of the ancients, *etc.*

c. *History of the medical sciences*

ALLBUTT, C., 1921: Greek medicine in Rome, 633 p. (London: Macmillan).—

A well-written historiography of the development of medicine in ancient Rome, the origins of Greek physiology, Alexandrian medicine, the settlement of Greek physicians in Rome, the Methodist, Pneumatic, and Eclectic Schools, Celsus, Musa, Pliny, Soranos, Rufus, Galen, doctrines of the pulse and of generation, hygiene, therapeutics, pharmacy, toxicology, infectious diseases, *etc.* It also contains essays on Byzantine medicine, on public health service and on the medical school of Salerno, in which Greek, neo-Latin and mediaeval medicine met. A French book dealing with the same period and topics is: ALBERT, M., 1894: Les médecins grecs à Rome, 320 p. (Paris: Hachette).

AMBER, R. B. & A. M. BABEY-BROOKE, 1966: The pulse in Occident and Orient: its philosophy and practice in India, China, Iran and the West, 210 p. (New York, N.Y.: Santa Barbara; London: Dawsons).—

Unfortunately I am unable to give further information about this book.

ARTELT, W., 1937: Studien zur Geschichte der Begriffe "Heilmittel" und "Gift". Urzeit-Homer-Corpus Hippocraticum, 101 p. (Studien Gesch. Med., Heft 23) (Leipzig: Barth).—

Ch. 1 deals with the concepts "Heilmittel" and "Gift" in preliterate societies, in Mesopotamia and Egypt (p. 1-37). Ch. II deals with the concept pharmacon in the Homeric poems in Hesiod's works and in Attic tragedies and comedies (p. 38-48). Ch. III deals with pharmacon in the Hippocratic Corpus (p. 49-95). Reprinted 1968 (Darmstadt: Wiss. Verlagsges.).

BARRAUD, G., 1954: Clio et Epidaure ou la médecine et l'humanisme chez les anciens, 282 p. (Paris: Sipuco).—

A (literary) historical review of the history of medicine from the earliest time to the Renaissance, composed of 24 chapters, each of which constitutes an essay dealing with a carefully selected theme, together illustrating the growth and development of medicine, but at the same time illustrating the situation of medical knowledge during the civilization or period considered. The book starts with an introductory chapter on prehistoric medicine and surgery, and it ends with an essay on medicine and poetry and an epilogue.

BERENDES, J., 1891: Die Pharmacie bei den alten Culturvölkern. Historisch-kritische Studien, 2 vols. Vol. I: 308 p.; Vol. II: 220 p. (Halle a.S.: Tausch & Grosse).—

The first part of vol. I deals with the history of pharmacy from ancient times up to Hippocrates: India (The Vedas, Suśruta, dietetics), Persia (Avesta, Greek influences), China, Egypt, Semitic countries, Greece (Homer, asclepiads, the Ionian philosophers, Pythagoras, Plato, Aristotle, Theophrastos). The second part deals with the period between Hippocrates and Galen (pharmacy in the Corpus Hippocraticum, the School of Alexandria, *e.g.,* Herophilos, Zeno, Demosthenes, Erasistratos, Serapion, Dionysios, Aristarchos, Mithridates, Nicomedes, Menecrates, Nicander, Dioscorides). The first part of vol. II is a continuation of the second part of vol. I and deals with Hellenistic and Roman pharmacy *(e.g.,* Asclepiades, Sextius Niger, Musa, Scribonius Largus, Soranos, Caelius Aurelianus, Celsus, Pliny, Aretaeus, Archigenes). The second part deals with Galen, and with Byzantine and Arab pharmacy (to quote some names: Serenus Samonicus, Africanus Sextus, Oribasios, Theodorus Priscianus, Aëtios, Alexander of Tralles, Paulos Aegineta, Geber, Rhazes, Mesuë the Younger, Avicenna, Abenguefit, Serapion jun., Ibn Zoar, Abulkasis, Maimonides, Ibn Baiṭār, Oseibiah). Reprinted in 1965 (Hildesheim: Olms).

BRAAMS, W., 1913: Zur Geschichte des Ammenwesens im Altertum, 31 p. (Jenaer med.-hist. Beiträge, Heft 5) (Jena: Fischer).—

Separate sections are entitled: Einleitung; II. Ansichten über die Zulässigkeit der Ammenernährung; III. Anforderungen an die Amme; IV. Verhalten der Amme sich selbst gegenüber während der Stillperiode; V. Verhalten der Amme gegenüber dem Kinde; VI. Die soziale und rechtliche Stellung der Amme.

BROTHWELL, D. R. & A. T. SANDISON, eds., 1968: Disease in antiquity: a survey of the diseases, injuries and surgery of early populations, 766 p. (Springfield, Ill.: Thomas).—

The book discusses two important sources of information about diseases of antiquity. The first source is represented by the Egyptian custom of embalming the dead, which has supplied us with a wealth of information. The book contains a study of mummy tissue by A. T. SANDISON, from which study he has been able to discuss the occurrence of some skin diseases prevalent in ancient Egypt. A. W. PIKE found and describes some parasitic eggs in the kidneys of some mummies, and in a mediaeval latrine at Winchester, England. MØLLER-CHRISTIENSEN has studied the incidence of leprosy in ancient Egypt, and he also examined some 700 Neolithic skeletons from France, and many mediaeval skeletons. D. BROTHWELL studied the occurrence of cancer of the bone in ancient skeletons. The second source is represented by the written texts of the Chinese, Egyptian, Greek and other civilizations. In the present book, J. V. KINNIER WILSON describes some mental diseases of ancient Mesopotamia, LU GWEI-DJEN & J. NEEDHAM discuss some diseases, remarkably well-described in old Chinese medical texts, and R. HARE tries to reconstruct the spread of smallpox from ancient China *via* the Near East to Europe.

BULLOUGH, V. L., 1966: The development of medicine as a profession: the contribution of the medieval to modern medicine, 125 p. (Basel: Karger).—

For more details, *vide* section History of the medical sciences, subsection d2.

CHOULANT, L., ed., 1956: Handbuch der Bücherkunde für die ältere Medicin. Zur Kenntniss der griechischen, lateinischen und arabischen Schriften im ärztlichen Fache und zur bibliographischen Unterscheidung ihrer verschiedenen Ausgaben, Uebersetzungen und Erläuterungen, 434 p. (Graz: Akad. Druck- und Verlagsanstalt).—

For more details, *vide* section Bibliographies, subsection e.

CORLIEU, A., 1885: Les médecins grecs depuis la mort de Galien jusqu'à la chute de l'empire d'orient, 208 p. (Paris: Baillière).—

A first chapter (p. 14-103) deals with anatomy, physiology, pathology, surgery, therapeutics, hygiene, *etc.*, in Greek medicine after Galen's death. A second chapter deals with the physicians, their scriptures and doctrines during that period. Among the physicians considered are: Philagrios, Oribasios, Nemesios, Palladios, Aëtios, Alexander of Tralles, Theophiles Protospatharios, Philotheos, Stephanos of Athens, Paulos of Aegina, Damascios, Meletios, Nonnos, Psellos, Seth, Joannes Actuarios, Hierophilos, Demetrios Pepagomenos, Nicholas of Myrepse, Maximos Planudes.

CREUTZ, W., 1934: Die Neurologie des 1.-7. Jahrhunderts n. Chr. Eine historisch-neurologische Studie, 106 p. (Leipzig: Thieme).—

In a first section the author considers the neurological theories of: Celsus, Soranos, Galen, Aretaios of Cappadocia, Cassios Iatrosophista, Oribasios, Aëtios of Amida, Alexander of Tralles, Paulos of Aegina. In a second section the author elucidates the anatomical and physiological knowledge of the brain and the other parts of the nervous system in the authors mentioned and their knowledge of the pathological conditions of the diseases of the nervous system.

DAWSON, W. R., 1930: The beginnings: Egypt and Assyria, 86 p. (Clio Medica, No. 1) (New York, N.Y.: Hoeber).—

This booklet contains the following chapters: 1. Primitive ideas of disease and death; 2. Averting death and prolonging life; 3. The magician; 4. The first medical books; 5. Ancient Egyptian medicine; 6. The "Pothecary": drugs and doses; 7. Assyrian medicine; 8. The legacy of the past: conclusion. The booklet can be considered as a more popular edition of the author's "Magician and leech", 159 p. (London: Methuen).

DIEPGEN, P., 1937: Die Frauenheilkunde der alten Welt, In: W. STOECKEL, ed., Handbuch der Gynäkologie, Vol. XII, pt. 1: Geschichte der Frauenheilkunde, 358 p. (Munich: Bergmann).—

The first part covers pre-classical civilizations of the Near East, the Far East, and primitive civilizations in general. The greater part (p. 97-321) deals with the history of gynaecology among the Greeks and Romans down to 400 A.D. Within the respective sections the material is arranged according to the various disciplines, *viz.*, anatomy and physiology, obstetrics, pathology, diagnosis, therapeutics, and hygiene. Each section is accompanied by a discussion on the social position of women and of the sources consulted. The book has essentially been written for physicians.

——, 1963: Frau und Frauenheilkunde in der Kultur des Mittelalters, 242 p. (Stuttgart: Thieme).—

>After a general introduction giving a general background of the mediaeval period, the author considers the development of gynaecology of the Byzantines, of the Muslims, and of the West-Europeans. The author gives many details of theoretical as well as of practical nature; special sections are devoted to personal hygiene, and to the various professional and other personnel concerned with gynaecological and obstetrical conditions, and with the influence of Christianity.

EDELSTEIN, L., 1967: Ancient medicine: selected papers, 496 p. (Ed. by O. & C. L. TEMKIN) (Baltimore, Md.: Johns Hopkins Press).—

>A series of publications originally published in specialized journals or other publications, by the late Ludwig Edelstein, classicist, medical historian, and philosopher. It is a collection of contributions to the history of ancient medicine and science, dealing with, *e.g.*, the Hippocratic Oath; Greek medicine in relation to religion; magic and philosophy; the professional ethics of the Greek physician; the humanism of Vesalius. Six essays appear in English for the first time; they have been translated from the German.

ESSER, A. A. M., 1961: Das Antlitz der Blindheit in der Antike. Die kulturellen und medizinhistorischen Ausstrahlungen des Blindenproblems in den antiken Quellen, ed. 2, 192 p. (Janus, Suppl. IV) (Leiden: Brill).—

>First published in 1939 (Stuttgart: Enke). An attempt to consider a medical problem within the scientific and cultural framework of the time. The author writes in his preface: "Die vorliegende Arbeit stellt den Versuch dar, alle aus der Blindheit in der Antike sich ergebenden Gesichtspunkte einheitlich zusammenzufassen und zu betrachten, soweit sie rein aus den Quellen selbst fliessen."

FLASHAR, H., 1966: Melancholie und Melancholiker in den medizinischen Theorien der Antike, 145 p. (Habil.-Vortrag, erw. Fassung) (Berlin: de Gruyter).—

>A review of the theories concerning origin, characteristics, progression, cure, *etc.*, of melancholy. In an introductory chapter the author considers contemporary ideas; other chapters deal with the Hippocratic conception of melancholy and with the ideas of Diocles of Carystos, Aristotle and his School, Celsus, Aretaios, Soranos, Rufus of Ephesus, Galen, Poseidonios, and Alexander of Tralles.

FRINGS, H. J., 1959: Medizin und Arzt bei den griechischen Kirchenvätern bis Chrysostomos, 128 p. (Diss. Univ. Bonn).—

>The book describes the early development of Christian Greek medical literature from the second to the fourth century, and the author compares this literature with the pagan literature of earlier Greek medical writers. It appears that Greek medicine changed only little throughout these centuries. The subject matter has been divided into two parts: at first the judgment on the medical art and secondly the evaluation of the physician and his activities. The book elucidates the kind of medicine of the early Greek Fathers, the reactions of the patient to disease and cure, and it gives an impression of the medical situation of those days.

GORDON, B. L., 1949: Medicine throughout antiquity, 818 p. (Philadelphia, Pa.: Davis).—

>A historical summary of medicine as it was conceived, developed and practised by the various peoples of antiquity. It considers the diseases of early man, the origins of medicine, prehistoric medicine, primitive concepts of life and death, nature worship and medicine, medicine in Assyro-Babylonia and in ancient Egypt, ancient Hebrew medicine, medicine in ancient Persia, India, China, Japan, medicine among the prehistoric American Indians, medicine during the Graeco-Roman period, Talmudic medicine, diagnosis and treatment. Index. The book ends with the 5th century A.D. Each chapter is supplied with a long list of references to original sources.

GUPTA, A. K., 1963: Physical, mental and social fundamentals of ancient Indian and Chinese medicine, 72 p. (Inaug. Diss., Univ. Bern) (Calcutta: Truth Press).—

>In this study oriental medicine has been considered in its physical, mental, and social aspects. The first section attempts to

trace in India and China the continuation from philosophy and religion to personal health as well as to social structure, security and public health. The second section gives an exposition of the fundamentals of Indian medicine and its curative aspects, and the third section discusses some fundamentals of Chinese medicine. The whole is followed by a brief comment and by notes.

HOPF, L., 1904: Die Heilgötter und Heilstätten des Altertums. Eine archäologisch-medizinische Studie, 69 p. (Tübingen: Pietzcker).—

The author stresses the role played by mineral springs in ancient healing cultures, and he describes how ancient hospitals were situated in the neighbourhood of these springs. He discusses such locations in ancient Mesopotamia, Asia Minor, Israel, the Arabian world, India, Japan, Egypt, Greece, Rome and with the Etruscans, Celts, and Germanics, and ancient hospitals in India, Ceylon, Greece and in the Roman-Byzantine empire. The priests should act as an intermediary between the gods and Man; priests were enveloped in a veil of mystery, but sometimes they also used drugs, the curative activities of which were known by experience.

JAYNE, W. A., 1962: The healing gods of ancient civilizations, 569 p. (New York, N.Y.: University Bks).—

This book is a reprint of 1925. It is an encyclopaedic work dealing with the healing gods of the Egyptians, Babylonians, Indians, Iranians, Greeks, Romans, and Celts. Each part is preceded by a section describing the regional pantheon, which is followed by a more detailed consideration of the part played by the individual gods. The author protests against scientific scepticism and the increasing influence of materialism on modern medicine.

KIRFEL, W., 1951: Die fünf Elemente insbesondere Wasser und Feuer. Ihre Bedeutung für den Ursprung altindischer und altmediterraner Heilkunde. Eine medizingeschichtliche Studie, 48 p. (Beiträge zur Sprach- und Kulturgeschichte des Orients, Heft 4) (Walldorf-Hessen: Verlag für Orientkunde).—

In this study the author traces back the concept of the four or five elements and their relationship to the various parts

of the body and he tries to understand where these ideas have their origin. He especially compares ancient Greek and Chinese sources.

MAGNUS, H., 1901: Die Augenheilkunde der Alten, 691 p. (Breslau/Wrocław: Kern).—

The text is in five parts, of which the largest part (p. 41-650) is devoted to classical antiquity, dealing respectively with: pt. 1 (p. 1-21) Egyptian ophthalmology (esp. as it occurs in Papyrus Ebers); pt. 2 (p. 22-34) Jewish ophthalmology (esp. dealing with Biblical and Talmudic ophthalmology); pt. 3 (p. 35-40) Indian ophthalmology; pt. 4 (p. 41-650) Greek and Roman ophthalmology (separate sections deal with: Greek ophthalmology from earliest times to Thales, p. 44-54; *idem* from Thales to the School of Alexandria, p. 55-202; *idem* from Alexandria to Galen, p. 203-413; and *idem* from Galen up to Paulos of Aegineta, p. 414-650); pt. 5 (p. 651-668) deals with ophthalmological instruments. Index of subjects and of persons.

MANI, N., 1959: Die historischen Grundlagen der Leberforschung. Pt. 1: Die Vorstellungen über Anatomie, Physiologie und Pathologie der Leber in der Antike, 112 p. (Basler Veröff. Gesch. Med. Biol., Fasc. IX) (Basel & Stuttgart: Schwabe).—

This book is devoted to an investigation of the varying concepts of the structure, the function and the diseases of the liver as held throughout antiquity. The author discusses those observations which were made exclusively for mantic and religious purposes, as they were practised by Babylonians and Assyrians, but also in Greece and even during the Roman Empire; but he also considers the writings of leading Greek and Roman physicians whose interests were of a more clinical character. The culmination of this ancient clinical knowledge he finds in Galen's work. Extensive appendixes containing references, bibliography, personal and geographical names, indexes of quotations and subject headings. *Cf.* also section History of the medical sciences, subsection c7.

MEYER-STEINEG, T., 1912: Chirurgische Instrumente des Altertums. Ein Beitrag zur antiken Akiurgie, 52 p. + 68 figures (Jena. med. hist. Beitr., vol. 1) (Jena: Fischer).—

A general review of age, origin, and fabrication of Greek surgical instruments, and a description of probe-instruments, spoons, spatulas, knives, forceps, clamps, hooked and tube-shaped instruments, needles, instruments to treat bones, pestles, instrument cupboard.

NEUBURGER, M., 1910-1925: History of medicine, 2 vols. Vol. I (1910); Vol. II (1925), 135 p. (Oxford: U.P.).—

> This is a partial and revised English translation of Neuburger's "Geschichte der Medizin" in 2 vols. (Stuttgart: Enke, 1906-1911). Unfortunately this work was never completed and comes to an end with the fifteenth century. There are no references, bibliographical notes or index. From a philosophical point of view this is the best history of medicine of the period covered.

O'BRIEN-MOORE, A., 1924: Madness in ancient literature, 228 p. (Diss. Princeton Univ.) (Weimar: Wagner).—

> This is a study of the concept of madness as it is represented in ancient literature. Although the author starts this study by giving a review of popular and medical conceptions of madness, popular, medical, social, and legal aspects are considered only as far as they may serve as a kind of a scientific background. It is stressed that the concept of madness as we use it to-day cannot be the same as that used in the past.

RIST, E., 1966: Histoire critique de la médecine dans l'Antiquité, 276 p. (Publié par Les amis d'Édouard Rist) (Paris: Firmin-Didot).—

> "A l'occasion du dixième anniversaire de sa mort, ses amis se sont chargés de publier la partie déjà rédigée et qui a trait à l'Antiquité. Médecine de l'homme primitif, médecine des Chaldéo-assyriens et celle du peuple hébreu, médecine égyptienne, médecine grecque et hippocratique, médecine romaine sont ainsi passées en revue et soumises à une analyse méthodique. Rist en arrive à l'oeuvre de Galien dont il fait une judicieuse critique et termine par une évocation de la profession médicale à Rome et dans l'Empire." (From: Monspelliensis Hippocrates 10, No. 37).

SAUNDERS, J. B. de C. M., 1963: The transitions from ancient Egyptian to Greek medicine, 40 p. (Lawrence, Kans.: Kansas U.P.).—

> The text of the Logan Clendening lectures on the history and philosophy of

medicine. Separate chapters deal with: early Graeco-Egyptian relations, incubation, external reputation of Egyptian medicine, scientific examples of transmission, rationalism in Egyptian medicine, Egyptian theoretical system of medicine and its influence. *Cf.* STEUER, R. O. & J. B. de C. M. SAUNDERS, *vide infra*.

SCHMIDT, A., 1924: Drogen und Drogenhandel im Altertum, 136 p. (Leipzig: Barth).—

> From a wide variety of sources (*e.g.*, cuneiform texts, papyrus texts, ancient botanical, medical, and geographical texts, poems, philological studies, *etc.*), the author tries to reconstruct the usage of drugs in medicine, technics, magic, cults, and as cosmetics, poisons, and spices (p. 5-62). From the data discovered in this way the author arrives at some general conclusions concerning origin, production, trade, storage, packing, prices, tolls, monopolies, falsifications, trade routes, *etc.*, of drugs.

SIGERIST, H. E., 1955: A history of medicine. Vol. I: Primitive and archaic medicine, 564 p. (New York, N.Y.: Oxford U.P.).—

> For more details, *vide* section Prehistoric and primitive biology and medicine, subsection c2.

——, 1961: A history of medicine. Vol. II: Early Greek, Hindu, and Persian medicine, 352 p. (London & New York, N.Y.: Oxford U.P.).—

> This vol. has been published posthumously. In it the author studies the medical developments of Greece, India and Persia in close connection with the cultural background of these countries. Starting with archaic medicine in Greece, the author illustrates the state of medical knowledge with the aid of the Homeric legends; other sections deal with the cult of Aesclepios, and with the pre-Socratic medical schools. Then he examines Hindu medical schools and their interrelation with philosophy; interesting in this context is the parallel study of Greek and Indian medicine. After considering medicine in ancient Persia, the author returns to Greece in Hippocratic times, during which period the separation between empirical methods on the one hand and religious and magical methods on the other hand becomes established.

SOULÉ, A., 1913: Histoire de l'art dentaire dans l'Antiquité, 87 p. (Paris: Jouve).—

Separate sections deal with dentistry of prehistoric Man, the Egyptians, Chinese, Greeks, and Romans. *Cf.* also GRAWINKEL, C. J., 1906: Zähne und Zahnbehandlung der alten Ägypter, Hebräer, Indier, Babylonier, Assyrer, Griechen und Römer. (Diss. Erlangen).

STEUER, R. O. & J. B. de C. M. SAUNDERS, 1959: Ancient Egyptian and Cnidian medicine: the relationship of the aetiological concepts of disease, 90 p. (Berkeley, Calif.: Univ. California Press).—

The authors study the influence of ancient Egyptian medicine on Greek medical science and practice. Special attention has been paid to the exact meaning of some medical terms as they were used by the Egyptians and the Greeks respectively. The book is of equal value to historians of medicine, to philologists and to Egyptologists. *Cf.* SAUNDERS, J. B. de C. M., 1963, *vide supra.*

TABANELLI, M., 1963: La medicina nel mondo degli Etruschi, 132 p. (Firenze: Olschki).—

Concerned with Etruscan anatomy, pathology, surgery, odontology, hygienics, medical botany, *etc.*, based on a compilation of all the Greek and Latin references to Etruscan medicine, on archaeological evidence and on Etruscan art. A special chapter deals with anatomical ex-votos, *i.e.*, models of a part of the body. This topic has been dealt with in more detail by DÉCOUFLÉ, P., 1964: La notion d'ex-voto anatomique chez les Etrusco-Romains. Analyse et synthèse, 41 p. (Collection Latomus, 72) (Brussels: Latomus, Revue d'études latines).

TEMKIN, O., 1932: Geschichte des Hippokratismus im ausgehenden Altertum, 80 p. (Kyklos 4: 1-80).—

The following topics are considered: 1. Der Hippokratismus im 2. Jahrhundert; 2. Das 3. Jahrhundert und der lateinische

Westen; 3. Hippokratismus und Galenismus bis zum Ausgang der Schule von Alexandria; 4. Die Kanonisierung von Hippocrates und Galen.

TOEPLI, R. von, 1898: Studien zur Geschichte der Anatomie des Mittelalters, 121 p. (Leipzig & Vienna: Deuticke).—

For more details, *vide* section Middle Ages in the West, subsection c.

THORWALD, J., 1963: Science and secrets of early medicine: Egypt, Mesopotamia, India, China, Peru, 331 p. (London: Thames & Hudson; New York, N.Y.: Harcourt, Brace).—

A popular introduction into the history of medicine in the countries mentioned in the title. The book is especially valuable for its many fine illustrations (more than 340, of which 8 in full colour). Originally published in German: Macht und Geheimnis der frühen Ärzte. Ägypten. Babylonien. Indien. China. Mexiko. Peru, 1962, 331 p. (Munich & Zurich: Knaur). Also in French translation: Histoire de la médecine dans l'antiquité, 331 p. (Paris: Hachette).

WATSON, J., 1856: The medical profession in ancient times, 222 p. (New York, N.Y.: Baker & Godwin).—

In this book the author considers the condition of medicine in the earliest organisations of society (the Druids of Europe, the Vaidhyas of India, the Lamas of Central Asia, the Tla-quill-aughs of America, the priests of Egypt), and the origins of medicine among the Greeks (*e.g.*, Pythagoras, Democedes, the aesclepiads, Hippocrates and his immediate successors) with the Schools of Pergamon, Alexandria, Smyrna, and Epidaurus, with the Schools of Rome and the Greek contemporary writers and teachers, with Galen and subsequent Latin and Greek medical writers, and with laws and customs of the Roman empire in relation to the medical profession.

2. THE LIFE AND MEDICAL SCIENCES IN PREHISTORIC TIMES (INCL. PALAEOPATHOLOGY, FOLK MEDICINE, ETHNOBIOLOGY, AND SOME FOLKLORISTIC ASPECTS OF BIOLOGY)

a. *General*

BREUIL, H. & R. LANTIER, 1965: The men of the Old Stone Age: palaeolithic and mesolithic, 272 p. (London: Harrap).—

A translation from the French: "Les hommes de la pierre ancienne", 1961 (Bibliothèque Scientifique) (Paris: Payot). Very useful introduction. Special attention has been paid to Palaeolithic cave art and the implements of Old and Middle Stone Age men. It contains an index (which the French edition lacks) and useful footnotes. A study of man in prehistoric Europe in relation to his environment from the Upper Palaeolithic up to the Iron Age is: CLARK, J. G. D., 1952: Prehistoric Europe: the economic basis, 349 p. (New York, N.Y.: Philosophical Library). With good bibliography. Reprinted 1966 (Stanford, Calif.: U.P.). Another recent publication, of which I do not possess further information, but probably dealing with the same subject is: LOMMEL, A., 1966: Prehistoric and primitive man, 176 p. (New York, N.Y.: McGraw-Hill). Still another comparable study seems to be: MELLERSH, H. E. L., 1959: The story of man: human evolution to the end of the Stone Age, 256 p. (London: Hutchinson).

BREWER, E. C., 1923: A dictionary of phrase and fable, new ed., 1158 p. (London: Cassell).—

Contains a history of the chief figures mentioned in the mythologies of the world; a record of superstitions and customs, ancient and modern; etymological information; a glossary of scientific, historical, political and archaeological terms, local and national legends, *etc.* Very useful. This book was originally published in 1870 under the title: "Dictionary of phrase and fable, giving the derivation, source, or origin of common phrases, allusions, and words that have a tale to tell", and in the edition of 1887 was added "a concise bibliography of English literature, based upon the larger work... by W. Davenport Adams, with additions", 1061 p. In 1952 a revised and enlarged edition appeared, 977 p. (London: Cassell). *Cf.* JOBES, G., 1961; and LEACH, M. & J. FRIED, 1950, *vide infra.*

BUDGE, E. A. W., 1930: Amulets and superstitions, 543 p. (London: Oxford U.P.).—

Its contents may become clear from its subtitle: The original texts with translations and descriptions of a long series of Egyptian, Sumerian, Assyrian, Hebrew, Christian, Gnostic and Muslim amulets and talismans and magical figures; with chapters on the evil eye, the origin of the amulet, the pentagon, the swastika, the cross (pagan and Christian), the properties of stones, rings, divination, numbers, the kabāllāh, ancient astrology, *etc. Cf.* HANSMANN, L. & L. KRISS-RETTENBECK, 1966, *vide infra.*

CATALOG OF FOLKLORE and folk songs. Cleveland public library, John G. White department, 1965, 2 vols. (Boston, Mass.: Hall).—

The White Collection is one of the greatest book collections of the world in this

field. In 1964 the collection had over 110,000 volumes with more than 7,000 languages and dialects represented. "The term 'folklore' has been interpreted by John Griswold White in a broad sense approximating the German term 'Volkskunde', and includes folk tales, riddles, proverbs, folk songs and ballads, fables, chapbooks, romances, works on superstition, magic and witchcraft, and studies on folk habits, beliefs and customs." This Folklore Catalog has been extracted from the general dictionary catalogue of the J. G. White Collection and includes *ca.* 25,000 entries.

CATALOGUE of the library of the PEABODY MUSEUM of archaeology and ethnology, Harvard University, 1963, 26 vols. (authors) + 27 vols. (subjects) + index to chapter headings. (Boston, Mass.: Hall).—

The author-section of the catalogue includes personal authors, editors, translators, museums, societies and other institutions, main entries for journals, and contents of monograph series; included are journal articles. The subjects covered in the subject-section are general and physical anthropology, ethnology, and prehistoric archaeology. The arrangement is primarily geographical, with topical subdivisions. The index to chapter headings offers a complete list of headings used and cross-references to them.

CHRISTIAN, P., 1870: Histoire de la magie du monde surnaturel et de la fatalité à travers les temps et les peuples, 668 p. (Paris: Furne & Jouvet).—

The whole work consists of 7 books, *viz.*, 1. Les portes du monde surnaturel; 2. Les mystères des pyramides; 3. Les oracles antiques, les Sibylles et les Sorts; 4. La magie depuis l'ère chrétienne jusqu'à la fin du Moyen-Âge; 5. Curiosités des sciences surnaturelles; 6. Théorie générale de l'horoscope; 7. Clefs générales de l'astrologie. An English translation of the original French text is: The history and practice of magic. Newly transl. by J. Kirkup & J. Shaw, ed. by R. NICHOLS, 1952, 2 vols., 324 and 297 p. (London: Forge Press). A German standard text dealing with the same topics is: LEHMANN, A., 1925: Aberglaube und Zauberei, von den ältesten Zeiten bis in die Gegenwart, ed. 3, 752 p. (Bearbeitet von D. PETERSEN) (Stuttgart: Enke).

CLARK, G., 1967: The stone age hunters, 143 p., 25 colour plates, 112 black-and-white plates. (Library of the early civilizations) (London: Thames & Hudson).—

In this study the author evaluates recent researches in human palaeontology and Palaeolithic cave art, and shows how they have strongly affected our views on the culture of early men. The author also draws many parallels between these early men and those people who still live under largely Stone Age conditions. *Cf.* GRAZIOSO, P., 1960; and LOMMEL, A., 1965, *vide infra*.

DAWSON, W. R., 1930: The bridle of Pegasus: studies in magic, mythology and folk-lore, 203 p. (London: Methuen).—

This book consists of 8 separate and independent studies of subjects concerning magic, mythology, and folk-lore, which all have in common attempts of primitive man to control, by divine or magical act, the forces of nature. The studies included are 1. The Amphidromia rite; 2. Harpies and bats; 3. A man who became a God (Imhotep); 4. Nose-rubbing and salutations; 5. Mouse eating; 6. The lore of the hoopoe; 7. Birthworts: a study in the progress of medical botany through 23 centuries; 8. Mummy as a drug. Good bibliography.

EBERT, M., 1924-1932: Reallexikon der Vorgeschichte, 15 vols. (Berlin: de Gruyter).—

Standard book of reference on the subject of prehistoric archaeology. The articles have been written by specialists; they carry bibliographies which sometimes are very extensive. Each vol. is about 400 to 500 pages in length and has about 130 plates and maps. Vol. 15 is the index vol. (515 p.).

ELIADE, M., 1951: Le chamanisme et les techniques archaïques de l'extase, 444 p. (Paris: Payot).—

The author discusses shamanism as it has occurred (and even still occurs) in parts of North-, Central- and South-West Asia, North- and South America, in Tibet and China. He deals with the ideology and techniques of shamanism as professed by the Indo-European peoples, with psychopathological phenomena of shamanism, the education of the shaman, the symbolic meaning of his clothes and his drum, diseases and dreams, *etc.* Also in English translation: Shamanism: archaic techniques of ecstasy, 1964, 610 p. (London: Routledge & Kegan Paul). *Cf.* LOMMEL, A., 1965, *vide infra*.

FORBES, T. R., 1966: The midwife and the witch, 196 p. (New Haven, Conn.: Yale U.P.).—

The book contains a record of a va-

riety of superstitions connected with reproduction and childbirth. It mainly deals with the period from the late Middle Ages to the 17th century. Separate sections deal with such subjects as: sex reversal, sexual anomalies in animals, fertility and pregnancy tests, sex prediction, good-luck charms employed during childbirth, the social status of the midwife, her role as medical and spiritual guide, her alleged relations with the powers of evil, the attempts made by both church and state in the later 16th century to raise the standard of her profession by licensing procedures. Valuable bibliography of over 900 items.

FRAZER, J. G., 1963: The golden bough: a study in magic and religion, ed. 3, 13 vols. (London: Macmillan).—

First published in 1890. This is the twelfth reprint of the 3rd edition of 1911. A very useful work on primitive superstition and religion. The 13 vols. have been divided into 9 parts as follows: pt. I: The magic art and the evolution of kings (in 2 vols.); pt. II: Taboo and the perils of the soul; pt. III: The dying God; pt. IV: Adonis, Attis, Osiris (in 2 vols.); pt. V: Spirits of the corn and of the wild (in 2 vols.); pt. VI: The scapegoat; pt. VII: Balder the Beautiful: the fire festivals of Europe and the doctrine of the external soul (in 2 vols.); pt. VIII: Bibliography and general index; pt. IX: Aftermath: a supplement to "The Golden Bough". Much about plants in folklore and superstition, *e.g.*, the worship of trees, the influence of the sexes on vegetation, the killing of the tree-spirit, *etc. Cf.* also: FRAZER, J. G., 1935: Creation and evolution in primitive cosmogonies and other pieces, 151 p. (New York, N.Y.: Macmillan).

GRAZIOSO, P., 1960: Palaeolithic art, 277 p. (London: Faber).—

As far as the editor is aware, the best reference work on this subject. After a short introduction to the study of palaeolithic art, a panoramic view of the artistic achievements of the Old Stone Age follows. The volume is richly illustrated with some 306 plates, many of them being coloured. *Cf.* CLARK, G., 1967, *vide supra*.

HANSMANN, L. & L. KRISS-RETTENBECK, 1966: Amulett und Talisman. Erscheinungsform und Geschichte, 270 p. (Munich: Callwey).—

A beautifully and profusely illustrated history of talismans and amulets. Separate sections deal with stones, trees and herbs, animals and Man, various forms and situations. *Cf.* BUDGE, E. A. W., 1930, *vide supra;* and: SELIGMANN, S., 1927; VILLIERS, E., 1927, *vide infra.*

HAWKES, J., ed., 1963-1964: The world of the past, 2 vols. Vol. I: 602 p.; Vol. 2: 709 p. (London: Thames & Hudson; New York, N.Y.: Knopf).—

An anthology of archaeological history; the great archaeological discoveries are rendered in the words of those who made or interpreted them. Among these persons are lay travellers, poets and men of letters. Extensive introductory notes. The text is in 4 parts. The first part deals with Asia Minor, Greece and Italy: the classical world and its background; the second part (p. 233-318) with India and China; the third part with Europe (p. 319-498); and the fourth part with the Americas (the Mayas, Aztecs, Incas, and North American Indians).

HOLE, F. & R. F. HEIZER, 1965: An introduction to prehistoric archeology, 306 p. (New York, N.Y.: Holt, Rinehart & Winston).—

This book is an attempt to explain to the college student as well as to the layman, how archaeology operates. Its first part is introductory, its second part deals with excavation techniques, its third part with dating of material and its fourth part with interpretation. A very useful introduction to prehistoric archaeological methods and techniques.

JOBES, G., 1961: Dictionary of mythology, folklore and symbols, 2 vols., 1759 p. (New York, N.Y.: Scarecrow Press).—

This is primarily a dictionary of symbolism. The pattern of the more general items, such as animals, gems, plants, *etc.,* follows, where possible, this form: universal and popular symbolism; dream significance; significance in freemasonry; heraldic significance; occult significance; word explanation; cognates or comparisons; mythological and religious significance. In treating deities, wherever possible, the information given is: genealogy, function, explanation of activities and behaviour, attributes or emblems, steeds, how depicted in art, and parallel deities. *Cf.* BREWER, E. C., 1923, *vide supra;* and LEACH, M. & J. FRIED, 1950, *vide infra.*

KOTY, J., 1934: Die Behandlung der Alten und Kranken bei den Naturvölkern, 373 p. (Forschungen zur Völkerpsychologie und Soziologie, XIII) (Stuttgart: Hirschfeld).—

A monograph concerning the bad treatment of old and of sick people as it has occurred and still occurs with some primitive tribes. The author tries to analyse the biological *(e.g.,* hunger), psychological *(e.g.,* religious and/or magical imaginations) and social *(e.g.,* nomadism) motivations of this treatment, criticizes existing theories, and makes comparisons with some aspects of animal life. *(Cf.* SIMMONS, L. W., 1945, *vide infra).*

LEACH, M. & J. FRIED, eds., 1950: Funk & Wagnalls' standard dictionary of folklore, mythology and legend, 2 vols., 1196 p. (New York, N.Y.: Funk & Wagnalls).—

In this book "the folk stories and songs, the gods, heroes, fairies and demons, angels and devils, ogres, guardian spirits, witches, vampires, ... of many different cultures - and in their many varying cultural forms - come to life in 4000 entries." It also includes Assyrian, Babylonian, Egyptian, and Hebrew religious beliefs. *Cf.* BREWER, E. C., 1923; and JOBES, G., 1961, *vide supra.*

LÉVY-BRUHL, L., 1963: Le surnaturel et la nature dans la mentalité primitive, nouv. éd., 526 p. (Paris: Presses Univ. de France).—

An approach to magic, shamanism, sorcery, magical performances, *etc.,* from the psychological rather than from the medical point of view.

LOMMEL, A., 1965: Die Welt der frühen Jäger. Medizinmänner. Schamanen. Künstler, 196 p. (Ed. by B. S. MYERS and J. THIERRY) (Munich: Callwey).—

In his introduction the author tries to give a definition of shamanism, and to indicate in which characteristics the shaman is to be distinguished from the medicineman. Ch. 1 deals with shamanism and hunting; ch. 2 with the main characteristics of the shaman; ch. 3 with his activities, his position in primitive society, with witchcraft in general, *etc.;* ch. 4 with shamanism and art, the shaman's customs, clothes, instruments, *etc.;* and ch. 5 deals with the shaman as a creative artist. Beautifully illustrated; good bibliography (p. 186-196). Also in English translation: The world of the early hunters, 1968, 175 p. (London: Evelyn, Adams & Mackay). An American ed. appeared under the title: Shamanism:

the beginnings of art, 1968, 175 p. (New York, N.Y.: McGraw-Hill). *Cf.* also: CLARK, J., 1967; and ELIADE, M., 1951, *vide supra.*

PEUCKERT, W. E., 1967: Gabalia. Ein Versuch zur Geschichte der magia naturalis im 16.-18. Jahrhundert, 578 p. (Berlin & Munich: Schmidt).—

    An introduction into magico-hermetical literature. The central theme is Paracelsus and his influence.

RADIN, P., 1953: The world of primitive man, 370 p. (New York, N.Y.: Schuman).—

    This book is an attempt to evaluate the contributions made by aboriginal theorists and philosophers to the history of thought. It has been divided into three parts. The first one deals with general aspects of non-literate cultures; the man of action and the thinker; the religious and non-religious man; the interrelations between economy and religion; rites of passage. Part two deals with government, law, social and personal status, and part three with man and his world in myth, literature, and philosophy.

ROBBINS, R. H., 1959: The encyclopedia of witchcraft and demonology, 571 p. (New York, N.Y.: Crown).—

    The author considers witchcraft to be a Christian heresy, and the subject therefore is limited to Western Europe from the beginning of the 15th century up to the 18th century. Witchcraft is considered to be a part of theology; sorcery as it is practised in Africa, Central- and South America, or elsewhere, is not treated in this volume.

SCOTT, G. R., 1951: Phallic worship: a history of sex and sex rites in relation to the religions of all races from antiquity to the present day, 319 p. (London: Torchstream Bks.; New York, N.Y.: Anglobooks).—

    The text is in two parts. The first part is entitled: "The nature and evolution of phallic worship", and deals with such subjects as: the creation of the gods; sun, moon and nature worship; the birth of phallicism; the phallic factor in sexual promiscuity; the connection between serpent-worship and phallicism; the relation between witchcraft and phallicism. The second part (p. 117-268) deals with such subjects as: phallicism in the religions of savage and primitive races; phallicism in the Bible, in ancient Greece and Rome, in Egypt, Persia, Assyria,

etc.; China and Japan; the phallic gods of India; phallic worship in Great Britain, France and other parts of Europe; phallicism in relation to Christianity. A glossary deals with the principal gods and goddesses mentioned in the book. Bibliography and index.

SELIGMANN, S., 1927: Die magischen Heil- und Schutzmittel aus der unbelebten Natur, mit besonderer Berücksichtigung der Mittel gegen den bösen Blick. Eine Geschichte des Amulettwesens, 309 p. (Stuttgart: Strecker & Schröder).—

    Contains a summing-up of all known inorganic substances that have been used as fetish, amulet or talisman. Extensive bibliography and index. A study by the same author, especially dealing with the evil eye: SELIGMANN, S., 1910: Der böse Blick und Verwandtes. Ein Beitrag zur Geschichte des Aberglaubens aller Zeiten und Völker, 2 vols. Vol. I: 88 + 406 p.; Vol. II: 526 p. (Berlin: Barsdorf). This last study will be reprinted by Olms (Hildesheim). *Cf.* HANSMANN, L. & L. KRISS-RETTENBECK, 1966, *vide supra.*

SIMMONS, L. W., 1945: The role of the aged in primitive society, 317 p. (New Haven, Conn.: Yale U.P.; London: Oxford U.P.).—

    This book is a report on the status and treatment of the aged within a worldwide selection of primitive societies. More specifically it deals with the question what securities for long life may be provided by the various social milieus and what may the aged do as individuals to safeguard their interests? The chapter headings are: The assurance of food; Property rights; Prestige; General activities; Political and civil activities; The use of knowledge, magic and religion; The functions of the family; Reactions to death. Extensive bibliography. *Cf.* KOTY, J., 1934, *vide supra.*

SUMMERS, M., 1965: The history of witchcraft and demonology, 354 p. (London: Routledge & Kegan Paul; New York, N.Y.: Univ. Bks.).—

    Reissue of the original 1926 edition. Separate chapters deal with: 1. The witch: heretic and anarchist; 2. The worship of the witch; 3. Demons and familiars; 4. The sabbat; 5. The witch in holy writ; 6. Diabolic possession and modern spiritism; 7. The witch in dramatic literature. Useful and extensive bibliography. Index.

THOMPSON, C. J. S., 1932: The hand of destiny: the folk-lore and superstitions of everyday life, 303 p. (London: Rider).—

This book deals with the folk-lore of birth and infancy, childhood, love and courtship, betrothal and marriage, the body, the hand, the face and features, the hairs, nails and teeth, the folk-lore of apparel, food, everyday life, healing, death and burial, skulls and bones, the folk-lore of sailors and fishermen, birds and insects, plants and flowers, colours, letters and numbers, drinking and drinking vessels, and it deals with the lore of amulets, talismans, mascots, healing-stones, games, and with superstition and witchcraft in everyday life. Illustrations and index.

THOMPSON, S., 1955: Motif-index of folk-literature: a classification of narrative elements in folktales, ballads, myths, fables, mediaeval romances, exempla, fabliaux, jest-books, and local legends, rev. ed., 6 vols. (Bloomington, Ind.: Indiana U.P.; Copenhagen: Rosenkilde & Bagger).—

In the author's own words, the purpose of the present study has been to arrange in a single logical classification the elements which make up traditional narrative literature. Stories that have formed part of a tradition, whether oral or literary, find a place here. The subject matter has been classified in 23 divisions. Vol. 1 contains the sections A (Creation and the nature of the world, creation of living nature, etc.), B (Animals, incl. mythical animals and totemism), and section C (Taboo); vol. 2: D (Magic objects and powers, transformation, etc.), E (Ideas about the dead, ghosts, reincarnation, the nature of the soul); vol. 3: F (Journeys to other worlds, extraordinary creatures, marvellous persons and events), G (Ogres, witches, etc.), H (Tests, e.g., tests of cleverness, of identity, etc.); vol. 4: J (Wisdom, cleverness, foolishness), K (Deceptions); vol. 5 contains some smaller chapters, dealing with such subjects as: reversal of fortune, ordaining the future, chance and fate, society, rewards and punishments, captives and fugitives, unnatural cruelty, sex, the nature of life, religion, traits of character, humour, formulas, symbolism, heroes, horror stories, etc. etc. Vol. 6 contains an elaborate index (892 pages). *Cf.* BÄCHTOLD-STÄUBLI, H., 1927-1942, *vide* subsection d*.

VILLIERS, E., 1927: Amulette und Talismane und andere geheime Dinge: eine volkstümliche Zusammenstellung von Glücksbrin-

gern, Sagen, Legenden und Aberglauben aus alter und neuer Zeit, 314 p. (Munich: Drei Masken Verlag).—

The book contains a more or less complete alphabetical list of the most customary objects incl. numbers and colours to which is ascribed a magic power to bring good luck or to ward off or neutralize evil, as they have been and still are used all over the world, together with an attempt to analyse their historical and/or legendary background. This German edition has been revised by A. M. PACHINGER. *Cf.* also LAARSS, R. H., 1932: Das Buch der Amulette und Talismane. Talismanische Astrologie und Magie, ed. 3, 304 p. (Leipzig: Hummel). *Cf.* HANSMANN, L. & L. KRISS-RETTENBECK, 1966, *vide supra.*

WAGNER, R. L., 1939: "Sorcier" et "magicien". Contribution à l'histoire du vocabulaire de la magie, 292 p. (Paris: Droz).—

In the introduction (p. 9-36), the author discusses such subjects as: the magical vocabulary, the various kinds of magic, the magical vocabulary of H. de Balzac. The first chapter (p. 37-158) discusses the predecessors of the magician, the sorcerer and the singer or chanter. The second chapter deals with the birth of the magician. Useful bibliography. Many historical notes.

WEBSTER, H., 1942: Taboo: a sociological study, 393 p. (Stanford, Calif.: U.P.).—

This book consists of a collection of the most important cases of taboo and taboo transgression. Chapters having special value for the biohistorian and the medical historian are those which deal with: reproductive life, separation of sexes, sexual intercourse, death and the dead, illnesses and dying people, birth accidents, the therapeutic use of diet and confession, the purificatory function of emetics and purgatives, etc.

——, 1948: Magic: a sociological study, 524 p. (Stanford, Calif.: U.P.).—

This book is a kind of a compendium of all that is known of the customs and beliefs which we usually classify under the term of magic, and an attempt to analyse this knowledge in terms of psychological meanings and social functions. Among the topics discussed are such as: the meaning of the concept of the occult in primitive societies, magical techniques and procedures, spells and charms, the personality of the magician, his schooling and his function, and witchcraft and the defence against it (fetishes, amulets, etc.).

ZEUNER, F. E., 1958: Dating the past: an introduction to geochronology, ed. 4, 516 p. (London: Methuen).—

The book describes the various techniques available to determine passed events prior to the time of the historic calendars, especially as they are applied in prehistoric archaeology and human palaeontology. Separate sections deal with tree-ring analysis (back to about B.C. 1000), with the analysis of varved clay (back to about 15,000 years ago), with dating the Old Stone Age, the phases of the ice age and the pluvial phases of the warmer countries (p. 110-306), and with dating the history of the earth and of life before the arrival of Man (back to about 3500 million years ago). Valuable bibliography. Index.

b. Prehistoric and primitive biology
(incl. some folkloristic aspects)

AIGREMONT, 1919: Volkserotik und Pflanzenwelt, ed. 2, 2 vols., 165+121 p. (Leipzig: Krauss).—

Its contents are described by the subtitle: "Eine Darstellung alter wie moderner erotischer und sexueller Gebräuche, Vergleiche, Benennungen, Sprichwörter, Redewendungen, Rätsel, Volkslieder, erotischen Zaubers, und Aberglaubens, sexueller Heilkunde, die sich auf Pflanzen beziehen." Vol. I deals with the trees of the wood, with fruit trees, cultivated shrubs and trees, herbs for the kitchen, and with mushrooms. Vol. II deals with herbs and flowers, with aphrodisiacs and with plants whose names have been derived from parts or functions of the female or the male genital organs. Within each section the plants have been arranged in alphabetical order according to their German name.

BURDICK, L. D., 1905: Magic and husbandry: the folklore of agriculture, 315 p. (Binghamton, N.Y.: Otseningo).—

A book which according to the subtitle deals with "rites, ceremonies, customs, and beliefs connected with pastoral life and the cultivation of the soil; with breeding and the care of cattle; with fruit-growing, bees, and fowls." No further information can be given.

CLAUSEN, L. W., 1954: Insect fact and folklore, 194 p. (New York, N.Y.: Macmillan).—

A rather popular attempt to assemble the widely scattered information about

"insect folklore, products, uses, and other less known associations with man ... against just enough of a background of scientific detail, such as classification and nomenclature, to enable the reader to find his way later through the standard texts and reference works". Much in it is of interest from the literary-historical point of view. Valuable bibliography.

CORNWALL, L. W., 1968: Prehistoric animals and their hunters, 214 p. (London: Faber).—

A semi-popular introduction, describing the animal environment of early man with emphasis on the mammals. The book is primarily intended for students. Much information concerning environment, hunting techniques, *etc.*, of palaeolithic man. *Cf.* LOMMEL, A., 1965, *vide* subsection a.

DELATTE, A., 1938: Herbarius, recherches sur le cérémonial usité chez les anciens pour la cueillette des simples et des plantes magiques, ed. 2, 177 p. (Liège: Bibliothèque Fac. Philos. Lettres Univ. de Liège, fasc. 81).—

The first edition appeared in the Bull. Acad. roy. Belgique (Cl. Lettres) 22: 227-348). In ancient times gathering of herbs or digging of roots were considered dangerous occupations, and therefore, gathering of these herbs, needed for food, drugs, magical or religious rites was accompanied by appropriate ceremonies. Some other rites were performed in order to preserve or to augment the desired properties. In the present book these ceremonies and rites have been described. Many of them persisted for very long periods and probably they have played a role in many of the practices of folk medicine. *Cf.* OHRT, F., 1929, *vide infra.*

DIMBLEBY, G. W., 1967: Plants and archaeology, 187 p. (London: Baker).—

The book is in three parts. The first part contains a survey of the many uses man has made of plants and their products; the second part contains an account of the ways in which different parts of plants may be preserved and discovered, and the third part contains an indication of the kind of information that may be derived from the discoveries. Many literature references (p. 169-176) and very useful illustrations (23). Many examples of changes of vegetation caused by Neolithic Man. A study especially dealing with this last aspect is: IVERSEN, J., 1949: The influence of prehistoric man on vegetation (Danmarks Geol. Undersøgelse 4, Raekke 3: 1-25).

DYER, T. F. T., 1889: The folk-lore of plants, 328 p. (London: Chatto & Windus).—

The author attempts to give a systematic summary of the many branches into which the subject naturally subdivides itself. This book deals with primitive and savage notions respecting plants, plant worship, lightning plants, plants in witchcraft, demonology, fairy-lore, love charms, dream plants, plants and the weather, plant proverbs, ceremonial use, plant names and languages, fabulous plants, the doctrine of signatures, plants and the calendar, children's rhymes and games, sacred plants, plant superstitions, plants in folk-medicine, plants and their legendary history, and mystic plants. Reprinted 1968 (Detroit, Mich.: Singer Tree). *Cf.* LEYEL, C. F., 1932, *vide infra.*

ENGEL, F. M., 1966: Flora magica. Geheimnis und Wesen der Pflanze, 338 p. (Munich: Keysersche Verlagsbuchhandlung).—

A profusely illustrated (many coloured plates) history of plants and the relationship of these plants or their parts to demonology, myths, legends, art, and the science of botany.

GESSMANN, G. W., 1899: Die Pflanze im Zauberglauben. Ein Katechismus der Zauberbotanik. Mit einem Anhang über Pflanzen-Symbolik, 252 p. (Vienna: Hartleben).—

This book consists of the following sections: 1. Die Pflanze im Zauberglauben; 2. Alphabetisch geordnetes Verzeichnis der zu Zauberzwecken verwandten Pflanzen, nebst Beschreibung derselben; 3. Die Stellung der Pflanzen in der Astrologie; 4. Zaubersalben und Räuchermittel; 5. Magische Behandlung der Pflanzen; Appendix: Die Symbolik der Pflanzen. *Cf.* ENGEL, F. M., 1966, *supra.*

LEHNER, E. & J., 1960: Folklore and odysseys of food and medicinal plants, 128 p. (New York, N.Y.: Tudor).—

"In this rare and fascinating work, two of the world's foremost collectors of herbal lore and pictorial symbols proceed to tell of the many voyages, expeditions, intrigues and wars it took to bring to our doorsteps and backyards those plants and foodstuffs of daily use which we have learned to take as a matter of course." Out of these stories the authors collected a body of food- and plant folklore around our commonest foods and herbals. A comparable book written by the same authors is: Folklore and symbolism of flowers, plants and trees, 1960, 128 p. (New York, N.Y.: Tudor), a book devoted to flower symbolism, with explanations of their religious, magical, and legendary significance. With 200 illustrations.

LEYEL, C. F., 1932: The magic of herbs: a modern book of secrets, 320 p. (London: Cape).—

The book deals with the herbs in medicine before the Christian era, in Arabian and European mediaeval medicine, with the great herbals, occult herbalists, herbs in magical rites, with love powders, potions, philtres, poisons and narcotics, recipes of famous cosmetics, with the history of the distillation of aromatic oils and waters, perfumes, with lavender, rosemary, mint, miraculous and magical scents, quacks and their herbal nostrums, with the history of some remedies and the shops and gardens of early apothecaries. *Cf* MAVÉRIC, J., 1935, *vide infra.*

MACLEISH, K. & H. E. HENNEFRUND, eds., 1940: Anthropology and agriculture: selected references on agriculture in primitive cultures, 134 p. (Agricultural Economics Bibliography, No. 89) (Washington, D.C.: U.S. Dept. Agric.).—

A selected list of references to general books and articles in the field of anthropology and to works on the culture of individual peoples and communities, particularly those in which their agriculture is discussed and the man-land relationship is brought out.

MAVÉRIC, J., 1935: La médecine hermétique des plantes ou l'extraction des quintessences par art spagyrique, ed. 2, 216 p. (Paris: Dorbon-Aînée).—

The contents of this booklet may be made clear by its subtitle: Synthèse de la génération universelle, classification et correspondances astrales des plantes, exposé rationnel des vibrations astrales, la chimie spagyrique, détail des opérations les plus secrètes concernant l'extraction des quintessences avec leur administration selon des tempéraments et maladies. Among the many persons considered are: Albert the Great,

R. Lull, Paracelsus, van Helmont, Sylvius, Johannes Actuarios, Dioscorides, Avenzoar, Abulcasis, Celsus, Oribasios, Pierre d'Alban, and others. *Cf.* LEYEL, C. F., 1932, *vide supra.*

OHRT, F., 1929: Herba, gratiâ plena. Die Legenden der älteren Segenssprüche über den göttlichen Ursprung der Heil- und Zauberkräuter, 30 p. (F. F. Communications, No. 82) (Helsinki: Acad. Sci. Fenn.).—

> This short publication deals with the ideas (imaginations) and legends about the divine origin of herbs and their healing or magic properties. *Cf.* DELATTE, A., 1938, *vide supra.*

ROLFE, R. T. & F. W., 1925: The romance of the fungus world: an account of fungus life in its numerous guises, both real and legendary, 309 p. (London: Chapman & Hall).—

> "This treats in a popular way of the group of the fungi, discussing references to them in folk-lore and fiction, describing their morphology, the damage they cause, and also their uses in medicine, in the arts, and as food. Poisonous fungi, the study of fungi as a hobby, and the derivation of fungus names are among other subjects treated." (From: Bot. Abstr. 15: 374, 1926).

SCHMIDT, A. M., 1958: La mandragore, 123 p. (Collection Symboles) (Paris: Flammarion).—

> Table of contents: Cueillir des enfants, des bêtes et des filles; Absorber la mandragore; Enfanter la mandragore; Déterrer la mandragore; Cajoler la mandragore; Raconter la mandragore; Conclusions. *Cf.* THOMPSON, C. J. S., 1934, *infra.*

THOMPSON, C. J. S., 1934: The mystic mandrake, 253 p. (London: Rider).—

> This booklet deals with such topics as: the name, description, and habitat of the mandragora; the mandrake of the Bible; the mandrake of the Hebrews, the Egyptians, Assyrians, Persians, Greeks, Romans; Dioscorides and the mandrake; the mandrake legends in China; mandrake in the Middle Ages; the mandrake in Britain, Germany (Alraun), France, Italy, Armenia; ceremonies in gathering mandrakes; the mandrake in drama, poetry and story; the mandrake in the herbals of the 16th and 17th centuries; the medical and occult properties

attributed to the mandrake, *etc.* A very valuable German contribution to this topic is: STARCK, A.T., 1917: Der Alraun. Ein Beitrag zur Pflanzensagenkunde, 85 p. (New York Univ., Ottendorfer Memorial Series of Germanic Monographs, 14) (Baltimore, Md.: Furst). A more recent (French) publication is: SCHMIDT, A. M., 1958, *supra.*

c. *Prehistoric and primitive medicine*

c₁. *Palaeopathology*

JARCHO, S., ed., 1966: Human palaeopathology. Proceedings of a Symposium held in Washington, D. C., Jan. 14, 1965, under the auspices of the Subcommittee on Geographic Pathology, National Academy of Sciences - National Research Council, 182 p. (New Haven, Conn.: Yale U.P.).—

> An introductory section deals with general problems in human palaeopathology and in the pathology and palaeopathology of the skeleton; a second section deals with the conclusions which may be drawn from findings at specific excavation sites. The symposium was entirely devoted to North American palaeopathology. A Russian book, dealing with the same subject: ROHLIN, D. G., 1965: Bolezni drevnik lyudei kosti lyudei razlitchnyh epohnormalnye i patologitcheski izmenennye, 303 p. (The diseases of fossil men: human bony remains normal and with pathological deformities from various periods) (Moscow & Leningrad: Izdatel'stvo Nauk).

MOODIE, R. L., 1923: Paleopathology: an introduction to the study of ancient evidences of disease, 567 p. (Urbana, Ill.: Univ. of Illinois Press).—

> A very complete survey of all materials available concerning palaeopathology, ranging from Algonkian bacteria down to pre-Columbian and Inca ossements and accompanied by many very beautiful figures. Contains much material concerning the evolution of disease and much that is of interest to any study of prehistoric medicine. After a general introduction in which the subject has been defined, the author gives a historical account of the development of palaeopathology, tabulates all geological evidences of disease, reviews such topics as the pathological conditions of fossil plants; fractures and callus formation, deforming arthritides, caries and alveolar osteitis, chronic infections, and opisthotonos in fossil vertebrates; parasitism among fossil animals; bacteriology of past geological ages;

the extinction of races. The last four chapters have been devoted to palaeoanthropology and deal with: Pathology of the early human races; Diseases of the ancient Egyptians; Disease among the pre-Columbian Indians of North America; Diseases of the ancient Peruvians.

PALES, L., 1930: Paléopathologie et pathologie comparative, 352 p. + 63 plates. (Paris: Masson).—

Separate sections deal with: material and techniques; dystrophias, (congenital malformations, bone diseases, *etc.); traumatic lesions (especially of the skull and of the extremities); lesions of the jaw and teeth; spondylosis; osteo-arthritis; ossification of muscles; unspecific infectious lesions; prehistoric syphilis; prehistoric tuberculosis; cranial osteo-periostitis; tumours of bones. The bibliography contains some 660 items.

TASNÁDI-KUBACSKA, A., 1962: Paläopathologie. Pathologie der vorzeitlichen Tiere, 269 p. (Jena: Fischer).—

This is the first volume of a planned series of three volumes; the other two will deal with human pathology. The present book contains a compilation of all Hungarian palaeopathological material, together with a summary of material gathered from literary sources.

WELLS, C., 1964: Bones, bodies and disease: evidence of disease and abnormality in early man, 288 p. (London: Thames & Hudson).—

This book deals primarily with the history of disease as evidenced by surviving human remains and by ancient arts and artifacts. The author stresses that from the facts discovered in this way conclusions can be drawn about their way of life. The following diseases and abnormalities have been discussed in more or less detail: congenital disease, injury, degenerations, new growths, non-specific infections, specific infections, endocrine and metabolic disorders, poisons, diseases of unknown origin, deficiency diseases, dental diseases, mental diseases. The book includes also subjects such as: skeletal adaptations, cannibalism, trepanning, and artificial deformations. A special section has been devoted to the author's radiographic technique for investigating the frequency of disease in ancient peoples. Good bibliography, classified according to the subjects considered. A standard work on cranial deformation is: DINGWALL, E. J., 1931: Artificial cranial

deformation: a contribution to the study of ethnic mutilations, 313 p. (London: Bale & Danielson). *Cf*. MOREL, C., 1960, *vide* subsection d*.

c2. *Primitive medicine* (incl. such aspects as: shamanism, fetishism, sorcery, amulets, and some other aspects of folk medicine, rational as well as magical)

ARNOLD, D., 1927: Frauenheilkunde bei den primitiven Völkern der Jetztzeit, 21 p. (Diss. Univ. Freiburg i. Br.) (Stettin: Saran).—

A review of primitive anatomy and physiology in general and primitive anatomy and pathology of the female genital organs in particular, discussing such subjects as: gynaecological therapy, prevention of pregnancy, sexual life and hygiene, *etc*. A supplementary study is: BÜGGE, 1927: Die rationell-empirischen Elemente in der Geburtshilfe bei den Primitiven (Diss. Univ. Freiburg i. Br.).

BACKMAN, E. L., 1955: Religious dances in the Christian Church and in popular medicine, 364 p. (London: Allen & Unwin).—

In this study the author makes an effort to discover an explanation of the role which religious dances have played in the history of medicine and in the popular treatment of disease. This has been done from a more general study of the appearance and significance of religious dances in the Christian Church and in Christian Society. Special attention has been paid to the mediaeval dance epidemic. Very detailed accounts have been given of the methods of demon-exorcisms, which, together with the art of healing, are treated as two branches of the same tree.

BALDINGER, M., 1936: Aberglaube und Volksmedizin in der Zahnheilkunde, 70 p. (Diss. Univ. Basel) (Basle: Helbing & Lichtenhahn).—

Separate sections deal with such subjects as: The tooth in superstition (*e.g.,* the place of the teeth, dropping out of the teeth, teeth as amulets, the golden tooth); Teething and shedding of teeth (vegetable, animal and mineral remedies relieving and stimulating teething; amulets relieving teething; the period of teeth eruption; children born with teeth); Remedies against toothache (teeth saints and other religious invocations; vegetable, animal and mineral remedies, amulets, *etc.;* teeth-picking; fixing of teeth

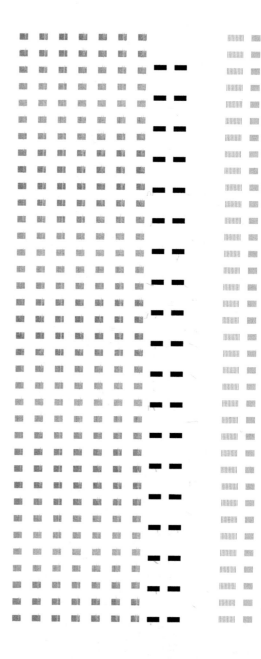

with wedges, spells, and prayers against toothache); Hare-lip; Care of the teeth. Another dissertation dealing with the same kind op topics is: BLÜTHNER, G., 1936: Beiträge und kritische Betrachtungen zur Volksmedizin in der Zahnheilkunde, 30 p. (Diss. Leipzig).

BARTELS, M., 1893: Die Medicin der Naturvölker. Ethnologische Beiträge zur Urgeschichte der Medicin, 361 p. (Leipzig: Grieben).—

One of the first attempts to enrich our knowledge of prehistoric medicine by means of a comparative study of medical practice in primitive races. Many topics have been discussed in order to elucidate medical life of primitive people. To mention some of them: the way in which primitive man reacts to his disease; his beliefs about the causation of the disease; the social position of the physician; natural and supernatural diagnostics; medicines and medical prescriptions used; many examples of surgical intervention. *Cf.* BUSCHAN, G., 1941, *vide infra.*

BOUTEILLER, M., 1950: Chamanisme et guérison magique, 377 p. (Diss. Univ. Paris) (Paris: Presses Univ. de France).—

This is a well-documented essay on primitive culture, chiefly from the psychological point of view *(cf.* LÉVY-BRUHL, L., 1963, *vide supra,* subsection a). Two-thirds of the text are concentrated on the study of shamanism as it has occurred and still occurs in S. Siberia and with the American Indians. It is supposed that the shaman acts by, and on behalf of, society; his curative activities are compared with contemporary physicians as they work in modern France. Part of the book is reserved for a discussion of the techniques of the medicine man whose main procedure is sorcery or magic. A rich and well-classified bibliography has been added. *Cf.* LOMMEL, A., 1965, *vide* subsection a. *Cf.* NIORADZE, G., 1925, *vide* subsection d*.

BROCKBANK, W., 1954: Ancient therapeutic arts, 162 p. (London: Heinemann).—

The text of the Fitzpatrick lectures delivered in 1950 and 1951 at the Royal College of Physicians. Unfortunately I cannot give any information concerning the contents of this book.

BUSCHAN, G., 1941: Ueber Medizinzauber und Heilkunst im Leben der Völker. Geschichte der Urheilkunde, ihrer Entwicklung und Ausstrahlung bis in die Gegenwart, 816 p. (Berlin: Arnold).—

Modern medicine is rooted in prehistoric medicine, and the principal method of unravelling its history is, according to the author, the study of primitive people still living under stone-age circumstances, and the study of old remedies as they are still used in the countryside. In this book the author discusses such topics as: the role of demons both in the causation of and in the defence against, diseases; witchcraft, fetishism, and shamanism in primitive medicine; cure by means of plants and by homeopathic methods; old surgical methods and techniques.

CHAUVET, S., 1936: La médecine chez les peuples primitifs (préhistoriques et contemporains), 143 p. (Paris: Maloine).—

A very readable attempt at writing a history of prehistoric and primitive pathology and therapy. It discusses internal and external pathology and deals with such topics as: sorcery, fetishism, prophylaxis, healing of fractures, trepanations, sexual rites and tattooing. Comparable, but more concise studies, analysing character and techniques of archaic medicine are: ACKERKNECHT, E. H., 1946: Natural diseases and rational treatment in primitive medicine (Bull. Hist. Med. 19: 467-497), and TEMKIN, O., 1930: Beiträge zur archaischen Medizin (Kyklos 3: 90-135).

CLEMENTS, F. E., 1932: Primitive concepts of disease, 67 p. (Univ. Calif., Publ. in Amer. Archaeol. Ethnol. 32: 185-252).—

The author gives a description, classification and discussion of the five main types of disease-concepts of primitive medicine, *viz.,* sorcery, breach of taboo, disease-object intrusion, spirit intrusion and soul loss. It is his aim to obtain an insight into the geographical distribution of these concepts, into their relative antiquity, probable origin, and historical connection. In a large table he summarizes the distribution of these main disease-concepts over the world. Bibliography of 229 items. According to Sigerist this is an important contribution.

DE FRANCESCO, G., 1937: Die Macht des Charlatans, 258 p. (Basle: Schwabe).—

A history of quackery and alchemy with bibliography and index. Many illustrations. *Cf.* JAMESON, E., 1961, *vide infra.*

FILLIOZAT, J., 1943: Magie et médecine, 148 p. (Paris: Presses Univ. de France).—

Separate sections deal with such subjects as: physicians in antiquity, indirect medical magic (divine and demoniacal actions, possession, demoniacal etiology of organic diseases, diagnostic and prognostic, preventive practices, purification, antidemoniacal precautions, curative practices), direct medical magic (etiology, diagnosis and prognosis, preventive and curative practices), the conquest of soul and body by magic, the development and diffusion of magic. *Cf.* RIVERS, W. H. R., 1924, *vide infra.*

FÜHNER, H., 1902: Lithotherapie. Historische Studien über die medizinische Verwendung der Edelsteine, 150 p. (Berlin: Calvary).—

The first part briefly reviews the history of lithotherapy, considering the role of lithotherapy in ancient India, China, Egypt, Mesopotamia, Israel, Greece, Rome, and with the Arabs, in the Salernitan literature, and in the Middle Ages. The second part considers some 52 drugs, arranged in an alphabetical way, and the author shows that most of them had only a suggestive function.

GRABNER, E., ed., 1967: Volksmedizin. Probleme und Forschungsgeschichte, 575 p. (Wege der Forschung, 63) (Darmstadt: Wiss. Buchges.).—

A collection of articles by specialists, published previously in a less accessible form. The editor attempts to determine how much of folk medicine is and has been valid in medical treatment. *Cf.* MAGNUS, H., 1905; and STEMPLINGER, E., 1925, *vide infra.*

GUIARD, E., 1930: La trépanation cranienne chez les néolithiques et chez les primitifs modernes, 126 p. (Paris: Masson).—

Trephining was a cult widely spread over the world during antiquity, a cult still being followed by some peoples. Since trephining was practised on living individuals as well as on the dead, and since the "rondelles" sometimes were perforated and used as necklaces (amulets?) it seems plausible to think of some magico-religious function as well. This is a standard work on the subject, with a bibliography of 242 items. A more recent study of the problem is: JENKNER, F. L., 1966: Prähistorische und präkolumbianische Schädeltrepanation. Kultisch-theurgische oder rationell-medizinische Handlung?, 31 p. (Paracelsus Schriftenreihe der Stadt Villach, No. 11) (Klagenfurt: Geschichtsverein für Kärnten im Landesmuseum für Kärnten). With 5 figures, 7 tables, and bibliography. Another general discussion (in Spanish) can be found in VARA LOPEZ, R., 1949: La craniectomía a través de los siglos, 148 p. (Valladolid: S.R. Cuesta); this book contains many fine illustrations. *Cf.* also LASTRES, J. B. & F. CABIESES, 1960, *vide infra,* subsection d**.

HAMPP, I., 1961: Beschwörung. Segen. Gebet. Untersuchungen zum Zauberspruch aus dem Bereich der Volksheilkunde, 284 p. (Stuttgart: Silberburg).—

This book essentially consists of a collection of 3,000 spells, embracing a period of *ca.* 5000 years. The authoress attempts to make a clear distinction between spell and prayer. A special section (p. 31-109) has been devoted to the medical element in the spell. Other sections deal with spells and magic, and with the various types of spells.

HOVORKA, O. VON, 1915: Geist der Medizin. Analytische Studien über die Grundideen der Vormedizin, Urmedizin, Volksmedizin, Zaubermedizin, Berufsmedizin, 364 p. (Vienna: Braumüller).—

A rather popular general survey of the subjects mentioned in the title. It discusses prehistorical animal and human medicine, protomedicine, popular medicine, magical medicine and the principles and the spirit of professional medicine. The bibliography contains a list of *ca.* 200 books. *Cf.* SIGERIST, H. E., 1955, *vide infra.*

——, & A. KRONFELD, 1908-1909: Vergleichende Volksmedizin. Eine Darstellung volksmedizinischer Sitten und Gebräuche, Anschauungen und Heilfaktoren, des Aberglaubens und der Zaubermedizin, 2 vols. Vol. I: 459 p.; Vol. II: 960 p. (Stuttgart: Strecker & Schröder).—

The book deals with folk-medicine from a comparative point of view, and is mainly restricted to Europe. The first volume deals with causes, nature, and healing of sickness and consists of a list of catchwords (including the historical, cultural and literary implications). In the second volume the material has been arranged according to modern principles, considering such subjects as: diseases of the respiratory-, circulation-, excretory-, nervous-, *etc.* systems; surgery, gynaecology and obstetrics; paediatrics; dermatology; ophthalmology; dentistry. A separate chapter has been devoted to magic medicine. Extensive indexes and many illuminating illustrations.

JAMESON, E., 1961: The natural history of quackery, 224 p. (London: Joseph).—

This book deals especially with the bizarre in medical quackery and contains many anecdotes of famous quacks. The author has chosen some typical representatives of quackery and describes the life and practices of the persons considered. *Cf.* also: CRAMP, A. J., 1923: Nostrums and quackery, 2 vols. Vol. I: 708 p.; Vol. II: 832 p. (Chicago, Ill.: Amer. Med. Assn.), a book of which I am unable to give further information.

MCKENZIE, D., 1927: The infancy of medicine: an enquiry into the influence of folklore upon the evolution of scientific medicine, 421 p. (London: Macmillan).—

A very readable introduction into the history of the beginnings of medicine and the role of this medicine in primitive society, its relation to religion and magic. The book gives very good lists of modern botanical remedies emanating from folk medicine and a list of poisonous herbs recognized as such by folk-lore. There is also a discussion of primitive surgery, major and minor, and of counter-irritation. Extensive bibliography and index.

MADDOX, J. L., 1923: The medicine man: a sociological study of the character and evolution of shamanism, 330 p. (New York, N.Y.: Macmillan).—

This is a comparative study of the position and the role of the medicine man in many countries. The author discusses such subjects as: the training of the medicine man, his social position, functions, fees, methods, remedies, *etc.;* medicine women; the history of some special remedies; the role of charlatans; *etc. Cf.* BOUTEILLER, M., 1950, *vide supra,* and LOMMEL, A., 1965, *vide* subsection a; and CORLETT, W. T., 1935, *vide* subsection d**.

MAGNUS, H., 1905: Die Volksmedizin, ihre geschichtliche Entwicklung und ihre Beziehungen zur Kultur, 112 p. (Abh. Gesch. Med., Heft XV) (Breslau: Kern).—

The first four chapters deal with folk medicine in its relation to primitive and

Christian philosophy. Ch. 5 deals with literary sources of folk medicine, ch. 6 with the circumstances promoting the existence of folk medicine, ch. 7 with treatments employed and medicines used in folk medicine, and ch. 8-13 deal with such subjects as: the role of water, fire, and earth in folk medicine, number and folk medicine, *etc. Cf.* SIGERIST, H. E., 1955, *vide infra;* and GRABNER, E., ed., 1967, *vide supra.*

PRECOPE, J., 1954: Medicine, magic and mythology, 284 p. (London: Heinemann).—

This book contains the history of irrational medicine of pre-Hellenic (Egyptian, Chaldean, and Minoan) and Hellenic times. The author shows that these forms of irrational medicine still exist in our days in many parts of the world, even in the civilized parts of it. The author makes a clear distinction between rational and irrational medicine.

RIVERS, W. H. R., 1924: Medicine, magic, and religion, 147 p. (London: Kegan Paul).—

The author deals with a rather large number of concepts of primitive medicine from the ethnological point of view *(e.g.,* the concept, causation and ascription of disease, magical action on victim's body, treatment, disease and taboo, diagnosis and prognosis, religious elements, leech and priest, rationality of leech-craft, review of primitive medicine in different parts of the world, mind and medicine), and draws certain conclusions as to the historical relationships between various peoples. A book probably dealing with the same kind of subjects, but of which I cannot give further information is: THOMPSON, C. J. S., 1947: Magic and healing, 176 p. (London: Rider). *Cf.* also: FILLIOZAT, J., 1943, *vide supra.*

SAINTYVES, P., 1920: Les origines de la médecine. Empirisme ou magie?, 98 p. (Paris: Nourry).—

The author stresses the role of instinct in the discovery of medicine. He discusses such topics as: magical therapeutics and its religious connections, spirits, the meaning of the soul, sacerdotal medicine, medical mythology, the extasis of the magician, and the empirico-rational elements of mystical medicine. *Cf.* SIGERIST, H. E., 1955, *vide infra.*

SIEBENTHAL, W. von, 1950: Krankheit als Folge der Sünde, 99 p. (Heilkunde und

Geisteswelt, 2) (Hannover: Schmorl & v. Seefelt).—

The author attributes the readiness to view disease as a consequence of sin to a general belief in man's dependence on a higher order; somatic disorder should be a reflection of the disturbance of this order, caused by committing sin. In the present study the author tries to analyse historically the forms in which this belief manifested itself. The five stages distinguished are: primitives; ancient India; Mesopotamia; the Hebrews; the Christian Western civilization. The latter stage is divided into: Jesus of Nazareth; patristic and mediaeval period; Paracelsus; romanticism; development up to the present.

SIGERIST, H. E., 1955: A history of medicine. Vol. I: Primitive and archaic medicine, 564 p. (New York, N.Y.: Oxford U.P.).—

This is an attempt to write a history of medicine in which all human activities directed towards the promotion of health, the prevention of disease, and the restoration and rehabilitation of the sick, are examined in their relation to social, philosophic, economic, geographic, educational, *etc.*, factors, characteristic for the period considered. This is the first volume of the planned 8 volumes, of which, owing to the premature death of its author, only two volumes appeared. It starts with a long introductory chapter, in which the author defines the term medical history used by him, in which he discusses the conceptions of disease in space and time and in which he elaborates his general methodology. One chapter deals with primitive medicine (presenting the medicine of primitive peoples as an expression of their general behaviouristic or cultural pattern), another with medicine of ancient Egypt (in which parallels are established between religion, magic and medicine); and another chapter deals with Mesopotamian medicine (which shows many parallels with Egyptian medicine, however a rational theory is lacking). At the end four appendixes have been added: 1. A list of books on the history of medicine; 2. A list of source books of medical history; 3. A list of museums of medical history; 4. A list of literature dealing with palaeopathology, published since 1930. Sigerist's book was reprinted in 1967. Also in German translation: SIGERIST, H. E., 1963: Anfänge der Medizin. Von der primitiven und archaischen Medizin bis zum Goldenen Zeitalter in Griechenland, 783 p. (Zurich: Europa).

STEMPLINGER, E., 1925: Antike und moderne Volksmedizin, 120 p. (Das Erbe der Alten, 2. Reihe, X) (Leipzig: Dieterich).—

It is shown that folk medicine, as it survives at the present time, is a continuation of ancient occultism, as becomes apparent in its theory and practice. This kind of medicine maintained itself by oral and written tradition during the centuries apart from empirico-rational medicine, that is, it developed in its own specific way. *Cf.* GRABNER, E., ed., 1967, *vide supra.*

d. *Some regional histories on primitive biology and medicine*
d*. *Europe (incl. the Asiatic part of Russia)*

BÄCHTOLD-STÄUBLI, H., ed., 1927-1942: Handwörterbuch des deutschen Aberglaubens, 10 vols. (Berlin & Leipzig: de Gruyter).—

The purpose of the book is described by the editor in the following words: "Das eine (Ziel) ist, die in zahllosen, oft seltenen und entlegenen Publikationen zerstreuten Materialien über die einzelnen abergläubischen Ueberlieferungen zusammenzufassen; das andere, Ursprung und Bedeutung des einzelnen Aberglaubens darzulegen, so weit das uns heute möglich ist ... (Wir haben versucht) ... bei seltener vorkommenden abergläubischen Erscheinungen möglichst alle Belege, die uns bekannt sind, mitzuteilen, dagegen bei solchen die sich häufig finden, oder gar allgemein verbreitet sind, meist nur ihre typischen Formen und als Belege solche Werke zu geben, die leicht zu beschaffen sind und ihrerseits wieder weitere Literaturangaben bieten, so dass der Benützer durch sie den Kreis seiner Belege nach Bedürfnis erweitern und die Verbreitung eines Aberglaubens auch geographisch verfolgen kann. Grundsätzlich hielten wir aber dafür, dass es eher zu viel Literatur mitgeteilt worden solle als zu wenig." Volume 10 contains the index, compiled by G. LÜDTKE.

BOUTEILLER, M., 1966: Médecine populaire d'hier et d'aujourd'hui, 369 p. (Paris: Maisonneuve & Larose).—

This book deals with the whole field of folk medicine as it is and as it was practised in France. The book is especially valuable for its bibliography (exclusively containing French references!). It consists of the following sections: I. Folklore médical, XIXe et XXe siècles; II. Traités de vulgarisation médicale; III. Histoire de la médecine; IV. Phytothérapie; V. Précis de thérapeutique; VI. Le problème des guérisseurs, ses aspects psychologiques, psychosomatiques et psychiatriques; VII. Philosophie générale, anthropologie structurale; VIII. Évolution économique, sociale, religieuse; IX. Radiesthésie, magnétisme, guérison "mystique".

CLARK, J. G. D., 1952: Prehistoric Europe: the economic basis, 349 p. (New York, N.Y.: Philosophical Library).—

    A study of Man in prehistoric Europe from the Upper Palaeolithic to the Iron Age from the ecological point of view, *i.e.,* in relation to his environment. Very good bibliography.

DIEPGEN, P., 1935: Deutsche Volksmedizin, wissenschaftliche Heilkunde und Kultur, 136 p. (Stuttgart: Enke).—

    "Fesselnde und leicht verständliche Darstellung über die Verbundenheit der deutschen Volksmedizin mit der wissenschaftlichen Heilkunde, über ihre Wurzeln im deutschen Volkstum und in der deutschen Kultur von den alten Germanen bis zur Gegenwart ... Von besonderem Interesse sind die deutlich hervortretenden Beziehungen des magischen und religiösen Bedürfnisses der Volksseele zu dem magisch-religiösen Weltbild der wissenschaftlichen Medizin und der grosse Einfluss der körperlichen und seelischen Volkskrankheiten auf das volksmedizinische Denken. Beides wird neben den Erfahrungselementen und dem, was sich aus den Standesverhältnissen des Heilpersonals ergibt, ausführlich behandelt. Ueberall ergeben sich Beziehungen zum Volkstum und zu schwebenden Fragen der Gegenwart." (From Isis 24: 285). A comparable booklet, suffering from the same nationalistic bias is: JUNGBAUER, G., 1934: Deutsche Volksmedizin. Ein Grundriss, 216 p. (Berlin: de Gruyter).

ERIXON, S. E., ed., 1960 → : International dictionary of regional European ethnology and folklore. Vol. 1 (1960): 282 p.; Vol. 2 (1965): 364 p. (Copenhagen: Rosenkilde & Bagger).—

    This terminological dictionary of regional European ethnology and folklore is published by CIAP (International Commission on Folk Arts and Folklore), under the auspices of the International Council for Philosophy and Humanistic Studies, and will consist of 12 vols. Chairman of the editorial committee: S. E. Erixon; chief editor: A. Hultkrantz. The first vol. of this dictionary (ed. by A. HULTKRANTZ), deals with general concepts, schools and methods. The second vol. (ed. by L. BØDKER), deals with Germanic folk literature. The scope of the dictionary is restricted to the scientific terminology employed by experts in the fields of ethnology and the different branches of folklore.

HÖFLER, M., 1908: Die volksmedizinische Organotherapie und ihr Verhältnis zum Kultopfer, 305 p. (Stuttgart, Berlin & Leipzig: Union dtsch. Verlagsges.).—

    Review of the treatment of human diseases by means of animal organs (brain, liver, heart, spleen, lungs, kidneys, *etc.)* especially as they were practised in German folk medicine, and the relationship between these organs and primitive magic and religion.

——, 1908: Volksmedizinische Botanik der Germanen, 125 p. (Quell. Forsch. dtsch. Volkskunde, V) (Vienna: Ludwig).—

    "Die volksmedizinische Botanik ... hat besonders dann ein Interesse, wenn (man) Freude hat an dem Rückblicke auf den kulturgeschichtlichen Hintergrund, auf dem ungezählte Generationen in ihrer Denk- und Vorstellungsweise sich die Wirkung solcher Heilkräuter zurechtlegten, und wenn (man) dabei den Entwicklungsgang aus den Urzeiten wenigstens zu ahnen vermag." The author considers only those plants which are endemic in the areas formerly occupied by the Germanic peoples. Popular introduction.

KEMP, P., 1935: Healing ritual: studies in the technique and tradition of the southern Slavs, 335 p. (London: Faber).—

    This book deals with folk-psychology, -physiology, and -pathology, the ritual of healing, the elements of a folk-Christianity and its relation to magic, the sources of ancient magic and medicine, the folk-doctor and his patrons, and with therapy, technique, and tradition in folk medicine. Bibliography and index.

KRONFELD, M., 1898: Zauberpflanzen und Amulette. Ein Beitrag zur Culturgeschichte und Volksmedicin, 84 p. (Vienna: Perles).—

    The author discusses the occult and magic powers in health and disease ascribed to the most common (Middle) European plants and their application as amulets to ward off diseases. The plants have been arranged according to their Latin names. A list of German folk-names has been included.

LELAND, C. G., 1963: Etruscan magic and occult remedies, new ed., 385 p. (New York, N.Y.: Univ. Bks.).—

This study is mainly based on the pagan beliefs of Tuscan peasantry. Up to the days when Leland studied these beliefs (*ca.* 1880) Tuscany was relatively isolated. In the first part of this book the author tells about Tuscan peasants and their real priests, their witches and warlocks, their gods and goblins. In the second part he tells about their incantations, divination, medicine and amulets.

MANNHARDT, W., 1904-1905: Wald- und Feldkulte, ed. 2. Vol. I: Der Baumkultus der Germanen und ihrer Nachbarstämme. Mythologische Untersuchungen, 648 p.; Vol. II: Antike Wald- und Feldkulte aus nordeuropäischer Ueberlieferungen erläutert, 40+359 p. (Berlin: Borntraeger).—

Vol. 1 contains the following chapters: 1. Die Baumseele; 2. Die Waldgeister und ihre Sippe; 3. Die Baumseele als Vegetationsdämon; 4. Anthropomorphische Wald- und Baumgeister als Vegetationsdämonen; 5. Vegetationsgeister: Maibrautschaft; 6. Vegetationsgeister: Sonnenzauber; 7. Vegetationsdämonen: Nerthus; Appendix: Baumgeist und Korndämon. Vol. 2 contains the following chapters: 1. Dryaden; 2 and 3. Die wilden Leute der griechischen und römischen Sage (p. 39-211); 4. Erntemai und Maibaum in der antiken Welt; 5. Persönliche Vegetationsgeister in Jahrfestgebräuchen; 6. Sonnenwendfeuer im Altertum. Index.

MANNINEN, I., 1922: Die dämonistischen Krankheiten im finnischen Volksaberglauben. Vergleichende volksmedizinische Untersuchung, 254 p. (F. F. Communications 45) (Helsinki: Acad. Sci. Fenn.).—

I. Die Krankheiten nach ihrem Ursprung (p. 13-150). 1. Krankheiten die von den Toten herrühren; 2. Idem, die von den Erdgeistern und der Erde herrühren; 3. Idem, die von den Waldgeistern und dem Walde herrühren; 4. Idem, die von den Wassergeistern und dem Wasser herrühren; 5. Idem, die vom Winde herrühren; 6. Idem, die vom Feuer herrühren; 7. Idem, die von den Haus- und Badstubengeistern herrüh-

ren; 8. Idem, die von spezialisierten Gottheiten und aus verschiedenen Ursachen hervorgerufen sind; 9. Die Krankheitsdämonen. II. Die Krankheiten nach ihrer Erscheinungsweise (p. 151-197). 1. Das Besessenwerden als Ursache der Krankheiten; 2. Äussere Angriffe von Seiten der Geister als Ursache der Krankheiten; 3. Anstecken-Angreifen. Valuable bibliography (p. 228-251).

MARZELL, H., 1938: Geschichte und Volkskunde der deutschen Heilpflanzen, 2. Aufl. von "Unsere Heilpflanzen", 312 p. (Stuttgart: Hippokrates).—

This book contains folkloristic information on about 80 German medicinal plants, chiefly based on the study of original source material such as ancient herbals and garden books. It is a book of reference; excluded are theorizing discussions and speculations. Good bibliography and index. A more specialized study of the role of plants in German folklore and folkbelief is: MARZELL, H., 1922: Die heimische Pflanzenwelt im Volksbrauch und Volksglauben. Skizzen zur deutschen Volkskunde, 133 p. (Wissenschaft und Bildung, No. 177) (Leipzig: Quelle & Meyer). The same author also wrote: Bayrische Volksbotanik. Volkstümliche Anschauungen über Pflanzen im rechtsrheinischen Bayern, 1926, 252 p. (Nuremberg: Spindler); reprinted in 1968 (Munich: Fritsch). Another thorough study of folkloristic botany of Germany is: NIESSEN, J., 1935-1937: Rheinische Volksbotanik. Die Pflanzen in Sprache, Glaube und Brauch des rheinischen Volkes, 2 vols. Vol. I: 276 p.; Vol. II: 341 p. (Bonn: Dümmler). *Cf.* also PRITZEL, G. & C. JESSEN, 1882, *vide infra,* and KROEBER, L., 1934-1935: Das neuzeitliche Kräuterbuch. Die Arzneipflanzen Deutschlands in alter und neuer Betrachtung, 3 vols. Vol. I (ed. 4, 1948): 454 p.; Vol. II (ed. 3, 1947): 336 p.; Vol. III (ed. 2, 1949): Giftpflanzen, 476 p. (Stuttgart: Hippokrates).

MOREL, C., 1960: La médecine et la chirurgie osseuses aux temps préhistoriques dans la région des Grands Causses, 128 p. (Paris: La Nef de Paris).—

A study on human palaeopathology, based on regional findings. The greater part of this study deals with trepanning, and a new hypothesis to explain its function has been put forward. It also deals with such subjects as vertebral malformations, osteomyelites, wounds, and fractures of bones. *Cf.* also: LEHMANN-NITSCHE, R., 1898: Beiträge zur prähistorischen Chirurgie nach Funden aus deutscher Vorzeit. (Diss. Univ. Munich).

NIORADZE, G., 1925: Der Schamanismus bei den sibirischen Völkern, 121 p. (Stuttgart: Strecker & Schröder).—

The author states that formerly shamanism had a very wide distribution in Asia, and that now nearly all shamans have been baptized. The author discusses the principles of shamanism, the meaning of death, spirits, the connection between spirits and earthy things, plants and animals, the causes of diseases. Concerning the shaman himself a variety of topics have been discussed, *e.g.,* his psychology, education, inauguration, clothes, ceremonies, *etc.,* and his social position. Another study dealing with shamanism in Siberia is: CZAPLICKA, M. A., 1914: Aboriginal Siberia: a study in social anthropology, 374 p. (Oxford: Clarendon Press). One section (p. 307-325) gives a systematic account of that mental defect that can be designated by the term "Arctic hysteria"; other sections deal with such subjects as: marriage, customs and beliefs connected with birth, death, burial, future life, ancestor worship (p. 23-165) and with religion, particularly with shamanism (p. 166-306). Good bibliography concerning Russian and other literature on shamanism (p. 331-351). Glossary and extensive index. *Cf.* BOUTEILLER, M., 1950, *vide* subsection C₂.

PRITZEL, G. & C. JESSEN: 1882: Die deutschen Volksnamen der Pflanzen. Neuer Beitrag zum deutschen Sprachschatze. Aus allen Mundarten und Zeiten zusammengestellt, 2 vols. Vol. I: 465 p.; Vol. II: 241 p. (Hannover: Cohen).—

An alphabetically arranged list of plant names according to the Latin name. Under each of them the German folk-names have been given. Vol. I contains an alphabetical list of folk names, followed by the Latin name. Reprinted 1967 (Amsterdam: Schippers). *Cf.* also MARZELL, H., 1938, *vide supra.*

QVIGSTAD, J., 1932: Lappische Heilkunde, 270 p. (Oslo: Inst. for comparative studies of culture; Cambridge, Mass.: Harvard U.P.).—

Lappish medical traditions are comparable to those which occurred amongst the hordes of barbarians, such as Huns, Slavs, and Goths between the 4th and 10th century, and many of their superstitions may be derived from those of the pre-Vikings. The author gives much information concerning some woman-healers, and he discusses their form of treatment of patients

and the therapeutics they used. The author shows that many points of agreement exist with folk medicine of the Far East, especially concerning some obstetric methods and ceremonies.

RANTASALO, A. V., 1919-1925: Der Ackerbau im Volksaberglauben der Finnen und Esten mit entsprechenden Gebräuchen der Germanen verglichen, 537 p. (F. F. Communications 30(1919): 1-95; 31(1919): 1-142; 32(1920): 1-36; 55(1925): 164 p.) (Helsinki: Acad. Sci. Fenn.).—

The first part deals with such subjects as: reclamation of land, digging of ditches, fencing, manuring, ploughing, harrowing; the second part with: seeding time, the times of sowing and planting, the weather, bewitching of the seeds; the third part with: sacrificial rites accompanying sowing and planting, various precautionary measures concerning sowing and planting, sowing and ploughing feasts; the fourth part deals with: bewitching of strange cultures and removal of the bewitching, the wreaking of vengeance upon the bewitcher, protection of the crops. *Cf.* MANNHARDT, W., 1904-1905, *vide supra.*

——, 1945-1953: Der Weidegang im Volksaberglauben der Finnen, 886 p. (F. F. Communications 134 (1945): 130 p.; 135 (1947): 328 p.; 143 (1953): 248 p.; 148 (1953): 180 p. (Helsinki: Acad. Sci. Fenn.).—

The first part ("Die Vorbereitungen für das Viehaustreiben") deals with such subjects as: the first day of driving the cattle out of the stable; bewitching of the grazing-land; the cow-bell. The second part ("Die Hinausführung des Viehes auf die Weide") deals with such subjects as: the cattle drover; the letting loose of the cattle and the driving out of the stable; protection of the herd by means of charms; bewitching of the cattle in order to make them return from the grazing-land. The third part ("Viehhüten und Weidegang") deals with such subjects as: the shepherd, his attributes, and his festivals; the ghosts living on the grazing-land and the protection of the cattle against these ghosts. The fourth part ("Das Zurückführen des Viehes im Herbst in den Viehstall") deals with such subjects as: the day of return; the driving in and tying up the cattle; bewitching of the stable; bewitching of the animals when entering the stable; feeding of the cattle in autumn. Bibliography and valuable index of subjects.

ROLLAND, E., 1877-1916: Faune populaire de France, 12 vols. (Paris: Maisonneuve).—

Each volume considers the popular names, old sayings, proverbs, legends, narratives and superstitions of the animals included. Vol. 1 (1877) deals with wild mammals; vol. 2 (1879) with wild birds; vol. 3 (1881) with reptiles, fishes, molluscs, crustaceans and insects; vol. 4 (1881) with domestic mammals; vol. 5 (1882) also with domestic mammals; vol. 6 (1883) with domestic birds and falconry; vols. 7 (1906) and 8 (1908) are supplementary to vol. 1 and also deal with wild mammals; vols. 9 (1911) and 10 (1915) are supplementary to vol. 2 and also deal with wild birds; vols. 11 and 12 are supplementary to vol. 3; vol. 11 (1916) deals with reptiles and fishes; and vol. 12 (1909) with molluscs, crustaceans, arachnids, and annelids.

——, 1914: Flore populaire ou histoire naturelle des plantes dans leurs rapports avec la linguistique et le folklore, vol. I (1896): 256 p.; vol. II (1899): 268 p.; vol. III (1900): 264 p.; vol. IV (1903): 254 p.; vol. V (1904): 416 p.; vol. VI (1906): 308 p.; vol. VII (1908): 262 p.; vol. VIII (1910): 218 p.; vol. IX (1912): 282 p.; vol. X (1913): 226 p.; vol. XI (1914): 261 p. (Paris: Maisonneuve).—

This work has been set up in the same way as the preceding one. Vols. VIII-XI have been edited by H. GAIDOZ. The whole work was reprinted in 1967 (Paris: Maisonneuve & Larose).

SEBILLOT, P., 1904-1907: Le folk-lore de France. Vol. III: La faune et la flore, 541 p. (Paris: Guilmoto).—

A thorough study of French folk lore of animals, trees and herbs, including folk medicine, folk tales, folk beliefs, etc. Important as a bibliographical source. Cf. ROLLAND, E., 1877-1916 and 1914, supra.

WILKE, G., 1936: Die Heilkunde in der europäischen Vorzeit, 418 p. (Leipzig: Kabitzsch).—

Separate sections deal with such subjects as: anatomical knowledge (head, eye, heart, lungs, spleen, genitals, extremities, etc.), the concept of disease and ideas about the causation of disease (diseases caused by witchcraft, demons, sin, etc.), diagnostics and the knowledge ancient people had of some diseases and their treatment (rheumatoid arthritis, infectious diseases, tuberculosis, jaundice, diseases of the heart, the stomach, the urogenital tract, eyes, ears, etc.), fecundation, pregnancy, childbirth, female diseases (incl. menstruation), diseases of the child (incl. child sacrifices), surgery (wounds caused by implements of war, by animals, tumours, ulcers, operations, fractures of bones or joints), dentistry, magical medicine (shamanism, amulets, defence against demons, witchcraft, etc.), murder on sick and old people, healing baths, etc.

d**. America

BRANDT, D. D., ed., 1936: Symposium on prehistoric agriculture, 72 p. (Univ. New Mexico Bull., No. 296) (Albuquerque, N.M.: Univ. New Mexico Press).—

After a brief introduction by the editor, there are chapters on the origin of the maize plant and maize agriculture in ancient America, on maize as a measure of Indian skill, on the utilization of maize among the ancient Pueblos, on prehistoric irrigation in the Salt River Valley, on the Snaketown canal, on aboriginal cotton in the Southwest, and on southwestern agricultural history. A study especially dealing with the history of maize is: WEATHERWAX, P., 1954: Indian corn in old America, 253 p. (New York, N.Y.: Macmillan), and a very useful bibliography of these topics is: EDWARDS, E. E., 1932: Agriculture of the American Indians: a classified list of annotated historical references, with an introduction, 89 p. (Bibliographical Contributions, U. S. Dept. Agric. Library, No. 23). This is a mimeographed issue published by the U.S.D.A. Library, considering the following topics: Agriculture of the American Indians: general historical references; Agriculture of particular regions and tribes; Specific crops, miscellaneous; Agriculture on Indian reservations in the United States; Uncultivated plants used by the American Indians (food and industrial plants; medicinal plants).

CASTETTER, E. F., et al., 1935-1941: Ethnobiological studies in the American Southwest, 480 p. (Univ. New Mexico Bull., Nos. 266, 275, 297, 307, 314, 335, 372) (Albuquerque, N.M.: Univ. New Mexico Press).—

The contents of this series of papers may be illustrated by giving its subtitles: 1. Uncultivated native plants used as sources of food (Bull. 266, 1935); 2. The ethnobiology of the Papago indians (in collaboration with R. M. UNDERHILL; Bull. 275, 1935);

3. The ethnobiology of the Chiricahua and Mescalero Apache: A. The use of plants for foods, beverages and narcotics (in coll. with M. E. OPLER; Bull. 297, 1936); 4. The aboriginal utilization of the tall cacti in the American southwest (in coll. with W. H. BELL; Bull. 307, 1937); 5. The utilization of mesquite and screwbean by the aborigines in the American Southwest (in coll. with W. H. BELL; Bull. 314, 1937); 6. The early utilization and distribution of agave in the American southwest (in coll. with W. H. BELL and A. R. GROVE; Bull. 335, 1938); 7. The utilization of yucca, sotol, and beargrass by the aborigines in the American southwest (in coll. with W. H. BELL; Bull. 372, 1941).

CHAVEZ, I., 1947: México en la cultura médica, 187 p. (Mexico, D. F.: Ed. Colegio Nacional).—

This is a study to evaluate Mexico's place in the world of medicine. The history of Mexican medicine begins with that of the Aztecs, Toltecs and Maya, and this form of medicine reminds us in many ways of Egyptian and Babylonian medicine; the main difference is that there are no written documents. The only thing Mexican medicine could contribute to the old world was a series of new spices, drugs, and foods, but no new theories or techniques. During the colonial period (1521-1821) there was a great Spanish influence: hospitals, leprosaria, schools, and even a university were established, and by 1536 European medicine was taught officially; but much attention was paid to native medicine, too, and so the famous Badianus ms. could originate (cf. EMMART, E. W., 1940, vide infra). But the development remained behind and in 1829 Hippocrates, Galen and Avicenna were still the official textbooks of medicine. In 1833 a reform movement began and many Mexican physicians went to Europe for study and training. Another new period began in 1920, the period of specialization. This is, in short, the history described in this book. Another study dealing with the history of medicine of the Aztecs (of which - unfortunately - I possess no further details) is: GALL, A. von, 1939-1940: Medizinische Bücher der alten Azteken aus der ersten Zeit der Conquista. (Quell. Stud. Gesch. Med., vol. 7, Nos. 2-5). Cf. GERSTE, A., 1910, vide infra.

CORLETT, W. T., 1935: The medicine-man of the American Indian and his cultural background, 369 p. (Springfield, Ill.: Thomas).—

This book extends the scope of STONE's book (vide infra) since it includes the rest of America. The author shows the fundamental similarities of medical practice among the New World aborigines, and emphasizes the close interconnection between Indian religious beliefs and medical practice. The text has been divided into five parts. Part I deals with, e.g.: the origin, races, culture of American Indians; Indian diseases past and present; religion, medicine men and disease. Part II deals with the medicine men of the New World; the Eskimos, and the different Indian tribes of N. and S. America. Part III deals with childbearing; part IV with foods and materia medica, and part V with the American Indian's recessional. An extensive bibliography has been included.

COURY, C. & M. D. GRMEK, 1969: La médecine de l'Amérique précolombienne. 351 p. (Paris: Dacosta).—

A beautifully-illustrated history of pre-Columbian American medicine. Separate sections deal with ancient civilizations, the magico-religious and empirical aspects of medicine, knowledge of anatomy, physiology, and pathology, infectious and parasitic diseases, endemics and epidemics, deformities, surgery, public hygiene, the medical profession, therapy. An appendix (by M. D. GRMEK) deals with medical subjects in the iconography of ancient Mexican manuscripts (p. 233-252). Bibliography (p. 333-350). Cf. STONE, E., 1962, vide infra.

d'HARCOURT, R., 1939: La médecine dans l'ancien Pérou, 248 p. (Paris: Maloine).—

After a brief introduction, the author discusses various aspects of old Peruvian folk medicine. Some remedies are discussed in some detail, e.g., the coca, the datura, the ayahuasca, and the yaje. The author also considers some old-Peruvian diseases (e.g., uta and verruga, and syphilis), surgical practices (trepanation, amputation, mutilation), and some rituals with medical implications, such as those relating to skull deformation, child care, marriage, the attainment of adolescence, etc. A more recent study of ancient Peruvian medicine is to be found in: LASTRES, J. B., 1951: Historia de la medicina Peruana, Vol. I: La medicina Incaica, 352 p. This book has been described in the section History of the medical sciences α , subsection b.

EMMART, E. W., ed., 1940: The Badianus manuscript (Codex Barberini, Lat. 241) Vatican Library. An Aztec herbal of 1552, 341

p. + 118 plates in colour. (Baltimore, Md.: Johns Hopkins U.P.).—

A very beautiful facsimile reproduction and translation of a brilliantly illustrated Aztec medical herbal containing coloured pictures of some 183 Mexican plants. The original was written in 1552 by two Aztec Indians at the College of Santa Cruz in Tlaltelulco; one of them, Joannes Badianus, translated the ms. into Latin with the exception of the plant names (at that time these plants had no Latin names). The plants were arranged according to their curative properties, and the medicine involved is purely Indian, still uninfluenced by the Spanish conquerors. In an introduction, the editor places the contents of this herbal in its proper historical setting. The Badianus ms. is incorporated in the Vatican Library, and was discovered there by 1929. An English translation of this same herbal has been prepared by GATES, W., 1939. The De la Cruz-Badiano Aztec herbal of 1552: translation and commentary, 144 p. (Baltimore, Md.: Maya Society). In 1964 appeared, under the editorship of Efrén C. DEL POZO, a Spanish facsimile edition with many commentaries and many illustrations: Libellus de medicinalibus indorum herbis. Manuscrito Azteca de 1552 según traducción latina de Juan Badiano, 394 p., 133 pages facsimile, 179 coloured plates and 3 figs. (México: Inst. Mexicano de Seguro Social).

GERSTE, A., 1910: Notes sur la médecine et la botanique des anciens Mexicains, ed. 2, 191 p. (Rome: Impr. Polyglotte Vaticane).—

The rich and many sided contents of this book may become evident from the chapter headings: 1. La médecine indigène au XVIe siècle; 2. La médecine précolombienne; 3. La magie médicale; 4. La thérapeutique; 5. La botanique indigène; 6. Science rudimentaire des végétaux; 7. Iconographie conventionelle; 8. Iconographie figurative; 9. Taxonomie végétale; 10. Classifications diverses; 11. Ébauche de géographie botanique; 12. Les fleurs dans la poésie Nahua; de quelques travaux récents sur la botanique et la médecine des anciens Mexicains. It contains much that is of ethnobotanical value. Cf. CHAVEZ, I., 1947, vide supra.

HILL, W. W., 1938: Agricultural and hunting methods of the Navaho Indians, 194 p. (New Haven, Conn.: Yale U.P.).—

This book deals inter alia with: territory, annual cycle and daily life, field location, ownership of the land, preparation for planting, planting, cultivation of crops, harvesting, storage, crop utilization, the culture of non-food plants and of introduced plants, agricultural rituals (e.g., rain ceremonies), the mythological background of hunting, education in ritual hunting, nonritual hunting, the ritualization of everyday behaviour, and with Navaho culture in its relationship to neighbouring cultures.

KLUCKHOHN, C. K. M., 1944: Navaho witchcraft, 149 p. (Papers of the Peabody Museum of American Archaeology and Ethnology, XXII, No. 2) (Cambridge, Mass.: Peabody Museum).—

The contents have been divided into three parts. The first part contains many facts of witchery, sorcery, wizardry, and frenzy witchcraft, terms which are defined in this study. The second part "An essay in structural dynamics", contains a theoretical discussion of witchcraft and its psychological role in Navaho society; and the third part consists of translated interviews and folklore materials.

LASTRES, J. B. & F. CABIESES, 1960: La trepanación del cráneo en el antiguo Perú, 207 p. (Lima: Imp. Univ. San Marcos).—

The first half of the book serves as a background for a general discussion of trephinations in pre-Columbian Peruvian societies. The second half deals with the technique of trephining, the instruments used, etc. The authors conclude from this study that the defects were made for therapeutic reasons, although these peoples had no special knowledge of the brain and its functions. Many fine illustrations. A table of cases of putative trephining from North America, arranged in a chronological order, can be found in: STEWART, J. D., 1957: Stone age skull surgery: a general review, with emphasis on the New World. (Ann. Rep. Smithsonian Inst. for 1957: 469-491). With bibliography.

LEIGHTON, A. H. & D. C., 1945: The Navaho door: an introduction to Navaho life, 149 p. (Cambridge, Mass.: Harvard U.P.).—

This book is primarily meant for Indian service workers, but because of its thoroughness it is of general value to anyone interested in the Indian way of life. It gives a description of life and work of the Navaho, the way they look at things, and a special study has been made of health conditions. The Navahos looked at disease as a social responsibility and distinguished between 3 types of healing personnel, *viz.*, the diagnostician, the curer, and the singer or chanter. Two chapters have been devoted to the Navaho way in medicine and the influence of the European immigrants and one to the Navaho conditions of health (p. 54-94). About the Navahos and their medicine, *cf.* KLUCKHOHN, C. K. M. & K. E. SPENCER, 1940: A bibliography of the Navaho Indians, 93 p. (New York, N.Y.: Augustin). *Cf.* also KLUCKHOHN, C. & D. LEIGHTON, 1962: The Navaho, ed. 2, 355 p. (Garden City, N.Y.: Doubleday). *Cf.* also: HILL, W. W., 1938; and KLUCKHOHN, C. K. M., 1944, *vide supra*.

MACGOWAN, K., 1950: Early man in the New World, 260 p. (New York, N.Y. & London: Macmillan).—

A rather popular but yet scientifically sound work on New World prehistory. There are also chapters on the beginning of agriculture. It contains a large body of information.

MOONEY, J. & F. M. OLBRECHTS, 1932: The Swimmer manuscript: Cherokee sacred formulas and medicinal prescriptions, 319 p. (Smithsonian Inst., Bur. Amer. Ethnology, Bull. 99) (Washington, D.C.: Govt. Printing Office).—

This book is in two parts. The first part (p. 1-165) contains an elaborate account of Cherokee views on disease and therapeutics, discussing such subjects as: the medicine man, child-birth, views on pregnancy and its care, care for children, raising a child to become a witch, twins, death and after-life, *etc.* The second part contains the Cherokee text with English translation.

MORLEY, S. G., 1946: The ancient Maya, 32 + 520 p. (Stanford, Calif.: Stanford U.P.).—

According to Sarton in Isis 37: 245 an admirable synthesis of Maya knowledge. Also in Spanish translation: La civilisación maya. Versión española de Adrián Recinos, 1947, 577 p. (Mexico, D. F.: Fondo de Cultura Economica). A rather popular history concerning Maya civilization is: THOMPSON, J. E. S., 1966: The rise and fall of Maya civilization, ed. 2, 344 p. (Norman, Okl.: Oklahoma U.P.). A summarily review, based upon six of seven major classics on the subject, has been given by GALLENKAMP, C., 1959: Maya: the riddle and rediscovery of a lost civilization, 240 p. (New York, N.Y.: McKay). Also 1960 (London:

Muller). *Cf.* also: PENNACCHIA, T., 1960; and ROYS, R. L., 1931, *vide infra*.

PARDAL, R., *ca.* 1937: Medicina aborigen americana, 377 p. (Humanior, Biblioteca del Americanista moderno, sección C: Patrimonio cultural indiano, No. 3) (Buenos Aires: Anesi).—

The text is in four parts. The first part deals with medical ethnology, showing that medical knowledge of the Indians was based on magic and therapeutical empirism; the second part deals with medicine in ancient Peru and Mexico, with special reference to the practice of trephining and to the representation of some diseases, especially of syphilis, on pottery; the third part deals with stimulating, narcotic, and hallucinating drugs, especially with coca, maté and peyotl, with the balsams of Tolu and Peru, with guiacum, cinchona, and some other drugs; the fourth part deals with the introduction of modern American drugs and medicines. *Cf.* COURY, C. & M. D. GRMEK, 1969, *vide supra*.

PENNACCHIA, T., 1960: La storia della medicina Maya, 160 p. (Pisa: Scientia Veterum).—

This study on the pathology, therapeutics, and surgery of the Maya has been based on the collected archaeological material, gathered in Honduras by F. Lunardi and preserved at Genoa. Many of the original pieces of the collection have been reproduced on 35 plates.

PÉREZ DE BARRADAS, J., 1957: Plantas mágicas Americanos, 342 p. (Madrid: Consejo superior de investigaciones cientificas, Instituto "Bernardino de Sahagun").—

Chapter headings are as follows: 1. De cómo los españoles descubrieron la medicina de los Indios; 2. Chamanismo, magia y medicina primitiva; 3. Chamanes, médicos brujos y curanderos americanos; 4. Las plantas medicinales mágicas y fantásticas de la América indigena; 5. Plantas mágicas excitantes y estimulantes mentales; 6. La coca, planta mágica, eufórica y dinamógena; 7. El peyotl, la planta que produce sueños en color; 8. El yagé, planta mágica fantástica; 10. Los borracheros, plantes mágicas alucinantes. Indexes of authors, geographical terms, and names of plants.

ROYS, R. L., 1931: The ethno-botany of the Maya, 359 p. (Tulane Univ. Louisiana Middle American Research Series, Publ. 2)

(New Orleans, Dept. Middle Amer. Research, Tulane Univ.).—

With the Maya Indians the study of medicinal plants and their properties was a specialized science confined to a priestly class which has survived in the persons of the herb-doctors, or yerbateros of today. The purpose of the present book is to offer a survey of his extensive knowledge of medical applications of plants. Among the topics discussed are, *e.g.*, the treatment of aches and pains; asthma, colds and diseases of the lungs and breathing passages; birth, obstetrics and diseases peculiar to women; bites and stings of animals; bleeding; bowel complaints; burns, chills, and fever; convulsions; nervous complaints, irritability, loss of speech, nightmare, depression; dislocations and complaints of the bones; ear and eye complaints; hair and diseases of the scalp; complaints of the head; inflammation; jaundice; complaints of the mouth, tongue and nose; poisoning; skin diseases, ulcers, abscesses, cancer and tumours; teeth and germs; throat and neck; the urine; wounds, cuts, bruises and ruptures. A section has been devoted to charms and magic, and another to cupping.

SAPPER, C., 1936: Geographie und Geschichte der indianischen Landwirtschaft, 98 p. (Hamburg: Ibero-amerikanisches Institut).—

The author gives lists of plants growing in different regions of the New World according to altitude, *etc.,* and he discusses the development of agriculture before Columbus, the spread of old Indian plants through Europe and America, and the effect of New World products on its immigrants. A thorough study of Indian agricultural techniques and methods is: CASTETTER, E. F. & W. H. BELL, 1951: Yuman Indian agriculture, 274 p. (Albuquerque, N. M.: Univ. New Mexico Press). The authors made a study - partly in the field, partly from books - of the agricultural methods of the Cocopa, Yuma, Mohave, and Maricopa Indians of the Lower Colorado and Gila rivers. The authors demonstrate that the agricultural techniques employed by these Indians are largely determined by cultural factors rather than by environmental ones.

STONE, E., 1962: Medicine among the American Indians, 139 p. (Clio Medica, No. VII) (New York, N.Y.: Hafner).—

This is a reprint of the first edition (1932). It is a readable and concise introduction into the medical practices of the

North American Indians, based on tales of pioneers, travellers, explorers and missionaries and on descriptions of ethnologists and physicians. The booklet deals with the theory of medical practices; the medicine men, their societies and equipment; supernatural, ceremonial, and legitimate therapeutics; treatment of surgical, gynaecological and obstetrical conditions. Bibliography has been added. The various drugs used for different medical purposes have been summarized in some 15 tables. *Cf.* COURY, C. & M. D. GRMEK, 1969, *vide supra.*

TANTAQUIDGEON, G., 1942: A study of Delaware Indian medicine practice and folk beliefs, 91 p. (Harrisburg, Pa.: Pennsylvania Hist. Comm.).—

This study is devoted to medical beliefs and practices, to herbal remedies, witchcraft, belief in dreams, natural signs, omens, and food resources of the Delaware Indians, and deals *inter alia* with such subjects as: theories on the causes of disease, the importance of dream vision in curation, Delaware practitioners, love charms, food taboos, divinatory practices, pregnancy, childbirth, the medicine bundle, the medicine stone, *etc.* and with maize, wild vegetable foods and animal foods.

TOWLE, M. A., 1961: The ethnobotany of pre-Columbian Peru, 180 p. (Chicago, Ill.: Aldine).—

This book provides a systematic reconstruction of the ethnobotany of the prehistoric cultures of the Peruvian Central Andes. Here, according to the authoress, we find one of the sources of New World agriculture. The study is based upon plant remains found in archaeological sites, surveys of botanical and ethnological literature, and field studies of modern plant utilization. The plant species found are fully described, and the last part of the book gives a chronological description of the use of wild and cultivated plants against a general cultural background of the relevant period.

WISSLER, C., 1938: The American Indian: an introduction to the anthropology of the New World, 466 p. (New York, N.Y.: Oxford U.P.).—

This is the third edition of the standard anthropological treatise on the American Indian; it has been very appreciably enlarged since the first and second editions were issued respectively in 1917 and 1922, and brought up to date in the light of the most recent researches bearing upon every possible aspect of the life and culture of the American Indian. Invaluable introduction to the study of the American Indian. (From Isis 31: 227). A reprint of this third edition appeared in 1950 and again in 1966 (Magnolia, Mass.: Smith). A study especially dealing with the South American Indian is: STEWARD, J. H., ed., 1946: Handbook of South American Indians. Vol. 1: The marginal tribes, 624 p.; Vol. 2: The Andean civilizations, 33 + 1035 p. (Washington, D. C., Smithsonian Inst., Bur. Amer. Ethnology, Bull. 143). The whole work will consist of 5 vols.; each of them will be devoted to one of the four cultural divisions into which South America and certain regions of the north have been divided. Vol. I deals with marginal and hunting tribes from Tierra del Fuego up to north eastern Brazil; Vol. 2 with the Andean civilizations to the West; Vol. 3 with the tribes of tropical forests and savannahs in the great central areas of the sub-continent and on the east coast; Vol. 4 with the circum-Caribbean cultures to the north and up the Isthmus to Honduras and along the Antilles to Cuba. The fifth volume will deal with the comparative anthropology of the South American Indians, and will contain general summaries and comparisons of the various aspects of the cultures considered. More than a hundred contributors have cooperated in producing this work. A study especially dealing with North American Indians is: HODGE, F., 1907-1910: Handbook of American Indians north of Mexico, 2 vols. (U.S. Bur. Amer. Ethnology, Bull. 30) (Washington, D.C.: Govt. Printing Office). This book contains descriptions of the stock, confederacies, tribes, tribal divisions, and settlements of the Indians north of Mexico, together with sketches of their history, archaeology, manners, customs, and institutions. *Cf.* also: FREEMAN, J. F., ed., 1966: A guide to manuscripts relating to the American Indian in the library of the American Philosophical Society, 491 p. (Mem. Amer. Phil. Soc., Vol. 65) (Philadelphia, Pa.: Amer. Philos. Soc.). A bibliography of the large and important collection of manuscript materials relating to the American Indian. It amounts to about 50,000 items in 300 separate collections, all of them catalogued, and many analyzed. The bibliography is classified by titles, languages and regions, and copiously indexed.

d***. Other parts of the world

BEST, E., 1942: Forest lore of the Maori: with methods of snaring, trapping and preserving birds and rats, uses of berries, roots, fern-root, and forest products, with mythological notes on origins, kariaka used, *etc.*,

503 p. (Dominion Museum Bull., 14) (Wellington: Skinner).—

Separate sections deal with such subjects as: the Maori and the forest, forest products, Polynesian plant names, trees and ceremonial, paths and travelling, seasons, tree dwellings, food supplies, *etc.*, obtained from the forest (hinan, tawe, karaka, tutu, titoki, small berries), various oils and gums, masticatories, edible herbs, fungi, flax, bark and its uses, the rata tree, bird lore (the Maori as a fowler, mythical birds, the arts of the fowler, bird-taking implements, how birds were taken, how the Maori climbed trees, the wood-pigeon, the parson-bird, the parakeet, the bell-bird), the kiore or native rat, *etc.* The same author also wrote an essay on Maori agriculture: The cultivated food plants of the natives of New Zealand, with some account of native methods of agriculture, its ritual and origin myths, 1926, 172 p. (Melbourne: Whitcombe & Tombs; also in J. Polyn. Soc. 39 (1930): 346-380, and *Idem* 40 (1931): 1-20). A general study of Maori mythology is: BEST, E., 1924: Maori religion and mythology: being an account of the cosmogony, anthropology, religious beliefs and rites, magic and folklore of the Maori folk of New Zealand, 264 p. (Dominion Museum Bull., 10) (Wellington: Skinner).

BRANDL, L., 1966: Aerzte und Medizin in Afrika, 200 p. (Pfaffenhofen, Ilm: Afrika Verlag).—

The author tries to give an overall survey of medicine in Africa. The book deals rather extensively with Egyptian and Arabian medicine. A large part of the book deals with "Ethnomedizin" (native medicine), and still another part deals with the introduction of European medicine. No division into chapters, no register or index.

BRYANT, A. T., 1966: Zulu medicine and medicine-men, 115 p. (Cape Town: Struik).—

A special study of the healing-methods and medicines used by the Zulu medicine-man; the author made a more special study of the botanical materia medica. There is a table of Zulu medicinal plants arranged in botanical order (p. 86-115).

BURKILL, I. H. & M. HANIFF, 1930: Malay village medicine, 156 p. (Gardens' Bull., Straits Settlements Vol. 6, part 2: 165-321).—

On a tour through the Malay Peninsula, the authors asked the "bomor" (physician of the native school) and the "bidan" (midwife), to bring specimens of plants in illustration of their simples. In this way, for each of the plants considered (1,675 in number), the following characteristics have been given: the botanical name; the Malay name as the informant used it; the name of the most important place in the neighbourhood of the informant's dwelling; the complaint for which it is used, and the way in which it is used. Glossary of vernacular names. *Cf.* also GIMLETTE, J. D. & I. H. BURKILL, 1930, *infra.*

GELFAND, M., 1964: Witch doctor: traditional medicine man of Rhodesia, 191 p. (London: Harvill Press.).—

A study of Shona native doctors, the ethics governing their professional behaviour, the medical value of some of their herbal remedies, the way he inspires his patients, and his other social functions, *e.g.,* giving religious guidance, protection of the property of individuals, detection of criminals, his keeping the village safe from witchcraft. A study especially dealing with Shona witchcraft is: CRAWFORD, J. R., 1967: Witchcraft and sorcery in Rhodesia, 312 p. (Oxford U.P.). It describes some 100 cases of witchcraft, and contains an up-to-date bibliography and rather useful index.

——, 1964: Medicine and custom in Africa, 174 p. (Edinburgh & London: Livingstone).—

A series of lectures given to first-year students in the Faculty of Medicine of the University College of Rhodesia and Nyasaland. Chapter headings are: 1. Early man and the first doctor; 2. The earliest doctors; 3. The witchdoctor; 4. The witchdoctor in practice; 5. The witchdoctor as a herbalist and preventive medicines; 6. The African child and its environment; 7. Food and dietary habits; 8. Major events in life; 9. Shona hygiene; 10. What we can learn from the African; 11. The African's contact with Western culture; 12. Social medical effects of urbanisation on Africans living in urban and rural social systems.

——, 1967: The African witch, 227 p. Edinburgh & London: Livingstone).—

A companion to the two above-mentioned volumes. The book deals, almost exclusively with the Shona people and its contents are based on information from patients, medicine men, police and court records.

GIMLETTE, J. D. & I. H. BURKILL, 1930: The medical book of Malayan medicine, 152 p. (Translated by Insche'Ismail, Munshi, possibly in Penang, circa 1886, now edited with medical notes by J. D. Gimlette and determinations of the drugs by I. H. Burkill) (Gardens' Bull., Straits Settlements, vol. 6, part 3: 323-474).—

This is a new edition of a ms. in the possession of the Pharmaceutical Society of Great Britain, containing some 543 prescriptions for diseases and enumerating various drugs, many of them prepared from plants. It also includes fanciful remedies and cures by suggestion. Some light is also thrown upon native surgery. *Cf.* also: GIMLETTE, J. D., 1939: A dictionary of Malayan medicine, 259 p. (Edited and completed by H. W. THOMSON) (London & New York, N.Y.: Oxford U.P.). According to Sarton (in Isis 33: 130), this is an excellent and very valuable dictionary. *Cf.* also BURKILL, I. H. & M. HANIFF, 1930, *supra.*

GOLDIE, W. H., 1904: Maori medical lore: notes on the causes of disease and treatment of the sick among the Maori people of New Zealand, as believed and practised in former times, together with some account of various ancient rites, connected with the same, 120 p. (Trans. New Zealand Institute 37: 1-120).—

This is a series of notes collected and compiled by the author, dealing with the diseases which afflicted the Maori in past times, as also with those introduced by the Europeans, together with an attempt to explain the manner in which a primitive people looks upon disease, as to its origin and treatment. The book deals with such subjects as: classification and diagnosis of diseases, general treatment of the sick, legends concerning the origin of disease and death, disease gods, disease demons, sorcery, the healing rites, treatment of wounds, leprosy, fractures, burns and scalds, skin diseases, toothache, insanity, venereal diseases, epidemic diseases, the Maori's aversion to European doctors, menstruation, pregnancy, childbirth, medicinal plants, *etc.*

GREENWAY, P. J., 1937: A Swahili dictionary of plant names, 112 p. (Dar es Salaam: Govt. Printer).—

An accurate identification of the vernacular names of medicinal, food and other plants, used by East African natives. Under each native name the English equivalent, if any, is given, followed by a brief description and the scientific name and family name. Notes on the uses of the various species are given. Lists of native morphological terms and of botanical terms are included.

HARLEY, G. W., 1941: Native African medicine, 294 p. (Cambridge, Mass.: Harvard U.P.).—

A book on African medicine especially based on the author's personal observations of the Mano people living in Nigeria. From its contents we may mention: Medicine in general and its relationship with religion; the conception of disease; treatment of diseases, magical as well as rational; treatment of snakebite; black magic and poison; divination; special medicines and sacred objects; medicine as it is practised by secret societies. The book has been supplemented by a chapter on "Native medical practice in Africa as a whole" (p. 197-228) and an appendix on "Excerpts from the literature on African medicine" (p. 231-253); it includes a bibliography, a list of plants mentioned in the text, and a complete index.

HOMBURGER, L., 1929: Noms des parties du corps dans les langues négro-africains, 118 p. (Collection linguistique, No. 25) (Paris: Champion).—

A study devoted to the names of the parts of the body in various negro-African languages. Separate sections deal with African morphology in general: the body (bones, flesh, skin), the upper extremities (arm, hand, fingers), the lower extremities (feet, legs, knee, ankle, *etc.),* the head (eye, ear, nose, chin, cheek), oral cavity (teeth, tongue, throat), pectoral and costal regions (breast, flanks, hip, arm-pits, lungs, heart, liver, spleen), abdominal region (navel, belly, penis, testicles, vagina, *etc),* dorsal region. Indexes of French terms of bodily parts and of dialects. Bibliography.

JAP TJIANG BENG, 1965: Ueber indonesische Volksheilkunde an Hand der Pharmacopoeia Indica des Hermann Nikolaus Grim(m) (1684), 174 p. (Quell. Stud. Gesch. Pharm., Vol. 5) (Frankfurt a.M.: Govi).—

H. N. Grim(m) was a Swedish physician who made a study of Indonesian drugs. The first part of the present study is devoted to the history of Indonesia and to Indonesian folk medicine (this part of the study has been based on many Dutch

sources). The second part of this study contains a discussion of the Pharmacopoeia Indica (its contents, make-up, the drugs and instruments considered, *etc.),* and some biographical information about its author. The third part contains an attempt to identify the vegetable, animal and mineral drugs considered by Grim(m) and the author tries to relate them to drugs known in other parts of the world. A German translation of the Pharmacopoeia Indica, a bibliography, and indexes of persons and subjects complete this volume.

KLEIWEG DE ZWAAN, J. P., 1913: Die Heilkunde der Niasser, 292 p. (The Hague: Nijhoff).—

Separate chapters deal with such subjects as: the causation of diseases (the gods, the dead, evil spirits); the most common diseases *(e.g.,* malaria, dysentery, smallpox, skin diseases, abscesses, struma, epilepsy, *etc.);* diseases of the lungs; fractures, luxations, burns, cauterization; pregnancy (incl. menstruation, fecundation, coitus); pregnant women and evil spirits; childbirth; venereal diseases; the child; death and the soul, dreams. Bibliography and glossary.

MALINOWSKI, B., 1935: Coral gardens and their magic: a study of the methods of tilling the soil and of agricultural rites in the Trobriand Islands, 2 vols. Vol. 1: The description of gardening, 500 p.; Vol. 2: The language of magic and gardening, 350 p. (London: Allen & Unwin).—

The book is mainly of linguistic interest, but, besides, it also contains much that is of value to the history of agriculture, *e.g.,* some thoughts on the cultivation of plants, on growth, life, and reproduction.

MARWICK, M. G., 1966: Sorcery in its social setting: a study of the Northern Rhodesian Cêwa, 339 p. (Manchester: U.P.).—

The Cêwa are spread over parts of Mozambique, Malawi and Zambia. In the book some 194 cases of sorcery are analysed. The first part of the book consists of a general survey of Cêwa culture. The main body of the work is entitled "The contexts of Cêwa Sorcery", an analysis of Cêwa social structure and of Cêwa sorcery. Some other studies of religion, folklore, magic, and medicine of some African Negro peoples are: FIELD, M. J., 1937: Religion and medicine of the Gā people, 214 p. (New York, N.Y.: Oxford U.P.). A study of the religion and of the magical practices and beliefs of the Gã people of Ghana, West Africa: HEWAT, M. L., ca. 1906: Bantu folklore: medical and general, 112 p. (Cape Town: Miller; London: Churchill); and KOUADJO-TIACOH, G., 1950: La médecine des guérisseurs noirs de l'Ouest africain, 83 p. (Diss. Univ. Paris) (Cf. also HARLEY, G. W., 1941, vide supra).

RODINSON, M., 1967: Magie, médecine et possession en Ethiopie, 203 p. (The Hague & Paris: Mouton).—

A thorough study of Ethiopian medicine and therapy. There is much of interest to the history of ethnobotany; other topics considered are: medical magic, demoniacal possession, fees of the physician, the origin of Ethiopian medicine, Graeco-Arabian influences, the causes of diseases, some surgical treatments (e.g., circumcision and other ritual operations, etc.).

SPENCER, D. M., 1941: Disease, religion and society in the Fiji Islands, 82 p. (Diss. Univ. Pennsylvania) (Monographs Amer. Ethnol. Soc. III).—

This monograph contains the results of field work done in the district of Namatuku, and the authoress concludes that disease functions foremost as a religious sanction. She distinguishes three categories of disease, viz., "natural diseases", diseases caused by spirits, and diseases caused by sorcery. Diseases are treated by lay herbalists and by the medicine men. Therapeutic procedures consist of a combination of herb lore, propitiation and confession. Diagnosis is obtained by touch, crystalgazing and the like, in order to discover the agent causing the disease.

WECK, W., 1937: Heilkunde und Volkstum auf Bali, 248 p. (Suttgart: Enke).—

The author based this study on his experiences as a government physician in

the former Dutch East Indies, and on his knowledge of native documents and customs. The subject is divided as follows: Literaturverzeichniss, Einleitung, Die balischen Aerzte, Die medizin-philosophischen Lehren der Balier, Anatomie, Physiologie, Ehe und Schwangerschaft, Die Krankheiten, Cholera, Lepra, Pemali, Pocken, Kropf, Aerztliche Diagnostik, Desti (Krankheitszauber), Heilmittel, Yoga, Der menschliche Körper als Mikrokosmos, Sasirep atangi, Die Gifte. No index.

WINSTEDT, R. O., 1951: The Malay magician, being "shaman, saiva and sufi", revised and enlarged with a Malay appendix, 160 p. (London: Routlegde & Kegan Paul).—

The first edition appeared in 1925. This book deals with the magic, occurring within the Federation of Malaya and within Patani, a northern Malay state belonging to Siam. This system of magic has persisted for thousands of years and has assimilated many Hindu and even Muslim elements. Among the subjects discussed are: the primitive magician, animism, primitive gods, spirits and ghosts, Hindu influence, the ritual of the rice-field, the séance of the Shaman, sacrifice, magician and sufi, Muslim magic, magic in daily life. Good bibliography and index.

WIRZ, P., 1941: Exorzismus und Heilkunde auf Ceylon, 292 p. (Bern: Huber).—

This study is based on personal experience, and describes a kaleidoscopic variety of ceremonies which the author was able to see in various places, as well as the explanations and the legends on which they are based. It is an attempt to make the Western mind familiar with the world of thought of the Sinhalese people and their medicine men. The descriptions sampled primarily deal with the art of healing in primitive medicine and with sexual life. Also in English translation: Exorcism and the art of healing in Ceylon, 1954, 255 p. (Leiden: Brill).

3. LIFE AND MEDICAL SCIENCES IN EGYPT

a. *History of science and culture in general*

BREASTED, J. H., 1927: A history of Egypt from the earliest time to the Persian conquest, ed. 2, 634 p. (London: Hodder & Stoughton).—

This book gives a review of Egyptian history from ancient times up to 525 B.C.

The book is a classic, giving much information concerning daily life of the kings and the people, enlightening many cultural aspects (e.g., mummification, religion, language, script, death rituals, etc.). Also in German translation: Geschichte Aegyptens, 1936. (Zurich: Phaidon). Cf. GARDINER, A., 1961; MONTET, P., 1958; and MURRAY, M. A., 1949; vide infra.

BUDGE, E. A. W., 1899: Egyptian magic, ed. 3, 234 p. (London: Paul, Trench & Trübner).—

A book, dealing with the antiquity of magical practices in Egypt, magical stones and amulets, magical figures, pictures, formulae, spells, names, and ceremonies, demoniacal possession, dreams, ghosts, lucky and unlucky days, horoscopes, prognostications, transformations, the worship of animals, and with the power of the priest who was skilled in the knowledge of magic and who could heal the sick and cast out the evil spirits which caused pain and suffering. For a more extensive study of these topics cf. LEXA, F., 1925, vide infra; and PETRIE, W. M. F., 1917, vide subsection b.

ERMAN, A., 1923: Aegypten und ägyptisches Leben im Altertum, 692 p. (Tübingen: Mohr).—

A rather extensive review of the history of land, people, culture and customs of ancient Egypt, discussing such topics as e.g., administration and government, legislation, education, death-cults, clothes, tattooing, make-up, housing, daily life, traffic and transport, war, hunting and fisheries, agriculture and husbandry, food and drink, trade and industry, family relations, religion, science, literature, plastic arts, etc. A book of the same character, stressing the cultural aspects is: WIEDEMANN, A., 1920: Das alte Aegypten, 442 p. (Heidelberg: Winter).

GARDINER, A., 1961: Egypt of the Pharaohs: an introduction, 461 p. (Oxford: Clarendon Press).—

Another publication, dealing with the same subjects as BREASTED's book (vide supra). The book is in three parts: the first part (p. 1-71) deals with such subjects as: Egyptology ancient and modern, the Egyptian language and writing, the land, its neighbours and resources, methods of dating, the nature of Egyptian history. In the second part (p. 72-383), separate sections deal with the Old Kingdom, the rise and fall of the Middle Kingdom, the Theban supremacy, the religious revolution and after, the Ramesside period (the 19th and 20th dynasties), Egypt under foreign rule and the last assertions of independence. The third part (p. 384-428) deals with the prehistory and with Manetho's first two dynasties. An appendix contains a list of the kings of Egypt (p. 429-453). Also in German translation: Geschichte des alten Aegypten, 1965, 556 p. (Stuttgart: Kröner).

LEXA, F., 1925: La magie dans l'Egypte antique de l'ancien empire jusqu'à l'époque copte, 3 vols. Vol. I: Exposé, 220 p.; Vol. II: Les textes magiques, 237 p.; Vol. III: Atlas. (Paris: Geuthner).—

A more extensive study concerning the same topics as BUDGE (vide supra). Vol. I deals with magic formulae, remedies images and statues, amulets, and rites, with the relationship between magic and religion, magic and science, Coptic magic, and with the relations between Egyptian and Greek magic in the Graeco-Roman period. Vol. II gives French translations of magical passages from the Pyramid texts, tomb and coffin inscriptions, the papyri thus far known (including the medical papyri), and some other sources. Vol. III is a collection of 71 plates showing various Egyptian amulets, sculptures, mannikins, and tables of hieroglyphs which seem to be connected with the practice of magic.

MASSOULARD, E., 1949: Préhistoire et protohistoire d'Egypte, 568 p. (Travaux et mémoires de l'Institut d'Ethnologie, Vol. 53) (Paris: Inst. d'Ethnologie).—

A summary of the history of the origin and development of civilization in the Nile Valley before written records, from Palaeolithic times down to the end of the Second Dynasty. It gives many details and abundant references.

MONTET, P., 1958: Everyday life in Egypt in the days of Ramesses the Great, 365 p. (New York, N.Y.: St. Martin's Press).—

A review of Egyptian institutions, practices, customs, and beliefs based upon evidences of buildings, tombs, and papyri, relating to Egyptian life in the 13th- and 12th centuries B.C. It is intended for the general reader. The French original is entitled: La vie quotidienne en Egypte au temps de Ramsès (XIIIe - XIIe siècles avant J. C.). (Paris: Hachette, 1947, 348 p.).

MURRAY, M. A., 1949: The splendour that was Egypt, 354 p. (New York, N.Y.: Philosophical Library).—

A well-written comprehensive survey of ancient Egyptian culture and civilization, written mainly for the general reader. Coptic survivals from ancient Egyptian culture are included. The first two chapters give a survey of ancient Egypt from prehistoric times to the Ptolemaic period. Other chapters deal with social conditions, religion, art and science, language and literature, *etc.* There are over 200 illustrations, in line, half-tone, and colour. According to a review in Isis 42: 347, it is the best one-volume survey of the main elements of Egyptian culture in the English language. A book on a more advanced level, and stressing philosophic and speculative thinking in ancient Egypt is WILSON, J. A., 1951: The burden of Egypt: an interpretation of ancient Egyptian culture, 332 p. (Chicago: U.P.).

OTTO, E., 1964: Beiträge zur Geschichte der Stierkulte in Aegypten, 60 p. (Beitr. Gesch. u. Altertumskunde Aegyptens, 13) (Hildesheim: Olms).—

A reprint of the 1938 edition (Leipzig: Hinrichs). In his preface the author describes the purpose of this monograph as follows: "In dieser Arbeit wird versucht, eine äusserlich gleichförmige Gruppe ägyptischer Götter auf Grund einheimischer wie auch antiker Quellen möglichst vielseitig darzustellen. Dabei handelt es sich nur um stiergestaltige Gottheiten, die an einem bestimmten Ort verehrt wurden; beiseite gelassen sind also alle Dämonen, kosmische und astrale Mächte, Verkörperungen von Naturkräften, die in der Vorstellung der Aegypter Stiergestalt annahmen, aber keinen Lokalkult besassen." *Cf.* HOPFNER, T., 1914, *vide infra,* subsection b.

PRATT, J. A., 1925: Ancient Egypt: sources of information in the New York Public Library, 486 p., and supplement: Ancient Egypt, 1925-1941, 340 p. (New York, N.Y.: Public Library).—

Among the subjects of interest to both the historians of medicine and biohistorians, we mention: Bibliography (p. 1-2, suppl. p. 1-3); periodicals and collections (p. 2-7, suppl. p. 3-8); science incl. astronomy, geology, botany, zoology, medicine and meteorology (p. 220-236, suppl. p. 168-180); divination and magic (p. 257-259, suppl. p. 193-195); papyri (p. 332-350, suppl. p. 225-245); scientific Coptic literature (p. 394-395). Extensive index. Reprinted in 1967 (Detroit, Mich.: Gale).

ROEDER, G., 1952: Volksglaube im Pharaonenreich, 273 p. (Stuttgart: Spemann).—

A book mainly concerned with religious belief in Ancient Egypt. It sets out to show the why and how of the people's cherished beliefs, their superstitions, local deities, and their adherence to age-old traditions. It illustrates how this depends on climate and landscape and how it influenced the Near East, Greece, Rome and Christianity. Sacred plants and animals are considered.

b. History of the plant and animal sciences

BOESSNECK, J., 1953: Die Haustiere in Altägypten, 50 p. + 22 plates. (Veröff. zool. Staatsamml., München, No. 3) (Munich: Pfeiffer).—

This publication deals with cattle, goat, sheep, pig, ass, horse, mule, dog, cat, camel, with semi-domesticated animals, and with poultry, goose, crane, doves, and ducks. Interesting bibliography.

GAILLARD, C., 1923: Faune égyptienne antique. Recherches sur les poissons représentés dans quelques tombeaux égyptiens de l'Ancien Empire, 136 p. (Cairo: Inst. français archéol. orientale).—

This book contains descriptions of fishes pictured on old Egyptian monuments. They are compared with the fishes actually living in the Nile to-day near Cairo. Fine illustrations elucidate the text.

——, & G. DARESSEY, 1905: La faune momifiée de l'antique Egypte, 159 p. + 64 plates. (Cat. gen. des ant. égypt. du musée du Caire, Vol. 25) (Cairo: Inst. français archéol. orientale).—

The present book is a catalogue of the collection of some 334 animal mummies of the Museum of Cairo: *e.g.,* mummies of bulls, dogs, cats, sheep, birds (esp. birds of prey), serpents, crocodiles, scarabs, *etc.* It gives minute descriptions of the specimens considered.

GOMPERTZ, M., 1927: Corn from Egypt: the beginning of agriculture, 88 p. (London: Howe; New York, N.Y.: Morrow).—

A brief, popular, and well-written narrative of the development of agriculture through Egyptian and Babylonian times. From a comparative study the author concludes that agriculture should have originated in Egypt. (Another study, especially dealing with Egyptian wheat, is HOHLWEIN, N., 1938: Le blé d'Egypte, 87 p. (Et. papyrologie 4: 33-120).

HARTMANN, F., 1923: L'agriculture de l'ancienne Egypte, 332 p. (Thèse Univ. Paris) (Paris: Impr. Réunies).—

The introduction deals with climate, the Nile valley, and agriculture in palaeolithic and neolithic times. The study has been divided into two parts. The first part (p. 17-177) deals with the plants, wild as well as cultivated, used by the Egyptians, with agricultural implements, agrarian technique, viticulture, etc. The second part deals with the capture and breeding of animals, with wild animals and with those selected for taming, the methods and instruments to catch them, the attention given to them, their diseases and treatment, etc. Very useful bibliography and a still more useful "Répertoire des principaux thèmes de la vie agricole".

HOHLWEIN, N., 1939: Palmiers et palmériers dans l'Egypte romaine, 74 p. (Et. papyrologie 5: 1-74).—

A historical study restricted to the date-cultures of Roman Egypt, because, according to the author, there are not enough data available for earlier periods. The first chapter deals with the date-palm in general, the second chapter deals with existing varieties, the third with its usage, the fourth with its culture (irrigation, fecundation, date-picking, etc.), the fifth and the sixth with its economic and legal aspects. Cf. also WALLERT, I., 1962, vide infra.

HOPFNER, T., 1914: Der Tierkult der alten Aegypter nach den griechisch-römischen Berichten und den wichtigeren Denkmälern, 201 p. (Denkschr. Akad. Wiss., Wien, phil.-hist. Kl., 57, No. 2).—

"An elaborate survey of this subject, which may interest the historian of zoology. The main subdivision is zoological, 36 successive chapters being devoted to as many species (no. 19 is devoted to the okapi)." (Sarton in Isis 4: 613).

KEIMER, L., 1924: Die Gartenpflanzen im alten Aegypten, 188 p. (Aegyptol. Studien Bd. I) (Hamburg: Hoffmann & Campe).—

This book is the first and only volume of a planned series of 3 volumes concerning the agricultural history of Egypt. The botanical material has been supplied by G. SCHWEINFURTH who was responsible for the determination of most botanical remains from ancient Egypt. Some 44 plants are considered; a short description of each of them is given, together with a discussion of the information available concerning authentic material of it which has been found, its usage, its representation in ancient Egyptian art, and the meaning of its name in ancient Egypt. From this material, Keimer gives a picture of Egyptian horticulture, and tries to reconstruct the distribution of cultivated plants in remote times. Reprinted 1967 (Hildesheim: Olms). Cf. also LORET V., 1887; and WOENIG, F., 1886, vide infra.

——, 1938: Insectes de l'Egypte ancienne, 172 p. (Cairo: Inst. français archéol. orientale).—

A valuable contribution to the nattural history of pharaonic Egypt. The contents of the book consist of a series of papers originally published between 1931 and 1937 in the "Annales du Service des Antiquités de l'Egypte".

——, 1947: Histoires des serpents dans l'Egypte ancienne et moderne, 111 p. (Mémoires de l'Institut d'Egypte 50) (Cairo: Inst. français archéol. orientale).—

This study brings together all that is known about snakes in ancient and modern Egypt, and deals in particular with the mystery of the snake-charmers. Valuable contribution to Egyptian folklore.

LORET, V., 1887: La flore pharaonique d'après les documents hiéroglyphiques et les spécimens découverts dans les tombes, 64 p. (Paris: Baillière).—

Short descriptions of some 136 plants of which remains have been found in Egyptian tombs. The author succeeded in determining the names of some 50 plants with certainty, and for each of the plants mentioned he gives much secondary information. An attempt to reconstruct a flora of ancient Egypt. A second edition appeared in 1892, 145 p. (Paris: Louvre). Cf. also KEIMER, L., 1924, vide supra.

MOLDENKE, C. R., 1886: Ueber die in altägyptischen Texten erwähnten Bäume und deren Verwerthung, 149 p. (Diss. Univ. Strasbourg) (Leipzig: Breitkopf & Härtel).—

A philologic study dealing with the trees of ancient Egypt and their role in religion, magic, feeding, medicine, technique, etc. Besides, it tries to give information concerning the parks around the palaces in ancient Egypt.

PETRIE, W. M. F., 1917: Scarabs and cylinders with names, 48 p. + 58 p. + 72 plates. (London: School of Archaeology in Egypt).—

The book deals with the little amulets of beetle form, many of them bearing names of kings. It also gives much information concerning the religious aspects, the varieties and the preparation of scarabs, the materials used, and a chronology. It is mainly based upon the Egyptian collection in University College, London.

WALLERT, I., 1962: Die Palmen im alten Aegypten. Eine Untersuchung ihrer praktischen, symbolischen und religiösen Bedeutung, 159 p. (Münchener Aegyptologische Studien, 1) (Berlin: Hessling).—

A monograph devoted to the following species of date-palms: *Phoenix dactylifera, Hyphaene thebaica, Medemia argun.* Separate sections deal with the meaning in daily life, the uses of the different parts, the date-palm as a motive in ancient Egyptian art, the date-palm in the landscape, in the garden, and in the cemetery; holy date-palms and their connections with Thot, Hathor, Thoeris, Min and Rē. Indexes and bibliography. *Cf.* also HOHLWEIN, N., 1939, *vide supra.*

WIT, C. DE, 1951: Le rôle et le sens du lion dans l'Egypte ancienne, 37 + 473 p. (Leiden: Brill).—

An exhaustive monograph elucidating the meaning and function of the lion in ancient Egyptian civilization. Section headings are as follows: I: Lion et sphinx; II. Dieux en rapport avec le lion; III: Déesses en rapport avec le lion; IV: Varia; V: Le lion dans la géographie; VI: Le lion dans la langue égyptienne. It is a mine of information containing an immense amount of textual material referring to the lion, derived from pyramid texts and temple inscriptions. A study dealing with lion hunting is: WRESZINSKI, W., 1932: Löwenjagd im alten Aegypten, 27 p. (Morgenland. Darstellungen aus Geschichte und Kultur des Ostens, 23) (Leipzig: Hinrichs).

WOENIG, F., 1886: Die Pflanzen im alten Aegypten, ihre Heimat, Geschichte, Cultur, und ihre mannigfache Verwendung im sozialen Leben, in Cultur, Sitten, Gebräuchen, Medizin, Kunst, 425 p. (Leipzig: Friedrich).

A classic in this field, containing much information concerning the history of cultivated plants. Separate sections deal with such topics as: bog-plants *(e.g., Lotus, Papyrus);* agriculture; cereals and the baking of bread; the cultivation of flax; vegetables and their production *(e.g., Allium,* melons, asparagus, artichokes, leguminous, plants, radish, beetroot, cabbage, and salad); spice-plants; the architecture of gardens; garden flowers and flowers for garlands; viticulture; trees and shrubs; medicinal plants; plants in Egyptian works of art. A second edition appeared in 1897, 426 p. (Leipzig: Heitz). *Cf.* KEIMER, L., 1924; and LORET, V., 1887, *vide supra.*

c. *History of the medical sciences*

BASLEZ, L., 1932: Les poisons dans l'antiquité égyptienne, 58 p. (Paris: Le François).—

A review of the poisons and some drugs used in ancient Egypt, such as: animal substances and products, vegetable poisons, some mineral poisons (they had some knowledge of mercurials and of arsenic, they knew of lead colic, and they used copper sulphate), some vegetable drugs *(e.g.,* nepenthe, coriander, carob, hemlock, Indian hemp), snake poisons, excrements and putrefying substances, *etc.* The book is severely criticized in a review in Bull. Hist. Med. 4: 250, 1939. There exists a more elaborate study considering the same topics, but of which I possess no further information, *viz.,* GEORGIADÈS, N., 1906: La pharmacie en Egypte, 230 p. (Thèse Univ. Bordeaux).

BREASTED, J. H., ed., 1930: The Edwin Smith surgical papyrus: published in facsimile and hieroglyphic transliteration with translation and commentary. Vol. I: Hieroglyphic transliteration and commentary, 596 p.; Vol. II: Facsimile plates and line-for-line hieroglyphic transliteration, 16 p. (Univ. Chicago Oriental Institute Publications, Vols. III and IV) (Chicago, Ill.: U.P.; Cambridge: U.P.).—

This papyrus is a fragment (in all probability) of a manual of surgery for the instruction of surgeons, written *ca.* 1600 B.C., but based on much older sources. It is largely without reference to magical and speculative elements, but deals mainly with surgical matters. It contains the description of 48 cases: injuries, wounds, dislocations, fractures, and tumours. The cases are listed according to a certain pattern: each case has a title followed by a list of symptoms, then the diagnosis follows and finally the treatment. It also contains eight incantations against plague, a prescription for a woman's disease, and recipes for an ailment of the anus and for the magical transformation of an old man into a youth. A long review of Breasted's book by G. Sarton can be found in Isis 15: 355-367. A modern German translation of the Edwin Smith surgical papyrus appeared in 1966 in Huber's series "Klassiker der Medizin und der Naturwissenschaften", vol. IX. It is edited by W. WESTENDORF and entitled: Papyrus Edwin Smith. Ein medizinisches Lehrbuch aus dem alten Aegypten. Wund- und Unfallchirurgie, Zaubersprüche gegen Seuchen, verschiedene Rezepte, 119 p. (Bern: Huber). With commentaries. *Cf.* also EBBELL, B., 1939, *vide infra.*

EBBELL, B., 1937: The papyrus Ebers: the greatest Egyptian medical document, 135 p. (Copenhagen: Munksgaard).—

This papyrus stems from the first half of the 16th century B.C., and has been based on still older sources. It is a complete compendium of ancient Egyptian medicine, a collection of monographs and excerpts, primarily dealing with internal medicine. A large group of texts consists of collections of recipes with prescriptions for the treatment of internal diseases, diseases of the eye, of the skin, of women, and other ailments. Other texts deal with surgical problems or are of a didactic character, describing diseases, giving diagnoses and treatments. Two treatises on the heart and the vessels are of a theoretical and physiological nature; they are a first attempt to explain the phenomena of life in terms of speculative philosophy. A special study devoted to the diseases of the eye is: EBERS, G., 1889: Papyrus Ebers. Die Maasse und das Kapitel über die Augenkrankheiten (Abh. sächs. Ges. Wiss., phil.-hist.Kl., XI: 133-366). From this study it becomes clear that the Egyptians have known and treated such eyediseases as blepharitis, chalazion, trichiasis, ectropion, pinguecula, pterygium, night blindness, inflammation, haemorrhage, leucoma, iritis, cataract, granulations probably due to trachoma, and perhaps also hydrophthalmus, which findings have been confirmed by later research. *Cf.* also HIRSCHBERG, J., 1889, *vide infra),* and MEYERHOF, M., 1940: Eye diseases in ancient Egypt. (Ciba Symposia I: 305-310).

——, 1938: Altägyptische Bezeichnungen für Krankheiten und Symptome, 65 p. (Skr. norske Vidensk.-Akad. II. Hist.-filos. Klasse, 1938, No. 3).—

This is an attempt to explain Egyptian medical terminology, and to identify the diseases mentioned in the Egyptian medical papyri. This study has been written by a physician.

——, 1939: Die alt-aegyptische Chirurgie. Die chirurgischen Abschnitte der Papyrus E. Smith und Papyrus Ebers uebersetzt und mit Erläuterungen versehen, 92 p. (Skr. norske Vidensk-Akad. II. Hist.-filos. Klasse, 1939, No. 2).—

This study contains a new German translation of the Edwin Smith Papyrus, together with the surgical sections of the Ebers Papyrus, with commentaries; it is a welcome supplement to BREASTED's translation *(vide supra),* for it has been written from the medical, rather than from the philological, point of view. The many medical notes can be considered as medical commentaries on the texts translated by philologists.

ERMAN, A., ed., 1901: Zaubersprüche für Mutter und Kind. Aus dem Papyrus 3027 des berliner Museums, 52 p. (Abh. preuss. Akad. Wiss., phil.-hist. Kl., 1901: 1-52).—

A transcription and translation of, and commentary on, a magico-medical papyrus, written at the end of the Hyksos period or at the beginning of the New Empire *(i.e.,* 16th century B.C.). It is a compilation from two sources; the first consists of a collection of incantations against two diseases of infants (which cannot be identified); the second was a book that began with charms to fascilitate childbirth and continued with prescriptions and incantations for the protection of infants.

FOURNIER, R. L. P., 1933: La médecine égyptienne dès origines à l'école d'Alexandrie, 84 p. (Thèse Univ. Bordeaux) (Bordeaux: Delmas).—

O. Temkin wrote about this book: "René Fournier published a book on Egyptian medicine in which he tried to give a general outline of our knowledge of all its branches... Fournier believes that dissection of human bodies had been performed for anatomical studies. He estimates the Egyptian materia medica as numbering more than five hundred substances, of which some were magic, others empiric. He sees a close relationship between magic and science and thinks Egypt the origin of medicine, from which the Greeks borrowed extensively... on the whole the book is well written and gives a fair picture of our knowledge at the time of its publication." (Bull. Hist. Med. 4: 254, 1939).

GHALIOUNGUI, P., 1963: Magic and medical science in ancient Egypt, 189 p. (London: Hodder & Stoughton).—

> An account for the general reader and for the physician who is curious about the infancy of his science, written not from the philological, but from the medical point of view. It is stressed that medical science in Ancient Egypt was neither wholly obscure nor wholly based on religious belief, but Egyptian empirical science may even have had a great influence on the beginnings of Greek medicine. A beginning has been made with a comparison between popular therapeutics actually practised in Egypt to-day and the treatments prescribed in Pharaonic time; probably in the future this method may prove to be valuable in deciphering old texts.

——, & Z. EL DAWAKHLY, 1965: Health and healing in ancient Egypt: a pictorial essay, 55 + 3 p. + 176 illust. (Cairo: Dar al Maaref).—

> A pictorial collection of the most important epigraphic documents, statues, stone reliefs, and human remains, relating to medicine. The text accompanying the illustrations is both in English and in Arabic. A valuable supplement to any other book on Egyptian medicine.

GOLDSTEIN, M., 1933: Internationale Bibliographie der altägyptischen Medizin, 1850-1930, 24 p. (Berlin: Aegyptologischer Verlag Miron Goldstein).—

> A (not very complete) bibliography containing 243 items of books and publications in scientific journals, arranged by subject.

GRAPOW, H., 1935; 1936: Untersuchungen über die altägyptischen medizinischen Papyri, I and II, 111 + 138 p. (Mitt. vorderasiat. Ges., Vol. 40, No. 1, 1935 and Vol. 41, No. 2, 1936) (Leipzig: Hinrichs).—

> A general discussion of the Egyptian medical papyri as a whole, a basic study for all work on Egyptian medical literature. Vol. I gives an analysis of the contents of the 7 medical papyri known thus far (i.e., Pap. med. Kahun, Pap. veter. Kahun, Pap. Edwin Smith, Pap. Ebers, Pap. Hearst, Pap. Berlin, Pap. London), discusses the origin of compendia and the position of the physician and of the patient. Vol. II mainly deals with diagnostics, recipes, the denomination of diseases, the names of the drugs used, and spells.

GRAPOW, H., 1954-1962: Grundriss der Medizin der alten Aegypter, 8 vols. Vol. I (1954): Anatomie und Physiologie, 102 p.; Vol. II (1959): Von den medizinischen Texten, 149 p.; Vol. III (1956): Kranke, Krankheiten und Arzt, 168 p.; Vol. IV, 1 (1958): Uebersetzung der medizinischen Texte, 319 p.; Vol. IV, 2 (1958): Erläuterungen zu diesen Texte, 257 p.; Vol. V (1958): Die medizinischen Texte in hieroglyphischer Umschreibung autographiert, 549 p.; Vol. VI (1959): Wörterbuch der ägyptischen Drogennamen, 604 p. (With the assistance of H. VON DEINES); Vol. VII (1961/62): Wörterbuch der medizinischen Texte, 1109 p. (ed. by H. VON DEINES & W. WESTENDORF); Vol. VIII (1962): Grammatik der medizinischen Texte, 399 p. (ed. by W. WESTENDORF). (Berlin: Akademie Verlag).—

> This is a monumental study of old Egyptian medicine, based on a thorough philological study of the original texts as far as they are known to us. Vol. I contains a general review of Egyptian thought on the anatomy and physiology of the body; it starts with an introductory chapter concerning the philological difficulties occurring in Pharaonic medical science, and the larger part is devoted to a discussion of Egyptian anatomical and physiological nomenclature. Vol. II gives an analysis of the contents, the language, and the style of the old texts; discusses magical formulae, diagnostics, and medical prescriptions; acknowledges the origin of the existing papyri, and gives an analysis and a review of their contents. Vol. III re-publishes medical texts, provided with annotations and discusses the relationship physician-patient and disease-cure. Vol. IV consists of two supplementary parts: the first contains a translation of the original Egyptian texts and the second contains the notes and annotations belonging to the translation. Vol. V gives the same text as Vol. IV, but in hieroglyphic symbols. Vol. VI gives many particulars concerning the application, etc., of drugs which consist of, or are derived from, inorganic, vegetable or animal substances. Vol. VII contains a dictionary of medical terms used in this work, and Vol. VIII is of only philological importance.

GRIFFITH, F. L., ed., 1898: The Petrie papyri: hieratic papyri from Kahun and Gurob (principally of the Middle Kingdom), 2 vols. Vol. I: Text, 114 p.; Vol. II: Plates. (London: Quaritch).—

It contains English translations of: 1. The veterinary papyrus of Kahun: a short fragment giving documentary evidence of the existence of veterinary medicine as early as 1900 B.C. which was of the same character as human medicine. The fragment deals with diseases of various animals, particularly of the dog and the bull. *Cf.* also NEFFGEN, H., 1904: Der Veterinär-Papyrus von Kahun. Ein Beitrag zur Geschichte der Tierheilkunde der alten Aegypter, 1904, 23 p. (Berlin: Calvary). Contains a German translation from the English with important veterinary comments. 2. The gynaecological papyrus of Kahun, a fragment of three pages of which the first two are devoted to (17 cases of) diseases of women and their treatment, and the third page to matters of pregnancy. *Vide* also REINHARD, F., 1917: Gynäkologie und Geburtshilfe der altägyptischen Papyri, 66 p. (Arch. Gesch. Med. 9: 315-344; 10: 124-161), a thorough study of the gynaecological and obstetrical contents of the old Egyptian medical papyri and an attempt to translate the cases mentioned into modern medical terminology.

HIRSCHBERG, J., 1889: Aegypten. Geschichtliche Studien eines Augenarztes, 116 p. (Leipzig: Thieme).—

The contents of this booklet consist of the text of three lectures: 1. Aegypten als klimatischer Kurort; 2. Ueber die Augenheilkunde der alten Aegypter; 3. Ueber die aegyptischen Augenentzündung. A more recent publication is: KRAUSE, A. C., 1933: Ancient Egyptian ophthalmology. (Bull. Inst. Hist. Med. 1: 258-276).

HURRY, J. B., 1928: Imhotep: the vizier and physician of King Zoser and afterwards the Egyptian God of medicine, ed. 2, 211 p. (London: Oxford U.P.).—

The author defends the hypothesis that Imhotep was vizier of King Zoser, chief architect of the court, builder of the step-pyramid at Sakkara and the temple at Edfu, astrologer, magician, and physician of great renown, who was heroized during his life, became a demigod after his death, and still later the healing God, identified with Aesculapius by the Greeks. This is an attempt to analyse the forces which resulted in such an exceptional occurrence as the deification of an ordinary mortal. Moreover, this book contains much that is of medical historical importance, with chapters on *e.g.,* incubation and the medical library of the asklepieion at Memphis. A critical study, denying most of the theses put forward by Hurry, is: GARRY, J. G., 1931: Egypt: the home

of the occult sciences with special reference to Imhotep, the mysterious wise man and Egyptian god of medicine, 93 p. (London: Bale & Danielson). In order to find out the personality and identity of Imhotep and his influence on medicine, the author starts from a study of old-Egyptian magic and magical ceremonies.

IVERSEN, E., 1939: Papyrus Carlsberg No. VIII with some remarks on the Egyptian origin of some birth prognoses, 31 p. (K. danske Vidensk. Selsk. Skr., Hist. filolog. Med. XXVI, No. 5) (Copenhagen: Munksgaard).—

Text and translation of the remnants of two pieces of a papyrus deposited in the Egyptological Inst., Univ. of Copenhagen, of which one side contains fragments of a treatise on diseases of the eye (the text of which can be found almost word for word in Pap. Ebers), and of which the other side deals with gynaecological matters, *e.g.,* with pregnancy, childbirth, birth prognoses, and diseases of women. The text could be reconstructed with the aid of similar prescriptions occurring in the Kahun gynaecological papyrus and the Berlin papyrus. The author also points to some parallels existing between some Egyptian birth prognoses and those described in the Corpus Hippocraticum and those in Western mediaeval literature and in later European folk medicine, thus illustrating the spread of ancient Egyptian medicine throughout Europe.

JONCKHEERE, F., 1944: Une maladie égyptienne. L'hématurie parasitaire, 63 p. (La médecine égyptienne, No. 1) (Brussels: Fond. Egyptol. Reine Elisabeth).—

This study contains a collection of passages derived from Pap. Ebers, Pap. Hearst, Pap. Berlin, and Pap. London, which deal with the presence of blood in the urine, caused by parasites. The author attempts to describe the therapeutical measures of the ancient Egyptians, and he makes clear that this is rather difficult, because many of the drugs used cannot be identified.

——, 1947: Le papyrus médical Chester Beatty, 79 p. (La médecine égyptienne, No. 2) (Brussels: Fond. Egyptol. Reine Elisabeth).—

A French translation of the Chester Beatty Papyrus, written at the time of the XIXth or XXth Dynasty (*i.e.,* 13th or 12th century B.C.). It is a fragment of a monograph on "Remedies for diseases of the anus", from which we learn something about ancient Egyptian medical specialists. It contains 41 prescriptions.

———, 1958: Les médecins de l'Egypte pharaonique. Essai de prosopographie, 172 p. (La médecine égyptienne, No. 3) (Brussels: Fond. Egyptol. Reine Elisabeth).—

A posthumously published prosopography or index of names of those persons bearing the title "sinw" (=physician) during the Pharaonic period. In this way the author collected the names of almost a hundred individuals. There are alphabetical and chronological lists of names, additional titles borne by the named physicians, descriptions of the social conditions of the physicians, an iconographic list of 30 of the physicians listed, *etc.* The book gives an insight into the position occupied by physicians, and their status.

LEAKE, C. D., 1952: The old Egyptian medical papyri, 108 p. (Lawrence, Kansas: Kansas U.P.).—

Besides a general review of medical papyri, this volume contains a description and analysis of the Hearst Papyrus. Separate chapters deal with: the chief Egyptian medical papyri, old Egyptian weights and measures, drug measurement in the old Egyptian medical papyri, ancient Egyptian therapeutics, the Hearst medical papyrus, its organization, and the diseases and ingredients described in it.

LEFEBVRE, G., 1956: Essai sur la médecine égyptienne de l'époque pharaonique, 212 p. (Paris: Presses Univ. France).—

This book contains much information on philological, medical, therapeutical, and pharmaceutical aspects of Pharaonic medicine. Many quotations of Egyptian texts are given in French translation, and attempts are made to identify the plants mentioned in the old papyri. The book contains a chapter on the medical papyri known thus far, and their relationship to religion and magic; a discussion of the organization of the medical profession; a chapter on anatomy and physiology; 9 chapters on diseases and therapeutics of the separate organs of the human body.

LEIGH, R. W., 1934: Notes on the somatology and pathology of ancient Egypt, 54 p. (Univ. Calif. Publs. Amer. Archaeol. Ethnol. 34, No. 1).—

This publication deals with such topics as mandibular measurements, dental index, gnathic index, anomalies of cranial sutures, tooth morphology, cusps, roots, attrition, dental caries, periapical osteitis, osteoarthritis, syphilis, rachitis, lesions on parietal bosses, fractures, dental operative interference. The study is based on an examination of the Egyptian skeletal collection in the Museum of Anthropology, Univ. of California.

MAHFOUZ, N. B., 1935: The history of medical education in Egypt, 121 p. (Egyptian Univ., Faculty of Medicine, Publ. No. 8) (Cairo: Govt. Press).—

Except the first chapter which deals with ancient Egyptian medicine (9 p.) all the rest of the book is concerned with Islamic Egypt. Ch. 2 deals with Islamic medicine before the 19th century and the rest of the book deals with modern Egyptian medicine.

PIANKOFF, H., 1930: Le "coeur" dans les textes égyptiens depuis l'Ancien jusqu'à la fin du Nouvel Empire, 128 p. (Diss. Univ. Paris) (Paris: Geuthner).—

The heart played an important role in ancient Egyptian moral and religious life. The present publication is a philological study, mainly dealing with the religious aspects and giving many quotations both in hieroglyphs and in French translation. A short chapter (p. 14-18) deals with a medical text concerning the heart.

RIAD, N., 1955: La médecine au temps des Pharaons, 319 p. (Paris: Maloine). —

A French history of ancient Egyptian medicine, discussing such topics as *e.g.,* chronology, race, and customs in ancient Egypt, old medical documents (papyri, mummies, the interrelation between art and medicine), hygiene, medicine and physicians, knowledge of anatomy and physiology, surgery, pharmacy and therapeutics, dental care, obstetrics, *etc.,* during Pharaonic time. A French study concerning Egyptian anatomical knowledge is: LEFEBVRE, G., 1952: Tableau des parties du corps humain mentionnées par les Egyptiens, 73 p. (Cairo: Inst. français archéol. orientale).

RUFFER, M. A., 1921: Studies in the paleopathology of Egypt (ed. by R. L. MOODIE), 372 p. (Chicago, Ill.: U.P.).—

A collection of a series of papers written by M. A. Ruffer on the palaeopathology of Egyptian mummies; this collection of papers is one of the great classics on the subject.

SCHERING Corporation, 1955: Medicine and pharmacy: an informal history. 1. Ancient Egypt, n.p. (Bloomfield, N.Y.: Schering Corporation).—

A well-illustrated semi-popular introduction.

STEUER, R. O., 1948: (Whdw) Aetiological principle of pyaemia in ancient Egyptian medicine, 36 p. (Suppl. Bull. Hist. Med., No. 10) (Baltimore, Md.: Johns Hopkins Press).—

Based upon a careful study of existing medical papyri, the author analyses the meaning of the medical term "whdw" which plays such an important role in Egyptian medicine. This study implies that theoretical thinking in Egyptian medicine stood at a much higher level than is generally believed.

WALKER, J., 1934: Folk medicine in modern Egypt: being the relevant parts of the Tibb al-rukka or Old wives' medicine of 'Abd al-Rahmān Ismā'īl, 128 p. (London: Luzac).—

The text deals with medical and other superstitions; as such it is a valuable contribution to the literature on Egyptian folklore.

WATERMANN, R., 1958: Bilder aus dem Lande des Ptah und Imhotep. Naturbeobachtung, Realismus und Humanität der alten Aegypter, besprochen an zahlreichen Darstellungen alter, kranker, und körperbehinderter Menschen und an missgebildeten Göttern, 151 p. (Cologne: Balduin Pick).—

A collection of representations of sick and crippled persons, persons suffering from fatty degeneration, anthropomorphic gods, etc., as they occur on ancient Egyptian works of art. With discussions of the diseases considered.

WEINDLER, F., 1915: Geburts- und Wochenbettdarstellungen auf altägyptischen Tempelreliefs, 41 p. + 28 photographs. (Munich: Beck).—

Excellent, mostly full-page, illustrations with explanatory text.

WRESZINSKI, W., ed., 1909: Der grosse medizinische Papyrus des Berliner Museums (Pap. Berl. 3038), 142 p. (Leipzig: Hinrichs).—

A facsimile of the papyrus, with transcription, German translation, commentary and glossary. The papyrus was in all probability written during the XIXth Dynasty (i.e., between 1350 and 1200 B.C.). It contains 204 recipes and tests to be used in order to ascertain whether a woman will have a child or not and it also contains a good version of the "Book on the vessels". This is primarily a book on pathology, for it deals with the system of vessels of the human body as being the seat and the origin of all diseases.

——, ed., 1912: Der Londoner medizinische Papyrus (Brit. Museum, Nr. 10059) und der Papyrus Hearst in Transkription, Uebersetzung und Kommentar. Mit Faksimile des Londoner Papyrus, 239 p. (Leipzig: Hinrichs).—

A facsimile reproduction of two medical papyri with transcription, German translation and commentaries. The first text is predominantly magical in its contents and was written at the end of the XVIIIth Dynasty (i.e., middle 14th century B.C.). It contains 61 prescriptions for the treatment of a variety of diseases, and it ends with two prayers to Amon that have no connection with the rest of the book. The Hearst Papyrus is much more rational and was written during the first half of the 16th century B.C. It is a collection of 260 recipes; roughly one third of its contents can also be found in the Ebers Papyrus; moreover, it contains an interesting series of charms. An (older) English translation of the Hearst Papyrus has been prepared by REISNER, G. A., 1905: The Hearst medical papyrus: with introduction and vocabulary, 48 p. (Univ. Calif. Publ. Egyptian Archeology, Vol. I) (Oxford: U.P.; Leipzig: Hinrichs).

d. History of Coptic medicine

CHASSINAT, E., 1921: Un papyrus médical copte, publié et traduit, 395 p. (Mém. Inst. français Archéol. orient. 32) (Paris: de Boccard).—

A large manuscript of the 9th or 10th century in which ancient Egyptian medical knowledge has been preserved in the Coptic language. It contains 237 recipes, almost 100 of which are for diseases of the eye. The prescriptions follow very closely the pattern found in the ancient Egyptian papyri, and the drugs are in many cases the same, but there are also Greek and Arabic influences. Long historical introduction and indexes of Coptic, Greek and Arabic words on medical matters.

TILL, W. C., 1951: Die Arzneikunde der

Kopten, 153 p. (Berlin: Akademie Verlag).—

An elaborate analysis of the medical contents of Coptic medical texts, chiefly of the late Coptic period. Among the topics discussed are: words to designate drugs; weights and measures; different diseases; Coptic anatomy; and a discussion of (174) drugs. German, Coptic, Egyptian, Greek, Latin and Arabic indexes.

4. LIFE AND MEDICAL SCIENCES IN MESOPOTAMIA

a. History of science and culture in general (incl. literature on divination, omens, incantations, *etc.*)

CONTENAU, G., 1940: La divination chez les Assyriens et les Babyloniens, 379 p. (Paris: Payot).—

The first part gives a historical review of divination from antiquity to the present and a thorough discussion of the role of divination in Babylon and the practice of divination. The second part deals with *inter alia:* mantic inspiration, oracles, necromancy, behaviour, and instinctive reactions of animal and man, the behaviour of plants and inorganic bodies, physiognomy, astrology, and omens derived from monstrous animals. A separate section deals with hepatoscopy and the role of the intestines as omens; the liver was considered as the seat of the soul and the centre of life and thus played an important role in prediction practices. More special studies are: DILLON, H., 1932: Assyrio-Babylonian liver-divination, 50 p. (Rome: Pontificium Institutum Biblicum); and NOUGAYROL, J., 1941-1946: Textes hépatoscopiques d'époque ancienne conservés au Musée du Louvre (Rev. Assyr. 38 (1941): 67-88; 40 (1945/'46): 56-98), and MEISSNER, B., 1934: Omina zur Erkenntnis des Opfertieres (Arch. Orientforsch. 9: 118-122).

——, 1947: La magie chez les Assyriens et les Babyloniens, 298 p. (Paris: Payot).—

After an introductory chapter on oriental magic in antiquity in general, the rest of the book deals with magic and religion in Babylon. It discusses such topics as: the position of the magician, his clothes and ritual, and the parts played by plants, music, and dancing; exorcism; sorcery; medical applications of magic; preventive magic *(e.g.,* amulets, talismans, tattooing); the evil eye; votive spells, *etc.*

——, 1954: Everyday life in Babylon and Assyria, 324 p. (London: Arnold).—

This book is an English translation of "La vie quotidienne à Babylone et en Assyrie" (1954) and gives a popular description of daily life in ancient Mesopotamian civilization during the period 700-530 B.C. It contains much information of bio-historical interest, *e.g.,* on fishing and hunting activities; gardens and "hanging gardens"; agriculture and irrigation; livestock; cattle, goat, sheep and milk industry; meals, drinks and vegetables; magic and medicine. The agricultural backbones were the date-palm and the rich crops of cereals. In its northern parts the country mainly consisted of pastures inhabited by nomads and their cattle.

FALKENSTEIN, A., 1931: Die Haupttypen der sumerischen Beschwörung literarisch untersucht, 104 p. (Leipziger semitische Studien, N.F., Vol. I) (Diss. Univ. Leipzig) (Leipzig: Hinrichs).—

To obtain success, witchcraft has to be destroyed and demons have to be expelled, and this could be performed in a magical way with incantations. This book gives the text of the oldest Sumerian incantations we have; and makes an attempt to bring some order into these early texts by analysing their literary genre. It consists of 40 short texts written on small tablets, and it can be traced to the IIIrd Dynasty of Ur. Reprinted 1968 (Leipzig: Zentralantiquariat). A publication of the same type: KUNSTMANN, W. G., 1932: Die babylonische Gebetsbeschwörung, 114 p. (Leipziger semitische Studien, N.F., Vol. II) (Leipzig: Hinrichs). Reprinted 1968 (Leipzig: Zentralantiquariat).

FOSSEY, C., 1912-1913: Présages tirés des naissances, 256 p. (Babyloniaca V: 1-256).—

Abnormal human and animal births were considered to be very portentous, and, therefore, birth omens were believed to be an important group of signs. Some of them were of great medical importance and had to be interpreted correctly. The present book gives a transcription and French translation of those passages of cuneiform tablets that deal with these phenomena. A study of the same type: JASTROW, M., 1914: Babylonian-Assyrian birth-omens and their cultural significance, 86 p. (Religionsgeschichtliche Versuche und Vorarbeiten XIV: 5). The author makes many comparisons of the role of birth-omens with the Romans and Greeks, discusses the relationship with fabulous creatures in Babylonian-Assyrian literature and in Greek mythology, with Egyptian sphinxes, and with animals in fairy tales and the belief in monsters. Still another comparable work is: DENNE-FELD, L., 1914: Babylonisch-Assyrische Geburts-Omina. Zugleich ein Beitrag zur Geschichte der Medizin, 232 p. (Leipzig: Hinrichs).

HARTMAN, L. F. & A. L. OPPENHEIM, 1950: On beer and brewing techniques in ancient Mesopotamia, according to the XXIIIrd tablet of the series Ḫar-ra = ḫubullû, 56 p. (Suppl. J. Amer. orient. Soc., No. 10) (Baltimore, Md.: Amer. orient. Soc.).—

A description of the technology of brewing as it was practised in Mesopotamia with transliteration, translation, *apparatus criticus,* index of Akkadian and Sumerian words and 4 pages with illustrations.

HUNGER, J., 1909: Babylonische Tieromina nebst griechisch-römischen Parallelen, 176 p. (Mitt. vorderasiat. Ges. XIV, 3) (Leipzig: Hinrichs).—

Many animal omens played a very important role in Babylonian divination, and the author discusses many of them, citing many passages in German translation. Many comparisons with usage in Greek and Roman divination.

KRAMER, S. N., 1963: The Sumerians: their history, culture, and character, 355 p. (Chicago, Ill.: Chicago U.P.).—

The first chapter is introductory in character, giving archaeological evidence, the decipherment of the cuneiform script, *etc.* Ch. 2 deals with the history of Sumer from prehistory to the early second millennium B.C., when the Sumerians ceased to exist as a political entity. Ch. 3 deals with social, economic, legal, and technical aspects of Sumerian life, ch. 4 and 5 deal with religion and literature, ch. 6 and 7 with education, and ch. 8 sketches the "legacy of Sumer". Appendixes deal with Sumerian script and language, votive inscriptions, the sequence of Sumerian kings, letters, the Lipit-Ishtar law code, and with the "farmer's almanac". Bibliography and index. Also in French translation: L'histoire commence à Sumer, 315 p. (Grenoble: Arthaud).

KRAUS, F. R., 1935: Die physiognomischen Omina der Babylonier, 106 p. (Mitt. Vorderasiat.-Aegypt. Ges., 40) (Leipzig: Hinrichs).—

The general constitution of the parts of the body and the special features present on the surface of the body should reflect the character and general psychosomatic constitution of the individual and should make possible the prediction of his future.

MEISSNER, B., 1920-1924: Babylonien und Assyrien, 2 vols. Vol. I: 466 p.; Vol. II: 493 p. (Heidelberg: Winter).—

A book which is indispensable for anyone interested in Babylonian and Assyrian history. Mesopotamian culture is of Sumerian origin and has highly influenced surrounding peoples. The first volume contains, *inter alia,* chapters dealing with agronomy, hunting and fisheries, trade, traffic, and industry. Vo' II deals with the interrelationship between science and religion, and the author makes it clear that Mesopotamian life was strongly dominated by religious superstition and that philosophy, medicine, and astronomy can scarcely be separated from theology. A long chapter (p. 283-323) on magic and medicine, and a chapter on natural and exact sciences (p. 380-418). Many illuminating illustrations.

OPPENHEIM, A. L., 1964: Ancient Mesopotamia: portrait of a dead civilization, 433 p. (Chicago, Ill.: Chicago U.P.).—

According to the author the portrait of Mesopotamia ought to be given by "comprehending, reducing, and rendering in a more or less readable manner a characteristic selection of the staggering mass of diversified and very often unrelated facts which philologists and archaeologists alike have extracted from the tablets and sherds, the ruins and images of Mesopotamia and have labeled and arranged in innumerable ways." It is a general account, and some sections are of special biohistorical value, *e.g.,* those on the care and feeding of the gods, Mesopotamian psychology, the arts of the diviner, medicine and psysicians, craftsmen and artists. Appendix on Mesopotamian chronology of the historical period. Glossary of names and terms. Bibliography and index.

PFEIFFER, R. H., 1935: State letters of Assyria, 265 p. (American Oriental Series, Vol. VI) (New Haven, Conn.: Amer. Oriental Soc.).—

A very attractive selection of the royal correspondence of the Assyrian empire, containing much correspondence (both in transcription and in English translation) between the king and his physicians, thus giving much "inside" information concerning medical matters (incl. magical ceremonies, incantations, expiatory rites), concerning agriculture and commerce (incl. delivery of horses, husbandry, shepherds, agricultural produce), and concerning animal omens and their interpretation.

PRATT, J. A., 1917: Assyria and Babylonia: a list of references in the New York Public Library, 112 p. (Bull. New York Publ. Library 21: 748-810; 840-890).—

For botany, zoology and medicine, see p. 799-800. Reprinted in 1967 (Detroit, Mich.: Gale).

TALLQVIST, K. L., 1894: Die assyrische Beschwörungsserie Maglû nach den Originalen im British Museum herausgegeben, 2 vols. Vol. I: Einleitung, Umschrift, Uebersetzung, Erläuterungen und Wörterverzeichnis, 180 p.; Vol. II: Keilschrifttexte, 98 p. (Acta Soc. Sci. Fenn. 20: No. 6).—

A series of incantations and rites, mostly of an imitative magic character, using fire to destroy evil. The first volume gives a transcription and a German translation on the opposite page; the second volume contains the cuneiform text.

b. *History of the plant and animal sciences*

BONAVIA, E., 1894: The flora of the Assyrian monuments and its outcomes, 215 p. (London: Constable).—

Starting from the Assyrian flora, the author attempts to interprete certain symbols found woven in with this, and to throw some light on some other features which seem to be affiliated to those symbols. Spe-

cial attention has been paid to the sacred trees (date palm, vine, pomegranate, fir tree), the cone-fruit, the lotus, the evil eye and to the trident.

DANTHINE, H., 1937: Le palmier-dattier et les arbres sacrés dans l'iconographie de l'Asie occidentale ancienne, 2 vols. Vol. I: Texte, 279 p.; Vol. II: Album, 206 plates with 127 illustrations. (Bibliothèque archéologique et historique, 25) (Paris: Geuthner).—

Separate sections deal with the botanical aspects of the date-palm (its culture, reproduction, geographical distribution, *etc.*), with the different ways of artistic representation of sacred trees in general and of the date palm in particular, with descriptions of different scenes in which the date palm plays a role *(e.g.,* as an element in the landscape, in hunting and fighting scenes, date-picking, divinities associated with the date-palm, artificial fecundation, adoration scenes, *etc.),* with the vegetation gods, and with possible interpretations of the date-palm cult. The last chapter (p. 165-209) contains a comparative study considering the role of sacred trees in Mesopotamia, Egypt, Cyprus and with the people living around the Aegean Sea.

DELITZSCH, F., 1874: Assyrische Studien. Heft 1: Assyrische Thiernamen, mit vielen Excursen und einem assyrischen und akkadischen Glossar, 190 p. (Leipzig: Hinrichs).—

A philological study giving explanations of the names of animals, *i.e.,* of mammals, insects, fishes, and birds. *Cf.* LANDSBERGER, B. & I. KRUMBIEGEL, 1934, *vide infra.*

HOLMA, H., 1911: Die Namen der Körperteile im Assyrisch-Babylonischen. Eine lexikalisch-etymologische Studie, 183 p. (Ann. Acad. Sci. Fenn., Ser. B, VII, No. 1).—

An Assyrio-Babylonian nomenclature of bodily parts, both of man and animals, incl. such parts as blood, flesh, *etc.,* together with quotations of passages in which the terms were used. The subjectmatter has been divided as follows: the head and its parts; the parts between the head and the body; the body excl. the genitals; the upper and lower extremities; special animal parts (spines, tail, *etc.*). Another study devoted to Assyrio-Babylonian anatomical nomenclature is: DHORME, E., 1963: L'emploi métaphorique des noms des parties du corps en hébreu et en akkadien,

183 p. (Paris: Geuthner). A reprint of a 1923 publication. With tables considering: 1. The parts of the body, 2. Assyrian terms, 3. Hebrew terms, 4. A list of biblical quotations.

HROZNÝ, F., 1913: Das Getreide im alten Babylonien. Ein Beitrag zur Kultur- und Wissenschaftsgeschichte der alten Orient, part 1. Mit einem botanischen Beitrage von F. v. FRIMMEL "Ueber einige antike Samen aus dem Orient", 216 p. (S.B. Kgl. Akad. Wiss., Wien, phil.-hist. Kl., 173, No. 1).—

A philological study which, after a general review of the cultivation of corn in antiquity, deals particularly with the culture of emmer wheat *(Triticum dicoccum)* which supplied people with bread, beer, *etc.* This species is still cultivated in large parts of Abyssinia, Egypt and Arabia.

JONES, T. B., 1952: Ancient Mesopotamian agriculture (Agric. Hist. 26: 46-52).—

A summary review of Mesopotamian agriculture and agricultural economics, written by a specialist in these fields. The study has been based on material remains and written records, such as law codes, letters, the "farmer's almanac", and actual business records written on clay tablets. The principal field crops were: barley, wheat, emmer, sesame, onions, peas, and beans; the gardens produced dates, pomegranates, and figs. The author states that much transliteration work has to be done, before we can get a true picture of Mesopotamian agriculture and horticulture. *Cf.* HROZNÝ, F., 1913, *supra.*

LANDSBERGER, B. & I. KRUMBIEGEL, 1934: Die Fauna des alten Mesopotamien nach der 14. Tafel der Serie Ḫar-ra = ḫubullû, 158 p. (Abh. sächs. Akad. Wiss., phil.-hist. Kl., Vol. 42, No. VI) (Leipzig: Hirzel).—

Tablet enumerating hundreds of animals, except most domestic animals, birds and fishes. In the first part the names are given in two columns, the first giving the Sumerian term and the other its Accadian equivalent; the second part gives many quotations of passages in which the animals have been described. A study dealing with the domestic animals according to the 13th tablet of the same series has been published by: OPPENHEIM, A. L. & L. F. HARTMAN, 1945: The domestic animals of an-

cient Mesopotamia according to the XIIIth tablet of the series Ḫar-ra = ḫubullû (J. Near Eastern Stud. 4: 152-177). *Cf.* DELITZSCH, F., 1874, *vide supra;* and VAN BUREN, E. D., 1939, *vide infra.*

SALONEN, A., 1955: Hippologica accadia, 318 p. (in German) (Ann. Acad. Sci. Fenn., Ser. B, 100).—

The scope of this publication is fully covered by its subtitle: "Eine lexikalische und kulturgeschichtliche Untersuchung über Zug-, Trag-, und Reittiere, ihre Anschirrung, Aufzäumung, Besattelung, Bepanzerung und Pflege, sowie über die Gespanne und Karawanen, die Besatzung und Mannschaften der Wagen, über die Reiterei, das Pflegepersonal, usw. bei den alten Mesopotamiern samt einem Verzeichnis der hippologischen Termini und Redewendungen."

THOMPSON, R. C., 1924: The Assyrian herbal: a monograph on the Assyrian vegetable drugs, 294 p. (London: Luzac).—

A monograph on about 250 Assyrian vegetable drugs based on a thorough examination of all known medical texts and of more than 120 fragments of cuneiform plant lists, including chiefly plants with medicinal value and often including short descriptions of the plants considered. The work has been written mainly from the philologist's point of view. It gives a very interesting insight into the Assyrian arrangement of plants. Assyrian, Syriac, Hebrew, Aramaic, Arabic, Persian, Greek, Latin, and English indexes have been included. There is no historical synthesis of the material discussed.

——, 1949: A dictionary of Assyrian botany, 405 p. (London: British Academy).—

Aims and methods of this posthumously published book are explained in the introduction by the following words: "The method used in this dictionary for rehearsing and identifying the names known to the Assyrians is, first, to quote the passages where the respective words occur in the bilingual or explanatory botanical lists, and then to seek the identity of the plant not only from the data of these lists, but by the aid of other cuneiform texts, principally the medical prescriptions and magical formulae. Philological evidence is then adduced, and often ancient, medieval, or modern science and practices in the Oriental lands are compared." Sumerian, Accadian, Hebrew, Aramaic, Syriac, Arabic, Persian, Greek, Latin, and English indexes have been included. As such the book is comparable to the author's "The Assyrian herbal", *supra*.

VAN BUREN, E. D., 1939: The fauna of ancient Mesopotamia as represented in art, 113 p. (Rome: Pontificium Institutum Biblicum).—

Intended for scholars who wish "to learn whether a particular animal was known in Mesopotamia, and how and when it was represented." This is a catalogue of such natural animals as are known in art (excl. fantastic or monstrous creatures). No discussion of the significance of animals in religion or magic. *Cf.* LANDSBERGER, B. & I. KRUMBIEGEL, 1934, *vide supra*.

c. History of the medical sciences

BIGGS, R. D., 1967: Š.À.ZI.GA. Ancient Mesopotamian potency incantations, 86 p. (Texts from Cuneiform Sources, Vol. II) (Locust Valley, N.Y.: Augustin).—

Among the rituals and incantations familiar to the Mesopotamian medicine-man there was a small group aiming at restoring lost sexual potency. This group, called Š.À.ZI.GA., helped the medicine-man to find the material necessary to reconstitute the lost power. The substances used include some animal parts having a reproductive function. To enhance the power of the substances, various spells could be recited over them before they were used.

CONTENAU, G., 1938: La médecine en Assyrie et en Babylonie, 230 p. (Paris: Maloine).—

A very readable book intended for the historian of medicine and for the educated layman. From the archaic script and language of the medical documents it can be concluded that medical science has a high antiquity. In its beginnings, medicine was a part of the religious system, but gradually more exact observations, a better insight into the nature of disease, and a better understanding of therapy developed, but most Babylonian medicine remained sacerdotal and magical in its nature. Consequently, the greater part of the book is devoted to medicine as it was practised by the priests: sickness is the punishment for sin. There are long lists containing the old Sumerian names of the diseases and their translation into Assyrian language and attempts to give proper diagnoses of the diseases. There is an illuminating general historical introduction, and some sections have

been devoted to more or less general topics, such as: medicine and art, medicine and law, medical schools and books, physician and society, the possible relations between Babylonian medicine on the one hand, and the medicine of the Egyptians, Greeks, and Christian Syrians on the other hand. Exhaustive bibliography.

JONG, H. M. W. DE, 1959: Demonische ziekten in Babylon en bijbel, 131 p. (Leiden: Brill).—

The author considers many facets of Biblical and Babylonian (incl. Sumerian) demonic medicine in the ancient literature, and as such the book gives a good review of protohistoric medicine and the mixture it contains of magico-religious and empirico-rational elements. The author gives a review of the various types of demons, and the role of the Evil Spirit idea in relation to medical prognosis, diagnosis, and therapeutics. It includes some interesting accounts of the demonic medicine of Jesus, Saul, Sarah, Paul, and that found in Flavius Josephus.

KÜCHLER, F., 1904: Beiträge zur Kenntnis des assyrisch-babylonischen Medizin. Texte mit Unterschrift, Uebersetzung und Kommentar, 154 p. (Assyrologische Bibliothek XVIII) (Leipzig: Hinrichs).—

A transcription, translation and discussion of old cuneiform medical texts, mainly belonging to the Konyunjik Collection of the British Museum, that is, the tablets from the library of Ashurbanipal, 7th century B.C., but much of its contents has been copied from much older sources. CIVIL, M., 1960 (Rev. d'Assyriol. 54: 57-72) gives a transcription and translation of a Sumerian medico-pharmaceutical text dating from *ca.* 2100 B.C.

LABAT, R., 1951: Traité akkadien de diagnostics et pronostics médicaux, 2 vols. Vol. I: Transcription et traduction, 49 + 247 p.; Vol. II: 68 plates (Coll. Trav. Acad. intl. Hist. des Sciences, No. 7) (Leiden: Brill).—

A very important text of Mesopotamian medicine based on fragments, dispersed in many libraries and ranging in date from *ca.* 710 to 453 B.C., comprising many older elements. The treatise is made up of 40 tablets which can be divided into 5 groups: I: "When the incantation priest goes to the house of a sick man" . . ., this text deals with the omens observed on the way to the sick, around the house, or in the sick room; II: "When you approach a sick man"..., deals with prognoses arrived at from a systematic observation of the patient; III: "If being ill for a day"..., this text deals with the patient's condition and behaviour from the first to the sixth day of illness, and thereafter, the symptoms observed, the patient's desires, *etc.;* IV: The title is somewhat obscure, it lists symptoms caused by various demons; V: "The pregnant woman, if her forehead is yellow...", a divination text, giving information concerning the child to be born. The same author gives a semi-popular historical review in: LABAT, R., 1953: La médecine babylonienne, 23 p. (Conférences du Palais de Découverte, Serie D, No. 22) (Paris: Univ. de Paris).

LE PORT, L. R., 1925: Les causes morales du mal physique dans la médecine assyro-babylonienne (Contribution à l'histoire de la pathologie générale), 104 p. (Thèse Univ. Montpellier) (Montpellier: Causse, Graille & Castelnau).—

The book has been divided into three parts. I: General introduction, concerning Assyrio-Babylonian thought on nature, man, and his gods. II: Illness; the priest-magician *(âshipu),* his theoretical views and his methods of treatment; the physician *(asû)* and his knowledge of anatomy, physiology, obstetrics, surgery, therapeutics, ophthalmology, hygiene, and legal medicine. III: Death and survival.

LEVEY, M., 1961: Some objective factors of Babylonian medicine in the light of new evidence. (Bull. Hist. Med. 35: 61-70).—

According to the author, charms, incantations, and purification rites should be considered as mystical or magical medical treatments. Demon causation and "sympathetic" medicine, however, should be constituents of an "empirico-rational" treatment. Other studies dealing with rational elements of Mesopotamian medicine are: KRAUSE, A. C., 1934: Assyrio-Babylonian ophthalmology (Ann. Med. Hist., N.S., VI: 42-55), and LABAT, R., 1954: A propos de la chirurgie babylonienne (J. asiat. 1954: 207-218). This publication deals with an (isolated) passage that speaks of the lancet in connection with eye diseases. Although - as the author makes clear - the Code of Hammurabi shows that surgery was practised, it remains curious that thus far none of the other practices referred to in the Code are ever mentioned in medical texts.

THOMPSON, R. C., 1903-1904: The devils and evil spirits of Babylonia: being Baby-lonian and Assyrian incantations against the demons, ghouls, vampires, hobgoblins, ghosts, and kindred evil spirits, which attack mankind, 2 vols. Vol. I: "Evil Spirits", 65 + 211 p.; Vol. II: "Fever sickness" and "Headache", 54 + 179 p. (Luzac's Semitic Text and Translation Series XIV-XV) (London: Luzac).—

These volumes give transliterations, notes and a vocabulary, together with an English translation from the original cuneiform texts of three major series of magic texts. They present copies of the exorcisms and spells which the Sumerian and his Babylonian successor employed, and they make it clear that medicine (including its rational elements) has to be fitted into a religious system. Sickness was considered to be a form of punishment sent by the gods, directly or through the medium of demons, *etc.,* so that the patient had to be submitted to all kinds of magic and religious myth. Both volumes have long introductions. *Cf.* CONTENAU, G., 1938, *vide supra.*

——, 1934: Assyrian prescriptions for diseases of the urine, *etc.,* 152 p. (Babyloniaca: études de philologie assyro-babylonienne 14: 57-190).—

Contains transliterations and translations of cuneiform tablets dealing with remedies for urinary and similar diseases, *e.g.,* gonorrhoea, retention of urine, discharges of pus and blood, stone, prolapse of intestines, texts relative to copulation and love charms, methods of treatment of urinary troubles either by sensible potions, or by the introduction into the urethra, usually by a tube of copper or bronze, of various drugs, or by ointments,... THOMPSON (London, 1923, 107 p.), edited his "Assyrian medical texts" from the originals in the British Museum, comprising the bulk of the medical tablets from Ashurbanipal's library at Niniveh, 7th cent. B.C., and he has since published a series of papers in which he has transcribed and edited parts of these Assyrian texts. The one considered here is one of them, others are: Assyrian medical texts (Proc. roy. Soc. med. 17 (1924): 1-34; 19 (1926): 29-78, dealing with diseases of the head, of the eyes, and of the mouth; Assyrian prescriptions for treating bruises or swellings (Amer. J. semitic Lang. 47 (1930): 1-25); Assyrian medical prescriptions against simmatu "poison" (Rev. d'Assyriol. 27 (1930): 127-135); Assyrian prescriptions for diseases of the chest and lungs *(idem,* 31 (1934): 1-29); Assyrian prescriptions for diseases of the ears (J. roy. Asiatic Soc. 1931: 1-25); Assyrian prescriptions for the "Hand of a Ghost" *(idem,* 1929: 801-823); Assyrian prescriptions for diseases of the feet *(idem,* 1937: 265-286). *Cf.* also THOMPSON, R. C., 1924, *vide* subsection b.

5. LIFE AND MEDICAL SCIENCES IN INDIA

a. History of science and culture in general

BODDING, O., 1925: Studies in Santal medicine and connected folklore. Part I: The Santals and disease; Part II: Santal medicine; Part III: How the Santals live. (Mem. Asiat. Soc. Bengal X, Nos. 1, 2, and 3, 502 p.).—

> In the first two parts the author discusses the medicine used by the Santals, their application and administration. He deals with the ideas of the Santals as to the origin and causation of diseases, their superstitions and fears, their medicine man and his doings and magic. The third part contains descriptions of Santal villages, agriculture, cereals prepared, food, vegetables, leaves and plants, mushrooms, fruits, fowls and birds, catching of animals, milk, honey, fishes and fishing, *etc.*

CROOKE, W., 1926: Religion and folklore of Northern India, new ed., 471 p. (Oxford: U.P.).—

> The following chapter-headings may give an insight into those parts of the book which are of a biohistorical interest: The godlings of disease (p. 114-145); Fertility and agricultural rites (241-275); The evil eye (276-307); Omens and divination (308-316); Animal worship (348-382); Serpent worship (383-399); Tree and plant worship (400-418).

DE BARY, T., S. HAY, R. WEILER & A. YARROW, eds., 1958: Sources of Indian tradition, 962 p. (New York, N.Y.: Columbia U.P.).—

> Part 1 deals with Brahmanism, the Vedic hymns and the Upaniṣads; part 2 with Jainism and Buddhism, their philosophy, politics, ethics, *etc.;* part 3 with Hinduism, its philosophy, hymns, aesthetics, *etc.,* and the four ends of man; part 4 with Islam in medieaval India; part 5 with Sikhism; part 6 with modern India and Pakistan. In its totality the book gives a picture of the development of Indian thought since earliest times in order to provide an understanding of contemporary civilization in India (and Pakistan).

ELIADE, M., 1960: Le yoga. Immortalité et liberté, 428 p. (Paris: Payot).—

> A comparative study of Yoga theories and practices, not only in India but all over the world, including the yoga system of Patañjali, the technique of meditation, liberation and re-integration, the history of yoga practice, Buddhist yoga, Haṭha-yoga, alchemy, mystic erotics, shamanism.

HAUER, J. W., 1958: Der Yoga. Ein indischer Weg zum Selbst. Kritisch-positive Darstellung nach den indischen Quellen mit einer Uebersetzung der massgeblichen Texte, ed. 2, 487 p. (Stuttgart: Kohlhammer).—

> A historical review in which the author discusses such subjects as: the beginnings of yoga in the Vedic age, yoga in the Upaniṣads, in Buddhism and Jainism, yoga in the Mahābhārata, and in the Rāma Upaniṣads, the history and the texts of the Pātañjala-yogasūtram and its later developments. The last part (p. 274-450) deals with yoga as medical treatment in East and West in which the author defends the thesis that yoga is of equal value to all Indo-European peoples. The first edition of this book appeared under the title: Der Yoga als Heilweg, nach den indischen Quellen dargestellt, 1932, 159 p. (Stuttgart: Kohlhammer). *Cf.* ELIADE, M., 1960, *vide supra.*

MACKAY, E., 1948: Early Indus civilization, ed. 2, 169 p. (London: Luzac).—

> An excellent and well-written introductory survey of ancient Indus civilization, discussing such topics as: architecture and masonry, religion, dress and personal ornaments, copper and bronze, household equipment, tools and weapons, arts and crafts, customs and amusements, *etc.,* together with a chronology in which the connections with other countries have been made clear. *Cf.* MASSON-OURSEL, P., 1933: l'Inde antique et la civilisation indienne, 497 p. (Paris: La Renaissance du Livre). Also in English translation: Ancient India and Indian civilization, 1933, 497 p. (London: K. Paul, Trench & Trubner). Reprinted 1967. *Cf.* also: MAJUMDAR, R. C. & A. D. PUSALKER, eds., 1951, *vide infra.*

MAJUMDAR, G. P., 1938: Some aspects of Indian civilization (in plant perspective), 450 p. (Calcutta: Author).—

> This treatise is an attempt to show how the "indebtedness of Indian civilization

in all its various aspects to plants and plant-life ... (and) ... to indicate how far plants and plant-products have served as a basis of certain material aspects of Indian civilization." Its contents can be read from the chapter-headings which are as follows: 1. Knowledge of plants; 2. Food and drinks; 3. Dress and other personal requisites; 4. Toilet; 5. Furniture; 6. Conveyances; 7. Trade and commerce; 8. Health and hygiene; 9. Hearth and home; 10. Domestic rites and rituals; 11. Odes to plants.

MAJUMDAR, R. C. & A. D. PUSALKER, eds., 1951 →: The history and culture of the Indian people in 10 vols. Vol. I (1951): The Vedic age, 565 p.; Vol. II (1953): The age of imperial unity, 733 p.; Vol. III (1954): The classical age, 754 p.; Vol. IV (1955): The age of imperial Kanauj, 585 p.; Vol. V (1958): The struggle for empire, 940 p.; vol. VI (1961): The Delhi sultanate, 882 p.; Vol. IX, 1 (1963): British paramountcy and Indian renaissance, 1205 p. (Bombay: Bharatiya Vidya Bhavan).—

A planned ten-volume history of India in which the (Indian) authors try to make a distinction between what is really old in Indian culture and what is of a more recent date, with the aid of inscriptions, monuments, coins, archaeological findings, *etc.* All volumes contain chapters on general and regional historiography, and chapters on such subjects as: language and literature, political theory, law, religion and philosophy, art, social conditions, education, economic life, colonial and cultural expansion, *etc.,* for each of the periods considered. Hardly anything about the history of science. A comparable, but older survey is RAPSON, E. J., ed., 1922-1932: The Cambridge history of India, 6 vols. (Cambridge: U.P.). A more handsome edition is: DODWELL, H. H., ed., 1934: The Cambridge shorter history of India, 970 p. (Cambridge: U.P.). A very good survey is also: SMITH, V. A., 1958: The Oxford history of India, ed. 3, 898 p. (Oxford: Clarendon Press). *Cf.* also: MACKAY, E., 1948, *vide supra;* and RENOU, L. & J. FILLIOZAT, 1947, 1953, *vide infra.*

MEYER, J. J., 1937: Trilogie altindischer Mächte und Feste der Vegetation, 238 p. (Kāma) + 267 p. (Bali) + 399 p. (Indra) in one volume. (Zurich: Niehans).—

A copious illustrated series of essays devoted to the Indian deities of vegetation and fertility Bali, Kāma, Indra, and Varuṇa. The author tries to explain the meaning of old Indian nature-myths and forms of nature

worship. A book known to me only by title, but probably of the same character, is: RELE, V. G., 1931: The Vedic gods as figures of biology, 134 p. (Bombay: Taraporevala).

PATHI, A. L., ed., *ca.* 1962: A textbook of Āyurveda, ed. 2, Vol. I, Sec. I: Historical background, 636 p.; Vol. II, Sec. II: Philosophical background, 624 p. (Jamnager: Jain Bhaskarodaya Press).—

The historical volume discusses such subjects as: the Hindu Dharma, ancient India and its universities, history of Āyurveda, Vrikṣāyurveda, ancient town planning, civic administration in ancient India, and present methods in Hindu medicine. In the other volume the author gives the philosophical background of Āyurveda, *e.g.,* the Nyāya system, Saṅkhya, Yoga psychology, Pūrva-Mīmāṃsā, Vedānta, Cārvāka, Jainism, and many other theoretical problems related to Indian science and medicine.

PRAKASH, O., 1961: Food and drinks in ancient India, 341 p. (Delhi: Lal).—

"This monograph on food and drinks in ancient India is mainly a study of the food habits of Indians from the earliest times to *ca.* 1200 A.D. in which I have tried to reconstruct the picture on the basis of all available sources - literary, epigraphic and archaeological." The author starts his study with prehistoric civilizations; other chapters deal with food and drink during the Vedic, Sūtra, Maurya, Suṅga, Kuṣāṇa, Saka Sātavāhana, and Gupta periods, and with early Buddhist and Jain works, the epics and Manusmṛti. Appendices deal with: frying in ancient India up to *ca.* 500 A.D., sugar industry, betel-chewing, and smoking in ancient India, antiquity of certain food articles in India (cereals, oil seeds, fruits, vegetables, spices), with food preparations, beverages, books on food and drinks in India, and with articles in journals on food and drinks in ancient India.

RENOU, L. & J. FILLIOZAT, 1947, 1953: L'Inde classique. Manuel des études indiennes, 2 vols. Vol. I: 699 p.; Vol. II: 758 p. (Vol. I: Paris: Payot; Vol. II: Paris: Imprimerie Nationale).—

Vol. I deals with such topics as: the geography, races, languages, historiography, and politics of India, with the Vedas, and with Brahmanism. Vol. II deals *inter alia* with the philosophy of Brahmanism, with old Indian literature and theatre, with Buddhism and Jainism. A special chapter (p. 138-

194) deals with science: medicine (hygiene, pathology, therapeutics, physiology, the treatises of Suśruta and Caraka, the doctrines of the Āyurveda, the Bower manuscript, yoga, Arabic influences); veterinary medicine; physical and natural science; chemistry; mathematics; astronomy.

SEAL, B., 1915: The positive sciences of the ancient Hindus, 295 p. (London & Madras: Longmans, Green).—

According to the author, the main body of positive knowledge presented in this book may be assigned to the millenium 500 B.C.-500 A.D. It contains much material that is of interest to the historian of biology and medicine, *e.g.,* chapters on: chemistry in the medical schools of ancient India (p. 56-85); Hindu ideas about plants and plant-life (169-176); Hindu classification of animals (177-201); Hindu physiology and biology (202-243); Hindu doctrine of scientific method (244-295).

VOGEL, J. P., 1962: The goose in Indian literature and art, 74 p. (Memoirs of the Kern Institute, No. 11) (Leiden: Brill).—

This study is especially devoted to the figure of the haṃsa which played an important role in Indian literature and art, and which the author proves to be the Indian goose (and not a swan). The work rests on a rather sound biological basis. Subject headings are as follows: Introduction; The goose in the epics; The goose in Buddhist literature; The goose in Indian fables and fairy-tales; The goose in Indian art.

——, 1926: Indian serpent-lore of the Nāgas in Hindu legend and art, 318 p. (London: Probsthain).—

A study on serpent worship in Indian literature, folklore, and art. In this volume the author collected the legends relating to the Nāgas which are found in the Brahmanical and Buddhist literature of India.

b. *History of the plant and animal sciences*

AIYER, A. K. Y. N., 1949: Agricultural and allied arts in Vedic India, 69 p. (Bangalore: Bangalore Press).—

This study has been based upon the hymns or Saṃhitā portion of the Ṛg-, Yajur-, Sāma-, and Atharvavedas and not on their elaboration as contained in the Brāhmaṇas or Upaniṣads. The author tries to give an idea about agricultural conditions in those days, relying on the numerous similes and illustrations of which the hymns contain so many. *Cf.* MORELAND, H. W., 1929, *vide infra.*

BURKILL, J. H., 1965: Chapters on the history of botany in India, 245 p. (Delhi: Govt. of India Press).—

A history of Indian botany from its earliest beginnings up to *ca.* 1900, originally published in chapters in the J. of the Bombay Natural History Society. The term "India" in the title includes Burma and Ceylon. Burkill sums up the effort of 457 persons to whom, according to the author, the formation of Indian botany is to be attributed; at the Rijksherbarium of the University of Leiden, an index was prepared to the names as they occur in the text as it was published in the J. of the Bombay Natural History Society. *Cf.* MAHESHWARI, P. & R. N. KAPIL, 1963: Fifty years of science in India: progress of botany, 178 p. (Calcutta: Indian Science Congress Assn.).

CHAKRABERTY, C., n.d.: The cultivated plants of India: their history and their uses, 128 genera - 230 species, 50 p. (Calcutta: Vijaya Krishna).—

An enumeration of those plants which can serve or formerly served as food, with many historical notes and brief descriptions.

EDGERTON, F., ed., 1931: The elephant-lore of the Hindus. The elephant-sport (Mataṅga-līlā) of Nilakantha, 129 p. (Transl. from the original Sanskrit with introduction, notes, and glossary) (New Haven, Conn.: Yale U.P.).—

This book is of importance to veterinary medicine; mythological arguments are restricted to a minimum. Starting from the assumption that the physiology of the elephant does not essentially differ from that of man, the theory of Indian (human) medicine is adapted to elephants: diseases are attributed to disturbances of the equilibrium of the three bodily humours: wind, gall and phlegm. The book has been divided into 12 chapters dealing with: 1. The origin of elephants; 2 and 3. favourable and unfavourable marks; 4. marks of longevity; 5. marks of the stages of life; 6. measurements; 7. prices; 8. marks of character; 9. must (Sanskrit: mada); 10. capture; 11. to keep them in good health, description of some diseases, together with therapeutic indications; 12. on the qualities of elephant drivers. A publication dealing with Indian veterinary medicine is: KRISHNASWAMI, A. A., 1939: Tierheilkunde und tierärztliche Instrumente im alten Indien (Beitr. Gesch. Vet. Med. 2: 75-82). *Cf.* ZIMMER, H. R., ed., 1929, *vide infra.*

GIBOIN, L. M., 1949: Epitome de botanique et de matière médicale de l'Inde et spécialement des établissements français dans l'Inde, 387 p. (Contribution à l'étude de la pharmacopée et de la médecine ayurvédique) (Thèse Fac. Méd., Marseille) (Pondichéry: Ashram).—

A very valuable study of medicinal botany. The plants have been summed up alphabetically according to the genera, many illustrations of the plants mentioned are added, the medicinal properties are discussed and the role they play in Āyurvedic medicine is stressed. Glossaries of names in French, Latin, Sanskrit, Tamil, Bengal, Telugu, and Hindi. A comparable study is: CHAKRABERTY, C., 1923: A comparative Hindu materia medica, 213 p. (Calcutta: Author). It deals with some 800 plant species belonging to 190 genera; they are arranged in the alphabetical order of the Sanskrit names and are accompanied by brief botanical descriptions, Latin, European, Bengal and Hindi synonyms, medical and other remarks. Indexes in English and Sanskrit. A more recent study is: CHOPRA, R. N., S. L. NAYAR & I. C. CHOPRA, 1956: Glossary of Indian medicinal plants, 330 p. (New Delhi: Council of Scientific and Industrial Research).

MAHESHWARI, P. & U. SINGH, 1965: Dictionary of economic plants in India, 197 p. (New Delhi: Indian Council of Agricultural Research).—

"The dictionary lists over 1,700 species of economic plants, in alphabetical sequence of their scientific names. The name of the family is given after each plant and then the English and the Hindi names (in Roman script). This is followed by brief information on habit, distribution and uses. An index of English and Hindi names included at the end will prove useful to lay readers." (From a book review in: Current Science 35 (15): 399).

MAJUMDAR, G. P., 1927: Vanaspati. Plants and plant-life as in Indian treatises and traditions, 254 p. (Calcutta: U.P.).—

This book contains a collection of Sanskrit texts pertaining to botany. The book has been written by a botanist. Its contents are: Introduction; Botany and philosophy (incl. such topics as germination, external and internal morphology, plant physiology, ecology, taxonomy, evolution and heredity); Botany and medicine (incl. such topics as the use of plants in Atharvaveda and the development of medical science in Caraka and Suśruta); Botany and agriculture (incl. such topics as Vedic agriculture, Kṛṣi-Parāśara, a treatise on agriculture, meteorological observations, soil selection, sowing, planting, reaping, *etc.);* Indexes. The author has not been able to give the Latin name of all plants mentioned. *Cf.* also: MAJUMDAR, G. P., 1938; and MEYER, J. J., 1937, *vide* subsection a.

——, 1935: Upavana-Vinoda: a Sanskrit treatise on arbori-horticulture, 128 p. (Calcutta: Indian Research Institute).—

The Upavana-Vinoda is the arbori-horticultural part of a great encyclopaedic work, the Śārṅgadhara-paddhati, an anthology compiled by Śārṅgadhara. It deals with the glory of trees, good and evil omens, selection of soil, sowing of seed, planting, watering, protection, nutrition, treatment of diseases, *etc.,* of plants and trees. There is an historical introduction, followed by the Sanskrit text, an English translation, a bibliography and a list of plants.

MORELAND, W. H., 1929: The agrarian system of Moslem India: a historical essay with appendices, 296 p. (Cambridge: Heffer).—

"Chapter I deals with the antecedents of the Moslem Agrarian System and its relation to the Hindu Sacred Law. Succeeding chapters discuss the 13th and 14th centuries, the Sayyid and Afghan Dynasties, the Reign of the Akbar and the 17th century. The body of the work closes with a consideration of Northern India, the Deccan, and Bengal. Extensive appendices explain the technical terms employed, amplify points mentioned in the body of the book, and give the list of authorities cited." (From Biol. Abstr. 6: 340). *Cf.* AIYER, A. K. Y. N., 1949, *vide supra.*

MUKERJI, B. & S. PRADHAN, 1963: Fifty years of science in India: progress of physiology, 168 p. (Calcutta: Indian Science Congress Assn.).—

Unfortunately I am unable to give further information about this publication.

MÜLLER, R. F. G., 1955: Altindische Embryologie, 52 p. (Nova Acta Leop. Carol., 17) (Leipzig: Barth).—

An attempt to elucidate ancient Indian ideas concerning foetal development as they are expressed in the treatises of Suśruta, Caraka and Vāgbhaṭa. Chapter headings are as follows: Männlicher Zeugungsstoff, Zeugungsanteile des männlichen Körpers, Fortpflanzungsanteile des weiblichen Körpers, weiblicher Fortpflanzungsstoff, Bildung des Embryos, Geschlechtsbestimmung, Bemerkungen zur Ausbildung von Besonderheiten, Einfluss von Schwangerschaftsgelüsten, Grundsätzliche Beziehungen, Die "Herabkunft" des Keimes, Erkenntnis-Grundsätze, Begriff einer sogenannten "Seele".

RAYCHAUDHURI, S. P., 1964: Agriculture in ancient India, 167 p. (New Delhi: Indian Council of Agricultural Research).—

A study of agriculture and husbandry of the ancient Indians as it is expressed in Vedic literature and commented upon by Caraka, Suśruta, Kāśyapa, Parāśare, Varāhamihira and others. It considers such topics as classification of land, irrigation and drainage, tree planting, tillage and tillage implements, ploughs, manuring, cultivation of crops, vegetables and fruits, protection of crops from disease and pests, sowing of seeds, meteorology, livestock, cattle, cows, bulls, and the treatment of diseases of cattle.

SIMOONS, F. J. & E. S., 1968: A ceremonial ox of India: the mithan in nature, culture, and history, 323 p. (Madison, Wisc.: Univ. Wisconsin Press).—

To quote from the author's preface: "While collecting information from the literature on the hill peoples of Assam and adjoining areas, we became aware of the existence among them of a strange-looking domesticated bovine animal - the mithan (Bos frontalis) - which was not milked. The mithan, sometimes also referred to in the literature as "gayal", is little known to the outside world ... though our initial effort was intended only to present a brief statement for the dairying study, we became aware of the need for someone to collect the widely scattered material on the animal. This book springs from that awareness." The first part of this book (p. 1-36) deals with the mithan in nature, the second part (p. 37-162) with the mithan in selected cultures, the third part (p. 163-210) with the mithan in society and economy, and the fourth part (p. 211-265) with the domestication of the mithan and of common cattle. Glossary, references, and index.

STEBBING, E. P., 1922-1962: The forests of India, 4 vols. Vol. I (1922): 1796-1864, 548 p.; Vol. II (1923): The development of the Indian forest service, 1864-1900, 633 p.; Vol. III (1926): The progress of conservancy and the development of research in forestry 1901-1925, including brief reviews of the progress of conservancy in the several presidencies and provinces between 1871 and 1900, 705 p.; Vol. IV, ed. by H. CHAMPION & F. C. OMASTON, 1962: The history from 1925 to 1947 of the forests now in Burma, India and Pakistan, 485 p. (I-III: London: Lane; IV: London: Oxford U.P.).

—

The first volume deals with the early history of the forests in India and goes on to the position and treatment of the forests during the period 1796-1850. After that comes the first beginnings of forest conservancy 1850-1857 and the initiation of forest conservancy 1858-1864. The second volume is in two parts: the inauguration of the Indian Forest Service, and a scientific conservancy of the forests, and the progress of forest conservancy and the development of the forest department in India, 1871-1900. The third volume describes the progress of forest conservancies in the several presidencies and provinces between 1871 and 1900 and the inauguration of forest research work in India and Burma 1901-1925, concluding with the effects of the Great War and of the constitutional reforms on forest policy. The fourth volume is in two parts: the general progress of forest conservancy between 1925-1947 and: the progress of forest administration in the provinces 1925-1947. (For this information I am much indebted to Miss Katharine M. Davidson, librarian of the Dept. of Forestry and natural Resources of the Univ. of Edinburgh).

ZIMMER, H. R., ed., 1929: Spiel um den Elefanten. Ein Buch von indischer Natur, 184 p. (Munich: Oldenbourg).—

This book contains a German translation of the Mataṅga-līlā (Elephant sport), and an analysis of a much longer treatise: The Hastyāyurveda (Treatment of disease in elephants). The introduction deals with elephant-lore in general, and the text deals with the mythological origin of elephants, their "castes" (types), "birthmarks"; but also with practical matters: to capture them, train them, keep them in good health, etc. The book deals with the same topics as that of F. EDGERTON, 1931 (vide supra), but much more stress has been laid on metaphysical and mythological arguments.

c. History of the medical sciences

BODDING, O., 1925: Studies in Santal medicine and connected folklore, 3 parts, 502 p. (Mem. Asiat. Soc. Bengal, 10, Nos. 1, 2, and 3).—

> For more details, *vide* subsection a.

CALAND, W., 1900: Altindisches Zauberritual. Probe einer Uebersetzung der wichtigsten Theile der Kauśika Sūtra, 196 p. (Verh. Kon. Ned. Akad. Wetenschappen, Afd. Letterk., N.R. III, 2).—

> A partial German translation of the Kauśika Sūtra, a commentary of the Atharvaveda, our chief medical source of Vedic medicine which is of particular importance since it indicates the manual rites that had to be performed when hymns were recited. A reprint has been announced (Wiesbaden: Sändig). *Cf.* also: CALAND, W., 1968: Altindische Zauberei. Darstellung der altindischen "Wunschopfer", ed. 2, 143 p. Reprint by Sändig (Wiesbaden).

Caraka (fl. *ca.* 150 B.C.) - MEHTA, P. M., ed., 1949: The Caraka Samhita. Expounded by the worshipful Atreya Punarvasu, compiled by the Great Sage Agnivesa and redacted by Caraka and Dṛdhabala, with translation in Hindi, Gujarati and English, 6 vols. Vol. I: 4 + 32 + 625 p.; Vol. II: 28 + 969 p.; Vol. III: 22 p. + p. 970-1920; Vol. IV: 25 p. + p. 1921-2881; Vol. V: 46 + 1051 p.; Vol. VI: 6 + 445 p. (Jamnagar: Shree Gulabkunverba Āyurvedic Society).—

> The Caraka Saṃhitā is the earliest known written treatise by an Indian physician. An editorial board headed by P. M. Mehta prepared a new text containing many explanations to be used by those who have no appropriate knowledge of Sanskrit or of Indian cultural history. Vol. I provides the reader with the background information needed for an understanding of Caraka's work; it contains a historical review of medicine in ancient India and an analysis of the philosophical concepts in Caraka, leading to a discussion of general pathology. Vols. II, III and IV contain the text, together with the translations and explanatory footnotes. Vol. V contains the complete text and table of contents in English, and Vol. VI contains indexes for the entire work, lists of diseases, drugs, recipes, sketches and pictures of the flora and fauna mentioned by Caraka. A scientific synopsis of the con-

tents of the Caraka Saṃhitā can be found in: RAY, P. & H. N. GUPTA, 1965: Caraka Saṃhitā, 120 p. (New Delhi: Nat. Inst. of Sciences of India). Most of the material in it has been arranged in tabular form. Latin equivalents of all Sanskrit names and terms have been given.

DASTUR, J. F., 1960: Everybody's guide to Āyurvedic medicine, 316 + 85 p. (Bombay: Taraporevala).—

> This is, as the subtitle announces, a repertory of therapeutic prescriptions based on the indigenous systems of India. Appendix 1 gives explanations of Āyurvedic terminology, appendix 2 describes the standard preparations mentioned in the text, and appendix 3 contains a glossary of the drug plants mentioned in the text, in Latin, together with Sanskrit and/or Hindi equivalents. *Cf.* also: PATHI, A. L., ed., *vide* subsection a.

DWARKANATH, C., 1959: Introduction to kāyachikitsā, 399 p. (Bombay: Popular Book Depot).—

> Kāyachikitsā means internal medicine. This book presents the physiological doctrines and concepts of Āyurveda in order to elucidate their role in the theories of pathogenesis and therapeutics. The book has been written for under- and post-graduate students of medicine. Separate chapters have been devoted to the analysis of one of the principal concepts of Indian medicine.

ESSER, A. A. M., 1930-1932: Die Ophthalmologie des Bhāvaprakāśa. I. Anatomie und Pathologie, 55 p. (Studien zur Geschichte der Medizin, Heft 19.); II. Die ophthalmologische Therapie des Bhāvaprakāśa, 29 p. (Arch. Gesch. Med. 25: 184-213).—

> The beginning of the first article gives a good physiological introduction to Hindu pathology and therapeutics in general and to that of the eye in particular. On p. 13 is a short review of the contents of the text. On p. 22-34 the text follows (in transcription), and then the translation. The second article contains a critical analysis of the relevant textparts, the technical measures, the ointments applied, *etc.* in ophthalmological therapy.

FILLIOZAT, J., 1949: La doctrine classique de la médecine indienne, ses origines et ses parallèles grecs, 230 p. (Paris: Imprimerie Nationale.).—

An elaborate study of ancient Hindu medicine, derived from the original texts. The author points to parallels with Greek medicine. Ch. 1 deals with the Āyurveda; ch. 2 with pre-Aryan and Indo-Iranian medical ideas; ch. 3, 4 and 5 deal with pathology, anatomy, and physiology respectively in the Vedic Saṃhitās, including a glossary of anatomic terms; ch. 6 with Veda and Āyurveda; ch. 7 with Āyurvedic ideas on wind and Greek pneumatism; ch. 8 with Plato's Timaeos; ch. 9 with communications between India and Greece before Alexander. Index is included. In 1964 there appeared an English translation: The classical doctrine of Indian medicine: its origins and Greek parallels, 298 p. (New Delhi: M. Manoharlal).

GUPTA, K.V.N.S., 1906-1909: The Āyurvedic system of medicine, or an exposition, in English, of Hindu medicine as occurring in Charaka, Suśruta, Vāgbaṭa, and other authoritative Sanskrit works, ancient and modern, 3 vols. Vol. I (1909): 29 + 54 + 421 p.; Vol. II (1906): 65 + 776 p.; Vol. III (1907): 723 p. (Calcutta: Chatterjee).—

Vol. I consists of two parts. The first part deals with health, diagnosis of disease, examination of the pulse, of the urine, of the eyes and of the tongue, and with the classification of diseases. The second part deals with fevers and their treatment, with diarrhoea, dysentry, haemorrhoids, indigestion, cholera, worms, jaundice, bronchitis, asthma, vomiting, intoxication, epilepsy, diseases of the nervous system, leprosy, tumours, heart-disease, diabetes, obesity, oedema, measles, small-pox and a lot of minor diseases, with diseases of the mouth, the ear, the nose, the eye, with diseases of women, children, etc. Vol. II contains a pharmacopoeia, discussing the methods of purifying minerals, etc., methods of boiling, roasting, etc., different kinds of vessels used, with technical names and with the preparation of diets for patients. The second part of this volume deals with fevers and with a great many diseases. Volume III contains a glossary with the names of all the Indian plants and metals that are useful to the students of Āyurveda. In this list the Sanskrit names, the synonyms, the vernacular, and the scientific names of the plants considered have been given. Cf. PATHI, A. L., ed., ca. 1962, vide subsection a; also DASTUR, J. F., 1960, vide supra.

HOERNLÉ, A. F. R., ed., 1893-1913: The Bower Manuscript. Facsimile leaves, Nāgarī transcript, romanised transliteration and English translation with notes, 95 + 406 p. (Calcutta: Office of Superintendent of Govt. Printing).—

Fragments on medical literature, consisting of 7 parts. The contents of part 1 are of a miscellaneous nature; the pharmaceutical characteristics of garlic, some pharmaceutic directions regulating digestion, aphrodisiac formulae, formulae for eye lotions, face plasters, remedies for the hair. Part 2 and 3 contain a practical formulary, or handbook of prescriptions covering the whole field of internal medicine; parts 4 and 5 contain two short manuals dealing with the art of foretelling a person's fortune; part 6 and 7 contain two different portions of the same text referring to a charm, protecting against snakebite and other evils. A study especially dealing with ophthalmology is: ESSER, A. A. M., 1942: Die Ophthalmologie im Bower Manuskript (Sudh. Arch. Gesch. Med. 35: 28-42).

——, 1907: Studies in the medicine of ancient India. Vol. I: Osteology or the bones of the human body, 264 p. (Oxford: Clarendon Press). — (No other volume published).—

Useful study of Hindu osteological doctrines, a first attempt to explain Hindu anatomy and physiology. After a general discussion of ancient Indian medical authors, their works and their terminology, the author compares the different systems, viz., those of Ātreya, Caraka, Suśruta, Vāgbhaṭa and of the Vedas. In a next section he tries to give a detailed identification of the bones which compose the human skeleton, and the last section contains a critical apparatus.

JOLLY, J., 1951: Indian medicine. Supplemented with notes by C. G. KASHIKAR, 239 p. (Poona: C. G. Kashikar).—

A translation from JOLLY, J., 1901: Medicin, In: Grundriss der Indo-Arischen Philologie und Altertumskunde, Vol. III, Heft 10, 140 p. It describes in great detail the ideas contained in the principal Sanskrit treatises, chiefly those that relate to the pathology and nomenclature of the diseases. It contains much information, taking into account the entire literature on medicine from the Vedas down to the Bhāvaprakāśa. Separate chapters deal with: Sources (p. 1-29); physicians and therapy (p. 30-58); theoretical notions (p. 59-72); the theory of development and gynaecology (p. 73-100); internal diseases and their treatment (p. 101-136); external diseases (p. 139-165); diseases of the head (p. 166-174); nervous and mental diseases and toxicology (p. 175-183). Supplementary notes by the translator, Sanskrit index and general index.

KUTUMBIAH, P., 1962: Ancient Indian medicine, 14+54+225 p. (Bombay: Orient Longmans).—

A very good introduction to the classics of ancient Indian medicine in which the relevant philosophical and medical problems are elucidated. Separate chapters deal with ancient Indian anatomy, physiology, the doctrine of tridoṣa, aetiology, classification and pathology of diseases, diagnosis and prognosis, materia medica, treatment, surgery and ophthalmology, and with obstetrics, gynaecology and paediatrics. Notes, references and index. A short review of Indian medicine can be found in: REHM, K. E., 1969: Die Rolle des Buddhismus in der indischen Medizin und das Spitalproblem, 57 p. (Zürcher Medizingeschichtl. Abh., N. R., No. 65) (Zurich: Juris).

MÜLLER, R. F. G., 1951: Grundsätze altindischer Medizin, 163 p. (Acta Historica Scientiarum Naturalium et Medicinalium, Vol. 8) (Copenhagen: Munksgaard).—

The book mainly consists of an attempt to outline the influence of treatises of the "Ancient Trio" Caraka (on early Buddhistic medicine) Suśruta (especially on surgery) and Vāgbhaṭa (on the principles of medicine) on the formation of the basic principles and further development of early Indian medicine. Whereas sensory perception was one of the main problems of Vedic medicine, much stress has been laid on the diffusion of this principle in Indian medicine. Other topics discussed *inter alia* are: the relationship between priestly and lay medicine in Vedic antiquity; the transmission of ideas on the wind and its medical effects; old Indian concepts of space and time which stem from earlier metaphysical principles; the soul-image emerging from the doctrine of Indian surgery. A more recent introduction into Indian medicine published by the same author and containing a critical survey of the whole subject in the light of the very comprehensive knowledge of the author is: Medizin der Inder in kritischer Uebersicht, 1965, 121 p. (Indo-Asian Studies, Part 2: 3-124) (New Delhi: Internatl. Acad. of Indian Culture).

MUKHOPĀDHYĀYA, G., 1913, 1914: The surgical instruments of the Hindus, with a comparative study of the surgical instruments of the Greek, Roman, Arab and the modern European surgeon, 2 vols. Vol. I: 444 p.; Vol. II: plates. (Calcutta: U.P.).—

This study commences with an evaluation of the ancient medical authors and their works. Thence chapters follow on hospitals and dispensaries, the materials of the instruments used, the classification and description of the instruments, the hygienic appliances, hospital requisites, and the relation of Hindu to Greek, Persian, Arabian, Chinese, Tibetan and modern European medical science. The author follows closely the classical Hindu medical texts.

——, 1923-1929: History of Indian medicine: containing notices, biographical and bibliographical, of the Āyurvedic physicians and their works on medicine from the earliest ages to the present times. Vol. I (1923): 172 p. + p. 1-204; Vol. II (1926): 99 p. + p. 205-518; Vol. III (1929): 20 + 14 p. + p. 519-868. (Calcutta: U.P.).—

The first volume contains a long introduction (p. 1-172) in which the author gives a general background, and in which he discusses and evaluates work done by former medical historians. Next comes the text of the book, entitled "Notices, biographical and bibliographical, of the Āyurvedic physicians and their works on medicine" (that means including the account of the gods and sages who took part in the development of the healing art in India, for, as the author states, to know the history of medicine in Ancient India is to know the entire domain of indology). It contains a detailed study of the works of Āyurvedic physicians with translated excerpts. Every chapter has as its heading the name of the physician whose life is described; it is an index of Sanskrit medical work. This study is continued in vols. II and III. Vol. II also contains a long introduction mainly dealing with the present situation of Āyurvedic medicine (*ca.* 1925!); it also includes a bibliography of Āyurvedic books, on general medicine, materia medica, anatomy and surgery, history of medicine and cognate sciences.

RAY, D.N., 1937: The principles of tridoṣa in Ayurveda, 188 p. in English, 168 p. in Sanskrit. (Calcutta: Banerjee).—

The author himself is a practitioner of Ayurveda, a medical system based on the theory of tridoṣa, comparable with the Greek system of the four humours. The particularities of these principles are explained in detail, as well as their applications to the understanding of digestion, heredity, temperament, pathology, and therapeutics. In order to do this, a study of Hindu physics and metaphysics has been added. Each doṣa exists in five different forms and the contents of the Āyurveda are derived from the consideration of the normal and abnormal interactions of those forms. When the equilibrium between them is disturbed, it can sometimes be reestablished by appropriate drugs, by physical or psychical means. *Cf.* KIRFEL, W., 1951, *vide* section Antiquity in general, subsection c.

SAMBOO, G., 1963: La médecine de l'Inde autrefois et aujourd'hui, 285 p. (Paris: Ed. du Scorpion).—

    A French history of Indian medicine. The first part deals with the history of Indian medicine in general, the second part contains short chapters on Indian botany, agricultural science, zoology, and chemistry, the third part deals with the different aspects of old Indian medicine and the fourth part deals with present day Indian medicine. *Cf.* NEELAMEGHAN, A., 1963: Development of medical societies and medical periodicals in India, 1780-1920, 120 p. (Iaslic special Publ., No. 3) (Calcutta: Oxford Book Co.).

SANYAL, P. K., 1965: A story of medicine and pharmacy in India. Pharmacy 2000 years ago and after, 224 p. (Calcutta: Sanyal).—

    A short history of the four systems of medicine that are practised in India today, *viz.,* the Āyurvedic, the Ynani, the European, and the homoeopathic system. The author also describes Arabic medical science which came to India in the 11th century, and how it fused with existing Indian medicine. Many illustrations.

SHARPE, E., 1937: An eight-hundred year old book of Indian medicine and formulas, translated from the original very old Hindi into Gujarati character and thence into English, 135 p. (London: Luzac).—

    A translation of the only extant ms. written by the pupil of the great Jain priest Hemacandra. The text deals with the various kinds of diseases and their remedies. Separate sections deal with powders, pills, ointments, and oils. Very useful index and an additional list of Indian drugs, woods and dyes with their English equivalents have been added.

SINGHAL, G. D. & D. S. GAUR, 1963:

Surgical ethics in Āyurveda, 99 p. (Varanasi: Chowkhamba Sanskrit Series Office).—

    This book is intended for students of Āyurveda, medical historians, and modern surgeons and physicians. It deals especially with the ideas of Suśruta, but also with Caraka and Vāgbhaṭa, and it contains many quotations from their works, both in Sanskrit and in English translation. The ethical principles have been placed into nine groups: general ethics, professional and academic ethics, pre-operative ethics, operative ethics, post-operative ethics, experimental surgery ethics, quacks, ethics towards the dying, ethics in emergency surgery.

SRIVASTAVA, G. P., 1954: History of Indian pharmacy. Vol. I., ed. 2, 276 p. (Calcutta: Pindars).—

    Only the first volume of the planned two volumes has been published. It deals with ancient and mediaeval pharmacy. After an introductory chapter, chapter 2 deals with mythology, describing the heavenly origin of medicine, ch. 3, 4 and 5 deal with the pre-Caraka-, the Caraka-, and the post-Caraka period, in which light has been thrown on the important pharmaceutical personages of India and their works. Ch. 6 deals with the mediaeval period, and ch. 7, 8 and 9 are devoted to science and technique of pharmacy as practised by the Indians through the ages. The last chapter relates Indian pharmacy to the pharmacy of other countries, esp. Greece and Arabia.

Suśruta (6th cent. B.C.) — BHISHAGRATNA, K. K. L., ed., 1907-1916: An English translation of the Sushruta Samhita based on original Sanskrit texts, 3 vols. Vol. I (1907): Sutrasthānam, 4+67+12+571 p.; Vol. II (1911): Nidāna-sthāna śārira-sthāna, chiksita-sthāna, and kalapa-sthāna, 5+17+20+762 p.; Vol. III (1916): Uttara-tantra, 4+14+416 p. (Calcutta: Bhaduri).—

    The Suśruta Saṃhitā is the most representative work of Āyurveda; it not only deals with the essentials of Indian therapeutics, but it also embraces the whole range of the science of Āyurveda as it was understood and practised in the Vedic ages. The first volume opens with a general review of the Āyurveda, followed by chapters dealing with *e.g.,* surgical measures, the influence of the seasons on health and drugs, surgical instruments and practice, cauteries, leeches, functions of chyle, blood, and semen, swellings, ulcers, classification of diseases, extraction of splinters, prognoses of omens, curable diseases, classification of drugs, specific properties of drugs and flavours, purgatives. The second volume deals *inter alia* with: diseases of the nervous system, diseases of the urinary tract, mammary glands, *etc.*, tumours, fractures and dislocations, pregnancy, the anatomy of the human body, vascular system, venesection, medical treatment of ulcers, sores, fractures, nervous disorders, haemorrhoids, fistulae, cutaneous infections, abscesses, *etc.*, elixirs, poisons, and the medical treatment of snake- and insect-bites, treatment with the sounds of a drum. The third volume deals with diseases of the eye, the ear, the nose, the head, symptoms and therapeutics of the diseases of the female organs of generation, of fever, of diarrhoea, of *gulma,* of heart-diseases, jaundice, alcoholism, vomitting, asthma, cough, worms, and of diseases brought on by superhuman influences, rules of health. Suśruta's work is especially important from the surgical point of view; it describes a number of operations, explains the particularities of many special instruments, and illustrates the training needed for surgeons. Full attention is paid to careful diagnosis, diet and bathing. Some 760 medicinal plants are mentioned. A reprint of this edition appeared in 1963 (Varanasi, India: Chowkhamba Sanskrit Series Office). For a German translation of that part of the Suśruta Saṃhitā that deals with eye disease, *cf.* ESSER, A. A. M., 1934: Die Ophthalmologie des Susruta, textkritisch bearbeitet, übersetzt und mit Concordanztabellen zu Bhāvamiśra versehen, 84 p. (Stud. Ges. Med., Heft 22) (Leipzig: Barth).

(Vāgbhaṭa *ca.* 650 A.D.) HILGENBERG, L. & W. KIRFEL, 1941: Vāgbhata's Aṣṭāṅgahṛdaya saṃhitā. Ein altindisches Lehrbuch der Heilkunde. Aus dem Sanskrit ins Deutsche übertragen, mit Einleitung, Anmerkungen und Indices, 52+4+885 p. (Leiden: Brill).—

A systematic and comprehensive book on Hindu medicine. Its contents have been divided as follows: I: Sūtrāsthāna. Theoretical introduction, in 30 chapters (161 p.) including: tridoṣa, diet and regimen, surgery, cauterization, *etc.* II: Sarīrasthāna. Anatomy, in 6 chapters (51 p.), including: conception, embryology, obstetrics, parts of the body, dreams. III: Nîdānasthāna. Aetiology, in 16 chapters (73 p.). IV: Cikitsāsthāna. Therapeutics, in 22 chapters (200 p.). V: Kalpasthāna. Preparation of remedies, in 6 chapters (31 p.). VI: Uttarasthāna. Final part, in 40 chapters (220 p.), dealing with a number of special diseases or ailments, toxicology, elixirs, aphrodisiacs. The book includes a glossary (21 p.) of Sanskrit plant names and an extensive general index of 94 p. There also exists an English translation of the first five chapters: VOGEL, C., ed., 1965: Vāgbhaṭa's Aṣṭāṅgahṛdayasaṃhitā. The first five chapters of its Tibetan version, with the original Sanskrit, accompanied by a literary introduction and a running commentary on the Tibetan translating-technique, 298 p. (Abh. Kunde Morgenland. 37, No. 2) (Wiesbaden: Steiner).

ZIMMER, H. R., 1948: Hindu medicine, 72 + 203 p. (Baltimore, Md.: Johns Hopkins Press).—

This book contains the text of two lectures. In the first lecture entitled "Medical tradition and the Hindu physician", the author deals with medical ideas found in Vedic literature, *viz.*, in the Atharvaveda and in the Ṛgveda, and he shows the interconnections between the procedure of the Hindu physician and the Buddhist method of salvation. The second lecture "The human body: its forces and resources" deals with the main theories of Hindu physiology, such as the theory of the parallelism between micro- and macrocosmos as it has been developed in the Vedas and Upaniṣads, the theory of the three humours, the yoga theory of respiration, and with anatomy and embryology. Comparison of Hindu and Greek medicine is attempted. *Cf.* HAUER, J. W., 1958, *vide* subsection a.

6. LIFE AND MEDICAL SCIENCES IN THE FAR EAST

a. History of science and culture in general

CHANG KWANG-CHIH, 1963: The archaeology of Ancient China, 346 p. (New Haven, Conn.: Yale U.P.).—

A history of the cultural growth of China from *ca.* 15000 B.C. to the founding of the Ch'in in 221 B.C. It describes the development of human culture in China during the late prehistoric and early historic periods. It is of a great biohistorical interest for it is mainly devoted to the following topics: the hunter-fishers of the Mesolithic culture, the first farmers of the Huangho and the Jangshao; the spread of agriculture during the Neolithic period; the emergence and further development of civilization in North China; the farmers and nomads of the Northern Frontier and the early civilizations in South China.

CORDIER, H., 1904-1908: Bibliotheca sinica. Dictionnaire bibliographique des ouvrages relatifs à l'empire chinois, ed. 2, 4 vols. (Paris: Geuthner). In 1924 a supplement and index were published, and in 1953 an "Author index to the Bibliotheca Sinica of Henri Cordier (2nd edition, 4 vols., Paris 1904-1908. Supplement, 1 vol., Paris, 1924)", distributed by the East Asiatic Library of Columbia University Libraries, New York, 84 p.—

> The whole work has been divided into 5 parts, viz., La Chine proprement dite; Les étrangers en Chine; Relations des étrangers avec les Chinois; Les Chinois chez les peuples étrangers; Les pays. For the present purpose the following sections are the most valuable: Vol. I, section 4: Ethnographie et anthropologie (p. 359-374); section 6: Histoire naturelle (p. 387-527) divided as follows: zoology p. 390-442, botany p. 442-507, geology p. 507-527; section 10: Histoire (p. 558-695); Vol. II, section 12: Sciences et arts (p. 1363-1576), esp. the part dealing with medicine (incl. surgery, anatomy, the pulse, acupuncture, pharmacology, medical botany, hygiene, therapeutics, infectious diseases, parasitology, folklore, dental medicine, medical education) (p. 1462-1498) and the part dealing with agriculture (p. 1498-1538). The second part (vol. III, p. 1917-2287), deals with the knowledge of foreign people about China, and with trade. The third part deals with the contacts, influences, etc. between China and Portugal, Spain, the Netherlands, England, Russia, France, the Scandinavian countries, the United States, Germany, etc. Parts 4 and 5 have no direct relevance to the topics considered in this guide. An unaltered reprint, including the supplementary vol. appeared in 1966 (Taipei: Ch'eng-Wen).

EBERHARD, W., 1948: Chinas Geschichte, 404 p. (Bern: Francke).—

> This is a short history of China from prehistoric times to the end of World War II. The author shows how politics, economics, science, literature and art are closely interwoven. This is a very good one-volume history, containing a selected and annotated bibliography and a detailed index. Cf. HUARD, P. & M. WONG, 1960, vide infra.

FAIRSERVIS, W. A., 1959: The origins of oriental civilization, 192 p. (New York, N.Y.: Mentor Books).—

> A paperback, containing a semi-popular description of the evolution of culture in China, Japan, Korea, Manchuria, Mongolia and Siberia, and the history of ancient man in Asia. It is shown that the development of those old cultures was closely bound

to the means and methods of obtaining food, and one of the oldest methods is that of agriculture which originated initially in the Near East and moved from there towards the East, bringing profound changes in those regions.

FORKE, A., 1925: The world-conception of the Chinese: their astronomical, cosmological and physico-philosophical speculations, 300 p. (London: Probsthain).—

> The work has been divided into four books: 1. The universe; 2. Heaven; 3. Yin and Yang; 4. The five elements. It is essentially based upon the Chinese sources; the relevant texts are quoted both in Chinese script and in translation. This book is essentially philosophical in character, and according to Sarton, it is an important contribution to knowledge of Chinese thought.

GOODRICH, L. C., 1959: A short history of the Chinese people, ed. 3, 295 p. (New York, N.Y.: Harper).—

> A comprehensive history of the Chinese people and their civilization, with emphasis on their means of livelihood, religious and moral ideas, government, literature, and fine arts. It includes much literature for supplementary reading. It contains also information on agriculture, medicine, and science in general. Excellent maps and useful tables. According to Sarton this short history of China contains a surprising amount of information not available in much larger works.

HUARD, P. & M. WONG, 1960: Chine d'hier et d'aujourd'hui. Civilisation-arts-techniques, 271 p. (Paris: Horizons de France).—

> A popular and richly illustrated history of China. It contains also a chapter (p. 178-197) on Chinese science and technology, incl. Chinese astronomy, mathematics, physics, chemistry, alchemy, geology, botany, zoology, medicine. Cf. EBERHARD, W., 1948, vide supra.

HUMMEL, A. W., ed., 1943-1944: Eminent Chinese of the Ch'ing period (1644-1912). Vol. I (1943): A-O, 604 p.; Vol. II (1944): P-Z, p. 605-1103. (Washington, D.C.: U.S. Govt. Print. Office).—

> This biographical encyclopaedia deals with eminent Chinese, Manchus, Mongols, Muslims, and Koreans who lived between

1644 and 1912. Most of the persons included are of politico-historical interest, but some of them were famous scientists (*e.g.,* agriculturists, geographers, encyclopaedists). Vol. II also contains indexes of names, books and subjects.

LI CH'IAO-P'ING, 1948: The chemical arts of old China, 215 p. (Easton, Pa.: J. chem. Educ.).—

> Separate sections deal with such subjects as: alchemy, metals, salt, ceramic industries, lacquer and lacquering, gunpowder, colours and dyes, Chinese ink, vegetable oils and fats, incense, essential oils, cosmetics, sugars, paper, leather and glue, soybean products, alcoholic beverages and vinegar. One appendix contains a table of the Chinese dynasties, and another a table of Chinese weights and measures.

NEEDHAM, J., 1954 →: Science and civilization in China. With the research assistance of WANG LING. Vol. I (1954): Introductory orientations, 38 + 318 p.; Vol. II (1956): History of scientific thought, 697 p.; Vol. III (1959): Mathematics and the sciences of the heavens and the earth, 47 + 874 p.; Vol. IV: Physics and physical technology, Part 1 (1962): Physics, 34 + 434 p. (to be continued) (Cambridge: U.P.).—

> The first volume contains geographical and general historical introductions and discusses the characteristics of the Chinese language. It gives a review of what contacts there were between east and west, what Chinese culture received from the outside world, and what the world learned from the Chinese. The central theme of the second volume is why science in China did not evolve as rapidly as it did in the West. A passage from the dust cover is informative about its contents: "Beginning with ancient times, it (*i.e.* the second volume) describes the Confucian milieu in which arose the organic naturalism of the great Taoist school, the scientific philosophy of the Mohists and Logicians, and the quantitative materialism of the Legalists. Thus we are brought on to the fundamental ideas which dominated scientific thinking in the Chinese Middle Ages. The author opens his discussion by considering the remote and pictographic origins of words fundamental in scientific discourse, and then sets forth the influential doctrines of the Two Forces and the Five Elements. Subsequently he writes of the important sceptical tradition, the effects of Buddhist thought, and the Neo-Confucian climax of Chinese naturalism.

Last comes a discussion of the conception of laws of nature in China and the West." Vol. III contains chapters, *inter alia,* on meteorology, geography, cartography, and geology, incl. palaeontology. Vol. IV (1) contains chapters on Chinese optics, acoustics, and magnetism: branches well developed in Chinese physical science.

NOTT, S. C., 1947: Voices from the flowery kingdom, 278 p. (New York, N.Y.: The Chinese Culture Study Group of America).—

> This book aims at "being an illustrated descriptive record of the beginning of Chinese cultural existence incorporating a complete survey of the numerous emblematic forces selected from nature by the ritualistic leaders of the Chinese throughout the ages." It deals with such subjects as: archaic Chinese funeral devices, the six sacrificed objects, spears and arrowheads, and the dental formula of animals in Chinese art, the worship of the ancestors, seasonal festivities, the twelve animals of the duodenary cycle (horse, goat, rat, dog, cock, tiger, serpent, hare, monkey, pig, buffalo, dragon), the five symbolically animated animals of the Chinese (bat, eagle, deer, fish, lion), and the eight felicitous animals of the Chinese (ram, elephant, rhinoceros, tapir, bear, fox, camel, leopard). A complementary volume, "being an illustrated descriptive record of the meaning of emblematic and symbolic designs personified in the arts of China throughout the ages", written by the same author is: Chinese culture in the arts, 1946, 134 p. Topics of special biohistorical interest discussed in this volume are *e.g.,* fruits, flowers, berries, blossoms, tree from, *etc.,* in Chinese art, and those parts dealing with the dragon, the tortoise, the buffalo, the duck, and the bat.

OSGOOD, C., 1951: The Koreans and their culture, 387 p. (New York, N.Y.: Ronald Press).—

> The subject matter has been divided into 5 parts as follows: 1. A contemporary Korean village (the village and its environment, its social organisation, economic life, the life of the individual, death and religion); 2. The Korean capital and the ruling class; 3. The origins and chronological development of the Korean nation; 4. A résumé of the cultural history of Korea; 5. Modern Korea.

SOWERBY, A. de C., 1940: Nature in Chinese art, 203 p. (New York, N.Y.: Day).—

> An attractively illustrated and authoritative discussion of the interpretation of

nature by Chinese artists and art-craftsmen from the earliest times. It is an attempt to identify many of the natural forms portrayed by these artists. It deals with birds, the Chinese lion and other mammals, domestic animals, reptiles, fishes, invertebrates, flowers, trees, rocks, agriculture, *etc.*

STEIN, R. A., 1962: Civilization tibétane, 269 p. (Paris: Dunod).—

A review of the history of Tibet and its people, from the 7th century up to recent times. It describes the different peoples, their customs, religious beliefs, family life, agriculture, art and letters (literature). Less about the history of Tibetan science.

VISSER, M. W. de, 1913: The dragon of China and Japan, 242 p. (Verh. Kon. Ned. Akad. Wet., Amst., Afd. Letterkunde. Nieuwe Reeks, Vol. 13, No. 2).—

The most familiar creature to Far Eastern art and literature is the dragon. It plays a role comparable with the Indian serpent. There are different kinds of dragons, but they all belong to the class of rain bestowing, thunder- and storm-arousing gods of the water. Many dragon legends have been formed, and in the first part of this book the most interesting quotations have been collected, selected from Chinese literature. The second part deals with the dragon in Japanese literature. A reprint has been announced by Sändig (Wiesbaden).

VOLKER, T., 1950: The animal in Far Eastern art and especially in the art of the Japanese netsuke with references to Chinese origins, traditions, legends, and arts, 191 p. (Leiden: Brill).—

The greater part of the decorative images, generally used in Japan, have a symbolic meaning, and those representing animal life usually contain a moral teaching, but not always. In this book the author tries to find, whenever possible, the deeper meaning of animal pictures in Japanese art. Because the symbolic meanings of many animals described in this book have their origin in China and in Chinese art, often Chinese names and traditions are added. The book consists of a general part (p. 1-11) and an alphabetical description of animals (more than 85). Good index and bibliography. *Cf.* SOWERBY, A. de C., 1940, *vide supra.*

WATERBURY, F., 1952: Bird-deities in China, 191 p. (Artibus Asiae, Suppl. X)

(Ascona, Switzerland: Artibus Asiae).—

Separate chapters deal with such subjects as: the pervasiveness of animal-worship and the concept of the soul; some representations of anthropomorphized bird-forms in the Palaeolithic and Neolithic eras and the Bronze Age; the widespread belief in a connection between birds and the spirit-world; the history of bird-deities in China (p. 73-140); two representations of bird-deities from Christian churches of the European Peninsula. List of references, extensive index, and some 60 plates, mainly of Chinese origin.

b. *History of the plant and animal sciences*

BARTLETT, H. H. & H. SHOHARA, 1961: Japanese botany during the period of wood-block printing, 271 p. (Los Angeles, Calif.: Dawson's Book Shop).—

The contents of this book are reprinted from Asa Gray Bull., N.S., 3: 289-561 (1961). It consists of two parts: the first part (p. 1-100) deals with the development of natural history, especially botany, in Japan, with the influence of early Chinese and Western contacts, and with Japanese books and wood-block illustration. The second part consists of a catalogue of an exhibition of Japanese books and mss., mostly botanical, held at the Clements Library of the Univ. of Michigan, in commemoration of the 100th anniversary (1954) of the First Treaty between the U.S.A. and Japan. The record of each exhibit in this catalogue consists of a) a Romanized bibliographic entry, b) a characteristic illustration, and c) a legend for the illustration. It contains among others: herbals, encyclopaedias, works on medicine, famine herbals, books on floristics, economic botany, agriculture, horticulture, geography, books on art historical aspects (*e.g.,* flower arrangement and garden design), and books showing the beginning of Western influence on Japanese botany.

BÖTTGER, W., 1960: Die ursprünglichen Jagdmethoden der Chinesen, nach der alten chinesischen Literatur und einigen paläographischen Schriftzeichen, 97 p. (Berlin: Akademie Verlag).—

This book deals with such subjects as: the meaning of hunting in ancient China, general notes on hunting technique (*e.g.,* hunting grounds, animals fit for hunting, equipment of the huntsman, hunting magic), old Chinese hunting techniques (such as the use of sporting dogs or fire, hunting by means of carts, traps, nets, of snares, application of baits and camouflage), prehistoric hunting techniques, and the hunting techniques of the surrounding peoples.

BRETSCHNEIDER, E., 1882-1895: Botanicon Sinicum: notes on Chinese botany from native and western sources I-III. (J. R. Asiat. Soc., N. China Branche, 16, 1881, No. III, 228 p.; *idem*, N.S., 25, 1892, 468 p.; *idem*, N.S., 29, 1895, 623 p.).—

The first part deals with the history of the development of botanical knowledge among Eastern Asiatic nations, Chinese literature on materia medica and botany, Chinese works on agriculture, Chinese geographical works containing botanical information, the acquaintance of the Chinese with Indian and Western Asiatic plants, the history of materia medica and botany in Japan, botanical knowledge of Koreans, Manchus, Mongols, and Tibetans, the scientific determination of the plants mentioned in Chinese books; it contains an alphabetical list of Chinese works, and an index of Chinese authors. Vol. II deals with the herbaceous plants and trees mentioned in Rh Ya and with the cereals, vegetables, cultivated cucurbitaceous plants, textile plants, tinctorial plants, water plants, fruits, trees, bamboos and various other herbaceous plants in the Shi King, the Shu King, the Li Ki, the Chou li, and other Chinese classical works; and the classification of Chinese names of plants. In volume III the author attempts to examine and identify the drugs of vegetable origin noticed in the earliest Chinese works on materia medica, *viz.*, the Shen nung Pen ts'ao King, the Herbal of the Emperor Shen Nung, and the Ming i pie lu, a supplement to the former, employed by eminent physicians in the Han and Wei periods.

COX, E. H. M., 1945: Plant-hunting in China: a history of botanical exploration in China and the Tibetan marches, 230 p. (London: Collins).—

A popular history of plant collecting in China and of the constant endeavour to bring live plants safely to the Western World. Reprinted 1961 (London: Selbourne Press). A more elaborate and extremely accurate study of the topic is: BRETSCHNEIDER, E. V., 1935: History of European botanical discoveries in China, 2 vols., 1167 p. (Unaltered reprint of the 1880 edition, published by Koehlers Antiquarium, Leipzig).

BULLET, G., ed., 1946: The golden year of Fan Cheng-ta. A Chinese rural sequence rendered into English verse, with notes and calligraphic decorations by Tsui Chi, 44 p. (Cambridge: U.P.).—

Fan Ch'êng-ta (1126-1193) was a geographer, botanist, lexicographer, poet, and official of the Sung dynasty. The present booklet contains a sequence of 60 poems, written probably *ca.* 1186, expressing the moods of a farmer-poet throughout the seasons of the year.

DUMONT, R., 1957: Révolution dans les campagnes chinoises, 463 p. (Paris: Ed. du Seuil).—

The author describes the agricultural revolution as it took place in China in 1956, and he places this revolutionary movement in a historical setting. *Cf.* also: DAWSON, O. L., 1970: Communist China's agriculture: its development and future potential, 334 p. (New York, N.Y.: Praeger).

FRANKE, O., 1913: Kēng tschi t'u. Ackerbau und Seidengewinnung in China. Ein kaiserliches Lehr- und Mahnbuch aus dem Chinesischen uebersetzt und mit Erklärungen versehen, 194 p., 102 plates. (Abh. hamburg. KolonInst., 11) (Hamburg: Friedrichsen).—

The pictures form the most important part of this edition. In the introduction, the author states that "Ackerbau und Seidengewinnung, gleichbedeutend mit Beschaffung von Nahrung und Kleidung, sind Urbestandteile des Chinesentums, sie gehören zu den Grundlagen nicht bloss des staatlichen Lebens, sondern der gesamten Kultur". This quotation expresses the contents of the book very well. From that starting point the author discusses mainly the ethical, religious, literary and aesthetic aspects, but there are also short chapters dealing with agriculture and the manufacture of silk as it was practised in ancient China.

GULIK, H. v., 1935: Hayagrîva. The Mantrayânic aspects of horsecult in China and Japan, 105 p. (Internationales Archiv für Ethnographie, Suppl. zu vol. 35) (Diss. Univ. Leiden) (Leiden: Brill).—

Hayagrîva "is the specialized and therefore continually changing aspect of a great, essentially never changing, organic unity: the horse-cult". This god is characterized by the horse-head.

HARADA, J., 1956: Japanese gardens, 160 p. (Boston, Mass.: Branford).—

A historical review of the development of Japanese gardens. The sections deal with: the pre-Kamakura period (-1183), the Kamakura and Joshinocho period (1184-1393), the Muromachi period (1394-1572), the Momoyama period (1573-1602), the early Edo period (1603-1680), the middle Edo period (1681-1778), the late Edo period (1779-1868), and the period since the Restoration. Many gardens belonging to the respective periods have been considered in some detail, and illustrations of them have been added. *Cf.* SAITO, K. & S. WADA, 1964, *vide infra.*

HERVEY-SAINT-DENYS, L., 1850: Recherches sur l'agriculture et l'horticulture des Chinois, 262 p. (Paris: Allouard & Kaeppelin).—

This book is in two parts. The first part (p. 1-217) deals with the general conditions of agriculture and horticulture in China, and these conditions are compared with those in Europe and North Africa. It also sums up the plants cultivated (cereals, vegetables, fruits, plants and trees cultivated for industry and building activities, medicinal and ornamental plants). The second part contains an analysis of the contents of the agricultural encyclopaedia Cheou chi thong Khao. *Cf.* KING. F. H., 1948, *vide infra.*

HUAN, N.T., 1957: Esquisse d'une histoire de la biologie chinoise dès origines jusqu'au IVe siècle, 37 p. (Rev. hist. Sci. 10: 1-37).—

The author summarizes his views as follows: "Nous pouvons dire qu'à la fin du IIIe siècle, la biologie chinoise a fait d'énormes progrès et qu'au point de vue scientifique et philosophique, existent trois courants de pensée qui s'interpénètrent et restent souvent confondus, à savoir: la pensée taoïste, essentiellement Chinoise; la pensée bouddhique, apport de l'Inde, et enfin le mouvement rationaliste, le plus près de la pensée scientifique, qui recrute ses croyants dans le groupe des adeptes de Confucius."

KAN-CHIH-LIU, G., 1950: Cicadas in Chinese culture (including the silver fish), 121 p. (Osiris 9: 275-396).—

"It is essentially a history of Chinese insects but, to study the Chinese people, this history of insects may be more helpful than a history of Chinese emperors." The author wanted to find out what his countrymen know about their insects. The term "Cicadas" includes also plant lice, scale insects, leaf-hoppers and some other homopterous insects. The book gives much biological information but the author also discusses such topics as: cicadas as food, or as drugs; cicadas for entertainment, in decoration, allegory, poetry, painting, love-making, augury, and mythology; cicadas as money-makers, and the festival cicadas. A study dealing with Chinese cricket-lore against the general cultural background is: LAUFER, B., 1927: Insect musicians and cricket champions of China, 27 p. (Anthropology Leaflet, No. 22) (Chicago, Ill.: Field Museum Nat. Hist.).

KATO, G., ed., 1965: Japanese physiology: present and past, 204 p. (Tokyo: XXIII Internatl. Congress of Physiol. Sciences).—

The text is in three sections, of which the first two are of a historical interest. The first section contains a synopsis of the history of Japan and Japanese medicine from its beginnings through the Edo Period (1867) (p. 1-32); the second section considers the development of physiology in Japan from the beginning of the Meiji Period (1868) to the present (dealing with, *inter alia,* the beginnings of modern physiology in Japan, the development of Japanese pharmacology and biochemistry). The third section (p. 69-192) deals with contemporary physiology in Japan, considering the individual university institutions, medical schools, staff members and their interest, *etc.* Index of names.

KING, F. H., 1948: Farmers of forty centuries, or, permanent agriculture in China, Korea and Japan, 379 p. (Emmaus, Pa.: Rodale Press).—

An account of the cropping practices, crop rotations, drainage, irrigation methods, and soil management procedures in the countries considered. The central theme is the maintenance of soil fertility as it has been practised by oriental farmers. It is a second edition of a book published in 1911; only slight additions have been made. There also exists an edition of 1927, published by Cape (London). A book, especially dealing with Japanese agriculture is: SMITH, T. C., 1959: The agrarian origins of modern Japan, 246 p. (Stanford, Calif.: Stanford U.P.). Unfortunately, I cannot give further information about this book. *Cf.* HERVEY-SAINT - DENYS, L., 1850, *vide supra.*

LAUFER, B., 1919: Sino-Iranica. Chinese contributions to the history of civilization in ancient Iran. With special reference to the history of cultivated plants and products, 455 p. (Field Museum Nat. Hist., Anthropol. Ser. 15, No. 3) (Chicago, Ill.: Field Museum Nat. Hist.).—

An encyclopaedia of Chinese botany in which the author shows that known Chinese importations of plants from Central Asia extended over a period of fifteen centuries. After a short introduction, a series of chapters follow, each of them being a monograph devoted to one or more plants. Special attention has been paid to the plants introduced by the Chinese from Iran and cultivated in their own country, and to those drugs and aromatics which were imported from Iran to China. The Iranians were "the great mediators between the West and the East, conveying the heritage of Hellenistic ideas to central and eastern Asia and transmitting valuable plants and goods of China to the Mediterranean area." Because the Chinese have cultivated so many useful plants from all over the world, this study also contains much useful material for elaborating a history of cultivated plants.

Li Shih chen — CHANG HUI-CHIEN, 1960: Li Shih-chen: great pharmacologist of ancient China, 68 p. (Peking: Foreign Language Press).—

For more details, *vide* CHANG HUI-CHIEN, subsection c.

LIOU-HO & C. ROUX, 1927: Aperçu bibliographique sur les anciens traités chinois de botanique, 39 p. (Lyon: Bosc & Riou).—

Separate sections deal with ancient treatises on botany (The Pen-tsao, the Tche-wou-ming-che-tou-kao, and some other botanical treatises, p. 5-15), with ancient treatises on agriculture (the Keng-tchi-thou-chi, the Thsi-ming-yao-chou, and some others, p. 15-23), with treatises dealing with artistic aspects of botany (p. 23-25), and with ancient treatises on fungiculture (p. 25-27). Useful bibliography containing 91 entries. *Cf.* BRETSCHNEIDER, E., 1882-1895, *vide supra;* READ, B. E., 1936 and 1946; and SHIH SHENG-HAN, 1958, *vide infra.*

MERRILL, E. D. & E. H. WALKER, 1938: A bibliography of Eastern Asiatic Botany, 42 + 719 p. (Jamaica Plain, Mass.: Arnold Arboretum of Harvard University).—

This bibliography contains over 21,000 author-entries and relates mainly to China, Japan, Formosa, Korea, Manchuria, Mongolia, Tibet, and less completely to the Philippines, Indo-China, Siam, Burma, India, and Central and Northern Asia. Only publications with distinct taxonomic, geographic, or economic significance are included, but the subject-index is very extensive (p. 593-719), so that biohistorians can use it with much profit *(e.g.,* by consulting the headings: history and progress of botany, biographies, collections, organizations, institutions, *etc.).* Over 1,200 serials are listed with annotations of general utility. Appended to the extensive "Index of authors and titles" is an annotated list of older Chinese works, a reference list of oriental serials, and a reference list of oriental authors. In 1960, E. H. WALKER published along the same lines a supplement to this Bibliography of Eastern Asiatic Botany in which the coverage of the original bibliography is extended through the year 1958. (Washington, D. C.: Amer. Inst. Biol. Sci.).

READ, B. E., 1936: Chinese medicinal plants from the Pen Ts'ao Kang Mu, ed. 3, 389 p. (Bull. Peking Soc. Nat. Hist. 36).—

A botanical, chemical, and pharmacological reference list. The book consists of the following parts: 1. A list in tabular form of the 898 vegetable drugs mentioned in the Pen Ts'ao Kang Mu (including the following columns: Latin name, Chinese name, parts used, constituents, habitat, reference, and remarks) (p. 1-288); 2. An index of romanized Chinese names in tabular form, alphabetically arranged, containing the Chinese name, serial no., and the reference in the Pen Ts'ao (p. 289-361); 3. An index of common English names; and 4. A Latin index. *Cf.* also: MOSIG, A. & G. SCHRAMM, 1955: Die Arzneiplanzen und Drogenschatz Chinas und die Bedeutung des Pen-Ts'ao Kang-Mu, 72 p. (Berlin). Both books are useful reference tools for studies in the history of Chinese botany and medicine. *Cf.* also READ, B. E., 1931, *vide* subsection c.

——, 1946: Famine foods listed in the Chiu-Huang Pen-ts'ao, 90 p. (Shanghai: Henry Lester Institute).—

In the beginning of the 15th century this book was compiled by Chou Ting-wang, a treatise on plants fit for food in times of famine. The book contains descriptions of 414 plants of which 358 have been identified. The present booklet lists the contents of the Chiu-Huang Pen-ts'ao in their original order, giving the Chinese name, the botanical identity, the English name, the chemical analysis when known, notes upon the use of the plants as food in other countries, and general information for consultation of more detailed sources.

ROI, J., 1955: Traité des plantes médicinales chinoises, 484 p. (Encyclopédie biologique, 47) (Paris: Lechevalier).—

Descriptions of some 1,500 plants growing in China, together with their medical properties. Of each plant the French (if possible), the Latin, and the Chinese (popular and scientific) names have been given, together with references to Chinese literature, the parts used, *etc.* Indexes of French and Latin plant names and of therapeutic usage. *Cf.* READ, B. E., 1936 and 1946, *vide supra.*

SAITO, K. & S. WADA, 1964: Magic of trees and stones: secrets of Japanese gardening, 282 p., 199 figures. (New York, N.Y. & Tokyo: The JPT Book Comp.).—

A handsomely illustrated account of Japanese gardening, indicating the theoretical and actual functions of the different elements, such as: stone for the shoes, stepping stones, stone pavements, a garden water basin, stone lanterns, ponds and waterfalls, stone- and plant arrangement and their symbolic meaning. The following types of gardens are considered in some detail: the front garden, the kitchen garden, the inner garden, the courtyard garden, the interior garden, the rooftop garden, the garden below the floor, the alleyway garden, and the tea garden. Japanese gardens are linked with more than thirteen centuries of Japanese history and culture; and the present book contains much information from both the historical and the cultural points of view. Two books of the same character are: KUCK, L. E., 1940: The art of Japanese gardens, 304 p. (New York, N.Y.: Day), and TAMURA, T., 1937: Jardins japonais. Ses origines et caractères, dessins et plans, 280 p. (Tokyo: Kokusai Bunka Shin Kokai). *Cf.* also: HARADA, J., 1956, *vide supra.*

SCHAFER, E. H., 1963: The golden peaches of Samarkand: a study of T'ang exotics, 399 p. (Berkeley & Los Angeles, Calif.: California U.P.).—

The book deals in a humanistic way with imports of exotic products in T'ang China. It largely rests on literary history, and the author shows that the products considered achieved a kind of a Platonic real-

ity in Chinese life. The book is of a strong biohistorical interest because half of the book deals with biological objects, thus: ch. 3 deals with domestic animals (horses, camels, cattle, sheep and goats, asses, mules and onagers, dogs); ch. 4 with wild animals (elephants, rhinoceroses, lions, leopards, gazelles, marmots, *etc*); ch. 5 with birds (hawks and falcons, peacocks, parrots, ostriches); ch. 6 with furs and feather deerskins, sealskins, skin of martens, leopards, lions, *etc.)*; ch. 7 with plants (preservation and propagation, date palms, narcissus, lotuses, water lilies, *etc.)*; ch. 8 with timbers; ch. 9 with foods (*e.g.,* grapes, vegetables, sugar); ch. 10 with aromatics, and ch. 11 with drugs.

SHIH SHENG-HAN, 1958: A preliminary survey of the book Ch'i Min Yao Shu, an agricultural encyclopedia of the 6th century, 107 p. (Peking: Science Press).—

The original text together with the English translation of an important agricultural classic "Essential ways for living of the ordinary people", the best-preserved text among the now existing Chinese classics devoted solely to agriculture. Written in the early 6th century A.D. by Chia Ssu-hsieh. It deals with such subjects as: land cultivation, varieties of crops, seed corn, sowing, fertilizing the ground, protective maintenance, culinary vegetables, fruit trees, timber woods, animal husbandry, domestic economy and other technical instructions for commodities of daily life.

SIRÉN, O., 1949: Gardens of China: an interpretation of China's garden art by one of the world's great authorities on Chinese art and civilization, 141 p. + 208 illus. (New York, N.Y.: Ronald Press).—

The book gives a description of Chinese gardens - mostly from Péking parks and the gardens of Suchou - both from the artistic and the historical point of view. The book is richly illustrated with over 200 photographs and coloured plates. Another volume by the same author (*viz.,* "China and gardens of Europe of the eighteenth century, 1950, New York, N.Y.: Ronald") is devoted to the Chinese influence upon European gardens.

STEIN, R., 1942: Jardins en miniature d'Extrême-Orient, 104 p. (Bull. Éc. franç. Extr. Orient 42: 1-104).—

Miniature gardens and their connections with philosophy, social life, foklore, magic, *etc.* An elaborate study.

c. History of the medical sciences

BÀNH DU'O'NG BÁ, 1947-1950: Histoire de la médecine du Viêtnam, 86 p. (Hanoi: Éc. franç. Extr. Orient).—

A review of the history of medicine in Vietnam from earliest times to the introduction of French medicine. Much Chinese influence on medical theory and practice can be found, *e.g.*, the necessary balance of the 5 elements for good health, the governmental organization of organs, reflecting the hierarchical structure of human society, the attention given to the pulse in medical theory and practice, and acupuncture as a basic method for cure. Besides there is some Indian influence especially on the culture of the western parts of Vietnam. The influence of religion (Taoism and Buddhism) on medicine has been elucidated and the state of various medical specialities practised locally has been considered. Brief biographical notes of some notable Vietnamese doctors and a review of the literature of the history and practice of Vietnamese medicine have been added. A bibliography, containing the original Vietnamese sources: DURAND, M., 1959: Médecine sino-vietnamienne (Bull. Éc. franc. Extr. Orient 44: 675-678); contains, however, no translation or commentary in any European language. *Cf.* CHUONG VAN-VINH, 1962, *vide infra.*

BURANG, T., 1957: Tibetische Heilkunde, 170 p. (Zurich: Origo).—

A popular introduction. From the table of contents: Die kosmischen Essenzen; Arzneimittel; Der Doppelkörper; Der Krebs: eine Viruskrankheit?; Seelenleiden als Besessenheit; Zusammenarbeit von abendländischer und asiatischer Wissenschaft. *Cf.* KORVIN-KRASINSKI, P. C. von, 1964; and VEITH, I., 1960, *vide infra.*

CHAMFRAULT, A. & UNG KANG SAM, 1954-1961: Traité de médecine chinoise, 4 vols. Vol. I (1954): Acupuncture, moxas, massages, saignées, d'après les textes chinois anciens et modernes, 986 p.; Vol. II (1957): Les livres sacrés de médecine chinoise, 575 p.; Vol. III (1959): Pharmacopée, 320 p.; Vol. IV (1961): Formules magistrales, 251 p. (Angoulême: Coquemard).—

The first volume gives a general review of Chinese medicine. An idea of its scope can be obtained by quoting the table of contents: Ch. I: Doctrine de la médecine chinoise (l'homme dans le cosmos, le Inn et le Iang, l'énergie dans le corps humain, les organes, les méridiens); Ch. II: L'examen du malade (étude des symptômes, examen du pouls, du teint du facies et des yeux, examen de l'abdomen); Ch. III: Éléments de pronostic; Ch. IV: La pratique de la médecine chinoise (technique de l'acupuncture, des moxas, des petites saignées des capillaires, et des massages, aperçu sur la pharmacopée chinoise); Ch. V: Les méridiens et leurs points; Ch. VI: Thérapeutique. The second part contains French translations of the Chinese medical classics: "So Ouenn" and "Neï King", the third and fourth volumes contain a pharmacopoeia.

CHANG HUI-CHIEN, 1960: Li Shih-chen: great pharmacologist of ancient China, 68 p. (Peking: Foreign Language Press).—

A short biographical review of Li-Shih-chen *(ca. 1518 - ca. 1593)*, the famous author of the Pen-ts'oa Kang-mu, "The text and commentary of the Great Herbal", consisting of 48 volumes devoted to materia medica, 2 volumes of theoretical discussion, 2 volumes of disease indications, and 3 volumes of woodcuts. It classifies some 1900 drugs. *Cf.* KAROW, O., ed., 1956; and READ, B. E., 1931, *vide infra.*

CHUONG VAN-VINH, 1962: Contribution à l'étude de l'histoire de la pharmacie au Viet-Nam, 377 p. (Thesis No. 17) (Thèse de Rennes) (Ronéotypée).—

This work is in two parts, one devoted to traditional Vietnamese pharmacy (110 pages), the other to modern Vietnamese pharmacy and their economic, commercial, legal, *etc.* aspects (267 pages). The first part considers such subjects as: the close relationship between Vietnamese pharmacy and Vietnamese medicine; Chinese influences; specific Vietnamese drugs; Vietnamese weights and measures. Most Vietnamese drugs are of a vegetable origin, and the author describes in detail their often complicated way of fabrication. Of much interest are the illustrations of the instruments used. The second part deals with the development of pharmacy in South Vietnam during the colonial and post-colonial periods, stressing Western influences. Important bibliography. *Cf.* BÁNH DU'O'NG BÁ, 1947-1950, *vide supra.*

CROZIER, R. C., 1968: Traditional medicine in modern China, 326 p. (Cambridge, Mass.: Harvard U.P.; London: Oxford U.P.).—

In this study the author describes how official Chinese government attitudes to traditional Chinese medicine have changed during the last 100 years of modernization in China. It is in three parts. The first part (p. 13-56) deals with the traditional medical system and the introduction and growth of modern medicine in China (1800-1949); the second part (p. 59-148) deals with national essence and national medicine, and with the rejection of national medicine and the introduction of Western medicine; the third part (p. 151-228) deals with the communist rehabilitation of Chinese medicine and the position of old medicine in the new society. Included are a comprehensive bibliography, a glossary, and index.

DORÉ, F. J., 1920: La thérapeutique et l'hygiène en Chine. De l'influence des superstitions sur le développement des sciences médico-pharmaceutiques, 221 p. (Paris: Vigot).—

Separate chapters deal with such subjects as: Why become a physician or a pharmacologist?, the most famous healers, medicine, pharmacy, superstition in medicine and hygiene, talismans, hygiene and epidemics. No index. Cf. NEEDHAM, J. & LU GWEI-DJEN, 1962, vide infra.

FUJIKAWA, Y., 1934: Japanese medicine, 128 p. (Clio medica, 12) (New York, N.Y.: Hoeber).—

An English translation of the short German edition: Geschichte der Medizin in Japan. Kurzgefasste Darstellung der Entwicklung der japanischen Medizin mit besonderer Berücksichtigung der Einführung der europäischen Heilkunde in Japan, 115 p. (Tokyo: Kaiserl. Japan. Unterrichtsministerium), distributed at the International Exposition of Hygiene at Dresden, 1911. This English translation has been brought up to date. It deals with the so-called mythical era of Japanese medicine, with Chinese, Portuguese, Dutch, and German influences and with the so-called National Era, the last period in which Japanese medical science again became national. The table of contents reads as follows: 1. The mythical period; 2. To the Nara period; 3. The Nara period; 4. The Heian period; 5. The Kamakura period; 6. The Muromachi period; 7. The Azuchi-Momoyama period; 8. The Yedo period; 9. The Meiji period; 10. The recent history of medicine in Japan (by K. W. AMANO). Appendix with chronological table of Japanese medicine, indexes of personal names and of subjects. A more recent publication dealing with the same topics and containing a very useful bibliography

is: HUARD, P. & Z. OHYA, 1963: Panorama de la médecine japonaise traditionelle, 110 p. (Biologie médicale, Numéro "Hors Série"), and a study especially dealing with the impact of Western medicine upon old Japanese medical traditions is: BOWERS, J. Z., 1965: Medical education in Japan: from Chinese medicine to Western medicine, 174 p. (New York, N.Y.: Hoeber Medical Division). Cf. also: MESTLER, G. E., 1964, vide infra.

GRMEK, M. D., 1962: Les reflets de la sphygmologie chinoise dans la médecine occidentale, 120 p. (Numéro hors série de la "Biologie Médicale") (Paris: Specia).—

A study of the Chinese theory of the pulse and its influence on the development of medicine in East and West. Separate chapters deal with such subjects as: the theory and the practice of the pulse doctrine; the original sources of the theory of the pulse in Western medicine: Galen; the sources of the Chinese theory of the pulse; the dispersion of the theory of the pulse in India, Persia, and the Arab countries; the first European printed publications dealing with the pulse (1622-1670); the first monograph concerning the theory of the pulse: Les secrets de la médecine des Chinois, consistant en la parfaite connaissance du Pouls (1671, Grenoble); practical applications of the theory of the pulse in Europe; John Floyer (1649-1734) and J. B. du Halde; increasing opposition against the practical implications of the pulse-theory; the theory of the pulse as subject of historical research. Cf. AMBER, R. B. & A. M. BABEY-BROOKE, 1966, vide section Antiquity in general, subsection c.

HARTNER, W., 1941-1942: Heilkunde im alten China, 110 p. (Sinica 16: 217-265; 17: 266-328).—

The first section of this series of articles on the art of healing in ancient China gives a chronological survey. The second section contains a study of the theory and practice of Chinese medicine, with special emphasis on the Nei Ching, China's oldest and most influential medical work. Many comparisons between Chinese medical theories on the one hand and those of the philosophers of the West and Near East on the other hand. Cf. HUARD, P., 1957, vide infra.

HOEPPLI, R., 1959: Parasites and parasitic infections in early medicine and science, 526 p. (Singapore: Malaya U.P.).—

The greater part of this study deals with the history of parasitology in China, and according to the author himself this is a "series of loosely connected essays, each dealing in a comparative way with a special branch of parasitology." The book has been divided into three parts. The first and the last part deal with the subject in a chronological way from ancient times to the middle of the 18th century; the greater part has been devoted to the pre-microscopic era. The second part deals with special parasitological subjects of historical interest (such as malaria, dysentery and leeches in Chinese medicine, Chinese anthelmintic prescriptions, the habit of eating lice, parasites and parasitic infections in religion). Many parallelisms of thought between Eastern and Western cultures have been noted.

HOOPER, D., 1929: On Chinese medicine: drugs of Chinese pharmacies in Malaya, 163 p. (Gardens' Bull., vol. 6, part 1).—

An attempt at identifying and recording the drugs to be found in Chinese pharmacies in Malaya. The number of species dealt with is 456, mostly of plant origin. The Chinese name of each drug is given, together with the romanised Mandarin transliteration. Wherever possible, the botanical source is mentioned, and a note as to the composition, uses, *etc.,* of the drug is added.

HUARD, P., 1957: Structure de la médecine chinoise, 91 p. (Conf. Palais de la Découverte, Ser. D, No. 49) (Paris: Presses Univ. de France).—

An introduction into the character of Chinese medicine. Its contents may be elucidated by means of the chapter-headings: 1. La doxologie médicale chinoise; 2. La médecine interne; 3. La pédiatrie; 4. La dermatologie et la vénéorologie; 5. La parasitologie; 6. La psychiatrie; 7. La médecine légale; 8. La chirurgie; 9. L'ophthalmologie; 10. Obstétrique et gynécologie; 11. L'odonto-stomatologie; 12. Les maladies carencielles; 13. Les matières médicales; 14. L'éthique médicale, la déontologie et l'organisation médicale; 15. L'acupuncture, les moxas et les massages; 16. La culture physique; 17. La gérontologie et la géronto-prophylaxie; 18. L'hygiène sexuelle et les traités chinois de la chambre à coucher. *Cf.* CHAMFRAULT, A. & UNG KANG SAM, 1954-1961, *vide supra;* HUME, E. H., 1940; and MORSE, W. R., 1934, *vide infra.*

——, 1957: Quelques aspects de la doctrine classique de la médecine chinoise, 119 p. (Biol. méd. 46: i-cxix).—

A short but very good review of Chinese medicine, covering a period of 25 centuries. The author discusses the oldest sources (the Nei King, *ca.* 300-200 B.C., and the commentaries of Nan King, *ca.* 275 B.C.). The author illustrates how the human body was considered as a microcosmic representation of the macrocosmos, an idea which - through the Arabian Kabbalists - came to Paracelsus. The author makes clear the special character of Chinese anatomy, and explains the theory of the pulse. A long section is devoted to therapeutics, in which the author discusses the herbal of emperor Chen Nong (2836-2698 B.C.), which herbal also contains many zootherapeutical recipes, *e.g.,* entomophagy (silk-worms, larvae of bees), the use of animal excrements, of stag-horn, of gelatine, of the skin of the elephant or buffalo, the application of perfume, and the use of fossil bones as amulets. *Cf.* HARTNER, W., 1941-1942, *vide supra.*

—— & M. DURAND, 1953: Lan-Ong et la médecine Sino-Vietnamienne, 72 p. (Bull. Soc. Étud. Indochin., N.S., 28, No. 3: 221-293).—

Lan-Ong (1720- *ca.* 1785) was the greatest representative of medicine in Vietnam before the introduction of Western medicine, and in later years he kept a kind of medical school. He studied Chinese medicine, and his writings are in Chinese, printed in 1866 and arranged in 10 volumes. The present work contains a brief analysis of these volumes, and comparisons with Chinese, Indian, and Western medical views. *Cf.* BÁNH DU'O'NG BÁ, 1947-1950, *vide supra;* and NGUYEN-TRAN-HUAN, 1951, *vide infra.*

—— & M. WONG, 1959: La médecine chinoise au cours des siècles, 192 p. (Paris: Dacosta).—

A well-illustrated semi-popular review of the development of Chinese medicine up to recent times. An analysis of Chinese influences on Japanese medicine has been given. Much has been said on acupuncture and its meaning for modern medical practice. Also in English translation: Chinese medicine, 1968, 256 p. (London: Weidenfeld & Nicolson). A more popular text is published by the same authors under the title: La médecine chinoise, 1964, 127 p. (Que sais-je, No. 1112) (Paris: Presses Univ. de France). *Cf.* also: Évolution de la matière médicale chinoise, 1948, 67 p. (Janus 47: 1-67). *Cf.* also MANN, F., 1962; and WALLNÖFER, H. & A. VON ROTTAUSCHER, 1959, *vide infra.*

HÜBOTTER, F., 1929: Die chinesische Medizin zu Beginn des XX. Jahrhunderts und ihr historischer Entwicklungsgang, 356 p. (Leipzig: Verlag Asia major).—

Based on personal observations in both China and Japan, the author sampled much material very useful to the historian of Chinese medicine. After some bibliographical information, the author starts his review with Chinese anatomy (incl. embryology, osteology, and myology). Chinese anatomical names do not refer to definite bones but to parts of the ossature which can be seen from the outside. Some organs (e.g., eye, ear, lung, large intestine, stomach, spleen, heart, bladder, kidney, liver and the san chiad) have been considered in more detail. Chinese psysiology is elucidated by means of extracts from the medical classics. A number of short chapters are devoted to special diseases and to special branches of medicine (e.g., dentistry, obstetrics, pediatrics, etc.). Short sections deal with forensic medicine, hospitals, and the medical profession. An altlas of medicine (p. 113-156) contains a great number of figures extracted from Chinese and Japanese books. A long section (p. 157-272) is devoted to diagnosis, which section also contains translations of two texts, viz., of the book Nan-Ching and of a text on the secrets of the pulse, Mai-chück. The chapter on therapeutics contains sections devoted to pharmacology, a list of the most useful recipes, brief accounts of massage and gymnastics and to acupuncture. A final chapter (p. 340-355) contains a historical sketch of Chinese medicine. A comparable study, also based upon personal observation (in Chengtu, Szechwan), is that of GERVAIS, A., 1933: Aesculape en Chine, 253 p. (Paris: Gallimard). Also in English translation: Medicine man in China, 1934, 336 p. (New York, N.Y.: Stokes). Cf. WONG, K. CHIMIN & WU LIEN-TEH, 1936, vide infra; cf. also AMBER, R. B. & A. M. BABEY-BROOKE, 1966, vide section Antiquity in general, subsection c.

——, 1957: Chinesisch-Tibetische Pharmakologie und Rezeptur, 180 p. (Ulm/Donau: Haug).—

A collection of recipes and drugs used in Chinese and Tibetan medicine.

HUME, E. H., 1940: The Chinese way in medicine, 189 p. (Baltimore, Md.: Johns Hopkins Press).—

An introductory text to the history of Chinese medicine, being the text of the Hideyo Noguchi lectures delivered at the Institute of the History of Medicine in Baltimore. The first lecture: The universe and man in Chinese medicine, gives the spiritual background of Chinese medicine; the second lecture: The founders and chief exemplars of Chinese medicine, is a historical sketch, dealing with the three legendary emperors Fu Hsi, Shên Nung, and Huang Ti, and with the physicians Pien Ch'iao (5th cent. B.C.), Chang-Chung-ching (2nd cent. A.D.), Hua T'o (3rd cent. A.D.), and Li Shih-chên (16th cent. A.D.); the third lecture is entitled: Some distinctive contributions of Chinese medicine. Cf. HUARD, P., 1957, vide supra.

KAROW, O., ed., 1956: Die Illustrationen des Arzneibuches der Periode Shao-hsing (Shao-hsing pen ts'ao hua-t'u vom Jahre 1159), 83 p. (Leverkusen: Farbenfabriken Bayer A.G.).—

The subject of this booklet is the most famous work on Chinese pharmacology, the Pên Ts'ao, or "Great Herbal", the authorship of which has been attributed to Shên-nung, one of the three legendary God-emperors of the third millenium B.C., the divine patron of makers and sellers of Chinese drugs. The editor has added a brief reconstruction of the actual history and contents of this work, and translations of the Chinese names of the plants and animals, together with summaries considering their pharmacological applications. Cf. CHANG HUI-CHIEN, 1960, vide supra.

KLEIWEG DE ZWAAN, J. P., 1917: Völkerkundliches und Geschichtliches über die Heilkunde der Chinesen und Japaner, mit besonderer Berücksichtigung holländischer Einflüssen, 656 p. (Natuurkundige Verh. Holl. Maatschappij der Wetensch., Haarlem, 3e Verzameling, Deel 7) (Haarlem: Loosjes).—

A history of Chinese and Japanese medicine in order to elucidate the influences of West-European medicine. The author bases his study not only on written sources but also on folk-medicine as it was still practised in his time.

KORVIN-KRASINSKI, P. C. von, 1964: Die tibetische Medizinphilosophie. Der Mensch als Mikrokosmos, ed. 2, 40 + 363 p. (Mainzer Studien zur Kultur- und Völkerkunde, 1) (Zurich: Origo).—

A thorough study of lamaistic medicine, especially in connection with philosophical and religious suppositions, and with mythological and cosmogenetical ideas. *Cf.* BURANG, T., 1957, *vide supra.*

LO, J. H., 1930: Schou schen hsiau bu (Kleine Hilfe zur Verlängerung des Lebens) von Wang Dui Me, 107 p. (Trans. med. Fac. Sun Yat Sen Univ., Canton 2: 19-126).—

A German translation of the gynaecological and obstetrical parts of a Chinese treatise ("Small help to longevity"), written in 1832 by Huang Tui-mei. The medical contents of this book is still almost uninfluenced by Western medicine.

——, 1938: Shou shih pao yuean (Zur Verlängerung des Lebens und zur Erhaltung der Gesundheit) von Kung Ting-Hsien, 174 p. (Arb. der deutsch-nordischen Gesell. für Gesch. der Med., der Zahnheilkunde und der Naturwissenschaften, No. 20).—

German translation of the Shou-shih-pao-yüan, in 10 yüan, a book on macrobiotics and hygiene, written by Kung T'ing Hsien, and first published in 1575.

MANN, F., 1962: Acupuncture: the ancient Chinese art of healing, 178 p. (New York, N.Y.: Random House).—

Acupuncture is a treatment consisting of pricking various strategic spots on the human body with a fine needle to obtain a curative effect. These spots are held to form a system based on meridians of the body, which in turn relate to the main internal organs. Acupuncture is a traditional form of Chinese medicine dating from prehistoric times that is now practised extensively in various parts of the world. Books dealing with the same topic are: LAVIER, J., 1964: Les bases traditionelles de l'acupuncture chinoise, 234 p. (Paris: Maloine), and LAVIER, J., 1966: Histoire, doctrine et pratique de l'acupuncture chinoise, 271 p. (Paris: Tchou). A book dealing with the application of acupuncture in Japan is: NAKAYAMA, T., 1934: Acupuncture et médecine chinoise vérifiées au Japon, 85 p. (Paris: Le François).

MASPERO, H., R. GROUSSET & L. LION, 1939: Les ivoires religieux et médicaux chinois, 96 p. (Paris: Ed. d'Art et d'Histoire).—

Consists of the following essays: Chinese ivories and the iconography of the three religions (by H. MASPERO); Ming ivories and the evolution of Chinese art (by R. GROUSSET); Study of the ivory statuettes of the Ming period (by L. LION);

Description of the Lion collection containing, *e.g.,* religious ivories, animals, cachets, *etc.*

MESTLER, G. E., 1964: An index to selected Japanese medical literature of pre- Meiji times. (Los Angeles, Calif.: Dawson's Book Shop).—

The contents of the book consist of the reprinted text of five successive papers originally published in the Bull. Med. Libr. Ass. Vols. 42-45 (1954-1957) under the general title "A galaxy of old Japanese medical books, with miscellaneous notes on early medicine in Japan". Separate papers deal with: Medical history and biography. General works. Anatomy. Physiology and pharmacology (40 p.). Acupuncture and moxibustion. Bathing. Balneotherapy and massage. Nursing, pediatrics and hygiene. Obstetrics and gynaecology (32 p.). Urology, syphilology and dermatology. Surgery and pathology (29 p.). Ophthalmology, psychiatry, dentistry (20 p.). Biblio-historical addenda. Corrections. Postscript. Acknowledgements (55 p.). These essays are preceded by a short title list, presenting a bibliographical review of medical literature of pre-Meiji Japan (*i.e.* before 1868). *Cf.* FUJIKAWA, Y., 1934, *vide supra.*

MORSE, W. R., 1934: Chinese medicine, 185 p. (Clio Medica, No. 11) (New York, N.Y.: Hoeber).—

A useful introduction to the subject. After a general introduction, discussing Chinese natural philosophy and cosmogony, and the Chinese gods of medicine, the author refers to old Chinese medical literature, and he explains Chinese pathology, anatomy, physiology and diagnosis. Then he discusses Chinese materia medica and therapeutics, the pulse, the Chinese practitioner of medicine, acupuncture, *etc.* A modern treatise dealing with the same topics is: PÁLOS, S., 1963: Chinesische Heilkunst. Rückbesinnung auf eine grosse Tradition, 206 p. (Munich: Delp'sche Verlagsbuchhandlung). Deals, according to its subtitle on the dust-cover, with acupuncture, moxibustion, remedial massage, -gymnastics, and -breathing, pharmacology. In his preface the author writes: "Die Herausgabe meines vorliegenden Buches zunächst in Ungarn, wie nun auch in Deutschland erscheint mir vornehmlich aus dem Grund gerechtfertigt zu sein, weil es nicht allein eine Uebersicht über die historischen Ueberlieferungen bringt, ... sondern auch die Weiterführung bewährter heilkundlicher Traditionen im Lichte der westlichen Wissenschaft aufzeigt." *Cf.* also: HUARD, P., 1957, *vide supra.*

NEEDHAM, J. & LU GWEI-DJEN, 1962: Hygiene and preventive medicine in ancient China. (J. Hist. Med. 17: 429-478).—

An attempt to render some information about the historical concepts of hygiene and preventive medicine in Ancient China, mainly covering the period down to the end of the Han dynasty (ca. 200 A.D.), i.e., the period before foreign importations in medical philosophy (esp. of Buddhism) entered China. The authors stress the close relationship between medical philosophy and the thoughts of the writers on philosophy, ethics, and logic. Separate sections deal with such subjects as: early concepts of prevention, ancient literature, the Yellow Emperor's treatise, mental and physical hygiene, nutritional regimen, cooking and nutritional hygiene, water and tea, personal hygiene, and with some specific diseases, i.c., rabies and smallpox. Added are a chronology of China and a list of Chinese characters. Cf. DORÉ, F. J., 1920, vide supra.

NGUYEN-TRAN-HUAN, 1951: Contribution à l'étude de l'ancienne thérapeutique viêtnamienne, 92 p. (Hanoi: Éc. franç. Extr. Orient).—

The first part of this book contains an analysis of the Nam duoc thān hiêu ("Book of marvellous recipes"), a purely Vietnamese pharmacopoeia written ca. 1400. It is a herbal dealing with the plants, animals, and minerals to be found in Vietnam, and was written by the physician Tué-tinh (fl. during the Trăn period, 1225-1414). This work was revised in 1761 by another Vietnamese physician, Lān-ōng (vide supra, HUARD, P. & M. DURAND, 1953) and biographies of both physicians have been included. The first part of this pharmacopoeia is translated and discussed; Chinese, Vietnamese, and Latin indexes of plant names are added.

READ, B. E., 1931: Chinese materia medica: animal drugs, 145 p. (Bull. Peking Soc. Nat. Hist., Vol. V, Pt. 4: 37-80 and Vol. VI, Pt. 1: 1-102).—

Deals with animal drugs from the Pen ts'ao Kang mu by Li Shih-chen, emanating from domestic animals, wild animals, fishes, snakes, molluscs, etc., rodents, monkeys, supernatural beings, and with man as a medicine. Other publications of the same author (known to the editor only as reprints without further details) deal with avian drugs (Bull. Peking Soc. Nat. Hist. VI, pt. 4, 112 p.), with drugs from dragons and snakes (idem., 166 p.), with turtle and shell-fish drugs (idem., 1937, 95 p.), and with fish drugs (idem., 1939, 136 p.). The part dealing with avian drugs is also of importance for the history of Chinese ornithology. Cf. also: READ, B. E., 1936, vide subsection b.

REGNAULT, J., 1902: Médecine et pharmacie chez les Chinois et chez les Annamites, 235 p. (Paris: Challamel).—

A review of the drugs used (especially the herbs) and the medical practice employed by the aboriginal physicans of the Tonkin valley. According to the author there was much resemblance with drugs used in, and medical practice of, China. Included are an index of French-Latin names of medicines, a Chinese pharmaceutical index, and a French-Chinese-Annamite lexicon of medicines used. Cf. SALLET, A., 1931, vide infra.

SALLET, A., 1931: L'officine sino-annamite en Annam. I. Le médecin annamite et la préparation des remèdes, 153 p. (Paris: van Oest).—

This booklet deals with such topics as: the native physician, the sorcerer, the drugs in the town, the village, and on the market, the preparation of the medicines and the instruments used, a comparison between the drugs of Annam and those of China, local drugs, disease and diet, etc. The last chapter, comprising nearly half the book, consists of notes. Bibliography (containing exclusively French references), no index. Cf. REGNAULT, J., 1902, vide supra.

SASSADY, K., 1962: Contribution à l'étude de la médecine laotienne, 142 p. (Thèse Univ. de Paris) (Ronéotypée).—

This is the first comprehensive study of Laotian medicine. In a first section the author deals with the anthropology and the medical geography of Laos. A second part deals with traditional Laotian medicines which are compared with those used in some neighbouring countries, such as: India, Siam, and Cambodia. A special section deals with traditional medical practice, the role of the physician, his knowledge of anatomy, physiology, pathology, and nosology; another section deals with the meaning of shamanism and animism in traditional medicine. Included are: an alphabetical table of symptoms of diseases and of materia medica of animal origin, a historical review of the introduction of European medical knowledge, a review of the present sanitary organization, a historical review of the Royal

College of Medicine at Vientiane, founded in 1957, and a useful bibliography.

STANDLEE, M. W., 1959: The great pulse: Japanese midwifery and obstetrics through the ages, 192 p. (Rutland, Vt.: Tuttle).—

The author makes a study of customs and usages associated with pregnancy and childbirth in Japan from earliest times onwards. The major part of the book deals with practices and ideas extending into antiquity, but it also contains much information about present-day obstetrics in Japan.

VEITH, I., 1966: Huang Ti Nei Ching Su Wên: the Yellow Emperor's classic of internal medicine. Chapters 1-34 translated from the Chinese with an introductory study, new ed., 260 p. (Berkeley, Calif.: Univ. Calif. Press).—

The book consists of a translation from the Chinese of the first 34 chapters of the ancient medico-philosophical classic "Huang Ti Nei Ching Su Wên", preceded by a critical analysis of its contents. The translator states in the preface that the work "represents the approach of a medical historian rather than of a Chinese philologist". This book is the only surviving one of the medical treatises of Ancient China, and this is the first time that it has been translated into a Western language. This treatise stands at the outset of a systematized and philosophically-founded art of healing in the Far East. First published 1949.

——, 1960: Medizin in Tibet, 44 p. (Leverkusen: Bayer, Pharm.-wiss. Abt.).—

Facsimile reproduction of 12 coloured plates with a short explanation by the authoress. Plate 1: integument and superficial vessels; 2: skull, teeth, skeleton; 3: rachis and splanchnology (kidney, lungs, heart, liver); 4, 5 and 6: vascular system (a theoretical construction, serving as a base for acupuncture); 7: points used for cauterization and moxa; 8: surgical instruments; 9 and 10: vegetables used in dietetics and therapeutics; 11 and 12 also deal with dietetic questions (fish, birds, fruits, scorpions, serpents, vegetables, *etc.*). *Cf.* BURANG, T., 1957, *vide supra*.

WALLNÖFER, H. & A. v. ROTTAUSCHER, 1959: Der goldene Schatz der chinesischen Medizin, 176 p. (Stuttgart: Schuler).—

A popular introduction to Chinese medicine, intended for the interested layman. This book is one-third folk medicine, one-third traditional rational medicine, and one-third romance. Fine illustrations, some coloured. A comparable booklet is: BEAU, G., 1965: La médecine chinoise, 190 p. (Paris: Ed. du Seuil). *Cf.* HUARD, P. & M. WONG, 1959, *vide supra*.

WARE, J. R., ed., 1966: Alchemy, medicine, religion in the China of A.D. 320: the Nei P'ien of Ko Hung (Pao-p'u tzu), 404 p. (Cambridge, Mass.: M.I.T. Press).—

The Pao P'u Tzu book is one of the central works of speculative Taoism, an "extraordinary amalgam of mystical insight, wild speculation, superstition and legend, disciplined observation, and intellectual control" (Isis 58: 62). It discusses, *inter alia,* the techniques of achieving longevity and immortality, and it contains a systematization of the knowledge of chemical operations. Chapters 4 and 16 describe the making of elixirs of life.

WONG, K. CHIMIN & WEI-KANG-FU, eds., 1963: Catalogue of publications on medicine in China in foreign languages 1656-1962, 104 p. (Shanghai: Shanghai Academy of Chinese Medicine, Medical History Museum).—

Contains a list of publications (in Chinese and Western languages) on the following topics: General medicine, medical history, the pulse, practical medicine, acupuncture and moxa, materia medica, hygiene and health, books and periodicals, biography.

—— & WU LIEN-TEH, 1936: History of Chinese medicine: being a chronicle of medical happenings in China from ancient times to the present period, ed. 2, 906 p. (Shanghai: Evening Post and Mercury Press).—

This is a very valuable review of the development of Chinese medicine. It consists of two parts. Part I (written by WONG) discusses such topics as: the ancient or legendary period (2697-1122 B.C.) (the beginnings of healing art, the founders of Chinese medicine, religion and medicine); the Golden period (1121 B.C.-960 A.D.) (philosophy of disease; influence of Taoism and Buddhism; the great trio: Ts'ang, Chang, and Hua), and the mediaeval or controversial period (961-1800 A.D.) (specialism, medical schools and sects; early obstetrics; gynaecology; ophthalmology; parasitology; leprosy; beri-beri; cholera, smallpox; syphilis; *etc.*). Part II (written by WU) contains much information concerning the history of Chinese medicine from the time of the first contacts

of China with western medicine up to 1936. The subject-matter of the first part is comparable with HÜBOTTER's work (1929), but the sources consulted differ essentially *(vide supra).*

7. LIFE AND MEDICAL SCIENCES OF THE HEBREWS
(incl. Biblical and Talmudic biology and medicine)

a. History of science and culture in general

FARBRIDGE, M. H., 1923: Studies in biblical and Semitic symbolism, 288 p. (London: Trübner).—

  This book deals with the following topics: development of biblical and Semitic symbolism; trees, plants and flowers; animals; symbolism of numbers (p. 87-156); symbolical representations of the Assyrio-Babylonian pantheon; burning and mourning customs. Index.

FRAZER, J. G., 1918: Folk-lore in the Old Testament: studies in comparative religion, legend and law, 3 vols. Vol. 1: 594 p.; Vol. 2: 592 p.; Vol. 3: 584 p. (London: Macmillan).—

  An encyclopaedic study of Hebrew folklore. The work is in 4 parts, *viz.,* 1. The early ages of the world (the creation and fall of Man, the great flood, the tower of Babel); 2. The patriarchal age (Abraham, Jacob, Joseph); 3. The times of the Judges and the Kings (Moses, Gideon, Samson and Delilah, Solomon and the Queen of Sheba, bird sanctuary, Elijah and the ravens, sacred oaks, Jonah and the whale, Jehova and the lions); 4. The law. Elaborate index. The author also published an abridged edition: FRAZER, J. G., 1923: Folk-lore in the Old Testament, 476 p. (London: Macmillan), of which a French translation exists: Le folklore dans l'Ancien Testament, 1924, 448 p. (Paris: Geuthner). *Cf.* SAINTYVES, P., 1923, *vide infra.*

FRIEDREICH, J. B., 1966: Zur Bibel. Naturhistorische, anthropologische und medicinische Fragmente, 2 vols. Vol. I: 334 p.; Vol. II: 215 p. (Bad Reichenhall: Kleinert).—

  A reprint of the original edition (1848, Nuremberg). Vol. I deals with such subjects as: explanation of the names of animals, healing springs, nutrition, feeding laws, the Egyptian Plagues, childbirth, menstruation, aphrodisiacs, dreams, diseases and malformations. Vol. II deals with such subjects as: old age, suicide, circumcision, castration, raising from the dead, remarkable deaths, embalming of the dead, *etc.*

HUSIK, I., 1958: A history of mediaeval Jewish philosophy, 50 + 466 p. (New York, N.Y.: Meridian Bks.; Philadelphia, Pa.: Jewish Publ. Soc. of America).—

  A standard reference work, first published in 1916 (New York, N.Y.: Macmillan); in 1930 the bibliography was brought up to date by the author, and this bibliography was again revised in 1941 (by H. A. WOLFSON). The present edition is an unaltered reprint of the later.

SAINTYVES, P., 1923: Essais de folklore biblique. Magie, mythes et miracles dans l'Ancien et le Nouveau Testament, 483 p. (Paris: Nourry).—

  This book considers the same kind of topics as FRAZER's book *(vide supra),* but Saintyves's philosophy differs widely from that of Frazer. Many comparisons between Jewish, Christian, and Arabic traditions. The book consists of the following parts: 1. Le feu qui descend du ciel et le renouvellement du feu sacré; 2. La verge fleurie d'Aaron ou le thème du bâton sec qui reverdit; 3. L'eau qui jaillit du rocher sous le bâton ou la flèche; Moïse, Dionysios et Mithra, Jésus et la source d'eau vive; 4. Le tour de la ville et la chute de Jéricho; 5. Les origines liturgiques du miracle de l'eau changée en vin; 6. Le miracle de la multiplication des pains; Le miracle de la marche sur les eaux; son origine et sa signification; 8. L'anneau de Polycrate et le statère dans la bouche du poisson; 9. *Deux thèmes de la passion et leurs significations symboliques.* Elaborate index.

SCHRIRE, T., 1966: Hebrew amulets: their decipherment and interpretation, 192 p. (London: Routledge & Kegan Paul; New York, N.Y.: Humanities Press).—

  This book, written by a South-African Jew, contains a history of the use of amulets bearing mystic names of God and the angels, as they were used particularly in the Oriental Jewish communities. It also contains a description of the various kinds of amulets and an explanation of their relation to the mystical doctrines of the Kabbala and Hasidism.

STEINSCHNEIDER, M., 1956: Die hebraeischen Uebersetzungen des Mittelalters und die Juden als Dolmetscher, 34 + 1077 p. (Graz: Akad. Druck- und Verlagsanstalt).—

> Photomechanical reprint of the 1893 edition. A very useful study. A special section deals with medicine (Alexander of Tralles, Dioscorides, Galen, Hippocrates, Jochanan Jerichoni, Paulos Aegineta, Plato, Soranos, Theophilos). The Wellcome Historical Medical Library, London, possesses a list of names of 2,168 Jewish physicians, compiled by M. STEINSCHNEIDER *Cf.* also: STEINSCHNEIDER, M., 1965-1966: Allgemeine Einleitung in die jüdische Literatur des Mittelalters. Zur pseudepigraphischen Literatur des Mittelalters. Vorlesungen über die Kunde hebräischer Handschriften, 359 p. (Amsterdam: Philo). A reprint. Originally published in 1902-1905 (152 p.); 1862 (97 p.); and 1897 (110 p.) resp. M. J. SCHLEIDEN devoted a study to the role of the Jews in the development of science during the Middle Ages: Die Bedeutung der Juden für Erhaltung und Wiederbelebung der Wissenschaften im Mittelalter, 1877, 41 p. (N.B. ed. 5, 1912, 54 p.). Also in English translation: The sciences of the Jews before and during the Middle Ages, 1883, 64 p. (Baltimore, Md.: Binswanger). Reprinted 1966 (New York, N.Y.: Da Capo).

——, 1964: Die arabische Literatur der Juden. Ein Beitrag zur Literaturgeschichte der Araber, grossenteils aus handschriftlichen Quellen, 54 + 348 + 32 p. (Hildesheim: Olms).—

> Originally published in 1902. (Frankfurt a. M.). This is a list of Jewish authors and the studies they wrote, together with biographical notes, *etc.*

UNGER, M. F., 1954: Archaeology and the Old Testament: a companion volume to Archaeology and the New Testament, 339 p. (London: Pickering & Inglis).—

> Much of the interest that attaches to biblical archaeology does of necessity spring from its connection with the Bible. The contributions of archaeology to the study of the Old Testament is the central theme of this book and a very interesting history of the Jewish people is the result of this

study. The companion volume, written by the same author, is entitled: Archaeology and the New Testament, 1964, 353 p. (London: Pickering & Inglis).

b. History of the plant and animal sciences

BODENHEIMER, F. S., 1960: Animal and Man in Bible lands, 232 p. (Leiden: Brill).—

> For more details, *vide* section Antiquity in general, subsection b.

DUNS, J., 1863-1868: Biblical natural science, 2 vols. Vol. I: 575 p.; Vol. II: 624 p. (London: Mackenzie).—

> Its contents may become clear from the subtitle: the explanation of all references in Holy Scripture to geology, botany, zoology and physical geography. Illustrated by maps and numerous wood-cuts.

DUSCHAK, M., 1870: Zur Botanik des Talmuds, 136 p. (Pest: Neuer).—

> Allusions to those passages of the Talmud which deal with botanical subjects. Separate sections deal with plants used in industry (flax, cotton, hemp), with vegetable products used in tanning, vegetable oils, wax, tartaric and oxalic acid, resins and gums, fruit trees, trees used for timber, cereals, leguminous plants, vegetables, preserved vegetables, spices, edible fungi, and with the flower garden. *Cf.* LÖW, I., 1924-1934, *vide infra*.

LEVYSOHN, L., 1858: Die Zoologie des Talmuds. Eine umfassende Darstellung der rabbinischen Zoologie, unter steter Vergleichung der Forschungen älterer und neuerer Schriftsteller, 400 p. (Frankfurt a. M.: Baer).—

> A compilation of references in the Talmud to animals. The first part (p. 1-63) deals with general zoology (*e.g.,* with the living organism, reproduction, generatio originaria, castration, crossing, the senses, instinct, the anatomical parts, *etc.*). The second part deals with the various animals (including many philological details) and the third part (p. 350-357) deals with fabulous animals. *Cf.* DHORME, E., 1963: L'emploi métaphorique des noms des parties du corps en hébreu et en akkadien, 183 p., *vide* HOLMA, H., 1911, section Mesopotamia, subsection b.

LÖW, I., 1924-1934: Die Flora der Jüden, 4 vols. Vol. I (1926/'28): 807 p.; Vol. II (1924): 532 p.; Vol. III (1924): 522 p.; Vol. IV (1934): 740 p. (Veröffentl. der Alexander Kohut Memorial Foundation) (Vienna & Leipzig: Löwit).—

A very useful and indispensable tool of botanical cultural history of the Jews, based on the Talmud, itineraries, and all sorts of learned books. The titles of the separate volumes are: Vol. I: Kryptogamae. Acanthaceae-Composaceae; Convolvulaceae-Graminaceae; Vol. II: Iridaceae-Papilionaceae; Vol. III: Pedaliaceae-Zygophyllaceae. The plants are considered in alphabetical order of family names. Vol. IV: Zusammenfassung. Nachträge. Berichtungen. Indizes. Abkürzungen. Reprinted 1967 (Hildesheim: Olms). It is a very elaborate reissue of the author's "Aramäische Pflanzennamen" of 1881 (Leipzig: Engelmann). *Cf.* MOLDENKE, H.N. & A. L., 1952, *vide infra*.

MACKAY, A. J., 1950: Farming and gardening in the Bible, 280 p. (Emmaus, Pa.: Rodale Press).—

A compilation of references in the Bible to farming, gardening, and rural life *(e.g.,* herbs, trees, fruits, the vine, flowers, vegetables, field crops, perfumes, spices, ointments, reeds, plant pests and diseases, flocks and herds, poultry, pigs, bees, *etc. Cf.* also: ROHDE, E. S., 1967: Garden-craft in the Bible and other essays, 242 p. (Freeport, N.Y.: Bks. for Libraries Press). A reprint of the 1938 edition (London: Jenkins); first published 1917. *Cf* also SHORT, A. K., 1938, *vide infra*.

MOLDENKE, H. N. & A. L., 1952: Plants of the Bible, 364 p. (New Series of Plant Sciences Bks., No. 28) (Waltham, Mass.: Chronica Botanica Co.).—

The most comprehensive treatise available on plants and plant products mentioned in the Holy Scriptures. It contains a historical sketch of biblical botany, a description of the land, and an alphabetical list of plants (242) arranged alphabetically according to their Latin name (p. 23-249). Each section is devoted to a plant; it opens with quotations from the Bible, referring to the plant considered and contains a summary of all that is known of that plant. The bibliography contains more than 600 publications on the subject published between 1566 and 1951. General index and index to Bible verses. A more popular and

pleasingly illustrated book (12 coloured plates) is: ANDERSON, A. W., 1957: Plants of the Bible, 72 p. (New York, N.Y.: Philosophical Library), and still another is: WALKER, W., 1957: All the plants of the Bible, 244 p. (New York, N.Y. & London: Harper & Row), containing a presentation of 114 plants of the Bible in full-page illustration with on the opposing page a short description of it, the most familiar Bible verse(s) in which the plant is mentioned, its English, Latin, and Hebrew names, its use in folklore, *etc. Cf.* LÖW, I., 1924-1934, *vide supra*.

PARMELEE, A., 1959: All the birds of the Bible, their stories, identification and meaning, 279 p. (London: Lutterworth Press).—

A collection of those biblical stories in which birds play a part, with identifications of the birds mentioned and discussions of their natural history. Special sections deal with the raven, dove, eagle, vulture, quail, sparrow and cock. *Cf.* WOOD, J. G., 1884, *vide infra*.

PETERSEN, W. W., 1928: Das Tier im Alten Testament. Ein Beitrag zur modernen Tierschutzfrage, 83 p. (Frankfurt a. M.: Kauffmann).—

A study concerning the meaning of the animal in biblical texts; more particularly it is an attempt to answer the question whether the Bible imposes upon Man certain duties in his contacts with animals. The author restricts his studies to the Old-Testament Books, *viz.*, the Books of Moses (Pentateuch), of Joshua, Samuel, Job, the Psalms of David, the Book of Proverbs and the Ecclesiastes of Solomon, the Books of Isaiah, Jeremiah, Ezekiel, Daniel, and of some other minor prophets.

RÜTHY, A. E., 1942: Die Pflanzen und ihre Teile im biblisch-hebräischen Sprachgebrauch, 82 p. (Diss. Univ. Basel) (Bern: Francke).—

A philological study dealing with trees, shrubs, and herbs, and their parts (roots, stem, leaf, flower, fruit, *etc.),* as they are used in Hebraic lexicography. *Cf.* LÖW, I., 1924-1934, *vide supra*.

SHORT, A. K., 1938: Ancient and modern agriculture, 158 p. (San Antonio, Tex.: Naylor).—

A compilation of biblical references to agriculture and its techniques, with annotations. The quotations are grouped around the subjects considered, such as: tillage, rotation, crops, gardens, herbs, orchards, vine yards, flowers, shrubs, weeds, domestic animals, agricultural equipment, game animals, and topics considering the social aspects of agriculture, *e.g.*, labour and market, buildings, the position of the labourers, *etc.* A study especially dealing with ancient Jewish agriculture is: NEWMAN, J., 1932: The agricultural life of the Jews in Babylonia between the years 200 C.E. - 500 C.E., 215 p. (London: Oxford U.P.). *Cf.* also MACKAY, A. J., 1950, *vide supra.*

TRISTRAM, H. B., 1868: The natural history of the Bible: being a review of the physical geography, geology, and meteorology of the Holy Land; with a description of every animal and plant mentioned in Holy Scripture, 518 p. (London: Society for Promoting Christian Knowledge).—

The author made a special study of the flora and fauna of the Holy Land. As to living nature, separate chapters deal with mammals, birds, reptiles, fish and fishing, invertebrate and articulate animals, trees and shrubs, and with herbs and flowers. A more recent study of animals mentioned in the Bible is: AHARONI, I., 1938: On some animals mentioned in the Bible (Osiris 5: 461-478). This study has been based upon the author's own observations of the animals in that region, as well as upon his study of biblical and talmudic literature. *Cf.* also FRIEDREICH, J. B., 1966, *vide* subsection a; DUNS, J., 1863-1868, *vide supra;* and WOOD, J. G., 1884, *vide infra.*

WOOD, J. G., 1884: Bible animals, new ed., 625 p. (London: Longmans, Green).—

A compilation of references in the Bible to animals. Mammals (ape, bat, lion, leopard, cat, dog, wolf, fox, hyena, weasel, ferret, badger, bear, hedgehog, porcupine, mole, mouse, hare, cattle, unicorn, bison, gazelle, sheep, chamois, goat, deer, camel, ass, mule, swine, elephant, and some others), birds (lämmergeier, vulture, eagle, hawk, owl, swallow, hoopoe, sparrow, cuckoo, dove, poultry, peacock, partridge, raven, ostrich, heron, crane, stork, swan, cormorant, pelican, and some others), reptiles and amphibians (tortoise, crocodile, lizard, gecko, serpents, frog), fishes and fishermen, invertebrates (molluscs, snail, pearl, oyster, insects, bee, ant, worms, moths, flies, gnats, louse, flea, scorpion, spider, horseleech, sponge, and coral). Some other books dealing with animals of the Bible are: FARB, P.,

1967: The land, wildlife, and peoples of the Bible, 171 p. (New York, N.Y.: Harper & Row); HAMER, G. T., 1962: Hamer's Bible animals, 301 p. (Rockford, Ill.: Remah House); PANGRITZ, W., 1963: Das Tier in der Bibel, 173 p. (Munich & Basle: Reinhardt); WILLS, G., 1962: Animals of the Bible, 64 p. (Sponsored by the Benedictine monks of Belmont Abbey) (Garden City, N.Y.: Doubleday). *Cf.* also: LEVYSOHN, L., 1858; TRISTRAM, H. H., 1868, *vide supra;* and BODENHEIMER, F. S., 1960, *vide* section Antiquity in general, subsection b.

c. History of the medical sciences

BRIM, C. J., 1936: Medicine in the Bible, 384 p. (New York, N.Y.: Froben Press).—

A thorough study of those passages in the Bible, and more especially in the Pentateuch, which contain allusions to medicine. The study is based upon the original Hebrew text of Rashi (= Rabbi Schlomo Izchaki, *ca.* 1040-1105). With notes, definitions, index, and many references to the Talmud. No bibliography. *Cf.* FRIEDREICH, J. B., *vide* subsection a. A comparable study considering the Cabbala is: PREIS, K., 1928: Die Medizin in der Kabbala, 20 p. (Schr. Ges. zur Förderung der Wiss. des Judentums, No. 35) (Frankfurt a.M.: Kauffmann). *Cf.* also: PREUSS, J., 1923, *vide infra.*

CANAAN, T., 1914: Aberglaube und Volksmedizin im Lande der Bibel, 153 p. (Abh. hamburg. KolonInst. 20, Reihe B, No. 12) (Hamburg: Friederichsen).—

An eye-witness of folk-medicine in Israel as it was practised some 50 years ago. The author discusses the aetiology, diagnosis, prognosis, prophylaxis and treatment of diseases. Much attention has been paid to the evil eye, fetishes, amulets and talismans. *Cf.* SCHRIRE, T., 1966, *vide* subsection a; *cf.* also: JONG, H. M. W. DE, 1959, *vide* section Mesopotamia, subsection c.

FENNER, F., 1930: Die Krankheit im Neuen Testament. Eine religions- und medizingeschichtliche Untersuchung, 116 p. (Untersuchgn. Neuen Testam., No. 18) (Leipzig: Hinrichs).—

This booklet deals with such topics as: the evaluation of New Testamentary passages containing allusions to diseases,

317

318

ideas concerning the origin of diseases, descriptions of diseases (psychical as well as physical), the spreading of diseases, the healing of diseases, Luke as physician, *etc.* Valuable list of references. *Cf.* BRIM, C. J., 1936, *vide supra.*

FRIEDENWALD, H., 1944: The Jews and medicine: essays, 2 vols., 817 p. (Baltimore, Md.: Johns Hopkins Press).—

A collection of 42 essays and studies dealing with the contributions of the Jews to the science of medicine. Friedenwald possessed a famous private collection of books and mss. on the subject (*cf.* FRIEDENWALD, H., 1946, *vide infra*). A very valuable chapter of the present book is ch. 8 of Vol. 1 (p. 99-145), containing a classified bibliography of ancient Hebrew medicine. Other chapters deal, *inter alia*, with the attitude of the Bible towards medicine, and with the medical knowledge of Isaac Judaeus (*ca.* 850 - *ca.* 950 A.D.).

——, 1946: Jewish luminaries in medical history and a catalogue of works bearing on the subject of the Jews and medicine from the private library of Harry Friedenwald, 199 p. (Baltimore, Md.: Johns Hopkins Press).—

A catalogue of the private book collection of Harry Friedenwald, probably the best collection dealing with the history of Jewish medicine. This publication can be considered supplementary to that of the preceding entry. It opens with an essay summarizing the Jewish contributions to medicine from Old Testament days up to Paul Ehrlich. The catalogue itself is alphabetically arranged and is divided into two parts, *viz.*, 1. writings of individual physicians and publications concerning them, and 2. works of reference.

FRIEDENWALD, H. M., 1967: The Jews and medicine and Jewish luminaries in medical history, 3 vols. Vol. I: 36 p. + p. 1-390; Vol. II: p. 391-817; Vol. III: 199 p. (Introd. by G. ROSEN) (New York, N.Y.: KTAV Publ. House).—

This is a reprint-edition of Friedenwald's books of 1944 and 1946, *vide supra.* *Cf.* also: KAGAN, S. R., 1952, *vide infra.*

GEMAYEL, A., 1932: L'hygiène et la médecine à travers la Bible, 296 p. (Paris: Geuthner).—

The separate books of the Bible are supplied with annotations from the medical

point of view by a Syrian physician who makes many comparisons with ideas, usages, customs, *etc.*, which could still be observed in his own days. The older literature on the subject, however, has been neglected. Valuable index.

JAKOBOVITS, I., 1959: Jewish medical ethics: a comparative and historical study of the Jewish religious attitude to medicine and its practice, 42 + 381 p. (New York, N.Y.: Philosophical Library).—

In the author's own words, the book is "a comparative and historical study of the Jewish religious attitude to medicine and its practice." It mainly deals with medico-moral problems. Nearly one-third of the book consists of notes and of a comprehensive bibliography; no index of subjects and authors.

KAGAN, S. R., 1952: Jewish medicine, 575 p. (Boston, Mass.: Medico-Historical Press).—

Contains chapters on biblical and talmudic medicine, Jewish mediaeval medicine, Jewish medicine in the Renaissance period, in the seventeenth and eighteenth centuries, and in the modern period. Dealing with the same kind of subjects is: FRIEDENWALD, H., 1944, *vide supra. Cf.* also: KAGAN, S. R., 1948: The bibliography of ancient Jewish medicine. (Bull. Hist. Med. 22: 480-485); and PREUSS, J., 1923, *vide infra.*

KRAUSS, S., 1930: Geschichte der jüdischen Aerzte vom frühesten Mittelalter bis zur Gleichberechtigung, 180 p. (Veröffentl. der A.S. Bettelheim-Stiftung in Wien, Vol. 4) (Vienna: Perles).—

Separate sections deal with the position of the Jews in mediaeval science and medicine in East and West, the Jewish physician in mediaeval Germany, Jewish superstition and its influence on the development of medicine, the Jewish physician and the common people, legislative and other measures of hostility and the defence of the Jews, the social differentiation of the Jewish physicians, the influence of the Jews on the progress of medicine. Index.

MARCUS, J. R., 1947: Communal sick-care in the German ghetto, 335 p. (The Ella H. Philipson Memorial Publication, Vol. 1) (Cincinnati, O.: The Hebrew Union College Press).—

This book discusses such subjects as: the employment of communal physicians, surgeons, midwives, the Jewish hospital, supervision of wet nurses, butchers, *etc.,* the qualification, the suppression, the fees, the economic conflicts with Christian doctors, with quacks, barbers, and druggists, *etc.,* the influence of the cabbalistic school, *etc.*

MÜNZ, I., 1922: Die jüdischen Aerzte im Mittelalter. Ein Beitrag zur Kulturgeschichte des Mittelalters, 175 p. (Frankfurt a. M.: Kauffmann).—

The author evaluates the scientific meaning of the Jewish physician during the Middle Ages in the Orient, in Spain, Germany, France, Turkey, Poland, and Italy. He also discusses the inclination of the Jews towards medical practice during the Middle Ages, the attacks on their position and their defence of it. *Cf.* also: STEIN-SCHNEIDER, M., 1956, *vide* subsection a.

NOBEL, G., 1930: Zahnheilkunde und Grenzgebiete in Bibel und Talmud, 140 p. (Leipzig: Author).—

This booklet consists of a general introduction considering the literature on the history of dentistry in antiquity in general (Mesopotamia, Egypt), and on the history of Jewish dentistry in particular (p. 1-16). Sections follow on: anatomical knowledge (as it is expressed in the Talmud and by the prophets, by their knowledge of anatomical anomalies in phrases, their ideas about the meaning and production of saliva, their ideas concerning the set of teeth of animals in its relationship with their food, *etc.,* p. 16-31); physiology (considering such topics as: teeth; tongue, and the production of sound; the shedding of teeth; the hare-lip; teeth, saliva, and the digestion of food; the sense of taste, p. 32-50); the tooth-pick (p. 50-57); proverbs (p. 58-63); the legislative aspects of dentistry (p. 64-69); extraction and other minor surgical treatments (p. 70-82); pathology, therapeusis, dental hygiene, *etc.* (p. 83-104). P. 107-140 contain some 181 annotations.

PREUSS, J., 1923: Biblisch-talmudische Medizin. Beiträge zur Geschichte und der Kultur überhaupt, ed. 3, 735 p. (Berlin: Karger).—

The most elaborate treatise on the subject, dealing with it in a systematic way. Separate sections deal with: the physician and his assistants (p. 10-43); the parts of the body and their functions, *i.e.,* anatomy and physiology (p. 43-157); the sick and their cure: general pathology and therapeutics (p. 157-171); the diseases and their treatment: special pathology and therapeutics (p. 172-217); injuries and malformations: surgery (p. 218-300); ophthalmology (p. 300-329); dentistry (p. 329-333); otology (p. 333-339); rhinology (p. 339-341); nervous diseases (p. 341-356); psychical diseases (p. 356-369); skin diseases (p. 369-434); gynaecology (p. 434-440); obstetrics (p. 440-505); medicines (p. 505-519); forensic medicine (p. 519-588); hygiene (p. 588-653); dietetics (p. 653-688); bibliography. Other valuable studies of the same topics are: EBSTEIN, W., 1903: Die Medizin im Alten Testament, 184 p. (Stuttgart: Enke); reprinted in 1965 (Munich: Fritsch) and EBSTEIN, W., 1903: Die Medizin im Neuen Testament und im Talmud, 337 p. (Stuttgart: Enke); reprinted in 1965 (Munich: Fritsch).

SMITH, C. R., 1950: The physician examines the Bible, 394 p. (New York, N.Y.: Philosophical Library).—

Separate chapters deal with the following topics: etiology and diagnosis, medical subjects in the Old Testament (priest physicians, the serpent and the staff, God and disease, the anatomical parts of the body, diseases, pestilences and plagues, sex relations, medicines, gynaecology and obstetrics, *etc.),* medical notes on the apocrypha, alcoholic liquors and the Bible, New Testament medical references (medical notes on Christ's life, the miracles, the resurrection, demonology, psychology, Luke as physician, the scriptures in the atomic age, and the temple of the body. An approach from an endocrinologist's point of view: GREENBLATT, R. B., 1963: Search the scriptures: a physician examines medicine in the Bible, 127 p. (Philadelphia, Pa.: Lippincott).

SNOWMAN, J., 1935: A short history of Talmudic medicine, 94 p. (London: Staples Press).—

A brief sketch of Talmudic medicine, discussing such topics as: the environment of Talmudic medicine, the social status of the physician, anatomy, physiology, causation and cure of disease, types of disease, surgery, circumcision, venesection, *etc.,* gynaecology and obstetrics, embryology and pediatrics, eyes, teeth, ears, leprosy and skin lesions, comparative pathology. Mainly a summary in English of PREUSS's book *(vide supra).*

ZIMMELS, H. J., 1952: Magicians, theologians and doctors: studies in folk-medicine and folk-lore as reflected in the rabbinical Responsa (12th - 19th centuries), 293 p. (London: Goldston).—

The "Responsa" are to the Rabbi a guide for decisions in similar cases and to the historian they constitute a source of material for further research. The present book will be a contribution to folk-lore and folk-medicine as it can be derived from the "Responsa". Separate chapters deal with the education of doctors, their social status, and the evolution of medicine; physicians, leeches and quacks; anatomy, physiology, and bodily defects; obstetrics; theories of the causation and character of disease; some notes on disease; therapeutics; remedies; surgery. There are many notes. Good bibliography, glossary, and index.

d. Some individual scientists

Asaph Judaeus (7th century) — SIMON, J., 1933: Asaph Ha-Jehoudi. Médecin et astrologue du Moyen-Age, 98 p. (Paris: Lipschutz).—

This study has been based upon a careful examination of the Paris ms. of Asaph's work. From a minute analysis of the contents of this ms., the author concludes that Asaph lived in Palestine during the 7th century, and for some time was instructor in a medical school in Syria. His treatise on medicine deals with such subjects as: physiology, embryology, the four periods of human life, pathology, hygiene, medicinal plants, the medical calendar, *etc.* According to the author, the greatest merit of Asaph is to have stated, ten centuries before Harvey, that the blood circulates in the veins, and to have affirmed, twelve centuries before Mendel, that ailments are transmitted from parent to child at the moment of fecundation. It also contains the original Hebrew text. An older study dealing with Asaph's medical treatise is: VENETIANER, L., 1916-1917: Asaf Judaeus, der älteste medizinische Schriftsteller in hebräischer Sprache, 193 p. (Strasbourg: Trübner).

Gershon ben Shlomoh d'Arles (fl. *ca.* 1280) — BODENHEIMER, F. S., 1953: The gate of heaven (Shaar ha-Shamayim), 356 p. (Jerusalem: Kiryath Sepher).—

After a general introduction, containing much information about life and work of Gershon ben Shlomoh, the author gives a review of the contents of the book. Most of it deals with natural history. Next (from p. 89 onwards) the translation follows. The Sha'ar ha-Shamayim consists of 13 treatises: 1: on the elements and on the weather; 2: on minerals; 3: on plants; 4-7: on animals; 8: on the nature of Man, his shape and development; 9: on the organs of Man, his bones, flesh, vessels, and nerves; 10: on sleep and wakefulness; 11: on the soul and its forces; 12: on the separate intellects; 13: on astronomy.

Josephus, Flavius *(ca. 37 - ca. 98)* — NEUBURGER, M., ed., 1919: Die Medizin im Flavius Josephus, 74 p. (Bad Reichenhall: Buchkunst).—

Josephus was a famous Jewish historian. This study contains a collection of passages dealing with medical subjects derived from his works, *viz.,* "The history of the Jewish War", "The Jewish antiquities", his "Autobiography", and "Against Apion". The contents of these passages are discussed against the background of biblical and talmudic medicine in general.

Moses ben Maimon (1135-1204) — BARSELA, A., H. E. HOFF & E. FARIS, eds., 1964: Moses Maimonides' two treatises on the regimen of health: Fī Tadbīr al Siḥḥah, and Maqālah fī Bayān Ba'd al-A'raḍ wa-alǧawāb anha. Translated from the Arabic and edited in accordance with the Hebrew and Latin versions, 50 p. (Trans. Amer. Philos. Soc., N.S., 54, Pt. 4).—

This study contains English translations of "The regimen of health" (the contents of which is described below, *cf.* GORDON) and of "The treatise of accidents", originally composed for king al-Afḍal in response to a letter of the king in which he described all the accidents which had befallen him.

—— GORDON, H. L., ed., 1958: The preservation of youth: essays on health, 92 p. (New York, N.Y.: Philosophical Library).—

An English translation of "The regimen of health" (*cf.* BAR-SELA, *et al., vide supra),* originally composed in 1198 in Arabic. It is a treatise written for king al-Afḍal, dealing with the regimen of health in general and with that of the king in particular, with the care of the sick when a physician cannot be found, or when the physician available is unsatisfactory or is not to be trusted. It describes compound and simple drugs, purgatives and emetics, music as a therapeutic agent, and it contains directions for various pharmaceutical preparations. A special chapter is devoted to the mind-body problem.

—— GORLIN, M., ed., 1961: Maimonides "On sexual intercourse", 128 p. (transl. from the Arabic with introduction and commentary) (Medical Historical Studies of Medieval Jewish Medical Works, Vol. I) (Brooklyn, N.Y.: Ramdash Publ. Co.).—

In those days the science of sex and intercourse was considered as a branch of medicine. In a review of this book, M. Levey writes "The pharmacological notes are unreliable, the English is poor, and the remarks in the appendices on related literature are almost entirely without discrimination." (J. Hist. Med. 18: 306).

—— MEYERHOF, M., ed., 1940: Un glossaire de matière médicale de Maïmonide; édité et traduit, 76 + 258 p. + 69 p. Arab text. (Mém. Inst. Egypte, No. 41) (Cairo: Inst. français archéol. orientale).—

The edition and translation of the text is preceded by a long introduction in which are described the Dioscoridan tradition in Arabic, Maimonides's life and medical activities, and the ms. of the medical glossary, its contents, translation, and commentary, and in which is given a list of synonyms of drug names in Arabic. The book itself consists of an alphabetical glossary of drug names and their synonyms, divided into 405 entries.

—— MUNTNER, S., ed., 1963: Treatise on asthma, 115 p. (The medical writings of Moses Maimonides, No. 1) (Philadelphia, Pa.: Lippincott).—

This is the first volume of the first English translation of Maimonides's medical writings which will be published in 9 volumes under the auspices of the Israel Torah Research Institute, Jerusalem. The editor has inserted dates referring to writers mentioned in the text. Informative introductions and notes; useful index. The origi-

nal text served as a guide for the son of Sultan Saladin.

—— ——, 1966: Treatise on poisons and their antidotes, 39 + 77 p. (The medical writings of Moses Maimonides, No. 2) (Philadelphia, Pa.: Lippincott).—

This volume deals with poisons and the protection against deadly remedies. Of this book there also exists a French translation: RABBINOWICZ, I. M., 1935: Traité des poisons, ed. 2, 70 p. (Paris: Lipschutz). This translation is accompanied by an alphabetical list of Arabic and Hebraic pharmaceutical names. The zoological aspects of this treatise are considered by THÉODORIDÈS, J., 1956: Les sciences naturelles et particulièrement la zoologie dans le Traité des poisons de Maimonide (Rev. Hist. Med. hébr. 9).

—— ——, 1966: Regimen Sanitatis oder Diätik für die Seele und den Körper. Mit Anhang der medizinischen Responsen und Ethik des Maimonides, 208 p. (Basle & New York, N.Y.: Karger; Frankfurt a.M.: Akad. Verl. Ges.).—

This book contains a bibliographical review, an introduction describing the purpose and history of the "Regimen", a sketch of the historical background for Maimonides's dietetic theories, and an evaluation of its meaning for present-day biology. Then the German translation of the Regimen follows (p. 57-114). A second ed. appeared in 1968, 208 p. Same publishers.

—— WEIL, G., ed., 1953: Maimonides: Ueber die Lebensdauer. Ein unediertes Responsum, 55 p. (Basle & New York, N.Y.: Karger).—

In this little treatise which is a quotation from an anonymous commentary on chapter 10 of the Laws of the Foundations of the Torah of the Code of Maimonides, Maimonides expresses the meaning that the duration of Man's life is not predetermined and fixed in advance by fate. He supports this theory theologically as well as medically.

8. LIFE AND MEDICAL SCIENCES IN CLASSICAL ANTIQUITY

α. LITERATURE COVERING THE WHOLE PERIOD

a. History of science, philosophy, and culture in general

BIESE, A., 1882-1884: Die Entwicklung des Naturgefühls bei den Griechen und Römern, 147 + 210 p. (Kiel: Lipsius & Tischer).—

A discussion of the development of the use of nature-imagery in the Graeco-Roman literature. The first part contains a presentation of the use of nature-allusions by the Greeks from the earliest mythology, down to the latest productions of the Hellenistic period. The second part contains a similar history of the Roman attitude toward nature from the earliest extant writings in Latin down to the end of the 4th-century A. D. Mainly of literary historical interest. *Cf.* FAIRCLOUGH, H. R., 1963, *vide infra;* and GEIKIE, A., 1912, *vide* section γ, subsection a.

BOMMER, S. & L., 1943: Die Ernährung der Griechen und Römer, 121 p. (Planegg: Müllersche Verlagshandlung).—

An attempt to correlate food and culture in ancient Greece and Rome and to make comparisons with the food-situation in Europe during the last war. It is a popular account, written by a physician. Another study dealing with food habits in antiquity is: ARBESMANN, R., 1929: Das Fasten bei den Griechen und Römern, 131 p. (Giessen: Töpelmann). Other books dealing with the same topic are: VICKERY, K. F., 1936: Food in early Greece, 97 p. (Univ. Illinois Studies in the Social sciences, Vol. XX, 3); ANDRÉ, J., 1961: L'alimentation et la cuisine à Rome, 259 p. (Paris: Klincksieck); HAUSSLEITER, J., 1935: Der Vegetarismus in der Antike, 428 p. (Berlin: Töpelmann).

BUCHWALD, W., *et al.,* 1963: Tusculum-Lexikon griechischer und lateinischer Autoren des Altertums und des Mittelalters, 544 p. (Munich: Heimeran).—

For more details, *vide* section Antiquity in general, subsection a.

BURY, J. B., 1951: History of Greece, ed. 3, 925 p. (New York, N.Y.: Macmillan).—

A classic, first published in 1900. In this new edition (revised by R. MEIGGS), significant new facts and discoveries have been included. There are 205 figures, a chronological table, numerous notes and references, and an excellent index.

CARY, M., 1949: The geographic background of Greek and Roman history, 331 p. (Oxford: Clarendon Press).—

A study of the influence of the geographic environment on the world of ancient Greece and Rome. The following regions have been considered in more or less detail: Greece, Italy, the Asiatic Near East (Asia Minor, Syria, Armenia, Caucasus, Mesopotamia, Arabia), the Asiatic Middle East (Persia, the east Iranian lands, India), North Africa (the Red Sea border, Egypt, Cyrenaica and Tripolitania, N.W. Africa, W. Africa), Western Europe (the Iberian peninsula, Gaul, Britain), Central Europe (Germany, the Alpine lands, the middle Danube lands), Eastern Europe (the Balkan lands, Scythia).

CHAIGNET, A. E., 1966: Histoire de la psychologie des grecs, 5 vols., 2396 p. (Bruxelles: Culture et Civilisation).—

Photomechanical reprint of the 1887-1893 edition. The first volume deals with psychology of the Schools of the Stoics, Epicureans, and Sceptics, the third volume with the psychology of the New Academy and the Eclectic School, and the fourth and fifth volume with the psychology of the Alexandrian School.

CLAGETT, M., 1955: Greek science in antiquity, 217 p. (New York, N.Y.: Abelard-Schuman).—

For more details, *vide* section Antiquity in general, subsection a.

COHEN, M. R. & I. E. DRABKIN, 1948: A source book in Greek science, 579 p. (New York, N.Y., London & Toronto: McGraw-Hill).—

A collection of abstracts derived from many sources, which together give a picture of Greek science. They are arranged by subject. By inserting explanatory notes the authors try to overcome the disadvantages of offering passages abstracted from their context. The section on biology (p. 394-466) includes such topics as: purpose in nature, classification, structure and function, generation and embryology, ecology, pathology of plants and animals; the section on medicine (p. 467-529) includes such topics as: the rational spirit of Greek medicine, anatomy and physiology, diseases, diagnosis and prognosis, therapeutics and hygiene, surgery; the section on physiological psychology (p. 530-558) includes such topics as: traits and character of animals, the senses of animals, human psychology, sensation and perception, association of ideas, the interrelation of bodily and mental states, aberration of the senses, psycho-pathology.

DAREMBERG, C. & E. SAGLIO, eds., 1873-1918: Dictionnaire des antiquités grecques et romaines, d'après les textes et les monuments, 5 tomes in 9 vols. (Paris: Hachette).—

A large dictionary giving extensive explanations of many terms used in art, science, society and social life, war, navy, *etc.,* accompanied by some 3,000 figures. In a supplementary volume indexes have been added on subjects, Greek and Latin words, and collaborators.

FAIRCLOUGH, H. R., 1963: Love of nature among the Greeks and Romans, 270 p. (New York, N.Y.: Cooper Square).—

The author treats of the feeling of nature among the ancients and the treatment of nature in Greek and Roman literature. After a short prologue, containing a review of the literature, chapters follow on: Mythology and religion; Art; Agriculture and outdoor life (Hesiod); Homeric poetry; Lyric poetry; The Greek drama; The Alexandrian and later ages; Theocritus and the anthology; Roman literature; Epilogue. The original edition is of 1930 (London: Harrap). *Cf.* BIESE, A., 1882-1884, *vide supra;* SOUTAR, G., 1939, *vide infra;* and GEIKIE, A., 1912, *vide* section γ, subsection a.

FARRINGTON, B., 1940: Science and politics in the ancient world, 243 p. (London: Allen & Unwin).—

A very well-written, Marxist-inspired and non-conformist history of ancient classic philosophy in which many doubts concerning traditional interpretations of certain aspects of this philosophy are expressed. Farrington himself calls it a study in "popular superstition" in the ancient world, and he shows how most ancient philosophers supported some kind of superstition that was impressed upon the people. Thus doing, he settles with much modern preconditioned admiration, especially of Plato, but also many other thinkers; *e.g.,* Aristotle, Cicero, Varro, Epicuros and Lucretius have thus been re-interpreted. It is shown how only Epicuros and Lucretius proposed a way of

life which should be free of any form of superstition; and Farrington tries to evaluate the proper role of both these often neglected philosophers. A second ed. appeared in 1966, 243 p. (New York, N.Y.: Barnes & Noble). *Cf.* also: AFRICA, T. W., 1967: Science and the state in Greece and Rome, 128 p. (New York, N.Y.: Wiley), a book of which I can not give further information.

——, 1953: Greek science: its meaning for us, 320 p. (London: Penguin).—

A very clearly-written introductory text describing the various phases of the development of Greek science. The first part deals with the period from Thales to Aristotle, *i.e.,* the period during which the foundations of many of the chief branches of science were laid. The second part deals with the period between Theophrastos and Galen. The text was previously issued as two separate booklets in the Pelican series, published by Penguin Books in 1944 and 1949 respectively. Also in French translation: La science dans l'antiquité (Grèce-Rome), 1967, 317 p. (Petite Bibliothèque Payot, No. 94) (Paris: Payot).

FUCHS, J. W., n.d.: Klassiek vademecum, 236 p. (The Hague: van Goor).—

A dictionary of mythological, historical, literary, linguistical, sociological, art-historical, *etc.,* terminology of classical antiquity. In Dutch.

FUHRMANN, M., 1960: Das systematische Lehrbuch. Ein Beitrag zur Geschichte der Wissenschaften in der Antike, 192 p. (Göttingen: Vandenhoeck & Ruprecht).—

Although mainly of philological interest, there is much in it that may interest the medical or biological historian also. Some of the subjects considered are: Anaximenes's concept of *techne*, Varro's treatise of agriculture, its composition, methodology, *etc.,* Celsus's Libri medicinae. Other chapters deal with textbooks during the Hellenistic period, and with Roman textbooks based on Hellenistic examples *(e.g.,* the books of Cato, Varro, Celsus, and Cicero).

HALLIDAY, W. R., 1927: Greek and Roman folklore, 154 p. (Our debt to Greece and Rome series, No. 44) (London: Harrap).—

In this study the author aims at illustrating by some examples the character of the folklore elements in classical culture, and he discusses the relation of the legends, mythology, and fables of the Greeks and Romans to the folktales of the Indo-European area. The text is in three parts, *viz.*, a part dealing with superstitious beliefs and practices in classical antiquity, a part dealing with folktales and fables of classical antiquity, and a third part dealing with the relation between the classical and mediaeval traditions.

LAUFFER, S., 1956: Abriss der antiken Geschichte, 180 p. (Munich: Oldenbourg).—

A chronology of Greek and Roman history from 1200 B.C. up to 395 A.D., dealing mainly with political and cultural history. Appendixes deal with the history of science and technology and with the history of Graeco-Roman music. Lengthy index, and list of kings from 305 B.C. tot 395 A.D.

LESKY, A., 1947: Thalatta. Der Weg der Griechen zum Meer, 341 p. (Vienna: Rohrer).—

Although stress is on the art- and literary-historical aspects - for this book mainly deals with ornaments, fabulous animals, poems, epics, the influence of the sea in Hellenistic thought and fantasy - the book also contains much that is of interest from a biohistorical point of view *(e.g.,* concerning marine animals, esp. fishes and marine mammals, fishermen and fisheries and their economic implications).

LIVINGSTONE, R. W., ed., 1962: The legacy of Greece, 424 p. (Oxford: Clarendon Press).—

This collection of essays concerning the value of Greece to the future of the world was reprinted many times since its first appearance in 1921. There are two essays by C. SINGER on biology and medicine; both have been reprinted in Singer's booklet on: "Greek biology and Greek medicine" *(cf.* section β, b). Attention is directed to the anonymous work on generation (380 B.C.), and to later works by Aristotle, Theophrastos, Cratevas, Pliny, and Dioscorides.

PAULY, A. F. VON & G. WISSOWA, 1893 → : Pauly's Realenzyclopädie der classischen Altertumswissenschaft. Neue Bearbeitung hrsg. von G. WISSOWA, many volumes. (Stuttgart: Druckenmüller).—

The first series consists of 47 half volumes, Aal to Quosenus (1893-1963). The

second series, 18 half volumes Ra to Zenius, (1914-1967). Supplement 11 vols. (1903-1968). Comprehensive signed articles cover every aspect of classical literature, history and civilization. An indispensable work.

REHM, A. & K. VOGEL, 1933: Exakte Wissenschaften, ed. 4, 78 p. (In: GEREKE, A. & E. NORDEN, Einleitung in die Altertumswissenschaft, Vol. II, pars 5) (Leipzig & Berlin: Teubner).—

A review of the history of science. Separate sections deal with the history of geology, meteorology, astronomy, mathematics, zoology, botany, pharmacology, medicine in pre-Socratic Greece, during the Attic period, during Hellenism and during the Roman Empire. *Cf.* REYMOND, A. A., 1924, *vide infra.*

REYMOND, A. A., 1924: Histoire des sciences exactes et naturelles dans l'antiquité gréco-romaine: exposé sommaire des écoles et des principes, 238 p. (Paris: Blanchard).—

A very readable introduction to the principles and methods of the sciences of mathematics, astronomy, mechanics, chemistry, geology and biology from the 7th cent. B.C. up to the 6th cent. A.D. Also in English translation: History of the sciences in Greco-Roman antiquity, 1924, 245 p. (Reprinted in 1963, New York, N.Y.: Biblo & Tanner). A new French second edition appeared in 1955 (Paris: Presses Univ. de France). *Cf.* also: REY, A., 1930-1948: La science dans l'antiquité, 5 vols., *vide* section Antiquity in general, subsection a.

ROBIN, L., 1928: La pensée grecque et les origines de l'esprit scientifique, 480 p. (Paris: La Renaissance du Livre).—

The book mainly gives a review of the history of Greek philosophy from its earliest beginnings up to the closure of the School of Athens in 529. For our purpose the most important chapter entitled "Science and philosophy" (114 p.), deals with the beginnings of science and philosophy (which were closely intermingled), with the pre-Socratic period, the School of Miletos, the Pythagoreans, Heraclitos, the Eleatics, Empedocles, the School of Abdera, Anaxagoras. The latter part mainly deals with Socrates, Plato and Aristotle, their Schools, disciples, followers, and antagonists. Both, the ideas and the persons who expressed them, are considered in their social framework. Good bibliography. There also exists an English translation: Greek thought and the origins of the scientific spirit, 1928, 409 p. (London: Kegan Paul; New York, N.Y.: Knopf). A new French edition appeared in 1963, 544 p. (Paris: Michel). With a modernized bibliography compiled by P. M. SCHUHL.

SANTILLANA, G. DE, 1961: The origins of scientific thought: from Anaximander to Proclus, 600 B.C. - 500 A.D., 320 p. (Chicago, Ill.: Chicago U.P.).—

>Neglecting the technical details of Greek science, the author emphasizes the Greek scientific concepts and attitudes towards nature. He tries to elucidate their origin and to explain their ultimate fate during the decline and fall of ancient science. Also in paperback edition (New York, N.Y.: The New American Library).

SOUTAR, G., 1939: Nature in Greek poetry: studies partly comparative, 258 p. (London: Oxford U.P.).—

>A comprehensive study of the Greek attitude toward nature as revealed by poets. The author describes how nature sets the stage for epic sciences, and how the Alexandrian school developed a wider interest in nature than the Attic. *Cf.* FAIRCLOUGH, H. R., 1963, *vide supra*.

STRÖMBERG, R., 1944: Griechische Wortstudien. Untersuchungen zur Benennung von Tieren, Pflanzen, Körperteilen und Krankheiten, 119 p. (Göteborgs VetenskSamh. Handl., Ser. A, Vol. 2, No. 2) (Göteborg: Elander).—

>A lexicographical study of the names of beetles, cockchafers, centipedes, insects, spiders, worms, plants, parts of the body, diseases and symptoms. The part considering diseases and symptoms treats of fevers, diabetes, ailments of the bladder, eruptions, tumours, anginas, *etc.* Well indexed. *Cf.* also STRÖMBERG, R., 1940, *vide* subsection b.

TAYLOR, H. O., 1923: Greek biology and medicine, 155 p. (London: Harrap).—

>The popular series "Our debt to Greece and Rome", of which this booklet is the third volume, tries to assess the influence of classical antiquity on modern cultural life. This booklet is divided as follows: Early biology; the Hippocratics; Aristotle's biology; progress in anatomy and medicine; the final system: Galen; the link-

age with modern times. A brief chronology compiled by G. D. HADZSITS, showing the influence of Greek biology and medicine on Western culture down to recent times, has been added. Reissued 1963 (New York, N.Y.: Cooper Square).

THOMPSON, D'Arcy W., 1940: Science and the classics, 264 p. (St. Andrews Univ. Publ., No. 44) (London: Oxford U.P.).—

>A collection of 12 essays, originally published between 1919 and 1935, dealing with philological, archaeological and scientific matters. There is much in it that is of interest to the historian of biology, for the writer was a distinguished naturalist: *cf.* the biography written by his daughter, *vide* Appendix.

WOODCOCK, P. G., 1955: Concise dictionary of ancient history, 465 p. (New York, N.Y.: Philos. Library).—

>"The period covered is, roughly, from the beginning of recorded history in the Mediterranean world, to the fall of the Roman Empire, with the greater number of references applying to the Greek and Roman civilizations at the peak of their flowering. This means, of course, the exclusion of most Christian writers, except the very earliest church figures." (Quoted after Isis 47: 239).

ZELLER, E., 1955: Outlines of the history of Greek philosophy, 349 p. (New York, N.Y.: Meridian Books).—

>A pocket edition, containing an English translation of one of the standard surveys of Greek philosophy *(vide infra)*. The text has been prepared from the 13th German edition of 1928, prepared by W. NESTLE: Grundriss der Geschichte der griechischen Philosophie, 392 p. (Leipzig: Reisland). (N.B. The first edition is dated 1883). In a general introduction the meaning, sources, and periods of Greek philosophy are considered. Greek philosophy is here divided into 4 periods: 1. The Pre-socratic philosophy (p. 38-111); 2. The Attic philosophy and the Socratics, Plato, Aristotle (p. 112-224); 3. Hellenistic philosophy. The Stoa. The later cynicism. Epicureanism. Scepticism. Eclecticism (p. 225-284); 4. The philosophy of the Roman Empire (p. 285-338).

——, 1963: Die Philosophie der Griechen in ihrer geschichtlichen Entwicklung. Photomechanische Nachdruck der von W. NESTLE herausgegebene Auflage von 1919-1923. Three parts in six volumes, Part I: 1460 p.;

Part II (1): 1105 p.; Part II (2): 948 p.; Part III (1): 864 p.; Part III (2): 931 p. (Hildesheim: Olms).—

A classic. The first part contains a general introduction and a general review of the origin, character, and development of Greek philosophy. The first section deals with pre-Socratic philosophy. After a brief review of its general characteristics, the author discusses successively: The old Ionians (p. 253-361) (e.g., Thales, Anaximander, Anaximenes, Diogenes of Apollonia); Pythagoras and the Pythagoreans (p. 361-617) (incl. Alcmaeon); The Eleatics (p. 617-782) (e.g., Xenophanes, Parmenides, Melissos); Heraclitos (p. 783-939); Empedocles (p. 939-1038); Leucippos, Democritos, and the atomic theory (p. 1038-1194) (incl. its implications for organic nature, the soul, and the sense organs); Anaxagoras (p. 1195-1278); The Sophists (p. 1278-1459) (incl. Protagoras). Part II(1) starts with a general review of the development of Greek thought and culture during the 5th century B.C.; p. 44-388 deal with life and work of Socrates and his pupils (e.g., Xenophon), the Megarians, the schools of Elis and Eretria, the Cynic and Cyrenaic philosophers; p. 389-1049 deal with life and work of Plato, his academy, etc., supplemented by an essay of E. HOFFMANN on the present state of Platonic research. Part II(2) gives a general review of life, publications, philosophy, logic, methodology, metaphysics, ethics, aesthetics, and politics of Aristotle. Of special importance to our purpose are p. 479-563 which deal with his philosophy on organic nature (soul-body; teleology; principle of analogy; life and inorganic nature; plants, animals and their organs; origin of life; psychology; classification), and p. 563-607 which deal with problems of life, soul and psychology, etc., of man. On p. 806-946 the Peripatetic School has been considered, incl. sections on Theophrastos and his views on botany, zoology, and anthropology (p. 806-869); on Aristoxenos and Dicaearchos (p. 869-896) and on Strabon and his contemporaries and followers. Part III(1) deals with Zeno of Citium, Stoicism, Epicuros and his pupils, Eclecticism, Cicero, Varro, and Greek philosophy in the Roman Empire. Part III(2) mainly deals with Neoplatonism and the decline of Greek philosophy. For a pocket ed. in English, vide supra.

b. History of the plant and animal sciences

BILLERBECK, J., 1824: Flora classica, 286 p. (Leipzig: Hinrichs).—

This book sums up all plant names mentioned in the works of the classical Greek and Roman writers, together with noteworthy particulars of the plants occurring in these writings. The book is of particular interest to historians, botanists, and philologists. Announced facsimile reprint by Liebing, Würzburg, 1971.

BLERSCH, K., 1937: Wesen und Entstehung des Sexus im Denken der Antike, 104 p. (Tübinger Beiträge zur Altertumswissenschaft, No. 29).—

This publication deals with sex-determination in the embryo in Greek philosophy: the pre-Socratics (Alcmaeon, Cnidian School, Empedocles, Corpus Hippocraticum, Anaxagoras), Aristotle (the differentiation of the sexes, and the sexual organs as its expression), and Hellenistic science (esp. Galen and his supposition that the male and female genital apparatus are analogous). Cf. LESKY, E., 1950, vide infra.

BÖTTICHER, C., 1856: Die Baumcultus der Hellenen. Nach den gottesdienstlichen Gebräuchen und den überlieferten Bildwerken dargestellt, 544 p. (Berlin: Weidmann).—

This book deals with such topics as birth and education of the gods, their origin and their worship, in trees, offerings, famous sacred trees, the sacred tree as oracle, mutilations of sacred trees or woods, serpents as guards and protectors of sacred trees, statues of gods made of the wood of sacred trees, the sacred tree and the deaths, etc. Separate sections deal with the laurel (p. 338-384), oak, palm-tree, olive-tree, fig, poplar, myrtle, rose, apple, orange, pomegranate, and cypress. Short reviews of the tree-cults of the Egyptians, Indians, Assyrians, Persians, Hebrews, Celts, and Germans, and of the decline of the tree-cult in early Christianity. Cf. WENIGER, L., 1919, vide section β, subsection b.

DIERBACH, J. H., 1833: Flora mythologica oder Pflanzenkunde in Bezug auf Mythologie und Symbolik der Griechen und Römer. Ein Beitrag zur ältesten Geschichte der Botanik, Agricultur und Medicin, 218 p. (Frankfurt a.M.: Sauerländer).—

The similarity existing between many plant-names and Greek and Roman mythology clearly indicates an interconnection between them. But also general aspects of plant life and plant growth find expression in this mythology, while agriculture as well as the culture of plants of medical interest also are interwoven with Greek and Roman mythology. These and some other subjects form the contents of this book. A book of the same scope seems to be: DU MOLIN, J. B., 1856: Flore poétique ancienne ou études sur les plantes les plus difficiles à reconnaître des poètes anciens, grecs et latins. Ouvrage où l'on trouvera, en particulier l'explication botanique et critique du vers de Virgile... et d'un grand nombre d'autres, 320 p. (Paris: Baillière). *Cf.* also FRAAS, C., 1845, *vide infra,* and MURR, J., 1880, *vide* section β, subsection b.

FRAAS, C., 1845: Synopsis plantarum florae classicae oder: übersichtliche Darstellung der in den classischen Schriften der Griechen und Römer vorkommenden Pflanzen, nach autoptischer Untersuchung im Florengebiete entworfen und nach Synonymen geordnet, 39 + 320 p. (Munich: Fleischmann).—

> Characteristic of this study is, that it is based not only on the literature left behind by the classic writers themselves, but also on a thorough on-the-spot study of the native flora of the regions where those writers actually lived and worked. Agricultural, medical, and mythological details have been omitted. The author gives an extensive conspectus of preceding literature on the same subject. A second ed. appeared in 1870 (Berlin: Calvary). Particularly this second ed. seems to be the best general study of the identification of ancient plant names. *Cf.* also DIERBACH, J. H., 1833, *vide supra.*

HAGEN, H., 1961: Die physiologische und psychologische Bedeutung der Leber in der Antike, 127 p. (Diss. Univ. Bonn).—

> Discussion of the liver in the physiology of Hippocrates, Diocles, Aristotle, Herophilos, Erasistratos, Cicero, Galen, and of the liver as the seat of the psychical faculties. *Cf.* MANI, N., 1959, *vide* section Antiquity in general, subsection c.

HEITLAND, W. E., 1921: Agricola: a study of agriculture and rustic life in the Graeco-Roman world from the point of view of labour, 492 p. (Cambridge: U.P.).—

> In a review of Greek agriculture (p. 16-130), the works of old poets *(e.g.,* Homer and Hesiod), of historians *(e.g.,* Herodotos and Thucydides), of philosophers *(e.g.,* Plato and Aristotle), of artists, creators, *etc.,* are considered. The Roman period, which fills the greater part of the book, has been divided into many sections in which the same kind of topics are discussed. Also early

Christian writers (Lactantius, Sulpicius, Severus, Salvian, Apollinaris Sidonius) have been considered. Indexes have been added of subjects, words and phrases, passages cited, modern authorities, countries, places and peoples.

JASNY, N., 1944: The wheats of classical antiquity, 176 p. (Baltimore, Md.: Johns Hopkins Press).—

> The author, a linguist and classicist, as well as a professional agriculturist, who is well-acquainted with some aspects of agriculture and systematic botany, shows how many difficulties have to be overcome in determining what kind of wheat was bred by the Greeks. These embrace *e.g.,* the physical properties of the plants, milling properties of the grain, type of flour, suitability for bread-making, for porridge, climatic adaptation, colour of endosperm, yield per unit of cultivated ground, *etc.* All three groups of wheat *(i.e.,* einkorn, emmers, and spelts) were cultivated in the classical world, so that all surrounding countries must have contributed to the food production of Greece. *Cf.* JARDI, A., 1925, *vide* section b, subsection b.

LENZ, H. O., 1856: Zoologie der alten Griechen und Römer. Deutsch in Auszügen aus deren Schriften, 656 p. (Gotha: Becker).—

> Extracts from the zoological writings of classical antiquity with German translations of sources. The extracts are chronologically arranged and mainly derived from: Herodotos, Xenophon, Aristotle, Pliny, Strabon, Cato, Nicander, Varro, Cicero, Gratius, Virgil, Siculus, Columella, Plutarch, Arrianus, Pausanias, Oppianus, Aelianos, Athenaeos, Palladius. A short review is: DAHL, F., 1926: Zur Geschichte der Zoologie. Von Aristoteles bis Plinius, 42 p. (Sitzber. Naturf. Freunde, Berlin 192: 62-104). *Cf.* also DOUGLAS, N., 1928: Birds and beasts of the Greek anthology, 215 p.; and KELLER, O., 1963: Die antike Tierwelt, 2 vols., *vide* section Antiquity in general, subsection b.

——, 1859: Botanik der alten Griechen und Römer. Deutsch in Auszügen aus deren Schriften nebst Anmerkungen, 776 p. (Gotha: Thienemann).—

> Extracts from the botanical writings of classical antiquity with German translation of sources. The extracts are chronologically arranged, following a systematic order, from Graminae (p. 229) to Fungi (p.

753), and derived from: Cato, Nicander, Varro, Vergil, Columella, Strabon, Pliny, Athenaeos, Palladius, Hippocrates, Theophrastos, Celsus, Dioscorides, Arrianus, Galen, the Geoponica, and many other sources. A very good study, but a very incomplete index minimizes its value. Reprinted 1966 (Wiesbaden: Sändig).

LESKY, E., 1950: Die Zeugungs- und Vererbungslehren der Antike und ihr Nachwirken, 201 p. (Abh. Akad. Wiss., Mainz, Geistes- u. sozialwiss. Kl., No. 19) (Mainz: Verlag der Akad. der Wiss. u. Literatur).—

A detailed and critical study of the development of the hereditary concept in Greek thought and the influence of this ancient concept on later times. Among the topics considered are, *e.g.*, the encephalomyelogenic theory of Alcmaeon, the pangenesis theory of the atomists, the views held on sex determination, the Hippocratic writers and their ideas on heredity, the role of the pneuma, the ideas of Aristotle, the School of Alexandria, the Stoics and Galen concerning heredity and sex determination. A comparable study seems to be BALSS, H., 1936: Zeugungslehre und Embryologie in der Antike. Eine Uebersicht, 82 p. (Quell. Stud. Gesch. Naturw. Med. 5: 1-82). Another study dealing with Greek ideas concerning heredity, *etc.*, is: HAEDICKE, W., 1936: Die Gedanken der Griechen über Familienherkunft und Vererbung, 163 p. (Inaug. Diss., Univ. Halle) (Halle: Klinz). *Cf.* also GEURTS, P. M. M., 1941, *vide* section β, subsection b.

MAKKONEN, O., 1968: Ancient forestry, 84 p. (Acta For. Fenn. 82: 1-84).—

After a brief introduction, considering such subjects as: the most important ancient written sources of information in connection with forestry, and recent literature on forest history in antiquity, chapters follow discussing the structure, the vital functions (propagation and growth), and the factors affecting the growth of trees (soil, location and climate), and tree species mentioned in Greek and Latin literature. This is only part of a study which will be published under the title "The significance of forests to the peoples of ancient times". The whole work will be published in instalments, of which this is the first. The subtitle of the next instalment will be "The procurement and trade of forest products". I am not able to verify whether this part has been published.

RICHTER, G. M. A., 1930: Animals in

Greek sculpture: a survey, 87 p. + 236 illus. (New York, N.Y.: Oxford U.P.).—

Although primarily written from the art-historical point of view, this book contains much of interest to the historian of zoology as well. The author considers some 27 mammals, 11 birds, the snake, the lizard, some insects and arachnids, and some water animals (fishes, dolphin, seal, octopus, tortoise, lobster, frog). A book of comparable scope is: KÖHLER, C. S., 1967: Das Thierleben im Sprichwort der Griechen und Römer. Nach Quellen und Stellen in Parallele mit dem deutschen Sprichwort herausgegeben, 221 p. (Hildesheim: Olms). Originally published in 1881 (Leipzig: Fernau).

STRÖMBERG, R., 1940: Griechische Pflanzennamen, 190 p. (Göteborg Högsk. Årskr., 46) (Göteborg: Elander).—

The author expounds his aim in these words: "Das Schwergewicht dieser Arbeit ruht in dem Bemühen, die griechischen Pflanzen nach ihren Benennungsgründen anzuordnen und an Hand von sicher zu bestimmenden Beispielen einen festen Grund für die Etymologie und Morphologie ihrer Namen zu legen." To do this, the author considers a number of characteristics such as: form characteristics, *e.g.*, comparisons with animals, precious stones, colours, *etc.*; physiological characteristics, *e.g.*, smell, taste, poisonousness, *etc.*; medical characteristics, *e.g.*, usage as purgatives or as aphrodisiacs, their symbolical or mythological indication; practical characteristics, *e.g.*, their use for bows and arrows, for hedges, or as roofcover; geographical characteristics, mythological, etymological, *etc.* characteristics. A book serving the same (etymological) purpose is: STRÖMBERG, R., 1943: Studien zur Etymologie und Bildung der griechischen Fischnamen, 165 p. (Göteborg: Wettergren & Kerber). *Cf.* STRÖMBERG, R., 1944, *vide* this section, subsection a; and STRÖMBERG, R., 1937, *vide* Theophrastos, section β, subsection d. *Cf.* also: LANGKAVEL, B., 1964, Botanik der spaeteren Griechen, *vide* section Antiquity in general, subsection b; and CARNOY, A., 1959, section γ, subsection b.

TAYLOR, H. O., *ca.* 1923: Greek biology and medicine, 155 p. (London: Harrap).—

For more details, *vide* this section, subsection a.

THOMPSON, D'Arcy W., 1936: A glossary of Greek birds, ed. 2, 342 p. (St. Andrews Univ. Publ., No. 39) (Oxford: Clarendon Press).—

George Sarton writes about this book: "The title is far too modest, in fact, misleading, for we are given not simply a glossary, a very rich glossary, but in addition a treasury of Greek quotations and of folk-lore (largely but not exclusively Greek) concerning the Greek birds." This book is indispensable to anyone interested in the study of Greek or Roman ornithology and invaluable for studies in ancient symbolism in which birds play a role, *e.g.*, bas-reliefs, bird emblems of classical coinage, fables and myths. Reprinted 1966 (Hildesheim: Olms). Originally published in 1895. *Cf.* THOMP-SON's A glossary of Greek fishes, *infra.*

——, 1947: A glossary of Greek fishes, 302 p. (London: Oxford U.P.).—

This book has been set up along much the same lines as the glossary of Greek birds *(vide supra)*. Many references to other languages, such as: Egyptian, Coptic, Arabic, Hebrew, and Byzantine, Italian, and modern Greek dialects. It is not restricted only to true fishes, but includes many other creatures living in the water such as crustaceans, sponges, star-fishes, corals, squids, *etc.* Many references to culinary or medical uses, folklore, and literature.

WATKINS, M. G., 1885: Gleanings from the natural history of the ancients, 258 p. (London: Stock).—

Separate sections deal with such subjects as: a Homeric bestiary, Greek and Roman dogs, the cat, owls, pygmies, elephants, the horse, gardens, hunting, Virgil as an ornithologist, roses, wolves, ancient fish-lore, mythical animals, oysters and pearls.

c. History of the medical sciences

BROCK, A. J., 1929: Greek medicine: being extracts illustrative of medical writers from Hippocrates to Galen, 256 p. (London: Dent).—

After a general treatment of the subject, an anthology (in English translation) follows. Most passages are from Hippocrates (p. 35-96) and Galen (p. 130-244). Others are from Thucydides, Plato, Aristotle, Rufus of Ephesus (2), Diodoros, and Aëtios (2). Many annotations. Doe & Marshall state: "Dr. Brock has chosen his extracts admirably and they illustrate well some six centuries of Greek thought."

COHN-HAFT, L., 1956: The public physicians of ancient Greece, 91 p. (Northampton, Mass.: Smith College, Dept. History).—

A study in the history of the Greek organization of public medicine, mainly as it was employed in the Greek city-states, down to the foundation of the Roman empire. It discusses the civil status, training, social and economic status and professional recognition of these physicians, and discusses whether the public physicians were an institution for social welfare or for the general welfare. It has been emphasized that each case has to be considered within the framework of the ideas current at the time.

DEFRASSE, A. & H. LECHAT, 1895: Epidaure, 246 p. (Paris: Librairies imprimeries réunies).—

A large-sized and beautifully printed book containing many photographs and drawings of Epidaurus as it is now and as it has probably been. It gives the history of Epidaurus and its cult, the legend of Asclepios, and extensive descriptions of the different parts which together formed the Asklepieion. For comparable studies concerning the Asklepieion of Cos, *cf.* SCHAZMANN, P., 1932: Asklepieion. Baubeschreibung und Baugeschichte, 78 p. (In: R. HERZOG, ed., Kos, Ergebnisse der deutschen Ausgrabungen und Forschungen, Vol. I) (Berlin: Keller); *idem* of Pergamon, *cf.* DEUBNER, O., 1938: Das Asklepieion von Pergamon (Berlin: Verlag für Kunstwiss.); *idem* of Athens, cf. GIRARD, P., 1881: L'asclépieion d'Athènes, d'après de récentes découvertes (Paris: Thorin); *idem* of Corinth, *cf.* ROEBUCK, C. A., 1951: The Asklepieion and Lerna, 183 p. (Princeton, N. J.: Amer. School of Classical Studies). *Cf.* also HERZOG, R., 1931, *vide infra.*

EDELSTEIN, E. J. & L., 1945: Asclepius: a collection and interpretation of the testimonies, 2 vols. Vol. I: Testimonies, 470 p.; Vol. II: Interpretations, 277 p. (Baltimore, Md.: Johns Hopkins Press).—

The book gives an extensive collection of source-material about Asclepios and his cult published in the original language and in English translation. The material has been arranged so that the various aspects of the problem are illustrated. According to the authors, Asclepios originally was the blameless physician of the old. Later on, when medicine was still a secular craft, the physicians formed a guild whose members supposed that they were descendants of Asclepios (asclepiads), and that they were protected by him. Gradually the name of their patron became identified with medicine; and at last Asclepios became the chief healer, supplementing the work of the physician. Deification would have taken place *ca.* 6th cent. B.C. English translations of cases 1-43 of the inscriptions on the tables of Epidaurus have been added. A more general discussion of the problem is: KUTSCH, F., 1913: Attische Heilgötter und Heilheroen, 138 p. (Religionsgesch. Versuche und Vorarbeiten XII, H. 3) (Giessen: Töpelmann). A discussion of mythology and cultural remains of Heros Iatros, Aristomachos, Amynos, Asclepios, and Amphiarios. *Cf.* KERÉNYI, C., 1960, *vide infra*. *Cf.* also: SCHOUTEN, J., 1967, *vide infra*.

ELLIOT, J. S., 1914: Outlines of Greek and Roman medicine, 165 p. (London: Bale).—

A brief survey of the most important stages in the advancement of the healing art in Greece and Rome, written for medical students and the interested layman. It also includes some aspects of the influence of Christianity on Graeco-Roman medicine. *Cf.* LUND, F. B., 1936, *vide infra*.

FLASHAR, H., 1966: Melancholie und Melancholiker in den medizinischen Theorien der Antike, 145 p. (Berlin: de Gruyter).—

After a general introduction, considering the discussion concerning the concept of melancholy in present-day medicine, the author considers the opinions about this concept as they are reflected in the Corpus Hippocraticum, by Diocles of Carystos, Aristotle, Celsus, Aretaeos, Soranos, Rufus of Ephesus, Galen, Poseidonios, and Alexander of Tralles. Indexes of names and subjects.

GHINOPOULO, S., 1930: Pädiatrie in Hellas und Rom, 132 p. (Jenaer med.-hist. Beitr., Heft 13).—

Separate sections deal with such subjects as: the ideas of the ancients about the newborn child, nurses, diseases of the alimentary system, infectious diseases, diseases of the respiratory, circulatory, and urogenital organs, diseases of the nervous system, diseases of the skin, surgery, diseases of the ears and eyes of children.

HAUSMANN, U., 1948: Kunst und Heiltum. Untersuchungen zu den griechischen Asklepios reliefs, 191 p. (Potsdam: Stichnote).—

After a cure in the temples of Asclepios a fee or *ex voto* was offered, often in the form of an artistic presentation of what had happened. This book is a monograph about such votive offerings, found in places where temples of Asclepios have been excavated. It contains a wealth of annotations and a catalogue of votive reliefs. Illuminating photographs have been added. The author points to the magic significance of these thank-offerings. A large collection of them is to be found in the National Museum of Athens: reproductions can be found in the catalogue of J. N. SVORONOS, 1908-1911: Das Athener National Museum (Athens: Griech. Verlagsges.).

HERZOG, R., 1931: Die Wunderheilungen von Epidauros. Ein Beitrag zur Geschichte der Medizin und Religion, 164 p. (Philologus, Suppl. XXII, H. 3) (Leipzig: Dieterich).—

A philological study of the tables found at the asklepieion of Epidaurus. The complete text (as far as it is known) has been reproduced, together with a German translation. In Epidaurus, according to the author, the cult was of a religious character (in contradiction with those of *e.g.,* Cos or Pergamon where physicians intervened in the cult). The author stresses the role of psychogenic factors in the origin and cure of the diseases. Older booklets stressing the medical aspects are: DAUFRESNE, C., 1909: Epidaure. Les prêtres - les guérisons, 120 p. (Paris: Vigot) and CATON, R., 1900: The temples and ritual of Asklepios at Epidaurus and Athens, ed. 2, 49 p. (London: Clay). *Cf.* also DEFRASSE, A. & H. LECHAT, 1895, *vide supra*.

KERÉNYI, C., 1960: Asklepios: archetypal image of the physician's existence, 151 p. (London: Thames & Hudson).—

The author makes a stand against the assumption that Asclepios must once have been worshipped as a mortal hero, being elevated to divine rank only later on. The author starts from the proposition that, if we wish to know what role Asclepios really played in antiquity, we have to consult the old mythological tradition and to visit the sites where the cult of Asclepios was practised. Accordingly the book contains many illustrations of statues of Asclepios, showing different ancient interpretations. Extensive discussion of Homer's role in the historical interpretation of Asclepios. *Cf.* EDELSTEIN, E. J. & L., 1945, *vide supra*.

KLIPPEL, M., 1937: La médecine grecque dans ses rapports avec la philosophie, 79 p. (Paris: Ed. Hippocrate).—

The author especially tries to make clear how Greek medicine is closely connected with Greek philosophy. The first chapters deals with pre-Hippocratic medicine and shows how medicine became independent of sacerdotal prejudices. The second chapter deals with Hippocratic medicine and its philosophical sources, and the third chapter deals with post-Hippocratic medicine, the dogmatic, empiricist, methodist, and pneumatic schools, and it is shown how these different schools are linked with philosophical premises. *Cf.* PRECOPE, J., 1961, *vide* section β, subsection c.

KUDLIEN, F., 1968: Die Sklaven in der griechischen Medizin der klassischen und hellenistischen Zeit, 46 p. (Forschungen zur antiken Sklaverei, Vol. II) (Wiesbaden: Steiner).—

A study discussing the problem of the slaves in old Greek medicine, based on Greek literary sources, *e.g.,* the passage in the Hippocratic oath, referring to both free men and slaves, some passages of the Hippocratic books on the "Epidemics", and a reference in Plato's "Laws", where Plato has made a distinction between physicians for free men and for slaves. The author rejects the thesis that the slaves were treated in a more or less veterinarian way, and that there were slave-physicians (Servi medici, since the arguments for both these theses were unsatisfactory.

LUND, F. B., 1936: Greek medicine, 161 p. (Clio Medica) (New York, N.Y.: Hoeber).—

An introductory text. The author divides his subject into the following parts: 1. The Hippocratic Corpus; 2. The nature of humours; 3. Alexandrian era; 4. Empiric School; 5. Greek medicine in the Roman empire; 6. Methodist School; 7. Celsus and Pliny; 8. The Pneumatic and Eclectic Schools; 9. Aretaeos, Rufus, Soranos; 10. Galen; 11. Antyllos and general conditions in the later Roman empire; 12. Oribasios and medicine after Oribasios. *Cf.* ELLIOT, J. S., 1914, *vide supra*; also: DEICHGRÄBER, K., 1930; MEYER-STEINEG, T., 1916; and WELLMANN, M., 1895, *vide* section γ, subsection c.

MEYER-STEINEG, T., 1912: Kranken-Anstalten im griechisch-römischen Altertum, 46 p. (Jena: Fischer).—

This booklet deals with the following topics: a) Greece: The historical development of the treatment of the sick, the physician's house as hospital, and the role of the asklepeion as hospital; b) Rome: The treatment of the sick in the Roman Empire the slave-valetudinaries, and the Roman military hospital.

MÜRI, W., 1962: Der Arzt im Altertum. Griechische und lateinische Quellenstücke von Hippokrates bis Galen mit der Uebertragung ins deutsche, ed. 3, 508 p. (Munich: Heimeran).—

A collection of translations from 10 medical and 4 non-medical Greek and Roman writers. The original text and the translation are printed on facing pages. There are chapters on the duty and obligation of the physician, biographical sketches of individual doctors, the physician at the bedside, health and disease, anatomy and surgery, dietetics and drugs, and the borderlands of medicine. An appendix contains many notes to the selection; there is a glossary of individual names, and a small chronological table. First edition 1938.

SCHÖNER, E., 1964: Das Viererschema in der antiken Humoral-pathologie, 114 p. (Sudhoffs Arch. Gesch. Med., Beiheft 4) (Wiesbaden: Steiner).—

An analysis of the role of the doctrine of the four elements in classical antiquity. In ch. 1 the author considers the fragments of the pre-Socratic philosophers (more especially of Empedocles and Alcmaeon); in ch. 2 the author proves that this doctrine forms the basis of the theory of the Corpus Hippocraticum (p. 15-58). In ch. 3 the author considers Philiston of Locroi, Plato, Dexippos of Cos, Aristotle, Diocles of Carystos, Mnesitheos of Athens, Menecrates, and Praxagoras of Cos; ch. 4 considers the period between 300 and 50 B.C., ch. 5 considers the physicians of the Pneumatic School (Diocles of Carystos, Erasistratos and the Sicilian physicians), and ch. 6 deals with Galen. The final chapter elucidates the influence of this doctrine during the Middle Ages and Renaissance.

SCHOUTEN, J., 1967: The rod and serpent of Asklepios: symbol of medicine, 260 p. (Amsterdam: Elsevier).—

Separate sections of this book deal *inter alia* with: Asclepios the divine physician in Hellas and Rome; the effigy of Asclepios and his attributes in classical times; incubation in the temples of Asclepios; Hygieia; Asclepios in the Middle Ages; rod and serpent as medical symbols; Asclepios and his rod-and-serpent in some frontispieces of medical works, herbals, and pharmacopoeias; *etc.* With bibliography and index.

SOUQUES, A., 1936: Étapes de la neurologie dans l'antiquité grecque (d'Homère à Galien), 247 p. (Paris: Masson).—

The author considers such topics as: the impact of philosophy on neurology (Alcmaeon, Democritos), Hippocrates and the anatomy and physiology of the nervous system; Aristotle and his views on sensation; the anatomical discovery of the nerves and the position of the brain in the works of Herophilos and Erasistratos; Greek medicine in Rome and its influence on Celsus; Galen and his anatomical and physiological investigations of the brain; Galen's influence during the Middle Ages.

TEMKIN, O., 1932: Geschichte des Hippokratismus im ausgehenden Altertum, 80 p. (Kyklos 4: 1-80).—

For more details, *vide* section Antiquity in general, subsection c.

VAN BROCK, N., 1961: Recherches sur le vocabulaire médical du grec ancien. Soins et guérisons, 294 p. (Paris: Klinksieck).—

An elaborate philological study of medical terms.

β. ANCIENT GREECE

a. History of science, philosophy, and culture in general

BACCOU, R., 1951: Histoire de la science grecque de Thalès à Socrate, 257 p. (Paris: Montaigne).—

The present book contains the posthumously published series of lectures given by its author at the Institut Catholique de Toulouse. The author puts forward a personal view of the period and philosophers considered, based on a minute study of the extant texts. Separate sections deal with the origin of Greek thought and its roots in Assyrio-Chaldaic and Egyptian science, with the times of Homer and Hesiod, with Thales, Anaximander, Anaximenes, Pythagoras, Heraclitos, Xenophanes, Parmenides, Zeno of Citium, Empedocles, and Anaxagoras, with atomism and with Pythagorean speculation. *Cf.* BURNET, J., 1953, *vide infra.*

BONNARD, A., 1962: Greek civilization, 3 vols. Vol. I: From the Iliad to the Parthenon, 199 p.; Vol. II: From Antigone to Socrates, 248 p.; Vol. III: From Euripides to Alexandria, 288 p. (New York, N.Y.: Macmillan).—

A very useful general survey of Greek culture, paying much attention to the history of science in its relationship with philosophy, literature, art, and the organization of the state.

BURNET, J., 1953: Greek philosophy. I. Thales to Plato, 360 p. (All published) (London: Macmillan).—

This is a reproduction of the first ed. (1914). The book is in three parts. The first part (p. 17-101) deals with the Ionians, Pythagoras, Heraclitos, Parmenides, Empedocles, Anaxagoras, Leucippos, the Eleatics and the Pythagoreans. The second part (p. 105-201) deals with the Sophists, with the life, philosophy, and death of Socrates, and with the philosophy of Democritos. The third part deals with Plato, his life, philosophy, academy, politics *etc.* *Cf.* BACCOU, R., 1951, *vide supra.*

DIELS, H., 1956-1960: Die Fragmente der Vorsokratiker. Griechisch und deutsch. Ed. by W. KRANZ, 3 vols. Vol. I, ed. 9 (1960): 504 p.; Vol. II, ed. 9 (1959): 428 p.; Vol. III, ed. 10 (1960): 660 p. (Berlin: Weidmann).—

An attempt to illustrate, by giving the original sources, the advancement of Greek philosophy and science. The names of every person who is known, or thought, to have contributed to the progress of ancient knowledge have been arranged in chronological order. Under each name statements of ancient writers about the life and opinions of the thinker in question have been given, together with the remaining fragments, if any, of his works. Volumes I and II together contain fragments from some 80 writers; medicine has been considered as far as it is connected with physiology; for further particulars attention is directed to WELLMANN's collection of fragments (*vide* this section, subsection c). From the authors mentioned the following are of interest for our purpose: Thales, Anaximander, Anaximenes, Pythagoras, Democedes, Xenophanes, Heraclitos, Alcmaeon, Parmenides, Empedocles, Hippon, Philolaos, Anaxagoras, Diogenes of Apollonia, Democritos, Protagoras, and Hippias. Vol. III contains extensive indexes to facilitate reference to the text. Also in English translation: FREEMAN, K., 1948: Ancilla to the pre-Socratic philosophers: a complete translation of the fragments in Diels' "Fragmente der Vorsokratiker", 162 p. (Oxford: Blackwell). *Cf.* also FREEMAN, K., 1946; and TANNERY, P., 1930, *vide infra*.

FREEMAN, K., 1946: The pre-Socratic philosophers: a companion to Diels' "Fragmente der Vorsokratiker", 486 p. (Oxford: Blackwell).—

> The object of this companion is to offer a guidance to the study of the fragments collected by Diels, and accordingly the chapters follow the arrangement adopted by Diels. Each chapter at first tells what is known of the life of the philosopher, then provides a summary of his teaching. Every statement is supported by an exact reference either to the thinker's own words or to some exponent of his views. Greek quotations have been kept out of the text. *Cf.* DIELS, H., 1956-1960, *supra*.

GIGON, O., 1945: Der Ursprung der griechischen Philosophie. Von Hesiod bis Parmenides, 291 p. (Basle: Schwabe).—

> A study of historical continuity, and an attempt to investigate what any philosopher borrowed from his predecessors and what new elements he had added to existing knowledge. This is linked up with the question of the origin of philosophy. Moreover, it is an attempt to deduce, from the principle of continuity, the real meaning of the old philosophers. Discussed in this way are: Hesiod, Thales, Anaximander, Anaximenes, Pythagoras, Xenophanes, Heraclitos, Parmenides.

GOMPERZ, T., 1922-1931: Griechische Denker. Eine Geschichte der antiken Philosophie, ed. 4, 3 vols. Vol. I: 499 p.; Vol. II: 628 p.; Vol. III: 644 p. (Berlin & Leipzig: de Gruyter).—

> The first volume deals with the beginnings of Greek philosophy (Ionian philosophers; Pythagoras and the Pythagoreans), with the transition of metaphysics to positivistic science (Xenophanes, Parmenides, Anaxagoras, Empedocles), and with the period of enlightenment (atomic theory, the Sophists). The second volume is exclusively devoted to Socrates and his followers (p. 3-193) and Plato (p. 197-521) and has no special significance for our purpose. The third volume deals with Aristotle and his successors. This volume includes chapters on Aristotle's studies on organic nature (*e.g.*, on systematics, anatomy, physiology,

embryology) and four chapters on Theophrastos (of which one deals with his work on botany, p. 396-403). Extensive indexes (p. 517-663) of names, subjects, geographical names, *etc.* Also in English translation: Greek thinkers: a history of ancient philosophy, 1901-1912, 4 vols. (Transl. by L. MAGNUS) (New York, N.Y.: Scribner's).

GUTHRIE, W. K. C., 1962: A history of Greek philosophy, vol. I: The earlier pre-Socratics and the Pythagoreans, 539 p. (Cambridge: U. P.).—

> This is the first of two volumes (*vide infra*, GUTHRIE, 1965) of a comprehensive history of ancient Greek philosophy. This first volume deals with the period from the beginning of the 6th century to the middle of the 5th century B.C., a period during which no line can be drawn between philosophy, theology, and science. After a general introduction the author starts with a chapter on the beginnings of philosophy in Greece. Then follow, on p. 45-72: The Milesians (Thales); on p. 72-115: Anaximander (incl. a section on the origin of animals and human life); on p. 115-140: Anaximenes (incl. a section on air, life and divinity); on p. 146-336: Pythagoras and the Pythagoreans (*inter alia* on Philolaos and a section on Man and his place in nature and on the nature of the soul); on p. 341-359: Alcmaeon (incl. a discussion of the philosophical character of his work and his physiology); on p. 360-402: Xenophanes (incl. a section dealing with "all creatures born from the earth"); on p. 403-492: Heraclitos. Excellent index.

———, 1965: A history of Greek philosophy, vol. 2: The pre-Socratic tradition from Parmenides to Democritus, 554 p. (Cambridge: U.P.).—

> The main theme of the second volume is the emergence of philosophical problems. It deals with the Eleatics: Parmenides (p. 1-79); Zeno of Citium (p. 80-100); Melissos (p. 101-118), with Empedocles: *e.g.*, his personality, healing activities, his theory of mixture and its relationship to atomism, chance and necessity in nature, the formation of living creatures, the structure of animate nature, physiology, cognition, thought, sensation, *etc.* (p. 122-265), with Anaxagoras: life and writings, the problem of becoming, origin and nature of living things, sensation, *etc.* (p. 266-338), with Archelaos (p. 339-344), and Diogenes of Apollonia: life and writings, cosmogony, physiology, *etc.* (p. 362-381), and with the atomists of the fifth century (p. 382-507): Leucippos and Democritos: the fun-

damentals of the theory, general nature, motion, *etc.*, of the atoms, the four elements, soul, life and death, sensation, biology, physiology, and medicine. Man and the cosmos, the origin of life, *etc.* Very good bibliography and index.

JAEGER, W., 1939-1944: Paideia: the ideals of Greek culture, 3 vols. Vol. I (1939): 32 + 420 p.; Vol. II (1943): In search of the Divine Centre, 442 p.; Vol. III (1944): The conflict of cultural ideals in the age of Plato, 374 p. (London: Oxford U.P.).—

There exist two German editions under the title: Paideia. Die Formung des griechischen Menschen, ed. 1, 1934; ed. 2, 1936. (Berlin: de Gruyter). Mainly of literary importance, for it tries to evaluate the educational function of literature. Vol. I deals with Archaic Greece from Homer to Pindar, and Athens of the fifth century B.C. Vol. II deals with Socrates and Plato; it chiefly contains an exposition of Plato's chief works. Vol. III deals mainly with the intellectual conflict between Plato and Isocrates, but also with Xenophon and Demosthenes. One chapter deals with "Greek medicine as Paideia".

JONES, W. H. S., 1909: Malaria and Greek history. To which is added: The history of Greek therapeutics and the malaria theory, by E. T. WITHINGTON, 175 p. (Manchester: U.P.).—

The view is put forward by the writer that malarial infection was the cause of the decadence of the Greeks. (After Garrison-Morton, No. 5263).

KIRK, G. S. & J. E. RAVEN, 1957: The pre-Socratic philosophers: a critical history with a selection of texts, 487 p. (Cambridge: U.P.).—

This book is primarily designed for those who have more than a casual interest in the history of early Greek thought. The text has been adapted to those students of the history of philosophy and science who have no previous acquaintance with this period. Each chapter has been built up with the aid of original texts (in Greek). The book is in 5 parts. The index gives some doxographical and chronological information. Part 2 considers the cosmogonical and cosmological speculations of Homer and Hesiod. Part 3 considers Thales, Anaximander, Anaximenes, Heraclitos and Xenophanes. Part 4 considers the Pythagorean and

Eleatic movements. Part 5 deals with Pythagoras, Alcmaeon, Parmenides, Zeno of Citium, Melissos, Philolaos, Empedocles, Anaxagoras, Archelaos, Leucippos, Democritos, and Diogenes of Apollonia.

KOPP, J. V., 1939: Das physikalische Weltbild der frühen griechischen Dichtung. Ein Beitrag zum Verständnis der vorsokratischen Physik, 333 p. (Diss. Univ. Fribourg, Switzerland) (Fribourg: Paulusdruckerei).—

An attempt to investigate the origin and the background of early Milesian thought, and to analyse the world picture held by the common people of those days. In the introduction, the author formulates his aim as follows: "Diese Untersuchung stellt sich also die Aufgabe in philologischer Einzelinterpretation das frühgriechische physikalische Weltbild, wie es Homer und Hesiod bieten und wie es in den homerischen Hymnen, in den Resten des Kyklos und in der Lyrik nachklingt und weiterentwickelt wird, zu untersuchen und darzustellen. Dabei ist unter 'Weltbild' alles zu verstehen, was diese Dichter in physikalischem Sinne über den Makrokosmos, über die Erde, den Himmel, die Unterwelt, die Gestirne und die atmosphärischen Erscheinungen geäussert haben. Das Ziel der Arbeit ist, die rationalen Ansätze in den genannten physikalischen Vorstellungen der Dichter aufzudecken."

LURIA, S., 1963: Anfänge griechischen Denkens, 158 p. (Berlin: Akademie Verlag).—

A popular introduction into the history of Greek science and philosophy in which much attention has been paid to the influence of still older scientific achievements, of magic, and of religion on the formation of Greek thought. This booklet has been planned as a general introduction to the philosophy of Democritos; therefore, those achievements which contributed to Democritos's philosophy have been presented in some detail (contrary to many other introductions which more or less can be considered as introductions to Socrates and Plato).

NESTLE, W., 1929: Die Vorsokratiker. Auswahl mit Einleitungen, ed. 3, 264 p. (Jena: Diederichs).—

After giving a general review of the beginnings of Greek philosophy in general, the author briefly describes some representatives of this period (p. 1-105). The second part of this book gives fragments from most of these authors in German translation. For our purpose only some of them are of interest, *e.g.,* those of Anaximander, Alcmaeon, Xenophanes, Heraclitos, Parmenides, Melissos, Empedocles, Anaxagoras, Philolaos, Leucippos, Democritos, and Protagoras. A somewhat comparable study is: HOWALD, E., 1949: Die Anfänge der abendländischen Philosophie. Fragmente und Lehrberichte der Vorsokratiker, 263 p. (Zurich: Artemis).

SARTON, G., 1952: A history of science: ancient science through the golden age of Greece, 2 vols., 646 p. (Cambridge, Mass.: Harvard U.P.).—

    The volumes of this History of science series (as to the other volumes of this series, *cf.* the index of our Guide), are based on the author's Harvard lectures on the history of science. They do not try to give a mere chronology of scientific discoveries but they deal particularly with the cultural background leading to man's acquisition of positive knowledge. This first volume is in three parts. The first part deals with Oriental and Greek origins (incl. Egypt, Mesopotamia, Aegean culture, Homer and Hesiod, Assyrian science, Ionian science, and Pythagoras). The second part deals with the 5th century B.C. (Graeco-Persian wars, philosophy and science to the death of Socrates: Heraclitos, Anaxagoras, Eleatics, Parmenides, Empedocles, Atomists, Sophists, Hippocratic Corpus). The third part deals with the 4th cent. B.C. (Plato and the Academy, Xenophon, Aristotle and the Lyceum, natural sciences and medicine in Aristotle's time, theories of life and of knowledge, Stoic science and philosophy). Roughly a third of the book is devoted to each of the three parts. Paperback edition, 1965, 646 p. (New York, N.Y.: Wiley).

SCHUHL, P. M., 1949: Essai sur la formation de la pensée grecque. Introduction historique à une étude de la philosophie platonicienne, ed. 2, 482 p. (Paris: Presses Univ. de France).—

    An essential part of the book deals with foreign influences on the formation of Greek philosophy, thus giving a social and psychological background. The author describes the medium of superstition and irrationalism out of which Greek philosophy originated, and tries to explain them by comparison with the folklore of other nations. He considers the religious evolution down to Homer and the beginnings of positivist thought of the Ionian "physiologists". He describes more or less mythical cults,

e.g., the Pythagorean cults, discusses *inter alia* Xenophanes, Heraclitos, Parmenides, Empedocles, the Sophists, and the last part of the book is devoted to Plato. Many valuable notes and an extensive bibliographical index (p. 391-464) have been included.

TANNERY, P., 1930: Pour l'histoire de la science hellène. De Thalès à Empédocle, 535 p. (Paris: Gauthier-Villars).—

    When in 1887 the original edition appeared (Paris: Alcan), it took a non-conformist position compared with current treatises on the history of philosophy. It consists of a series of monographs on: Thales (p. 54-83), Anaximander (p. 84-122), Xenophanes (p. 123-149), Anaximenes (p. 150-171), Heraclitos (p. 172-205), Alcmaeon (p. 206-224), Parmenides (p. 225-254), Zeno of Citium (p. 255-270), Melissos (p. 271-283), Anaxagoras (p. 284-312), Empedocles (p. 315-347). At the end of each monograph fragments in French translation have been added with references to DIELS's "Fragmente" and "Nachweise" *(vide supra).* There is a very good bibliography containing the literature up to 1930. *Cf.* BACCOU, R., 1951, *vide supra.*

b. History of the plant and animal sciences

BJÖRCK, G., 1932: Zum Corpus Hippiatricorum Graecorum. Beiträge zur antiken Tierheilkunde, 91 p. (Uppsala Univ. Årsskr., 1932, No. 5).—

    Mainly of philologic interest. Proves the interconnections between the Corpus Hippocraticus and Arabian hippological literature. Discussion of the veterinary works of Theomnestos, Eumelos, and Apsyrtos. *Cf.* also BJÖRCK, G., 1944, this section γ, subsection b.

BRETZL, H., 1903: Botanische Forschungen des Alexanderzuges, 412 p. (Leipzig: Teubner).—

    The campaign of Alexander the Great led to an increasing knowledge both of new plant-forms and of the physiognomy of new landscapes, especially of mangrove woods. This caused a revival of Ionian plant-geography, the results of which have been preserved in the work of the famous Greek plant-geographer Theophrastos, who based his studies on the collections which had been concentrated in Babylon. Stress is laid on the fact that Greek plant-geography can be successfully understood only by starting from the flora of the Eastern Mediterranean area, because the Greeks based their geographical studies on this flora. Reprint announced by Olms (Hildesheim). Another important study of the same subject is: JORET, C., 1904: Les recherches botaniques de l'expédition d'Alexandre, 113 p. (J. Savants, 1904: 498-611). *Cf.* also SENN's studies on Theophrastos (1933 and 1956), *vide* this section, subsection d.

ECKELS, R. P., 1937: Greek wolf-lore, 88 p. (Philadelphia, Pa.: Pennsylvania U.P.).—

The chapters are titled as follows: 1. The wolf in Greek zoology; 2. Greek superstitions about the wolf, and something of their later history; 3. The werwolf and "lycanthropy"; 4. The wolf in Greek religion; 5. The wolf-nurse. Topographical and name indexes. Most widely feared as the wild animal is, he became the embodiment of all that is hostile, malignant, and terrible in the natural world. The same position is held by the wolf in the folklore of European civilization in general.

GEURTS, P. M. M., 1941: De erfelijkheid in de oudere Griekse wetenschap, 214 p. (Nijmegen & Utrecht: Dekker & v. d. Vegt). —

This study tries to give an insight into the views held by old Greek philosophers about genetic problems. The text is divided into three parts: the inheritance of somatic characters, the heredity of the soul, and problems connected with constitution, race, and eugenics. *Cf.* also LESKY, E., 1950, *vide* section α, subsection b.

JARDÉ, A., 1925: Les céréales dans l'antiquité grecque. La production, 237 p. (Paris: Boccard).—

Many problems are here discussed, *e.g.,* the species of cereals used, their amelioration, selection, growth, yield, value; technical farm equipment and work on the fields; characteristics of climate and soil, crop rotation and distribution of the cultures; property of land, surface of the area cultivated, population density, commerce; *etc.* Good bibliography.

KOCH, K., 1884: Die Bäume und Sträucher des alten Griechenlands, ed. 2, 290 p. (Berlin: Jacobsthal).—

An attempt at reconstructing the flora of trees and shrubs as it must have been in ancient Greece. The first edition appeared in 1879 (Stuttgart: Enke).

MURR, J., 1890: Die Pflanzenwelt in der griechischen Mythologie, 324 p. (Innsbrück: Wagner).—

A book of the same scope as DIERBACH's (*cf.* section α, subsection b), *viz.,* an attempt to elucidate the interconnections between plants and mythology. Much more attention, however, has been paid to source references, and to plants with magical or medicinal properties. Reprinted 1969 (Groningen: Bouma).

PALM, A., 1933: Studien zur Hippokratischen Schrift περὶ διαίτης, 127 p. (Inaug. Diss. Tübingen).—

The present study can be divided into two totally different parts; the first part deals with the history of zoology, and the second part with the fourth chapter of "On diet" (sleep and dreams). As to the first part (p. 1-42): the author considers the history of Greek zoology before Aristotle as it can be found in "On diet" and other Hippocratic writings; animal systematics of Diocles of Carystos and of Philyllios, zoological knowledge of the old Ionian philosophers, of Homer, and of the sophists, and the role played by Greek medicine in zoological systematics. A general review of pre-Aristotelian zoology gives: JANSSENS, E., 1933: La zoologie pré-Aristotélienne. (Rev. Univ. Bruxelles 38: 371-376).

SIKES, E. E., 1914: The anthropology of the Greeks, 112 p. (London: Nutt).—

A study of the speculations entertained by the Greek philosophers about the origin and development of their own species, their meaning of race, their methodology, and the philosophical implications.

SINGER, C. J., 1922: Greek biology and Greek medicine, 128 p. (New York, N.Y. & London: Oxford U.P.).—

A very good introductory text. The first part deals with Greek biology, and is divided into three sections: 1. Before Aristotle (14 p.); 2. Aristotle (37 p.); 3. After Aristotle (25 p.). The last 50 pages are devoted to Greek medicine. *Cf.* TAYLOR, H. O., *ca.* 1923: Greek biology and medicine, 155 p. (London: Harrap). For more details, *vide* section α, subsection a.

SKUPAS, M., 1962: Altgriechische Tierkrankheitsnamen und ihre Deutungen, 71 p. (Inaug. Diss., tierärztl. Hochsch. Hannover).—

After a short introduction discussing

antiquity, origin, influence, and literature concerning ancient Greek veterinary terminology, the author discusses some 133 of these terms, in the same way as it has been done by Petrus Ruellius in his "Rei veterinariae nomenclatura" (1530), the oldest veterinary glossary known.

WENIGER, L., 1919: Altgriechischer Baumkultus, 64 p. (Das Erbe der Alten, N. F., H. 2) (Leipzig: Dieterich).—

> The author writes in his preface: "Das altheilige Kranzeslaub der Hellenen steht als Sinnbild feinster Gedanken noch heut in Ehren. Aber nur wenige sind sich dessen bewusst, wie es zu solcher Auszeichnung gelangt ist. In der folgenden Darstellung wird der Versuch gemacht, dies an den edelsten dieser Pflanzensymbole, Eichenlaub, Lorbeer, wilder und zahmer Olive, nachzuweisen." Cf. BÖTTICHER, C., 1856, vide section α, subsection b.

c. History of the medical sciences

KUDLIEN, F., 1967: Der Beginn des medizinischen Denkens bei den Griechen. Von Homer bis Hippokrates, 174 p. (Zurich: Artemis).—

> An introduction to early Greek medicine from 8th-5th century B.C. The author is primarily interested in the irrational, prescientific elements of early Greek medicine, physiology, anatomy, pharmacology, and pathology. Separate chapters deal with: the physician-patient relationship, the emergence of medicine as an autonomous *techne,* the relationship of medicine to surgery, early concepts of disease and treatment. Interesting summary and index of names. The Greek quotations are accompanied by German translations.

MOLLET, M., 1906: La médecine chez les Grecs avant Hippocrate, 292 p. (Paris: Maloine).—

> After a general introduction considering the Greek gods of medicine, the author considers the medicine of Homer, Hesiod, the cult of Asclepios, religious medicine, the schools of Cos, Cnidos, and Rhodes, medicine and the Greek philosophers: Pythagoras, Democedes, Heraclitos, Anaxagoras, Empedocles, Hippon, Acron, Diogenes of Apollonia, Philistion, Democritos, and some others.

PANAYOTATOU, A. G., 1923: L'hygiène chez les anciens Grecs, 286 p. (Paris: Vigot).

> With the aid of quotations from the classic authors, Panayotatou gives a picture

of hygiene among the ancient Greeks. Included are such aspects as bath-houses, music, gymnastics, diet, and morals.

PRECOPE, J., 1961: Iatrophilosophers of the Hellenic states, 313 p. (London: Heinemann).—

> This book considers the lives and works of those philosophers who have shown a great interest in medicine. The interaction between medicine and philosophy has been made particularly clear. The author deals with priest-physicians (incl. Linus, Orpheus, Asclepios), wise men (Epimenides of Crete, Solon), physicists (incl. Thales, Anaximander, Anaximenes, Pythagoras, Alcmaeon, Xenophanes, Diogenes of Apollonia, Leucippos, Democritos), and sophists (incl. Protagoras, Gorgias, Socrates, Plato, Aristotle). The text is documented by numerous quotations.

SCHUMACHER, J., 1963: Antike Medizin. Die naturphilosophischen Grundlagen der Medizin in der griechischen Antike, ed. 2, 327 p. (Berlin: de Gruyter).—

> Separate sections deal with: the meaning of Greek science for the development of science in the West, philosophy and medicine, micro- and macrocosmos, teleology; Old-Ionian philosophy: Thales, Anaximander, Anaximenes; Pythagoras and the Pythagoreans, his doctrine of numbers, medicine, health, disease and therapy in Pythagorean philosophy; Alcmaeon, Ikkos of Tarentum, Herodikos of Selymbria; Heraclitos, his theory of the elements, his doctrine of contradiction, the healing power of nature; the Eleatics, Melissos and medicine; Empedocles and Anaxagoras, medicine, physiology, disease and healing; atomists: Leucippos and Democritos; Diogenes of Apollonia; the Corpus Hippocraticum (p. 177-211); Plato, his teleology and his ideas on medicine, health and disease, therapy, and physiology. Bibliography and indexes of names and subjects.

———, 1965: Die Anfänge abendländischer Medizin in der griechischen Antike, 160 p. (Urban-Bücher, No. 84) (Stuttgart: Kohlhammer).—

> After a general philosophical introduction, the author shows how the ideas expressed by Thales, Anaximander, Anaximenes, the Pythagoreans, Eleates, Heraclitos, Empedocles, Anaxagoras, Leucippos, and Democritos find their highest expression in the Corpus Hippocraticum.

WELLMANN, M., 1901: Die Fragmente der

sikelischen Aerzte Akron, Philistion und des Diokles von Karystos, 254 p. (Berlin: Weidmann).—

The book starts with a general introduction and the author assesses the connections of Acron (a pupil of Alcmaeon), Philistion (a contemporary of Plato) and Diocles (a famous physician living after Hippocrates) with the Corpus Hippocraticum. A chapter (p. 94-107) has been devoted to the peri kardiès. Fragments from Acron of Agrigentum are given on p. 108-109; from Philistion of Locroi on p. 109-116; from Diocles of Carystos on p. 117-207. The vindiciani fragmentum (cod. Bruxellensis n. 1342-50 fol. 48 ff) has been added. Numerous footnotes elucidate the text.

c* *Hippocratic medicine*

ADAM, F., ed., 1946: The genuine works of Hippocrates. Translated from the Greek, 374 p. (Baltimore, Md.: Williams & Wilkins).—

Contains English translations of: The oath, Ancient medicine, Airs, waters and places, Prognostics, Regimen in acute diseases, The epidemics, Injuries of the head, Surgery, Fractures, Articulations, Mochlicus, Aphorisms, The law, Ulcers, Fistulae, Haemorrhoids, and On the sacred disease.

ALEXANDERSON, B., 1963: Die hippokratische Schrift Prognostikon. Ueberlieferung und Text, 250 p. (Göteborg: Elander).—

According to a review of O. Temkin in Amer. J. Philology 87: 250-251, the Prognostic is one of the most important books of the Hippocratic Corpus. It has influenced many other books of the Corpus, but it also has had a great influence on Celsus, Galen, and Stephanos. The present study elucidates the textual history; the author has prepared a new edition of the Greek text, based on the existing mss., which, according to Temkin, is likely to supersede its predecessors, from which it differs in a great many instances.

BOURGEY, L., 1953: Observation et expérience chez les médecins de la collection hippocratique, 304 p. (Paris: Vrin).—

A very useful study based on Littré's Collection hippocratique *(vide infra),* with many quotations and a useful index. In a review of this book, Louis Millet writes (in Rev. Hist. Sci. 7: 189-190): "M. Bourgey nous présente le résultat de ses lectures et de ses méditations des 10 tomes de l'édition Littré ... L'idée directrice de l'auteur est la saisie d'une distinction de trois courants à l'intérieur de cette collection: une tendance théoricienne (iatrosophistes et médecins théoriciens), une tendance empiriste (école de Cnide) et une tendance qu'il nomme tantôt 'positive', tantôt 'rationelle' (école de Cos proprement dite). C'est donc à une synthèse des travaux particuliers consacrés surtout depuis une cinquantaine d'années aux différents livres ou aux différents aspects de la 'Collection' que M. Bourgey nous convie."

CAPELLE, W., ed., 1955: Hippokrates. Fünf auserlesene Schriften, 238 p. (Zurich: Artemis).—

After a long introduction, reviewing life and work of Hippocrates, translations in the German language have been given from: On the sacred disease; Airs, waters, and places; Prognostics; Epidemics I and III; The oath. The sections are preceded by a short introduction. Notes (p. 215-236) and a selective bibliography have been added. (Also as paperback: Frankfurt a.M.: Fischer, 1959, 196 p.).

CHADWICK, J. & W. N. MANN, eds., 1950: The medical works of Hippocrates: a new translation from the original Greek made especially for the English readers, 301 p. (Oxford: Blackwell).—

This volume gives new English translations of: The oath; Epidemics I and III; Coan prognosis; Diet in acute diseases; On the sacred disease and The aphorisms. The book is especially intended for students of medicine. Good index. A French translation of The aphorisms is: DAREMBERG, C. V., ed., 1961: Les aphorismes d'Hippocrate, 188 p. (Paris: Le Livre Club du Libraire); a German translation is: MENKE, F. A., 1844: Die Aphorismen des Hippocrates. Reprinted by A. Lorentz (Leipzig, 1931).

DEICHGRÄBER, K., 1933: Die Epidemien und das Corpus Hippocraticum. Voruntersuchungen zu einer Geschichte der Koischen Aerzteschule, 172 p. (Abh. preuss. Akad. Wiss., Phil.-Hist. Kl., 1933, No. 3) (Berlin: de Gruyter).—

A thorough analysis of the Hippocratic book On epidemics.

——, ed., 1935: Ueber Entstehung und Aufbau des menschlichen Körpers, 97 p. (Leipzig & Berlin: Teubner).—

The text has been divided into three parts. The first part (p. 1-23) contains the Greek text with the German translation on facing pages; the second part (p. 24-63) contains a general introduction to this work, an explanation of the different chapters, and an evaluation of this work in the light of modern medicine. The third part (by E. SCHWYZER) is exclusively of a philological interest.

DIERBACH, J. H., 1824: Die Arzneimittel des Hippokrates; oder Versuch einer systematischen Aufzählung der in allen hippokratischen Schriften vorkommenden Medikamente, 270 p. (Heidelberg: Groos).—

> As far as the editor is aware, by far the most complete survey of drugs in the Hippocratic collection, written by a competent botanist. Very good indexes. Reprinted 1969 (Hildesheim: Olms).

DILLER, H., ed., 1962: Hippocrates' Schriften. Die Anfänge der abendländischen Medizin, 277 p. (Reinbek/Hamburg: Rowohlt).—

> A pocket edition, containing full German translations of: The oath; Epidemics I and III; Prognostics; The physician; The law; Airs, waters and places; On the sacred disease; On breaths; The art; On ancient medicine. It contains German translations of some parts of: On fractures of bones; On internal ailments; Aphorisms; On the nature of man; On diet I and IV. Each text is preceded by a special introduction in which its characteristics are outlined.

EDELSTEIN, L., 1931: περι αὲϛων und die Sammlung der hippokratischen Schriften, 188 p. (Berlin: Weidmann).—

> In the first chapter the author analyses construction, meaning, etc., of this work, and according to the author it appears to belong to the prognostic works of the Corpus. In a second chapter the author explains this. A third chapter deals with the position of the Hippocratic physician in general and with his work as a surgeon, dietist, etc., in particular. In a final chapter the author tries to explain the literary position of this work in which the role played by Alexandrian and Roman philologists has been elucidated; this chapter is mainly of philological interest.

——, ed., 1943: The hippocratic oath: text, translation and interpretation, 64 p. (Supplements to the Bull. Hist. Med., No. 1) (Baltimore, Md.: Johns Hopkins Press).—

> Edelstein concludes that The oath was not composed before the 4th century

B.C., and that all the doctrines followed in the treatise are characteristic of Pythagoreanism. Although this oath became the nucleus of all medical ethics in all countries (or epochs) in which monotheism was the accepted creed, this oath - according to the author - can nevertheless not be considered to be the expression of an absolute standard of medical conduct. An older English edition of The oath is: JONES, W. H. S., 1924: The doctor's oath, 62 p. (Cambridge: U.P.); this publication contains the text of the Hippocratic oath and of Christian and Arabic versions, together with a full discussion.

ELLINGER, T. U. H., ed., 1952: Hippocrates on intercourse and pregnancy: an English translation of "On semen" and "On the development of the child", 128 p. (New York, N.Y.: Schuman).—

> Although not written by Hippocrates himself, both treatises present an interesting interpretation of medical knowledge of the 5th century B.C. Among the topics considered are: some aspects of the physiology of reproduction, heredity, embryology, sex determination, the connection between the reproductive tract and the central nervous system, and the causation of foetal abnormalities.

FASBENDER, H., 1897: Entwicklungslehre, Geburtshülfe und Gynäkologie in den hippokratischen Schriften. Eine kritische Studie, 300 p. (Stuttgart: Enke).—

> The classic book on Hippocratic gynaecology and obstetrics. The first part deals with Hippocratic medicine in general and the author tries to elucidate the older sources (Egyptian, Hebraic and/or Indian) which served as the basis for Hippocrates's knowledge of embryology, obstetrics and gynaecology (p. 1-70). Then an evaluation follows of Greek anatomical knowledge of the female genital organs, and of the physiology and pathology of pregnancy, (symptoms, diagnosis, sex of the foetus, etc.), the physiology and pathology of birth (incl. midwives, twins, position of the foetus) (p. 71-174). Other sections deal with obstetrics (incl. the instruments used), with physiology and pathology of childbirth (p. 175-210) and with gynaecology in the Hippocratic writings (menstruation, fecundity, diseases of the genital organs, etc.). Cf. BUCHHEIM, E., 1916: Die geburtshilflichen Operationen und zugehörigen Instrumente des klassischen Altertums, 46 p. (Jena: Fischer).

FESTUGIÈRE, A. J., ed., 1948: Hippocrate. L'ancienne médecine, 34 + 85 p. (Paris: Klincksieck).—

In his introduction, the editor gives a short review of Greek medicine in general and of the contents of "On ancient medicine" in particular, especially stressing the causes of the diseases mentioned in it (p. vii - xxxiv). Then the text follows both in the original Greek version (22 p.) and in French translation (22 p.) on pages opposite each other. A long series of notes and commentaries (48 p.) follows.

FUCHS, R., ed., 1895-1900: Hippokrates. Sämtliche Werke. Ins Deutsche übersetzt und ausführlich commentiert, 3 vols., 526 + 604 + 660 p. (Munich: Hippocrates Verlag).—

Vol. I contains German translations of the works concerning anatomy and physiology, dietetics, general pathology, and prognostics; Vol. II the works concerning special pathology and the Coan prognosis; Vol. III the works concerning therapeutics, surgery, ophthalmology and gynaecology.

GOMPERZ, T., 1910: Die Apologie der Heilkunst. Eine griechische Sophistenrede des 5. vorchristlichen Jahrhunderts, ed. 2, 182 p. (Leipzig: Veit).—

Gomperz shows that the author of "The art" was not a physician, and that this treatise is unique as an extant example of a speech by a sophist of the best period.

GRENSEMANN, H., 1968: Die hippokratische Schrift "Ueber die heilige Krankheit", 126 p. (Ars medica, II. Abt., Vol. 1) (Berlin: de Gruyter).—

A thorough study of this Hippocratic treatise. The book consists of the Greek text and a newly prepared German translation, preceded by an introduction, discussing the sources, various codices and the text of the book, and followed by valuable annotations.

JOLY, R., 1960: Recherches sur le traité pseudo-hippocratique du régime, 260 p. (Bibliothèque fac. philos. et lettres l'Univ. Liège, fasc. 156) (Paris: Les Belles Lettres).—

The author considers the history of the dietetic tradition in ancient medicine and particularly the role played by the "De

Virtu". This is considered to be the first treatise on preventive medicine and its scientific foundation lies in the concept of prodiagnosis (i.e., early recognition of an oncoming disease). The author assumes that its philosophical foundations can be derived from the fragments of Anaxagoras, and he elucidates the connexions with pre-Socratic speculation and Hippocratic tradition. The difference between this notion prodiagnosis and the diagnostic techniques employed in the hippocratic treatises are discussed in detail.

——, 1966: Le niveau de la science hippocratique. Contribution à la psychologie de l'histoire des sciences, 248 p. (Paris: Les Belles Lettres).—

After a general introduction (p. 1-69), French translations follow of parts of Diseases IV, Diet, Ancient medicine, The nature of Man, Airs, waters and places, On the sacred disease, The epidemics, Prognostics, On fractures. Cf. also JOLY, R., 1964: Hippocrate. Médecin grecque, 250 p. (Paris: Gallimard).

JONES, W. H. S., 1945: Hippocrates and the Corpus Hippocraticum, 23 p. (London: Oxford U.P.).—

The main thesis of the author is that no generally acceptable hypothesis with regard to the authorship of the Corpus can be deduced. This conclusion has been based on a discussion of the references to Hippocrates, from Plato to Galen.

——, 1946: Philosophy and medicine in ancient Greece: with an edition of περι ἀρχαίης ἰῆρίκῆς , 100 p. (Bull. Hist. Med., Suppl. VIII) (Baltimore, Md.: Johns Hopkins Press).—

In the first section (p. 1-25) the author points out the unique position of Alcmaeon in the history of thought; besides there are short essays on the Pythagoreans, the Work Sevens, the Sicilian School, Anaxagoras, Plato and the Hippocratic Corpus. Section II deals with hypothesis in Greek thought and philosophy and medical etiquette. Section III presents an introduction to "On ancient medicine", an edition of the Greek text, based on 2 eleventh-century mss., followed by a complete translation with commentaries. A thorough analysis of "On ancient medicine" in which the contents of this Hippocratic treatise are correlated with other literary achievements of the period, medical as well as non-medical, is: KÜHN, J. H., 1956: System- und Methodenprobleme im Corpus Hippocraticum, 160 p. (Hermes, Einzelschriften, H. 11) (Wiesbaden: Steiner).

——, ed., 1948-1952: Hippocrates, 4 vols. Vol. I (1948): 70 + 362 p.; Vol. II (1952): 66 + 336 p.; Vol. III (1948): 455 p.; Vol. IV (1953): 49 + 519 p. (Loeb Classical Library) (London: Heinemann; New York, N.Y.: Putnam).—

> The introduction to Vol. I contains a summary of our present Hippocratic knowledge. Each text is printed both in Greek and in English translation and is preceded by a special introduction wherein its characteristics are outlined and previous editions and translations are cited. Volume I contains the following texts: On ancient medicine; Airs, waters, places; Epidemics I and III; The oath; Precepts; Nutriment. Vol II contains: Prognostic; Regimen in acute diseases; On the sacred disease; The art; Breaths; Law; Decorum; Physician (ch. 1); Dentition. Vol. III (translations by E. T. WITHINGTON) contains: On wounds in the head; In the surgery; Fractures; Joints; Mochlicon. Vol. IV contains: Nature of Man; Regimen in health; Humours; Aphorisms; Regimen I, II, III; Dreams; and of Heraclitos: On the Universe (p. 449-509). A text especially dealing with dentistry is: RECH, W., 1920: Zahnärztliches aus dem hippokratischen Schriftenkorpus, 62 p. (Diss. Univ. Leipzig).

KAPFERER, R., 1951: Die anatomischen Schriften. Die Anatomie, das Herz, die Adern in der hippokratischen Sammlung, 55 p. (Suttgart: Hippokrates).—

> The most thorough study of Hippocratic anatomy. The author rearranged existing fragments of On anatomy, On the heart, and On the nature of bones. Based on the new arrangement of the texts, he believes that the Hippocratic physicians had some notion of a circulatory motion of the blood. Anyway the author tries to make clear that Hippocratic writers knew more about the vascular system than is commonly believed.

LITTRÉ, E., ed., 1961-1962: Oeuvres complètes d'Hippocrate. Traduction nouvelle avec le texte grec en regard collationné sur les manuscrits et toutes les éditions; accompagnée d'une introduction, de commentaires médicaux, de variantes et de notes philologiques; suivi d'une table générale des matières, 10 vols. Vol. I: 638 p.; Vol. II: 41 +

720 p.; Vol. III: 46 + 564 p.; Vol. IV: 672 p.; Vol. V: 736 p.; Vol. VI: 664 p.; Vol. VII: 61 + 616 p.; Vol. VIII: 40 + 676 p.; Vol. IX: 468 p.; Vol. X: 80 + 348 p. (Amsterdam: Hakkert).—

> This is the only complete French translation of the Hippocratic collection, and one of the most famous. The book gives the Greek text and French translations on pages facing each other. Each chapter is preceded by a special introduction wherein its characteristics are outlined. Vol. I contains a general introduction in which are discussed *inter alia:* Greek medicine before Hippocrates, his biography, the composition, chronology, transmission, editions, *etc.,* of the different parts of the collection, together with the text of On ancient medicine. Vol. II contains the texts of: Airs, waters, and places; Prognostics; Regimen in acute diseases with an appendix containing a collection of annotations both in the original Greek and in French translation; Epidemics I. Vol. III contains Epidemics III; On the wounds of the head; In the surgery; On fractures. Vol. IV contains: On joints; Instruments of reduction; Aphorisms; The oath; The law. Vol. V contains Epidemics II, IV, V, VI and VII; On humours; Prorrhetic I; Coan prenotions. Vol. VI contains: The art; On the nature of Man; On diet in acute diseases; On breaths; On the use of liquids; On diseases I; On ailments; On places in Man; On the sacred disease; The haemorrhoids; On fistulae; On diet I, II, III and IV. Vol. VII contains Diseases II and III; On internal ailments; On Cnidian medicine; On the nature of women; On the seven-months embryo; On the eight-months embryo; On generation; On the nature of the child; Diseases IV. Vol. VIII contains On women's diseases I and II; On sterile women (= On Women's diseases III); On the diseases of maidens; On superfoetation; On excision of the embryo; On anatomy; On dentition; On glands; On flesh; On periods of seven days. Vol. IX contains Prorrhetic II; On the heart; On nutriment; On vision; On the nature of bones; The physician; Decorum; Precepts; On crisis; On critical days; Letters; and a new text of "On periods of seven days", published and commented upon by Ch. DAREMBERG. Vol. X contains tables. There also exists a German translation of the Hippocratic collection, *viz.,* KAPFERER, R., 1933-1940: Die Werke des Hippokrates. Die hippokratische Schriftsammlung in neuer deutscher Uebersetzung. Unter Mitwirkung von G. STICKER, *et al.,* 5 vols. (Stuttgart: Hippokrates). German translations of the most important sections of this work are to be found in: KAPFERER, R., 1943: Hippokrates-Fibel. Auszüge aus der Schriftensammlung

"Die Werke des Hippokrates", 355 p. (Stuttgart: Hippokrates).

MICHLER, M., 1963: Die Klumpfusslehre der Hippokratiker. Eine Untersuchung von De articulis cap. 62, mit Uebersetzung des Textes und des galenischen Kommentars, 64 p. (Sudhoffs Arch. Gesch. Med. Naturw., Beiheft 2) (Wiesbaden: Steiner).—

The text contains a German translation of that part of the "De articulis" that deals with club-foot, and a German translation of Galen's commentary upon this part of the text. Separate chapters deal with practical treatment of club-foot (p. 17-41) and with theoretical interpretations (e.g., the problems of localization, causation, and of malformation in general, p. 42-56). The book includes a glossary of Greek technical terms, both Hippocratic and Galenic, and a list of sources from Aristophanes to Xenophon. Many footnotes and references.

MOON, R. O., 1923: Hippocrates and his successors in relation to the philosophy of their time, 171 p. (London: Longmans, Green).—

This booklet contains the text of a series of the 4 Fitzpatrick lectures. It is an attempt to conjure up the philosophic milieu in which Hippocrates lived and in which the medical schools immediately succeeding him flourished.

PETERSEN, W. F., 1946: Hippocratic wisdom: a modern appreciation of ancient scientific achievement, 263 p. (Springfield, Ill.: Thomas).—

A commentary on the Hippocratic texts written for young physicians and for medical students. After a general introduction, emphasizing the influence of the seasons, the author discusses Hippocrates's ideas concerning anoxia, reproduction, epilepsy, hydrophobia, the medical clinic (pneumonia, pleurisy, empyema, phthisis, the surgical treatment: the art, the skull, fractures and dislocations), and Hippocratic theory (the cosmic concept, the unstable equilibrium). An important part of the study is the "Notes and references" (p. 175-241). Glossary and index.

PÉTREQUIN, J. E., ed., 1877-1878: Chirurgie d'Hippocrate, avec des commentaires, notes et traductions, 2 vols. Vol. I: 565 p.; Vol. II: 651 p. (Paris: Imprimerie Nationale).—

In these volumes the following Hippocratic writings are considered: Vol. I: The oath (p. 171-198); The physician (p. 199-256); On ulcers (p. 257-328); On haemorrhoids and On fistulae (p. 329-412); On injuries of the head. Vol. II: In the surgery (p. 1-84); On fractures (p. 85-274); On the articulations (p. 275-548); Mochlicus (p. 549-635). Vol. I contains a long introduction (p. 1-170); and of each of the Hippocratic writings considered is given: the original Greek text, a French translation (both with extensive notes), a general introduction, and a commentary. A publication which I know only by title, but which might contain supplementary information is: ZERVOS, S., 1932: Les bistouris, les sondes et les curettes chirurgicales d'Hippocrate, 63 p. (Livre d'or du Dr. Théodore L. Papayoannou) (Naumburg: Lippert).

POHLENZ, M., 1938: Hippocrates und die Begründung der wissenschaftlichen Medizin, 120 p. (Berlin: de Gruyter).—

This book contains an analysis of Hippocrates's "Airs, waters, and places", esp. chapters 1-24, and of his On the sacred disease. After this analysis the author tries to reconstruct the personality of Hippocrates, his scientific influence, and his position as founder of scientific medicine. An authoritative German translation of Airs, waters, and places is: JACOBJ, G., 1930: Das goldene Buch des Hippocrates. Eine medizinische Geographie aus dem Altertum, 75 p. (Stuttgart: Orient-Occident Verlag).

ROSCHER, W. H., 1913: Die hippokratische Schrift von der Siebenzahl in ihrer vierfachen Ueberlieferung, 187 p. (Studien zur Geschichte und Kultur des Altertums VI, H. 3/4) (Paderborn: Schöningh).—

The number seven played an important role in the thinking of ancient peoples and of various medical schools. The present work deals with a treatise of the Hippocratic collection especially devoted to this subject. It was believed, for example, that children born in the seventh month survived; women menstruated at intervals of four times seven days; the child was born after seven times forty days, etc.

WELLMANN, M., 1931: Hippokratesglossare, 88 p. (Quell. u. Stud. Gesch. Naturw. u. Med., No. 2) (Berlin: Springer).—

A historical analysis. The first who wrote a collection of glosses on Hippocrates was Bakcheios (ca. 200 B.C.). These glosses were used by Lysimachos of Cos. According to the thesis of the author, the editor of the (incomplete) extant text, Erotianos, physician during Nero's reign, has made use of these glosses of Lysimachos together with the works of Antigonos the Grammarian, Tiberius, Artemidoros of Tarsus, and Sextius Niger.

d. Some individual philosophers and scientists

Anaxagoras of Clazomenae *(ca.* 499 - *ca.* 428 B.C.) — CLEVE, F. M., 1949: The philosophy of Anaxagoras: an attempt at reconstruction, 167 p. (New York, N.Y.: Kings Crown Press, Columbia Univ.).—

Basing his results on thirty years' research, the author tries "to construct a philosophic building in such a way that all the authentic material handed down can be fitted in." Of special importance for our purpose are p. 77-122 dealing with such topics as: the problem of generation, the meaning of the psyche, human perception, nutrition and digestion, sleep and death, the conscious and unconscious (in plants, animals and man). The last chapter deals with Anaxagoras's influence on Aristotle.

Anaximander of Miletos *(ca.* 610 - *ca.* 545 B.C.) — KAHN, C. H., 1960: Anaximander and the origins of Greek cosmology, 250 p. (New York, N.Y.: Columbia U.P.).—

It is the intention of the author to make clear that Anaximander created a Milesian cosmic world-picture which in essence was accepted by many subsequent pre-Socratic thinkers. Another study which seeks to establish Anaximanders' cosmology in Greek mythology is: SELIGMAN, P., 1962: The apeiron of Anaximander: a study in the origin and function of metaphysical ideas, 181 p. (London: Athlone Press).

ARISTOTLE (384 - *ca.* 322 B.C.). A series of volumes published in the Loeb Classical Library, 1937-1965. (London: Heinemann; Cambridge, Mass.: Harvard U.P.).—

All booklets of this series contain the original Greek text together with an authorized English translation on the opposite page, and many annotations. Those texts which are of great value to the history of biology are: a) Generation of animals (ed. by A. L. PECK, 608 p., supplied with a very clear introduction written by the translator, p. v - lxxviii); b) On the soul (ed. by W. S.

HETT, p. 1-203); Parva naturalia (ed. by W. S. HETT, p. 205-482); On breath (ed. by W. S. HETT, p. 483-517) (the part Parva naturalia deals with problems such as those of sense and sensation; memory, sleeping, waking and dreams; youth, old age, life and death; respiration), c) Parts of animals (ed. by A. L. PECK, p. 52- 433); Movements of animals (ed. by E. S. FORSTER, p. 440-480; Progression of animals (ed. by E. S. FORSTER, p. 484-541, with introductions and indexes); d) Minor works (containing *inter alia* the following chapters: On colours (p. 1-46); On things heard (p. 47-80); Physionomics (p. 81-138); On plants (p. 139-234); On marvellous things heard (p. 235-326); e) Historia animalium (ed. by A. L. PECK, 239 p.). In the long preface preceding the text and translation, the editor examines the question of what scheme of classification may underlie this "factual survey", and he discusses some terminological problems. Valuable French translations are: Les parties des animaux, ed. by P. LOUIS, 1956, 40 + 194 p. (Paris: Les Belles Lettres); De la génération des animaux, ed. by P. LOUIS, 1961, 233 p. (Paris: Les Belles Lettres); Histoire des animaux, vol. I: Livres I-IV, ed. by P. LOUIS, 1964, 343 p. (Paris: Les Belles Lettres); Histoire des animaux, ed. by J. TRICOT, 1957, 2 vols. (Paris: Vrin).

——, ALLEN, D. J., 1952: The philosophy of Aristotle, 220 p. (London: Oxford U.P.).—

A very useful introduction to the logic and philosophy of Aristotle. The book is in five parts. The first part, p. 1-30, deals with the life of Aristotle, the literary problem, and his criticism of the Platonists. The second part, p. 31-100, deals with the general principles of physics, the heavens and the unmoved mover, the sublunary region, soul and mind, Man and the lower animals. The third part, p. 101-124, deals with the idea of substance and with the divine mind. The fourth part, p. 125-162, deals with his formal logic, and contains a survey of Aristotle's theory of knowledge. The fifth and last part, p. 163-210, deals with his ethics, politic, and rhetoric. *Cf.* also: DÜRING, I., 1966: Aristoteles. Darstellung und Interpretation seines Denkens, 670 p. (Heidelberg: Winter).

——, BALSS, H., 1943: Aristoteles biologische Schriften. Griechisch und deutsch, 301 p. (Munich: Heimeran).—

A discussion of Aristotle's views on biology, illustrated by fragments which are given both in Greek and in German translation. Separate sections deal with: fundamental ideas in the study of nature, introduction to natural history, classification of animals, form and function of organs, how the animals live, soul and life, generation and growth, the state as an organism.

——, FLASHAR, H., 1962: Aristoteles: Problemata physica, 766 p. (In: GRUMACH, E., ed., Aristoteles Werke in deutscher Uebersetzung, Vol. 19) (Berlin: Akademie Verlag).——

The text consists of some 38 treatises in German translation (p. 7-292) and a great many annotations (the rest of the book). Some of the texts included which are of special interest to us may be given (in German translation): Was medizinische Fragen betrifft; Was den Schweiss betrifft; Was Weintrinken und den Rausch betrifft; Was den Geschlechtsverkehr betrifft; Was die Ermüdung betrifft; Was blutunterlaufene Stellen, Narben und Striemen betrifft; Was die Stimme betrifft; Was wohlriechende Dinge betrifft; Was übelriechende Dinge betrifft; Was beseelte (Gegenstände) betrifft; Was Sträucher und Kräutergewächse betrifft; Was Gerstenmehl, Gerstenbrot und dergleichen betrifft; Was das Obst betrifft; Was das Salzwasser und Meer betrifft; Was die Augen betrifft; Was die Ohren betrifft; Was die Nase betrifft; Was den Mund betrifft und das, was in ihm ist; Was das Gesicht betrifft; Was den ganzen Körper betrifft; Was die Hautfarbe betrifft.

——, GREENE, M., 1963: A portrait of Aristotle, 271 p. (Chicago, Ill.: Chicago U.P.).——

Aristotle is portrayed primarily as a biologist, and against this background his other works are discussed and connections have been constructed between Aristotle and Plato, Hume, the mechanistic systems of post-Renaissance thought, modern existentialism, and other trends and developments of the modern period.

——, JAEGER, W., 1934: Aristotle: fundamentals of the history of his development, 410 p. (Oxford: Clarendon Press).——

An attempt to show how Aristotle's philosophical ideas possessed the power of creating sciences. The central point of this philosophy is the concept of form, which concept developed gradually and this development was of ultimate influence to biology. This book is an English translation of JAEGER's: Aristoteles. Grundlegung einer Geschichte seiner Entwicklung, 1923, to which a number of annotations, additions,

etc. have been added. In 1955 a second (German) edition appeared, 446 p. (Berlin: Weidemann) in which the annotations, additions, etc., of the English translation have been included.

——, KALTHOFF, P., 1934: Das Gesundheitswesen bei Aristoteles, 372 p. (Berlin & Bonn: Dümmler).——

The rich contents of this book may be illustrated by the headings of the separate chapters which are as follows: 1. Forschung, allgemeine Anschauungen, Methodik; 2. Gesundheitsverwaltung, Statistik, Rechtsauffassung in medizinischen Dingen; 3. Soziale Hygiene (Unfall, Invalidität, Gewerbeschäden, Schädlingsbekämpfung usw.); 4. Leibesübungen und Lebensweise; 5. Wohnung und Hauseinrichtungen; 6. Kleidung; 7. Nahrung; 8. Die Milch; 9. Der Alkohol; 10. Kulturpflanzen und Zuchttiere; 11. Abfallstoffe; 12. Leichen; 13. Klima; 14. Die Luft; 15. Das Wasser; 16. Der Boden; 17. Ansteckenden Krankheiten; 18. Hautkrankheiten; 19. Krankheitsübertrager; 20. Krankheitserreger, Parasiten; 21. Fäulnis, Gärung, Mikroorganismen; 22. Konservierung, Desinfektion; 23. Anatomie, Entwicklungsgeschichte, Vererbungslehre; 24. Normale und pathologische Physiologie; 25. Pathologie; 26. Chirurgie; 27. Sexualität und Gesundheit; 28. Innere Medizin; 29. Innere Sekretion; 30. Psychiatrie; 31. Diagnostik; 32. Therapie und Prophylaxe; 33. Medizinisch bedeutsame Pflanzen und Tiere; 34. Hygienisch und medizinisch bedeutsame Kulturprodukte.

——, MANQUAT, M., 1932: Aristote naturaliste, 128 p. (Paris: Vrin).——

Chapter 1 contains biographical information, ch. 2 contains a French translation of the text of the history of animals. Other chapters deal with the area the fauna of which was studied by Aristotle, with Aristotle's sources: poets, philosophers, physicians, Herodotos, fishermen, hunters, veterinarians, apiculturists, stock- breeders, shepherds, artisans, travellers, with his personal works, his zoological resources, and with his methodology they contain some interesting details of his history of animals.

——, RANDALL, J. H., 1960: Aristotle, 309 p. (New York, N.Y.: Columbia U.P.).——

A rather popular and yet very sound introduction to the philosophy and scientific achievements of Aristotle. The problems are elucidated from a modern philosophical outlook, and attention is drawn to the role Aristotle played and still plays in the development of philosophy. This does not mean, however, that Aristotle is presented from a preconceived philosophical point of view. A clear explanation of the Aristotelian philosophy is given.

——, ROSS, W. D., 1959: Aristotle: a complete exposition of his works and thought, ed. 5, 320 p. (New York, N.Y.: Meridian Bks.).——

> This book deals with the life and works of Aristotle, his logic, philosophy of nature, biology, psychology, metaphysics, ethics, politics, rhetoric and poetics. Bibliography, chronology of the Peripatetic School, and index. This is a reprint of the 5th ed. (1949); ed. 1, 1923. Also in French translation: Aristote, 1930, 420 p. (Paris: Payot). It is an extract of Ross's classical work: ROSS, W. D., ed., 1909-1931: Aristotle: works in English translation, 11 vols. (London: Oxford U.P.).

——, SUNDEVALL, C. J., 1863: Die Thierarten des Aristoteles von den Klassen der Säugethiere, Vögel, Reptilien und Insekten, 242 p. (Stockholm: Samson & Wallin).——

> After a historical and general introduction (p. 1-38) an enumeration follows of the animals known to Aristotle and the places where they are discussed in Aristotle's works. They are considered in a special part: I. Mammals (p. 38-92: apes, bats, carnivores, rodents, bestiolae, ungulates, whales, fabulous mammals); II. Birds (p. 92-173: birds of prey, song-birds, crows, parrots, doves and fowl, stilt-walkers, ducks and geese); III. Reptiles (p. 173-188, incl. the amphibians); IV. Insects (p. 189-241). *Cf.* also: STEIER, A., 1913, *vide* section γ, subsection b.

Diocles of Carystos (fl *ca.* 325 B.C.) — JAEGER, W., 1963: Diokles von Karystos. Die griechische Medizin und die Schule des Aristoteles, ed. 2, 244 p. (Berlin: de Gruyter).——

> In this book the author tries to give a faithful picture of the famous Greek physician Diocles, based on a reconstruction of that part of his work that has been lost, together with an interpretation of that part of his work that is known by tradition. Diocles is a contemporary - partly at least - of Plato, Aristotle, Hippocrates and Philistion, and whereas his works contain elements

of the works of these contemporaries, a fairly complete picture of Diocles could be reconstructed. First edition, 1938.

Diogenes of Apollonia (fl. *ca.* 450 B.C.) — ZAFIROPULO, J., 1956: Diogène d'Apollonie, 207 p. (Paris: Les Belles Lettres).——

> This book gives the available biographical information. It contains a review of the writings of Diogenes, makes clear what he borrowed from his predecessors, and how he influenced his contemporaries. It gives a review of his physical theories, his teleology and his physiological theories (*e.g.*, the role of air and temperature, the nature of sensation, the structure of the eye, colour vision). The last chapter contains the Greek text of the remains of his works, with a French translation.

Empedocles of Acragas (*ca.* 490 - *ca.* 435 B.C.) — KRANZ, W., 1949: Empedocles. Antike Gestalt und romantische Neuschöpfung, 393 p. (Zurich: Artemis).——

> A useful study of Empedocles, elucidating his meaning as a physician, and containing a translation of the extant fragments. Other relevant studies are: SCHUMACHER, J., 1941: Der Physis-Begriff bei Empedocles (Sudhoffs Arch. Gesch. Med. Naturw. 34: 179-196), and VEAZIE, W., 1922: Empedocles' psychological doctrine in its original and its traditional setting, 27 p. (Arch. Philos., No. 14) (New York, N.Y.: Columbia U.P.), a study based upon Empedocles's fragments and the tradition of his doctrine as it was preserved by Plato, Aristotle, and some others.

Heraclitos of Ephesos (fl. *ca.* 470 B.C.) — SOLOVINE, M., 1931: Héraclite d'Ephèse. Doctrines philosophiques (traduites intégralement et précédées d'une introduction), 40 + 101 p. (Paris: Alcan).——

> The introduction gives a review of Heraclitos's philosophy (p. xvii-xl). A biography of Heraclitos follows (p. 1-18), incl. his correspondence with Darius. A summing-up of doxographical documents in French translation (p. 18-41), 135 original fragments in French translation, and a large series of notes complete this volume. A more "advanced" study is: KIRK, G. S., ed., 1954: Heraclitus: the cosmic fragments (introduction and commentary by the editor), 424 p. (Cambridge: U.P.). The author made a study of those fragments of Heraclitos of which the subject is the world as a whole. In securing his text, the author takes

into account all existing ancient testimonies. To each fragment he gives a literal translation and extensive commentaries. In the introduction he gives a short biography. Heraclitos's views on doctors are expounded on p. 88-93. An extensive general index has been added.

Herodotos of Halicarnassos *(ca.* 484 - *ca.* 425 B.C.)* — MOELLER, C., 1903: Die Medizin im Herodot. Für Mediziner und Philologen, 36 p. (Berlin: Karger).—

> A review of the medical contents of Herodotos's works. *Idem,* concerning the botanical contents: KANNGIESSER, F., 1910: Die Flora des Herodot (Arch. Gesch. Naturw. Tech. III, 2: 81-102).

Hesiod (8th cent. B.C.) — SINCLAIR, T. A., ed., 1932: Hesiod: works and days, 64 + 96 p. (London: Macmillan).—

> The work is intended mainly for the classical student, but it touches upon many topics which are of interest to the student of the history of (biological) science as well. This didactic poem gives knowledge of ancient peasant wisdom on common sense hygiene, on religious medicine, on old taboos and it describes the charm of the farm in the different seasons, and the influence of these seasons on farm life. Also of interest is the study of KÖRNER, O., 1933: Die zoologischen Kenntnisse in den Gedichten des Hesiod (Quell. Gesch. Naturw. 3, H. 4: 59-71).

Hippocrates, *vide supra,* subsection c*: Hippocratic medicine.

Homer *(ca.* 8th cent. B.C.) — DELEBECQUE, E., 1951: Le cheval dans l'Iliade, suivi d'un lexique du cheval chez Homère et d'un essai sur le cheval pré-homérique, 251 p. (Paris: Klincksieck).—

> The book has been divided into three parts. The first part deals with the horse in the "Iliad", with its role in many existing legends from before the outbreak of the Trojan war, and with the way in which Homer describes the horse and the role it played in the Trojan war. The second part gives a lexicographical review of the horse in Homer's writings; and the third part deals with the history of the Indo-European horse, its domestication, the way it has been used, and its relation to the heroes and the gods in Homer's "Iliad".

——, FELLNER, S., 1897: Die homerische Flora, 84 p. (Vienna: Hölder).—

The author gives a review of the flora of the Ionian coast of Asia Minor and of the eastern coast of Greece - the region in which Homer in all probability lived and wrote his epic poems. Roughly the first half of this booklet describes the flora of the coast, the mountains, the marshes, *etc.* of Asia Minor in some detail. The second half deals more particularly with plants cultivated in agriculture, viticulture, and fruit culture. The author also mentions such plants as oranges and citrus fruits not cultivated in that region in Homer's time.

——, KÖRNER, O., 1929: Die ärztlichen Kenntnisse in Ilias und Odyssee, 89 p. (Munich: Bergmann).—

> The author tries to evaluate medical knowledge during Homer's time, and tackles the problem from where this knowledge could stem. He considers anatomical knowledge *(e.g.,* problems of bodily beauty, heredity of bodily characters, gerontology, topographical anatomy), physiological knowledge *(e.g.,* problems of reproduction and birth, life and death, sleep, activity of the nervous system, respiration, speech), hygiene, physical and psychical diseases, and surgery (incl. supernatural healing of wounds). As far as the editor is aware the most complete and extensive review of Homeric medicine is: MICCA, A. B., 1930: Omero medico: medici, ferite e medicine in Omero (Homer as physician: physicians, wounds, and medicines in Homer), 237 p. (Viterbo: Agnesotti), of which Biological Abstracts (Vol. 8, No. 2138) writes: "The aspects of medical practitioners and practices, types of weapons and corresponding wounds, anatomy, physiology, surgery, obstetrics, hygiene, drugs as seen in the Iliad, Odyssey, Homeric hymns, and Batrachomyomachia, are discussed. Illustrative quotations from the poems are given (in Italian translation). Individual technical terms are frequently cited in the original Greek. There is a table of contents, but no index except of persons referred to". A study especially dealing with Homeric pharmacy is: SCHMIEDEBERG, O., 1918: Ueber die Pharmaka in der Ilias und Odyssee (Schr. wiss. Ges. Strassburg, 36, 29 p.). KÖRNER also wrote a study concerning sense perception: Die Sinnesempfindungen in Ilias und Odyssee, 1932, 62 p. (Jena. med. hist. Beitr., Heft 15) (Jena: Fischer). An old, but valuable study is: DAREMBERG, C., 1865: La médecine dans Homère ou études d'archéologie sur les médecins, l'anatomie, la physiologie, la chirurgie et la médecine dans les poèmes homériques, 96 p. (Paris: Didier).

—— ——, 1930: Die homerische Tierwelt, ed. 2, 100 p. (Berlin: Springer).—

The author describes and elucidates all animal stories out of Homer's work and gives much additional information on them. The booklet is especially intended for zoologists and philologists. A full bibliography, and indexes of animal names in Greek, of words elucidated, and of passages in the Iliad and Odyssey on which this treatise throws light, are added.

——, MUGLER, C., 1963: Les origines de la science grecque chez Homère. L'homme et l'univers physique, 243 p. (Études et commentaires, No. 46) (Paris: Klincksieck).—

Mainly of philosophical interest. It contains the following chapters: 1. Forces, vitesses et résistances (dealing *inter alia* with the muscular force of Man, forces localized in solid bodies, water, and wind); 2. Les phénomènes de l'atmosphère. L'osmose (wind, fog, precipitation, *etc.);* 3. L'univers sonore d'Homère (the human voice, voices of nature, and of animals, instruments of music); 4. Le feu et la lumière. L'énergie latente des aliments et des poisons (dealing *inter alia* with: warmth, fire, light, vision, chemical activities of matter, medicaments, poisons); 5. Réactions en chaîne et cycles fermés. La relation entre les dieux et les hommes (chains of cause and effect, closed cycles, direct intervention of the Gods); Conclusion; L'humanité homérique et l'homme grec. Index of passages quoted in the text.

——, WACE, A. J. B. & F. H. STUBBINGS, eds., 1962: A companion to Homer, 595 p. (London: Macmillan).—

The book is a mine of interesting information on Homer and his time. It discusses such topics as: physical geography of Greece and the Aegean Sea; lands and peoples in Homer; Homeric archaeology; the principal Homeric sites; polity and society; religion; burial customs; houses; palaces; dress; arms; food and agriculture; crafts and industries; communication and trade; all subjects which together give a picture of Homer and his time. As such it is of great interest for all interested in this period, not at least because of its many fine illustrations.

Plato (*ca.* 428 - *ca.* 348 B.C.) — KAPFERER, R. & A. FINGERLE, eds., 1952: Platons Timaios, oder die Schrift über die Natur, 112 p. (Stuttgart: Hippokrates).—

This is a translation of the Timaeus, prepared by medical men. According to the editors, for a full understanding of the Ti-

maeus, knowledge of the whole body of works of Hippocrates is a necessary presumption. This point they make clear in the introduction and in the notes to the translation in which they give many illustrations of Hippocratic analogies and influences. Some shorter publications dealing with Plato and medicine are: ABEL, K., 1957: Plato und die Medizin seiner Zeit (Gesnerus 14: 94-118); DOBROVICI, A., 1953: Les idées médicales de Platon (Act. Congr. intl. Hist. Sci., 1953(6): 592-600) (Also: Bull. scient. roum. 1: 90-98); KING, L. S., 1954: Plato's concepts of medicine (J. Hist. Med. 9: 38-48); OSLER, W., 1903: Physic and physicians as depicted by Plato, 20 p. (Boston, Mass.: Damrell & Upham). Another interesting study is: RITTER, C., 1919: Platons Stellung zu den Aufgaben der Naturwissenschaft, 119 p. (Sitzber. heidelb. Akad. Wiss., Phil.-Hist. Kl., 1919, Abh. 19) (Heidelberg: Winter).

——, TAYLOR, A. E., 1949: Plato: the man and his work, ed. 6, 562 p. (London: Methuen).—

An introduction to life and work of Plato intended for students and "readers with philosophical interest, but no great store of Greek scholarship."

—— ——, 1962: A commentary on Plato's Timaeus, 700 p. (Oxford: Clarendon Press).—

This book is intended as a commentary on the text of Burnet's edition of Plato and it is an attempt to throw light on the matter discussed in the dialogue and to furnish evidence about the stages by which Plato's text has been transmitted to us. *Cf.* BURNET, J., 1911, Plato. Opera. (Scriptorum classicorum bibliotheca oxoniensis). Many comparisons have been made with Aristotle's treatment of the same problems as are touched upon in the Timaeus. In the Prolegomena (p. 1-44) the author discusses such subjects as: the authenticity of the dialogue, the date of its composition, and its relationship to other dialogues. Indexes of personal names and of Greek words.

——,WUNDT, M., 1914: Platons Leben und Werk, 174 p. (Jena: Diederichs).—

"After a little essay on Plato and the problem of culture and a sketch of Socrates, the author treats simultaneously of Plato's life and work, which implies a chronological classification of his writings. The account is simple and clear and followed by a conclusion on Plato and the development of culture." (Sarton in Isis 3: 452).

Polybos of Cos (1st half fourth cent. B.C.) — GRENSEMANN, H., 1968: Der Arzt Polybos als Verfasser hippokratischer Schriften, 45 p. (Abh. Akad. Wiss. Litt., Mainz, Geistes- und Sozialwiss. Klasse) (Wiesbaden: Steiner).—

> Polybos, son-in-law of Hippocrates, was a Greek physician, probably the greatest of Hippocrates' immediate successors. In this publication the author has gathered all biographical information available, and according to the author the "De natura hominis" can be ascribed with certainty to Polybos. It would be almost certain that he also has written the "De octimestri partu"; both works belong to the Corpus Hippocraticum.

Praxagoras of Cos (fl. *ca.* 340 - 320 B.C.) — STECKERL, F., 1958: The fragments of Praxagoras of Cos and his school, 132 p. (Leiden: Brill).—

> In this work the extant remains of Praxagoras and his disciples Phylotimos, Plistonicus and Xenophon have been collected. Praxagoras's doctrines have been considered on p. 7-44, and the author compares them with those of Diocles of Carystos, Aristotle, and others.

Theophrastos of Eresos (*ca.* 372 - *ca.* 288 B.C.) — DENGLER, R. E., ed., 1927: Theophrastus: De causis plantarum. Book one: text, critical apparatus, translation, and commentary, 143 p. (Philadelphia, Pa.: Westbrook).—

> A thorough translation of this work of Theophrastos, prepared by a classicist. Greek text and English translation on opposite pages. Numerous footnotes.

——, HORT, A., ed., 1916: Theophrastus: enquiry into plants and minor works on odours and weather signs, 2 vols. Vol. I: 475 p.; Vol. II: 499 p. (Loeb Classical Library) (London: Heinemann).—

> The present book reviews extensively the contents of the "Historia plantarum". It contains the description of over 500 plants. It gives the Greek text and the English translation on facing pages. The first vol. contains the following books: I: Of the parts of plants and their composition. Of classification; II: Of propagation, especially of trees; III: Of wild trees; IV: Of the trees and plants special to particular districts and situations; V: Of the timber of various trees and its uses. Vol. II contains books VI: Of under-shrubs; VII: Of herbaceous plants … pot-herbs and similar wild herbs; VIII: Of herbaceous plants: cereals, pulses and 'summer crops'; IX: Of the juices of plants, and of the medicinal properties of herbs. Of the minor works are included: Concerning odours, and Concerning weather signs. An index of plants (p. 435-486) and lists of plants mentioned under botanical and under popular names are included.

——, SENN, G., 1933: Die Entwicklung der biologischen Forschunsmethode in der Antike und ihre grundsätzliche Förderung durch Theophrast von Eresos, 262 p. (Veröff. schweiz. Ges. Gesch. Med. Naturw., VIII) (Aarau: Sauerländer).—

> In this study the author surveys the methodology applied by the Greek philosophers, and he tries to evaluate its effect on the development of Greek biology. According to the author the first important step was the method of observation introduced by Alcmaeon, Hippocrates, Aristotle, and Theophrastos. The second step advancing Greek science was the introduction of systematic experimentation, and a third one the recognition of the value of logic and critical concepts (Socrates, Plato, Aristotle). According to the author it was Theophrastos who developed a well-balanced scientific system in which logic, observation, induction, and deduction are united in an appropriate way. Therefore he would have been the first to give a realistic explanation of natural phenomena.

——— ——, 1956: Die Pflanzenkunde des Theophrast von Eresos. Seine Schrift über die Unterscheidungsmerkmale der Pflanzen und seine Kunstprosa, 123 p. (Basel: Privately published).—

> A posthumously-published, very valuable study of Greek botany in which the author compares Theophrastos's botanical studies with modern botanical methodology, an attempt having been made to reconstruct the original form of Theophrastos's work.

——, STRATTON, G. M., 1917: Theophrastus and the Greek physiological psychology before Aristotle, 227 p. (London: Allen & Unwin).—

> This book contains the Greek text of the fragments on the senses together with an English translation, an introduction, and

notes. According to COHEN & DRABKIN (*vide* section α, subsection a) it is an important work.

——, STRÖMBERG, R., 1937: Theophrastea. Studien zur botanischen Begriffsbildung, 234 p. (Göteborgs VetenskSamh. Handl., Ser. A., Vol. 6, No. 4).—

> From the preface: "In diesem Buch verfolge ich als Ziel, nachzuweisen wie die griechische Botanik aus der Philosophie des Peripatos hervorwächst, ferner darzulegen, wie Theophrast eine vergleichende Morphologie der Pflanzen bildet und überhaupt die Grundlagen der Botanik als Wissenschaft neu schuf, und schliesslich, wie er seine Forschungen sprachlich zu fassen und zu prägen wusste." It contains a detailed study of Theophrastos's botanical vocabulary. Indexes of Greek words, topics, and plant groups, and a useful 18-page bibliography.

——, WOOD, J. G., 1894: Theophrastus of Eresus on winds and on weather signs, 97 p. (London: Stanford).—

> A translation with introduction and notes, and an appendix on the direction, number and nomenclature of the winds in classical and later times. In Theophrastos's weather forecasts, especially the behaviour of animals constituted essential signs.

Xenophon (*ca.* 430 - *ca.* 355 B.C.) — DELEBECQUE, E., ed., 1950: De l'art équestre. Texte et traduction avec introduction et notes, 195 p. (Annls. Univ. Lyon, fasc. 18) (Paris: Les Belles Lettres).—

> Xenophon was a famous Greek historian who wrote *inter alia* a treatise on horsemanship (De re equestri), of which this book contains the text, together with a general introduction, a French translation, and annotations. There also exists a Dutch translation: WOELDEREN, C. A. VAN, 1950: Paardrijden. Naar het Grieks van Xenophon, ed. 4, 118 p. (The Hague: v. Stockum). An authoritative German translation, accompanied by many annotations and a very useful instructive introduction has been published by WIDDRA, K., ed., 1965: Xenophon. Reitkunst, 116 p. (Schriften und Quellen der alten Welt, Vol. 16) (Berlin: Akademie Verlag). Also in English translation: MORGAN, M. H., ed., 1968: The art of horsemanship: a translation, 188 p. (London: Allen).—

λ. ROME AND HELLENISM

a. History of science, philosophy, and culture in general

BAILEY, C., ed., 1957: The legacy of Rome, 512 p. (Oxford: Clarendon Press).—

> "This book is an endeavour to trace in many fields the extent of the inheritance which the modern world owes to Ancient Rome." The subjects discussed are: the transmission of the legacy, the conception of Empire, administration, communications and commerce, the science of law, family and social life, religion and philosophy, science, literature, language, architecture and art, building and engineering, agriculture.

CARY, M., 1957: A history of Rome down to the reign of Constantine, ed. 2, 820 p. (London: Macmillan).—

> A general survey of Roman history. The first part (p. 3-28) deals with pre-Roman Italy (the early inhabitants in Italy, Greeks and Etruscans in early Italy). The second part (p. 29-140) deals with the Roman conquest of Italy, the third part (p. 141-280) with the conquest of the Mediterranean, parts four (p. 281-472), five (473-720), and six (p. 721-783) with the fall of the Republic, the consolidation of the Roman Empire, and the decline of this Empire, respectively. Much attention has been paid to economic life of the Roman world, art and literature, social life and religion. Appendixes deal with the Roman emperors from Augustus to Constantine and with the genealogy of the Julio-Claudian dynasty.

GEIKIE, A., 1912: The love of nature among the Romans during the later decades of the Republic and the first century of the Empire, 394 p. (London: Murray).—

> The author - a well-known geologist - selected some parts of the realm of nature, and discusses the literary and artistic treatments of them in Rome during the period from Lucretius to Statius. The book deals with such subjects as the charms of the Italian landscape, Pliny, summer migration from Rome, the "Divini Gloria Ruris": Lucretius, Virgil, Horace, rural scenes and the elegiac poets: Propertius, Ovid, religious use of flowers, extravagance in garlands, the love of gardens, trees and woodlands, groves set apart as sacred, flowers and foliage in Roman art, the animal world in Roman life, amphitheatre, arena, love of dogs and birds, game preservation, springs,

rivers and lakes, the seashore and the open sea, the underworld, *etc*. *Cf*. FAIRCLOUGH, H. R., 1963, section ϒ, subsection a.

HADAS, M., 1959: Hellenistic culture: fusion and diffusion, 324 p. (New York, N.Y.: Columbia U.P.; London: Oxford U.P.).—

>This book deals with the diffusion of Greek culture (language and literature, and such concepts as: love, prayer, religion and law) among the peoples of the East, and its influence on Rome. Not much that is of interest to the history of science.

KAGAN, D., 1966: Problems in ancient history. Vol. II: The Roman world, 431 p. (New York, N.Y. & London: Macmillan).—

>An anthology which must be considered as an attempt to meet several problems facing the college student beginning the study of ancient history. According to Kagan it is meant to be used in conjunction with a narrative history or some suitable substitute. Not of much interest to the history of science.

KORNEMANN, E., 1948: Weltgeschichte des Mittelmeer-Raumes. Von Philipp II. von Makedonien bis Muhammed, 2 vols. Vol. I: 509 p.; Vol. II: 564 p. (Munich: Beck).—

>The first volume deals with the period 359-331 B.C. In a general introduction the author considers some interconnections between Medes, Persians, and Assyrians on the one hand and Hellenes on the other. The first part of Vol. I (p. 62-346) deals with the disintegration of the Greek empire and the rise of Alexandria and Rome; the second part of this volume deals with the world-hegemony of the Romans and the struggle between Romanism and Hellenism. The first part of Vol. II (p. 1-275) is a continuation of this, dealing with the period 31 B.C. - 305 A.D. The second part of Vol. II deals with the period 305-640 A.D., the decline of the Roman Empire and the rise of the Germanic and Arabic peoples.

SARTON, G., 1959: A history of science: Hellenistic science and culture in the last three centuries B.C., 554 p. (Cambridge, Mass.: Harvard U.P.).—

>Because Hellenistic ideals were dominant in the culture of Rome, Eastern Europe, Egypt, and Western Asia, the book

deals with Roman culture and Latin literature as well as with Greek literature. The book is devoted to the three centuries which followed the death of Alexander the Great and Aristotle and preceded the rise of Christianity, and it tries to display as many facets as possible of Hellenistic science and culture. The book has been supplied with careful and detailed accounts of the transmission of the great classical works and their translation during the following centuries; the princeps edition of each important book has been given; next to this, the best edition, the most convenient edition for reference, and the first and best translation into English have been mentioned. According to the author the book is intended for men of science who are anxious to know the origins of their knowledge. Paperback edition 1965, 554 p. (New York, N.Y.: Wiley).

STAHL, W. H., 1962: Roman science: origins, development, and influence to the later Middle Ages, 308 p. (Madison, Wisc.: Univ. Wisconsin Press).—

>An attempt to reconstruct the place of the Romans in the story of ancient science. The text is in three parts; in the first part the author considers the Greek origins of what went under the name of science in Rome; in the second part the author gives a description of "Roman science" in the Republic and in the (Western) Empire, and he tries to prove that this Roman science is only a derivative of Greek science; in the third part the author deals with the influence of the Roman tradition in the later Middle Ages.

TARN, W. & G. T. GRIFFITH, 1959: Hellenistic civilisation, 372 p. (London: Arnold).—

>This book was first printed in 1927 (ed. 3, 1952) and has been reprinted many times. It is a comprehensive history of the period between the death of Alexander the Great and the establishment of the Roman Empire by Augustus. Separate sections deal with: monarchy, the Greek cities, Asia, Egypt, Hellenism and the Jews, trade and exploration, literature and learning (incl. the pastoral poetry of Theocritus), science and art (incl. medicine, zoology, and botany), philosophy and religion (incl. Epicuros).

b. History of the plant and animal sciences

ANDRÉ, J., 1956: Lexique des termes de botanique en Latin, 343 p. (Paris: Klincksieck).—

According to J. Stannard, by far the best, most reliable study of the identification of Latin plant names. (Verbal communication).

BEAURREDON, L'abbé, 1898: Voyage agricole chez les anciens ou l'économie rurale dans l'antiquité, 380 p. (Paris: Savaète).—

A thorough description of agriculture as it has been described by the Latin agronomists Cato, Varro, Columella, and Palladius, with short biographical and bibliographical notes. The book deals with such divergent topics as: rural architecture, the farm and its inhabitants, the preparation of the soil (drainage, manuring, *etc.*), ploughing, sowing, harvesting, distribution of cultures, animal husbandry, apiculture, aviculture, pisciculture, propagation and multiplication of fruit-trees, horticulture, food-conservation, cheese-making, *etc. Cf.* also NISARD, D., ed., 1844: Les agronomes latins, Caton, Varron, Columelle, Paladius, avec la traduction en français, 651 p. (Paris). A still older but very interesting study dealing with the same topics is: DICKSON, A., 1788: The husbandry of the ancients, 2 vols. Vol. I: 527 p.; Vol. II: 494 p. (Edinburgh: Dickson). Reprint announced (Groningen: Bouma). Also of interest are: BEHEIM-SCHWARZBACH, H., 1967: Beitrag zur Kenntniss des Ackerbaus der Römer, 142 p. (Wiesbaden: Sändig). A reprint of the 1866 edition; and DOHR, H., 1965: Die italienische Gutshöfe nach den Schriften Catos und Varros, 165 p. (Inaug.-Diss. Univ. Köln). *Cf.* also: HEITLAND, W. E., 1921, *vide* section α, subsection b.

BJÖRCK, G., 1944: Apsyrtus, Julius Africanus et l'hippiatrie grecque, 70 p. (Uppsala Univ. Årskr. 1944: 4) (Uppsala: Lundequist).—

This study deals with such topics as the problems relative to collections of writings in general and to those of the hippiatric collection in particular, with the tradition of Greek hippiatry during the middle ages in the West, the mss. of Greek hippiatry and the editions extant, and with hippiatric magic. Apsyrtos (fl. *ca.* 333) was a Greek veterinary surgeon who wrote a treatise on the veterinary art which is one of the main sources of the Hippiatrica; Sextus Julius Africanus was a Christian encyclopaedist (fl. *ca.* 222-235) who wrote an encyclopaedia dealing with such subjects as: agriculture, husbandry, natural history, medicine, *etc. Cf.* BJÖRCK, G., 1932, this section β, subsection b; also: SIMON, F., 1930: Das Corpus hippiatricorum Graecorum von E. Oder

und C. Hoppe in seiner Bedeutung als Sammelwerk griechisch-römischer Ueberlieferungen in griechischer Sprache über Heilbehandlung von Tieren in den nach-christlichen Jahrhunderten unter besonderer Berücksichtigung des damaligen Standes der Veterinär-Chirurgie, 80 p. (Diss. Univ. Munich) (Murnau: Fürst).

CARNOY, A., 1959: Dictionnaire étymologique des noms grecs des plantes, 277 p. (Louvain: Univ. de Louvain).—

An etymological lexicon, containing Hellenistic and Aegean plant names as they were used by the Greek authors, or as they have been conserved by Pliny the Elder and some other Roman writers. For the benefit of herborists, medical men and horticulturists a certain number of modern plant names have been included, together with an indication of their origin. *Cf.* STRÖMBERG, R., 1940, section α, subsection b.

DAUBENY, C., 1857: Lectures on Roman husbandry delivered before the University of Oxford; comprehending such an account of the system of agriculture, the treatment of domestic animals, the horticulture *etc.*, pursued in ancient times, as may be collected from the scriptores rei rusticae, the Georgics of Virgil, and other classical authorities, with notices of the plants mentioned in Columella and Virgil, 328 p. (Oxford: Parker).—

A detailed account of the system of agriculture pursued by the Romans, embodying the ideas entertained by the Roman writers comprehended under the title of the "Rei rusticae scriptores" (Cato, Varro, Palladius, Pliny, and Columella). The author confines himself chiefly to the system of agriculture presented in the treatise of Columella, being the latest published, and therefore embodying in itself what was noteworthy in the writings which preceded it. The author discusses a number of problems, such as culture of vineyard and orchard, agriculture, cultivation of gardens, crops cultivated, treatment of the soil, treatment of domestic animals, *etc. Cf.* SCHNEIDER, J. G., ed., 1968: Scriptores rei rusticae veterum latinorum, 5 vols., 3162 p. (Hildesheim: Olms). A reprint of the 1794-1797 edition. *Cf.* also: HAUGER, A., 1921; and WHITE, K. D., 1967, *vide infra*.

GRIMAL, P., 1943: Les jardins romains à la fin de la République et aux deux premiers siècles de l'Empire: essai sur le naturalisme romain, 577 p. (Paris: De Boccard).—

The subjectmatter has been divided into four parts. The first part (p. 23-106) deals with the origin of garden art (Rome et la "conscience italienne" au temps de la Guerre Sociale; Tradition romaine et jardins; Les apports helléniques). The second part (p. 107-212) deals with the gardens of Rome (Étude topographique; Les parcs publics de Rome: bois sacrés, promenades, thermes). The third part (p. 213-376) deals with garden architecture (La demeure et son jardin; Éléments architecturaux des jardins; Jardin et nature). The fourth part (p. 377-468) deals with gardens in Roman thinking and literature. In an appendix the garden plants of the Romans have been listed. Very good indexes of names and subjects.

HAUGER, A., 1921: Zur römischen Landwirtschaft und Haustierzucht, 134 p. (Hannover: Schaper).—

After a general review of Roman agriculture in general, separate sections deal with the economic aspects of agriculture (p. 12-29), and with animal husbandry (p. 30-129). This last section deals with horses and horse-breeding (p. 36-70), donkeys, asses, cattle, pigs, sheep, goats, and dogs, and with the production of milk and cheese. *Cf.* DAUBENY, C., 1857, *vide supra;* and WHITE, K. D., 1970 *vide infra.*

JENNISON, G., 1937: Animals for show and pleasure in ancient Rome, 209 p. (Manchester: U.P.).—

A thorough study of which the contents are indicated by the chapter headings: I. Tamed animals of the city-states of Greece; II. Zoological magnificence in Egypt under the Ptolemies; III. The animals of the Roman games (to 30 B.C.); IV. Shows under the early Empire (29 B.C. - A.D. 117); V. Shows from Hadrian to Honorius (117-410); VI. The amateur's menagerie: birds; VII. *Idem:* fishponds; VIII. *Idem:* Quadrupeds and reptiles; IX. Capture and transport; X. Development of the arena; XI. Provincial amphitheatres; XII. Stockyards for the beasts; XIII. The shows in the arena. Appendixes on the leopard, the date of Calpurnius, the gold-finding ants, the training of man-eaters; and on the African and Indian elephants. The original sources are quoted in the margin.

PAPASOGLI, G., 1942: L'agricoltura degli etruschi e dei romani, 293 p. (Roma: Fratelli Palombi).—

Chapter headings are as follows: I. Le origini gli Etruschi; II. Aspetti e sviluppi dell'economia agraria romana fino alla unificazione giuridica d'Italia; III. Ricchezza e povertà nell'Etruria e nel Lazio sotto i Romani; VI. La coltura del frumento; V. La vite; VI. L'olivo; VII. Frutticoltura, orticultura; VIII. Il bestiame; IX. La mano d'opera agraria; X. Una fattoria romana secondo Columella; XI. Luci ed ombre della civiltà agricola nell'Etruria e nel Lazio.

SAINT-DENIS, E. de, 1947: Le vocabulaire des animaux marins au latin classique, 32 + 121 p. (Paris: Klincksieck).—

In this booklet the author tries to identify the marine animals quoted by the classical ancient authors, translators, and lexicographers. In the introduction the author considers the role played by fishes as food of the Romans, and the vocabulary of marine animals in classical Latin.

STEIER, A., 1913: Aristoteles und Plinius. Studien zur Geschichte der Zoologie, 305 p. (Würzburg: Kabitzsch).—

The aim of this study is to investigate which additions Pliny made to zoology and in which respects he differed from Aristotle. The book consists of three essays reprinted from the "Zoologische Annalen", entitled (in English translation) "The classification of animals in the Historia naturalis of Pliny", "The animals known to Pliny", and "Zoological problems in Aristotle and Pliny".

WHITE, K. D., 1967: Agricultural implements of the Roman world, 232 p. (Cambridge: Cambridge U.P.).—

In this book a review has been given of the abundant literature dealing with the agricultural implements of the Roman world; this has been supplemented by archaeological evidence. The author deals with the tools the Romans used in all their variety and with the way they used them. The author treats of each implement in a separate article. In all, some 50 implements are discussed, accompanied by 119 illustrations. The descriptions are detailed and the implements described vary from shovels and spades and saws to ploughs, harrows and reaping implements. *Cf.* also: WHITE, K. D., 1970, *vide infra.*

——, 1970: Roman farming, 536 p. (Ithaca, N.Y.: Cornell U.P.).—

A detailed study of all aspects of Roman agriculture with special emphasis on the economic structure of the individual Roman farmer insofar as it can be reconstructed from the texts and inscriptions. *Cf.* BEAURREDON, L'abbé, 1898; DAUBENY, C., 1857; HAUGER, A., 1921; and WHITE, K. D., 1967, *vide supra*.

c. History of the medical sciences

ALLBUTT, C., 1921: Greek medicine in Rome, 633 p. (London: Macmillan).—

> For more details, *vide* section Antiquity in general, subsection c; also: CORLIEU, A., 1885, same section; and SCARBOROUGH, J., 1969, *vide infra*.

BRIAU, R., 1869: L'assistance médicale chez les romains, 111 p. (Paris: Masson).—

> Chapter headings are as follows: 1. Coup d'oeil sur la profession médicale à Rome; 2. Des médecins attachés aux jeux du cirque; 3. Des médecins de gladiature; 4. Des médecins de la maison de l'Empéreur; 5. Des médecins dans les fouilles d'esclaves; 6. Des médecins dans les associations d'artisans; 7. Des secours médicaux chez les indigents. *Cf.* MEYER, T., 1907, *vide infra*.

——, 1877: L'archiatrie romaine ou le médecine officielle dans l'empire romain. Suite de la profession médicale, 130 p. (Paris: Masson).—

> Deals with such subjects as: the position of the archiater in general, his position at the court, the municipal archiater, the archiater as teacher, the archiater of the xystus and the Vesta, and the public archiater in Rome and Constantinople.

CARRÉ, A., 1933: L'hygiène et la santé dans la Rome antique, 170 p. (Bordeaux: Delmas).—

> The book has been divided into three parts. The first part deals with public hygiene, endemic and epidemic diseases, the social position of the physician, fevers and their treatment, and with such diseases as: plague, phthisis, typhus, cholera, *etc.* The second part deals with personal hygiene, feeding habits, drink and food, aphrodisiacs, cutaneous diseases, bodily cleanness, *etc.* The third part deals with depopulation, its causes and effects, and the disastrous effects of great epidemics.

DEICHGRÄBER, K., 1930: Die griechische Empirikerschule. Sammlung der Fragmente und Darstellung der Lehre, 398 p. (Berlin: Weidmann).—

> The aim and meaning of this book can best be made clear from a quotation from the author's preface: "Der erste Teil der Arbeit, die Fragmentsammlung, beschränkt sich bewusst auf die Mitteilung des unbedingt sicher Empirischen; alles Zweifelhafte oder nur wahrscheinlich Empirische fehlt, z.B. auch so Wertvolles wie das von Max Wellmann auf Herakleides von Tarent zurückgeführte diätetische Material im Athenaios. Der zweite Teil, die Darstellung der Lehre, behandelt fast ausschliesslich die empirische Wissenschaftstheorie und berührt deshalb die so wichtige Praxis der empirischen Aerzte nur in Beispielen. Dem Medizinhistoriker gibt dieses Buch also nur das philologisch hergerichtete Quellenmaterial und einen philosophiegeschichtlichen Beitrag. Seine Aufgabe ist es nun, die Chirurgie und die übrigens auch volkskundlich interessante Pharmazie der Empiriker aufzubauen." In 1965 an anastatic reprint appeared (Berlin & Zurich: Weidmann), to which Deichgräber added some new material (p. 399-424).

EDELSTEIN, L., 1932: Die Geschichte der Sektion in der Antike, 56 p. (Quell. Gesch. Naturw. 3, H. 2: 50-106).—

> A study of human dissection during antiquity, taken to have begun in Alexandria and to have ended in the first century A.D.

GUMMERUS, H., 1932: Der Aerztestand im römischen Reiche nach den Inschriften, 103 p. (Soc. Sci. Fennica, Comm. Humanarum Litterarum III, 6).—

> A collection of 403 inscriptions concerning physicians. Excluded are those reliefs which depict a medical subject but lack an inscription. Among the inscriptions included are those depicting *e.g.,* votive offerings, medical instruments, hospitals, veterinary medicine, apothecaries, midwives, and the social position of the Roman physician.

LEWY, A., 1931: Ueber die Bedeutung des Antyllus, Philagrius und Posidonius in der Geschichte der Heilkunde, nach dem Manuscripte des verstorbenen Cand. med. A. Lewy bearbeitet von M. LANDESBERG, 76 p. (Henschel's Janus 2 (1847): 298-329, 744-771; 3 (1848): 166-184). Reprinted, 1931. (Leipzig: Lorentz).—

Antyllos (ca. 100-150) was a famous Greek physician and surgeon of the Pneumatic School of which some fragments are known (through Oribasios). Philagrios (ca. 350-400) was a Greek physician, famous for his diagnosis and treatment of diseases of the spleen. Posidonios was a brother of Philagrios and made a study of brain diseases and made a first attempt of localization of functions in the brain. Only fragments are extant. For Philagrios cf. T. PUSCHMANN's Nachträge zu Alex. Trallius, 1886, p. 74-128 (Berlin), vide section The Middle-Ages in the Near East, subsection α, c.

MEYER, T., 1907: Geschichte des römischen Aerztestandes, 85 p. (Habilitationsschrift, Univ. Jena) (Kiel: Handorff).—

Chapter headings are as follows: 1. Aelteste römische Medizin; 2. Sklavenmedizin (Hausmedizin); 3. Beginnende Entwicklung eines aerztlichen Berufsstandes; 4. Begriffliche Aussonderung der wirklichen "medici"; 5. Staatliche Anerkennung eines Aerztestandes. Approbation; 6. Rechtliche Stellung der Aerzte; 7. Soziale Stellung der Aerzte; 8. Beamtete Aerzte; 9. Aerztliche Vereinsbildungen; 10. Der medizinische Unterricht; 11. Aerztliche Hülfskräfte, Kurpfuscher und Spezialisten. A study dealing with the position of the physician in Roman law is: BELOW, K. H., 1953: Der Arzt im römischen Recht, 136 p. (Münchener Beiträge zur Papyrusforschung und antiken Rechtsgeschichte, 37) (Munich: Beck). Cf. also: BRIAN, R., 1869, vide supra.

MEYER-STEINEG, T., 1916: Das medizinische System der Methodiker. Eine Vorstudie zu Caelius Aurelianus "De morbis acutis et chronicis", 131 p. (Jena. med. hist. Beitr., Heft 7/8) (Jena: Fischer).—

Separate chapters deal with the following subjects: Asclepiades of Bythinia, the forerunner of the methodist school; Themison of Laodicaea, the founder of the methodist school; Thessalos of Tralles, the practician; Soranos of Ephesus, the accomplisher; Caelius Aurelianus, De morbis acutis et chronices libri VIII, and his general pathology, his therapeutic principles, his therapy, and his treatment.

MICHLER, M., 1968: Die alexandrinischen Chirurgen. Eine Sammlung und Auswertung ihrer Fragmente, 171 p. (Die hellenistische Chirurgie, Vol. I) (Wiesbaden: Steiner).—

In the present study 42 Alexandrian

surgeons have been listed from Herophilos and Erasistratos, the founders of the Alexandrian school of medicine, to Celsus. This is accompanied by indications of the places in the literature where they are mentioned. Included are several fragments in Greek or Latin with their translation in German. Other publications in this series have been planned, e.g., Die alexandrinische Chirurgie; Die pneumatischen Chirurgen; Die hellenistische Operationslehre.

OPPENHEIMER, H., 1928: Medical and allied topics in Latin poetry, 445 p. (London: Bale).—

A selection of passages relevant to medical material in the literature produced by the Latin poets, arranged to subject matter, provided by a current explanatory text and English metric translations. The subjects are: medical sociology, doctor and patient, medical doctrine and education, biology, physiology, surgery, diseases of the eye, diseases of the nose, throat and ear, infectious diseases, internal disorders, materia medica, dietetics, balneology and hydrotherapy, toxicology, alcoholism, neurology, sleep and insomnia, insanity, sexual life and aberrations, midwifery, monstrous births and malformations, dermatology, cosmetics, nursing, medical metaphors. A comparable study dealing with dentistry is: HEYNE, R., 1924: Zähne und Zahnärztliches in der schönen Literatur der Römer, 52 p. (Diss. Sudhoff Inst., Leipzig) (Leipzig: Zeugner).

ROUYER, J., 1859: Études médicales sur l'ancienne Rome, 239 p. (Paris: Delahaye).—

Separate chapters deal with public baths, magicians and philtres, abortion, eunuchs, infibulation, cosmetics and perfumes, and with women who practised medicine.

SCARBOROUGH, J., 1969: Roman medicine, 238 p. (London: Thames & Hudson).—

A study of the nature of medical theory and practice in the Roman world. Considered are such subjects as: the background of Hellenistic medicine and its influence in the Roman world; Cato, Varro, and Celsus; medical practice in the Roman army; Roman technical and hygienic achievements; the physician's place in society; Roman medical education; and the effectiveness of Roman medicine in Roman society. Appendixes deal with biographical sketches

(77 entries), with sources and problems, with human dissection in Roman medicine, and with Roman veterinary medicine.

SUDHOFF, K., 1908: Aerztliches aus griechischen Papyrus-Urkunden. Bausteine zu einer medizinischen Kulturgeschichte des Hellenismus, 296 p. (Leipzig: Barth).—

> The separate sections are entitled as follows: 1. Nahrungsmittel und Getränke, Nahrungsmittelhygiene; 2. Öle; 3. Wohlgerüche und Drogen; 4. Badewesen; 5. Barbierwesen, Haarpflege; 6. Sexuelles; 7. Ehe, Scheidung und Heiratsgut; 8. Sklavenwesen; 9. Ammenwesen; 10. Geburtsanzeigen; 11. Beschneidung; 12. Anmeldung von Sterbefällen; 13. Bestattungskosten, Mumienetiketten; 14. Testamente; 15. Krankheitszustände, erwähnt in Urkunden und Briefe; 16. Asklepieien, *etc.;* 17. Kriminelles, Gerichtsaerztliches; 18. Von den Aerzten selbst.

WELLMANN, M., 1895: Die pneumatische Schule bis auf Archigenes, in ihrer Entwicklung dargestellt, 239 p. (Berlin: Weidmann).—

> In this historical review, the author considers: Athenaeos of Attalia, Agathinos, Herodotos of Halicarnassos, Leonidas, Apollonios of Pergamon, Heliodoros the Surgeon, Archigenes, and some others. As to the sources of this school, Wellmann refers to Aretaeos, Galen, Oribasios, and Aëtios of Amida. In a second part the author discusses the physiology, pathology, dietetics, and therapeutics of the pneumatic school.

d. Some individual scientists and philosophers

Aelianos, Claudios (fl. 193-211) — SCHOLFIELD, A. F., ed., 1958-1959: On the characteristics of animals (with an English translation), 3 vols. Vol. I (1958): Bks. I-V, 359 p.; Vol. II (1959): Bks. VI-XI, 413 p.; Vol. III (1959): Bks. XII-XVII, 445 p. (The Loeb Classical Library) (Cambridge, Mass.: Harvard U.P.; London: Heinemann).—

> The "De natura animalium" of which this work contains the original text with an English translation on facing pages, is a miscellany of facts, genuine or supposed, told with an ethical purpose, gleaned by Aelian from earlier and contemporary Greek writers (no Latin writer is named).

To a limited extent he gives his own observations, but much is derived from mythology, mariner's yarns and superstitions and Aelian is much concerned to bring out the moral side of animal behaviour, especially stressing the good qualities, the devotion, courage, self-sacrifice, and gratitude of the animals concerned. Very good indexes. There exists also a German translation of the complete works of Aelian, ed. by C. A. WUNDERLICH & F. JACOBS, 9 vols., 1126 p., Stuttgart, Metzler, 1839-1842. A general review of the animals mentioned in Aelian is: GOSSEN, H., 1935: Die Tiernamen in Aelians 17 Bücher, 60 p. (Quell. Gesch. Naturw. Med. 4, H.3: 128-188).

Apollonius of Citium (fl. *ca.* 50 B.C.) — KOLLESCH, J. & F. KUDLIEN, eds., 1965: Apollonius von Kition. Kommentar zu Hippokrates über das Einrenken der Gelenke, 133 p. (Corpus Medicorum Graecorum XI, 1, 1) (Berlin: Akademie Verlag).—

> The Alexandrian physician Appollonius wrote a commentary on the book "On articulations", belonging to the Hippocratic Collection. The present book contains the Greek text and a German translation on facing pages, together with 30 full-page facsimile reproductions of Greek surgical illustrations.

Apuleius, pseudo (4th cent. A.D.) — GUNTHER, R. T., 1925: The herbal of Apuleius Barbarus from the early twelfth-century manuscript formerly in the Abbey of Bury St. Edmunds (Ms. Bodley 130), 36 + 148 p. (Oxford: Roxburghe Club).—

> Of the present edition, the first 34 pages contain an introduction, the story of the ms., and a description and review of the contents of the herbal of pseudo Apuleius (the "De herbarum virtutibus"), of the Book of extracts of Dioscorides, and of the Book of medicine from animals of Sextus Placitus. The text itself consists of a very clear and beautifully illustrated facsimile reprint of the herbarium of pseudo-Apuleius, and a list of herbs described in it.

——, HUNGER, F. W. T., 1935: The herbal of pseudo-Apuleius from the 9th-century manuscript in the Abbey of Monte Cassino (Codex Casinensis 97) together with the first printed edition of J. P. de LIGNAMINE (Editio princeps Romae, 1481) both in facsimile, described and annotated, 48 + 168 p. (Leiden: Brill).—

In this very fine volume, almost two feet high, two documents, both marking stages in the series of herbals, are photographically reproduced. Corresponding ms. and incunabular pages are facing each other. The editor demonstrates that the herbal underwent no change during the 600 years which elapsed between writing and printing. This "prescription-book", containing about 130 illustrations of herbs, was the most widely-used book of medicine during the Middle Ages. According to the editor it must have been first written in the 4th century A.D. About the author nothing can be stated with certainty. Appendix with table of the names of plants. A translation of the text in early Middle English: BERBERICH, H., 1902: Das Herbarium Apulei nach einer früh-mittelenglischen Fassung herausgegeben, 140 p. (Anglistische Forschungen, No. 5) (Heidelberg: Winter).

Aretaeos of Cappadocia (ca. 120 - ca. 200) —KUDLIEN, F., 1963: Untersuchungen zu Aretaios von Kappadokien, 86 p. (Abh. Akad. Wiss. u. Litt. Mainz, Geistes- und Sozialwiss. Kl., 1963, No. 11: 1151-1229) (Wiesbaden: Steiner).—

The author places Aretaeos and his medical knowledge in a historical setting. Aretaeos was a contemporary of Dioscorides; from his views about physiology and pathology, Aretaeos seems to have adhered to the pneumatic tradition. Cf. also: STANNARD, J., 1964: Materia medica and philosophic theory in Aretaeus (Sudhoffs Arch. 48: 27-53).

——, MANN, A., ed., 1838: Die auf uns gekommenen Schriften des Kappadocier Aretaeus, aus dem Griechischen uebersetzt, 229 p. (Halle: Pfeffer).—

The text consists of German translations of the following parts: the causes and indications of acute diseases (p. 1-43); the causes and indications of chronic diseases (p. 44-122); treatment of acute diseases (p. 123-189); treatment of chronic diseases. A Greek text with English translation has been published by F. ADAMS, 1856, 530 p. (London: Sydenham Society). Aretaeos was a Greek physician of the Eclectic School; his descriptions of the diseases are notably methodical and "Hippocratic" in character. Reprinted 1967 (Wiesbaden: Sändig).

Asclepiades of Bithynia (born ca. 124) — GREEN, R. M., 1955: Asclepiades, his life and writings: a translation of Cocchi's "Life of Asclepiades", and Gumpert's "Fragments of Asclepiades", 167 p. (New Haven, Conn.: Elisabeth Licht).—

Asclepiades of Bithynia was the first eminent Greek physician in Rome, and the founder of the Methodist School. In 1794 Chr. G. GUMPERT published a collection of notes and fragments concerning the life of this famous Greek medical reformer. The present book contains a reprint of an English translation of this work, together with a new English version of Ant. COCCHI's "Life of Asclepiades", published in 1762. Another treatise dealing with life and work of Asclepiades is: VILAS, H. v., 1903: Der Arzt und Philosoph Asklepiades von Bithynien, 82 p. (Vienna & Leipzig: Braumüller).

Athenaeos of Naucratis (fl. ca. 200) — GOSSEN, H., 1939: Zoologisches bei Athenaios, 41 p. (Quell. Gesch. Naturw. Med. 7: 221-282).—

Athenaeos of Naucratis was a Hellenistic historiographer, living at the beginning of the third century, author of an encyclopaedia wherein extracts from many hundred ancient writers are quoted on almost every subject, though chiefly on gastronomy. The present study deals with the zoological aspects of his work. A short chapter in E. H. F. MEYER's Geschichte der Botanik (Vol. II: 197-202, vide section History of the pure plant sciences, subsection a) has been devoted to Athenaeos's botanical knowledge.

Caelius Aurelianus (fl. 400-450) — DRABKIN, I. E., ed., 1950: Caelius Aurelianus: On acute diseases and on chronic diseases, 1019 p. (Chicago, Ill.: Chicago U.P.).—

Caelius Aurelianus, a Roman physician, and the greatest Latin medical writer after Celsus, prepared a Latin translation of two important treatises of Soranos which still are not available in their original Greek fashion. Soranos was a Greek physician belonging to the Methodist School, which School developed symptomatology and differential diagnosis to a high degree of perfection; and that obliged them to make a fairly sharp distinction between acute and chronic diseases. Whereas the mss. of both Latin texts are lost, the present text has been based on two early editions, viz., the "Chronic diseases" ed. by J. SICHART (Basel, 1529) and the "Acute diseases" ed. by J. WINTER (Paris, 1533). The English translation has been printed opposite the Latin text. The text of the treatise on acute diseases runs from p. 2-439 and the text of the treatise on chronic diseases from p. 440-1001. DRABKIN, M. F. & I. E., also prepared a new (Latin) edition of Caelius Aurelianus's translation of Soranos's "Gynaecia", in Bull. Hist. Med., No. 13, 1951, 136 p. In this case the original Greek text of Soranos is still extant (*cf*. O. TEMKIN's English translation and J. ILBERG's German translation, *vide* Soranos of Ephesus, *infra*). *Cf*. also MEYER-STEINEG's study (*vide* this section, subsection c); and SCHMID, P., 1942: Contributions à la critique du texte du Caelius Aurelianus, 111 p. (Diss. Univ. Neuchâtel).

Cato the Censor, or Cato, Marcus Porcius (234-149 B.C.) — HOOPER, W. D. & H. B. ASH, 1960: Marcus Porcius Cato on agriculture. Marcus Terentius Varro on agriculture, 543 p. (Loeb Classical Library) (London: Heinemann; Cambridge, Mass.: Harvard U.P.).—

Cato was a Roman statesman, moralist, and farmer, who wrote in his old age a treatise on farming, gardening, fruit growing, *etc.*, containing also valuable information on Roman medicine of those days. P. 1-158 present the text of Cato's "De agri cultura" in Latin with English translation on facing pages. Cato's "De agri cultura" resembles a farmer's note-book in which the author put down all sorts of directions for the care of the farm; therefore the text is difficultly to interpret: THIELSCHER's study (see below) contains many more annotations than the present edition. A somewhat older English translation, supplemented by a vivid description of rural life in the Roman Republic, can be found in: BRE-HAUT, E., 1933: Cato the Censor on farming, 45 + 156 p. (New York, N.Y.: Columbia U.P.); reprinted 1966 (New York, N.Y.: Octagon Bks.).

——, THIELSCHER, P., 1963: Des Marcus Cato Belehrung über die Landwirtschaft, 396 p. (Berlin: Duncker & Humblot).—

The first German translation of Cato's "De agri cultura". After a short introduction, summarizing the agricultural position during Cato's lifetime, the text follows, together with the German translation on opposite pages (p. 31-169). Then extensive notes and authoritative commentaries follow (p. 171-396) which are valuable, not only from the philological, but also from the agricultural point of view.

Celsus, Aurelius Cornelius (fl. 14-37) — SPENCER, W. G., ed., 1948-1953: Celsus:

On medicine, 3 vols. Vol. I (1948): 499 p.; Vol. II (1953): 67 + 291 p.; Vol. III (1953): p. 292-649. (Loeb Classical Library) (London: Heinemann; Cambridge, Mass.: Harvard U.P.).—

The "De medicina libri VIII" is the only extant part of a large encyclopaedia entitled "Artes". It is an indispensable source for the history of Alexandrian medicine. Vol. I summarizes the arguments for regarding Celsus as a medical practitioner; it gives a short bibliography, and the text of the books I-IV, together with a list of chapter headings of the whole work. Vol. II contains a list of medicaments and of weights, measures, and symbols. together with the text of the Books V and VI; vol. III contains the text of Books VII and VIII (dealing with surgery and containing many anatomical descriptions), a list of chapter headings, a summing-up of parallel passages in Hippocrates and Celsus, an index of proper names, and a general index. There also exists a French translation by A. DES ÉTANGS, 1859, 289 p. (Paris: Didot), and an authoritative German translation by E. SCHELLER (ed. 2 revised by W. FRIE-BOES), 1906, 42 + 862 p. (Braunschweig: Vieweg). Reprinted 1967 (Hildesheim: Olms). A short review, placing Celsus within the framework of his time, is: ILBERG, J., 1907: A. Cornelius Celsus und die Medizin in Rom, 35 p. (Neue Jb. für das Klass. Altertum, Gesch. u. dtsch. Lit. 19: 377-412).

Cicero, Marcus Tullius (106-43 B.C.) — MENIÈRE, P., 1862: Cicéron médecin. Étude médico-littéraire, 376 p. (Paris: Baillière).—

A booklet collecting those passages of Cicero's work which deal with health, disease, medicine and its applications. After the introduction, separate chapters deal with: Cicero's correspondence (p. 15-105), his rhetorics (p. 106-129), his pleadings (p. 130-153), his consular works (p. 153-192), and his philosophical treatises. Valuable bibliographical study (p. 307-365), and list of diseases considered are added.

——, ORTH, E., 1925: Cicero und die Medizin, 113 p. (Leipzig: Noske).—

Contains the following sections: Die Aerzte in Rom vor Cicero; Die Aerzte in Cicero's Werken; Aerzte die Cicero persönlich kennt; Aerzte die Cicero ohne persönliche Berührung, mit ihrem Namen nennt; Ein Bild aerztlicher Tätigkeit nach Ciceros Schriften; Die Medizin bei Cicero

(Das Wesen der Medizin: Anatomie, Physiologie); Allgemeine und besondere Krankheitslehre; Krankheiten des ganzen Körpers, *e.g.,* Geschwülste, Fieber, Wassersucht; Krankheiten einzelner Körperteilen, *e.g.,* Infektionskrankheiten, Augenleiden, Magen-, Darm-, *etc.* leiden; Hygiene und Diätetik; Therapie und Chirurgie; Die Quellen der medizinischen Kenntnisse Ciceros, Griechische Begriffe der Medizin, Asklepiades und Cicero.

Columella, Lucius Junius Moderatus (fl. *ca.* 50) — ASH, H. B., E. S. FORSTER & E. A. HAFFNER, eds., 1954: Lucius Junius Moderatus Columella: On agriculture (with a recension of the text and an English translation), 3 vols. Vol. I (1960): De re rustica I-IV, 461 p.; Vol. II (1954): De re rustica V-IX, 503 p.; Vol. III (1955): De re rustica X-XII; De arboribus, 435 p. (The Loeb Classical Library) (London: Heinemann; Cambridge, Mass.: Harvard U.P.).—

Vol. I, edited by the late H.B. ASH, contains an introduction, discussing life and work of Columella, the manuscripts extant and the editions published so far. Then the text of Bks. I-IV follows together with an English translation. Vol. II contains text *plus* translation of Bks. V-IX, of which Bks. VI-IX deal with farm animals such as: oxen, bulls, cows, horses, mules, asses, sheep, goats, pigs, dogs, birds and fishes, poultry, pigeons, ducks, bees; it contains much information concerning breeding, diseases of the animals, *etc.* Vol. III contains text *plus* translation of chapters X-XIII of the "De re rustica" and *idem* of the "De arboribus", the only extant book of the first version of the "De re rustica" (p. 341-412), together with the index.

——, MARSHALL, L. B., 1918: L'horticulture antique et le poème de Columelle, 162 p. (Thèse Univ. Paris) (Paris: Hachette).—

This study has been divided into two parts. The first part deals with the origin of ancient horticulture, with botany, pharmacy, medicine, gastronomy, with the trade in flowers, with the flower in Greek literature, and with the horticulture of Virgil's "Georgics". The second part deals with book X of Columella, its sources and general scheme, the nomenclature of the plants considered, the activities of the gardener, and it contains an explanation of the technical terms used in relation to the gardener's activities. It also contains a discussion of Columella's successors.

Cratevas (fl. *ca.* 100-50 B.C.) — WELLMANN, M., 1897: Krateuas, 32 p. (Abh. Kgl. Gesell. Wiss. Göttingen, Phil.-Hist. Kl., II).—

Cratevas wrote a herbal, containing illustrations which possibly were prototypes of those included in the famous 6th-century manuscript of Dioscorides kept in Venice. The present publication contains reproductions of two plants from this ms.; *cf.* also: WELLMANN, M., 1898: Das älteste Kräuterbuch der Griechen, in: Festschrift für Franz Susemihl (Leipzig).

Dioscorides of Anazarbos, Pedanios (fl. *ca.* 50) — JBLER, C. E., 1953 - 1959: La 'Materia Médica' de Dioscórides. Transmisión medieval y renacentista, 5 vols. Vol. I (1953): 73 + 333 p.; Vol. II (1952-1957): 187 + 625 p. in Arabic; Vol. III (1955): 616 p.; Vol. IV (1955): 366 p.; Vol. V (1954): 940 p.; Vol. VI (1959): 353 p. (Barcelona: Privately published).—

A useful and very satisfactory Spanish edition. An insight into the contents of the various volumes is supplied by the subtitles: Vol: I: La transmisión medieval y renacentista y la supervivencia de la medicina popular moderna de la 'Materia Médica' de Dioscórides, estudiada particularmente en España y Africa del Norte; Vol. II: La versión árabe (texto, variantes e indices); Vol. III La 'Materia Médica' de Dioscórides traducida y comentada por D. Andrés de Laguna; Vol. IV: D. Andrés de Laguna y su época; Vol. V: Glosario médico castellano del siglo XVI; Vol. VI: Prólogo de Gregorio Marañón; indices generales y léxico especial.

——, GUNTHER, R. T., ed., 1959: The Greek herbal of Dioscorides (illustrated by a Byzantine, A.D. 512; englished by John Goodyer, A.D. 1655; edited and first printed A.D. 1933), 701 p. (New York, N.Y.: Hafner).—

The encyclopaedia of materia medica of Dioscorides, dealing with all the medicines known in the first century A.D., was often published and commented upon, and it was frequently cited as a first-rate authority up to the 17th century. It consists of 5 parts, dealing respectively with: 1) aromatics, oils, ointments and trees; 2) milk and dairy products, cereals and sharp herbs; 3) roots, juices and herbs; 4) herbs and roots;

5) vines, wines, and metallic ores. An appendix with identifications of the (about 600) plants mentioned by Dioscorides has been added, together with Latin and English indexes. The present edition is a reprint of the 1933 edition, containing the first English translation, prepared by JOHN GOODYER in 1652-1655. A German translation with many authoritative commentaries and comparisons with modern achievements is: BERENDES, J., ed., 1902: Des Pedanios Dioskurides aus Anazarbos Arzneimittellehre in fünf Büchern, 572 p. (Stuttgart: Enke). A French study is: BLONDEL, R., n.d., Les causeries médicales de Dioscoride, 3 vols. Vol. I: 355 p.; Vol. II: 351 p.; Vol. III: 352 p. (Paris: Michel). An attempt to characterize the plants mentioned by Dioscorides: KILLERMANN, S., 1955: Die in den illuminierten Dioskurides-Handschriften dargestellten Pflanzen. Beitrag zur Geschichte der älteren Pflanzenkunde. (Denkschr. Regensb. Bot. Ges. 24, N.F. 18: 3-64). *Cf.* also: WELLMANN, M., 1898: Die Pflanzennamen des Dioskurides, 62 p. (Hermes 33: 360-422). The reproduction of a complete facsimile edition of the famous and very beautiful Vienna Dioscorides Ms. is in progress. (Cod. Med. gr. 1 of the Austrian National Library). It will be delivered in five single parts, of which up to now three parts have been published. Reproduction and printing by the Akademische Druck- und Verlagsanstalt, Graz. For a bibliography on Dioscorides, see: STANNARD, J., 1966: Dioscorides and Renaissance materia medica (Analecta Medico-Historica, Vol. 1: 1-21); about the illustrations, see: MIONI, E., 1959: Un ignoto Dioscoride miniato. (Il Codice Greco 194 del Seminario di Padova), 48 p. + 21 plates. (Padova: Antenore). See review Isis 53 (1962): 588.

Galen of Pergamon (129-199) — BEINTKER, E. & W. KAHLENBERG, eds., 1939-1954: Werke des Galenos. Vol. I (1939): Galenos Gesundheitslehre, Buch 1-3, 139 p.; Vol. II (1941): *Idem,* Buch 4-6, 143 p.; Vol. III (1948): Die Kräfte der Nahrungsmittel, Buch 1-2, 137 p.; Vol. IV (1952): *Idem,* Buch 3-6. Gute und schlechte Säfte der Nahrungsmittel. Die Säfteverdünnende Diät. Die Ptisane, 163 p.; Vol. V (1954): Die Kräfte der Physis (Ueber die natürlichen Kräfte), 133 p. (Stuttgart: Hippocrates).—

As to the contents of vols. I and II, *cf.* GREEN, R. M., 1951 (*vide infra*). In vol. III Galen tries to evaluate how food influences the humours. In the first book he considers cereals and leguminous plants, and in the second book the other vegetable

means of subsistence, fruits, and vegetables. In vol. IV he considers *e.g.,* foodstufs derived from animals, honey, wine, deficiency diseases, putrefaction of the water of the river in Rome, epidemic diseases, *etc.* Vol. V deals with physiological problems, with the four main forces constituting the human body, *viz.,* the attractive, the conservative, the transformative and the repulsive force respectively, on which the functioning of all organs should rest, and which should also be responsible for the origin, transformation, and growth of the organs.

——, BROCK, A. J., ed., 1952: Galen: On the natural faculties, 55 + 339 p. (Loeb Classical Library) (London: Heinemann; Cambridge, Mass.: Harvard U.P.).—

Reprint of the 1916 edition. Translation based upon K. G. KÜHN's edition, *vide infra.* Valuable introduction, in which the editor reviews the history of medicine in Greece, the introduction of Greek medicine into Rome, Byzantine and Arabian medicine down to the Renaissance. Then the author gives a short exposition of Galen's philosophy and a synopsis of chapters. Concerning the "Natural Faculties", the editor states: "If Galen be looked on as a crystallisation of Greek medicine, then this book may be looked on as a crystallisation of Galen. Within its comparatively short compass we meet with instances illustrating perhaps most of the sides of this many-sided writer. The 'Natural Faculties' therefore forms an excellent prelude to the study of his larger and more specialised works."

——, DAREMBERG, C., ed., 1854-1856: Oeuvres anatomiques, physiologiques et médicales de Galien, 2 vols. Vol. I: 706 p.; Vol. II: 786 p. (Paris: Baillière).—

The first volume consists of the following French translations: Que le bon médecin est philosophe; Exhortation à l'étude des arts; Que les moeurs de l'âme sont la conséquence des tempéraments du corps; Des habitudes; De l'utilité des parties du corps humain, livre I-XI. The second volume consists of the following translations: De l'utilité des parties du corps humain, livre XII-XVII; Des facultés naturelles; Du mouvement des muscles; Des sectes aux étudiants; De la meilleure secte, à Thrasybule; Des lieux affectés; De la méthode thérapeutique, à Glaucon.

——, DUCKWORTH, W. L. H., M. C. LYONS & B. TOWERS, eds., 1962: On anatomical procedures: the later books, 279 p. (Cambridge: U.P.).—

This book (translated by W. L. H. DUCKWORTH, edited by M. C. LYONS & B. TOWERS) is a supplement to C. SINGER's book *(vide infra),* and contains an English translation from chapter 6 of book IX up to book XV of the De anatomicis administrationibus of Galen. Almost half of its contents deals with the dissection and description of the nervous system. In contrast to Singer's translation of the first 9 books, there are no annotations. The English translation is based partly on a new translation from an Arabic text, partly on the following German edited: SIMON, M., ed., 1906: Sieben Bücher Anatomie des Galen. Zum erstenmale veröffentlicht nach den Handschriften einer arabischen Uebersetzung des 9. Jahrh. n. Chr. Ins Deutsche übertragen und kommentiert von M. Simon. Vol. I: Arabischer Text. Einleitung zum Sprachgebrauch. Glossar mit zwei Faksimiletafeln, 81 + 366 p.; Vol. II: Deutscher Text. Kommentar. Einleitung zur Anatomie des Galen. Sach- und Namenregister, 68 + 366 p. (Leipzig: Hinrichs).

———, ENGLERT, L., 1929: Untersuchungen zu Galens Schrift Thrasybulos, 103 p. (Stud. Gesch. Med., Vol. 18) (Leipzig: Barth).—

The "Thrasybulos" is a treatise dealing with the iatric theory. In the first part the author considers the origin of the concept of medicine, discussing, *inter alia,* Hippocrates, Plato, Aristotle, the dogmatic, pneumatic, empiric, and methodic schools. The second part (p. 32-86) is the main part of the book; it is entitled "Untersuchungen zu Galen's Schrift Thrasybulos", and deals with such subjects as: object and construction, theory, terminology, *etc.* of the treatise. Notes (p. 87-98), bibliography, and indexes of names, subjects and quotations.

———, GREEN, R. M., ed., 1951: A translation of Galen's Hygiene (De sanitate tuenda), 277 p. (Springfield, Ill.: Thomas).—

This translation is mainly based upon K. G. KÜHN's Greek-Latin edition, Vol. 6: 1-452, *vide infra.* Originally the book was intended for the ruling classes during Galen's time, in order to guide them in the techniques of bathing, of gymnastic excercise, of rest and recreation, and of massage. The work itself is divided into six books: I. The art of preserving health; II. Exercise and massage; III. Apothecary, bathing, and fatique; IV. Forms and treatment of fatique; V. Diagnosis, treatment, and prevention of various diseases; VI. Prophylaxis of pathological conditions. For a German translation of this text, *cf.* E. BEINTKER & W.

KAHLENBERG, 1939-1954, vols. I and II *(vide supra).*

———, HARKINS, P. W., ed., 1963: Galen on the passions and errors of the soul, 136 p. (Columbus, Ohio: Ohio State U.P.).—

The first English translation of Galen's "On the passions of the soul" and "On the errors of the soul", based on the critical edition of W. DE BOER, 1937, in "Corpus Medicorum Graecorum" (Leipzig & Berlin). W. RIESE provides this book with an introduction to Galen's life and work, with an interpretation of the treatises, and an evaluation of their influence on subsequent philosophers. *Cf.* HAUKE, E., 1968: Galen: Dass die Vermögen der Seele eine Folge der Mischungen des Körpers sind, 38 p. (Abh. Gesch. Med. Naturw., No. 21) (New York, N.Y.: Johnson). Originally published 1937 (Berlin: Ebering).

———, KOLLESCH, J., ed., 1964: Galen über das Riechorgan, 128 p. (Corpus Medicorum Graecorum, Vol. V) (Berlin: Akademie Verlag).—

In an introduction a review is given of extant mss., early editions, *etc.* Then the text and German translation follow on facing pages (p. 29-66), together with commentaries (p. 67-110) and indexes (p. 111-128).

———, KÜHN, K. G., ed., 1821-1833: Greek-Latin edition of Galen's works, 20 vols. (Leipzig).—

Still the most useful edition. The last volume contains an index of 676 pages, according to Sarton still the best available key to Galen. Vol. I contains an elaborate bibliography of 250 p., containing the editions appeared before 1821. Reprinted in 1965 (Hildesheim: Olms). Vol. 20 of the reprint contains a series of annotations with bibliographical notes compiled by K. SCHUBRING.

———, LYONS, M., ed., 1963: Galeni in Hippocratis de officina medici commentarii. Versio arabica. Edit. et in linguam anglicam vertit, 172 p. (Corpus Medicorum Graecorum) (Berlin: Akademie Verlag).—

This book contains the Arabic text together with an English translation of a mediaeval Arabian manuscript of Galen's "Commentary on Hippocrates, Qatîtrîûm". The introduction contains a study of references and previous research connected with this work. The book is of much importance to anyone studying the transmission of Greek medicine to Arabian physicians. Greek-Arabic and Arabic-Greek glossaries (p. 125-172).

——, MAY, M. T., ed., 1968: Galen on the usefulness of the parts of the body: an English translation of "De usu partium", 2 vols., 784 p. (Ithaca, N.Y.: Cornell U.P.).—

An English translation of the 17 books of the "De usu partium" in which Galen sets out with the teleological explanation of the relationship between anatomy and physiology. Galen's fundamental object was to demonstrate that the structure of the human body was the product of intelligent and divine design. In an introduction the authoress gives an analysis of the contents of the treatise and a review of the situation in medical science in the period just before and just after Galen's time. Many illuminating annotations. The only other translation in one of the Western vernaculars is C. DAREMBERG's French version (1854-1856), based on the KÜHN standard ed. of Galen, *vide supra*.

——, MEYERHOF, M. & J. SCHAFT, eds., 1931: Galen über die medizinischen Namen, Arabisch und Deutsch, 62 p. (Abh. preuss. Akad. Wiss., Phil.-Hist. Kl., No. 3) (Berlin: de Gruyter).—

According to Sarton, this book "is one of the most important of the 45 authentic Galenic writings which are lost in Greek but were known in Arabic in the ninth century. Ḥunain ibn Isḥāq translated three parts of it (out of five) from Greek into Syriac, and his nephew Ḥubaish ibn al-Ḥasan translated the first of these from Syriac into Arabic... That Arabic text represented by a single ms. (Leiden Or. 585) is here edited and translated into German." (Isis 18: 445).

——, RICHTER, P., 1913: De tumoribus praeter naturam. German translation: Ueber die krankhaften Geschwülste, 26 p. (Klassiker der Medicin, Vol. 21) (Leipzig: Barth).—

A German translation of Galen's views about tumours. The text was written probably between 169 and 180; it greatly influenced Arabic and West-European medicine up to the 19th century.

——, SARTON, G., 1954: Galen of Pergamon, 112 p. (Lawrence, Ka.: Univ. of Kansas Press).—

A well-written account of Galen and his work. Sarton begins with an informative description of Graeco-Roman life in Asia Minor. He considers Galen's education in the four orthodox systems of philosophy and his eclecticism, his anatomical interests and his opposition to the Methodist School, his activities as a physician of the gladiators both in Rome and Pergamon and as courtphysician in Rome. Besides his anatomical and medical activities, Galen was also engaged in physiology, pharmacy, philosophy, history, and philology; all these aspects have been considered. Together with the descriptions of his character, literary style, his religious beliefs, and a lot of other details, this booklet gives a very lucid picture of Galen, his work, and his influence.

——, SIEGEL, R. E., 1968: Galen's system of physiology and medicine: an analysis of his doctrines and observations on bloodflow, respiration, humors and internal diseases, 419 p. (Basle & New York, N.Y.: Karger).—

In the present book the author attempts to come to a reappraisal of Galen's work. He does so by analysing Galen's doctrines and observations on blood flow, respiration, humours and internal diseases.

—— ——, 1970: Galen on sense perception: his doctrines, observations and experiments on vision, hearing, touch and pain, and their historical sources, 216 p. (Basle & New York, N.Y.: Karger).—

Nearly half of the book deals with the eye. For each sense an account of contributions made before Galen's time are included, so that Galen's doctrines on sense perception are related with those of his predecessors. Of each of the senses considered, a description of its end organ and a detailed analysis of the doctrine of its function has been given. Many quotations from the original text and extensive bibliography.

——, SINGER, C., ed., 1958: Galen: On anatomical procedures. De anatomicis administrationibus. Translation of the surviving books with introduction and notes, 289 p. (London: Oxford U.P.).—

De anatomicis administrationibus, an elaborate guide to the dissection of animal bodies, chiefly of monkeys, consisted originally of 15 books. Because the last 6 books were not recovered until the end of the 19th century, they had no influence on the history of anatomy and physiology; therefore the editor restricted himself to the first 9 books which treat of the upper and lower limbs, the vessels and nerves of the extremities, the muscles of the head, neck, and torso, the alimentary organs, the cardiopulmonary system, the thorax and the brain. The various structures considered have been described in modern terminology and the insertion of explanatory notes greatly increases the readability of the book. For a translation of the other six books *cf.* W. L. H. DUCKWORTH, *et al., 1962 (vide supra).* What is - according to Sarton (Isis 4: 577) - a useful study of Galen's special dissection-techniques for various tissues and organs, of material and instruments used, nomenclature, vivisection, and physiological experiments, is: ULLRICH, F., 1919: Die anatomische und vivisektorische Technik des Galenos, 54 p. (Diss. Univ. Leipzig).

——, WALZER, R., ed., 1934: Galen: On medical experience. First ed. of the Arabic version with English translation and notes, 164 p. (London: Oxford U.P.).—

This text has been prepared from a newly-discovered Arabian text, which itself was a translation from the Syriac. In his preface, the editor gives some data about the history of the text and the composition and significance of the work. The text itself reproduces a discussion held between the dogmatist Pelops and the empiricist Philippos; this discussion gives a valuable insight into philosophical argumentation in Greek medicine of those days.

Herophilos of Chalcedon (fl. 300-250 B.C.) — MARX, K. F. H., 1838: Herophilus. Ein Beitrag zur Geschichte der Medizin, 103 p. (Karlsruhe: Marx).—

This booklet is an attempt to place the Coic physician and anatomist Herophilos within the framework of his time. It deals with his life, writings, pupils, adversaries, medical, anatomical and physiological achievements. Herophilos was the founder of anatomy as a scientific discipline; he was the greatest anatomist of antiquity. Flourished in Alexandria under Ptomely I. *Cf.* also: DOBSON, J. F., 1925: Herophilus of Alexandria, 12 p. (Proc. roy. Soc. Med., Hist. Sect. 18: 19-31).

Lucretius Carus, Titus (98- *ca.* 55 B.C.) — BAILEY, C., ed., 1947: Titi Lucreti Cari De rerum natura libri sex. With prolego-

mena, critical apparatus, translation, and commentary, 3 vols., 1785 p. (Oxford: Clarendon Press.).—

The first volume contains a short biography of Lucretius (p. 1-22), an introduction to his poem, its sources, structure and composition, its grammar (accidence and syntax, metric, style), and an introduction to Lucretius's philosophy, its canonization, moral, theological, and religious aspects. This is followed by the text, critical apparatus, and translation. Vol. II contains commentaries on Bks. I-III, and Vol. III contains commentaries on Bks. IV-VI, addenda et corrigenda, indexes and bibliography. A somewhat older, but according to Sarton (in his "Introduction") excellent edition is MUNRO, H. A. J., 1928: T. Lucreti Cari De rerum natura libri sex, ed. 4. Vol. I: text, 296 p.; Vol. II: Notes, with an introductory essay on the scientific significance of Lucretius by E. N. DA C. ANDRADE, 424 p.; Vol. III: English translation, 183 p. (Cambridge: Deighton Bell). A new English ed.: ROUSE, W. H. D., ed., 1966: De rerum natura, 538 p. (Loeb Classical Library) (London: Heinemann; Cambridge, Mass.: Harvard U.P.).

——, ERNOUT, A., ed., 1962: Lucrèce. De la nature, 2 vols. Vol. I: 154 + 154 p.; Vol. II: 150 + 150 p. (Paris: Les Belles Lettres).—

In a short introduction the author describes what we know about the life and work of Lucretius. Then comes the Latin text (based on the two Leiden manuscripts), together with a French translation. An edition and German translation: DIELS, H., 1923-1924: Lukrez von der Natur: Lateinisch und deutsch, 2 vols. (Berlin: Weidmann). A modern English translation is: HUMPHRIES, R., 1968: Lucretius: the way things are. The De rerum natura of Titus Lucretius Carus, translated, 255 p. (London & Bloomington, Ind.: Indiana U.P.).

——, GORDON, C. A., 1962: A bibliography of Lucretius, 319 p. (London: Rupert Hart-Davis).—

The bibliography has been divided into 7 sections: plain texts, annotated editions, pocket-editions, translations, illustrated editions, selections, ghosts. Within each section the arrangement is chronological.

——, HADZSITS, G. D., 1963: Lucretius and his influence, 372 p. (New York, N.Y.: Cooper Square).—

This is a reprint of the 1935 edition (New York, N.Y.: Longmans, Green). In order to give an insight into the contents of this book, we give the chapter headings: 1. Life of Lucretius (p. 3-7); II. Epicurus and Epicureanism in Athens (p. 8-15); III. Lucretius and the Roman epicureans (p. 16-27); IV. The "De rerum natura" and Rome of the first century B.C. (p. 28-61); V. Lucretius and the atom (p. 62-78); VI. L. and the soul (p. 79-102); VII. L. and religion (p. 103-123); VIII. L. and ethics (p. 124-159); IX. L. and the Roman Empire (p. 160-197); X. L. and the Middle Ages (p. 198-247); XI. L. and the Renaissance (p. 248-283); XII. The 17th and 18th century and L., and the present. For a more thorough treatment of Lucretius's influence on 20th-century thinking, *vide* DUDLEY, D. R., ed., 1965: Lucretius, 166 p. (London: Routledge & Kegan Paul), a series of 7 essays, written by: D. R. DUDLEY, B, FARRINGTON, O. E. LOWENSTEIN, W. S. MAGUINNESS, T. J. B. SPENCER, G. B. TOWNEND & D. E. W. WORMEL.

——, SINKER, A. P., 1962: Introduction to Lucretius, 139 p. (Cambridge: U.P.).—

"In order to read any part of the 'De rerum natura' with full appreciation it is necessary to have a knowledge of the whole, since all parts are mutually interdependent." This book is intended to supply that knowledge; and thus it is not an alternative but an introduction to a full reading of the "De rerum natura". A booklet with the same intention is: WINSPEAR, A. D., 1963: Lucretius and scientific thought, 156 p. (Montreal: Harvest House).

Martialis, Gargilius (*ca.* 40 - *ca.* 102) — PEYER, B & H. REMUND, 1928: Medizinisches aus Martial, mit Ergänzungen aus Juvenal und einem naturgeschichtlichen Anhang, 102 p. (Zurich: Füssli).—

A collection of those passages from Martial's poems which deal with diseases and medicine. Separate sections deal with the social position of the physician, diseases, therapy, baths, cosmetics, sexual life, and poisons. A section (p. 77-97) deals with natural history and it also contains much information on feeding habits of those days.

Menodotos of Nicomedia (fl. *ca.* 150) — FAVIER, A., 1906: Un médecin grec du IIe siècle, précurseur de la méthode expérimentale modere: Ménodote de Nicomédie, 387 p. (Diss. Univ. Paris) (Paris: Rousset).—

Menodotos was a Greek physician,

and according to Sarton (Introd. I: 308) the first, or one of the first, to syncretize the ideas of empirical and sceptical medicine. The contents of this book: Introduction; 1. Médicine dogmatique et médecine empirique (p. 21-100); 2. La méthode expérimentale moderne (p. 101-197); 3. Menodote (p. 198-326).

Mithridates Eupator (120-63 B.C.) — REINACH, T., 1890: Mithridate Eupator, roi de Pont, 494 p. (Paris: Firmin-Didot).—

Mithridates, King of Pontos, is well-known because of his pharmaceutical and toxicological investigations. About the present book, Sarton writes in his Introduction I, p. 214: "An apparently exhaustive and very illuminating study of one of the most extraordinary personalities of ancient history; the scientific work of Mithridates is hardly discussed but the fundamental facts are given p. 283-285. This book has been translated into German by A. GOETZ (Leipzig: Teubner, 1895). This is really a new edition, for the author has taken advantage of it to make many corrections of, and additions to the original text."

Nemesianus, Marcus Aurelius Olympius (fl. 282-283) — MARTIN, D., 1917: The Cynegetica of Nemesianus, 83 p. (Thesis of Cornell Univ.).—

Nemesianus was a Roman poet, author of poems on fishing and hunting. Cynegetica is a fragment of 325 hexameters still extant. The present booklet contains the (Latin) text of the poem together with a long introduction discussing the history of the mss., their composition and editions, the life of its author, *etc.* (p. 1-23), and some 325 notes (p. 36-83).

Nemesios of Emesa (fl. *ca.* 400) — ORTH, E., ed., 1925: Anthropologie. Vorwort des Nik. Alfanus und des Rich. Burgondio, 121 p. (Koblenz: Martental).—

Nemesios was a Christian philosopher, Bishop of Emesa. His "Anthropology" is a book on the nature of Man that was very popular during the Middle Ages, and contains interesting views on human physiology. This is a German translation of this book. According to Sarton (Introduction I: 374) there exists an English translation by G. WITHER (London, 1636) and a French translation by J. B. THIBAULT (Paris, 1844).

Nicander of Colophon (fl. *ca.* 275 B.C.) —
GOW, A. S. F. & A. F. SCHOLFIELD, eds.,
1953: Nicander: the poems and poetical
fragments, 247 p. (Cambridge: U.P.).—

The themes of his two extant poems,
the "Theriaca" and the "Alexipharmaca",
are medicine, zoology, botany, and mineralogy, poisons in general and poisonous animals, the effects of their venoms and their
antidotes in particular. In the introduction
(p. 3-25) the author gives a short biography
of Nicander and briefly considers the zoological (reptiles, frogs, toads, fish, scorpions,
spiders, and insects) and botanical subject-
matter (125 plants are mentioned) of the
poems. Then the text and translation of the
poems follow (p. 26-169). There are appendixes on the botanical drawings, weights
and measures, and on books and papers relating to Nicander; and indexes of fauna,
flora, *etc.*

Oppianus (fl. 204) — MAIR, A. W., ed.,
1958: Oppian, Colluthus Tryphiodorus, 80
+ 636 p. (Loeb Classical Library) (London:
Heinemann; Cambridge, Mass.: Harvard
U.P.).—

From this booklet the larger part:
80 + 531 p. has been devoted to Oppian. In
his introduction to Oppian's text, the editor
briefly considers zoology before Oppian,
hunting, fishing and fowling, the identification of certain fishes, and some animal idio-
syncrasies. Then he gives the Greek text
together with the English translation of:
Cynegetica, or the chase (Bks. I-IV); Ha-
lieutica, or fishing (Bks. I-V) and a classified zoological catalogue.

Oribasios (325-403) — BUSSEMAKER,
U. C. & C. DAREMBERG, eds., 1851-1876:
Oribasius. Oeuvres, texte grec, en grande
partie inédit, collationné sur les manuscrits
(trad. pour la première fois en français, avec
une introduction, des notes, des tables et des
planches), 6 vols. Vol. I: 60 + 692 p.; Vol.
II: 921 p.; Vol. III: 723 p.; Vol. IV: 720 p.;
Vol. V: 956 p.; Vol. VI: 811 p. (Paris:
Imprimerie Nationale).—

Oribasios, born in Pergamon, was an
eminent Greek encyclopaedist, who wrote
a medical encyclopaedia in 70 books of
which a third are still extant. His works
have a considerable historical value because
Oribasios quoted his authorities with great
care (Sarton). According to Sarton the work
under consideration is an excellent Greek-
French translation of Oribasios's extanding

works. The last volume (ed. by A. MOLI-
NER) contains the ancient Latin translation of the "Synopsis" (a summary of his
medical encyclopaedia) and the "Eupovista"
(a book of home medicine). For a systematic
survey of those passages in Oribasios's
works dealing with dentistry, *vide* HEINE-
CKE, W., 1922: Zahnärztliches in den Werken des Oreibasios, 21 p. (Diss. Leipzig).
Contains also a list of drugs used, and a
bibliography.

Palladius, Rutilius Taurus Aemilianus (fl.
ca. 330) — LODGE, B., 1873: Palladius on
husbondry, ed. from the unique ms. of about
1420 A.D. in Colchester Castle, 36 + 20
+ 387 p. (London: Trübner).—

Palladius was the last of the Roman
geoponists, and he wrote a farmer's calendar, based upon Gargilius Martialis, the
"De agricultura". It consists of 14 books, of
which the first is introductory; books II to
XIII deal with the duties of each month,
and book XIV is a poem on the art of grafting. The present edition contains an alphabetically-arranged table of contents on p.
xxi-xxxvi. Then the middle-English text is
given, and those passages which possibly
may not be clear have been explained in
modern English in the margin. The text has
been printed on p. 1-220, notes follow on
p. 221-233. Glossarial index and rhyme index on p. 255-378. There also must exist
a French edition, ed. by NISARD (Paris,
1877).

Philagrios of Thessalonica (fl. *ca.* 350-400)
— PUSCHMANN, T., 1963: Nachträge zu
Alexander Trallianus. Fragmente aus Philumenus und Philagrius, *etc. (cf.* Philumenos,
vide infra).

From the Greek physician Philagrios
it contains the following fragments, both in
Latin and in German translation (p. 74-129):
1. Ad splenum ("Ueber die Milzleiden");
2. De ventositate splenis ("Ueber die Auftrü-
bung der Milz"); 3. Signa phlegmones splenis, si de solo sanguine flat ("Ueber die Ent-
zündung der Milz"); 4. De scirro splenis
("Ueber den Skirrhus der Milz"). *Cf.*
LEWY, A., 1931, *vide supra,* subsection c.

Philumenos (fl. *ca.* 175) — PUSCHMANN,
T., 1963: Nachträge zu Alexander Trallianus.
Fragmente aus Philumenus und Philagrius
nebst einer bisher noch ungedruckten Ab-
handlung über Augenkrankheiten, 189 p.
(Amsterdam: Hakkert).—

411

412

A facsimile reproduction of the original publication of 1887 (In: Berliner Studien für class. Philologie, Vol. II). After a brief introduction, the author gives the Latin text together with a German translation of the following fragments of the Greek physician of the Eclectic School Philumenos (p. 16-73): De reumate ventris ("Ueber den Unterleibsfluss"); 2. De dysenteria reumatica ("Ueber die fluxionäre Ruhr"); 3. De coeliacis ("Ueber die Unterleibsleiden"); 4. De tenesmo ("Ueber den Stuhlzwang"). There is an important shorter publication: WELLMANN, M., 1908: Philumenos, 32 p. (Hermes 43: 373:404).

Pliny the Elder (23-79) — ANDRÉ, J., *et. al.*, 1947 →: Pline l'Ancien: histoire naturelle in ?7 vols. (Paris: Les Belles Lettres).—

The present edition, published under the auspices of the Association Guillaume Budé, is a more ambitious edition of this popular mediaeval treatise than he Loeb one, (*cf.* H. RACKHAM & W. H. S. JONES, 1938-1953, *vide infra*), because it leaves more room for learned discussions of the matter considered. Up to now the following volumes have been published: Livre I (1950, ed. by J. BEAUJEU), 161 p.; Livre II (1950, ed. by J. BEAUJEU), 282 p.; Livre VIII (1952, ed. by J. ERNOUT), 192 p.; Livre IX (1955, ed. by E. DE ST. DENIS), 157 p.; Livre X (1961, ed. by E. DE ST. DENIS), 171 p.; Livre XI (1947, ed. by A. ERNOUT & R. PÉPIN), 219 p.; Livre XII (1949, ed. by A. ERNOUT), 112 p.; Livre XIII (1956, ed. by A. ERNOUT), 122 p.; Livre XIV (1958, ed. by J. ANDRÉ), 167 p.; Livre XV (1960, ed. by J. ANDRÉ), 135 p.; Livre XVI (1962, ed. by J. ANDRÉ), 198 p.; Livre XVII (1964, ed. by J. ANDRÉ), 205 p.; Livre XIX (1964, ed. by J. ANDRÉ), 187 p.; Livre XX (1965, ed. by J. ANDRÉ), 229 p.; Livre XXI (1969, ed. by J. ANDRÉ), 173 p.; Livre XXII (1970, ed. by J. ANDRÉ), 133 p.; Livre XXVI (1956, ed. by A. ERNOUT & R. PÉPIN), 129 p.; Livre XXVII (1959, ed. by A. ERNOUT), 123 p.; Livre XXVIII (1962, ed. by J. ERNOUT), 181 p.; Livre XXIX (1962, ed. by A. ERNOUT), 141 p.; Livre XXX (1963, ed. by A. ERNOUT), 108 p.; Livre XXXII (1966, ed. by E. DE ST. DENIS), 149 p.; Livre XXXIV (1953, ed. by J. LE BONNIEC), 324 p. For a full review of the whole work, see Vol. I which contains the complete table of contents of all volumes planned - of volumes published as well as of volumes still to be published.

——, DANNEMANN, F., 1921: Plinius und seine Naturgeschichte in ihrer Bedeutung für die Gegenwart, 251 p. (Jena: Diederichs).—

The purpose of this book is to give in German translation those parts of Pliny's Natural History which might be of educational value at the present time. In a brief introduction the author surveys the interrelations of Greek and Roman elements in science of those days and from which authors Pliny borrowed his material for his Natural History. The greater part of the text (p. 53-245) contains sections from the "Historia Naturalis" dealing with geography and ethnology, zoology, botany, and mineralogy; each section is preceded by a special introduction.

——, LE BONNIEC, H., 1946: Bibliographie de l'histoire naturelle de Pline l'Ancien, 55 p. (Paris: Klincksieck).—

A bibliography of extant mss. and the various editions of the books written by Pliny and a useful list of scholarly articles written about Pliny.

——, RACKHAM, H. & W. H. S. JONES, eds., 1938-1953: Pliny: Natural History, 6 vols. Vol. I (1938): Praefatio, Libri I, II, 378 p.; Vol. II (1942): Libri III-VII, 664 p.; Vol. III (1940): Libri VIII-XI, 616 p.; Vol. IV (1945): Libri XII-XVI, 556 p.; Vol. V (1952): Libri XVII-XIX, 544 p.; Vol. VI (1951): Libri XX-XXIII, 532 p.; Vol. VII (1946): Libri XXIV-XXVII, 588 p.; Vol. VIII (1953): Libri XXVIII-XXXII, 596 p.; Vol. IX (1952): Libri XXXIII-XXXV, 421 p.; Vol. X (1952): Libri XXXVI-XXXVII, 344 p. (The Loeb Classical Library) (London: Heinemann; Cambridge, Mass.: Harvard U.P.).—

The first 5 volumes and vol. IX have been edited by H. RACKHAM, vols. VI-VIII bij JONES and vol. X by D.E. EICHHOLZ. Bk. I contains the table of contents of the remaining 36 books, the contents of each book being followed by a list of the previous writers used as authorities. Bk. II deals with cosmology, astronomy, meteorology, geography, geology; Bk. III with Southern Spain, Southern Gaul, Italy, the western Mediterranean, Ionian and Adriatic islands, and the countries around the north of the Adriatic; Bk. IV with Greece and the rest of the Balkan Peninsula, the islands of the Eastern Mediterranean, the Black Sea and the countries west of it, Northern Europe; Bk. V with North Africa, the Eastern Mediterranean and Asia Minor; Bk. VI with countries from the Black Sea to India; Persia, Arabia, Ethiopia, and the Nile valley; Bk. VII deals with the human race, its biology, physiology and psychology; Bk. VIII deals with various mammals, wild, domesticated and introduced; Bk. IX with aquatic animals, especially with fish and fisheries; Bk. X with ornithology: hawking, birds as omina, domestic birds, reproduction, *etc.;* Bk. XI with insects and with animal classification. Bks. XVII-XIX deal with arboriculture, cereal agriculture, the cultivation of flax and of other plants used for industry, and with vegetable gardening. Bks. XX-XXVII deal with the use of trees, plants and flowers, especially in medicine; Bks. XXVIII-XXXII deal with drugs obtained from animals; Bks. XXXIII and XXXIV deal with the properties of the metals; Bk. XXXV with painting, sculpture, varieties of earth; Bk. XXXVI with the nature of stones.

——, WETHERED, H. N., 1937: The mind of the ancient world: a consideration of Pliny's "Natural History", 302 p. (New York, N.Y.: Longmans, Green).—

A modern survey of Pliny's great encyclopaedia. It consists of nearly 500 selections quoted (with slight modernization) from HOLLAND's text of 1601, grouped under the headings of: man, the body and physic, animals, fabulous creatures, birds, fishes, insects, flowers and herbs, inventions, magic and religion, gold and silver, precious stones, painters, sculptors, architecture and the seven wonders, the universe, places and peoples. Appendix 1 deals with mediaeval natural history, mainly with bestiaries, 2 with ancient science in literature, and 3 lists the chapter and page of the quotation in the text from Holland's translation. A book with the same purpose is: TURNER, P., ed., 1962: Natural history (transl. by P. Holland), 496 p. (Carbondale, Ill.: Southern Illinois U.P.). *Cf.* also: STEIER, A., 1913, *vide* this section, subsection b.

Priscianus Theodorus (fl. 367-383) — MEYER, T., 1909: Theodorus Priscianus und die römische Medizin, 352 p. (Jena: Fischer).—

This book deals with Roman medicine before Theodorus Priscianus (p. 1-29), with his life and publications (p. 30-32), his pathology and therapeutics (p. 33-76). Then the German translation follows of his book of medicine, the Euporiston, chiefly a collection of therapeutic descriptions consisting of four books. Book I: External ailments (p. 77-162); Book II: Internal medicine (p. 163-277); Book III: Women's diseases (p. 278-297) and Book IV: Miraculous remedies. An alphabetically-arranged glossary of the drugs and foods used by Priscianus, and subject-indexes, are included.

Rufus of Ephesus (fl. *ca.* 100-150) — DAREMBERG, C. & E. RUELLE, 1879: Oeuvres de Rufus d'Ephèse. Texte collationné sur les manuscrits, traduit pour la première fois en français, avec une introduction, 56 + 678 p. (Paris: Imprimerie Nationale).—

This edition contains all the Greek works extant and fragments collected from Greek and Arabic authors. It consists of the following parts: (text + translation): Traité des maladies des reins et de la vessie; Sur la satyriasis et la gonorrhée; Du nom des parties du corps humain; Des os; De l'interrogation des malades; Traité abrégé sur le pouls (anonymous); Traité de la goutte; Fragments de Rufus d'Ephèse extraits de Galien; Fragments extraits d'Aétius, d'Alexandre de Tralles, de Paul d'Egina, et de Rhazes. It contains only the text of: Aétius, livre XI, parties à rapprocher des textes précédents de Rufus; Livre 1er des dénominations des parties de l'homme; Scholies sur le traité du nom des parties du corps; Etymologies de Soranus.

——, GÄRTNER, H., ed., 1962: Rufus von Ephesos. Die Fragen des Arztes an den Kranken, 122 p. (Corpus Medicorum Graecorum, Suppl. IV) (Berlin: Akademie Verlag).—

Rufus can be considered to be the greatest physician of the Roman Empire after Galen. He has made elaborate anatomical researches and has seen the functional importance of the nervous system. The present publication contains the text of "$\iota\alpha\tau\rho\iota\kappa\alpha\ \epsilon\xi\omega\iota\eta\mu\alpha\iota\alpha$" of Rufus of Ephesus, based on two extant mss. After a general introduction (p. 15-23) text and German translation follow (p. 24-47) to which extensive commentaries have been added. To give an insight into the contents of this work we quote chapter headings: 1. Allgemeine Grundsätze der Befragung; 2. Der Zeitpunkt des Beginns einer Krankheit und periodische Abläufe; 3. Individualität und Gewohnheit; 4. Innere und äussere Ursachen von Krankheiten; 5. Schlaf, Schlaflosigkeit und Träume; 6. Angeborene Krankheiten; 7. Diät während der Krankheit; 8. Die Bedeutung von Schmerzen und Schmerzäusserungen für die Diagnose; 9. Die Beschaffenheit des Leibes und die Verdauung; 10. Tierbisse, besonders Bisse tollwütiger Hunde mit nachfolgender Hydrophobie; 11. Kriegsverletzungen; 12. Geographische und ethnographische Besonderheiten; 13. Rufus und Hippocrates. *Cf.* also: ILBERG, J., 1930: Rufus von Ephesos. Ein griechischer Arzt in trajanischer Zeit, 53 p. (Sächs. Akad. Wiss.,

Phil.-Hist. Kl. 41, No. 1) (Leipzig: Hirzel).

Scribonius Largus (fl *ca.* 50) — SCHO-NACK, W., 1913: Die Rezepte des Scri-bonius Largus. Zum ersten Male vollständig ins Deutsche übersetzt und mit ausführlichen Arzneimittelregister versehen, 198 p. (Jena: Fischer).—

A German translation of the collec-tion of recipes of the Roman pharmacolo-gist Scribonius, the "Compositiones medica-mentorum", together with an (alphabetically arranged) list of drugs mentioned (p. 121-176). *Cf.* also: SCHONACK, W., 1912: Die Rezeptsammlung des Scribonius Largus. Eine kritische Studie, 95 p. (Jena: Fischer). A special study of his dental therapy is: TRILK, F., 1921: Die zahnärztliche Phar-makotherapie in den "Compositiones" des Scribonius Largus, 43 p. (Diss. Sudhoff Inst.).

Seneca, Lucius Annaeus of Cordova (4 B.C. — 65 A.D.) — MARX, K. F. H., 1877: Uebersichtliche Anordnung der die Medizin betreffenden Aussprüche des Philosophen Lucius Annaeus Seneca, 66 p. (Abh. Kgl. Ges. Wiss., Göttingen) (Göttingen: Diete-rich).—

A summary of those passages of Seneca's works which deal with health, disease, medicine and its application.

Serenus Samonicus, Quintus († 212) — PÉ-PIN, R., 1951: Quintus Serenus (Serenus Samonicus). Liber medicinalis (Le livre de la médecine). Texte établ, traduit et commenté, 48 + 124 p. (Paris: Presses Univ. de France).—

A long introduction concerning the author and his medical poem consisting of 1,115 hexameters, his sources, the chapter headings, extant mss., ancient editors, and style of the poem. Then the text of the "De medicina praecepta saluberrima" follows, together with the French translation, on pages opposing each other (p. 1-57); this is followed by commentaries (p. 59-96) and an elaborate index (p. 97-114). The text of the poem chiefly consists of a collection of popular descriptions for various ailments, and it contains much information on natural history, medicine, and superstition. There also exists an Italian translation: LOMBAR-DI, F., 1963: Il "Liber medicinalis" di Quinto Serono Sammonico, 43 p. (Pisa: Giardini).

Soranos of Ephesus (fl. *ca.* 98—138) — TEMKIN, O., ed., 1956: Soranus' "Gyne-cology", 49 + 258 p. (translated with an introduction by O. TEMKIN, with the as-sistance of N. J. EASTMAN, L. EDEL-STEIN and A. F. GUTTMACHER) (Balti-more, Md.: Johns Hopkins U.P.).—

The Greek anatomist and physician of the Methodist School, Soranos of Ephe-sos, had a very great influence upon Western European thought up to the 11th century. His works were widely read, translated and annotated, and this holds especially for his "Gynaecology". (*Cf.* also Caelius Aurelia-nus, *vide supra*). From the "Gynaecology" an authoritative critical edition has been published by ILBERG, J., 1910: Die Ueber-lieferung der Gynäkologie des Soranus, 122 p. (Sächs. Akad. Wiss., Phil.-Hist. Kl., 28). On Ilberg's text the present translation has been based. It is supplemented by an exten-sive introduction, footnotes, and glossaries.

Strabon *(ca.* 63 B.C. — *ca.* 20 A.D.) — MEYER, E. H. F., 1852: Botanische Erläu-terungen zu Strabons Geographie und einem Fragment des Dikaearchos, 222 p. (Königs-berg: Borntraeger).—

The fragment will be found on p. 185-192: it is a description of Mount Pelion. Dicaearchos of Messina was a Greek geo-grapher who flourished in the second half of the 4th century B.C. Reprinted, 1931 (Leipzig: Lorentz). *Cf.* AUJAC, G., 1966: Strabon et la science de son temps. Les sciences du monde, 326 p. (Paris: Les Belles Lettres); a thorough study of Strabon's geo-graphy. A complete ed. of Strabon's works: JONES, H. L., ed., 1950-1967: The geo-graphy of Strabo, 8 vols. (Loeb Classical Library) (London: Heinemann; Cambridge, Mass.: Harvard U.P.).

Theocritus (fl. 3rd cent. B.C.) — FÉE, A. L. A., 1832: Flore de Théocrite et des autres bucoliques grecs, 121 p. (Paris: Didot).—

This book gives a list of plant-names, in alphabetical order, based on those names mentioned in the works of the creator of pastoral poetry, Theocritus. These plant-names are compared with the names given by other classical writers, such as Theo-phrastos, Dioscorides, Nicander, Hippocra-tes, Virgil, *etc.* The book is of interest to historians, botanists, and philologists. *Cf.* also: LINDSELL, A., 1936/'37: Was Theo-critus a botanist? (Greece and Rome 6: 78-93).

Thucydides *(ca.* 460 — *ca.* 400 B.C.) — WEIDAUER, K., 1954: Thukydides und die hippokratischen Schriften. Der Einfluss der Medizin auf Zielsetzung und Darstellungsweise des Geschichtswerks, 88 p. (Heidelberger Forschungen) (Heidelberg: Winter).—

In this study the author tries to elucidate some passages of medical interest in the works of Thucydides by comparing them with certain passages in the works belonging to the Corpus Hippocraticum, esp. in Epidemics I and III. The study is mainly of philological interest.

Varro, Marcus Terentius (116—28 B.C.) — STORR-BEST, L., ed., 1912: Varro on farming. M. Terenti Varronis Rerum rusticarum libri tres, transl. with introd., commentary, and excurses, 375 p. (London: Bell & Sons).—

A translation prepared for use by students. The work is divided into 3 parts or books. Book I deals with agriculture, with the soil, farm land, farm buildings, farm equipment, instruments of production, crops, manuring, the growth and habits of plants, reaping and threshing, storage of hay, beans and grapes, wine, walnuts, dates and figs, produce for market, *etc.* Book II deals with cattle: sheep, goats, pigs, cows and oxen, asses, horses, mules, dogs, shepherds, milk and wool, and Book III deals with the smaller stock: peacocks, pigeons, poultry, geese, ducks, but also with wild boars, snails, bees, fish-ponds, *etc.* There also exists an English translation by W. D. HOOPER & H. B. ASH, 1960, in the Loeb Classical Library, *cf.* Cato *(vide supra).*

Vegetius, Publius Renatus (fl. 4th cent.) — ANONYMOUS, 1748: Of the distempers of horses. (London: Millar).—

Vegetius wrote the Mulomedicina, a work on veterinary art. It is a translation into rustic Latin of the Mulomedicina Chironis, a Greek treatise ascribed to Chiron the Centaur and Apsyrtos. This book presents an English translation of Vegetius's Mulomedicina. The full title of this booklet is: Of the distempers of horses, and of the art of curing them, as also of the diseases of oxen and of the remedies proper for them, and of the best method to preserve them in health and restore them when sick, and to prevent the spreading and communication of infectious distempers, according to the

practice of the ancient Romans. As far as the editor is aware, this is the only English translation. There also exists an old German translation by M. LECHTER, 1565: Von rechter und warhaffter Kunst der Artzeney, allerley Kranckheit und Schäden der Thier, als Pferd, Esel, Ochsen, Maulthier, sie seien ausswendig oder inwendig, mit Tranck, Saltung, Brennen, Lassen, und andrem zu heylen … etc. etc.

Virgilius Maro, Publius (70—19 B.C.) — ABBE, E., 1965: The plants of Virgil's "Georgics", 217 p. (Ithaca, N.Y.: Cornell U.P.).—

The more than 90 plants named in Virgil's Georgics are commented upon, their use in classical times is explained, and translations have been given of passages from the work of earlier authorities. For each plant the original descriptive reference is given in its context in the Virgilian passage, together with an English translation. 63 Fine drawings of the plants considered, and English, French, German, and Italian common names, have been given.

——, BILLIARD, R., 1928: L'agriculture dans l'antiquité d'après les Géorgiques de Vergile, 539 p. (Paris: de Boccard).—

In this book the author deals mainly with those agricultural problems which Virgil treated so well in his "Georgics", such as use and improvement of the soil, culture of corn and of wine, breeding of cattle and of horses, agriculture, veterinary pathology, *etc.* Six plates containing the miniatures of a manuscript of the 4th century belonging to the Vatican library.

——, KLINGNER, F., 1963: Virgils Georgica, 248 p. (Zurich: Artemis).—

From the author's preface: "Die Interpretation von Virgils "Georgica", die auf diesen Seiten vorgelegt wird, soll nicht die Arbeiten früheren Ausleger ersetzen. Die Absicht ist die, den Freunden der Dichtkunst und den Mitforschern Anteil an den zu geben, was sich mir in langem, mehr als drei Jahrzehnte langem Umgang mit dem Gedicht neu ergeben hat." The author places the "Georgics" against the background of Rome of those days.

——, LEWIS, C. D., 1947: The "Georgics" of Virgil, 83 p. (New York, N.Y.: Oxford U.P.).—

In his preface the author writes that

he has tried to render his translation as explicit as possible, because he made it chiefly for readers who have no knowledge of Latin and because classical allusions have ceased to be commonplaces for even highly-educated people. Another English translation, but less "popular", is: JERMIJN, L. A. S., 1947: The singing farmer: a translation of Virgil's 'Georgics', 133 p. (Oxford: Blackwell). A German translation with extensive commentaries is: RICHTER, W., 1957: Vergil: Georgica, 446 p. (Munich: Hueber).

———, ROYDS, T. F., 1914: The beasts, birds and bees of Virgil: a naturalist's handbook to the Georgics, 107 p. (Oxford: Blackwell).—

A useful commentary on the "Georgics" of an author who is well acquainted with farming and field natural history, and who, moreover, is well acquainted with earlier (literary) commentators.

9. LIFE AND MEDICAL SCIENCES IN THE NEAR EAST IN THE MIDDLE AGES
α. LIFE AND MEDICAL SCIENCES IN BYZANTIUM

a. History of science and culture in general

AMANTOS, C., 1969: Prolegomena to the history of the Byzantine Empire, 199 p. (Amsterdam: Hakkert).—

An introduction to the history of the Byzantine Empire, and a review of the causes which led to its establishment, and of its role as the transmitter of ancient Greek knowledge to the Latin West. Much has been included concerning the reign and influence of Constantin the Great (p. 306-337) who transferred the capital of the Roman Empire to Constantinople, thereby transplanting the Roman traditions to lands where language, literature and thought were Greek.

BAYNES, N. H. & H. St.-L.B. MOSS, eds., 1948: Byzantium: an introduction to East Roman civilization, 436 p. (Oxford: Clarendon Press).—

"No chapter deals with Byzantine science, very few references are made to the leaders of thought in medieval life. In other respects the book is remarkably well informed." (From Isis 41: 78).

HARDY, E. R., 1931: The large estates of Byzantine Egypt, 162 p. (New York, N.Y.: Columbia U.P.).—
Ch. 1 contains a review of political organization, taxes, government, social circumstances, etc. in Byzantine Egypt. Other chapters deal with the proprietors of the land (the Apion family, imperial property, church and monastery), with feudalism and serfdom (taxes, irrigation, legislation, weights and measures, prisons), with estate management (financial organization, transport, income from grain, wine, oil) and with the estates in the social and economic life of Egypt (irrigation, seed, fruit and vegetables, animals, vineyards, estate services such as baths, oil-presses, mills, bakeries, donations to churches, etc.). A book dealing with the same topics, but stressing the economic aspects, is: ROUILLARD, G., 1953: La vie rurale dans l'empire byzantin, 207 p. (Paris: Maisonneuve). This book seems to be reprinted recently, but, unfortunately, I am unable to find further details.

KRUMBACHER, K., 1891: Geschichte der byzantinischen Literatur, 495 p. (Munich: Beck).—

Although dealing mainly with literary matters, there are some sections of bio-historical interest, such as those on philosophy, on animal histories (physiologos, pulologos, porikologos, and some others), and on house-medicine books (Hausarzneibücher). Valuable are the references given at the end of each section. A second edition of the book appeared in 1897.

OSTROGORSKY, G., 1965: Geschichte des byzantinischen Staates, 569 p. (Munich: Beck).—

"Zugrunde liegt die dritte Auflage (1963) der 'Geschichte des byzantinischen Staates', die im Rahmen des 'Handbuches der Altertumswissenschaft', Abteilung 12, Teil 1 den Band 2 bildet. Im Handbuch begleiten zahlreiche Quellennachweise und Literaturangaben die Darstellungen, orientieren eine Einleitung über die Entwicklung der byzantinischen Forschung, eingehendere Übersichten über den Quellenstand zu den einzelnen Abschnitten. In der vorliegenden Sonderausgabe wird auf den wissenschaftlichen Apparat verzichtet; die eigentliche Darstellung bleibt aber nahezu unverändert." (From Deutsche Bibliographie, Heft 2: 210, 1966).

b. History of the plant, animal, and medical sciences

DIEPGEN, P., 1950: Zur Frauenheilkunde im byzantinischen Kulturkreis des Mittelalters, 14 p. (Abh. Akad. Wiss., Mainz, Geistes- und Sozialwiss. Abt., Jg. 1950, No. 1) (Wiesbaden: Steiner).—

In this study the author discusses such subjects as: Alexandria as centre of medical education, the legal aspects of gynaecology, midwives, sterility, *etc.* Special attention has been paid to the gynaecological sections of the works of Soranos, Oribasios, Paulos of Aegineta, Theophilos Protospatharios, Joannes Actuarios, Simeon Seth, and Nicolaos Myrepsos.

GEMOLL, W., 1883: Untersuchungen ueber die Quellen, die Verfasser und die Abfassungszeit der Geoponica, 280 p. (Berlin: Calvary).—

Philological study. Among the names mentioned are those of Hesiod, Homer, Plato, Theophrastos, Virgil, Aristotle, Cassianos Bassos, Oppian, Didymos of Alexandria, Diophanes of Nicaea, Varro.

MONZLINGER, E., 1922: Zahnheilkundliches bei Alexandros von Tralles und späteren Aerzten der Byzantinerzeit, 27 p. (Diss. Sudhoff Inst.).—

The main part of this study deals with Alexander of Tralles (p. 6-13). Shorter sections are devoted to: Meletios the Monk, Theophilos Protospatharios, Leon (of Thessalonica?), Theophanes Nonnos, Merkurios, Michael Psellos, Simeon Seth and Joannes Aktuarios. Index of Greek drugs.

STRZYGOWSKI, J., 1899: Der Bilderkreis des griechischen Physiologus des Kosmas Indikopleustes und Oktateuch, nach Handschriften der Bibliothek zu Smyrna, 130 p. + 40 plates. (Byzantinisches Archiv, Heft 2) (Leipzig: Teubner).—

Mainly a description of the pictures belonging to this manuscript. Good facsimile reproductions have been added. Certainly of biohistorical interest, esp. from the iconographical point of view. Reprinted 1969 (Groningen: Bouma). *Cf.* WELLMANN, M., 1930, *vide* section History of the life sciences in the Latin West, subsection b.

THOMSON, M. H., 1955: Textes grecs inédits relatifs aux plantes, 177 p. (Paris: Les Belles Lettres).—

This is a first result of a study dealing with the history of botany during the Byzantine period. The authoress collected as many texts as she could, in order to reconstruct the botanical knowledge of the physicians of old Byzantine hospitals. The present study contains the text of only 11 treatises, illustrating the various aspects of Byzantine botany, *viz.,* texts on botanical folk-lore, arboriculture, medico-astrology, medico-magic, pharmaceutics, dietetics, and some botanical lexicons. The texts have been given both in Greek and in French translations on facing pages. The publication of a more definitive study of these texts was promised: it will refer to some 500 fragments.

——, ed., 1960: Le jardin symbolique; texte grec tiré de Clarkianus XI, 97 p. (Paris: Les Belles Lettres).—

The book deals with the symbolism of plants, for the word "jardin" or garden has been used metaphorically. It treats of the different virtues; and the writer sets out to equate the virtue of each of the plants mentioned with a corresponding Christian one. The therapeutic use of plants also provides examples of symbolism. Most ailments referred to are those mentioned in earlier Greek writings. The text and the French translation are given on facing pages.

c. Some individual scientists

Aëtios of Amida (fl. 527-565) — HIRSCHBERG, J., 1899: Die Augenheilkunde des Aëtius aus Amida, Griechisch und Deutsch, 204 p. (Leipzig: Veith).—

Aëtios was physician to the Byzantine court and wrote a medical encyclopaedia the "Tetrabiblon", in 16 books, an eclectic compilation mainly based upon Galen and Archigenes. It contains many extracts from ancient medical writings about internal medicine, surgery, obstetrics, gynaecology, and ophthalmology. His book on ophthalmology (Book VII) is especially famous; it has been edited both in Greek and German by Hirschberg. A German translation of some parts of the fourth book of this encyclopaedia is: STEINHAGEN, H., 1938: Das vierte Buch des Tetrabiblon des byzantinischen Arztes Aëtios von Amida. Aus dem Griechischen ins Deutsche übertragen, 53 p. (Diss. Univ. Düsseldorf). The German titles of the translated parts are: 1. Aufziehung des Kindes und Kinderkrankheiten; 2. Diätetische Vorschriften für die Greise; 3. Lebensweise der Berufstätigen und Ermüdungskrankheiten; 4. Die verschiedenen Mischungen der Säfte im Körper und ihre Wirkung auf die einzelnen Organe und die Temperamente.

——, LEHMANN, A., 1921: Die zahnärztliche Lehre des Aëtios aus Amida, 48 p. (Diss. Sudhoff Inst.) (Halle/Saale: Hendrichs).—

A general review of Aëtios' dentistry. Chapter headings of this work are: Einleitung, Materia Medica, Dentition, Krankheiten der Zähne, Erkrankungen des Zahnfleisches, Abfeilen der Zähne, Extraktion, Allgemeiner Lehrgang über Anwendung aller Mundsalben, Literatur.

——, RICCI, J. V., 1950: Aëtios of Amida: the gynaecology and obstetrics of the VIth century A.D., 215 p. (Transl. from the Latin edition of Cornarius, 1542 and fully annotated) (Philadelphia, Pa.: Blakiston).—

Ricci prepared an English translation from a physician's point of view of Book XVI of the medical encyclopaedia of Aëtios of Amida, a Byzantine physician of the first half of the fourth century. The translation has been based on the Latin edition by G. Cornarius (Basle, 1542) and is nowhere referred to the Greek text (ed. by S. ZERVÓS, Leipzig, 1901). The translation has been supplemented by medical notes, by a list of authors referred to, and a list of the drugs mentioned. There also exists a partial German translation of book XIV by WEGSCHNEIDER, M., 1901: Geburtshilfe und Gynäkologie bei Aëtios von Amida, 136 p. (Berlin: Springer).

Alexander of Tralles (*ca.* 525-605) — BRUNET, F., 1933-1937: Oeuvres médicales d'Alexandre de Tralles, le dernier auteur classique des grands médecins grecs de l'antiquité, 5 vols. Vol. I (1933): Alexandre de Tralles et la médecine byzantine, 297 p.; Vol. II (1936): Traité des fièvres. Lettre sur les vers intestinaux. Livre premier des douze livres de médecine (affections de la tête), 259 p.; Vol. III (1936): Livre 2. Thérapeutique oculaire; Livre 3. Affections des oreilles et des régions parotidiennes; Livre 4. Affections angineuses; Livre 5. Affections pulmonaires; Livre 6. De la pleurésie; Livre 7. Affections gastriques, 254 p.; Vol. IV (1937): Livre 7. Affections gastriques; Livre 8. Affections intestinales; Livre 9. Affections hépatiques; Livre 10. Affections abdominales; Livre 11. Affections génito- urinaires; Livre 12. De la podagre, 292 p. (Paris: Geuthner).—

Alexander of Tralles was a Byzantine physician whose main work was a treatise on pathology and therapeutics. Brunet's work is a very fine French edition. For our purpose Vol. I is of special importance, because it contains a biography of Alex. of Tralles and a review of his works (p. 1-90); ch. 2 deals with the situation of biological and medical science in the Byzantine empire during the 6th century (p. 91-190), and ch. 3 deals with treatment, hygiene, materia medica, and pharmacy of the 6th century and with Alexander's influence on them (p. 191-296). Vol. II contains a treatise on fevers and a treatise on intestinal worms and the contents of bk. 1. As is clear from the titles, Vol. III contains the contents of bks. 2-7, and Vol. IV that of bks. 7-12. A fifth vol. contains the best Greek text available.

——, PUSCHMANN, T., ed., 1878-1879: Alexander von Tralles. Original-text und Uebersetzung nebst einer einleitenden Abhandlung. Ein Beitrag zur Geschichte der Medicin, 2 vols. Vol. I: 617 p.; Vol. II: 620 p. (Vienna: Braumüller).—

After a historical introduction (p. 1-75), Puschmann briefly discusses the medical writings of Alexander and summarizes his ideas on anatomy, physiology, pathology, therapeutics, fevers, on diseases of the nervous system, skin, hair, eyes, ears, respiratory and urogenital system (p. 108-286). Then the text of 11 books of Alexander follows, with the German translation on the facing pages. (Bk. I in vol. I, the other books in vol. II). Alexander's studies on fevers and on intestinal worms have been included. For his treatise on eye diseases, *vide* PUSCHMANN, T., 1887: Nachträge zu Alexander Trallianus. Fragmente aus Philumenos und Philagrios. (*cf.* Section Classical Antiquity Υ, subsection d). In 1963 Hakkert (Amsterdam) published a reprint edition.

Anthimus (fl. 493-534) — LIECHTENHAN, E., ed., 1963: Anthimi de observatione ciborum ad Theodicorum regem francorum epistula iteratis, edidit et in linguam germanicum transtulit, 86 p. (Corpus medicorum lat., 8, 1) (Berlin: Akad. Verlag).—

Anthimus was a Greek physician who also was ambassador to Theodoric, King of the Francs. He wrote a memoir to this king on dietetics and cookery, in which he dealt with the methods of preparation of various victuals and beverages, both animal and vegetable, of which the therapeutic values are indicated. The text is also of much importance for students of linguistics.

Clement of Alexandria (*ca.* 150 — *ca.* 220) — MURPHY, M. G., 1941: Nature allusions in the works of Clement of Alexandria, 124 p. (Diss. Catholic Univ. of America) (Washington, D.C.: Catholic Univ. America Press).—

Clement of Alexandria was a Greek Church Father. The present study deals with the treatment of nature in the Protrepticus, the Paedagogus, the Quis dives salvetur, the Excerpta ex Theodoto, the Eclogae Propheticae, and the Fragments. From these studies it appeared that Clement has made use of 227 distinct objects and phenomena as a basis for nature-allusions; most frequent are allusions to the universe, fire, sun, light, darkness, springs, streams, sea, horses, serpents, fish, birds, swine, dogs, trees, flowers, and husbandry. *Cf.* DECKER, A., 1936: Kenntniss und Pflege des Körpers bei Clemens von Alexandria, 74 p. (Veröff. Salzburger-Konföderation der Benediktiner u. Zisterzienser des deutschen Sprachgebietes, No. 21) (Innsbruck: Rauch).

Constantinus VII Porphyrogennetos (905-959) — RAMBAUD, A. N., 1870: L'empire grec au dixième siècle. Constantin Porphyrogénète, 551 p. (Paris: Franck).—

Constantinos was a Byzantine emperor, patron of arts, letters, and science. He caused many compilations to be made on law, history, husbandry, medicine, and zoology. P. 51-174 of Rambaud's book are devoted to an analysis of Constantinos' literary and scientific activities.

Cosmas Indicopleustes (fl. *ca.* 525-550) — WOLSKA, W., 1962: La topographie chrétienne de Cosmas Indicopleustès. Théologie et science au VIe siècle, 329 p. (Paris: Presses Univ. de France).—

Unfortunately only little can be found here of interest to the history of biology or medicine. Probably the list of references may serve as a starting point for serious biologico-historical research. *(Cf.* also STRZYGOWSKI, J., 1899, *vide supra,* subsection b).

Cyprianus of Carthage (d. 258) — BALL, M. T., 1946: Nature and the vocabulary of nature in the works of Saint Cyprian, 303 p. (Diss. Catholic Univ. of America) (Washington, D.C.: Catholic Univ. America Press).—

The author discusses St. Cyprian's allusions to nature and the vocabulary of

nature in the apologetic works, in the disciplinary works, and in the letters. The author summarizes Cyprian's views in the following words: "He showed how the Lord's own method of drawing proof of and illustration for His mighty truths, and striking lessons for our instruction from the familiar world about Him, was practical and effective in any day and in every land."

John the Grammarian, called Joannes Philoponos (first half 6th cent.) — BÖHM, W., ed., 1967: Johannes Philoponos Grammatikos von Alexandrien (6. Jh. n. Chr.). Christliche Naturwissenschaft im Ausklang der Antike, Vorläufer der modernen Physik, Wissenschaft und Bibel. Ausgewählte Schriften, 479 p. (Munich: Schöningh).—

Special chapters deal with biology (p. 256-277), considering such subjects as: unconscious purposiveness, the part and the whole, vitalism and mechanism; with physiology and chemistry (p. 278-299), considering such subjects as: the organism as a chemical system and the chemical composition of the body; and with psychology (p. 208-255), considering such subjects as: observation, sense, smell, taste, memory, and the nature of the soul. As to John's psychology, *cf.* VERBEKE, G., ed., 1966: Jean Philopon. Commentaire sur le "De anima" d'Aristote: traduction de Guillaume de Moerbeke. Édition critique avec une introduction sur la psychologie de Philopon, 120 + 172 p. (Centre de Wulf-Mansion, Corpus Latinum Commentariorum in Aristotelem Graecorum, Vol. III) (Louvain: Publ. Univ.; Paris: Béatrice-Nauwelaerts).

——, MEYERHOF, M., 1931: Joannes Grammatikos (Philoponos) von Alexandrien und die arabischen Medizin, 21 p. (Mitt. dtsch. Inst. Aegypt. Altertumsk. Kairo, Vol. II, pt. 1) (Augsburg: Filser).—

An attempt to elucidate the influence of Joannes on Arabian medicine. He wrote commentaries on Aristotle and Galen. His works were translated into Syrian, and afterwards into Arabic. *Cf.* also STEINSCHNEIDER, M., 1869: Joannes Philoponos bei den Arabern, 24 p. (Mém. Akad. imp. Sci. St. Petersbourg, IIIe Série, Vol. XIII, No. 4: 152-176). Contains much biographical information, together with a review and evaluation of his medical works.

Paulos Aegineta (fl. *ca.* 640) — ADAM, F., 1844-1847: The seven books of Paulus Aegineta. Translated from the Greek with a commentary: embracing a complete review of the knowledge possessed by the Greeks, Romans, and Arabians on all subjects connected with medicine and surgery, 3 vols. (London: Sydenham Society).—

English translation with introduction, commentary, and index. Paulos wrote a medical treatise in seven books, of which Bk. I deals with hygiene, gerontological and dietetic problems, the seasons, and the temperaments; Bk. II with fevers; Bk. III with tropical affections *a capite ad calcem;* Bk. IV with external pathological affections and parasitic worms; Bk. V with venoms and poisonous animals; Bk. VI with surgery; and Bk. VII with drugs and therapeutics. A special study dealing with Paulos's gynaecology and obstetrics is: JOANNIDES, D. C., 1940: La gynécologie et obstétrique de Paul d'Égine et son influence sur la médecine arabe, 56 p. (Cairo). Another study deals with his dentistry: STRAUBEL, K., 1922: Zahn- und Mundleiden und deren Behandlung bei Paulos von Aegina, 24 p. (Diss. Sudhoff Inst.). There exists a French translation of Paulos's surgery: BRIAU, R., 1855: Chirurgie de Paul d'Égine, 508 p. (Paris: Masson), containing an introduction, the Greek text, and the French translation.

——, BERENDES, I., ed., 1914: Paulos' von Aegina, des besten Arztes sieben Bücher. Uebersetzt und mit Erläuterungen versehen. Nebst einem Anhang: Die römischen Baeder, die bei Paulos vorkommenden älteren Aerzte, und zwei Tafeln, 890 p. (Leiden: Brill).—

Paulos Aegineta can be considered to be the latest representative of Greek medicine before Muslim supremacy. He wrote a medical encyclopaedia in seven books, largely based upon Galen and Oribasios. Berendes's book contains a German translation based on an older Greek text. The contents of the seven books are outlined on p. 3, and the contents of each separate book are given on several pages preceding the translation of that book. Good index. Berendes's translations of Paulos's treatise originally appeared in Janus XIII to XVII (1908-1912).

Psellos, Michael, the Younger, (1018 - *ca.* 1078) — ZERVOS, C., 1919: Un philosophe néoplatonicien du XIe siècle. Psellos. Sa vie, son oeuvre ses luttes philosophiques, son influence, 269 p. (Thèse Univ. Paris) (Paris: Leroux).—

Psellos was a Byzantine polymath and philosopher. Here is an elaborate study of his life, philosophy, scientific work, *etc.,* with valuable bibliography. One section deals with his encyclopaedic writings, incl. medicine and agriculture. E. Jeanselme translated some fragments of medical interest from Psellos's annals, *viz.,* JEANSELME, E., 1923: La maladie et la mort de Romain III Argyre, empereur de Byzance (1028-1034). (Bull. Soc. franç. hist. méd. 17: 309-319); and JEANSELME, E., 1924: La pleurésie du Basileus Isaac Commène (1059) d'après le récit de Psellos *(Idem,* 18: 89-97).

Timotheus of Gaza (fl. *ca.* 491-518) — BODENHEIMER, F. S. & A. RABINOWITZ, 1949: Timotheus of Gaza on animals: fragments of a Byzantine paraphrase of an animal book of the 5th century A.D., translation, commentary and introduction, 54 p. (Coll. Trav. Acad. intl. Hist. Sci., No. 3) (Paris: Acad. intl. Hist. Sci.).—

English translation of a book on exotic animals. The text was preserved in the Codex Augustianus (Munich, No. 514). The translation is made on the basis of M. HAUPT's edition in Hermes, vol. 3, 1869. A more general study of Byzantine zoology is: THÉODORIDÈS, J., 1953: Introduction à l'étude de la zoologie byzantine. (Actes 7e Congrès intl. Hist. Sci., Jerusalem, p. 601-608).

β. LIFE AND MEDICAL SCIENCES IN SYRIA

a. *History of the medical sciences*

BUDGE, E. A. W., 1913: Syrian anatomy, pathology and therapeutics, or "The book of medicine", 2 vols. Vol. I: Introduction, 178 p.; Syriac text, 612 p.; Vol. II: English translation and index, 804 p. (London: Oxford U.P.).—

This text is an illustration of Syriac medical literature as it flourished in the schools of the Nestorians on Mesopotamian soil. The text consists for the greater part of translations from Greek sources (*e.g.,* Galen, Dioscorides, Hellenistic astrological medicine), but it also includes many Oriental elements; it is obviously the Syriac translation of a series of lectures on human anatomy, pathology, and therapeutics, originally written in Greek. The first section of Budge's book consists of lectures upon human anatomy, pathology and therapeutics, to each of which is added a series of prescriptions which the author recommends to be administered in the treatment of the various diseases described in the preceding lecture. The second section of the book has an astrological character; this part includes many superstitious elements. The third part contains some 400 prescriptions illustrating the folk-lore of a part of Mesopotamia, and preserving a number of popular beliefs and legends about birds, animals, magical roots, *etc.* As such the book is an illustration of one of the channels through which Mesopotamian and Greek medical lore was transmitted to the Middle Ages. J. SCHLEIFER published a series of studies on the problem of deciding which parts of the Syriac text were borrowed from Galen and other Greek writers; his conclusion was that almost the whole of the general pathological-therapeutic portion is taken from various works of Galen; the several passages in Galen's works are equated with the parallel passages of the Syriac text. Moreover, Schleifer has subjected Budge's translation to a revision, suggesting improvements, adding annotations and supplementary explanations based on a comparison with the original Greek texts. For the relevant literature, *vide* SCHLEIFER, J., 1926: Zum syrischen Medizinbuch, 81 p. (Ztschr. Semitistik 4: 70-122; 166-195), discussing some general principles, and SCHLEIFER, J., 1942-1946: Zum syrischen Medizinbuch II, 150 p. (Rev. degli Studi Orientali, Vols. 18, 20, and 21). In this series he discusses chapters 3-5 of Budge's book in Vol. 18: 341-372; ch. 6-9 in Vol. 20: 1-32; ch. 9-14 in Vol. 20: 163-210; ch. 14-16 in Vol. 20: 383-398; and ch. 16-20 in Vol. 21: 157-182.

b. Some individual scientists

Ayyūb al-Ruhāwi al Abrash (= Job of Edessa, *ca.* 760 - *ca.* 835) — LEVEY, M., ed., 1967: Medical ethics of medieval Islam with special reference to Al-Ruhāwi's "Practical ethics to the physician", 100 p. (Trans. Amer. Philos. Soc., N.S., 57, pt. 3) (Philadelphia, Pa.: Amer. Philos. Soc.).—

The text of al-Ruhāwi's book is composed of 20 chapters constituting a collection of quotations and commentaries compiled primarily from texts of ancient Greek authors (*e.g.,* Hippocrates, Galen, Plato, and Aristotle), and deals with the relevance of religion, philosophy, hygiene, anatomy, physiology, therapeutics, legal regulations, *etc.,* to the subject of medical ethics. In his introduction the editor gives a review of the literature of mediaeval Islamic medical ethics.

——, MINGANA, A., ed., 1935: Encyclopaedia of philosophical and natural sciences as taught in Baghdad about A.D. 817, or Book of treasures by Job of Edessa, Syriac text edited and translated with a critical apparatus, 48 +470 p. (Vol. I of Woodbrooke scientific publications) (Cambridge: Heffer).—

Job of Edessa was a famous translator from Greek into Syriac, and also a philosopher and encyclopaedist. The "Book of treasures" is a scientific encyclopaedia which is of much value for the history of biology and of medicine. In his introduction, the editor examines briefly Job's views on: metaphysics, theology, psychology, biology, anatomy, physiology, medicine, chemistry, physics, music, mathematics, astronomy. His large ms. is reproduced in this edition accompanied by an English translation of 292 pages. The text is divided into six discourses. Discourse I deals with the elements, theology, and anatomy (ch. 11 to 33 are devoted to anatomy). Topics of much interest to biohistory are, *inter alia:* genesis of the three genera; animals, animal-plants, and plants; the four humours; how a consideration of the humours leads to anatomy and physiology (which is essentially Galenic). Discourse II deals with anatomy and zoology (heat and cold as active powers; humidity and dryness as passive powers; sleep; sexes; beard, hair; menstruation; teeth; anatomical differences according to the climates; animals, animal-plants; soul; species of animals; comparative anatomy). Discourse III deals with psychology and the senses; IV with chemistry and geology; V with meteorology and astronomy; and discourse VI deals with angelology and eschatology. Only a few critical notes, and no glossary.

Grīghŏr (Abū al-Faraj), called Bar-Hebraeus (1225-1286) — BAKOŠ, J., ed., 1930-1933: Le candélabre des sanctuaires de Grégoire Aboul-faradj dit Barhebraeus, 282 p. (Patrologia Orientalis 20: 489-628; *Idem,* 24: 297-440).—

Barhebraeus wrote a monumental encyclopaedia, a combination of creative Greek thinking, Christian religious belief and Oriental superstition. As to its title, Barhebraeus himself writes in his introduction (in the French translation of Bakoš): "Et comme dans le présent ouvrage la lampe, c'est-à-dire la vérité des saintes Écritures, est posée ainsi que sur un candélabre, il se nomme précisément 'Candélabre des Sanctuaires'." The whole work consists of twelve bases or fundamentals on which the

Church has been founded. Bakoš gives an edition and French translation of the first base (Of knowledge in general, p. 517-541), and of the second base (The nature of the universe in accordance with the six days of creation). Bakoš has also given an edition and French translation of the eighth base which deals with psychological matters *(cf.* BAKOŠ, J., 1948, *vide infra).* The other bases (not edited by Bakoš) deal with religious matters. As to our purpose especially the second base is of importance. This base is divided into 3 chapters, *viz.,* 1. the eternity of the world; 2. the disappearance of the universe; and 3. the description of the creation of the world in six days (covers 75% of the text). In accordance with this idea of creation this chapter is divided into six parts, *viz.,* 1. first day: heaven, earth, water, air, fire, light; 2. second day: the firmament; 3. third day: the seas and the surface of the earth, incl. the plants (Barhebraeus's knowledge of the plants was mainly based upon the pseudo-Aristotelian treatise "De plantis", the Geoponica, and upon Dioscorides); 4. fourth day: astronomy; 5. fifth day: animals in the water (fishes, whales, molluscs, crustacea, echinodermata, coelenterata, tortoises, frogs and others) and animals in the air (birds, bats, insects); 6. sixth day: reptiles, mammals (also discussing problems of generation, propagation, instinct, *etc.),* and the creation of Man (incl. a discussion of his reasonableness, a Galenic interpretation of his anatomy, and some medical information). Barhebraeus's main source is Aristotle; other sources from which he derived his knowledge are the Geoponica, Dioscorides, the Hexaëmeron of Moses bar Kēphā, Job of Edessa, Galen, Basil the Great, and al-Kazvīnī. A treatise especially dealing with the plants mentioned by Barhebraeus is: GOTTHEIL, R. J. C., 1866: A list of plants and their properties from the Menārtb Kuhše of Gregorius Bar 'Ebhrāya (privately printed).

—— ——, ed., 1948: Psychologie de Grégoire Aboulfaradj dit Barhebraeus d'après la huitième base de l'ouvrage Le Candélabre des Sanctuaires, 40 + 148 p. + 131 p. in Syriac. (Leiden: Brill).—

A Syriac edition and French translation of the eighth "base" of the Menarath qudshe, dealing with the reasonable soul. In his preface, the editor gives a summary of Barhebraeus's psychology. Abundant notes (p. 75-129), Syriac glossary and index of proper names. In his treatise Barhebraeus deals with some topics which are of bio-historical, or medical, importance, such as: definition of the soul; the heart as main organ of the soul; philosophic proofs of the union of soul and body; metempsychosis;

souls of animals; revelations, visions, and dreans.

Moses bar Kēphā (*ca.* 813-903) — BAKOŠ, J., 1930: Die Zoologie aus dem Hexaëmeron des Mōšē bar Kēp(h)ā, 65 p. (Archiv orientalni 2: 327-361; 460-491).—

The "Hexaëmeron" of Moses bar Kēphā consists of 5 books of which a part of the third book deals with zoological matters. Its main source is the Hexaëmeron of Jacob of Edessa, written in 708. The Hexaëmeron is a treatise dealing with the six days of creation, and Moses's book is strongly influenced by the philosophy of St., Basil. The present edition and translation have been based upon 2 mss. of the Bibliothèque nationale de Paris. It deals with such subjects as: the animals of the earth, their number, names, food, form, reproduction, *etc.* To mention some animals considered in some detail: the sponge, some birds (*e.g.,* partridge, stork, crane, goose, vulture, swallow, birds of prey), bees, cattle, dog, spiders, ants, reptiles, *etc.* In another study Bakoš analyses the sources of Moses bar Kēphā's Hexaëmeron in more detail, *viz.,* BAKOŠ, J., 1934: Quellenanalyse der Zoologie aus dem Hexaëmeron des Moses bar Kēphā (Archiv orientalni 6: 267-271).

Shem'on de Ṭaibūthā (fl. *ca.* 685-700) — MINGANA, A., ed., 1934: Medico-mystical work by Simon of Ṭaibūtheh (d.c. 680): Syriac with English translation and notes, 109 p. (Woodbrooke studies, Vol. VII: Early Christian mystics, p. 1-69; 280-320) (Cambridge: Heffer).—

Shem'on de-Ṭaibūthā was a physician who - to quote the editor - "was the only mystical writer who has been brought up in the school of the old masters of medical science, Hippocrates and Galen, and who had acquired the knowledge of healing both the body and the soul" (p. 2). His medical views are essentially Galenic.

Λ. **LIFE AND MEDICAL SCIENCES IN PERSIA**

a. History of the plant, animal and medical sciences

DONALDSON, B. A., 1938: The wild rue: a study of Muhammedan magic and folklore in Iran, 216 p. (London: Luzac).—

A full account of Muslim superstitions as they occur in Iran. Most of the material has been collected within the province of Khorasan, but since pilgrims come to the sacred city of Meshed from all over Iran, its population can - according to the author - be considered as a representative group. Special attention has been paid to the use of seeds of wild rue in protective incantations. Many of the superstitions considered belong to common beliefs in Islam.

ELGOOD, C., 1934: Medicine in Persia, 105 p. (Clio Medica, Vol. 14) (New York, N.Y.: Hoeber).—

Persian medical history can be divided into two periods, *viz.*, the pre-Muslim or Avestan period and the Muslim period. During the first period medicine was mainly based on the Avesta, although it was strongly influenced by Egyptian, Mesopotamian, Greek, Christian and Byzantine learning. In 642, after the battle of Nihawand, the Arabian or Islamic period began, mainly Greek in character. At the end of his historical review the author gives a table of political and medical dates of Persian history, with comparable events in Europe.

——, 1951: A medical history of Persia and the Eastern Caliphate from the earliest times until the year A.D. 1932, 617 p. (Cambridge: U.P.).—

The first two chapters deal with pre-Islamic Persian medicine. Chapter I deals with the Zoroastrian doctrine in medicine, wherein the relationship between ceremonial purity and the prevention of disease is emphasized; chapter 2 deals with its role of conservator and transmitter of classical Greek learning. Other chapters deal with such subjects as: the nature of Persian medicine as it can be understood from the Avesta, medical knowledge of the conquering Arabs, training of doctors, various kinds of physicians, their dress and fees, anaesthesia and surgery, anatomy, Arabian medical knowledge in theory and practice, the influence of Avicenna and Rhazes, veterinary medicine, Persian medicine under the Mongol domination, and the coming of the European physicians to Persia.

——, 1966: Safavid surgery, 83 p. (Analecta Historica, No. 2) (Oxford: Pergamon).—

A historical account of the practice of surgery in Persia from the early 16th century down to 1736, when the last Safavid king died. The work has been based on three mss. It does not contain case-histories but gives descriptions of *e.g.*, the treatment of abdominal wounds, abscesses, swellings, piles, varicose veins, hydrocoele, ascites, *etc.*

Probably the surgeons used some sort of anaesthesia for painful operations. Moreover, Elgood makes clear that the Persian physicians had a more exact idea of the function of the heart, lungs and blood than most European colleagues before Harvey, that castration must have been very common, both as a punishment and to provide eunuchs, and that blinding and amputation must have been used for punishment.

FICHTNER, H., 1924: Die Medizin im Avesta, 55 p. (Diss. Univ. Leipzig) (Leipzig: Pfeiffer).—

In the introduction the author briefly considers old Persian folk medicine in its relationship with Zarathustra and the main contents of the Avesta. The first chapter is entitled "Die medizinischen Gottheiten und Heroen", the second "Der Aerztestand" (deals with the social position of the priest-physicians), the third "Die Krankheitslehre und die allgemeinen medizinischen Kenntnisse" (medicine and religion, knowledge of anatomy, physiology, pathology, and symptomatology), the fourth, "Diagnose und Prognose" (diseases of the skin, mental disorders, malformations, *etc.),* the fifth "Therapie" (irrational as well as rational), the sixth "Die Hygiene" (dietetics, social life, *etc.).* The appendix contains some information concerning veterinary medicine. An elaborate study of Zoroaster and the Avesta can be found in: HERZFELD, E., 1947: Zoroaster and his world, 2 vols., 851 p. (Princeton, N.J.: U.P.).

FONAHN, A., 1910: Zur Quellenkunde der persischen Medizin, 152 p. (Leipzig: Barth).—

Excellent (though somewhat obsolete) catalogue of sources, and a preliminary review of the literature, about Persian medicine of the post-Islamic period as it has been accumulated in old manuscripts. The subjects considered are: anatomy and physiology; pathology; therapy; hygiene; medical works in poetical form; pharmacology; directions to veterinary literature; medicine in some Persian encyclopaedias; medical lexicography, -geography, -biography, letters and portraits. *Cf.* also: SIDDIQI, Z., 1959, *vide* section δ, subsection a.

FROEHNER, R., 1929: Zur persischen Hippologie und Hippiatrie des 11. Jahrhunderts, 97 p. (Abh. Gesch. Veterinärmed., pt. 20) (Leipzig: Richter).—

This is a study devoted to chapter 25 of the Qābūsnāma, a domestic encyclopaedia in 44 chapters composed in 1082/83 by 'Unsur al-Ma'ālī kaikā'ūs. Chapter 25 deals with horses. Froehner's memoir contains the German translation of H. F. VON DIEZ (Berlin, 1811, translated from a Turkish ms.), the French translation of A. QUERRY (Paris, 1886), a new German translation from a Persian ms., a facsimile of ch. 25 in a Turkish ms., and an elaborate bibliography of 181 items. A rich series of notes on: 1. colours and temperaments of horses, with comparisons with Hrabanus Maurus, Hildegard, Georg Leonhard Löneysen, etc.; 2. colours of horses, with abundant references to ancient and mediaeval writings; 3. different parts of the horse's body; 4. its diseases, giving a parallel glossary of Turkish, Persian, Arabic and French terms, together with many references to Greek and Latin terminology.

HOOPER, D., 1937: Useful plants and drugs of Iran and Iraq: with notes by H. FIELD, 168 p. (Botanical Series, Field Museum Natl. Hist., Vol. 9, No. 3: 73-241).—

    For more details, *vide* section δ, subsection b.

LAUFFER, B., 1919: Sino-Iranica: Chinese contributions to the history of civilization in ancient Iran. With special reference to the history of cultivated plants and products, 455 p. (Chicago, Ill.: Field Museum Natl. Hist.).—

    For more details, *vide* section Far East, subsection b.

NADJMABADI, M., ed., 1965: A bibliography of printed books in Persian on medicine and allied subjects. Vol. I: Titles of the books, 922 cols. (461 p.) (Tehran: Daneshkab Publication Co.).—

    The book is in Persian. The titles have been given in alphabetical order and were taken from library catalogue cards. The brief title is given, then the name of the author, place of publication, year, and number of pages. Many of the titles included are of interest for the history of science and medicine. The author plans to continue publication of this bibliography. *Cf.* also ISKANDAR, A. Z., 1967. *vide* section δ, subsection a; and AZEEZ PASHA, M., 1966, *vide* same section, subsection c.

b. *Some individual scientists*

Ahmad ibn 'Umar Niẓāmī, 'Arūẓī (d. *ca.*

1152) — BROWNE, E. G., 1921: Revised translation of the Chahar Maqāla ("Four discourses") of Niẓāmī-i-Arūẓī of Samarqand, followed by an abridged translation of Mīrzā Muhammad's notes to the Persian text, 184 p. (E. J. W. Gibb Memorial Series, Vol. XI, Pt. 2) (London: Luzac).—

    Niẓāmī was a Persian writer who wrote (in Persian) the "Four Discourses" dealing respectively with the four classes of men indispensable for the service of the kings, *viz.*, secretaries, poets, astrologers, and physicians. As a sort of introduction to the discourses, the author deals with the evolution of the mineral, the vegetable, and the animal kingdoms and the five external and the five internal senses, with the Nasnās or wild man, and the ascent of Man. Then the translations of the discourses follow of which the fourth deals with physicians; it discusses such topics as: how to study medicine, characteristics of the good physician, healing by prayer, cases of psycho-therapeusis by Rāzi and Avicenna, the author's successful treatment of a young girl, Galen "treats the root to cure the branch", a sick lover cured by Avicenna.

Ismā'il ibn Hasan (Zain al-Din Abu Ibrāhīm), al-Jurjānī (*ca.* 1130) — NAFICY, A., 1933: La médecine en Perse dès origines à nos jours. Ses fondements théoriques d'après l'Encyclopédie médicale de Gorgani, 142 p. (Paris: Véga).—

    This booklet mainly deals with the influence of Gorgani (= Ismā'il ibn Hasan al-Jurjānī) on the development of Persian medicine. His work marks the revival of an autonomous Persian medicine after the period of Muslim invasions. Much biographical information about al-Jurjānī.

Kāi'Kā'iūs ibn Iskander, called 'Unsur ul-Ma'ālī, Amir of Dailam (d. 1069) — LEVY, R., 1951: A mirror for princes. The Qābūs nāma, by Kāi Kā'iūs ibn Iskandar, Prince of Gurgān, 265 p. (London: Cresset).—

    The present book is a kind of pedagogical encyclopaedia, giving an insight into the general influence of science on higher education in 11th-century Persia. Medical, hygienic and kindred matters have been considered in chapters 10 (eating), 11 (drinking), 14 (love), 16 (bathing), 17 (sleep), 33 (medicine). Human physiology is discussed in chapters 9 (old age and youth), 23 (physiognomic details), 27 (the bringing-up of children); and chapter 25 is devoted to the characteristics of fine horses. The medical text contains many Greek elements; there are no annotations.

Muwaffiḳ ibn 'Alī ,Abū Manṣūr) Haravī (fl. ca. 961-976) — ACHUNDOW, A. C., 1893: Die pharmakologischen Grundsätze, Liber fundamentorum pharmacologiae, des Abu Mansur Muwaffak bin Ali Harawi zum ersten Male nach dem Urtext ins Deutsche übersetzt und mit Erklärungen versehen, 332 p. (Koberts historische Studien aus dem pharmak. Inst. Univ. Dorpat [Tartu] III: 113-414; 450-481).—

> Abū Manṣūr was a Persian pharmacologist who, between 968 and 977, wrote the Kitāb al-abniya 'an ḥaqā'iq al-adwiya, the "Book of the foundations of the true properties of the remedies", written in Persian, and comprising Greek, Syriac, Arabic, and Hindu elements. It deals with 585 remedies (of which 466 are derived from plants and 44 from animals), classified according to their actions; and it contains an outline of a general pharmaceutical theory. Reprinted 1968, 451 p. (Leipzig: Zentralantiquariat der D.D.R.).

δ. LIFE AND MEDICAL SCIENCES OF THE ARABS (INCL. SOME ISLAMIC ASPECTS)

a. History of science and culture in general

ADNAN, A., 1939: La science chez les Turcs Ottomans, 182 p. (Paris: Maisonneuve).—

> A history of science among the Ottoman Turks, *i.e.,* a history of Turkish mathematics, natural science, and medicine between ca. 1330 and the beginning of the 19th century. The author shows how Arab science persisted up to the 19th century, when modern science was introduced. The first two chapters, dealing with the period ca. 1330 down to the beginning of the 17th century (p. 10-90) have been published in Archeion Vols. 19 and 21 (1937 and 1938). A second, enlarged edition, supplied with much additional information has been published in the Turkish language: Osmanli Türklerinde Ilim, 1943, 225 p. (Istanbul).

BROCKELMANN, C., 1943-1949: Geschichte der arabischen Literatur, ed. 2, Vol. I (1943): 676 p.; Vol. II (1949): 687 p. (Leiden: Brill).—

> A mine of information. Vol. I, p. 265-282 and 635-652 and Vol. II, p. 170-173, 219,

242, 276-277, 302, 333, 344-345, 473-480, 545, 594-596, and 617 contain material of biohistorical interest (medicine, zoology, hunting, agriculture, *etc.*). Besides, these volumes contain much biographical information. There also exist three supplements: Suppl. I (1937): 973 p.; Suppl. II (1938): 1045 p.; Suppl. III (1942): 1326 p.

GABRIELI, G., 1916: Manuale di bibliografia musulmana. Pars 1: Bibliografia generale, 501 p. (Rome: Tip. dell' Unione editrice).—

> The contents of this book are devided into the following chapters: 1. Territorio musulmano; 2. Commercio libraio (a list of oriental booksellers); 3. Bibliografie generali e parziali. Enciclopedie; 4. Periodici e collezioni; 5. Orientalismo ed orientalisti (a list of orientalists, and a list of congresses and their publications); 6. Didattica e propedeutica islamica antica e moderna (teaching and schools, lists of grammars, and of dictionaries; also of Persian, Turkish, and Hindustani languages); 7. Manoscritti (list of collections of mss., classified by cities in alphabetical order, of private collections, *etc.); 8.* Libri (including a list of printers having oriental founts; list of catalogues of public and private libraries); 9. Monete (bibliography of Muslim numismatics and of public and private collections); 10. Altre fonte archeologiche (museology, medals, seals, amulets, scientific instruments, *etc.);* 11. Calendar.

GRANQVIST, H., 1947: Birth and childhood among the Arabs. Studies in a Muhammedan village in Palestine, 289 p. (Helsinki: Söderström).—

> This book deals with such subjects as: pre-natal customs, cohabitation, conception, pregnancy, advice for pregnant women, sex of foetus, childbirth, midwife, presence of angels, difficult birth, first attentions to mother and child, announcement of birth of child, feast for boy, dream revelations, treatment of mother and new-born child, food for mother and child, cutting the umbilical cord, afterbirth burial, child's first dress and bath, nursing, lullabies, boys' and girls' games, education, circumcision: preparations for festival, procession and ceremony of circumcision, expenses of celebration, *etc.*

HITTI, P. K., 1943: History of the Arabs, ed. 3, 767 p. (Princeton, N.J.: U.P.).—

> This is a standard work in this field. The first ed. appeared in 1937 and a fourth

appeared in 1949. The book is in 5 parts. Pt. 1: The pre-Islamic age (the Arabs as Semites, geography, bedouin life, old kingdoms, p. 1-108); Pt. II: The rise of Islam and Caliphal state (Mohammed and the Koran, conquest of Syria, Persia, Egypt, *etc.*, p. 111-186); Pt. III: The Umayyad and 'Abbāsid empires (intellectual life under the Umayyads, scientific and literary progress in the 'Abbāsid state, education, fine arts, sects, heresies, *etc.*, p. 189-489); Pt. IV: The Arabs in Europe: Spain and Sicily (political, economic and educational institutions, intellectual contributions, art and architecture, p. 493-614); Pt. V: The last of the mediaeval Moslem states (Shi'ite caliphate in Egypt, the Crusades, cultural contacts, intellectual and artistic activity, p. 617-705). Long and valuable index (p. 707-767). There exists an abridged edition: HITTI, P. K., 1949: The Arabs: a short history, 224 p. (Princeton, N.J.: U.P.). (1st ed. 1937). A very readable history of Muslim culture in the tenth century is: MEZ, A., 1922: Die Renaissance des Islams, 498 p. (Heidelberg: Winter). *Cf.* also: GRUNEBAUM, G. E. von, 1966: Der Islam in seiner klassischen Epoche, 319 p. (Zurich & Stuttgart: Artemis). A French equivalent may be: SEDILLOT, L. A., 1877: Histoire générale des Arabes, leur empire, leur civilisation, leurs écoles philosophiques, scientifiques et littéraires, ed. 2, 2 vols., 906 p. (Paris: Maisonneuve). Reprinted 1967. (Not found).

ISKANDAR, A. Z., 1967: A catalogue of Arabic manuscripts on medicine and science in the Wellcome Historical Medical Library, 256 p. (London: Wellcome Hist. Med. Library).—

A catalogue of 245 items of Arabic and Persian manuscripts present in the Wellcome Historical Medical Library. More than 200 of them deal with medical subjects (25 of them deal with Avicenna's "Canon of medicine"), the others with zoology veterinary, science, alchemy, physiognomy, cosmology, and agriculture. In an introduction of 72 pages, the author gives a very readable review of Arabian medicine, and he makes a thorough comparison between the "Continens" of Rhazes and the "Canon of medicine" of Avicenna.

LÉVI-PROVENÇAL, E., 1950-1953: Histoire de l'Espagne musulmane, new ed., 3 vols. Vol. I (1950): La conquête et l'Emirat hispano-umaiyade (710-912), 403 p.; Vol. II (1950): Le califat umaiyade de Córdoue (912-1031), 435 p.; Vol. III (1953): La siècle du Califat de Córdoue, 576 p. (Paris: Maisonneuve; Leiden: Brill).—

Extensive history of Muslim Spain with many illustrations; there is little to be found in it concerning the history of science proper, but the period is of great interest in the history of science. Chapter headings are as follows: Vol. I: 1. La conquête et l'islamisation de l'Espagne (710-756); 2. La fondation et les débuts de l'émirat umaiyade de Córdoue (756-822); 3. L'Espagne musulmane sous le règne de 'Abd al-Rahman II (822-852); 4. L'émirat hispano-Umaiyade de 852 à 912. Vol. II: 5. 'Abd al-Rahman III al-Nasir, émir et calife d'al-Andalus (912-961); 6. L'Espagne califienne de 961 à 1008; 7. La décadence et la chute du califat de Córdoue (1008-1031). Vol. III: 8. L'organisation politique d'Espagne califienne; 9. L'organisation militaire; 10. L'organisation judicaire; 11. La société andalouse; 12. L'essor économique; 13. Le développement urbain; 14. La vie privée; 15. La vie religieuse et intellectuelle. Vols. II and III contain extensive indexes and bibliographies.

MIELI, A., 1938: La science arabe et son rôle dans l'évolution scientifique mondiale, 388 p. (Leiden: Brill).—

After a brief introduction considering Chinese, Hindu, Egyptian, Mesopotamian and Hellenistic influences on Arab science, the author describes the development of Arab science from the 8th to the 13th century. Appendixes deal with: 1. Quelques savants arabes et quelques ouvrages à partir du XIVe siècle; 2. Premiers textes proposés par M. Meyerhof, J. Millás Vallicrosa et H. P. J. Renaud pour être publiés dans le "Corpus scriptorum arabicorum de scientia naturali et arte medica"; 3. Liste des membres de la commission pour la publication du "Corpus"; 4. Correspondances entre les années de l'ère chrétienne et celles de l'ère Musulmanne; 5. Bibliographie. An anastatic reprint, supplemented by a bibliography and an analytic index compiled by A. MAZAHÉRI, appeared in 1966 (Leiden: Brill).

NABAVI, M. H., 1967: Hygiene und Medizin im Koran, 104 p. (Stuttgart: Enke).—

Separate sections of this booklet deal with such subjects as: Mohammed, his life and work, composition and style of the Koran, natural philosophy of Islam, the creation of the world and of Man, anatomy and physiology, diseases, therapy, death, catastrophes, feeding, drinks, fasting, hygiene, cleaning and washing in Islam, hygiene as duty, sexual life and hygiene, birth-control in the Koran, *etc.*

NASR, S. H., 1968: Science and civilization in Islam, 384 p. (Cambridge, Mass.: Harvard U.P.).—

A one-volume survey of the development and achievements of the various branches of Islamic science. Separate chapters deal with cosmology, geography, natural history (p. 108-125), physics, mathematics, astronomy, medicine (p. 188-229), and alchemy. The chapter on medicine considers such subjects as: the historical background of Islamic medicine; medicine of the prophet; medicine after Avicenna; medicine in Egypt, Syria, Spain, the Maghrib, and the eastern lands of Islam; the philosophy and theory of Islamic medicine. Much biographical information concerning the great men of Islamic science. An introductory chapter deals with the basic religious doctrines of Islam, and the three last chapters of the book are devoted to Islamic philosophy, theology, and mysticism. The book as a whole is an attempt to understand Islamic science as an integral part of Islamic civilization and culture. Cf. also: NASR, S. H., 1964: An introduction to Islamic cosmological doctrines: conceptions of nature and methods used for its study by the Ikhwān al Safā', al-Bīrunī, and ibn Sīnā, 312 p. (Cambridge, Mass.: Belknap). A Persian version of this book was published in 1964 by the Tehran U.P. This version contains many notes and quotations in Arabic and Persian, not found in the English version.

O'LEARY, De Lacy, 1948: How Greek science passed to the Arabs, 196 p. (London: Routledge & Kegan Paul).—

This in fact is a continuation of a former study by the same author: "Arabic thought and its place in history", 1922 (London: Routledge & Kegan Paul) in which the transmission of philosophy and theology was emphasized. In the present book stress is laid on the transmission of Greek science to the Arabs which began early in the eighth century. Special attention has been paid to the Syriac version of Hellenism, the role played by the Nestorians and Monophysites as intermediaries in the process of transmission. In reviewing this book in Isis 41: 125-127, S. Gandz criticizes its accuracy. Probably more reliable is: MEYERHOF, M., 1930: Von Alexandrien nach Bagdad. Ein Beitrag zur Geschichte des philosophischen und medizinischen Unterrichts bei den Arabern, 43 p. (Stzber. preuss. Akad. Wiss., phil.-hist. Kl., Vol. 23) (Berlin: de Gruyter); a publication dealing with the direct path in the transmission of Greek science from the school of Alexandria to Baghdad. Cf. ROSENTHAL, F., 1965. infra.

ROSENTHAL, F., 1965: Das Fortleben der Antike im Islam, 407 p. (Zurich & Stuttgart: Artemis).—

Sections of special importance to the historian of biology and of medicine are those dealing with the translators and their translations, those containing the biographies of Theophrastos and Galen, and those dealing with medicine (Hippocrates, theory of humours, Galen, Dioscorides, Rufus of Ephesus, veterinary medicine). Cf. O' LEARY, De Lacy, 1948, supra.

SALE, G., n.d.: The Korān commonly called 'The Alcoran of Mohammed'. Translated into English from the original Arabic, with explanatory notes taken from the most approved commentators to which is prefixed a preliminary discourse, 187 + 508 p. (London: Warne).—

The text is accompanied by a table of the chapters of the Koran according to the Arabic text, with their order of date and numbers of verses. This book was first published in London in 1734, re-issued by J. WILCOX in 1764, and has had 14 other edns. up to and including that of 1927 (which seems to have been the last).

STEINSCHNEIDER, M., 1964: Die arabische Literatur der Juden. Ein Beitrag zur Literaturgeschichte der Araber, grossenteils aus handschriftlichen Quellen, 54 + 348 + 32 p. (Hildesheim: Olms).—

For more details, vide section Hebrews, subsection a.

WÜSTENFELD, F., 1877: Die Uebersetzungen arabischer Werke in das Lateinische seit dem XI. Jahrhundert, 133 p. (Göttingen: Dieterich).—

For more details, vide section Middle Ages in the West, subsection a.

b. *History of the plant and animal sciences*

FRANKL, T., 1930: Die Anatomie der Araber. I. Die Nomenklatur des Verdauungstraktes. Eine philologische und kulturhistorische Studie, 148 p. (Prague: Calve).—

The purpose of this book is an attempt to interpret the terminology used by the Arabs to describe the different parts of the alimentary system. The author shows that the same part may be indicated by a variety of terms. Moreover, the author attempts to illustrate how a change in terminology may reflect a change in ideas about the function of these parts.

HOOPER, D., 1937: Useful plants and drugs of Iran and Iraq: with notes by H. FIELD, 168 p. (Field Museum Nat. Hist., Bot. Ser., Vol. 9, No. 3: 73-241).—

The main part of the book deals with drugs of vegetable origin (p. 79-188), other parts deal with drugs of mineral (p. 189-193) and of animal origin (p. 194-199). It is a kind of an Islamic herbal; for each drug the Latin name is given, followed by the Persian and other names and a description. The last part consists of prescriptions collected in Iran which are reproduced in facsimile ms. and translated. Alphabetical list of native names.

MERCIER, L., 1927: La chasse et les sports chez les Arabes. Illustrations de l'auteur d'après des miniatures orientales, 256 p. (Paris: Rivière).—

Sections which are of much interest from the point of view of the history of biology are those dealing with Arabic horses, with falconry (which is essentially of Persian origin), with the diseases of falcons and their cure, and with Arab cruelty to animals. Mercier also devoted a special study to Arabic hippiatry which is at the same time a very valuable contribution to our knowledge of Muslim civilization, viz., La parure des cavaliers et l'insigne des preux, 1922, 98 p. This publication contains a French translation of an Arab treatise on hippiatry written ca. 1356.

MEYERHOF, M., 1934: Esquisse d'histoire de la pharmacologie et botanique chez les musulmans d'Espagne, 41 p. (Al-Andalus 3 (1935): 1-41).—

Pharmacology was very popular among the Arabs, especially since Ḥunain Ibn Isḥāq (d. 873) translated the works of Dioscorides and Galen into both Syriac and Arabic; these translations became the basis of a purely Arabic pharmacology and therapeusis, secondarily influencing the Latin West, e.g., by the Pandectus of Yuḥanna ibn Sarābiyun (Jean Sérapion). Separate chapters deal with: The primitive period in Spain; The Arabic translation of Dioscorides's "Materia medica" by Ibn Jūljūl in Spain; The golden age of pharmacology in Spain (al.Ghāfiḳī, Ibn al-Baiṭar, Averroës, Abulcasis, Yaḳūb al-Manṣūr, Abu-l-Ḥayyay,

Abu-l-'Abbas); The influence of Spanish pharmacology in East and West.

PERRON, A., 1852-1860: La Nâcéri. La perfection des deux arts; ou, traité complet d'hippologie et d'hippiatrie arabes, traduit de l'Arabe, 3 vols. (Paris: Bouchard-Huzard).—

According to Sarton, Introd. III (1): 829, this book seems to be rare. In spite of some disorder, use of poor Arabic sources, and occasional carelessness, this work is very important; it is the source of all later Western commentaries. Vol. I is a long introduction, and Vols. 2 and 3 contain a French translation of the Nāṣiri together with fragments translated from an earlier Arabic text of the same kind. Vol. 3, p. 348-424, contains fragments concerning mules, asses, camels, elephants and cattle derived from a work written by al-Mujāhid 'ali al-Rasūlī. For a German translation of the third volume, vide Abu Bekr ibn Bedr, this section, subsection d; Cf. also: MERCIER, L., 1922, vide supra; and: BJÖRCK, G., 1932, vide section Classical Antiquity β, subsection b.

RENAUD, H. P. J., 1935: La contribution des arabes à la connaissance des espèces végétales: les botanistes musulmans. (Bull. Soc. Sci. nat. Maroc., Vol. 15).—

"Exellent résumé contenant plusieurs détails intéressants." (From Isis 25 : 269). Cf. 'Abd Allāh ibn Aḥmad, called Ibn al-Baiṭar; and Aḥmad ibn Dā'ud al-Dīnawarī, vide subsection d.

RENAUD, H. P. J. & G. S. COLIN, 1934: Tuḥfatnal-aḥbāb. Glossaire de la matière médicale marocaine. Texte publié pour la première fois avec traduction, notes critiques et index, 34 + 218 + 75 (Arab) p. (Publ. Inst. hautes Études marocaines, 24) (Paris: Geuthner).—

An edition of an anonymous Moroccan treatise on materia medica, accompanied by a French translation and many annotations. The text consists of 462 items, arranged alphabetically, the subject-matter of which has been based mainly upon Dioscorides, Ibn Biklārish, and Ibn al-Baiṭar. Many Berber and Roman synonyms, philological, historical, medical and botanical notes, with French, Latin, and Arabic indexes. Cf. DUCROS, M. A. H., 1930, vide subsection c.

SCHWEINFURTH, G., 1912: Arabische Pflanzennamen aus Aegypten, Algerien und Jemen, 232 p. (Berlin: Reimer).—

A glossary of plant names, expressing the wanderings and changes these names underwent which at the same time may reflect botanical and medical knowledge. This book is of value equally to students of comparative linguistics, to philologists, and to students of biohistory.

TJERNELD, H., ed., 1945: Moamin et Ghatrif. Traités de fauconnerie et des chiens de chasse, 443 p. (Stockholm: Fritze).—

A new edition of a mediaeval falconry text (late second quarter of the 13th century). The text can be considered complementary to the "De arte venandi cum avibus" (cf. Frederick II of Hohenstaufen, vide section Middle Ages in the West, subsection d). It primarily deals with the medical and herbal lore of falconry. Moamin's treatise was written originally in Arabic; Ghatrif's treatise in Persian (43 p.). There are two Moamin-treatises dealing respectively with falconry and with hounds (together 168 pages).

c. History of the medical sciences

AZEEZ PASHA, M., 1966: Union catalogue of Arabic and Persian medical manuscripts in the libraries of Hyderabad, 46 p. (Hyderabad: Dept. Hist. Med., Osmania Med. Coll.).—

A check-list of Arabic and Persian medical mss. existing in six libraries in Hyderabad. The section covering Arabic mss. contains 188 items; that covering Persian mss. 416 items. The author gives his data in 5 columns: serial numbers, titles (with transliterations), English translations of titles, author's names, and names of libraries. Cf. DIETRICH, A., 1966, vide infra.

BLOOM, A., 1935: L'ostéologie d'Abul Qasim et d'Avicenne. Son origine talmudique, 71 p. (Paris: Lipschutz).—

In this study the author elucidates the Talmudic origin of Arab osteology, and he makes clear that Arab osteological knowledge was to a large extent due to Jewish acquisitions.

BROWNE, E. G., 1962: Arabian medicine, 138 p. (Cambridge: U.P.).—

This booklet is a reprint to the 1921 edition. It gives a historical review of Muslim medicine, dealing with such topics as: the transmission of Greek learning, Syrian and Persian contributions, the evolution of scientific terminology in Arabic, psychotherapeusis, the School of Toledo, dissections,

Persian medical literature from the 12th to the 14th century, biographical works of the 13th century, the introduction of European medicine to Muslim lands, Muslim hospitals, fees of physicians, dropsy cured by a diet of locusts, early tradition of anaesthesia. Also in French translation: La médecine arabe, 1933, 173 p. (Paris: Larousse). Cf. also: WHIPPLE, A. O., 1967: The role of the Nestorians and Muslims in the history of medicine, 113 p. (Princeton, N.J.: Princeton U.P.). Unfortunately I am unable to give further information about this book Cf. also: KHAIRALLAH, A. A., 1946, vide infra.

CAMPBELL, D., 1926: Arabian medicine and its influence on the Middle Ages, 2 vols. Vol. I: 208 p.; Vol. II: 235 p. (London: Kegan Paul, Trench & Trübner).—

The first volume deals with Greek medicine in its relation to the Arabs, Arabic medical mss., the historiography of Islam (esp. concerning medical literature), Arabic medical writers and their works (Eastern as well as Western Caliphate), the age of early Arabian rumours in the West, Arabism in the intellectual currents of mediaeval Europe, the Latin translators and the college at Toledo, Hellenism and Arabism in the 15th and 16th centuries, medical curricula of European universities in the later Middle Ages. The second volume consists of two appendixes, the first containing a list of Latin translators of the Arabic works (p. 3-12) and the second containing a list of dates and authorship of the Latin versions of the works of Galen (p. 13-220). Bibliography and index. Cf. also: KHAIRALLAH, A. A., 1946, vide infra.

DIETRICH, A., 1966: Medicinalia Arabica. Studien ueber arabische Medizin. Handschriften in türkischen und syrischen Bibliotheken, 258 p. (Abh. Akad. Wiss. Göttingen, phil.-hist. Kl., Folge 3, No. 66) (Göttingen: Vandenhoeck & Ruprecht).—

This book I have not seen, but in the "Deutsche Bibliographie", Heft 4/1967, I found the following description: "Die Handschriftenbeschreibung ist nach Sachgebieten geordnet, in der Regel nach Schriftkreisen. Im einzelnen werden behandelt: Hippocrates und Galen mit ihren arabischen Bearbeitern, Hunains Questiones medica, Rhazes und die Autoren von Rhazes bis Avicenna, Avicennas Canon und seine Bearbeiter bis ins 8./14. Jahrhundert, die von Avicenna unabhängigen Autoren von Ibn Gazla ... bis zur osmanischen Medizin des 12./17. Jahrhunderts, schliesslich die "Materia medica", zwei Werke der Hippiatrie sowie Sammelhandschriften ..." Cf. also: ISKANDAR,

A. Z., 1967, *vide* this section, subsection a; and AZEEZ PASHA, M., 1966, *vide supra.*

DUCROS, M. A. H., 1930: Essai sur le droguier populaire arabe de l'inspectorat des pharmacies du Caire, 165 p. (Mém. Inst. égypt., 15) (Cairo: Inst. français archéol. orientale).—

This book gives a description of 233 drugs which are available or at least were available not very long ago in Cairo; for many drugs illustrations have been given. Indexes of Arabic, Latin, and French names. It would be interesting to compare this popular pharmacopoeia with a scientific one, such as *e.g.,* that of Maimonides (*cf.* MEYERHOF, M., 1940, *vide* section Hebrews, subsection d). *Cf.* also: RENAUD, H. P. J. & G. S. COLIN, 1934, *vide* subsection b.

ELGOOD, C., 1962: Ṭibb-ul-Nabbi or medicine of the Prophet. Being a translation of two works of the same name. I. The Ṭibb-ul-Nabbi of Al-Suyūṭī. II. The Ṭibb-ul-Nabbi of Mahmūd bin Mohamed a Chaghhayni, together with introduction, notes, and a glossary, 159 p. (Osiris 14: 33-192).—

Pseudo-medical works, collections of sayings on medicine of the Prophet Mohammed. The greater part (p. 48-185) deals with the work of al-Suyūṭī. This part consists of three divisions. The first division contains 3 sections: 1. Theory of medicine (constitution of Man, the state of his body, aetiology of disease); 2. Practical rules of medicine (food, drink, movement and rest, excretion, venesection, cupping, baths, emotions); 3. Principles of treatment. The second division deals with the properties of foods and drugs, and consists of a list of them arranged according to the Arabian alphabet, with a summary of their properties, preparation, *etc.* The third division deals with diseases and their treatment, and consists of 21 chapters dealing with diagnosis, doctor's fees, the use of drugs, attention to the sick, treatment of various diseases, cauterization, the evil eye, embryology and anatomy, and many other things. The book of Mahmhūd consists of 140 very short statements, many of them of a moralizing character. To mention some of them: no. 23: Less food, less sin; 8. To eat in the bazaar in public is to behave like a wine jar; 85. To eat figs protects against colic, and 136: Fever unloads sins as a tree throws off leaves.

HAMARNEH, S., 1964: Bibliography on medicine and pharmacy in medieval Islam.

Mit einer Einführung: Arabismus in der Geschichte der Pharmazie von Rudolf SCHMITZ, 204 p. (Veröffentl. Intl. Ges. Gesch. Pharmazie, N.F., Vol. 25) Stuttgart: Wiss. Verlagsges.).—

This bibliography is in four parts, *viz.,* 1. Books on medicine and pharmacy written in mediaeval Islam (but printed or edited later); 2. Relevant and useful books on the history of Islamic civilizations; 3. Reference books, bibliographies, and dictionaries; 4. Current periodicals. Each of the items included is accompanied by (brief) annotations in English.

HILTON-SIMPSON, M. W., 1922: Arab medicine and surgery: a study of the healing art in Algeria, 96 p. (Oxford: U.P.).—

An eyewitness of medical treatment as it is practised by the Berber and Arab doctors of the Aurès Massif, Algeria, written by a layman. One part deals with surgery (*e.g.,* asepsis, anaesthetics, trepanning, removal and substitution of bone from limbs, fractures, dislocations, hernia, cauterization, obstetric surgery, cupping, snake- and scorpion-bites, dentistry, skin-grafting, *etc.*). Another part deals with medicine, *e.g.,* with purges and laxatives, colic, worms, jaundice, diarrhoea, cholera, fever, bronchitis, headache, rheumatism, syphilis, skin diseases, abscesses, smallpox, aphrodisiacs, rabies, burns and scalds, *etc.* Index of materia medica.

HIRSCHBERG, J., 1905: Die arabischen Lehrbücher der Augenheilkunde. Ein Capitel zur arabischen Literaturgeschichte. Unter Mitwirkung von J. LIPPERT und E. MITTWOCH, 117 p. (Abh. preuss. Akad. Wiss., 1905).—

Discusses many Arabian authors on ophthalmology, *e.g.,* Ḥunain ibn Isḥāk (= Johannitius), Ḥubaish ibn al-Ḥasan, Thābit ibn Ḵurrah, 'Alī ibn Isā, 'Ammār ibn 'Alī al-Mauṣilī, Zarrin Dast (a Persian oculist), Ibn Wafid (=Abengefid), Abū Bakr ibn Zuhr, Ḥalifa and Ṣalaḥ ad-Dīn ibn Yūsuf (a Syrian oculist), Fatḫ ad-dīn ... al Qaisī, Ibn al-Nafis, *etc.*

HIRSCHBERG, J., J. LIPPERT & E. MITTWOCH, eds., 1905: Die arabischen Augenärzte nach den Quellen bearbeitet, 2 vols. Vol. I: Ali ibn Isā: Erinnerungsbuch für Augenaerzte aus arabischen Handschriften uebersetzt und erläutert, 362 p.; Vol. II:

'Ammār b. Ali al-Mauṣilī: Das Buch der Auswahl von den Augenkrankheiten; Ḥalīfa al Ḥalabi: Das Buch vom Genügenden in der Augenheilkunde; Ṣalāḥ ad-Dīn: Licht der Augen. Aus arabischen Handschriften übersetzt und erläutert, 262 p. (Leipzig: Veit).—

'Alī ibn Isā (= Jesu Haly, first half 11th century) is the most famous Arab oculist. His "manual" is the oldest Arabic work on ophthalmology of which the original text is completely extant. It is in 3 books; the first deals with the anatomy and physiology of the eye; the second with the diseases externally visible, and the third with hidden diseases, dietetics, and general medicine from the oculistic standpoint. 130 eye diseases are carefully described; 143 drugs characterized. 'Ammār ibn 'Alī (=Canamusali, fl. 996-1020), the most original of Arab oculists, wrote a summary on the treatment of the eye (transl. in Vol. II, p. 1-152), containing many descriptions of diseases and treatments, arranged in logical order, together with a valuable surgical part. There also exist French, German, English, and Spanish translation of "Las operaciones de caterata de 'Ammār ibn 'Alī al-Mausilī oculiste de el Cairo", ed. by M. MEYERHOF, published in Barcelona in 1937 (117 p.). Vol. II, p. 153-194 contains German translations of the most important parts of a treatise written by Ḥalifa, containing very detailed descriptions of the surgical treatment of the eye and of the instruments used. Ṣalāh ad-Dīn wrote one of the most elaborate treatises on ophthalmology. The last part of Vol. II contains a review of those parts of his work which deal with the anatomy of the eye (Ṣalāh's first book). Ṣalāh's second book: "The theory of seeing" (Die Lehre vom Sehen) has here been fully translated, but from his eighth book only ch. 5 "The cataract" (Vom Star) has been given in translated form here. Cf. also: HIRSCHBERG, J., 1905, vide supra; and ISSA BEY, A., 1925, vide infra.

ISSA BEY, A., 1925: Al-ālāt at-ṭibb w'al-jirāḥa w'al-kiḥāla 'inda 'l-'Arab, 24 p. (The medical, surgical and ophthalmic instruments of the Arabs) (Cairo).—

I have not seen this publication (it is not in any of the Dutch libraries), but Sarton gives in Isis 8: 597 the following characteristics: "This is a compilation of all that is known about the instruments of the Arabs for medical purposes, extracted mainly from the Chirurgia of Abulcasis (Abū-l-Oāsim az-Zahrāwī), and from the publications of Sudhoff and Hirschberg. The author gives an alphabetical list of the instruments

and a reproduction of the plates of Abulcasis and Hirschberg. Moreover a photo of the instruments found during the recent excavations at Fustāt (Old Cairo). Nevertheless, I have doubts about the medical character of some of these instruments. Several of them are probably cosmetic tools. A more extended vocalisation of the names of instruments would have been useful."

——, 1929: Histoire des bimāristans (hôpitaux) à l'époque islamique, 128 p. (C.R. Congrès intl. méd. tropicale, Cairo, 1929, Vol. I: 81-209).—

During the Islamic period, hospitals were called bimāristans. They were philanthropic institutions, created by caliphs, sultans, kings, and benefactors in general, meant to serve humanity. They were not only established for the service of the sick, but they also were used as teaching institutions. The author considers different kinds of bimāristans, their organisation, and their educational function; some 30 of them are considered in some detail. Besides, the author discusses such topics as the medicines used, the fees of physicians and surgeons, medical examinations and medical inspection.

KAPPAUF, W., 1921: Aus der Zahnheilkunde der Araber in der Ueberlieferung des Abendlandes, 80 p. (Diss. Leipzig).—

A summary of Muslim dentistry, including many extracts from the sources and a bibliography. (From Isis 4: 619).

KHAIRALLAH, A. A., 1946: Outline of Arabic contributions to medicine and the allied sciences, 288 p. (Beirut: American Press).—

After a brief review of medical knowledge before and during the Islamic period, the author discusses such topics as: some medical historians, editors and translators, Arab hospitals, internal medicine, the humoral theory, therapeutics, anatomy and surgery, diseases of the eye, chemistry and pharmacy, botany and zoology, transmission to Europe (Gerard of Cremona, Constantine the African, et. al.), and gives a short chapter concerning Arabic medicine from the end of the Islamic period to the present. Much additional information is provided by the appendixes: 1. A list of the better-known Arab physicians; 2. Idem of Greek physicians and their medical books translated into Arabic; 3. A list of the better-known Arabic books that were translated into Latin; 5. A list of Latinized proper Arabic nouns and 6. A bibliography. *Cf.* also: BROWNE, E. G., 1962; CAMPBELL, D., 1926, *vide supra;* and LECLERC, L., 1876: WÜSTENFELD, F., 1840, *vide infra.*

KONING, P. de, 1903: Trois traités d'anatomie arabes par Muhammed ibn Zakariyyā al-Rāzi, 'Ali ibn al-'Abbās et 'Ali ibn Sinā, 830 p. (Leiden: Brill).—

From the first two works the Arabian text has been given together with the French translation on facing pages; from the last treatise only the French translation has been given because good editions of the Arabian text exist. The first text is an edition of the anatomical parts of the Kitāb al-Manṣūrī (Liber Almansoris), a smaller compilation in 10 books of Al-Rāzi's great encyclopaedia of medicine. The second text is an edition of discourses 2 and 3 of a medical encyclopaedia of Ali-ibn-Abbās, (d. 994), one of the greatest physicians of the Eastern Caliphate. The whole encyclopaedia, the Kitāb al-Māliki, the "Royal Book", consists of 20 discourses of which the first half deals with the theory and the second half with the practice of medicine. The third text (p. 432-781) consists of a French translation of the anatomical sections of Ibn Sinā's "Canon"', an immense medical encyclopaedia comprising the whole of ancient and Muslim medical knowledge.

LECLERC, L., 1876: Histoire de la médecine arabe. Exposé complet des traductions du grec. Les sciences en Orient, leur transmission à l'occident par les traductions latines, 2 vols. Vol. I: 588 p.; Vol. II: 527 p. (Paris: Leroux).—

This is the most exhaustive history of Arabian medical translations from West to East and *vice versa.* Bk. I "De la médecine arabe jusqu'à la chute des Ommiades", discusses the time of Mohammed, the connections between the School of Alexandria and the Arabs, and contains much biographical material on Persian and Arabian physicians and alchemists. Bk. II: "IXe siècle. Siècle d'el Mamoun ou siècle des traductions", discusses the School of Jundīshāpūr, the most famous translators and the authors whose work has been translated, translations from Persian, Indian, and Chaldaean sources, incl. works on the natural sciences and alchemy. Bks. III-VI discuss the 10th, 11th, 12th, and 13th century respectively (each of them dealing with Persia, Iraq, Egypt, Maghreb and Spain). Bk. VII: "Les siècles de décadence" deals with the 14th and 15th centuries and with Arabian medicine in Persia. Reprint edition, 1961: New York,

N.Y.: Burt Franklin. *Cf.* also: DALMA, J., 1964: Les árabes y la medicina: aspectos historicos y culturales, 94 p. (Buenos Aires: Ed. Médica Panamericana), a book about which I am unable to give further information. *Cf.* KHAIRALLAH, A. A., 1946, *vide supra.*

OPITZ, K., 1906: Die Medizin im Koran, 92 p. (Stuttgart: Enke).—

A compilation of those passages in the Koran which are of a medical importance or which may give an impression of Mohammed's knowledge of the human body and of life itself: anatomy, embryology, pathology, therapy, personal hygiene, epidemics, catastrophes, food and drink, sexual behaviour and rites, *etc. Cf.* also RASSLAN, W., 1934, *vide infra;* and NABAVI, M. H., 1967, *vide* subsection a.

RASSLAN, W., 1934: Mohammed und die Medizin nach den Ueberlieferungen, 51 p. (Abh. Geŝch. Med. und Naturw., Heft 1) (Berlin: Ebering).—

Chapter 1 deals with Arabic medical knowledge before and during Mohammed's life; ch. II with Mohammed and medicine (anatomy, embryology, pathology, therapy, hygiene, and the drugs mentioned by Mohammed himself); ch. III deals with Mohammed and the social position of the physician. Reprinted 1968 (New York, N.Y.: Johnson). *Cf.* also: OPITZ, K., 1906; and ELGOOD, C., 1962, *vide supra.*

SBATH, P. & C. D. AVIERINOS, 1953: Sahlān ibn Kaysān et Rašīd al-Dīn Abū Ḥulayqā. Deux traités médicaux, 88 p. (Cairo: Inst. français archeol. orientale).—

Text and French translation of two medical treatises, *viz.,* the "Précis sur les médicaments composés employés dans la plupart des maladies", mainly a list of drugs, with particulars as to their preparation and usage, composed by Sahlān ibn Kaysān (p. 1-75); and the "Petit traité sur les hiéras", a short treatise concerning preparation and application of the "hiéras", composed by Rašīd al-Dīn Abū Ḥulayqa, a Christian Melkite physician, who died in 1277.

SCHACHT, J. & M., MEYERHOF, 1937: The medico-philosophical controversy between Ibn Butlān of Baghdad and Ibn Ridwan of Cairo: a contribution to the history of Greek learning among the Arabs, 124 p. English text, 91 p. Arabic text (Egyptian Univ., Fac. arts, Publ. 13) (Cairo).—

Ibn Riḍwān (of Cairo) and Ibn Buṭlān (of Baghdad) belong to the greatest
physicians of the middle of the 11th century. Ibn Buṭlān spent three years in Cairo
(1049-1052) and during that time, between
him and Ibn Riḍwān originated a strong
rivalry, concentrated around the problem
whether the nature of a bird's young was
"warmer" than that of the adult or not.
They wrote 5 treatises dealing with the subject, and although the whole problem is of
minor importance; yet these treatises give
an insight into medical argumentation of
those days and as such it is an important
contribution to the history of medicine. The
present book contains the original Arabic
text of the treatises and also an English
translation. It also contains much biographical information on both authors, Ibn Rid-
wān and Ibn Buṭlān (esp. p. 33-69).

SIDDIQI, Z., 1959: Studies in Arabic and
Persian medical literature, 48 + 173 p. (Calcutta: U.P.).—

The author gives an account of the
early medical literature of Arabic and Persian origin. He makes clear that Arabian
medicine was not merely a slavish adoption
of Greek and Indian ideas; he stresses the
importance of the "Firdaus al-ḥikma" (Paradise of wisdom) written by 'Ali ibn Rabbān al-Ṭabarī of Baghdad, as the first independent Arabic medical compendium; and
gives a brief summary of its contents. The
Arabs were noteworthy as founders of hospitals and medical institutions; thus as early
as A.D. 707 an Arabic hospital was established at Damascus, and in Baghdad there
were as many as 60 medical institutions by
the year A.D. 1160.

STEINSCHNEIDER, M., 1960: Die arabischen Uebersetzungen aus dem Griechischen, 381 p. (Graz: Akad. Druck & Verlagsanst.).—

A reprint edition of a collection of
bibliographies originally published in: Beihefte zum Centralblatt für Bibliothekwesen
V (1889) and XII (1893); Zeitschr. deutschen
Morgenländischen Gesellschaft 50 (1896)
and in Archiv path. Anat. Physiol. 124, Folge XII, Vol. IV (1891).

STRAUSS, B., 1934: Das Giftbuch des
Ṣānāq. Eine literaturgeschichtliche Untersuchung, 64 p. + 66 p. in Arabic. (Quell.
Gesch. Naturw., Vol. 4) (Berlin: Springer).—

This booklet, dealing with poisons,
contains the Arabic text (64 p.) of the Kitāb

al-sumūn ascribed to Shānāq the Hindu.
This edition also contains a German translation (34 p.) and an elaborate study of
sources, development, etc. Shānāq, or Cā-
ṇakya, lived ca. 320 B.C. According to Sarton (Isis 23: 447) the Sanskrit book of poisons was translated into Persian by Mankah
(fl. ca. 767). The text was probably rewritten
or edited in Arabic by al-'Abbās ibn Sa'īd
al-Jauharī (9th century). To the old Hindu
text were added Greek and Arabic elements.

WÜSTENFELD, F., 1840: Geschichte der
ʾarabischen Aerzte und Naturforscher, 167 p.
(Göttingen: Vandenhoeck & Ruprecht).—

A very valuable and authoritative
work on Arabic medical literature. It covers
the period 1-1000 A.D. and it gives in a
chronological order short biographical notes
and excellent bibliographical information
concerning the Arabic physicians. Reissued
1963, 183 p. (Hildesheim: Olms). Cf. KHAI-
RALLAH, A. A., 1946, vide supra; also:
Aḥmād ibn Ḳāsām Muwaffaḳ al-dīn Abū-l-
'Abbās, called Ibn Abī Uṣaibi'ah, vide subsection d.

d. Some individual scientists

'Abd Allāh ibn Aḥmad, called Ibn al-Baiṭār
(d. 1248) — BASSET, R., 1899: Les noms
berbères des plantes dans le traité des simples d'Ibn el Beïtar, 14 p. (Giornale Soc.
asiat. ital. 12: 53-66).—

His main work has been "Traité des
simples", of which a French translation
exists (by LECLERC, vide infra). In this
work Ibn Baiṭār gives synonyms of plant
names in vulgar Arabian, Spanish Arabian,
Greek, Berber, and Persian, of the plants
collected by him during his many voyages.
The present publication is a study of these
old Berber names; the author compares
these 13th-century names with those still
used to-day.

——, LECLERC, L., 1877-1883: Traité des
simples par Ibn el Beïthar, 3 vols. 476 +
489 + 483 p. (Notices et extraits Vol. 23,
pars 1 (1877): 476 p.; Vol. 25, pars 1
(1881): 489 p.; Vol. 26, pars 1 (1883): 483
p.) (Paris: Inst. de France).—

Ibn al-Baiṭār was a Hispano-Muslim
botanist and pharmacist, the greatest of Islam and the Middle Ages. He herborized
in Spain, in the Near East, and in North
Africa. His main work is a discourse on
simples (which also deals with various spe-

cies of food) considering some 1,400 different items; some 150 authors of older works have been quoted, including 20 Greek authors. Of this work Leclerc gives a French translation. "Notices et extraits" Vol. 23 contains the names from Aaloussen, Alyssum to Hay el a'lem, Sempervivum; Vol. 25 the names from Khānek en-nemer, Doronicum pardalianches to A'ïtsām, plantane; and Vol. 26 contains indexes of Arabian, Latin, and French names.

——, SONTHEIMER, J. von, 1840-1842: Grosse Zusammenstellung über die Kräfte der bekannten einfachen Heil- und Nahrungsmittel von Abū Mohammed Abdallāh ben Ahmed aus Malaga, bekannt unter dem Namen Ebn Baithār, aus dem Arabischen uebersetzt, 2 vols. Vol. I: 593 p.; Vol. II: 787 + 70 p. (Stuttgart: Hallberger).—

From the preface: "Dieses Werk umfasst alle einfache Heil- und Nahrungsmittel, soweit solche von den frühesten Zeiten an bis zu Anfang des 13. Jahrhunderts, in welchem der Verfasser ... lebte, aus arabischen, persischen, syrischen, indischen und griechischen Handschriften, deren Namen und Werke Ebn Baithār bei jedem einzelnen Gegenstand erwähnt, bekannt sind. Die in diesem Werke enthaltenen Heil- und Nahrungsmittel sind alphabetisch geordnet, deren arabische, persische, syrische, indische und griechische Benennungen den Anfang eines jeden abgehandelten Heilkörpers machen, auf welche die Beschreibung desselben in Absicht seiner äusseren Form, seiner Kräfte, seiner durch Erfahrung bestätigten Wirkung auf den menschlichen Körper, seines Nutzens in Krankheiten, seiner Nachtheile und Beschränkung derselben, seine Dosen unter den verschiedenen Gebrauchsformen, und endlich der Substituierung der Arzneimittel für einander, wenn eines oder das andere nicht vorräthig ist, folgt." The text has been based mainly on Dioscorides and Galen. There are many notes, a very useful list of biographies of the physicians mentioned in this book and an Arabic-Latin index.

'Abd Allāh ibn Muslim, al-Dīnāwarī, called Ibn Ḵutaibah (ca. 828- ca. 889) — BODENHEIMER, F. S. & L. KOPF, eds., 1949: The 'Uyūn al-akhbār of Ibn Qutayba: the natural history section from a 9th century "Book of useful knowledge", 87 p. (Collection de travaux de l'Académie intl. d'Hist. des Sciences, No. 4) (Leiden: Brill).—

The 'Uyūn al-akhbār is a compilation of what had been known to earlier genera-

tions and is one of the earliest authentic sources for Arab traditions on animals and on animal lore in a concentrated form, and as such is of special historical interest. The whole work is divided into ten parts (books), dealing with various subjects; the present booklet contains a translation of a part of the fourth book entitled: "Things of nature and blameworthy traits of character in Man". This fourth book is in 35 chapters, of which only the chapters X - XXXIV have been chosen for translation, since the others have no bearing on natural science in the sense the term is used now.

'Abd al-Laṭīf ibn Yūsuf, al-Baghdādī, called Ibn al-Labbād (1162-1231) — DE SACY, S., 1810: Relation de l'Egypte, suivie de divers extraits d'écrivains orientaux et d'un état des provinces et des villages de l'Egypte dans le XIVe siècle: le tout traduit et enrichi de notes historiques et critiques, 752 p. (Paris).—

One of the best-known works of 'Abd al-Laṭīf is his "Account of Egypt". The text transmitted to us is divided into 9 chapters dealing respectively with generalities, plants, animals, ancient monuments, buildings and ships, cookery, the Nile, and the events of the year 597 (= 1200) and 598 (= 1202), including a description of the great plague and famine of 597. It also contains much biographical information. In the book under consideration a French translation of the "Account" is to be found. According to Sarton, Introduction II (2): 600, De Sacy's book (including its long notes and elaborate index) is important. Chapter 2 deals with the plants, and chapter 3 with the animals, of Egypt.

'Abd al-Mālik ibn Quraib al-Aṣma'i (ca. 739-831) — Al Aṣma'i wrote a number of works treating of animals; some of his texts have been edited, e.g., by GEYER, R. (Sitzb. Wien. Akad. Wiss., phil.-hist. Classe, Vol. 115, 1887, p. 353-420); and by HAFFNER, A. (Idem, Vol. 132, 1895, 62 p.).—

Geyer's text deals with animals of the desert that play a great part in Arabic poetry. Geyer gives a list of 11 poets, but, according to him, the book of al-Aṣma'i is the only one which is known in Europe to exist. The animals treated of are the ass, ox, antelope, mountain goat, ostrich, lion, wolf, hyena, fox, and hare. Verses are given from the poets illustrating the use of the names adduced. Unfortunately no full translation of the text is given; only the introduction (p. 353-357) and the notes (p. 392-420) are in German. Haffner gives an edition of the Kitāb al Ḳhail of Al-Aṣma'i, a treatise dealing with the horse. The names given to the horse are recounted with examples of their use extracted from the works of the poets. This is followed by a description of the desirable and undesirable qualities of the horse, its colours, etc. Only the introduction (p. 1-5) and the notes (p. 30-62) are in German; no full translation is given. Al-Aṣma'i also wrote treatises on the camel and the sheep.

'Abd al-Mālik ibn Zuhr (Abu Marwān), called Avenzohar (ca. 1092- ca. 1161) — COLIN, G., 1911: Avenzoar, sa vie et ses oeuvres, 199 p. (Thèse Univ. Paris) (Paris: Leroux).—

After a rather long description of the life, predecessors and works of this famous physician of Muslim Spain (p. 1-52), the author proceeds with a discussion of the following works: 1) The "Kitāb al-iqtiṣād", written ca. 1122, of which title the author gives the following French translation: "Traité premier du Livre d'Iqtiṣād, concernant la confortation des esprits et des corps." It is a summary of therapeutics and hygiene, composed for the benefit of lay readers; 2) The "Kitāb al-taisīr", Avenzohar's main work, the "Book of simplification concerning therapeutics and diet", a study of pathological conditions and relevant therapeutics. This work has been translated into Latin during the Middle Ages, and of this work a list of chapter headings has been given in Latin, in Arabic, and in French; 3) The "Kitāb al-aghdhiya", the "Book of foodstuffs", with a short summary of its contents. In this book Avenzohar treats of various kinds of food and their use according to the seasons, simple drugs, and hygiene.

'Abd al-Raḥmān ibn Muḥammad, called Ibn Wafid (997 - ca. 1074) — FARAUDO DE SAINT-GERMAIN, L., 1943: El "Libre de les medecines particulars." Versión catalana trescentista del texto árabe del Tratado de los medicamentos simples de Ibn Wāfid, autor médico toledano del siglo XI. Transcripción, estudio proemial y glosarios, 199 p. (Barcelona: Real Academia de Buenas Lettras de Barcelona).—

Ibn Wāfid was a Hispano-Muslim physician and pharmacologist who wrote a work on simple drugs (De medicamentis simplicibus, or Kitāb al-adwiya al-mufrada), based on Dioscorides, Galen, and personal observations. It is an important treatise on materia medica, translated into Latin by Gerard of Cremona. There also exists a Catalan translation, prepared in the 14th century, of which this book contains an edition (p. 1-173). This edition is followed by a Catalan index of pharmaceutical items, 361 in all, of which 300 are of botanical origin, 28 of mineral, and 33 of animal origin. Ibn Wāfid also wrote a treatise on agriculture, of which a Catelan translation has been found in the National Library, Madrid. This text has been edited by MILLÁS VALLICROSA, J. M., 1943: La traducción castellana del "Tratado de Agricultura" de Ibn Wāfid, 51 p. (Al Andalus 8: 281-332).

Abi Ja'far Aḥmed ibn 'Ali ibn Moḥammed ibn 'Alī ibn Khātimah (fl. ca. 1350) — DINANAH, T., 1927: Die Schrift von Abi Ja'far Aḥmed ibn 'Alī ibn Mohammed ibn 'Alī ibn Khātimah aus Almeriah über die Pest, 54 p. (Arch. Gesch. Med. 19: 27-81).—

This publication contains a German translation of an Arabic treatise dealing with the plague which occurred in Almeria, Andalusia, in 1348. Its contents may become clear from the German chapter headings, viz., 1. Wesen der Pest; 2. Allgemeine und spezielle Ursachen; 3. Weshalb befiel die Pest gewisse Leute, verschonte andere trotz enger Nachbarschaft?; 4. Die Ansteckung; 5. Vorbeugung, Verhütung; 6. Therapie. It is one of the oldest pest treatises ever written. Cf. ANTUÑA, M. M., 1928: Abenjátima de Almeria y su tratado de la peste, 22 p. (Religión y Cultura 1, No. 4: 68-90).

Abu Bekr ibn Bedr al-dīn Ibn al-Mundhir al Baiṭār (fl. ca. 1293 - ca. 1340) — FROEHNER, R., 1931: Die Tierheilkunde des Abu Bekr ibn Bedr, 150 p. (Abh. Gesch. Veter-Med., Heft 23) (Leipzig: Richter).—

Abu Bekr ibn Bedr wrote the "Kamil assanaatin", a large treatise dealing with the breeding and training of horses and with horse diseases and their cure. The present German translation is chiefly a translation of those parts which deal with hippiatry. For a full translation of Abu Bekr's treatise, cf. PERRON, M., 1852-1860, vide subsection b. The present German translation is based mainly on Perron's third volume.

Abū-l-Haṣan al Mukhtār ibn al-Ḥasan ibn 'Abdūn ibn Sa'dūn ibn Buṭlān (= Elluchasem Elimithar, d. ca. 1063) — ASÍN PALACIOS, M., ed., 1943: Glosario de voces romances registradas por un botánico anónimo hispano-musulmán (siglos XI-XII), 54 + 420 p. (Madrid-Granada: Consejo superior de investigaciones cientificas).—

Glossary belonging to an Arabic manuscript of the Gayongos Collection and which, according to the editor, has to be attributed to the famous physician Abū-l-Ḥaṣan al Mukhtār ibn 'Abdūn of Baghdad. (Note: I am not sure that this person is the same as the one mentioned by SCHACHT, J. & M. MEYERHOF, 1937, subsection c). This manuscript contains a voluminous dictionary of materia medica of a vegetable nature, in alphabetical order. Extensive indexes have been added (p. 389-420). The flora described is largely Andalusian. In the text are many references to Ibn Baṣṣāl and Ibn al-Luengo.

Abū Ja'far Aḥmad ibn Ibrāhim ibn abī Khālid ib al-Jazzār (= Algizar Algazirah, d. 1009) — DUGAT, G., 1853: Études sur le traité de médecine d'Abou Djāffar, intitulé Zad al-Moçafir, "La provision du voyageur", 67 p. (Paris: Impr. Impériale).—

The "Zad al-musafir" (= "Traveller's provisions") was enormously popular and has been translated into Latin (by Constantinus Africanus), into Greek, and into Hebrew. It contains, inter alia, remarkable descriptions of smallpox and measles.

Aḥmad ibn 'Abd Allāh (Abu al-'Alā) 'al-Ma'arri (d. ca. 1130) — COLIN, G., 1911: La Tedkira d'Abū 'l-'Alā, publiée et traduite pour la première fois, 79 p. (Publ. de l'École supérieure des Lettres, Univ. dAlger, Vol. 45) (Paris: Leroux).—

Contains a general introduction, the Arabian text, a French translation and an index of technical terms of the "Reminder", a booklet which Abū al-'Alā wrote for his son Avenzohar when the latter was travelling in Morocco. It is a practical guide containing special references to climatological and pathological conditions in Marrākush, and also deontological advice.

Aḥmad ibn 'Abd al Wahhāb (Shihāb al-Dīn) al Baḥri Al Kindi Al Panni Al-Kurashi, commonly called Al-Nuwairī (1279-1332) — WIEDEMANN, E., 1918: Ueber den Abschnitt über die Pflanzen bei Nuwairi (Sitzb. phys.-medizin. Ges., Erlangen 48: 151-176); Ueber von den Arabern benutzten Drogen (Idem, 48-49: 16-60).—

Al-Nuwairī wrote an enormous encyclopaedia, the "Aim of the intelligent in the arts of letters", divided into 5 parts dealing respectively with: 1. Heavens and earth (cosmology, geography); 2. Man; 3. Animals (e.g., wild beasts, horses, cattle, mules, asses, venomous animals, birds, fishes, hunting, fishing, etc.); 4. Plants (e.g., the soil they need, food plants, trees, fruits, perfumed flowers, gardens, aromatics, drugs); 5. History. In his "Introduction" Vol. III (1): 620-621, Sarton gives a review of the contents of the different volumes. The only translations I could find in a modern West European language of those parts which are of interest from the biohistorical point of view, are these two papers of Wiedemann.

Aḥmad ibn Abi Bakr ibn Naṣr (Ḥamd Allāh) al-Mustaufi, al Ḳazwīnī (1203-1283) — STEPHENSON, J., ed., 1928: The zoological section of the Nuzhātu-l-Oulūb of Ḥamdullāh al Mustaufi al-Qazwīnī: a Persian compendium of science, 1340 A.D., 100 + 127 p. (Oriental Translation Fund, New Ser., 30, pt. 1) (London: Royal Asiatic Soc.).—

Al-Kazwīnī was a Persian encyclopaedist writing in Arabic. He has been called the Muslim Pliny, and he is author of two large compilations, one on cosmography, another on geography. The first, the Nuzhātu-l-Qulūb (Heart's Delight), deals inter alia, with minerals, plants, animals, and Man. The introduction of Stephenson's edition deals with the spheres, heavenly bodies, elements, and climates. The body of the Nuzhātu is divided into three parts, the first dealing with the mineral, vegetable and animal kingdoms, the second with Man, his bodily structure, his faculties and moral qualities, and the third with geography. In Stephenson's book only the zoological section has been given. The animals are classified as follows: 1. Animals of the land; a) domestic; b) wild; c) beasts of prey; d) poisonous animals and creeping things; e) animals some of whose members resemble Man; 2. Animals of the sea; 3. Animals of the air. This classification agrees with the scheme of the book. Separate paragraphs refer to the animals dealt with; in each of the several sections these paragraphs are arranged according to the alphabetical order of the Arabic name of the animals. Sometimes Persian, Turkish, or Mongolian equivalents of the names are added. There also exists a shorter treatise written by the same author to which the same title has been given in Isis 9: 285-315. This is a more general discussion, dealing with such topics as: the life of the author, the place of the Nuzhātu in the history of zoology, zoological sources of the Nuzhātu oral tradition and common knowledge, comparison with the "Physiologus", Arabic and Persian zoology after the Nuzhātu, the Nuzhātu in relation to medicine, the diseases mentioned, the animal remedies, the parts used, and magical uses of animals and various parts thereof.

——, WIEDEMANN, E., 1918: Ueber die Kriechtiere nach al-Qazwīnī nebst einigen Bemerkungen über die zoologischen Kenntnisse der Araber, 57 p. (Sitzb. phys.-mediz. Ges., Erlangen 48 : 228-285).—

This publication consists of the following sections: I. Einleitung (containing general remarks on Arabian mineralogy, botany, zoology, veterinary science, animal species known by the Arabs, and a review of Arabian sources of zoology); II. al-Quazwīnī über Kriechtiere und Insekten (with translations and comments); III. Stellen aus al-Qazwīnī über Wassertiere und al-Dīnawari über Insekten; IV. Beziehungen zwischen Tier und Mensch. From WIEDEMANN also came a publication on plants of al-Ḳazwīnī: Uebersetzung und Besprechung des Abschnittes über die Pflanzen von Qazwīnī (Idem, 48: 286-321).

Aḥmad ibn 'Alī, called Ibn Waḥshīya (fl. ca. 900) — LEVEY, M., 1966: Medieval Arabic toxicology: the book on poisons of Ibn Waḥshīya and its relation to early Indian and Greek texts, 130 p. (Trans. Amer. Philos. Soc., N.S., 56, pt. 7).—

A translation of the Kitāb al-sumūm. Ibn Waḥshīya was born of a Nabataean family; in this book he tried to demonstrate that the Nabataeans had a great civilization and had contributed greatly to human progress. The present book contains a study of his work on poisons and theriacs, together with commentary and translation, based on a ms. copied ca. 1500. Levey describes Ibn Waḥshīya's reference to various poisonous substances derived from plant, animal, and mineral origins, also antidotes; much of it was influenced by Eastern folk medicine. Moreover, the book contains a brief summary of Arabic toxicological literature from the 9th to the early 13th century, an explanation of chemical theory and practice in Ibn Waḥsīya's work, and a glossary of technical terms. Ca. 904 Ibn Waḥshīya wrote the "Kitāb al-falāḥa al-nabatiya", the so-called "Nabataean agriculture", an alleged translation from ancient Babylonian sources, which contains valuable information on agriculture and superstition. Cf. GUTSCHMID, A. von, 1861: Die nabateïsche Landwirtschaft mit ihren Geschirren (Ztschr. dtsch. Morgenl. Ges. 15: 1-110, and: Kleine Schriften, Vol. 2: 568-716). PLESSNER, M., 1928: Der Inhalt der nabatäischen Landwirtschaft. Ein Versuch Ibn Waḥshīya zu rehabilitieren (Ztschr. Semitistik 6: 27-56). Cf. WIEDE-

MANN, E., 1922: Zur nabataeïschen Landwirtschaft von Ibn Waḥschīja (Ztschr. Semitistik 1: 201-202).

Aḥmād ibn Dā'ud (Abū Ḥanīfah) al-Dīnawarī (ca. 820-895) — SILBERBERG, B., 1910: Das Pflanzenbuch des Abū Hanīfa Ahmed ibn Dā'ud ad Dīnawarī. Ein Beitrag zur Geschichte der Botanik bei den Arabern, 41 p. (Diss. Univ. Wrocklaw).—

About this publication Sarton writes in his Introduction I, p. 615: "Important. Silberberg has apparently collected all the fragments of the Kitāb al-nabāt, together with many other relevant texts and he gives an analysis of the work; various samples of Abū Hanīfa's manner and a good deal of information on early Muslim botany." The Kitāb al-nabāt" or "Book of plants" itself is a philological study which, however, contains much that is of interest to the historian of botany. It also has something to say about agriculture. This study has also been edited by SILBERBERG in Ztschr. für Assyrologie 24 (1910): 225-265; 25 (1911): 39-88). Quite recently a new edition appeared, with introduction, notes, indexes and a vocabulary: LEWIN, B., ed., 1953: The book of plants of Abū Hanīfa ad-Dīnawarī: part of the alphabetical section, 52 p. (Uppsala Univ. Årsskr. 1953, No. 10).

Aḥmad ibn Ḳāsam Muwaffaḳ al-dīn Abū-l-'Abbās, called Ibn Abī Uṣaibi'ah (1203-1270) — JAHIER, H. & A. NOUREDDINE, 1958: Ibn abi uçaibi'a (1203-1270) 'Uyūn al-Anbā fī i'abaqat al'Atibbā. Sources d'informations sur les classes des médecins, XIIIe chapitre: Médecins de l'occident musulman, 183 p. (Algiers: Ferraris).—

Ibn Abī Uṣaibi'ah was a Muslim-Syrian physician and historian of medicine. His main work was the "Sources of information on the classes of physicians", a series of bio-bibliographies of the most eminent physicians from the earliest times to his own, among which ca. 400 Arabic physicians. The present publication is a translation of Ch. XIII of the "Sources" which is entitled "Des médecins qui ont exercé dans l'Occident musulman et y ont séjourné". It contains the biographies of three Ifrīqiya physicians and of 85 Andalusian physicians. Arabic text and French translation on facing pages. Cf. also: WALY, H., 1910: Drei Kapitel aus der Aerztegeschichte des Ibn Abu 'Uṣaibi'a (Berlin: Schade). Unfortunately I do not possess further information about this book. A valuable review of Ibn Abī Uṣaibi'ah's' "Sources" was given by MÜLLER, A., 1884:

Ueber Ibn Abī Oçeibi'a und seine Geschichte der Aerzte. (Congrès des orientalistes de Leide, Vol. II: 259-280). A list of the Syrian and Muslim physicians dealt with was published by WÜSTENFELD, F., 1840, p. 132-144, *vide* subsection c.

Aḥmad ibn Muḥammad al Ghāfiqī (d. 1165) — MEYERHOF, M. & G. P. SOBHY, 1932-1940: The abridged version of "The book of simple drugs" of Aḥmad ibn Muḥammad al Ghāfiqī by Gregorius Abu'l-Farag (Barhebraeus): edited from the only two known manuscripts with an English translation, commentary and indexes, 588 p. (+ 131 p. Arab text). (Publ. Fac. Med. Egypt. Univ., No. 4) (Cairo: Govt. Press).—

Of this undertaking only 4 fascicules have appeared, which is at least partly due to the fact that two mss. of al-Ghāfiqī's original book of simple drugs have come to light, and these original works show remarkable illustrations and many original botanical observations which were omitted in the abridged edition of Barhebraeus. (*Cf.* MEYERHOF, M., 1940/'41: Deux manuscrits illustrés du Livre des simples d'Aḥmad al-Ghāfiqī, in: Bull. Inst. d'Egypte 23: 13-29). In order to publish the remainder of the abridged text, including commentaries and indexes, 15 more fascicules would be needed. *Cf.* also: STEINSCHNEIDER, M., 1879-1881: Gafikī's Verzeichniss einfacher Heilmittel (Virchows Archiv path. Anat. Physiol. 77: 507-548; 85 (1881): 132-171; 355-370). Contains much that is of interest for the history of Arab materia medica. Separate sections deal with what al-Ghāfiqī borrowed from the Greek and the other Arab writers.

'Ala al-dīn (Abū-'l-Ḥasan), Ibn al-Nafīs (*ca.* 1208-1288) — CHÉHADÉ, A. K., 1955: Ibn an-Nafis et la découverte de la circulation pulmonaire, 54 p. (Damascus: Institut français de Damas).—

This booklet contains a facsimile reproduction and French translation of that part of Ibn al-Nafis's text which contains his critical commentary on Ibn Sīnā's Galenic interpretation of the circulation in heart and lungs; in fact this meant the discovery of the pulmonary circulation. It also contains a valuable bibliography and much biographical information concerning Ibn al-Nafis. A somewhat older study dealing with the same problem is: MEYERHOF, M., 1935: Ibn an Nafis und seine Theorie des

Lungenkreislaufs (Quellen und Studien Gesch. Naturwiss. Med., Vol. 4) (Berlin: Springer).

'Alī ibn Isa, al Kaḥḥal of Baghdad (= Jesu Haly, *ca.* 940-1010) — WOOD, C. A., 1936: Memorandum book of a tenth-century oculist. For the use of modern ophthalmologists: a translation of the Tadhkirat of 'Alī ibn Isa of Baghdad (*ca.* 940-1010 A.D.), the most complete, practical and original of all early textbooks on the eye and its diseases, 39 + 232 p. (Chicago, Ill.: Northwestern Univ.).—

This is an English translation of "The oculist's memorandum book", the most famous ophthalmological textbook written before the 18th century. The present text has been translated from the German version of the book published by J. HIRSCHBERG, J. LIPPERT & E. MITTWOCH: Alī ibn Isa Erinnerungsbuch fuer Augenaerzte (Leipzig, 1905) (*vide* subsection c.) 'Alī ibn Isa was a Christian oculist living in Baghdad. His book was very popular and has been drawn upon and translated many times. It also appeared in Latin. The treatise consists of three books; the first book deals with the anatomy and physiology of the eye, the second with the diseases externally visible, and the third with hidden diseases, dietetics and general medicine from the oculistic standpoint. 130 eye-diseases are carefully described and 143 drugs characterized.

'Alī ibn Rabbān al-Ṭabarī (fl. 847-861) — SIDDIQI, M. Z., ed., 1928: Firdausu 'l-Hikmat, or Paradise of Wisdom by 'Alī B. Rabban aṭ Tabarī, 32 + 620 + 15 p. (Berlin: Sonne).—

'Alī al-Ṭabarī was a Muslim physician, whose main work, the "Paradise of Wisdom" seems to have been the very first medical compendium written in Arabic. It also deals with philosophy, meteorology, zoology, embryology, psychology, and astronomy. This is an (Arabic) edition of the whole work, accompanied by a short English preface and a very elaborate Arabic introduction. In 1931, M. MEYERHOF devoted a special study to this book: 'Alī aṭ-Ṭabarī's "Paradise of wisdom", one of the oldest compendiums of medicine. (Isis 16: 6-54). This study contains English translations of the 360 chapterheadings; sometimes information about the contents of the chapters have been added. Glossaries of technical terms, of names, of drugs, and of remedies are included. The "Paradise of Wisdom" partly follows the Greek compendia of *e.g.*, Oribasios and Paulos of Aegina; it also contains about 120 quotations from Hippocrates (more than 60 of them from the Aphorisms), some 20 quotations from Galen, and 13 from Dioscorides's "Materia Medica". It contains a sketch of Indian medicine which follows, *inter alia,* the books of Charaka and Suśruta. A. SIGGEL prepared German translations of certain parts of the "Paradise of Wisdom", *viz.,* 1941: Gynäkologie, Embryologie und Frauenheilkunde, 56 p. (Quell. und Studien Gesch. Naturwiss. Med., Vol. 8: 216-272); 1951: Die indischen Bücher, 55 p. (Abh. Akad. Wiss., Mainz, Abt. Geistes- und Sozialwiss. Kl., Jg. 1950, No. 14: 1097-1152). This last-mentioned publication contains a general introduction to the "Paradise of Wisdom" and a translation of those (34) chapters which deal with Indian medicine. According to Siggel, these chapters are an interesting example of an attempt at assimilating Indian medical thought into a system dominated by Greek concepts. In 1953 SIGGEL published: Die propädeutischen Kapitel (*Idem,* Jg. 1953, No. 8: 357-463), which contains a German translation of the parts dealing with al-Ṭabarī's philosophical arguments, and with his ideas about the origin of Man, the organs of the body, the soul, and the sense organs. A study containing much information concerning historical background, life and writings of 'Alī al-Ṭabarī is: MEYERHOF, M., 1931: 'Alī ibn Rabban aṭ-Ṭabarī, ein persischer Arzt des 9. Jahrhunderts n. Chr. (Ztschr. dtsch. Morgenl. Ges. 10: 38-68).

'Amr ibn Baḥr, called al-Jāḥiz (d. *ca.* 868) — LÖFGREN, O., 1946: Ambrosian fragments of an illuminated manuscript containing the zoology of al-Gāhiz, with 24 facsimile plates edited with an introduction and philological notes, with a contribution: the miniatures, their origin and style by C. J. LAMM, 39 p. + 24 plates. (Uppsala Univ. Årsskr. 1946, No. 5) (Uppsala: Lundqvist).—

The text of fragments of an illuminated ms., discovered in the Ambrosian Library at Milan, containing parts of the zoology (Kitāb al-Ḥayawān) of al-Jāḥiz. It contains very beautiful phototype plates, picturing many animals, commented upon from an art-historian's point of view. It is a compilation of animal knowledge, the purpose of which is moral and folkloric rather than scientific. The fragments are translated into English, p. 25-33. Another study dealing with life and philosophy of al-Jāḥiz and with scientific evolution and knowledge of nature in general at the time of the Abbassides, is: VLOTEN, G. VAN, 1918: Ein arabischer Naturphilosoph im 9. Jahrhun-

dert (El-Dschahiz), 47 p. (Stuttgart: Heppeler). This text was originally published in Dutch in the "Tweemaandelijksch Tijdschrift", May 1897.

——, PELLAT, C., 1967: Arabische Geisteswelt. Ausgewählte und übersetzte Texte von Al-Gahiz (777-869). Unter Zugrundelegung der arabischen Originaltexte aus dem französischen übertragen von Walter W. Müller, 477 p. (Die Bibliothek des Morgenlandes) (Zurich: Artemis).—

In the first part of this vol. the author gives a review of the life and works of one of the most famous physicians and oculists of that age. These works deal with numerous subjects, among them: philosophy, botany, zoology, anthropology, sociology, and education. Although the present vol. does not pay particular attention to the life sciences, there is much in it that is of value to the historian of biology and medicine.

'Arīb ibn Sa'id al-Kātib al-Qurṭubī (*ca.* 918-980) — JAHIER, H. & A. NOUREDDINE, 1956: 'Arīb ibn Sa'id al-Kātib al Qurṭ-ubi. Kitāb Khalq al-Janīn wa-Tadbīr al Ḥ'abālā wa'l-Mawlūdīn. Le livre de la génération du foetus et le traitement des femmes enceintes et des nouveau-nés, 105 p. in French + 100 p. in Arabic. (Algiers: Ferraris).—

'Arīb ibn Sa'id was a Hispano-Muslim historian and physician who wrote *inter alia* a treatise on gynaecology and obstetrics. This treatise deals with such subjects as: pregnancy, twins and their causes, amelioration of semen, the virgin, love-making, the description of male and female genital organs, conception, menstruation, coitus, the function of the semen, foetal development, childbirth, feeding of mother and child, the consultation of astrologers, puberty, *etc.* The present book contains an Arabic edition of the text, together with a French translation. *Cf.* also H. GRANQVIST, 1947, *vide* subsection a.

Ḥunain ibn Isḥāq al-Ibadi (= Joannitius, *ca.* 809-877) — BERGSTRÄSSER, G., 1925: Ḥunain über die syrischen und arabischen Galen-Uebersetzungen, 116 p. (of which 15 + 48 p. in German) (Abh. Kunde Morgenl.) (Leipzig: Brockhaus).—

Ḥunain ibn Isḥāq was the foremost translator of Greek medical works into Arabic. He translated a great many of Galen's works, various writings of Hippocrates, Plato, Aristotle, and Dioscorides. The present text, written by Ḥunain in 856 and represented by a single ms., is extremely important, for it contains a list of all the Galenic works known to Ḥunain, 129 in number, together with mention and criticism of the Syriac and Arabic translations. In 1932 BERGSTRÄSSER wrote a merely philological supplement to this publication, based upon another ms., including Galenic apocrypha, *viz.*, Neue Materialen zu Ḥunain ibn Isḥāq's Galen-Bibliographie, 108 p. (Leipzig: Brockhaus). Of both these publications of Bergsträsser (1925-1932) reprint editions were published by Kraus (New York, N.Y.) in 1966. Still another important study by BERGSTRÄSSER is: Ḥunain ibn Isḥāq und seine Schule. Sprach- und literaturgeschichtliche Untersuchungen zu den arabischen Hippokrates- und Galenübersetzungen, 1913, 81 p. (Arabic text) (Leiden: Brill). *Cf.* also: MEYERHOF, M., 1928: New light on Ḥunain ibn Isḥāq and his period, 39 p. (Isis 8: 685-724).

——, MEYERHOF, M., ed., 1928: The book of the ten treatises on the eye ascribed to Ḥunain ibn Isḥāq (809-877 A.D.): the earliest existing systematic textbook of ophthalmology. The Arabic text edited from the only two known manuscripts, with an English translation and glossary, 53 + 227 p. + 230 p. Arabic text. (Cairo: Govt. Press).—

In the introduction the editor sums up some 17 early Arabic ophthalmological treatises. One of them is "The book of Ḥunain ibn Isḥāq on the structure of the eye, its diseases and their treatment according to the conceptions of Hippocrates and Galen, in ten treatises". The text is essentially derived from Galen. It deals *inter alia* with: the anatomy of the eye, description of the brain, the optic nerves, the phenomenon of vision, causes of eye diseases, nosology, etiology, symptomatology, properties of simple remedies, treatment of eye diseases. To the text are added many notes derived from comparisons with other texts, Arabic and Greek indexes, a general index and a glossary of medical terms in Arabic, Greek, and English.

——, SA'DI, L. M., 1934: A bio-bibliographical study of Ḥunayn ibn Isḥāq al-Ibadi (Johannitius) (809-877 A.D.), 37 p. (Bull. Inst. Hist. Med. 2 : 409-446).—

After an introduction, considering the life and work of Ḥunain, a list of translations prepared by him follows, divided in

the following way: I. Ḥunain's non-medical translations: Plato (4), Aristotle (11), miscellaneous (9), translations of Galen's philosophical works (11); II. Ḥunain's medical translations: Hippocrates (15), Galen (90), miscellaneous (9); III. Ḥunain's original non-medical works (26), his original medical works (46). All (221) titles are in English translation.

Ḥusain ibn'Abd Allāh (Abū 'Ali), called Ibn Sīnā (= Avicenna, 980-1037) — AFNAN, S. M., 1958: Avicenna: his life and works, 298 p. (London: Allen & Unwin).—

An attempt to present to the general reader the life and works of Avicenna against the background of the Persian Renaissance of the 10th century. Separate chapters deal with Persia in the 10th century; life and works of Avicenna; problems of logic, of metaphysics, of psychology and of religion; medicine and natural sciences; Avicenna in East and West. A somewhat older, but - according to Sarton, Introd. I: 712 - clearly and beautifully written elaborate study of Avicenna is: CARRA DE VAUX, B., 1900: Avicenne, 310 p. (Paris: Alcan). A more popular biography, supplemented by summaries from the first book of the Qānūn is: SOUBIRAN, A., 1935: Avicenne, prince des médecins. Contribution à l'étude de sa vie et de sa doctrine, 176 p. (Paris: Lipschutz) *(vide infra). Cf.* also: KRAUS, P., 1932: Eine arabische Biographie Avizennas. (Klin. Wschr. 11: 1880-1884). An elaborate bibliography of the Avicennian mss. (of which some 1,500, many of which are still unpublished, are kept in 56 Istanbul libraries) is: ANAWATI, G. C., 1950: Essai de bibliographie avicennienne, 20 p. in French, 435 p. in Arabic. (Cairo: Dar al-Maaref).

——, BACOŠ, J., 1956: Psychologie d'Ibn Sīnā (Avicenne) d'après son oeuvre aṣ-Ṣifā, 1. Texte arabe, 270 p.; 2. Traduction et notes, 245 p. (Prague: Acad. Tchécoslovaque des sciences).—

The "Shifā" is a very famous encyclopaedia of learning and the most complete treatise of the Peripatetic School in Islam, and this is its first translation into a European language. The work is in 5 chapters, dealing with the definition of the soul as a substance and its faculties, with the vegetative soul and the senses, with the nature of light, colours and sight, with the internal senses of the animal soul, and with the nature of the human souls and intelligences. Generally speaking, with Avicenna psychology means forces moving things, and it embraces elements of the physical domain as well as elements concerning the relation of Man to God and the universe. Abundant footnotes have been added.

——, GRUNER, O. C., 1930: A treatise on the canon of medicine of Avicenna, incorporating a translation of the first book, 612 p. (London: Luzac).—

> The canon (Qānūn) is Avicenna's most important work. It is an immense medical encyclopaedia, comprising the whole of ancient and Muslim medical knowledge, and containing many new medical facts and observations: its materia medica contains some 760 drugs. In the preface of the present study the author states that the purpose of his book is two-fold: (1) to furnish a translation of the first Book of the Canon of Medicine of "Avicenna", in which the section on anatomy has been omitted in favour of the first half of the "De viribus cordis", and (2) to present a study of its mystical philosophy (tassawuf), especially showing where this and modern biological knowledge are reciprocally illuminative. A French discussion of the gynaecological part of the Qānūn is to be found in: MEYERHOF, M. & D. JOANNIDES, 1938: La gynécologie et l'obstétrique chez Avicenne (ibn Sīnā) et leurs rapports avec celles des Grecs, 80 p. (Cairo: Schindler).

——, HIRSCHBERG, J. & J. LIPPERT, 1902: Die Augenheilkunde des Ibn Sina, übersetzt und erklärt, 194 p. (Leipzig: Veit).—

> A German translation of Qānūn Book III, section III, consisting of 4 treatises: 1. Vorbemerkungen über das Auge und über Augenentzündung (with general remarks on anatomy, infections, therapy, etc. of the eye); 2. Von den übrigen Erkrankungen des Auges, hauptsächlich von denen der Zusammensetzung und des Zusammenhangs; 3. Von den Erkrankungen des Lids und Ihren Begleiterscheinungen; 4. Von den Zuständen der Sehkraft und ihren Tätigkeiten.

——, JAHIER, H. & A. NOUREDDINE, eds., 1956: Avicenna (370-426 Hégire). Poème de la médecine. Al-Ḥusayn ibn 'Abd Allāh ibn Sīnā, Urǧūza fī 'ṭ-ṭibb (Cantica Avicennae). Texte arabe, traduction française, traduction latine du XIIIᵉ siècle, avec introductions, notes et index, 209 p. (Paris: Les Belles Lettres).—

> This poem ('Arǧūzat fi-l-ṭibb) was intended to be studied by highranking lay-men. It covers the whole realm of medicine. The present publication contains an Arabic edition of this poem in juxtaposition with a French translation. This is followed by a reprint of a Latin translation prepared about 1284 by Armengaud Blaisse as it was published in 1556 by Hervagius in Basle. Valuable introductions to the different texts. An English translation of this poem can be found in: KRUEGER, H. C. & R. C. MAJOR, eds., 1963: Avicenna's poem on medicine, 112 p. (Springfield, Ill.: Thomas). This translation is accompanied by a review of the life and achievements of Avicenna and by a survey considering the value of the poem during Avicenna's own time and the following six centuries. Although Avicenna himself possessed much original clinical knowledge, his train of thought is entirely in keeping with that of Galen; therefore it could be considered a general practical manual during the Middle Ages in East and West. A German translation of the poem has been published by OPITZ, K., 1939: Das Lehrgedicht über die Heilkunde (Canticum de medicina), 69 p. (Quell. und Studien Gesch. Naturwiss. Med. 7: 151-220).

——, SHAH, M. H., ed., 1966: The general principles of Avicenna's "Canon of Medicine", 40 + 459 p. (Karachi: Naveed Clinic).—

> The "Canon" was the authoritative medical encyclopaedia in Iran (Persia) and neighbouring countries from the 11th century onwards. (Cf. ISKANDAR, A. Z., 1967, this section, subsection a, vide supra). In Arab countries as well as in Western Europe it was studied and commented on for several centuries. The present vol. contains an introduction and a translation of most of Book I of Avicenna's "Canon"; the text deals with diseases of individual organs of the body from the head to the feet. Another general discussion of Avicenna's "Canon of medicine" is: EDDÉ, J., 1889: Avicenne et la médecine arabe. (Paris). Unfortunately I do not possess further information about this book. A list of Western commentaries of the "Canon" has been given by ECKLEBEN, W., 1921: Die abendländischen Avicenna-Kommentare, 20 p. (Diss. Univ. Leipzig).

——, SOUBIRAN, A., 1935: Avicenne, prince des médecins. Contribution à l'étude de sa vie et de sa doctrine, 176 p. (Paris: Lipschutz).—

> An introduction into Avicenna's life and medical works, in which the author tries to measure the influence of Hippocrates and Galen on Avicenna's medical teachings. The

text is in two parts. The first part contains much biographical information, and the second part contains a French translation of the first book of the "Canon of medicine", with chapters on the definition of medicine, on disease, the preservation of health, and general therapeutics. The author also discusses many drugs of animal origin employed by Avicenna.

Ibn Sarābi (= Serapion junior, fl. *ca.* 1150) — GUIGUES, P., 1895: Les noms arabes dans Serapion, 137 p. (Paris: Leroux).—

Serapion, a physician who wrote in Arabic, but of whom nothing is known otherwise, wrote a treatise on simples, an elaborate compilation derived from Byzantine and Muslim sources. The original was Latinized by Simon Januensis, and this translation was very popular during the Middle Ages. According to Sarton (Introd. II (1): 229), the edition under consideration is very important; 544 drugs are discussed, there is a good bibliography, with French and Arabic indexes. It is a reprint of the J. asiat., mai - août, 1895. A new Italian edition appeared in 1962, ed. by G. IN-EICHEN: El libro agregà de Serapiom. Volgarizzamento di Frater Jacobus Philippus de Padua (Venezia: Ist. per la colleborazione culturale). The text of this ms. has been based upon the Latin text of Simon Januensis and has been prepared by a Paduan friar, *ca.* 1390. Of much interest are the illustrations included in this ms., which are reproduced in this Italian edition (12 of them in colour). A second vol. was promised; in this second vol. some iconographical and philological aspects of this Italian ms. will be considered.

Ishāq ibn Sulaimān (Abū Ya'qūb) al-Isra'ili (= Isaac Judaeus or Isaac Israel the Elder, *ca.* 830-932) — ALTMANN, A. & S. M. STERN, 1958: Isaac Israeli: a neoplatonic philosopher of the early tenth century: his works translated with comments and an outline of his philosophy, 226 p. (Oxford: U.P.).—

Isaac Judaeus was a Jewish physician and philosopher writing in Arabic, one of the first who directed the attention of the Jews to Greek science and philosophy. The present book contains the following texts in English translation: 1. The book of definitions; 2. The book of substances; 3. The book on spirit and soul; 4. The Mantua text; 5. An excerpt from the book on the elements. This is followed by a philosophical discussion (p. 151-218), an index of names and a subject-index. This study is mainly of phil-

osophical interest. But Isaac Judaeus composed many medical writings in Arabic which were translated into Latin by Constantinus Africanus. His "Guide to the physicians" has been translated into German by KAUFMANN, D., 1884. (Mag. Wiss. Judentums 11: 97-112); his treatise "On fevers" exists in a Spanish translation: LLAMAS, P. J., 1945: Tratado de las fiebres, 32 + 302 p. (Madrid & Barcelona: Inst. "Arias Montano"), and a German translation of his "On urine" can be found in: PEINE, J., 1919: Die Handschrift des Isaac Judeaus, 78 p. (Diss. Sudhoff Inst.).

Jābir ibn Ḥayyān, al Ṭarasūsī (= Yabir, Gabir, or Geber, fl. *ca.* 776) — KRAUS, P., ed., 1942/'43: Jābir ibn Hayyān. Contribution à l'histoire des idées scientifiques dans l'Islam, 2 vols. Vol. I (1943): Le Corpus des écrits jabiriens, 45 + 214 p.; Vol. II (1942): Jābir et la science grecque, 406 p. (Mémoires présentés à l'Institut d'Egypte, vols. 44 and 45) (Cairo: Inst. d'Égypte).—

In an introduction, the editor discusses the bibliography of the works ascribed to Jābir. The books of Jābir form a rather strange mixture of science, mysticism, exorcism, and magic. The main part of the first vol. consists of an enormous critical bibliography of the Jābir-collection; then follows the "Book of Mercy", the "112 Books", the "70 Books", several minor collections appended to the 70 Books, the "114 Books of Balances", the " 500 Books", "The book of the seven metals", and a series of books on theurgy, magic, physics, medicine, and pharmacology. The second vol. consists of six chapters dealing with, *inter alia,* Jābir's alchemy, the elixir, his classification of minerals; the science of specific properties, *i.e.* virtues ascribed to minerals, plants, and animals and their use in technique and medicine; artificial creation; Jābir's cosmology; the theory of balance; the origins of Jābir's science.

——, SIGGEL, A., 1958: Das Buch der Gifte des Gābir ibn Ḥayyān. Arabischer Text in Faksimile, 223 p.; German text, 194 p. (Veröffentl. Orient. Kommission Akad. Wiss., Mainz, Vol. 12) (Wiesbaden: Steiner).—

After a brief introduction, considering Jābir and the contents of his book, the German translation follows (p. 10-201). Indexes of the names of plants, animals, minerals, foodstuffs, perfumes, and the Arabic names of the diseases considered. According to the review in Isis 51: 356-358 the trans lation is not fully reliable. Jābir ibn Ḥayyān was the most famous Arabic alchemist; and probably was the alchemist Geber of the Middle Ages. His alchemical doctrines were very anthropomorphic and animistic. He also showed much interest in the technological aspects of chemistry. For more particulars concerning his alchemical activities, cf. DARMSTAEDTER, E., 1922: Die Alchemie des Geber, 202 p. (Berlin: Springer), or HOLMYARD, E. J., ed., 1928: The works of Geber, englished by Richard Russell, 1678, in a new edition with introduction, 264 p. (London: Dent).

Khalāf ibn al'Abbās, called Abulcasis al-Zahrawi (d. ca. 1013) — HAMARNEH, S. K. & G. SONNEDECKER, 1963: A pharmaceutical view of Abulcasis al-Zahrawi in Moorish Spain with special reference to the "Adhan", 176 p. (Janus, Suppl. 5) (Leiden: Brill).—

The introduction of this publication contains a review of Arabic culture in Spain during the time of Abulcasis, an informative biography of Abulcasis, and an evaluation of his influence on the West. Then the editing, translation, and analysis follow of a part of the 25th of the 30 treatises of Abulcasis's medical encyclopaedia, the "Kitab al-Tasrif". This part contains descriptions of fixed and volatile oils, their uses, and the techniques of extracting and preparing them. Besides, it contains much information on the drugs and simples available at the time of Abulcasis. Many annotations (relating Abulcasis's knowledge to previous and later Arabic writers and to Dioscorides), and valuable bibliography. Well indexed. The introduction contains much information about life, education, and activities of Abulcasis, and the cultural, social, and political circumstances of his time.

——, LECLERC, L., 1861: La chirurgie d'Abulcasis, 342 p. (Paris: Baillière).—

Abulcasis was the greatest Muslim surgeon. His medical work can be divided into a theoretical and a practical part, each consisting of 14 volumes. The last volume of the practical part deals with surgery. The first book translated by Leclerc deals with cauterization (p. 9-57); the second book with incisions, affections of the head, of the genital organs, etc. with tumours, surgical instruments, hernias, fistulae, and worms; the third book with fractures and dislocations. Abulcasis's surgery was very important for the development of mediaeval surgery. It was translated into Latin by Gerard of Cremona, and it deeply influenced such

men as Roger of Parma, Lanfranc, William of Saliceto, and Guy de Chauliac. The surgical portion of Abulcasis's encyclopaedia was translated into Turkish by Charaf Ed-Din, in 1465. From this work a French translation has been published, edited by HUARD, P. & M. D. GRMEK, 1960: Le premier manuscrit chirurgical turc, 139 p. (Paris: Dacoste). In this edition the text of Abulcasis has not been reproduced but is replaced by brief commentaries placed in a historical perspective. This edition, however, is of great value from the iconographical point of view, for it is illustrated by some 140 miniatures as full-page illustrations. The "Kunsthistorisches Hofmuseum" at Vienna contains a ms. of a Latin translation of Abulcasis's work on dietetics with reproductions of the illustrations. An essay concerning this ms. was written by: SCHLOSSER, J. von, 1895: Ein veronesisches Bilderbuch und die höfische Kunst des XIV. Jahrhunderts, 86 p. (Jb. der Kunsthist. Samml. des allerhöchsten Kaiserhauses 16: 144-230). Cf. also: MAKHLUF, T., 1930: L'oeuvre chirurgicale d'Abul Cassim Khalaf Ibn Abbas (Paris: Lac). Unfortunately I am unable to give further details about this book.

——, SPINK, M. S. & G. L. LEWIS, eds., 1968: Abulcasis on surgery and instruments: a definitive edition of the Arabic text, with English translation and comment, 600 p. (Berkeley, Calif.: Univ. California Press).—

Abulcasis's books on surgery were extremely influential throughout the Middle Ages; this is the first English translation of his treatise on surgery. The text has been compiled from the best of the surviving mss. and has been accompanied by extensive commentaries and notes. The text incorporates Abulcasis's illustrations of surgical instruments. The Arabic text and the English translation and commentary are printed on facing pages.

Maḥmūd ibn Ilyās al-Shīrāzī (d. 1330) — GUIGUES, P., 1902: Le livre de l'art du traitement de Najm ad-Dyn Mahmoud; remèdes composés. Texte, traduction, glossaires précédés d'un essai sur la pharmacie arabe, 562 p. (240 of them in Arabic). (Thèse Univ. Paris) (Printed at the author's expense).—

Maḥmūd composed a medical encyclopaedia consisting of 5 parts: 1. generalities; 2. fevers; 3. external infirmities; 4. simple drugs; 5. composite drugs. This last part includes more than 650 recipes; it is a kind of codex, wherein drugs are classified according to their pharmaceutical affinities. Sarton (Introd. III (1): 898) remarks on the book of Guigues: "This is the edition of part 5 based on the ms. of St. Joseph College in Bairut. Includes Arabic-French and French-Arabic glossaries; moreover, the author has added Latin synonyms found in the translation of Serapion Senior, Synonima Serapionis, by Gerard of Cremona; in the translation of Serapion Junior, De simplici medicina, by Simon of Genoa; in the Pandectae of Matthias Sylvaticus; and in the commentaries on Dioscorides by Pier Andrea Mattioli (1500-77)."

Mesuë the third (fl. *ca.* 1250) — PAGEL, J. L., 1893: Die angebliche Chirurgie des Joh. Mesuë jun. nach einer Handschrift der Pariser Nationalbibliothek zum ersten Male, theils herausgegeben, theils analysiert nebst einem Nachtrag zur Chirurgie des Heinrich von Mondeville, 146 p. (Berlin: Hirschwald).—

> From Sarton, Introd. II (2): 662-663 I quote: Mesúë the third is an unknown Arabian who composed a treatise on surgery divided into five books: 1. De anathomia et primo de anathomia membrorum consimilium (bones, cartilage, vessels, nerves, *etc.*); 2. De anathomia membrorum officinalium (separate parts and organs; in reality this book contains a list of simple medicines); 3. De curis omnium aegritudinum a causa antecedente provenientium cum medicinis et cauteriis et instrumentorum formis; 4. De cura omnium . . . sanguissugis; 5. Antidotarium. Pagel's work contains the German translation of the first three books only; translations of book 4 were published in Berlin theses by F. A. STERNBERG (1893, 51 p.), and W. SCHNELLE (1895, 31 p.) and a translation of book 5 similarly by H. BROCKELMANN (1895, 38 p.).

Muḥammad ibn Aḥamad, al-Bīrūnī (973-1048) — MEYERHOF, M., ed., 1932: Das Vorwort zur Drogenkunde des Bīrūnī. Eingeleitet, übersetzt und erläutert, 52 + 18 p. (Quell. Stud. Gesch. Naturw. Med., Vol. 3, pt. 3) (Berlin: Springer).—

> Al-Bīrūnī wrote a pharmacopoeia, the "Kitāb as-ṣaidana fi-ṭ-ṭibb" which seems to be far superior to those composed by Ibn al-Baiṭār or al-Ghāfiqī, but of which only an incomplete ms. exists. Fortunately the very interesting introduction to this pharmacopoeia still exists, and Meyerhof's study contains an edition, German translation, and many valuable annotations to this ms. The introduction itself contains much biographical information but also much that is

of interest to the historian of pharmacy. A brief review of its contents has been given by G. Sarton in Isis 20: 453-454.

——, SUTER, J. & E. WIEDEMANN, 1920-1921: Ueber al-Bīrūnī und seine Schriften, 45 p. (Beitr. Gesch. Naturwiss., No. 60) (Sitzb. phys.-med. Ges., Erlangen, 1920-1921, p. 52-96).—

> An elaborate account of the life and works of al-Bīrūnī, one of the greatest scientists of all times who is also of some interest to the historians of biology and medicine. *Cf.* WIEDEMANN, E., 1912: Ueber al-Bīrūnī. (Mitt. Gesch. Med. 11: 313-321); and WIEDEMANN, E., 1920: Ueber Gesetzmässigkeiten bei Pflanzen. (Biol. Zbl. 40: 113-116).

Muḥammad ibn Aḥmad al-Khwārizmī (= al-Kitāb, fl. *ca.* 976) — SEIDEL, E., 1914: Die Medizin im Kitāb mafātīh al-'ūlūm, 79 p. (Sitzb. phys.-med. Ges., Erlangen, No. 47).—

> Al-Khwārizmī was a Persian encyclopaedist who wrote (in Arabic) the "Keys of the Sciences" (Māfatīḥ al-'ūlūm), a book of great interest for the historian of science. (Maqāla II, Bāb 3). It consists of the following parts: 1. Anatomie; 2. Erwähnenswerte Krankheiten und Leiden; 3. Über die Nahrungsmittel; 4. Über die einfache Arzneimittel; 5. Über einfache Arzneimittel mit dunklen Namen; 6. Über die zusammengesetzten Arzneimittel; 7. Über Medizinalgewichte und Masse; 8. Über Besonderheiten.

Muḥammad ibn Aḥmad, called Ibn Rushd (= Averroës, 1126-1198) — KURLAND, S., 1958: Averroës on Aristotle's "De generatione et corruptione". Middle commentary and epitome. Translated from the original Arabic and the Hebrew and Latin versions, with notes and introduction, 245 p. (Cambridge, Mass.: Medieval Acad. of America).—

> The "De generatione et corruptione" was translated into Arabic in the very first stages of the assimilation of Greek philosophical literature by the Arabs. Averroës wrote his "Middle Commentary" on the works of Aristotle in 1172; the date of the composition of the "Epitome" is unknown to us. The "Epitome" is an independent brief restatement of the contents of the original, preceded by a few remarks. The "De generatione" of Aristotle is of importance to the biohistorian, because in it Aristotle discusses

problems of growth, form, function, generation, and nutrition from a philosophical point of view. About the form of the commentary: quoting or summarizing a short portion of the Aristotelian text, Averroës proceeds to explain and to clarify it, either by referring to other works, or by including an example, or by adducing arguments and views from post-Aristotelian sources, *etc.*

——, BLUMBERG, H., 1961: Averroës: Epitome of "Parva naturalia", transl. from the original Arabic and the Hebrew and Latin versions, with notes and introduction, 130 p. (Cambridge, Mass.: Medieval Acad. of America).—

On the "Parva naturalia" there only exists a "Short Commentary". As to the purpose and character of such a commentary, *cf.* KURLAND *(vide supra)*. The contents of this epitome are as follows: Introduction. Purpose of the work: discussion of the particular faculties of animals. The work is divided into three books: 1) sense and its objects; 2) memory and recollection; sleep and waking, dreams; 3) length and shortness of life.

Muḥammad ibn Ibrāhīm, called Ibn al-Baṣṣāl — MILLÁS VALLICROSA, J. M. & M. AZIMAN, eds., 1955: Ibn Baṣṣāl: libro de agricultura (Trad. y anotado), 231 p. in Spanish, 182 p. in Arabic. (Teṭūan: Inst. Muley el-Hasan).—

Ibn al-Baṣṣāl was an agriculturist in charge of the royal botanical garden in Toledo. In 1942 a mediaeval Castilian translation of his lost treatise was discovered *(cf.* MILLÁS VALLICROSA, J. M., 1948: La traducción castellana del "Tratado de Agricultura" de Ibn Baṣṣāl, in: Al-Andalus 13: 347-430). The text itself is divided into 16 chapters (On water, the good earth; manure; selection and preparation of land; the planting of various trees; propagation; pruning of trees; grafting; cultivation of herbs, grains and legumes; spices; cucumbers, melons, *etc.*; garden plants; aromatic plants; various advice to farmers). The book was intended for the (practical) farmer. No glossary or index.

Muḥammad ibn Qassūm ibn Aslam al-Ghāfiqī (d. *ca.* 1165) — MEYERHOF, M., 1933: (Al-morchid fi'l-Kohhl) ou Le guide d'oculistique. Ouvrage inédit de l'oculiste arabe-espagnol Mohammad ibn Quassoūm ibn Aslam al-Ghāfiqī (XIIᵉ siècle). Traduction des parties ophthalmologiques d'après

le manuscrit conservé à la bibliothèque de l'Escurial, 225 p. (Barcelona: Masnou).—

We have no biographical information of al-Ghāfiqī, only that he lived at Cordoba and that he seems to have had a practice in that city. The al-Morchid as a whole contains a summary of all knowledge (philosophical as well as medical) that the oculist should have; only the 6th and last section of it deals with ophthalmology proper, and it is mainly from this section that French translations have been given. Chapter 4 of section 6 deals with eye diseases of children and chapter 5 of section 6 contains a discussion of eye diseases and their treatment. This latter section constitutes the greater part of Meyerhof's translation (p. 22-158).

Muḥammad ibn Zakarīyā (Abū Bakr) al-Rāzī, commonly called Rhazes (*ca.* 850-923) — ARBERRY, A. J., ed., 1950: The spiritual physick of Rhazes, 110 p. (London: Murray).—

Abū Bakr, also called al-Rāzī or Rhazes, was a famous Arabian physician, physicist and alchemist, the greatest clinician of Islam and the Middle Ages. His most important work is the "Kitab al-hawī" (The Continens), an enormous encyclopaedia of medicine of which quite recently (1955) an Arabic edition has been published under the auspices of the Ministry of Education, Government of India, published by the Osmania Oriental Publ. Bureau (Hyderabad-Deccan). The present booklet by Arberry, the "Spiritual physick", belongs to the realm of popular ethics; it makes possible a clear view of the philosophical background of Rhazes's thought and it gives a synthesis of his scientific and metaphysical ideas. Besides, there is much in it that is of biohistorical interest, *e.g.*, those parts dealing with psychological problems, drunkenness, sexual intercourse, the fear of death, *etc.* Some other translations existing in one of the Western European languages are: BOER, T. J. DE, 1920: De "Medicina mentis" van den arts Rāzī (Med. Kon. Ned. Akad. Wetensch., afd. Letterkunde, Vol. 53, Ser. A, 17 p.). The first 9 pages contain a summary review of some aspects of the "Medicina mentis", the other pages contain notes. His ophthalmology exists in a German translation: BRUNNER, W., 1900: Die Augenheilkunde des Rhazes. (Diss. Univ. Berlin). Of his famous monograph on smallpox and measles the following translations exist in English: KELLY, E. C., 1939: A treatise on the small-pox and measles by Rhazes. (Med. Classics, Vol. 4, No. 1) (Baltimore, Md.: Williams & Wilkins); in French: PAULET, J. J., 1768: Histoire de la petite vérole, avec les moyens d'en préserver les enfants et d'en arrêter la contagion en France; suivi d'une traduction française du traité de la petite vérole de Rhazes. (Paris: Ganeau) (and another by LECLERC & LENOIR, Paris, 1866); and in German: OPITZ, K., 1911: Ueber den Pocken und den Masern, in: Klassiker der Medizin, Vol. 12, 39 p. (Leipzig: Barth). GUIGUES, P., 1904, published the text with French translation and notes of "La guérison en une heure par Rhazes", 22+13 p. (Beirut). Vol. I. of the first book of the "Liber Almansoris" (a smaller compilation of his encyclopaedia of medicine) has been translated into French by KONING, P. DE (1903) in his "Trois traités d'anatomie arabe", vide subsection c. M. NADJMALBADI translated some of Rhazes's books into Persian; these appeared in the Univ. of Tehran Publications.

——, KONING, P. DE, ed., 1896: Traité sur le calcul dans les reins et dans la vessie par Abū Bekr Muhammad ibn Zakarīyā al-Rāzī, suivie de parties d'al fahir (Liber pretiosus de morbis particularibus membrorum a vertice usque ad pedes), 285 p. (Leiden: Brill).—

This is an Arabic edition of a monograph of Rhazes with a French translation, followed by relevant texts extracted from the Fākhir and two papers by two other Arabian medical writers. The author himself summarizes the contents of this book with the following words: "À ce traité j'ai ajouté le texte et la traduction des chapitres traitant le calcul des reins et de la vessie, contenus dans les ouvrages suivants, pas encore imprimés, dont se trouvent des manuscrits dans la collection du Legatum Warnerianum de la bibliothèque de Leyde. 1. Le Fākhir (Livre précieux) par Rhazes; 2. Le Malakī (Livre royal) par 'Ali ibn al-'Abbās (p. 124-185); 3. Le Mokhtār fi'ibn al-ṭibb (Livre de ce qu'il y a de meilleur dans la médecine) par 'Ali ibn al-Hubal."

——, RUSKA, J., ed., 1935: Das Buch der Alaune und Salze. Ein Grundwerk der spätlateinischen Alchemie, übersetzt und erläutert, 127 p. (Berlin Verlag Chemie).—

This publication contains the text of the Arabic original, commonly attributed to al-Rāzī, from the fragmentary Berlin ms. Sprenger, 1908, together with the Latin version known as the "De mineralibus liber" of Joannes de Garlandia, and a German version thereof.

Najīb al-Dīn al-Samarqandī (d. 1222) — LEVEY, M. & N. AL-KHALEDY, 1967:

The medical formulary of al-Samarqandī and the relation of early Arabic simples to those found in the indigenous medicine of the Near East and India, 382 p. (Philadelphia, Pa.: Univ. Pennsylvania Press).—

In a general introduction (p. 13-52) the authors consider such subjects as: problems in mediaeval Arabic pharmacology, al-Samarqandī and his work, his travels, Indian, Greek, and Babylonian influences, his pharmaco-therapy, methods and rationale of compounding, Muslim materia medica in contemporary indigenous medicine, drugs in the Aqrābādhīns of al-Kindī and al-Samarqandī. Then the translation of al-Samarqandī's Aqrābādhīn follows; his medical formulary demonstrates the high development of pharmacology among the Arabs in the Middle Ages. This is the first complete translation of the work. With notes, comments, Arabic-English glossary, selected bibliography, Greek, general, and botanical indexes.

Pseudo-Mesuë (= ? Māsawaih al-Mardini, Mesuë the Younger, 925-1015) — VANDEWIELE, L. J., 1962: De Grabadin van Pseudo-Mesues (XIe-XIIe eeuw) en zijn invloed op de ontwikkeling van de farmacie in de Zuidelijke Nederlanden, 352 p. (Thesis Univ. Gent) (Gent: Author).—

The Grabadin is a combination of the "Antidotarium" and the "De Appropriatis" (or "Practica medicinarum particularium"), two books ascribed to Pseudo-Mesuë, an Arabian physician and pharmacist. In his study the author tries to prove that especially the Antidotarium-part of the Grabadin must have been the primary source of inspiration for the mediaeval books of recipes and the pharmacopoeia in the Low Countries. In order to illustrate this thesis, the author discusses many similarities in Pseudo-Mesuë's Antidotarium and the mediaeval pharmaceutical literature used in the Low Countries. This is accompanied by a translation of the Antidotarium in Dutch.

Thābit ibn Ḳurrah, al-Ḥarrānī (d. 901) — SOBHY, G., ed., 1928: The book of al-ḏakhīra, 18 + 44 p. in English; 186 + 6 p. in Arabic. (Cairo: Govt. Press).—

The greater part of the English text (43 pages) consists of a glossary of the technical terms. There is a very brief introduction and a summary of the text in only 3 pages.

——, WIEDEMANN, E., 1922: Ueber Thabit ibn Qurra, sein Leben und Wirken, 30 p. (Beitr. Gesch. Naturwiss., 64) (Sitzb. phys.-med. Ges., Erlangen 52 : 189-219).—

Thābit ibn Ḵurrah was physician, mathematician and astronomer, and one of the greatest translators from Greek and Syriac into Arabic, founder of a school of translators. The present publication contains an elaborate study of Thābit's life and works. These works are classified under the following headings: mathematics, astronomy, geography, music, physics and natural history, meteorology, agriculture, medicine.

Usāmah ibn Murshid (Mu'aiyid al-Daulah), called Ibn Munḵid (1095-1188) — DERENBOURG, H., 1895: Souvenirs historiques et récits de chasse, par un Emir syrien du douzième siècle. Autobiographie d'Ousāma ibn Mounkidh intitulée: L'instruction par les examples. Trad. française d'après le texte arabe, 238 p. (Paris: Leroux).—

This is a translation of an incomplete autobiography of a Syrian emir who was born at the time when Pope Urban II inaugurated the crusading movement at the Council of Clermont. It provides an illuminating account of the private life of a typical Arab chieftain, dealing with education, with the large part played in it by hunting and by exercise in the open air. His main interests were in hunting and fighting, so we find much in it about the pursuit of lions, and of the practice of falconry, but it also throws some light on medicine and surgery. Of this work an English translation exists by POTTER, G. R., 1929: The autobiography of Ousāma (Ousāma ibn Mounḵidh, 1095-1185). (London: Routledge); also: The story of Ousāma. By himself. Retold by M. WEST, based on the autobiography of Ousāma, 1953, 63 p. (London: Longmans & Green); also in a German translation: Memoiren eines syrischen Emirs, 1905, 299 p., by SCHUMANN, G. (Innsbruck).

——, HITTI, P. K., 1929: An Arab-Syrian gentleman and warrior in the period of the crusades. Memoirs of Usāmah ibn-Munqidh (Kitāb al-i'tibār), 265 p. (New York, N.Y.: Columbia U.P.).—

This is an English translation of the Kitāb al-i'tibār, "Learning by example", an (incomplete) autobiography of a Syrian emir who lived during the years of the greatest activity in the Crusades (1095-1291). He lived at Antioch, a crusading centre, and moreover, he spent much time at Jerusalem, Damascus, Cairo, etc., so that this book gives a good picture of the period. The most valuable part of this book, however, is the abundant information it contains about hunting and falconry. Besides, it contains many medical anecdotes. He also describes different ways of fishing. There also exists an older and less reliable French translation of this book by DERENBOURG, H., 1895 (vide supra).

Yaḥyā ibn Muḥammad, called Ibn al-'Awwām — CLÉMENT-MULLET, J. J., 1864-1867: Le livre de l'agriculture d'Ibn-al-Awan (Kitāb al-Felāḥah), trad. de l'arabe, 2 vols. Vol. I (1864): 657 p.; Vol. II, pars 1 (1866) : 460 + 18 p.; Vol. II, pars 2 (1867) : 293 p. (Paris: Franck).—

Ibn al-'Awwām was a Hispano-Muslim agriculturist flourishing at Seville at the end of the 12th century. He wrote the Kitāb al-falāḥah, the most important treatise on agriculture of the Moslem period and during the Middle Ages as well. The first 30 chapters (out of 35) deal with agriculture proper, the last four with cattle, poultry raising, and apiculture. The main literary source was probably Ibn Waḥshīya. It is based on Greek and Arabic writings and on practical experience, deals with 585 plants and explains the cultivation of more than 50 different fruit trees; separate sections deal with different kinds of soils (ch. 1), seeds (ch. 2), various methods of grafting (ch. 8), irrigation (ch. 12), the signs of some plant-diseases and their control (ch. 14), with different kinds of manure, sympathies and antipathies between plants, etc. Two chapters deal with the horse (ch. 32 and 33, more than 200 pages in Clément's text), its training, use, diseases, etc.

Ya'ḵub ibn Isḥaq, called al-Kindī (= Alkindus, ca. 800-873) — LEVEY, M., ed., 1966: The "Medical formulary" or "Aqrābādhīn" of al-Kindī: transl. with a study of its materia medica, 410 p. (Madison, Wisc.: Univ. Wisconsin Press).—

This is an English translation of a ms. in the Aya Sofia Library in Istanbul, accompanied by annotations, an introduction, an etymological and philological interpretation of the drugs and simples, indexes, and a selected bibliography. In his introduction, the editor gives a review of Arabic literature on pharmacology. There is a thorough discussion concerning identification and arrangement of the materia medica (p. 225-345). As to the authenticity of al-Kindī's authorship, some reservations are to be made. Al-Kindī was the first great Arab philosopher; he was deeply influenced by Aristotle and he had considerable knowledge of Greek science and philosophy. *Cf.* FLUEGEL, G., 1857: Al-Kindī genannt "Der Philosoph der Araber" (Abh. Kunde Morgenl.); reprinted 1966 (New York, N.Y.: Kraus); see also RESCHER, N., 1964: Al-Kindī: an annotated bibliography, 55 p. (Pittsburgh, Pa.: U.P.). *Cf.* also: GARBERS, K., ed., 1948: Kitāb kimyā 'al-'iṭr wat taṣ 'idāt. Buch über die Chemie des Parfüms und die Destillationen (Abh. Kunde Morgenl., No. 30). Reprinted 1966 (New York, N.Y.: Kraus).

Yuḥannā ibn Māsawaih (= Mesuë the Elder, 777-857) — PRUEFER, C. & M. MEYERHOF, 1916: Die Augenheilkunde des Juḥanna ibn Māsawaih, 52 p. (Der Islam 6 : 217-268; 7 : 108).—

Ibn Māsawaih was a Christian physician who wrote medical treatises in Arabic.

He also translated Greek medical works into Syriac. Dissected apes. Of his many medical works the "Disorder of the eye" (Daghal al-'ain) is a famous systematic treatise on ophthalmology in Arabic. According to Sarton (Introd. I: 574), this study of Pruefer & Meyerhof is very important. It contains a complete analysis of the "Disorder of the eye" and of a smaller book, a regular cram-book of ophthalmology, and also a study of early Syriac and Arabic ophthalmology. He was also one of the earliest in the Arabic world to write on pharmacology: LEVEY, M., 1962: Ibn Māsawaih and his treatise on simple aromatic substances: studies in the history of Arabic pharmacology (J. Hist. Med. 16: 394-410). This publication is based on one single ms. and contains an English translation of Ibn Māsawaih's treatise dealing with odoriferous materials in pharmacology. The aromatics dealt with are to be found in the Greek, Indian, and Babylonian pharmacopoeias.

10. LIFE AND MEDICAL SCIENCES IN THE LATIN WEST IN THE MIDDLE AGES (*ca.* 500-1450)

a. History of science and culture in general

BERNHEIMER, R., 1952: Wild men in the Middle Ages: a study in art, sentiment and demonology, 224 p. (Cambridge, Mass.: Harvard U.P.).—

Feral humans, raised by kindly animals, have been reported from the earliest times. After having traced the natural history of wild men and after having dealt with his mythological personality, the author considers his role in heraldry, in literature, and particularly he deals with the iconography of the wild man through mediaeval paintings, tapestries, cabinet carvings, sculpture, illuminated Bibles, printer's colophons, *etc.*

HARRISON, F., 1947: Mediaeval man and his notions, 276 p. (London: Murray).—

This is a scholarly study of mediaeval daily life. Special sections have been devoted to mediaeval medicine and to the position of the doctor and the surgeon. The book also deals with such subjects as: the schoolboy and his teacher, travelling, family life, meals and drinks, *etc.* Many fine illustrations.

HASKINS, C. H., 1927: Studies in the history of mediaeval science, ed. 2, 411 p. (Cambridge, Mass.: Harvard U.P.).—

The author approaches the history of 12th- and early 13th-century European science from two different points of view. At first: the recovery and assimilation of the

science of antiquity - mainly by means of the preparation of translations - and the rôle played by Spain, Sicily, and northern Italy in spreading the knowledge of the Arabs, Greeks, and Byzantines respectively. Secondly: the advance of knowledge by means of observation and experiment on plants and animals (esp. dogs, hawks, horses), treatment of diseases, and geographical exploration. The court of Frederick II is described as meeting-point of these Greek and Arabic currents of thought, at the same time serving as a centre of inquiry and experiment. The book is of much biohistorical value (considering, *inter alia,* the history of falconry, hunting, and medicine).

JANSON, H. W., 1952: Apes and ape lore in the Middle Ages and the Renaissance, 384 p. (London: Warburg Institute, Univ. London).—

A useful reference tool, written by a historian of art. It contains some 180 illustrations taken from mediaeval manuscripts, ornaments and sculptures of old buildings such as cathedrals, paintings, and early books. It deals with a lot of topics, such as: the ape in early Christianity, the Fall of Man, the sexuality of apes, the ape as sinner, the ape as an object of science, the fettered ape, and the ape in Gothic marginal art.

JONES, C. W., ed., 1950: Medieval literature in translation, 1004 p. (New York, N.Y.: Longmans, Green).—

"One will find here great excerpts of the Christian Tradition (St. Augustine, Boethius' hymns and liturgies), Old Irish literature, Bede and Beowulf, the Deeds of Charlemagne and some of Peter Abelard's own story, the legends of King Arthur and related tales, the Nibelungen literature and old German lyrics, the Song of Roland, the Cid, Aucassin and Nicolette, the Romance of the Rose, much of Dante, all of this interspersed with samples of song, ballad, drama, prayers, secular poems of wit, love and life - all of which renders this book a great boon to any student and any home." (From Isis 41: 377).

POUCHET, F. A., 1853: Histoire des sciences naturelles au Moyen Âge, ou Albert le Grand et son époque, considérés comme point de départ de l'école expérimentale, 656 p. (Paris: Baillière).—

For more details, *vide* section Antiquity in general, subsection a.

PREVITÉ-ORTON, C. W., ed., 1952: The shorter Cambridge medieval history, 2 vols., 1202 p. (Cambridge: U.P.).—

For more details, *vide* section Antiquity in general, subsection a.

STEINSCHNEIDER, M., 1956: Die europäischen Uebersetzungen aus dem Arabischen bis Mitte des siebzehnten Jahrhunderts, 84 + 108 p. (Graz: Akad. Druck- und Verlagsanstalt).—

The text was originally published in Sitzber. Kaiserl. Akad. Wiss., Wien, Phil.-hist. Kl., 149 and 151, 1904-1906. It is a valuable tool for the historian of science and an invaluable tool for the historian of medicine, the material being dominated by medicine. *Cf.* WÜSTENFELD, F., 1877, *vide infra;* and subsection d: Constantine the African.

TAYLOR, H. O., 1949: The mediaeval mind: a history of the development of thought and emotion in the Middle Ages, ed. 4, Vol. I: 603 p.; Vol. II: 620 p. (Cambridge, Mass.: Harvard U.P.).—

This is a reprint of the 4th ed. (1925; 1st ed. 1911). The work is a synthesis of Western mediaeval thought from its beginnings to Dante. Emphasis has been laid on belles lettres, philosophy, social life and the humanities in general.

THORNDIKE, L., 1944: University records and life in the Middle Ages, 476 p. (New York, N.Y.: Columbia U.P.).—

An anthology containing 176 notes or documents in chronological order from the 12th to the 17th century, most of them dealing with the 13th and 14th centuries. The first appendix contains the text of the "De commendatione cleri", discussing educational ideals and practice about the middle of the 14th century; and the second one deals with the foundation and location of colleges at Paris during the later Middle Ages.

——, 1963: Science and thought in the fifteenth century: studies in the history of medicine and surgery, natural and mathematical science, philosophy and politics, 387 p. (New York, N.Y. & London: Hafner).—

This is a photo-reprint of the 1929 edition. It will be of interest to every student of the period of the Italian Renaissance, and consists of a collection of independent studies on a number of separate subjects; much unpublished ms. material has been used. Its subject matter has been divided as follows: 1. Introduction: the study of Western science of the 14th and 15th centuries; 2. Medicine *versus* law at Florence; 3. The ms. text of the "Chirurgia" of Leonard of Bertipaglia; 4. A "Practica cirurgie" ascribed to John Braccia of Milan or to Peter of Tossignano; 5. Some minor medical works written at Florence; 6. A 15th-century autopsy; 7. Nicholas of Cusa and the triple motion of the earth; 8. Peurbach and Regiomontanus; their great reputation reëxamined; 9. The arithmetic of Jehan Adam, A.D. 1475; 10. Niccolò da Foligno's treatises on ideas: a study of scholasticism and Platonism in the 15th century; 11. Some Renaissance moralists and philosophers; 12. The "De constitutione mundi" of John Michael Albert of Carrara and its relation to similar treatises; 13. "Lippus Brandolinus de comparatione reipublicae et regni": a treatise in comparative political science.

WÜSTENFELD, F., 1877: Die Uebersetzungen arabischer Werke in das Lateinische seit dem XI. Jahrhundert, 133 p. (Göttingen: Dieterich).—

Some of the translators included are: Constantine the African (14 translated works mentioned), Adelard of Bath (4); Johannes Hispanus (20), Dominic Gundisalvo (5), Gerald of Cremona (71), Alfredus Anglicus (2), Joh. el-Gāfiki (1), Armengandus

Blasii (5), Michael Scot (6), Farag called Faragut (4), Marc of Toledo (5), Arnold of Villanova (5), Andreas Alpagus Bellunensis. A more recent book which seems to deal with the same kind of subjects, but of which I do not possess further details is: FÜCK, J., 1955: Die arabischen Studien in Europa bis in den Anfang des 20. Jahrhunderts, 355 p. (Leipzig: Harrassowitz). *Cf.* also STEIN-SCHNEIDER, M., 1956, *vide supra*.

ZWEIG, F. M., 1949: Wunder und Zeichen. Grosse Gestalten des Hochmittelalters, 256 p. (Esslingen, Württ.: Bechte).—

This history of the Middle Ages deals especially with the 13th century. Separate chapters deal with such topics as: mediaeval intellect between past mystery and future enlightenment, Bernard of Clairvaux, master of military technique, Saladin and Richard Coeur de Lion, Emperor Frederick II, Francis of Assisi, *etc.*

b. History of the plant and animal sciences

ABEL, W., 1955: Die Wüstungen des ausgehenden Mittelalters, ed. 2, 180 p. (Quellen und Forsch. zur Agrargeschichte, vol. 1) (Stuttgart: Fischer).—

According to the author, the 15th century is a century of agricultural decline, and the author analyses data showing the high incidence of abandoned holdings (Wüstungen) nearly everywhere in Europe, followed by a serious decline in population and in economic life in general. The causes of this decline are analysed, such as: high mortality, low reproduction rate, the effects of war, money shortage, *etc. Cf.* CLAPHAM, J. H. & E. POWER, 1941; and GRAND, R. & R. DELATOUCHE, 1940, *vide infra*.

AMSLER, H., n.d. (*ca.* 1925): Ein handschriftlicher illustrierter Herbarius aus dem Ende des 15. Jahrhunderts und die medizinisch-botanische Literatur des Mittelalters, 95 p. (Diss. Univ. Zurich).—

Rather extensive description of the Codex Thuriensis and its usefulness in suggesting possible relationships between three famous herbaria, *viz.,* the "Herbarius latinus", the "Hortus sanitatis" and the "Gart der Gesundheit". It also contains a brief outline of mediaeval botanical literature (p. 5-19), and a study of the medico-botanical literature of the 15th century (p. 20-55).

BEAUJOUAN, G., Y. POULLE DRIEUX & J. M. DUREAU - LAPEYSSONNIE, 1966: Médecine humaine et vétérinaire à la fin du Moyen-Âge, 473 p. (Geneva: Droz; Paris: Minard).—

For more details, *vide infra,* subsection c.

BELOW, G. v., 1937: Geschichte der deutschen Landwirtschaft des Mittelalters in ihren Grundzügen, 114 p. (Jena: Fischer).—

Discussion of some problems (especially those of landownership, property, and some aspects of rural economy) during ancient German agricultural history. Introductory chapter concerning these problems under Germanic conditions, but a more profound discussion of these topics (ch. II and ch. III) in the period between the rise of the Carlovingian dynasty and the end of the Middle Ages. A second ed. appeared in 1966, 114 p., ed. by F. LÜTGE (Quellen und Forsch. zur Agrargeschichte, vol. 18) (Stuttgart: Fischer). A history of German agricultural history from the 11th up to the 13th century is: DOPSCH, A., 1964: Herrschaft und Bauer in der deutschen Kaiserzeit, ed. 2, 272 p. (Quellen und Forsch. zur Agrargeschichte, vol. 10) (Stuttgart: Fischer). This is an unaltered re-issue of the original 1938 edition.

BEHLING, L., 1957: Die Pflanze in der mittelalterliche Tafelmalerei, 221 p.; and BEHLING, L., 1964: Die Pflanzenwelt der mittelalterlichen Kathedralen, 227 p. (Cologne & Graz: Böhlau).—

For more details, *vide* section History of the plant sciences, subsection a.

CARMODY, F. J., 1953: Physiologus: the very ancient book of beasts, plants, and stones, translated from Greek and other languages, 375 p. (San Francisco, Calif.: Book Club of California).—

This is an English translation of the "Physiologus" based on the Greek and other versions, but the edition was limited to only 325 copies. *Cf.* also: MCCULLOCH, F., 1962, *vide infra;* and subsection d: Theobald.

CLAPHAM, J. H. & E. POWER, eds., 1941: The Cambridge economic history of Europe from the decline of the Roman Empire. Vol. I: The agrarian life of the Middle Ages, 650 p. (Cambridge: U.P.).—

For more details, *vide* section Antiquity in general, subsection b.

CRIPPS-DAY, F. H., 1930: The manor farm: to which are added reprint-facsimiles of "The Boke of Husbondry" an English translation of the XIIIth-century tract on husbandry by Walter of Henley ascribed to Robert Grosseteste and printed by Wynkyn de Worde, *ca.* 1510 and "The Booke of Thrift", containing English translations of the same tract and of the anonymous XIIIth-century tract "Hosebonderie" by James Bellot printed in 1589, 38 + 114 p. (London: Quaritch).—

The text of this book is taken from 3 old tracts, giving practical details of the management of a small estate under the manorial system, of which "Walter of Henley" *(ca.* 1221) is the most important one, being probably the first original contribution to agricultural literature that was not borrowed from the Latin writers. Included is a translation from "Fleta", written in Latin *(ca.* 1289), which is a combination of two of the tracts, *viz.,* "Walter of Henley" and "Seneschausie"; to this translation two reprints have been added, one of the "Booke of Thrift", consisting of translations from the text of "Walter of Henley" and the third tract, *viz.,* "Hosebonderie", the other of the "Boke of Husbondry", a 16th-century version of a translation of "Walter of Henley" ascribed to Grosseteste. Reprint-facsimiles of this last reprint and of the "Booke of Thrift" have been added. *(Vide* also subsection d: Walter of Henley). Long introduction, giving a historical and scientific framework for the rest of the text.

CRISP, F., 1924: Mediaeval gardens, "Flowery medes" and other arrangements of herbs, flowers and shrubs grown in the Middle Ages, with some account of Tudor, Elizabethan and Stuart gardens, 2 vols. Vol. I: 140 p. + 225 figs.; Vol. II: 314 figs. (London: Lane).—

These volumes mainly consist of a collection of illustrations. They are preceded by a general introduction into mediaeval gardens, their plants, herbs, flowers, seedbeds, special features, *etc.* A facsimile-reprint of the original ed. appeared in 1966 (2 vols. in one, ed. by C. C. PATERSON) (New York, N.Y.: Hacker).

DAVIS, J. I., ed., 1958: Libellus de natura animalium: a fifteenth-century bestiary. Reproduced in facsimile with an introduction, unnumbered facsimile pages (London: Dawson).—

The facsimile pages number 64 and there are 57 woodcuts of various animals, birds, insects and fabulous monsters (incl. a mermaid). The text contains a statement of the nature of the animal considered and the pious moral to be drawn from it. *Cf.* MCCULLOCH, F., 1962 ,*vide infra.*

FISCHER, H., 1929: Mittelalterliche Pflanzenkunde, 326 p. (Munich: Münchner Drucke).—

This book mainly deals with mediaeval botany in Germany, but it contains much very interesting information of a more general interest. It has been divided into the following sections: I: Botany in monasteries and medical schools (p. 6-62, considering *e.g.,* Is. of Sevilla, Hrabanus Maurus, Platearius, Hildegard of Bingen, Albertus Magnus, Conrad of Megenberg, and some early mss.); II: Early printed books (p. 63-113, considering the Latin Dioscorides, Simon Januensis, Matthaeus Sylvaticus, botanical incunabula, Circa instans); III: Botanical iconography (p. 114-126); IV: Mediaeval agriculture (p. 127-184, considering monastic and other gardens, introduction of oriental plants, agricultural theory of Alb. Magnus and Petrus de Crescentius); V: Pharmaceutical botany (p. 185-235); VI: Agricultural expansion in Western Europe (introduction of new plants, deforestation, *etc.).* Very valuable and extensive list of synonyms of Latin plant names followed by their synonyms in mediaeval writings (p. 254-289). Glossaries of plant names of Roman and of German origin have been included. Reprinted 1967 (Hildesheim: Olms). *Cf.* HEILMANN, K. E., 1966, *vide* section History of the plant sciences, subsection a.

FREEMAN, M. B., 1943: Herbs for the mediaeval household for cooking, healing and diverse use, 48 p. (New York, N.Y.: Metropolitan Museum of Art).—

Based on original sources, such as Grete Herball (1526), Bancke's Herbal (1525), and Le menagier de Paris *(ca.* 1393), this booklet contains short chapters dealing with: herbs for cooking, for healing, for poisoning pests, and herbs with a sweet smell. Within each chapter the herbs are arranged alphabetically, provided with appropriate quotations from the old sources and by a statement of their modern use, if any. Excellent reproduction of wood-cut illustrations, many of them derived from the "Hortus sanitatis". A German counterpart is: SCHIWON, W. J., 1926: Gebräuchliche Heilkräuter am Ausgang des Mittelalters und ihre heutige Verwendung, 80 p. (Diss. Univ. Würzburg (Beuthen).

FRISK, G., 1949: A middle English translation of Macer Floridus De viribus herbarum, 338 p. (Diss. Uppsala).—

De viribus herbarum is a Latin poem of 2,269 lines and it has been composed between 849 and 1112. It is generally believed that Odo de Meung was its maker. From this poem eight English mss. still exist. Although the present study is mainly of linguistic interest, it nevertheless contains much information valuable to historians of botany and pharmacy.

GRAND, R. & R. DELATOUCHE, 1940: l'Agriculture au Moyen Âge de la fin de l'Empire romain au XVIe siècle, 740 p. (l'Agriculture à travers les âges, III) (Paris: de Boccard):—

This is a continuation of the late SAVOY's work "l'Agriculture à travers les âges" (vide section: History of the plant sciences β, subsection a). It also has been divided according to subjects, and stress has been laid on economic rather than on technical aspects. The subject matter has been divided as follows: Où placer le début du Moyen Âge?; De l'Antiquité au Moyen Âge ou période de formation; l'Homme; Le domaine; Le mode d'existence; La technique agricole (la culture, l'élevage, la pisciculture et la pêche, le gibier et la chasse); l'Industrie agricole; Le régime économique de l'agriculture médiévale; La fin du Moyen Âge et la Renaissance. No index. Cf. also: ABEL, W., 1955; CLAPHAM, J. H. & E. POWER, 1941, vide supra; and NEILSON, N., 1936, vide infra.

HENNEBO, D., 1962: Garten des Mittelalters, 196 p. (Geschichte der deutschen Gartenkunst, vol. 1) (Hamburg: Broschek).—

"Portions of this book relate directly to medieval botany. The short sections on Charlemagne's Capitulare de villis, and on Walahfrid Strabus, Macer Floridus, Albertus Magnus, Crescentius, et al., are dull but by copious citation from Old High German texts, accompanied by well-chosen illustrations, an informative account is given of the

many purposes served by a garden and what was grown therein. The provenance of the plates is often incomplete, the bibliography of 242 items contains several errors, and worst of all, there is no register ..." (From: Isis 56: 554). The whole work consists of three vols. As to the other vols., vide section: History of the plant sciences β, subsection b; cf. also: ABEL, W., 1955; CLAPHAM, J. H. & E. POWER, 1941 vide supra.

HENSLOW, G., 1899: Medical works of the fourteenth century together with a list of plants recorded in contemporary writings, with their identifications, 278 p. (London: Chapman & Hall).—

This work contains transcripts 1) of an old English ms. (which was in the possession of the author), mainly restricted to that part of the ms. which deals with medical recipes (= p. 159-211 of the ms.); 2) of selected portions from ms. Harl., 2378; 3) of ms. Sloane, 2584; and 4) of ms. Sloane, 521. The last three mss. are in the British Museum. These transcripts are followed by a vocabulary of the names of plants and vegetable products used as drugs, etc., in the fourteenth century.

HERON-ALLEN, E., 1928: Barnacles in nature and in myth, 180 p. (London: Oxford U.P.).—

A nicely-illustrated volume, divided into three parts. The first part contains the natural history of Lepas anatifera and of Balanus balanoides. The second part deals with the myth relative to Lepas anatifera. In this part the author analyses the statements given by mediaeval writers (e.g., Alexander Neckam, Gerald the Welshman, Pietro Damiani). The third part is devoted to the barnacle myth of Mycenaean times (9th century B.C.), as it has come to us from Mycenaean pottery, and to the transmission of the myth which is a mystery, for the myth occurs neither in Greek nor in Roman lore.

HUDSON, N., ed., 1954: An early English version of Hortus Sanitatis: a recent bibliographical discovery, 16 + 164 + 14 p. (London: Quaritch).—

In 1520 a Dutch book on natural history was printed by Jan van Doesburgh at Antwerp. From this book sprang an English translation by Lawrence Andrewe under the title "The noble lyfe & natures of man of bestes, serpentys, fowles & fishes yt be moste knowen". This book contains - in shortened form - all the zoological chapters of "Hortus Sanitatis", illustrated with copies of the woodcuts used in the Latin edition printed in Germany. The present book contains a facsimile reproduction of "The Noble Lyfe", together with some appendixes dealing with the medical side, the woodcuts and the textual discrepancies among the extant texts. *Cf.* also SCHREIBER, W. L., 1924, *vide* section: History of the plant sciences α, subsection a.

IVES, S. A. & H. LEHMANN-HAUPT, 1942: An English 13th-century bestiary: a new discovery in the technique of medieval illumination, 45 p. (New York, N.Y.: Kraus).—

This monograph "introduces a remarkable new edition to the forty odd known English bestiaries of the 12th and 13th centuries. The illuminated codex .... with its carefully written text apparently belongs to the first half of the 13th century. Mr. Ives gives an analysis of the text; Mr. Lehmann-Haupt discusses the miniatures. The history of the codex remains to be written." (From a thorough discussion of this booklet in Isis 34: 366-367).

KOSMINSKII, E. A., 1956: Studies in the agrarian history of England in the thirteenth century, 370 p. (London: Blackwell).—

This book has been translated from the Russian by R. KISCH. It contains mainly economic agrarian history, dealing with such topics as: manorial structure in 13th-century England, labour rent and money rent, economic and social differentiation among the English peasantry, small land-owners, the supply of labour on the English manor, *etc.* A complementary study dealing with the legal aspects is: AULT, W. O., 1965: Open-field husbandry and the village community: a study of agrarian by-laws in medieval England, 102 p. (Trans. Amer. Phil. Soc., N.S., 55, Pt. 7) (Philadelphia, Pa.: Amer. Phil. Soc.).

LANGLOIS, C. V., 1911: La connaissance de la nature et du monde au Moyen-Âge, d'après quelques écrits français à l'usage des laïcs, 401 p. (Paris: Hachette).—

Chapter headings are as follows: 1. Philippe de Thaon; 2. l'Image du monde *(cf.* Walter of Metz, *vide* subsection d); 3. Barthélemy l'Anglais, le maître des propriétés des choses; 4. Le roman de Sidrach *(cf.* Sarton, Introduction II (2): 589); 5. Placides et Timéo, ou le livre des secrets au philosophes; 6. Le livre du Trésor *(cf.* Sarton, Introduction II (2): 927). Useful bibliography.

LEY, W., 1948: The lungfish, the dodo, and the unicorn: an excursion into romantic zoology, ed. 3, 361 p. (New York, N.Y.: Viking Press).—

The book has been divided into three parts. The first part, entitled "Myth?" deals with legendary animals with accounts of the unicorn, giants, dragons, the basilisk, vegetable animals, the kraken, and sea serpents. In this part the author tries to discover what real animals are possibly meant. The second part, entitled "Extinct", deals with the aurochs, wisent, European bison, wild horse, geirfugel, giant sloth, and dodo. The third part, entitled "Witnesses of the past", deals with some relic species, the so-called living fossils, such as: the horse-shoe crab *(Limulus),* the platypus, the lungfish, the kiwi, *etc.* A profusely illustrated account of the history of the unicorn can be found in: BOULLET, J., 1959: La merveilleuse histoire de la Licorne (Aesculape 1959: 3-62).

LUDVIK, D., 1960: Untersuchungen zur spätmittelalterlichen deutschen Fachprosa (Pferdebücher), 181 p. (Diss. Laibach) (Ljubljana: Natisnila Univerzitetna založba).—

This book contains an analysis of three mss. dealing with the treatment of diseases of the horse. These texts are presumably independent of those used by Albrant in his "Rossarzneibuch" *(vide* subsection d). Moreover, this book contains a valuable review of veterinary science (especially concerning the horse) during the Middle Ages.

MCCULLOCH, F., 1962: Mediaeval Latin and French bestiaries, rev. ed., 212 p. (Chapel Hill, N.C.: Univ. of North Carolina Press).—

In her preface, the authoress describes the purpose of this book as follows: "The present monograph although treating the (religious) element only in a very brief manner, is intended to describe the nature of the contents of the 'Physiologus' in the animal realm and to clarify the complicated manuscript tradition." The study begins with a short survey of the hypothesis regarding the background of the Greek "Physiologus" from which the earliest Latin versions were translated; next the question of the various families of Latin mss. is reviewed. Then the French bestiaries of Philippe de Thaon, Gervaise, Guillaume le Clerc and Pierre de Beauvais are discussed and the larger part - and for our purpose the most valuable part - contains a general analysis of the principal subjects treated in Latin and French bestiaries. Very valuable bibliography! *Cf.* STRZY-GOWSKI, J., 1899, *vide* section Middle Ages in the Near East α, subsection a. *Cf.* also: CARMODY, F. J., 1953; DAVIS, J. I., 1958, *vide supra;* and WELLMANN, M., 1930; WHITE, T. H., 1954, *vide infra.*

MAURER, F., ed., 1967: Der altdeutsche Physiologus (Physiologus, lateinisch, althochdeutsch und mittelhochdeutsch). Die Millstätter Reimfassung und die Wiener Prosa (nebst dem lateinischen Text und dem althochdeutschen Physiologus), 95 p. (Altdeutsche Textbibliothek, No. 67) (Tübingen: Niemeyer).—

> A critical edition. Included are a facsimile-edition of the Millstätter manuscript, and fragments derived from mss. from Vienna and Munich, the text of the Old High German Physiologus according to the text of Steinmeyer, and the Latin text on which the German tradition has been based. *Cf.* SEEL, O., 1960, *vide infra; cf.* also subsection d: Philip of Thaon.

MOULÉ, L., 1913: Glossaire vétérinaire médiéval, 65 p. (Janus 18: 265-272; 363-379; 439-453; 507-535).—

> An alphabetical list of terms of animal pathology; an attempt to identify medical terms appearing in mediaeval veterinary treatises, manuscripts, incunabula and books printed before 1500. With bibliography. The same author also wrote a history of veterinary medicine in Europe during the Middle Ages: La médecine vétérinaire en Europe au Moyen Âge (Paris, 1900). Unfortunately, I do not possess further information about this book. *Cf.* G. BEAUJOUAN, *et al.,* 1966, *vide* subsection c.

NEILSON, N., 1936: Medieval agrarian economy, 106 p. (New York, N.Y.: Holt).—

> This booklet is intended for students in the field of history; it treats of manorial organisation, cultivation of the soil, homes of the people, courts and justice, the relation of the village to the church, *etc. Cf.* CLAPHAM, J. H. & E. POWER, 1941, *vide supra.*

POULLE-DRIEUX, Y., 1966: l'Hippiâtrie dans l'occident latin du XIIIe siècle (Une mémoire de volume "Hautes études médiévales et modernes"), 160 p. (Geneva: Droz).—

> "L'auteur a pu reconstituer là une histoire de l'hippiâtrie très instructive par les rapprochements de pathologie générale

qu'il permet d'établir entre la médecine vétérinaire et la médecine humaine." (From: Monspeliensis Hippocr. 10 (37): 40). *Cf.* also BEAUJOUAN, G., *et al.,* 1966, *vide* subsection c.

SEEL, O., 1960: Der Physiologus. Uebertragen und erläutert, 103 p. (Zurich: Artemis).—

> The text of the Physiologus is a paperback edition (p. 3-51), with postscriptum (p. 53-72) considering origin, translations, style, meaning *etc.,* notes (p. 73-95), and bibliographical information (p. 96-101). Another translation from Greek into German is: PETERS, E., 1921: Der Physiologus. Aus dem griechischen Original übertragen. Mit einem Nachwort versehen von Friedrich WÜRZBACH. Mit 174 Federzeichnungen von Flora Palyi, 152 p. (Munich: Musarionverlag); *cf.* also: MAURER, F., 1967; and MCCULLOCH, F., 1962, *vide supra.*

SHAFFER, E., 1957: The garden of health. An account of two herbals: the Gart der Gesundheit and the Hortus Sanitatis, 42 p. (San Francisco, Calif.: Printed for the Book Club of California).—

> This very beautiful edition has been embellished with 38 reproductions of some of the woodcuts in those works. Included is a list of 42 editions printed before 1550 (compiled by H. J. HEANEY). *Cf.* HUDSON, N., ed., 1954, *vide supra.*

THÉODORIDÈS, J., 1958: La zoologie au Moyen Âge, 34 p. (Conf. Palais de la Découverte, Sér. D, No. 55) (Paris: Presses Univ. de France).—

> The contents of this little book is very valuable from the historical point of view. The author's main thesis is that investigations of scientific interest to the history of biology during the Middle Ages in West and East are to be found in travel books, books on hunting and books on agriculture. According to the author, Frederick II has to be considered as the greatest zoologist of his time. Moreover, the author points to the importance of iconological studies for the history of mediaeval biology.

TILANDER, G., ed., 1963: Dancus rex, Guillelmus Falconarius, Gerardus Falconarius: les plus anciens traités de fauconnerie de l'occident publiés d'après les manuscrits connus, 294 p. (Cynegetica IX) (Lund: Blom).—

In this volume three works are edited, *viz.,* those of King Dancus, and of William and Gerard the Falconers. According to Tilander these treatises belong to the five earliest treatises on Western falconry; they are not influenced by Arabian and Persian traditions. The treatises can be considered to be a sort of concise, practical veterinary vademecum. Each of the works is treated in the same way, and at the end is an extensive glossary with many names of herbs, drugs and other medicaments used in the medical treatment of hawks and falcons.

WELLMANN, M., 1930: Der Physiologos. Eine religionsgeschichtlich-naturwissenschaftliche Untersuchung, 116 p. (Philologus, Suppl. 22, pars 1) (Leipzig: Dieterich).—

A very important study on Timotheus of Gaza, Pseudo-Solomon, Horapollon, Bolos-Democritus, Anaxilaos, Didymos, and some others. From this, Wellmann concludes that the Physiologus must have been written probably *ca.* 370, and that its composition must have taken place not in Alexandria but in Palestine. An authoritative study of the Physiologus and its composition is: SBORDONE, F., 1936: Ricerche sulle fonti e sulla composizione del Physiologus greco, 109 + 332 p. (Milan: Soc. Dante Alighieri). *Cf.* MCCULLOCH, F., 1962, *vide supra;* and STRZYGOWSKI, J., 1899, *vide* section: The history of the life and medical sciences in the Near East during the Middle Ages δ, subsection a.

WERNER, K., 1964: Psychologie des Mittelalters, 148 + 117 + 62 p. (Amsterdam: Bonset).—

This book consists of a series of three reprints of publications originally in the Sitzber. Kaiserl. Akad. Wiss., Wien, phil.-hist. Kl., *viz.,* 1. Der Averroismus in der christlich-peripathetischen Psychologie des späteren Mittelalters (Sitzber. vol. 98, 1881); 2. Die nominalisirende Psychologie der Scholastik des späteren Mittelalters (Sitzber. vol. 99, 1881); 3. Die augustinische Psychologie in ihrer mittelalterlich-scholastischen Einkleidung und Gestaltung (Sitzber. vol. 100, 1882).

WHITE, T. H., ed., 1954: The book of beasts: being a translation from a Latin bestiary of the twelfth century, 296 p. (New York, N.Y.: Putnam).—

An English translation of a 12th-century ms., with numerous illustrations. An appendix places this bestiary in its historic setting. *Cf.* MCCULLOCH, F., 1962, *vide supra.*

WINGATE, S. D., 1967: The mediaeval Latin versions of the Aristotelian scientific corpus, with special reference to the biological works, 136 p. (Dubuque, Iowa: Brown).—

Originally published 1931 (London & Leamington: Courier Press) as a dissertation, Univ. of London. After a discussion of some preliminary considerations (discussing, *e.g.,* works in possession of the Latins before the new translations, the Arabic and the Byzantine Aristotle), chapters follow on: Aristotle in the West (considering, *e.g.,* the historical setting of the translations, early evidences of diffusion of nature-history works, the beginnings of the mediaeval translating movement in the Sicilies, the Arabic and Byzantine Near East, and Aragon and Castille); 12th-century versions of Aristotle (considering the biological works from the Arabic: De generatione et corruptione, De sensu et sensato; De memoria et reminiscentia, and from the Greek: De generatione et corruptione, and the Parva naturalia); 13th-century versions of Aristotle (considering the biological works from the Arabic: the De plantis and the De animalibus of Michael Scot, and from the Greek: De animalibus, Parva naturalia, and Physiognomia and other versions by the School of Bartholomew of Messina); the 13th-century translators (evidence of Roger Bacon); and on versions and commentaries (Arabian and Greek). The last chapter deals with some later Latin versions of the Aristotelian works.

c. *History of the medical sciences*

ALLBUTT, C., 1905: The historical relations of medicine and surgery to the end of the sixteenth century: an address delivered at the St. Louis Congress in 1904, 125 p. (New York, N.Y.: Macmillan).—

Considered by Garrison to be the best history of mediaeval surgery in English.

AUDUREAU, C., 1892: Étude sur l'obstétrique en occident pendant le Moyen Âge et la Renaissance, 195 p. (Dyon: Darantière).—

Discusses the history of obstetrics from the end of the Roman Empire up to Paré. Special attention has been paid to the School of Salerno (Constantinus Africanus, Trotula). The section considering the Middle

Ages deals with, *e.g.*, Albert the Great, Roger of Parma, Bernard Gordon of Montpellier, John of Gaddesden, and Guy de Chauliac. Other physicians considered are, *e.g.*, Bertruccio, Savonarola, Benivieni, and Mondino.

BEAUJOUAN, G., Y. POULLE-DRIEUX & J. M. DUREAU-LAPEYSSONNIE, 1966: Médecine humaine et vétérinaire à la fin du Moyen-Âge, 473 p. (Hautes études médiévales et modernes, vol. 2) (Geneva: Droz; Paris: Minard).—

This book consists of three separate sections. The first section (by Y. POULLE-DRIEUX, p. 11-170) deals with hippiatry in the Latin West from the 13th up to the 15th century. In an introductory chapter the various hippiatric treatises are discussed; then chapters follow on anatomy and teratology, general pathology and therapeutics, medical and surgical pathology, parasitology, and materia medica. The second section (by J. M. DUREAU-LAPEYSSONNIE, p. 171-368) deals with the works of the 15th-century Catalan physician Antoine Ricart. It consists of three parts, *viz.*, 1. a study of his life and works (p. 177-205); 2. a discussion and analysis of his "Compendium secundi operis de certe graduandi medicinas compositas"; and 3. an analysis and review of existing mss. of Ricart's treatise "Libellus de quantitatibus et proportionibus humorum". The last section (by C. BEAUJOUAN) considers the library and medical school of the monastery of Guadalupe, discussing such subjects as: medicine and surgery, hospitals, medical books, manuscripts, *etc.*

BECCARIA, A., 1956: I codici di medicina del periodo presalernitano (secoli IX, X e XI), 500 p. (Roma: Ed. di Storia e Letteratura).—

This work "describes - and to a limited extent analyses - the volumes preserved in various European libraries, which contain Latin manuscripts written in the period from the Carolingian Renaissance to the beginning literary influence of Salerno... The texts range from Celsus 'De medicina' to the Latin translation of Joannitius' 'Isagoge...'." (From: Bull. Hist. Med. 32: 574).

BONSER, W., 1963: The medical background of Anglo-Saxon England: a study in history, psychology, and folklore, 228 p. (London: Wellcome Hist. Med. Library).—

The present study considers such aspects as the records on epidemics, accounts of cures by Saints and leeches as far as they have been preserved in the chronicles, the general state of health of the people, the interpretation of the various Anglo-Saxon words which relate to disease, methods of diagnosis, *etc.* Thus the book contains matter of interest to the physician, the historian, the philologist, the archaeologist and the folklorist. The subject matter has been divided into 10 parts as follows: pt. 1: general introduction (documents and research material, and the sources of Anglo-Saxon knowledge of medicine); pt. 2: historical (epidemics, hospitals, surgery); pt. 3: the pagan background; pt. 4: the church as physician (healing by holy men, and by means of relics); pt. 5: magic as an adjunct to medicine (things possessing magic properties, taboos, protective magic, sympathetic magic); pt. 6: diseases and conditions treated by magical means; pt. 7: remedial measures (*e.g.*, blood-letting, herb remedies, animal and mineral remedies); pt. 8: food, drink, and diet; pt. 9: organic diseases and their treatment; pt. 10: veterinary and agricultural magic. Good bibliography (p. xxi-xxxv) and index (p. 441-448). *Cf.* TALBOT, C. H., 1967, *vide infra*.

BRODMANN, C., 1931: Deutsche Zahntexte in Handschriften des Mittelalters, 71 p. (Diss. Sudhoff Inst.) (Wittenberg: Herrosé & Ziemsen).—

A reproduction of 8 manuscript texts on dentistry with annotations, technical index and bibliography.

BRUNNER, C., 1922: Ueber Medizin und Krankenpflege im Mittelalter in schweizerischen Landen, 158 p. (Veröff. schweiz. Ges. Gesch. Med. Naturw. 1) (Zurich: Füssli).—

After a brief introduction, considering medical conditions in the time of the introduction of Christianity into Switzerland, chapters follow on clerical medicine (describing St. Gall, Reichenau, Walafrid's Hortulus, blood-letting, medical practice of the monks), on lay physicians and surgeons (detachment of medicine from the church, early laws of medical interest, quacks, apothecaries, obstetrics, sanitary regulations), on the foundation of hospitals (their organization, kinds of hospices, leper-houses), on knightly and other orders to caring for the sick (Johannites, Templars, Lazarites, Antonites, Beguines, *et al.*), and on epidemics (pox and plague).

CLAY, R. M., 1966: The mediaeval hospitals of England , 357 p. (London: Methuen;

New York, N.Y.: Barnes & Noble).—

Separate chapters deal with such topics as: hospitals for wayfarers and the sick, homes for the feeble and destitute, homes for the insane, the Lazar-House, the leper in England, founders and benefactors, hospital inmates, hospital dwellings, the household and its members, care of the soul and of the body, hospital funds, relations with church and state, decline of the hospitals, the dissolution of religious houses and its effect upon hospitals, hospital patron-saints. In an appendix a tabulated list of foundations is added. Bibliography and index. Reprint of the 1909 edition. *Cf.* also MERCIER, C., 1915; and TALBOT, C. H., 1967, *vide infra.*

COCKAYNE, T. O., ed., 1961: Leechdoms, wortcunning and starcraft of early England, being a collection of documents, for the most part never before printed, illustrating the history of science in this country before the Norman conquest, 3 vols. (London: Holland Press).—

A modernized reappearance of the original text of this book, published in 1864-1866 (in 3 vols. of 405, 415, and 445 pages resp.). According to Singer in his introduction, these volumes must be considered not as the beginnings of modern medicine, but as the final aspects of all Greek medical practices in the Western world before the rise of scholasticism. Vol. 2 is entirely devoted to the book of Bald *(cf.* WRIGHT, C. E., 1955, *vide infra),* with a glossary and an English translation. Vol. 3 contains, *inter alia,* the text and translation of Lacnunga *cf.* J. H. G. GRATTAN & C. SINGER, 1952, *vide infra.* Again reprinted in 1964 (New York, N.Y.: Kraus).

DAEMS, W. F., 1967: Boec van medicinen in Dietsche. Een middelnederlandse compilatie van medisch-farmaceutische literatuur, 361 p. (Janus, suppl. vol. VII) (Leiden: Brill).—

A critical edition of a 12th-century medico-pharmaceutical compilation. The greater part of the text consists of a Middle-Dutch text which itself is an adaptation of the "Circa instans". This text is preceded by a scholarly introduction considering its sources and the influence of this work during the Middle Ages; it also gives a review of mediaeval medico-pharmaceutical literature. The last part of the book contains a review of the knowledge of medicines and their preparation as it can be deduced from the text of this book, a review of the materia medica

vegetabilis, a list of Middle-Dutch plant names, together with their synonyms, an alphabetical index, a list of modern scientific nomenclature, and an explanatory list of Middle-Dutch words. *Cf.* VANDEWIELE, L. J., 1965, *vide infra.*

DAWSON, W. R., ed., 1934: A leechbook: or collection of medical recipes of the 15th century: the text of ms. No. 136 of the Medical Society of London, together with a transcript into modern spelling, 344 p. (London: Macmillan).—

A valuable study of mediaeval medical ideas and practice of Europe in general and of England in particular. In the introduction the editor reveals, *inter alia,* how leechbooks were compiled and to what extent they owe their origin and their contents to Greek and Latin writers on medicine, who in their turn drew upon the Egyptians and to a lesser extent upon the Assyrians. Probably the ms. has been compiled in 1443-1444. In the present edition the editor transcribes, and renders into modern English, the original text; both texts being printed on opposite pages. *Cf.* COCKAYNE, T. O., 1961, *vide supra;* and TALBOT, C. H., 1967, *vide infra.*

DIEPGEN, P., 1912: Traum und Traumdeutung als medizinisch-naturwissenschaftliches Problem im Mittelalter, 43 p. (Berlin: Springer).—

An attempt to elucidate the mediaeval ideas concerning dreams und their explanation from the medical and scientific point of view *(i.e.,* not from the theological point of view). Considered are *e.g.,* the ideas of Hildegard of Bingen, Honorius of Antun, William de Congenis, Barth. Anglicus, Vincent of Beauvais, and more especially, the ideas of Alb. Magnus and Arnald of Villanova.

DUPOUY, E., 1888: Le Moyen Âge médical, 372 p. (Paris: Meurillon).—

The text of this book has been divided into four parts. The first part deals with mediaeval medicine proper, its development from the Greeks, Romans, and Arabs, its philosophy, and the way in which it transmitted classical knowledge to modern knowledge. The second part deals with the great mediaeval epidemics, especially with plague, leprosy, scurvy, and syphilis. The third part deals with those magical subjects which are of a typical mediaeval character, *viz.,* demonomania, sorcery, and spiritism. The fourth part tries to give an impression of the impact of medicine on mediaeval society, and the way in which that was expressed by mediaeval literature.

GORDON, B. L., 1960: Medieval and renaissance medicine, 843 p. (London: Owen).—

A comprehensive account of medical practice during the Midddle Ages and early Renaissance. The larger part of the book (p. 1-580) deals with mediaeval medicine. The author elucidates the role played by the Arabs in the conservation, translation and distribution of Greek medical knowledge in the Middle East and the role played by the Jewish physicians of Spain, Portugal, and Italy, whereby this Arabian knowledge was brought to the Western part of Europe. The restricting influence of the Church is emphasized, but also the never-ceasing revolt of individual scientists against ecclesiastical suppression. The larger part of the book contains biographical and bibliographical information.

GRATTAN, J. H. G. & C. SINGER, 1952: Anglo-Saxon magic and medicine: illustrated specially from the semi-pagan text "Lacnunga", 234 p. (London: Oxford U.P.).—

The essential part of this book is a new edition, prepared by the late J. H. G. GRATTAN, of the text of Lacnunga, an Anglo-Saxon ms. of the 11th century, containing much purely pagan material. Lacnunga is a book of prescriptions, magical formulae, and methods of treatment of various diseases. This new edition is preceded by a detailed introduction by C. SINGER, giving a general survey of magico-medical practice in Anglo-Saxon England. The book is of interest to biohistorians, students of medical history, and philologists. *Cf.* COCKAYNE, T. O., ed., 1961, *vide supra*; and TALBOT, C. H., 1967, *vide infra*.

HECKER, J. F. C., 1859: The epidemics of the Middle Ages, ed. 3, 360 p. (London: Trübner).—

A collection of three monographs originally published separately, dealing with the history of the plague, the dancing mania, and the sweating sickness, respectively. In an appendix are added "A boke, or council against the disease commonly called the Sweate, or sweating sickness" by John Caius; and an essay on pilgrimages. There are a chronological survey and a good bibliography. Originally published in 1835; reprinted in 1837, 1844, 1846, and 1859. Also in German translation: Die grossen Volkskrankheiten des Mittelalters (Berlin, 1865). Many references.

HUARD, P. & M. D. GRMEK, 1966: Mille ans de chirurgie en occident: V^e - XVe siècles, 82 p. text + 171 plates and photographs (Paris: Dacosta).—

A very well-illustrated history of mediaeval surgery. The most important part of the book are the illustrations, many of them consisting of full-page colour plates. The first chapter deals with Graeco-Latin and Arabic sources of mediaeval surgical texts, the second with the School of Salerno, the third with medicine in Italy in, the 13th century, the fourth with the beginnings of surgery in France, the Low Countries and England, the fifth with surgery in the 15th century, and the sixth chapter deals with practical mediaeval surgery. *Cf.* MOULIN, D. DE, 1964; SUDHOFF, K., 1914-1918, *vide infra*.

HUGHES, M. J., 1943: Women healers in medieval life and literature, 180 p. (New York, N.Y.: King's Crown Press).—

This book has been written from the point of view of a student of literature, but contains much that is of value to the medical historian as well. It mainly "is concerned with the woman healer and her practices from the eleventh through the fifteenth century, with special emphasis upon the English women." It deals with famous women healers mentioned in literature, with actual contributions of them, with practitioners, midwives and nurses; and the author describes them against the background of lay and academic medicine as they were practised during the period under discussion.

KOTELMANN, L., 1890: Gesundheitspflege im Mittelalter. Kulturgeschichtliche Studien nach Predigten des 13., 14. und 15.-Jahrhunderts, 276 p. (Hamburg: Voss).—

An attempt to use the text of mediaeval sermons as sources of medical history. Separate chapters deal with: food and drink, *e.g.,* table-luxuries, fasting, dipsomania; clothes, care of skin and hair, bathing, make up, furnishing of the house, *etc.;* prostitution and obscenity, *e.g.,* brothels, immoral behaviour of women, priests, and nuns, *etc.;* bodily exercises, *e.g.,* dances, gymnastics, athletics; medical treatment: physicians, quacks, the physician and the patient, the apothecary, healing and magic; nursing; burial ceremonies.

KÜHNEL, H., 1965: Mittelalterliche Heilkunde in Wien, 114 p. (Studien zur Geschichte der Universität Wien, No. 5) (Graz:
Böhlau).—

A historical review of the development of and the problems connected with
medicine in Vienna during the period between the priest-physicians of the 12th and
13th centuries and the beginnings of humanism of the Renaissance. Valuable bibliography (p. 104-107).

LARSEN, H., 1931: An old Icelandic medical miscellany, 328 p. (Oslo: Norske Vi-
denskaps-Akademi).—

A curious mixture of superstition
and medical knowledge. It has been edited
from a 15th-century ms. found in Dublin.
The text shows the far-reaching influence of
the School of Salerno. The contents are as
follows: 1. Charms against haemorrhages
and fevers; 2. A short chapter on the depth
of the sea; 3. A book of simples (the longest and most important part of the manuscript); 4. An antidotarium; 5. A lapidary;
6. A leechbook; 7. A cookbook. The text
and translations are preceded by some chapters considering the sources of the different
parts of the book. Cf. subsection d: Hrafn
Sveinbjarnarson.

LAWN, B., 1963: The Salernitan questions:
an introduction to the history of medieval
and Renaissance problem literature, 240 p.
(Oxford: U.P.).—

This is a monograph on mediaeval
and Renaissance question literature. It deals
with questions about various facets of anatomy, anthropology, astronomy, medicine,
physics, physiology, and zoology; a large
portion of them deals with fabled attributes
of mammals, birds, reptiles, and fishes.
Their concise nature made them particularly
suitable for teaching purposes. The author
makes clear that the Salernitan School gave
fresh impulses to the Galenic and Hippocratic theories, adding Arabic concepts to
them, and he shows the continuity of mediaeval science with its Greek and Roman
antecedents, a process which was continued
up to the 17th century. A supplement to
Lawn's book is: LIND, L. R., ed., 1968:
Problemata varia anatomia: the university
of Bologna ms. 1165, 100 p. (Univ. Kansas
Publ., Humanistic Studies, No. 38) (Lawrence, Ka.: Univ. Kansas Press). This is a
text belonging to one of the most popular
of the collections considered by Lawn.

MACKINNEY, L. C., 1937: Early medieval
medicine with special reference to France
and Chartres, 247 p. (Publ. Inst. Hist. Med.
Johns Hopkins Univ., Ser. 3, Vol. 3) (Baltimore, Md.: Johns Hopkins Press).—

The book consists of the text of three
lectures delivered at the Institute of the History of Medicine, Johns Hopkins Univ., 1936.
The first lecture: "The dark age concept and
early medieval medicine", mainly deals with
two types of medicine: supernatural and
human. Supernatural healing comprised the
use of saintly relics, charms (pagan as well
as Christian), and incantations (a method
generally used by the Church Fathers).
Human healing was applied by lay physicians, and includes the use of drugs, minor
surgery and diet. The second lecture: "Medicine in Merovingian and Carlovingian
France" shows the influence of classical
authorities on lay physicians, and how gradually a change took place from superstition
to lay medicine. Medical education becomes
part of the regular course of all clergymen.
The third lecture: "Medical progress at
Chartres in the tenth and eleventh centuries", deals with medical education at one
of the most important medical centres of
North Europe. A study especially devoted
to this last aspect is: TRIBALET, J., 1936:
Histoire médicale de Chartres jusqu'au XIIe
siècle. Sur un texte inédit Chartrain du Xe
siècle "Horus isagoge Sorani", 154 p. (Paris: Vigot). Cf. SEIDLER, E., 1967; and
WICKERSHEIMER, E., 1936, vide infra.

——, 1965: Medical illustrations in medieval manuscripts. Part I: Early medicine in
illuminated manuscripts; Part II: Medical
miniatures in extant manuscripts: a checklist
compiled with the assistance of T. HERN-
DON, 263 p. (London: Wellcome Hist. Med.
Library).—

This is a selection of 104 miniatures,
of which 18 in full colour, representing a
cross-section of the mediaeval medical il-
lustrator's art and providing a picture of
medical practice not only of the Middle
Ages, but also of that of Ancient Greece and
Rome which constitute the base of mediaeval knowledge of surgery and medicine.

MERCIER, C., 1915: Leper houses and
mediaeval hospitals, 47 p. (London:
Lewis).—

The FitzPatrick Lectures delivered before the Royal College of Physicians, London, 5th and 10th November, 1914. Starts
from the establishment of the leper house
of Zodicus (early in the 4th century). Very

readable story dealing mainly with the situation in England. *Cf.* also CLAY, R. M., 1966, *vide supra.*

MOULIN, D. DE, 1964: De heelkunde in de vroege middeleeuwen, 166 p. (Leiden: Brill).—

The author deals with the history of surgery from the 7th up to the 11th century. He divided his matter into the following sections: physicians, literature, surgical texts, surgical illustrations, surgical anaesthesia, instruments and bandages, and applications, such as the healing of various wounds, fractures, *etc.* The transcribed surgical texts are: the pseudo-Galenic Introductio sive Medicus (9th cent., Reichenau), the Epistula de fleatomia, the Epistula de incisione, and the Epistula Apollo de incisione (from Brussels), the Liber cyrurgie Ypocrates (from Paris) and parts of some other minor mss. English summary on p. 155-159. *Cf.* SUDHOFF, K., 1914-1918, *vide infra;* and HUARD, P. & M. D. GRMEK, 1966, *vide supra.*

NORRBOM, S., ed., 1921: Das Gothaer mittelniederdeutsche Arzneibuch und seine Sippe, 240 p. (Mittelniederdeutsche Arzneibücher, Vol. I) (Hamburg: no publisher mentioned).—

The Gothaer mnd. Arzneibuch is a receptary of the 14th century; it comprises the Düdesche Arstedie and the Practica Bartholomaei. It consists of a critical edition of the text based on 4 mss. (Gotha, Copenhagen (2), and Rostock). The Düdesche Arstedie was a popular medical manual containing many remedies of vegetative or animal origin, many of them were used in folk-medicine. As such it is a useful contribution to the study of Germanic medicine. The Practica Bartholomaei is a learned work, describing various diseases, and drugs obtainable in the apothecary's shop. The text of two still older German receptaries have been published by PFEIFFER, F., 1863: Zwei deutsche Arzneibücher aus dem 12. und 13.Jahrhundert, 90 p. (Sitzber. Kgl. Akad. Wiss., Wien, phil-hist. Kl. 42: 110-200). With glossary (p. 163-200).

RIESMAN, D., 1935: The story of medicine in the Middle Ages, 402 p. (New York, N.Y.: Hoeber).—

A very good and readable introductory history of mediaeval medicine dealing with such topics as: The Greek inheritance, monastic and clerical medicine, the School of Salerno, Arabian medicine, the Jewish physicians of the Middle Ages, Scholasticism and medicine, astrology, alchemy, the rise of the universities in general and those of Montpellier, Bologna, Padua, Paris, Oxford, Cambridge in particular, anatomy, Vesalius, surgeons and barbers, baths and mediaeval hygiene and sanitation, medicine and the guilds, mediaeval diseases and epidemics, leprosy, sweating sickness, epilepsy, plague, syphilis, dancing mania, medical treatment, uroscopy, textbooks, hospitals, Paracelsus, *etc.*

RUIZ MORENO, A., 1946: La medicina en la legislación medioeval Española, 202 p. (Buenos Aires: El Ateneo).—

A historical review of medicine in the legislation of mediaeval Spain based on an analysis of mediaeval municipal statutes, chronicles, romances, histories, and other literary materials of mediaeval Spain. The book deals with: royal physicians, medical education, medical practice, fees, surgeons, apothecaries, hospitals, military medicine, prostitution, rape, pregnancy, abortion, infanticide, castration, impotence, wet nurses, personal hygiene, public health, mental illness, the blind, the deaf and the mute, poisoning, hermaphroditism, marriage, *etc.* For a full history of Spanish medicine, *vide* section History of the medical sciences α, subsection b.

SCHIPPERGES, H., 1964: Die Assimilation der arabischen Medizin durch das lateinische Mittelalter, 240 p. (Sudh. Arch. Gesch. Med., Beiheft 3) (Wiesbaden: Steiner).—

This very valuable study deals with the influence of Arabian medical literature on the West during the 12th and 13th centuries (the time of Constantine the African and Gerard of Cremona), when these Arabian sources became available by Latin translations. The subject matter is in two parts. The first part deals with the available Latin mss., considering such topics as: Constantinus Africanus and the Corpus Constantinus; the reception of Aristotle via Arabian translations from the Greek, esp. of his physical, cosmological, psychological, and biological ideas, and the influence of these ideas upon medicine; the assimilation of Graeco-Arabian medicine (of *e.g.,* Avicenna, Abulcasis, *etc.*) in mediaeval Spain, especially Toledo. The second part deals with persons and centers of special value in the process of assimilation, *viz.,* with mediaeval France (Chartres, Toulouse, Paris, William of Congenis, the role of the Jews, *etc.*); with mediaeval England (*e.g.,* Adelard of Bath, Walcher of Malvern and the Lotharingean

School, Robertus Ketenensis and the School of Chartres, Daniel of Morley and the School of Toledo, Oxford and Roger Bacon); with south Italy *(e.g.,* Palermo, Frederick II of Hohenstaufen, Michael Scot and the "Secreta naturae" and Petrus Hispanus and Scholasticism). As a kind of introduction to this study can be considered: SCHIPPERGES, H., 1961: Ideologie und Historiographie des Arabismus, 76 p. (Sudh. Arch. Gesch. Med., Beiheft 1) (Wiesbaden: Steiner). *Cf.* WÜSTENFELD, F., 1877, *vide infra.*

————, 1964: Die Benediktiner in der Medizin des frühen Mittelalters, 62 p. (Leipzig: Benno).——

After a general introduction on mediaeval medicine, chapters follow on: medicine in accordance with the Regula Benedicti, the medical literature of the encyclopaedists (esp. Cassiodorus Senator, Isidore of Seville, and Hrabanus Maurus), and on medicine and the Benedictine way of life.

SEIDLER, E., 1967: Die Heilkunde des ausgehenden Mittelalters in Paris. Studien zur Struktur der spätscholastischen Medizin, 162 p. (Sudh. Arch. Gesch. Med., Beiheft 8) (Wiesbaden: Steiner).——

An attempt to elucidate the history of 14th-century medicine, illustrated by means of the situation at the University of Paris during this century. The first part of the text (p. 1-42) deals with the situation of medical education in the faculty of medicine of the Paris university, political and social influences; the second part with the literary background, considering the possessions of the royal library, the libraries of Sorbonne and other Paris institutions; the third part (p. 79-133) considers the situation in Paris against the background of the development of European late scholasticism in general. *Cf.* WICKERSHEIMER, E., 1915: Commentaires de la faculté de médecine de l'université de Paris (1395-1516), 561 p. (Paris: Impr. Nationale). *Cf.* also: WICKERSHEIMER, E., 1936, *vide infra;* and MACKINNEY, L. C., 1937, *vide supra.*

SIGERIST, H. E., 1923: Studien und Texte zur frühmittelalterlichen Rezeptliteratur, 220 p. (Stud. Gesch. Med., No. 13) (Leipzig: Barth).——

The book contains the text of 7 mediaeval antidotaria, *viz.,* those of London, Bamberg, Reichenau, Berlin, St. Gall, Glasgow, and Cambridge, five of them being of

the IX-Xth centuries, and one a century older, and another a century younger; and the author shows that they are seemingly independent publications, though based, to a large extent, upon the materia medica of the VI-VIIth centuries. The author also discusses such problems as: types of drugs, diseases and their treatment, sources, their influence on the Salernitan antidotarium. Text of the antidotaria in Latin. A continuation of this study is: JOERIMANN, J., 1925: Frühmittelalterliche Rezeptarien, 181 p. (Beiträge zur Geschichte der Medizin, Vol. 1) (Zurich: Füssli). It contains the text of three 9th-century antidotaria (two of St. Gall, and one of Bamberg), together with a discussion of their form and contents. Index of drugs.

SUDHOFF, K., 1908: Ein Beitrag zur Geschichte der Anatomie im Mittelalter, speziell der anatomischen Graphik nach Handschriften des 9. bis 15. Jahrhunderts, 94 p. + 24 plates (Stud. Gesch. Med., No. 4) (Leipzig: Barth).——

The purpose of the author is to show "dass die wissenschaftlichen Fachillustrationen . . . in den gedruckten medizinischen Werken am Ende des 15. Jh. nicht ad hoc hergestellte Originalzeichnungen sind, . . . sondern dass diese in ihrer ganz überwiegenden Zahl . . . genau wie der Text dieser Kompendien auf langer handschriftlicher Tradition beruhen . . . Es sollte ferner gezeigt werden, dass sich mit Hilfe dieser Untersuchungsreihen der Zeitpunkt und oft auch der Ort genau bestimmen lässt, wo die eigene Naturbeobachtung wach wird, . . . und dem eigenen sehen vertraut, dass damit der wirkliche Beginn der Renaissance der Naturwissenschaften in den Grenzen der Heilkunde blossgelegt wird . . .". Separate sections deal, *inter alia,* with pictures describing the posture of the foetus, derived from mss. of Soranos of Ephesos, and pictures belonging to Henri de Mondeville's anatomical treatise. *Cf.* TOEPLI, R. von, 1898, *vide infra.*

————, 1908: Deutsche medizinische Inkunabeln, 278 p. (Stud. Gesch. Med., Nos. 2/3) (Leipzig: Barth).——

The text consists of the following parts: 1. Books on folk-medicine *(e.g.,* the "Regimen sanitatis Salernitanum", the "Regimen sanitatis" of Rudolf von Hochenburg, texts of Heinrich Louffenberg, Ortolff von Bayerland, Johann Tollat von Vochenberg, Barthol. Metlinger of Augsburg, Albrecht von Eybe); 2. The writings of Hieronymous Brunschwig; 3. Popular books on natural history, lexica (Conrad of Megenberg's "Buch der Natur", the "Gart der Gesundheit", Petrus de Crescentius' "Liber ruralium commodorum", Albrecht's "Rossarznei", Barth. Anglicus, *etc.*); 4. Dietetics and physical therapy *(e.g.,* books on nutrition, fishing, preparation of beverages and brandy, on gymnastics, bathing, *etc.*); 5. Books on plague and syphilis (*e.g.,* pest-tractates of Heinrich Steinhöwel, Ulrich Ellenbog, Conrad Schwestermulner, Valescus de Taranta, Philipp Culmacher von Eger, Ambrosius Jung, Hier. Brunschwig, and a treatise on syphilis of Master Josef Grumpeck von Burckhausen; 6. Monstrosities, ghosts and witches; 7. Death and death-dances; 8. Calendars (medical calendars, blood-letting calendars, prognostications and planet-calendars).

——, 1914-1918: Beiträge zur Geschichte der Chirurgie im Mittelalter. Graphische und textliche Untersuchungen in mittelalterlichen Handschriften, 2 vols. (Stud. Gesch. Med., Nos. 10-12). Vol. I (1914): 224 p.; Vol. II (1918): 36 + 685 p. (Leipzig: Barth).——

A large collection of original texts and illustrations pertaining to mediaeval surgery. These documents are classified as follows: 1. Operationsbilder; 2. Lehr- und Merkschemata für die Beurteilung der Schwere von Verletzungen; 3. Abbildungen von Instrumenten; 4. Lateinische chirurgische Texte des Mittelalters aus Italien und Südfrankreich; 5. Chirurgische Texte aus Deutschland. Bibliography and indexes of subjects and of personal names. Among the texts considered are those of: Roger of Salerno, William of Saliceto, Guy de Chauliac, John Arderne, William of Congenis, Johannes Jamati, Peter of Spain, Bongianus de Orto, William of Brescia, Peter of Tussignano, Jacobus de Prato, Bruno of Longoburgo, Lanfrank, Henri de Mondeville, Peter of Argellata, Nikolaus of Montpolir, Scellinc, Ulrich Eberhards von Konstanz, Pankratius Sommers von Hirschberg, Joannes de Ketham, Johannes Beris, Heinrich von Pfalzpeunt, Johann Schenck von Würzburg, Hans Suff von Göppingen, Peter von Ulm, and others. *Cf.* HUARD, P. & M. D. GRMEK, 1966, *vide supra.*

TABANELLI, M., 1965: La chirurgia italiana nell'alto medioevo, 2 vols. Vol. I: Ruggero, Rolando, Theodorico, 495 p.; Vol. II: Guglielmo, Lanfranco, p. 500-1075 (Florence: Olschki).——

The first part of this study considers the surgical works of Roger of Salerno, Roland of Parma, Ugo of Borgognoni, and of Theodoric, son (or probably student) of Ugo of Borgognoni. The second part considers the surgical works of William of Saliceto and of Lanfranchi who introduced Italian surgical tradition into France. For all the persons considered much (and often original) biographical information is given, together with an enumeration of extant mss., printed editions, and an evaluation of the practical and theoretical value of their works. This is followed by Italian translations of summaries of the surgical aspects of the works of the authors mentioned.

TALBOT, C. H., 1967: Medicine in medieval England, 222 p. (London: Oldbourne).——

This valuable book deals with such subjects as: the intellectual links between early mediaeval England and Ireland and Gaul, early medical schools, Greek, Latin and Arabic sources which were studied by Anglo-Saxon leeches, Anglo-Saxon medical sources, King Alfred and the revival of medical education, the use of magic, amulets and charms in Anglo-Saxon medicine, the universities of Salerno and Montpellier and their influence on mediaeval England, the separation of surgery from medicine, medical education and degrees, the works of Gilbertus Anglicus, John of Gaddesden and others, Roger Bacon's attacks on the physicians of his time, mediaeval surgery, anatomy, hygiene, hospitals, mediaeval practitioners, medical ethics, epidemics, *etc. Cf.* BONSER, W., 1963; CLAY, R. M., 1966; COCKAYNE, T. O., 1961: DAWSON, W. R., 1934; GRATTAN, J. H. C. & C. SINGER, 1952, *vide supra;* and WRIGHT, C. E., 1955, *vide infra.*

—— & E. A. HAMMOND, eds., 1965: The medical practitioners in medieval England: a biographical register, 503 p. (London: Wellcome Hist. Med. Library).——

The purpose of this bibliography is simply "to bring together in convenient form all discoverable biographical information on the members of the medical profession in medieval Britain, and thereby to supply the basis for a clearer understanding of the social, economic and intellectual aspects of medicine and surgery in the period." For the period considered all names of medical men have been included, no matter how early they might occur; the end of the period has been set by MUNK's "Roll of the Royal College of Physicians of London", of which the starting point is 1518. *Vide* MUNK, section Biographical dictionaries, subsection c.

TOEPLI, R. von, 1898: Studien zur Geschichte der Anatomie des Mittelalters, 121 p. (Leipzig & Vienna: Deuticke).—

A useful study of mediaeval medical literature, containing much information. Its subject matter is divided as follows: 1. Galen's inheritance (p. 1-10, considering the anatomists living in ancient Greece, Alexandria, Galen's anatomical treatises and extant translations, pseudo-Galenic treatises, the Anatomia vivorum); 2. Byzantine anatomists (p. 20-60, considering, *inter alia,* Oribasios, Gregorius of Nyssa, Nemesios, Miletios, Theophilos); 3. Arab anatomists (p. 61-76, considering, *inter alia,* Mesuë the Elder, Abu Oseibia, Thābit ben Korra, Abu Bakr, Avicenna, Muhammed el-Gāfiqi, Avenzoar, Averroës); 4. Roman anatomists (p. 81-121, considering, *inter alia,* Isidore of Seville, Constantinus Africanus, Salernitan anatomy, William of Saliceto, Richard the Englishman, Henri de Mondeville, Thomas of Cantimpré, Bartholomaeus Anglicus). *Cf.* SUDHOFF, K., 1908, *vide supra.*

VANDEWIELE, L. J., ed., 1965: De "Liber magistri Avicenne " en de "Herbarijs", middel-nederlandse handschriften uit de 14e eeuw, 510 p. (Verh. Kon. Vlaamse Acad. Wetensch., Lett. en Schone Kunsten, Jaarg. 27, No. 83).—

An edition with commentaries on two 14th-century Middle-Dutch mss. dealing with materia medica, present in the Royal Library of Brussels. *Cf.* DAEMS, W. F., 1967, *vide supra.*

VIEILLARD, C., 1903: l'Urologie et les médecins urologues dans la médecine ancienne. Giles de Corbeil. Sa vie, ses oeuvres, son poème des urines, 391 p. (Paris: De Rudeval).—

A history of the doctrine of urology during the Middle Ages, dealing with such subjects as: urine and the pulse, the nature of urine, examination, colour and quantity of urine, the composition of urine and the substances it contains, the urological pharmacopoeia, urological physicians, urological iconography, the urologist in the literature, Bernard of Gordon and urology, Giles de Corbeil; life and works (p. 209-266), and his poem (p. 267-316); the urinary tract of John of Cuba (p. 317-377). Bibliography of 6 pages. *Cf.* also subsection d: Giles of Corbeil.

WALSH, J. J., 1911: Old-time makers of medicine: the story of the students and teachers of the sciences related to medicine during the Middle Ages, 446 p. (New York, N.Y.: Fordham U.P.).—

This book is a very useful addition to the other existing histories of mediaeval medicine. It deals with such topics as: Great physicians in early Christian times, great Jewish physicians, Maimonides, great Arabian physicians, the medical school at Salerno, Constantinus Africanus, mediaeval women physicians, Mondino and the medical school of Bologna, great surgeons of the medical universities, Guy de Chauliac, mediaeval dentistry and Giovanni of Arcoli, Cusanus and the first suggestion of laboratory methods in medicine, Basil Valentine (last of the alchemists, first of the chemists). Appendixes deal with St. Luke the physician, with science at the mediaeval universities, and with mediaeval popularization of science.

——, 1920: Medieval medicine, 221 p. (London: Black).—

A history of medicine from the deposition of Romulus Augustulus (476) up to the fall of Constantinople (1453). This is a brief history of medicine, surgery, and medical education during this period. Separate chapters deal with: early mediaeval medicine, Salerno and the beginnings of modern mediaeval education, Montpellier and medical education in the West, later mediaeval medicine, mediaeval surgeons, oral surgery and the minor surgical specialities, medical education for women, mediaeval hospitals, medical care for the insane. Appendix I contains the "Law of the Emperor Frederick II (1194-1250) regulating the practice of medicine", and Appendix II the "Bull of Pope John XXII, issued February 18, 1321, as a charter for the Medical Department of the University of Perugia". In a review of this book in Isis 3: 308, C. Singer makes some very critical remarks. A study particularly dealing with medical care for the insane during the Middle Ages is: GRAHAM, T. F., 1967: Medieval minds: mental health in the Middle Ages, 112 p. (London: Allen & Unwin). Unfortunately, I do not possess further information. *Cf.* also: SCHUMACHER, J., 1937: Die seelischen Volkskrankheiten im deutschen Mittelalter und ihre Darstellungen in der bildenden Kunst, 77 p. + 42 illus. (Berlin: Junker & Dünnhaupt).

WICKERSHEIMER, E., ed., 1936: Dictionnaire biographique des médecins en France au Moyen Âge, 2 vols., 867 p. (Paris: Droz).—

This dictionary is an indispensable source of biographical information concerning the physicians, surgeons, barbers and empirics, which have been cited inside of the present (1936) frontiers of France, from the fifth century on to the end of the fifteenth. The names have been given in French translation and are arranged in an alphabetical order according to the baptismal name; however, there is an index of family names which facilitates searching. Each item contains biographical as well as bibliographical information. *Cf.* MACKINNEY, L. C., 1937, *vide supra.*

WRIGHT, C. E., ed., 1955: Bald's leechbook: British Museum Royal Manuscript 12 D. xvii, 256 p. in collotype plus an introduction of 32 p. (Early English Manuscripts in facsimile, vol. V) (Copenhagen: Rosenkilde & Bagger; London: Allen & Unwin; Baltimore, Md.: Johns Hopkins Press).—

Bald's leechbook is of special interest to the study of the history of Anglo-Saxon medicine, being an outstanding example of the considerable amount of medical material which survived the Norman Conquest. *Cf.* COCKAYNE, T. O., 1961; and TALBOT, C. H., 1967, *vide supra.*

WÜSTENFELD, F., 1877: Die Uebersetzungen arabischer Werke in das Lateinische seit dem XI. Jahrhundert, 133 p. (Göttingen: Dieterich).—

For more details, *vide supra,* subsection a.

c*. Salernitan medicine

CAPPARONI, P., 1923: "Magistri salernitani nondum cogniti": a contribution to the history of the medical school of Salerno, 68 p. + 27 plates (Research Studies in Medical History of the Wellcome Hist. Med. Museum, No. 2) (London: Bale & Danielson).—

An attempt to elucidate the beginnings of this school or medical guild, founded in the 12th century and suppressed by Napoleon in 1811. Relying upon two old mss. containing the names of the brethren of the gild and an obituary of the gild, the author succeeded in the addition of many new names to the list of the Magistri Salernitani, together with much additional biographical information. Very nice illustrations. A somewhat older history of the School of Salerno is: BECAVIN, G., 1888: L'école de Salerne et les médecins salernitains, 127 p. (Paris: Baillière). Also in

English translation: The school of Salerno and the Salernitan physicians, 1902, 37 p. (Reprint Cincinnati Lancet-Clinic).

CORNER, G. W., 1927: Anatomical texts of the earlier Middle Ages: a study in the transmission of culture, 112 p. (Washington, D.C.: Carnegie Inst.).—

In the introduction the author considers Salernum before the arrival of Constantine the African, the influence of Constantine, mss. and printed editions of his works, the literature of Salernum, and the "Pantegni", a complete system of medical theory and practice, composed by Ali ibn al-Abbas, a Persian physician, and translated by Constantine. Then follows a chapter on 12th-century texts; the first Salernitan anatomical demonstration (Anatomia Cophonis, Anatomia parva Galeni), the second demonstration (Anatomia Mauri), together with an analysis of data and sources of these texts, and the Anatomia Ricardi (Salernitani) and the Anatomia Magistri Nicolai. This last-mentioned work is ascribed by Sarton to Nicholas II of Salerno. It is possible, Sarton writes in his Introduction II (1): 437, that both texts, *viz.,* the Anatomia Ricardi and the Anatomia Nicolai, are derived from the same original lectures of a Salernitan master called Richard or Nicholas. The second chapter concludes with a section on scholasticism in mediaeval anatomy. A third chapter deals with the Anatomia Vivorum (Anatomia Ricardi Anglici), a 13th-century text with a discussion of date and sources. Generally, this text is ascribed to Richard of Wendover or Richard the Englishman. Full English translations of the Anatomia Cophonis, the second Salernitan demonstration, the Anatomia Magistri Nicolai, and excerpts from the Anatomia Vivorum. Index and useful bibliography containing further references to, *e.g.,* Maurus, Archimatthaeus, Thomas of Brabant, Ricardus, and the School of Salerno in general. According to Sarton in his Introduction II(1): 437/438, Urso of Calabria may have been the author of another Salernitan anatomical treatise, which would be more concerned with physiology and pathology, rather than anatomy proper. According to Sarton it must be dated somewhere between the Anatomia Ricardi and the Anatomia Vivorum. For more particulars, *vide* Urso (subsection d).

——, 1937: On early Salernitan surgery and especially the "Bamberg surgery": with an account of a previously undescribed manuscript of the Bamberg surgery in the possession of Dr. Harvey Cushing, 32 p. (Bull. Inst. Med. 5: 1-32).—

According to the author the text of

this anonymous ms. is of an earlier date than Roger's surgical text, it being simpler, less comprehensive, and less orderly in its arrangement than that of Roger; and its contents can be derived partly from the writings of Constantinus Africanus, and partly from pre-Salernitan sources.

HARINGTON, J., F. R. PACKARD & F. H. GARRISON, 1920: The School of Salernum, 'Regimen sanitatis salernitanum', English version by Sir John Harington. History of the School of Salernum by Francis R. Packard and a note on the prehistory of the 'Regimen sanitatis' by F. H. Garrison, 215 p. (New York, N.Y.: Hoeber).—

In an introductory essay, Packard gives a historical review of the school of Salernum, followed by an essay by F. H. GARRISON considering the prehistory of the Regimen Sanitatis. Then an English translation of the "Regimen" follows prepared by J. HARINGTON in 1608 under the title: "The Englishmans doctor, Or, the Schoole of Salerno. Or, physicall observations for the perfect preseruing of Man in continuall health". This is followed by the original Latin text with notes and subject-index. Pleasing illustrations. An older book with the same intention, but more illustrations, is CROKE, A., 1830: Regimen sanitatis salernitanum: a poem on the preservation of health in rhyming Latin verse. Addressed by the School of Salerno to Robert of Normandy, son of William the Conqueror, with an ancient translation; and an introduction and notes, 199 p. (Oxford: Talboys). Harington's text has been reprinted by the Ente provinciale per il turismo at Salerno (1953). Also in German: "Die Kunst sich gesund zu erhalten" by R. SCHOTT, 1954 (Stuttgart: Kohlhammer). A fine German translation of the poem can be found in TESDORPF, P. & T. TESDORPF-SICKENBERGER, eds., 1915: Das medizinische Lehrgedicht der Hohen Schule zu Salerno. Aus dem Lateinischen ins Deutsche übertragen, unter Beifügung des lateinischen Textes, und mit Wiedergaben von Holzschnitten aus der Frankfurter Ausgabe des Regimens vom Jahre 1568, 96 p. (Berlin: Kohlhammer). A French translation with elaborate commentaries: MEAUX-SAINT-MARC, C., 1880: L'école de Salerne, 609 p. (Paris: Baillière). Introduction p. 1-50; text p. 53-271; commentary p. 275-585. *Cf.* also: PARENTE, P. P., 1967: The regimen of health of the medical school of Salerno, 94 p. (New York, N.Y.: Vantage Press).

HARTMANN, F., 1919: Die Literatur von Früh- und Hochsalerno und der Inhalt des "Breslauer Codex Salernitanus" mit erstmaliger Veröffentlichung zweier Traktate aus dieser Handschrift: "De morbis quattuor regionum corporis" und "De saporibus et numero eorundum"; samt Wiederabdruck der Schrift "De observatione minutionis", 70 p. (Diss. Leipzig) (Borna-Leipzig: Noske).—

In 1837 T. Henschel discovered in Breslau a Compendium Salernitanum from about 1160-1170, containing 35 treatises. The present work contains a useful summary of Salernitan medicine, deals briefly with the main personalities of the Salernitan School, gives a table of contents of the treatises included in the Breslau ms., a catalogue of Salernitan writings classified by subject, and the text of two treatises of which the first is anonymous and the second is attributed to Urso. Another study devoted to this Breslau ms. is: SUDHOFF, K., 1920: Die Salernitaner Handschrift in Breslau. Ein Corpus medicinae Salerni (Arch. Gesch. Med. 12: 101-148, 191). *Cf.* also subsection d: John of Saint Paul.

HIERSEMANN, C., 1921: Die Abschnitte aus der Practica des Trottus in der salernitanischen Sammelschrift De aegritudinum curatione, 37 p. (Diss. Sudhoff Inst.).—

The "De aegritudinum curatione" contained in the Breslau Salernitan ms. (*cf.* HARTMANN, F., 1919) is divided into two main parts. The first part, dealing with general diseases, is the work of a single anonymous author. The second part, dealing with local diseases arranged *a capite ad calces,* is a compilation from the works of seven authors, *viz.,* 1. Matthaeus Platearius (*vide* subsection d); 2. Copho (*vide* subsection d); 3. Petronius (*cf.* BLOEDNER, K., 1925: Petronus, Petronius, Petroncellus, ein salernitaner Arzt aus der Mitte des 12. Jahrhunderts (gest. 1197), sein klinisches Schriftwerk und der Autor der Uebergangszeit Petricellus, 59 p. (Diss. Sudhoff Inst.)); 4. Bartholomew of Salerno (*vide* subsection d); 5. Johannes Afflacius (*cf.* CREUTZ, R., 1930: Der Cassinese Johannes Afflacius Saracenus, ein Arzt aus "Hochsalerno" (Stud. und Mitt. zur Gesch. des Benediktinerordens 48: 302-324)); 6. Ferrarius (*cf.* FRANKE, J., 1925: Der salernitaner Magister Ferrarius und eine bisher nicht veröffentlichte Summa de purgatione quator humorum unter seinem Namen, 27 p. (Diss. Sudhoff Inst.)); 7. Trot'. Hiersemann publishes in his study all the texts ascribed to this mysterious Trot', but he could not succeed in establishing a relation between these texts and those in Trotula's "De mulierum passionibus" (*cf.* subsection d).

KRISTELLER, P. O., 1945: The School of Salerno, its development and its contribution to the history of learning, 56 p. (Bull. Hist. Med. 17: 138-194).—

A very interesting study of the history of the School of Salerno from its origin in the 10th century up to 1812. The author discusses such topics as the history of the School of Salerno, its origin as a group of medical practitioners whose medical teaching, at first purely practical, became increasingly theoretical, the development of the scientific method during the 12th century, its scientific decline in the 14th century, and the reorganization of the School as a city-university, its local revival in the 16th century, and the influence of scholasticism towards the end of the 12th century, mainly through the method of using standard texts for the medical curriculum as appears first in the commentaries of Maurus and through the close alliance between medicine and natural philosophy as appears in the works of Urso. A well-informed summary history of the School of Salerno is: SINGER, C. & D., 1923: The origin of the medical school of Salerno, the first university: an attempted reconstruction, 18 p. (Zurich: Seldwayla). In this study the authors show that the four cultural influences, Greek, Latin, Hebrew, and Arabic, welded together to form the first university in Europe. Cf. also: RENZI, S. DE, 1857: Storia documentata della scuola medica di Salerno, ed. 2, 608 + 184 p. (Napoli: Nobile). Recently reprinted (1967) (Milano: Ferro).

d. *Some individual scientists*

Adelard of Bath (fl. 1116-1142) — MÜLLER, M., ed., 1934: Die Quaestiones naturales des Adelardus von Bath, herausgegeben und untersucht, 92 p. (Beiträge zur Geschichte der Philosophie und Theologie des Mittelalters, vol. 31, pars 2).—

Adelard was an English philosopher, mathematician, and scientist and one of the earliest translators from Arabic into Latin. He wrote the "Quaestiones naturales", a dialogue divided into 76 chapters, each of which deals with a scientific question, the whole purporting to expound Arabic knowledge on these questions. The present edition is based primarily upon Latin ms. 2389 of the Bibliothèque Nationale, Paris. P. 72-91 contain a brief biography of Adelard and a synopsis of the "Quaestiones". A thorough study of Adelard is: BLIEMETZRIEDER, F. J. P., 1935: Adelhard von Bath. Blätter aus dem Leben eines englischen Naturphilosophen des 12. Jahrhunderts und Bahnbrechers einer Wiederentdeckung der griechischen Antike. Eine kulturgeschichtliche Studie, 395 p. (Munich: Hueber).

Adam of Cremona (fl. *ca.* 1227) — HÖNGER, F., ed., 1913: Aerztliche Verhaltungsmassregeln auf dem Heerzug ins Heilige Land für Kaiser Friedrich II. geschrieben von Adam von Cremona, 120 p. (Leipzig).—

This is a treatise on the hygiene of a crusading army or a large body of pilgrims: an elaborate treatise in three books, the first dealing with diet and sleep, camping, exercising, delousing, bathing, bloodletting and cupping, sea sickness, *etc.,* the second with fatigue and rest, the care of feet, and the third with the religious purpose of a crusade. The first book contains 86 out of 96 pages.

Albertus Magnus (*ca.* 1193-1280) — BALSS, H., 1947: Albertus Magnus als Biologe. Werk und Ursprung, 307 p. (Grosse Naturforscher, Vol. 51) (Stuttgart: Wiss. Verlagsges.).—

The text has been divided into three parts. The first part deals with the history of biology in antiquity and during the Middle Ages (Aristotle, Theophrastos, Dioscorides, Pliny, Galen, Isidore of Seville, the Physiologus, Hrabanus Maurus, Walahfrid Strabo, Wandalbert of Prüm, Hildegard of Bingen, Frederick II, Barth. Anglicus, Vincent of Beauvais, Thomas of Cantimpré. The second part deals with life and works of Albertus in general (p. 55-65), and the third part deals with his work in the natural sciences: physics, chemistry, astronomy, geography (p. 67-74), and biology: botany (morphology, ecology, systematics, cultivation, p. 75-187) and zoology (systematics, anatomy, physiology, heredity, ecology, faunistics, and animal psychology). Alphabetical list of plant and animal names, bibliography, index. A very interesting study of Albertus' "Liber de animalibus" (especially of his ornithological knowledge) is to be found in: LINDNER, K., 1962: Von Falken, Hunden und Pferden. Deutsche Albertus-Magnus-Uebersetzungen aus der ersten Hälfte des 15. Jahrhunderts, 231 p. (Quellen und Studien zur Geschichte der Jagd, Vol. VII) (Berlin: de Gruyter).

——, FELLNER, S., 1881: Albertus Magnus als Botaniker, 90 p. (Jb. Kais.-Kön. Ober-Gymnasiums zu den Schotten in Wien, p. 1-90) (Vienna: Hölder).—

After a brief historical introduction (p. 1-10), considering Albert's botanical sources (Theophrastos, Pliny, Isidore of Seville, Hrabanus Maurus, Nicholas Damascenus, Galen, Alex. of Aphrodisias, Palladius, Ishaq Israeli, Avicenna), separate sections deal with his organography (p. 11-31), treating such subjects as taxomony, plant-forms, anatomy, *etc.*, and with plant physiology (p. 31-82), incl. sections discussing the soul of the plant, assimilation, colours, taste, smell, *etc.*, of the plants, propagation, generation, natural and artificial transformation, *etc.*

——, GEYER, B. & E. FILTHAUT, eds., 1955: Albertus Magnus. Opera omnia, tomus XII: Liber de natura et origine animae; Liber de principiis motus processivi; Quaestiones super de animalibus, 48 + 360 p. (Münster: Aschendorff).—

The first treatise (ed. by B. GEYER) gives a clear expression of Albert's philosophical doctrine of the rational soul and its intellectual operation, being very similar to the doctrine expressed by his pupil Thomas Aquinas. The second treatise (ed. by B. GEYER) is largely a paraphrase of Aristotle's "De motu animalium". Both these treatises are edited from the Cologne autograph manuscript in which they occur as Books 20 and 22 respectively of the "De animalibus". The third treatise (ed. by E. FILTHAUT) is a set of 19 questions on Aristotle's "Historia animalium", "De partibus animalium" and "De generatione animalium", and is here published for the first time. Each treatise is preceded by a prolegomena and is followed by indexes both of authors and subjects.

——, MEYER, E., 1836/'37: Albertus Magnus. Ein Beitrag zur Geschichte der Botanik im dreizehnten Jahrhundert, and: Ein zweiter Beitrag zur erneuerten Kenntniss seiner botanischen Leistungen, 150 p. (Linnaea 10: 641-741; 11: 545-595).—

Our knowledge of the botanical work of Albertus is due mainly to these publications. The author starts his work with a biographical review of Albertus and the rest of his work has been devoted to a thorough analysis of his "De vegetabilibus libri VII". (For a critical re-issue of this work in Latin see: MEYER, E. & C. JESSEN, 1867: Alberti Magni de vegetabilibus libri VII, 52 + 751 p., Berlin). The "De vegetabilibus" consists of 7 books, of which the first five are of a theoretical (Aristotelean) nature; the sixth book contains descriptions of individual medicinal and economic plant species, the plants being arranged in alphabetical order;

the seventh book deals with agriculture and horticulture. Meyer considers Albertus' botanical work as the centre of crystallization of mediaeval botanical knowledge. In his second paper Meyer reviews other publications concerning Albertus' achievements and he gives a thorough description of the wood mentioned in the first section of book 6. A modern attempt to evaluate Albertus' botanical achievements in the light of present knowledge is: SPRAGUE, T. A., 1933: Plant morphology and botanical terms in Albertus Magnus (Kew Bull., 1933: 431-459); this publication contains a glossary of botanical terms used by Albertus.

——, PITZL, H., 1959: Albertus Magnus Tierforschung. Tierheilkundiges und Nutzanwendung der Haustiere, 57 p. (Inaug. Diss., Munich) (Munich: Uni Druck).—

Brief biographical and bibliographical introduction. Considered are: horse, ass, cattle, goat, pig, dog, cat, birds, goose, duck, dove, fowl, and bees. The bibliography contains many interesting items on the history of veterinary science during the Middle Ages and on Albert the Great.

——, SCHNEIDER, A., 1903: Die Psychologie Alberts des Grossen. Nach den Quellen dargestellt, 559 p. (Beitr. zur Gesch. der Phil. des Mittelalters, Vol. IV, pt. 5) (Münster: Aschendorff).—

The study has been divided into three parts, treating of the influence of the Peripatetic School, of Neoplatonism, and of St. Augustine's doctrine respectively.

——, STRUNZ, F., 1926: Albertus Magnus. Weisheit und Naturforschung im Mittelalter, 187 p. (Vienna & Leipzig: König).—

This booklet gives a portrait of Albertus against the background of mediaeval life. It considers him primarily as a natural scientist, and, according to the author, it is an attempt to free his life-history from the many myths and legends which enwrap his personality. As a scientist, Albertus was primarily concerned with alchemy, but he also worked in the fields of botany (incl. its medical implications), agriculture, and zoology (esp. embryology); and the author makes clear that he borrowed his scientific ideas chiefly from Aristotle as becomes especially clear in his cosmological speculations. The book illustrates how in those days magic and medicine were closely interwoven.

——, WILMS, H., 1930: Albert der Grosse, 237 p. (Munich: Kösel & Pustet).—

An evaluation of Albert the Great as a scientist, philosopher and theologian. After a biographical introduction, separate sections deal with Albert as a natural scientist (Albert and the plants, Albert and the fauna: mammals, fishes, birds, insects, Albert and the other divisions of natural science) with Albert as a philosopher (his connections with Aristotle and Plato, his metaphysics and psychology), and with Albert as a theologian (exegete, moralist, mystic, and dogmatist). The last section deals with Albert as a priest and religious man. Also in English translation: Albert the Great, saint and doctor of the church, 1933. (London: Burns).

Albrant (fl. *ca.* 1240-1265) — EIS, G., ed., 1939: Meister Albrants Rossarzneibuch im deutschen Osten, 160 p. (Schriften dtsch. wiss. Ges. Reichenberg, pt. 9) (Reichenberg: Kraus).—

About this book Sarton writes in Isis 33: 94: "Study of the text, and tradition in the German East, of a mysterious treatise on the veterinary art ascribed in the mss. and early editions... to one Master Albertin = Albrecht = Albrant, said to have been marshal to Frederick the Great (d. 1250) later to Pope Clement (Clement IV, 1265-1268) ..."

Albrecht van Borgunnien (fl. *ca.* 1425-1450) — WARDALE, W. L., ed., 1936: Treatise on medicine (Sloane ms. 3002, British Museum), 47 + 80 p. (London: Oxford U.P.).—

An English translation of a 15th-century medico-astrological treatise attributed to a certain Albrecht van Burgonnien, written in a Saxon dialect, typical of the Baltic Colonial Area, 1425-1450. As to the writer nearly nothing is known. The text has been given in the original language. Of much interest are the recipes. Glossary and bibliography. The work is mainly of a philological importance.

Aldobrandino of Siena (d. 1287) — LANDOUZY, L. & R. PÉPIN, eds., 1911: Le régime du corps, de Maîstre Aldebrandin de Sienne. Texte français du XIIIe siècle. Publié pour la première fois avec variantes, glossaire et réproductions de miniatures, 78 + 261 p. (Paris: Champion).—

The "Régime du corps" is divided into four main parts dealing respectively with:

1. General hygiene (treating of such subjects as: climate, eating, drinking, sexual life, bathing, blocd-letting, purgation, use of cupping glasses and leeches, hygiene of travellers, *etc.);* 2. Special hygiene of various organs (hair, eyes, ears, teeth, face, stomach, liver, heart); 3. Dietetics (cereals, beverages, meat, birds, beans, fruits, herbs, fish, *etc.);* 4. Physiognomy. The whole work relies heavily upon Arabic sources. The book under consideration is a critical edition of the original French text, with an elaborate introduction, elaborate glossary, and illustrations.

Alexander   Neckam   (1157-1217)   — WRIGHT, T., ed., 1863: Alexandri Neckam "De naturis rerum libri duo", with the poem of the same author, "De laudibus divinae sapientiae", 78 + 521 p. (London: Longmans).—

The long preface contains much information about Neckam's life, time, and work. The "De naturis rerum" is a popular encyclopaedia of scientific knowledge, divided into 5 books. It consists of two very distinct parts; the first two books form a sort of a manual of natural science as it was then thought, and the other three books form a commentary on the book of Ecclesiastes. Chapter 23 of the first book deals with natural history; much in it is taken from Solinus, Cassiodorus, Aristotle, and Pliny. Many animals have been considered, wild as well as domesticated, incl. mammals, birds, toads, serpents and even mystic animals (barnacle-goose, phoenix). Also plants, fruit trees, agriculture, and domestic implements are considered. The introduction contains short summaries of all the chapters included. Then the "De laudibus divinae sapientiae", a poetic paraphrase on the "De naturis rerum" follows. Reprinted in 1964 (New York, N.Y.: Kraus). S. GASELEE (1936) published a lecture based on the "De naturis rerum": Natural science in England at the end of the twelfth century, 21 p. (London).

Arnald of Villanova (1240-1311) — DIEPGEN, P., ed., 1922: Des Meisters Arnald von Villanova Parabeln der Heilkunst. Aus dem Lateinischen übersetzt, erklärt und eingeleitet, 67 p. (Leipzig: Barth).—

The "Parabels of health" is a treatise of medicine in condensed form. It is divided into seven doctrines which read in Diepgen's translation as follows: 1. Regeln welche die Seele des Arztes zu nützlichem Vorgehen instand setzen (1 Kap.); 2. Regeln, die besten Behandlungsmittel auszuwählen und zur Anwendung zu bringen (1 Kap.); 3. Regeln über die Abschätzung des Kräftezustandes des Kranken... (1 Kap.); 4. Regeln über die Behandlung der krankhaften Veränderungen des Temperaments (21 Kap.); 5. Regeln über die Behandlung der Krankheiten, welche die Struktur des Körpers betreffen (21 Kap.); 6. Ueber die Behandlung der zusammengesetzten Krankheit (1 Kap.); 7. Ueber das Regimen der Rekonvaleszenten (3 Kap.). *Cf.* also: STRAUSS, P., 1963: Arnald von Villanova. Deutsch unter besonderer Berücksichtigung der "Regel der Gesundheit", 197 p. (Inaug. Diss. Heidelberg).

——, VERRIER, R., 1947-1949: Études sur Arnauld de Villeneuve (1240?-1311) — Vol. I (1947): 88 p.; Vol. II (1949): 170 p. (Leiden: Brill).—

    Vol. I contains much biographical information concerning Arnald of Villanova and some of his relatives, particularly of his two nephews Jean and Armengaud Blaisse, of whom the first became a famous physician, and the second became one of the pioneer translators of Arabic and Hebrew medical books. Vol. II deals with the authorship of the "Breviarium practicae" and with the question of Arnald's studies at Naples. Besides, much biographical detail is given of John of Casamicciola, one of the leading physicians of that time and possibly one of the teachers of Arnald. For a list of works and translations ascribed to Arnald, *cf.* Sarton's Introduction II (2): 894-897, and BATLLORI, P. M., 1947: Arnau de Villanova. Obres catalanes, Vol. II: Ecrits medics, 276 p. (Barcelona: Barcino).

Arnoldus Doneldey *(ca.* 1342-*ca.* 1395) — WINDLER, E., ed., 1932: Das Bremer mittelniederdeutsche Arzneibuch des Arnoldus Doneldey. Mit Einleitung und Glossar, 83 p. (Niederdeutsche Denkmäler, No. 7) (Neumünster: Wachholtz).—

    Arnoldus Doneldey wrote his "Arzneibuch" in 1382. The present booklet contains an introduction, discussing the ms. and sources of the text. The conclusion of the editor is that this Arzneibuch has been composed of some high German sources, more especially those of Bartholomaeus. A separate chapter deals with the relationship of the Middle-Low-German pharmacopoeias to mediaeval medical literature.

Augustine (354-430) — KEENAN, M. E., 1936: Augustine and the medical profession, 22 p. (Trans. Amer. Phil. Assn. 67: 168-190).—

    A collection of those passages in the work of St. Augustine that contain allusions to the medical profession. A collection of those passages in his work that contain allusions to biology are assembled in another publication of the same authoress: St. Augustine and biological science (Osiris 7: 588-608, 1939).

Bartholomaeus Anglicus (d. *ca.* 1250) — STEELE, R., 1905: Mediaeval lore from Bartholomew Anglicus, 195 p. (London: Moring).—

    Bartholomew wrote an encyclopaedia, the "De proprietatibus rerum", an encyclopaedia of similes for the benefit of the preaching village friars. It was written to explain the allusions to natural objects met with in the scriptures; it was immensely popular during about three centuries. The present book contains a selection of passages from the work for modern readers, and the text is somewhat adapted to this purpose, *e.g.,* by modernizing the spelling, by the introduction of modern grammatical forms, by the substitution of modern words for obsolete words, and by the inclusion of a glossary. Introduction, considering the book and its object, its popularity during the Middle Ages, its previous editions, sources, *etc.* Separate sections deal with science, manners, medicine, geography, and natural history (of trees, birds, fishes and other animals), during the Middle Ages. Reprinted in 1966 (New York, N.Y.: Cooper Square). As to the medical part of this encyclopaedia, *cf.* WALSH, J. J., ed., 1933: De proprietatibus rerum (Book seventh - on medicine): annotated with an introductory essay, 143 p. (Medical life 40: 453-496; 499-544; 547-602).

Bartholomew of Salerno (1st half 12th cent.) — HAUPT, J., 1872: Ueber das mitteldeutsche Arzneibuch des Meisters Bartholomaeus, 115 p. (Sitzb. Akad. Wiss., Wien, Phil. Kl., 71: 451-566).—

    Bartholomew was the author of a "Practica", a treatise on pathology and therapeutics which enjoyed great popularity in Western Europe during the Middle Ages. The text of this "Practica" can be found in: RENZI, S. DE, 1856, vol. 4: 321-406. *(Vide* subsection c).

Benevenutus Grassus (fl. first half 12th century) — WOOD, C. A., 1929: Benevenutus Grassus of Jerusalem "De oculis eorumque egritudinibus et curis", transl. with notes and illustrations from the first printed edition,

Ferrara, 1474 A.D., 101 p. (Stanford, Calif.: Stanford U.P.).—

Benevenutus Grassus was the most famous non-Muslim oculist of mediaeval times. His "De oculis" was for over 500 years the most popular ophthalmic manual of the Middle Ages, and some 40 texts of it still exist. After some biographical information, the text of the "De oculis" follows in English translation (p. 27-83). Included are a catalogue of the codices and printings of the "De oculis" (mss., printed editions, and reprints), and a bibliography.

Cassiodorus *(ca.* 490-*ca.* 580) — JONES, L. W., ed., 1946: An introduction to divine and human readings, by Cassiodorus Senator. Translation, with an introduction and notes, 233 p. (New York, N.Y.: Columbia U.P.).—

The introduction, discussing life, work, *etc.* of the Ostrogothic statesman and scholar is followed by a translation of the "Institutiones divinarum et humanarum litterarum"; they were meant as a general introduction for the reading of divine and secular letters. A short chapter deals with medicine (Dioscorides, Hippocrates, Galen, Caelius Aurelianus). This is followed by a summary of the seven liberal arts. The book must have been written sometime after 551. (According to Sarton, Isis 39:74).

Charlemagne *(ca.* 742-814) — GAREIS, K., ed., 1895: Die Landgüterordnung Kaiser Karl des Grossen (Capitulare de villis vel curtis imperii), 68 p. (Berlin: Guttenberg).—

Text, notes, and introduction. This "Capitulare" (=ordinance) dates probably from 812 and is very important for the history of agriculture. There also exists a newer German translation: FLEISCHMANN, W., 1919, 76 p. (Berlin) (not seen). An insight into pharmaceutical knowledge of those days is given by STICKER, G., 1924: Die gebräuchlichen Heilkräuter in Deutschland zur Zeit Karls des Grossen. (Janus 28: 21-41).

Chaucer, Geoffrey *(ca.* 1340-1400) — CURRY, W. C., 1960: Chaucer and the mediaeval sciences, 367 p. (London: Allen & Unwin).—

„This volume is the result of an attempt to follow Geoffrey Chaucer in his studies of the mediaeval sciences and to indicate with what degree of success he has employed scientific materials in the creation of his poetical works." There is much in it that is of interest for the history of medicine (one chapter deals with the doctor of physic and mediaeval medicine), alchemy, astrology, and the interpretation of dreams.

Conrad of Megenberg (1309-1374) — PFEIFFER, F., ed., 1962: Das Buch der Natur von Konrad von Megenberg. Die erste Naturgeschichte in deutscher Sprache, 52 + 807 p. (Hildesheim: Olms).—

A reprint of the original edition of 1861. (Stuttgart: Aue). The introduction contains a review of life and work of Conrad of Megenberg and a general discussion of the underlying scheme of the book. "Das Buch der Natur" is a free translation of the "De natura rerum" of Thomas of Cantimpré. Each of the 8 chapters into which the book is divided is preceded by an introduction containing moralizations and theological ideas. The general scheme of the book under consideration is as follows: 1. Vom Menschen im Allgemeinen (p. 4-54); 2. Von den Himmeln und den sieben Planeten (p. 55-118); 3. Von den Thieren im Allgemeinen (von den vierfüssigen Thieren, p. 119-162; vom Geflügel, p. 166-230; von den Meerwundern, p. 231-243; von den Fischen, p. 244-261; von den Schlangen, p. 262-286; von den Würmern, p. 287-310); 4a. Von den Bäumen (p. 311-353); 4b. Von den wohlriechenden Bäumen (p. 354-379); 5. Von den Kräutern (p. 380-430); 6. Von den Edelsteinen (p. 431-473); 7. Von den Metallen (p. 474-481); 8. Von den wunderbaren Gewässern (p. 482-494). Elaborate critical apparatus and glossary (p. 495-807). There exists another German edition: SCHULZ, H., ed., 1897: Das Buch der Natur von Conrad von Megenberg. Die erste Naturgeschichte in deutscher Sprache. In neu hochdeutscher Sprache bearbeitet und mit Anmerkungen versehen, 445 p. (Greifswald: Abel).

———, IBACH, H., 1938: Leben und Schriften des Konrad von Megenberg, 185 p. (Neue Deutsche Forschungen, No. 210) (Berlin: Dünnhaupt).—

This book contains an elaborate sketch of the life and work of Conrad, the southern German scientist, theologian and historian. He was the first great scientific writer in German and he did much to help educate the women and the common people. The present book places Conrad within the framework of his time and it includes a list of the 28 writings ascribed to him.

Constantine the African (d. 1087)—STEINSCHNEIDER, M., 1866: Constantinus Africanus und seine arabischen Quellen, 79 p. (Virchows Archiv 37: 331-410).—

Constantinus was the first great translator of Arabic literature into Latin. A great number of medical treatises were translated by him, and though Muslim influences in the School of Salerno were accidental and limited at the beginning, they were considerably increased by these activities of Constantine, especially because he stayed for a while in Salerno. See also: SUDHOFF, K., 1932: Constantin, der erste Vermittler muslimischer Wissenschaft ins Abendland und die beiden salernitaner Fruehscholastiker Maurus und Urso als Exponenten dieser Vermittlung (Archeion 14: 359-369); and CREUTZ, R., 1929: Der Arzt Constantinus Africanus von Montekassino. (Studien u. Mitteilungen zur Geschichte des Benediktinerordens, Neue Folge, Vol. 16, pars 1: 1-44). Constantine's dentistry is dealt with in: NORD, K., 1922: Zahnheilkundliches aus den Schriften Konstantins von Afrika, 31 p. (Diss. Sudhoff Inst., Leipzig).

Copho (ca. 1060) — CREUTZ, R., ed., 1938-1941: Der Magister Copho und seine Stellung im Hochsalerno, 98 p. (Sudhoffs Arch. Gesch. Med. Naturw. 31 (1938): 51-60; 33 (1941): 249-338).—

The first publication (1938) contains a brief introduction to the text of the "Practica Cophonis" as it can be found in ms. M.p. med. Q 2 (Sacc. XIII) fol. 85a - 103a Würzburg; which text was published in 1941. In his introduction Creutz states that only the "Practica Cophonis" can be considered as having been written by Copho. The Würzburg ms. consists of two parts, the first dealing with fevers (in 61 chapters), the second with diseases a capite ad calcem in 85 chapters. Copho was a contemporary of Bartholomaeus, Ferrarius, and Petronius, and a pupil of Constantinus Africanus and probably also of Johannes Platearius II.

Cyprianus of Carthage (d. 258) — BALL, M. T., 1946: Nature and the vocabulary of nature in the works of Saint Cyprian, 303 p. (Diss. Catholic Univ. America) (Washington, D.C.: Catholic Univ. America Press).—

The author discusses St. Cyprian's thoughts about nature and the vocabulary of nature in the apologetic works, in the disciplinary works and in the letters. Ball summarizes Cyprian's views in the following words: "He showed how the Lord's own method of drawing proof of and illustration for His mighty truths, and striking lessons for our instruction from the familiar world about Him, was practical and effective in any day and in every land."

Dante (1265-1321) — HOLBROOK, R. T., 1902: Dante and the animal kingdom, 376 p. (New York, N.Y.: Columbia U.P.).—

"This book aims to set forth Dante Alighieri's whole philosophy of the animal kingdom, to show from what sources he derived his knowledge, and to what ends his knowledge is employed." After a brief introduction considering the mediaeval animal kingdom, and the animals in mediaeval art, the author proceeds to the position of man, the angels, and the devil and his brood (Charon, Minos, Pluto, the Furies, Minotaur, Centaurs, Harpies, Siren, giants, Lucifer). Among the beasts discussed are: monkey, ounce, lion, wolf, dog, fox, panther, cat, mouse, mole, bear, horse, mule, ass, cattle, swine, sheep, goat, deer, beaver, otter, elephant, whale, dolphin, frog, fish, sponge, griffin, kite, eagle, crow, lark, nightingale, dove, starling, crane, stork, pelican, swan blackbird, magpie, rook, phoenix, swallow, goose, cock, snail, serpent, scorpion, worm, caterpillar, butterfly, fly, flea, wasp, grasshopper, spider, ant, and bee. Other short chapters deal with lower animals, Dante's meeting with the three beasts, fowling and falconry. Good index. Reprinted in 1965 (New York, N.Y.: Ams Press). There also seem to exist two studies concerning Dante and medicine, viz., DRURY, G., 1908: Dante physician, 90 p. (Cincinnati, O.); and GIUFFRE, L., 1924: Dante e le scienze mediche, 194 p. (Bologna: Zanichelli); titles which I could not verify.

——, KUHNS, L. O., 1897: The treatment of nature in Dante's "Divina commedia", 208 p. (London: Arnold).—

In this study the author aims at giving a picture of all those aspects of animate and inanimate nature which Dante has made use of in the "Divina commedia". Chapter-headings are as follows: 1. Dante's conception of nature; 2. Dante's conventional treatment of nature; 3. The different aspects of nature as seen in the "Inferno", the "Purgatorio", and the "Paradiso"; 4. Italy in the "Divina commedia"; 5. The physical geography of the "Divina commedia"; 6. Atmospheric phenomena; 7. The flora of the "Divina commedia"; 8. The fauna of the "Divina commedia"; 9. The heavenly bodies; 10. Light, fire, and colour; 11. General discussion of Dante's attitude toward nature. Index.

Daude de Pradas (first half 13th century).—
Vide Frederik II of Hohenstaufen, infra.

Eberhard von Wampen (fl. ca. 1325) —

BJÖRKMAN, E., 1902: Everhards von Wampen Spiegel der Natur, ein in Schweden verfasstes mittelniederdeutsches Lehrgedicht, 84 p. (Uppsala Universitets Årsskrift).—

The "Spegel der Naturen" (Speculum naturae) is a poem in Low German of which 1775 lines are extant. It is divided into 4 books containing the following topics: Bk. I: an introduction, explaining the doctrine of the four elements, their qualities and the temperaments relying upon them; Bk. II: the ailments relative to each temperament, their causes and remedies; temperaments and seasons, ages, celestial, *etc.* conditions; signs of the zodiac; food and drugs, *etc.;* Bk. III: the properties of animals, herbs and stones, including various dietetic and medical rules; Bk. IV: rules for the preservation of health. Bks. III and IV are incomplete.

Frederick II of Hohenstaufen (1194-1250) — WOOD, C. A. & F. M. FYFE, 1943: The art of falconry, being the "De arte venandi cum avibus" of Frederick II of Hohenstaufen, 110 + 637 p. (Stanford, Calif.: Stanford U.P.; London: Oxford U.P.).—

A very beautiful translation of the old mss. of Frederick II. It gives a very good picture of Frederick's ornithological knowledge; abundant footnotes give additional information. There are 186 (for the greater part admirable) illustrations, including reproductions of miniatures and drawings from the various existing mss. Complete and annotated bibliography of ancient, mediaeval, and modern falconry. A second printing appeared in 1955 (Boston, Mass.: Branford; London: Oxford U.P.). Reissued in 1961 by Stanford U.P. A complementary text is: SCHUTZ, A. H., ed., 1945: The romance of Daude de Pradas called Dels Auzels Cassadors, 225 p. (Columbus, Ohio: Ohio State U.P.). This is an elaboration of Daude's 3792-line poem on falconry, a text of the late second quarter of the 13th century. The study is especially of philological importance. For a study dealing with falconry in the near East, *vide* TJERNELD, H., 1945, section The Middle Ages in the Near East δ, subsection b.

Gilbertus Anglicus (fl. *ca.* 1250) — HANDERSON, H. E., 1918: Gilbertus Anglicus: medicine of the XIIIth century, with a biography of the author, 77 p. (Cleveland, Ohio: Cleveland Med. Library Assn.).—

Sarton writes about this book (Isis 3: 325): "The book is scholarly and thorough without being heavy." Gilbertus Anglicus

wrote a compilation of Salernitan and Arabic medicine, dealing with diseases of the head, the hair, the nerves, the eyes, the face, the skin, the external members, the urogenital system, fevers, gout, cancer, poisons, hygiene, surgery, internal diseases, *etc.* A study especially dealing with dentistry in Gilbertus "Compendium" is: SEIDEMANN, M., 1922: Zahnärztliches in den Werken des Gilbertus Anglicus, 22 p. (Diss. Sudhoff Inst.). This study includes a brief summary of general knowledge about Gilbertus, and a list of mss.

Giles of Corbeil (d. *ca.* 1222) — VIEILLARD, C., 1909: Essai sur la société médicale et religieuse au XIIe siècle. Gilles de Corbeil, médecin de Philippe-Auguste et chanoine de Notre Dame, 475 p. (Paris: Champion).—

Giles of Corbeil was a French physician, who studied in Salerno and who later on became archiater to King Philip Augustus. In the first part of the present book (p. 1-336), the author places Giles of Corbeil within the framework of his time, considering his life and work, his medical teachings, his work as a physician, his relationship to the School of Salerno, the medicines used by him, *etc.* It also deals with his religious ideas and with the position of the "Hierapigra" in this connection. The second part (p. 337-412) has extracts from his medical poems, containing interesting information on the medical customs of his time, such as the "De urinis", a popular textbook on uroscopy, the "De pulsibus", and the "De laudibus et virtutibus compositorum medicaminum"; it also contains long extracts from the "Hierapigra" in French translation. An appendix contains an essay in which Giles defends the study of medicine and another deals with the physician's attitude to his patient. *Cf.* also: d'IRSAY, S., 1925: The life and works of Gilles de Corbeil (Ann. Med. Hist. 7: 362-378); and SUDHOFF, K., 1929: Commentatoren der Harnverse des Gilles de Corbeil (Archeion 11: 129-135). *Cf.* VIEILLARD, C., 1903, *vide* subsection c.

Guy de Chauliac (fl. *ca.* 1320) — NICAISE, E., 1890: La grande chirurgie de Guy de Chauliac, chirurgien, maistre en médecine de l'université de Montpellier, composée en l'an 1363, 191 + 747 p. (Paris: Alcan).—

In his general introduction the editor considers the interrelations between science and religion during the Middle Ages on the one hand, and the position of medicine and surgery during this period on the other hand. Then follows a discussion of Guy de Chauliac's sources (Hippocrates, Galen, Arabic influences, Schools of Salerno and of Bologna); list of authors *(ca.* 90) quoted by Guy de Chauliac; medical education in Montpellier and Paris during the Middle Ages; medical pharmacy. Biography of Guy de Chauliac (30 p.) and bibliography (mss. extant, printed editions, *etc.,* 86 p.). Then the French translation follows (p. 1-668), followed by glossaries concerning the therapeutics and instruments used, anatomical and pathological terms, and subjects considered. Reprint edition, 1965 (New York, N.Y.: Johnson). A part of the text exists in English translation: BRENNAN, W. A., ed., 1923: Wounds and fractures, 152 p. (Chicago, Ill.: Author). An evaluation of Guy de Chauliac's surgery within the framework of mediaeval medical science. *Cf.* also BRUNN, W. von, 1920-1921: Die Stellung des Guy de Chauliac in der Chirurgie des Mittelalters, 56 p. (Arch. Gesch. Med. 12: 85-100; 13: 65-106).

——, WALLNER, B., ed., 1964: The middle English translation of Guy de Chauliac's Anatomy, with Guy's essay on the history of medicine, 36 + 250 p. (Lunds Univ. Årsskrift, N.F., Avd. 1, Vol. 56, No. 5) (Lund:Gleerup).—

The "Anatomy" is the first of the seven treatises Guy wrote for his "Chirurgia magna". This edition includes a long introduction, containing a short sketch of Guy's life and work, and a review of the extant mss., their relationship, and the various dialects in which they were written.

Henri of Mondeville (d. *ca.* 1325) — NICAISE, E., 1893: Chirurgie de Maître Henri de Mondeville, chirurgien de Philippe le Bel. Traduction française avec des notes, une introduction et une biographie, 82 + 903 p. (Paris: Alcan).—

Henri of Mondeville was one of the leading French surgeons. He wrote a textbook on surgery, consisting of 5 treatises. The first treatise deals with anatomy, the second with the treatment of wounds, ulcers, contusions, *etc.,* the third with special surgical pathology and therapeutics (smallpox, measles, blood-letting, amputations, abcesses), the fourth with fractures and luxations, and the fifth treatise consists of an antidotary. Although containing many original observations, applications, *etc.,* it also assembles much of the knowledge of Hippocrates, Aristotle, Galen, Mesuë, Serapion, al-Rāzī, Avicenna, Theodoric Burgogni, and many others. About the book under consideration, Sarton writes in his "Introduction" Vol. III

(1): 872: "This is a modern translation with valuable notes, a study of surgical instruments used in the Middle Ages, and an additional glossary of drugs and their synonyms by Dr Saint-Lager." In a series of dissertations prepared under guidance of J. Pagel, parts of the "Cyrurgia" have been translated into German. A list of them can be found in Sarton *l. c.,* p. 872, and in PAGEL, J., 1896: Neue literarische Beiträge zur mittelalterliche Medizin, p. 195 (Berlin: Reimer). Also published: BOSSHARD, J. A., 1963: Psychosomatik in der Chirurgie des Mittelalters, besonders bei Henri de Mondeville, 39 p. (Inaug. Diss. Univ. Zurich) (Zurich: Juris). There also exists a French edition by A. BOS, 1898: La chirurgie de Maître Henri de Mondeville, 2 vols., 48 + 287 p. and 340 resp. This edition was reprinted in 1965 (New York, N.Y.: Johnson).

Henricus Breyell (fl. *ca.* 1450) — BESSLER, O., 1952: Das deutsche Hortus-Manuscript des Henricus Breyell, 73 p. (Nova Acta Leopoldina, N. F., Vol. 15, No. 107).—

A table elucidates the relationship of Breyell's botanical knowledge with that of Matthaeus Sylvaticus, William of Saliceto, Vincent of Beauvais, Barth. Anglicus, Albertus Magnus, Gerard of Cremona, the "Circa instans", the "Herbarius Apulei Platonici", the "Gart der Gesundheit" and the "Hortus Sanitatis". The ms. itself consists of 4 parts: a herbal, a receptary, a treatise dealing with "gebrannte Wässer", and a treatise dealing with wines of medical importance. In the present study only the first part has been discussed in some detail. This work was written *ca.* 1511 in a Rhineland dialect. Much biographical information.

Herrad of Landsberg (d. 1195) — STRAUB, A. & G. KELLER, 1899: Herrade de Landsberg. Hortus deliciarum, 113 plates. (Strasbourg: Imp. Strasbourgeoise).—

Herrad of Landsberg was a German nun who, for the instruction of her nuns, composed a sort of popular encyclopaedia, called the Hortus deliciarum. It is largely of a theologico-philosophical character. The present book is mainly a facsimile reproduction of the illustrations and is very useful from the point of view of Christian iconography. The introduction contains a review of Herrad of Landsberg, her life and work.

Hieronymus Brunschwig (1450-1512) — SIGERIST, H. E., ed., 1923: The book of cirurgia by Hieronymus Brunschwig (Strassburg, Johann Grüninger, 1497), with a study on Hieronymus Brunschwig and his work, 272 + 16 p. (Milan: Lier).—

The first 272 pages consist of a beautiful facsimile edition of Hier. Brunschwig's classical treatise on surgery. Hieronymus was the first German surgeon to write an important manual that far surpassed the average productions, and to take advantage of the recently-invented printing-press. The last 16 pages of the book consist of a short biography of Hieronymus, a commentary on the text, and a short bibliography. A somewhat older facsimile reproduction with introduction, *etc.,* is: KLEIN, G., ed., 1911: Das Buch der Cirurgia des Hieronymus Brunschwig. Strassburg, Johann Grüninger, 1497, 272 + 38 p. (Alte Meister der Medizin und Naturkunde, No. 3) (Munich: Kuhn).

Hildegard von Bingen (1098-1179) — RIETHE, P., ed., 1959: Naturkunde. Das Buch von dem inneren Wesen der verschiedenen Naturen in der Schöpfung. Nach den Quellen übersetzt und erläutert, 176 p. (Salzburg: Müller).—

This book is a translation of one of the two parts of the "Liber subtilitatum" (*cf.* SCHIPPERGES, H., 1957, *vide infra*) and is internationally known by the title: "Liber simplicis medicinae" or "Physica". It deals mainly with plants and animals, but also with minerals, stones, and metals, and emphasizes medical applications. It is composed of 9 books each of which is preceded by a short and very helpful introduction written by the translator, and some of the books are preceded by a preface by Hildegard in which she explains her ideas about the origin and characteristics of the elements mentioned. Although much in this work has been copied from already existing writings, Hildegard nevertheless has - according to the editor - to be valued for making the first attempt at critical and independent observation during the Middle Ages, and thereby she foreshadowed a new epoch.

——, SCHIPPERGES, H., ed., 1957: Heilkunde. Das Buch von dem Grund und Wesen und der Heilung der Krankheiten. Nach den Quellen übersetzt und erläutert, 332 p. (Salzburg: Müller).—

This book is a translation of the "Liber compositae medicinae" (also known as "Causae et Curae"), the other part of the "Liber subtilitatum diversarum naturarum creaturum" (*cf.* RIETHE, P., 1959, *vide supra*). In order to comprehend Hildegard's

views on diseases and their cure of human beings, one must be aware that these views cannot be separated from her visionary, cosmological, and theological ideas. This the translator fully realizes; in a rather extensive introduction, and in critical discussions at the end of each chapter, he pays full attention to these aspects. The text is translated from a symbolic mediaeval language (which - because it starts from the unity of science, theology, and mysticism - is very difficult to follow for a scholar trained in the methodology of modern science) into the modern language of science. Another German translation of the same text, but without such extensive annotations is: SCHULZ, H., 1955: Hildegard von Bingen. Ursachen und Behandlung der Krankheiten (causae et curae), 373 p. (Ulm: Haug).

——, 1965: Welt und Mensch. Das Buch "De operatione Dei" von Hildegard von Bingen aus dem Genter Kodex übersetzt und erläutert, 358 p. (Salzburg: Müller).—

In the "De operatione Dei" a series of 10 visions have been described. They are titled as follows: Ursprung des Lebens; Bau der Welt; Natur des Menschen; Gliederung des Leibes; Stätten der Läuterung; Sinn der Geschichte; Vorbereitung auf Christus; Wirken der Liebe; Vollendung des Kosmos; Ende der Zeiten. There is much in it that is of interest to the historian of medicine and of anthropology. Together they give an impression of 12th-century cultural life.

——, SCHRÄDER, M. & A. FÜHRKÖTTER, 1956: Die Echtheit des Schrifttums der heiligen Hildegard von Bingen. Quellenkritische Untersuchungen, 208 p. (Cologne & Graz: Böhlau).—

Critical evaluation of the sources, which led the authoresses to the conclusion that the authenticity of Hildegard's writings has been proved.

Hrafn Sveinbjarnarson (13th cent.) — TJOMSLAND, A., ed., 1951: Hrafns saga sveinbjarnarsonar: the saga of Hrafn Sveinbjarnarson, the life of an Icelandic physician of the thirteenth century with translation, introduction, and notes, 65 p. (Cornell Univ. Library, Islandica, Vol. 35) (Ithaca, N.Y.: Cornell U.P.).—

This book contains the life history of Hrafn, an Icelandic physician, as it is transmitted by a saga. This saga is discussed from the medical point of view but much attention has been paid to the cultural, historical, and literary points of view as well. The pilgrimages of Hrafn are considered and also his visits to the medical centres of Salerno and Bologna and the influences on his medical teachings.

Isidore of Seville *(ca.* 560-636) — SHARPE, W. D., ed., 1964: Isidore of Seville: the medical writings, 75 p. (Trans. Amer. Phil. Soc., N.S., 54, pt. 2).—

> An English translation of the medical and anatomical sections of Isidore's great encyclopaedia, with many annotations. In an introduction the editor relates Isidore's work to that of his predecessors, in which he not only considers purely medical authors, but also examines the views of the Church Fathers. Appendixes deal with the pulse, frenesis, iliac passion, plague, and undulant fevers. Valuable bibliography. A biography mainly dealing with Isidore as a theologian is: PÉREZ DE URBEL, J., 1945: Isidor von Sevilla, sein Leben, sein Werk, seine Zeit, 285 p. (Cologne: Bachem).

——, FONTAINE, J., ed., 1960: Isidore de Sevilla: Traité de la nature, 466 p. (Bordeaux: Féret).—

> The first translation of the "De rerum natura" in any modern language. The author considers the mss. still extant, the diffusion of Isidore's work through Europe (elucidated by a map illustrating the geographical and chronological diffusion), the Latin text (on pages to the right) and French translation (on pages to the left). *Cf.* also FONTAINE, J., 1959: Isidore de Seville et la culture classique dans l'Espagne wisigothique, 2 vols. (Paris: Études Augustiniennes). Not much of a biohistorical interest.

Jan Yperman *(ca.* 1270- *ca.* 1330) — LEERSUM, E. C. van, 1912: De "Cyrurgie" ·van Meester Jan Yperman, naar de handschriften van Brussel, Cambridge, Gent en Londen, 43 + 286 p. (Leiden: Sijthoff).—

> A critical edition in the Dutch language of Jan Yperman's book on surgery. Jan Yperman was a Flemish surgeon, the founder of surgery in the Netherlands. He mainly followed Lanfranchi's surgery. Only four mss. of his surgery are known. The work has been divided into 7 books, *viz.,* 1. head (30 chapters); 2. eyes (25 ch.); 3. nose (7 ch.); 4. mouth (20 ch.); 5. ears (9 ch.); 6. neck and throat (12 ch.) 7. rest of the body (40 ch.). The present edition is based on all four mss., contains an elaborate

introduction, notes, bibliography and glossary (p. 234-280). Besides this book on surgery, Yperman also wrote a book on practical medicine, including chapters on dropsy, rheumatism, apoplexy, epilepsy, frenzy, lethargy, lung abscesses, and on the treatment of haemorrhages by ligatures and torsions of the arteries; *cf.* BROECKX, C., 1867: Traité de médecine pratique de maître Jean Yperman, publié pour la première fois de la copie flamande de la Bibliothèque royale de Bruxelles, 147 p. (Antwerp: Buschmann).

Joannes de Ketham Alemanus (15th cent.) — SINGER, C. & K. SUDHOFF, eds., 1924: Joannes de Ketham Alemanus. Fasciculus Medicinae, 1491. Facsimile of the first edition with an historical introduction and notes by K. Sudhoff, translated and adapted by C. Singer, 55 p. (Monumenta Medica, Vol. I) (Milan: Lier).—

> This volume contains a complete facsimile of the incunabulum, including its illustrations which are of a didactical sort. The introduction contains a very complete study of the fasciculus itself, of the author, and of the ms. antecedents and illustrations. A pleasing Italian edition is: MANCINI, C., *et al.,* 1964: Il "Fasciculus medicinae" di Giovanni da Ketham (1495), 177 p. (Scientia Veterum. Collana di Studi di storia della medicina) (Pisa: Gardini). (*Cf.* also SINGER, C., 1925, *vide infra*).

——, SINGER, C., ed., 1925: The Fasciculo di Medicina, Venice 1493, 2 vols. Vol. I: Atlas of 90 illustrative figures from manuscript and printed sources with explanatory legends, 112 p.; Vol. II: Facsimile, 104 p. (Monumenta Medica, Vol. II) (Florence: Lier).—

> This is a facsimile of the second edition of Joannes de Ketham's "Fasciculo" (*cf.* C. SINGER & K. SUDHOFF, *vide supra*). This edition includes a lucid introduction and an English translation of Mondino's "Anathomia". Also reprinted in 1967: BOTTASSO, E., 1967: Fasciculo de medicina, Venice 5 Feb. 1493, 116 p. (Torino: Vita Farmaceutici). Bibliographical essay, p. 105-116.

Johannes Jacobi (d. 1384) — BLOEDNER, A. E., 1926: Das Secretarium practicae medicinae des Johannes Jacobi von Montpellier, 34 p. (Diss. Leipzig).—

> This is an analysis of the "Secretarium" (*ca.* 1378), which is an elaborate com-

pilation, together with an indication of its contents and a discussion of its sources. According to Bloedner, Johannes' compilation was largely based upon the "Passionarius" of Gariopontus, a Salernitan physician (d. *ca.* 1050). This "Passionarius" itself is a medical encyclopaedia, containing a collection of extracts from the late Greek, Byzantine, and Roman writers.

John of Arderne (1307-1380) — POWER, D'Arcy, 1922: De arte physicali et de cirurgia of Master John Arderne, surgeon of Newark, dated 1412. Transl. from a transcript made by E. Millar from the replica of the Stockholm ms. in the Wellcome Historical Medical Museum, 60 p. (London: Bale). —

John of Arderne was the first to revive surgery in England; he was essentially an operating surgeon whose practice lay amongst the nobility. He invented the cure of fistulae, and knew the literature of his time very well. His medical treatment was mainly that of Saxon leeches. The present edition contains many fine reproductions of anatomical drawings.

John of Gaddesden *(ca.* 1280-1361) — CHOLMELEY, H. P., 1912: John of Gaddesden and the Rosa medicinae, 184 p. (Oxford: Clarendon Press).—

John wrote his "Rosa medicinae" about 1314, a medical treatise which contains many mystical elements and also very good clinical observations. A small section is devoted to surgery, his antidotarium contains a large number of prescriptions. The "Rosa" gives us a valuable picture of 14th-century English folk remedies, superstitions, *etc.* Much of his knowledge John borrowed from Bernard of Gordon, Gilbert the Englishman, Peter of Spain, Hippocrates, Dioscorides, Galen, Avicenna, Constantine the African, Platearius, Giles of Corbeil, and others.

John Mandeville (d. 1372) — LETTS, M., 1949: Sir John Mandeville: the man and his book, 192 p. (London: Batchworth Press).—

Mandeville's travels perhaps was the most popular book of the later Middle Ages. The present booklet consists of three parts. The first part deals with Mandeville, the man (an English nobleman and physician), the times, his predecessors, and with the problem whether his travelbook is fictitious or not. The second part deals with the travels as such, the Near East, the route to

Cathay, Cathay and the Great Chan, Prester John, giants, Brahmans, golddigging ants, the earthly paradise, *etc.* The third part deals with such matters as: manuscripts and printed editions, translations, the transformation of place-names, errors in translation and the alphabets. A Latin-mediaeval English translation is: SEYMOUR, M. C., 1963: The Bodley version of Mandeville's travels, 188 p. (London: Oxford U.P.). Based on an exhaustive study of the mss., this edition presents the findings of modern scholarship which seeks to restore the book to its proper place in English literature. There also exists a German translation of Mandeville's travels: STEMMLER, T., ed., 1966: Die Reisen des Ritters John Mandeville durch das Gelobte Land, Indien und China. Bearbeitet nach der deutschen Uebersetzung des Otto von Diemeringen, 210 p. (Bibliothek klassischer Reiseberichte) (Stuttgart: Steingrüben). With 92 woodcuts from the Strasburg-edition of 1499.

John of Saint Amand (fl. *ca.* 1275-1312) — GÜNTHER, K., 1922: Johannes de Sancto Amando und sein Aderlasstraktat unter seinem Namen, 36 p. (Diss. Leipzig, Sudhoff Inst.) (Zeulenroda: Oberreuter).—

This booklet contains an edition of the "De flebotomia", the contents of which are an extract from the "Exposition". John of St. Amand was, according to Pagel, the main transmitter of Arabicized Greek medicine, especially for France. His largest work is the "Revocativum memoriae"; it is published in various theses of Pagel's pupils (Berlin, 1892-1895); other works of him have been edited by Pagel himself. A review can be found in Sarton's Introduction II (2): 1089-1091.

John of Saint Paul (fl. *ca.* 1175) — KROEMER, G. H., 1920: Johanns von Sancto Paulo Liber de simplicium medicinarum virtutibus und ein anderer salernitaner Traktat: Quae medicinae pro quibus morbis donandae sunt, nach dem Breslauer Codex herausgegeben, 86 p. (Diss. Sudhoff Inst.) (Borna-Leipzig: Noske).—

The "Liber de simplicium" is a collection of medical and chemical short recipes. The Breslau ms. (*cf.* HARTMANN, F., 1919, *vide* subsection c) was written *ca.* 1170, and this part of it is ascribed to Joannes de Sancto Paulo. Kroemer's study contains an elaborate bibliography and a dietetic-culinary-medical-pharmacological glossary. Another dissertation of the Sudhoff Institute deals with dietetics as discussed in a ms. which has also probably been written by Joannes: OSTERMUTH, H. J., 1919: Flores diaetarum, eine salernitanische Nahrungsmitteldiätetik aus dem XII. Jahrhundert verfasst vermutlich von Joannes de Sancto Paulo, 58 p. (Leipzig: Borna). This publication contains a technical glossary and bibliography. Of Joannes de Sancto Paulo we know hardly anything.

Lanfranchi (d. *ca.* 1306) — FLEISCH-HACKER, R. v., ed., 1894: Lanfrank's "Science of cirurgie", edited from the Bodleian Ashmole ms. 1396 (ab. 1380 A.D.) and the British Museum additional ms. 12.056 (ab. 1420 A.D.), 360 p. (London: Kegan Paul, Trench, Trübner).—

> Lanfrank was a disciple of William of Saliceto and may be called the founder of French surgery. His teaching seems to have been a real clinical teaching. He wrote a "Chirurgia magna", divided in 5 treatises as follows: 1. Definition of surgery, qualities of the surgeon, deontology, purposes of surgery; 2. Wounds of special parts, *a capite ad calcem,* together with the anatomy of these parts; 3. Other medical treatments, not necessarily surgical; 4. Fractures and luxations; 5. Antidotary. Fleischhacker's work is an edition of this work in archaic English. A more modern evaluation of Lanfrank is: MACDONALD, A. J., 1926: Lanfranc, a study of his life, work and writings, 307 p. (London: Milford). Unfortunately I am not able to give details of this book. A good review of the novelties included in the "Chirurgia magna" is given by Sarton: Introduction (2): 1080.

Macer, A. (fl. end 11th century) — FRISK, G., ed., 1949: A middle English translation of Macer floridus de viribus herbarum, 338 p. (Uppsala: Almqvist & Wiksells).—

> The "Macer floridus de virtutibus herbarum" is a mediaeval poem describing in 2,269 hexameters the medical properties of 77 herbs and roots. The herbal is based upon Pliny, Dioscorides, Galen, Oribasios, Gargilius Martialis, Palladius, Constantinus Africanus. It is one of the earliest documents indicating a revival of interest in botany. In Frisk's edition, the general introduction contains a review of the botanical and medical background, a description of the English translations of Macer, a comparison between the various extant mss., and philological remarks (p. 9-55). Next comes the text (p. 56-202), followed by notes, a glossary, a summary, an index of personal names, and a bibliography. Some authors believe that a certain Odo of Meung was the compiler of the "Macer floridus", *cf.*: RESAK, C.,

1917: Odo Magdunensis, der Verfasser des "Macer floridus" und der deutsche Leipziger Macer Text, 49 p. (Diss. Sudhoff Inst.) (Leipzig: Borna).

Marbode (Marbodus Redonensis) (1035-1123) — ERNAULT, L., 1890: Marbode, évêque de Rennes, sa vie et ses oeuvres (1035-1123). Extrait des Mémoires de la Soc. archéologique d'Ille-et-Vilaine, 261 p. (Rennes: Caillière).—

> According to Sarton, an important study. Marbode composed the "Liber lapidum" in which he described the medical and magical properties of some 60 precious stones. It consists of 743 hexameters which have been translated in many vernaculars. Most European lapidaries are derived from Marbode. A scientific edition with many notes and a glossary of a number of Anglo-Norman lapidaries, in prose and in verse, derived from Marbode's: STUDER, P. & J. EVANS, 1924: Anglo-Norman lapidaries, 404 p. (Paris: Champion).

Martin de Saint-Gille (fl. 1362-1365) — LAFEUILLE, G., ed., 1954: Les amphorismes Ypocras de Martin de Saint-Gille 1362-1365, 165 p. (Geneva: Droz).—

> This is a first attempt to translate a mediaeval Latin text into a vernacular. It consists of a French translation (of a part of the text) of Hippocrates' "Aphorisms", prepared by Martin de Saint-Gille in Avignon between 1362 and 1365, and according to Sarton in his preface, this event was of much historical interest, comparable with the importance of the translations of Oresme's works to the history of astronomy. This book is supplemented by a large introduction (40 p.) in which the editor tries to reconstruct life and activities of the author, by a glossary (p. 139-162), and by a larger study of the topic: "Les commentaires de Martin de Saint-Gille sur les amphorismes Yprocras, 1964, 388 p. (Geneva: Droz).

Matthaeus Platearius (d. 1161) — DORVEAUX, P., 1913: Le livre des simples médecins. Traduction française du Liber de simplici medicina dictus Circa instans de Platéarius tirée d'un manuscrit du XIIIe siècle et publiée pour la première fois, 280 p. (Paris: Soc. d'histoire de la médecine).—

> This Circa instans is a commentary on the "Antidotarium" of Nicolaus Praepositus (= Nicholas of Salerno, *vide infra*). The present ms. consists of 273 chapters

(more ample editions contain 432 chapters). Each chapter treats of a simple or other drug. They are arranged in an alphabetical order according to the Latin names of the drugs, and for each of them is given a description, mode of application, action, signs of purity, falsifications, distinctions of various kinds. A more or less specialized study is: ULLMANN, M. A., 1926: Geflügel, Eier, Fische, Früchte und Gemüse im Circa instans des Codex Salernitanus in Breslau, 28 p. (Diss. Sudhoff Inst.).

Maurus (fl. *ca.* 1160; d. 1214) — PLOSS, W. L. H., 1921: Anatomia Mauri, eine bisher unbekannte salernitaner Skizze vom Bau des Menschen auf Grundlage einer Zergliederung des Tierkörpers, herausgegeben nach einer weiland Heidelberger Handschrift des 12. Jahrhunderts im Vatikan zu Rom (Pal. lat. 1097, Bl. 122), 14 p. (Diss. Sudhoff Inst.) (Leipzig: Noske).—

Maurus was an anatomist and physician whose principal work was the "Anatomia Mauri", one of the earliest Latin texts on anatomy. It treats of the anatomy of the pig and it was strongly influenced by Constantinus Africanus. The present edition is based on a text dating from the second half of the 12th century. Another treatise composed by Maurus deals with venesection, *cf.:* BUERSCHAPPER, R., 1919: Ein bisher unbekannter Aderlasstraktat des salernitaner Arztes Maurus: De flebotomia, 38 p. (Diss. Sudhoff Inst.) (Borna-Leipzig: Noske). In this publication two texts are published *in extenso* in parallel columns *(viz.,* the ms. Dresden Db 91 and ms. Brussels 14324-14343), together with free translation and commentary.

Michael Scot (d. *ca.* 1235) — THORNDIKE, L., 1965: Michael Scot, 151 p. (Edinburgh: Nelson).—

According to Thorndike, Michael Scot may be regarded as the leading intellectual in Western Europe during the first third of the 13th century, one of the greatest transmitters of Aristotelian and Arabic knowledge to Western Europe. Thorndike has compiled a variety of scientific observations and speculations from works ascribed to Michael Scot, and has arranged them in some 8 chapters, one of them dealing with medicine (his medical reputation, uroscopy, pills ascribed to him, astrological medicine). There also are some remarks on his thoughts about plants, animals and Man. A valuable bibliography is: FERGUSON, J., 1931: A short biography and bibliography of Michael Scotus, 27 p. (Glasgow: Bibliograph. Soc.).

Mondino de Luzzi *(ca.* 1275-1326) — SIGHINOLFI, L. & G. VIOLA, 1930: Mondino de' Liucci. Anatomia. Riprodotta da un codice bolognese del secolo XIV e volgarizzata nel secolo XV, 197 p. + 18 p. facsimile reproduction of the original text. (Bologna: Capelli).—

Mondino was called the restorer of human anatomy whose chief work was a compendium of anatomy, the "Anatomia mundini", a practical textbook, arranged like a manual of dissection. The organs are dealt with in the following order: 1. abdominal cavity; 2. thoracic cavity; 3. head; 4. bones, spinal column, extremities. It is essentially Galenic in character. *Cf.* also: WICKERSHEIMER, E., 1926: Anatomies de Mundino de Luzzi et de Guido de Vigevano, 92 p. (Documents scientifiques du XVe siècle, part 3) (Paris: Droz).

Nicholas of Cues (1401-1464) — CREUTZ, R., 1939: Medizinisch-physikalisches Denken bei Nikolaus von Cues und die ihm als "Glossae Cardinalis" irrig zugeschriebenen medizinischen Handschriften, 34 p. (Cusanus-Studien, 4) (Sitzber. heidelb. Akad. Wiss., phil.-hist. Kl., 1938/39, pt. 3).—

A study concerning Cusanus' medical ideas and his relationship with Hippocrates, Galen, Asklepiades, Erasistratos, and the School of Salerno, especially Urso. The author makes it clear that the "Glossae Cardinalis" are wrongly ascribed to Cusanus.

——, HERON, F. G., ed., 1954: Of learned ignorance, 174 p. (New Haven, Conn.: Yale U.P.).—

Cardinal Cusanus was one of the first scientists to formulate non-scholastical ideas on the structure of the universe and man's place therein, albeit his ideas were based on mystical speculations. The present book reflects some of these ideas and is a translation of the "De docta ignorantia" (1440) into lucid English; it is intended for the educated general reader. Therefore, stress has been laid on modernity of language rather than on faithfulness to medical terminology and explanations; additional notes are lacking. *Cf.* also: LÜBKE, A., 1968: Nikolaus von Kues. Kirchenfürst zwischen Mittelalter und Neuzeit, 440 p. (Munich: Callwey); and WILPERT, P., ed., 1967: Nikolaus von Kues. Werke, 2 vols.

Vol. I: 336 p.; vol. 2: 770 p. (Quellen und Studien zur Geschichte der Philosophie, vols. 5 and 6) (Berlin: de Gruyter). A reissue of the Strasbourg-edition of 1488.

Nicholas of Salerno (= Nicolaus Praepositus, fl. *ca.* 1150) — DORVEAUX, P., 1896: L'antidotaire Nicolas. Deux trad. françaises de l'Antidotarium Nicolai, l'une du XIVᵉ siècle suivie de quelques recettes de la même époque et d'un glossaire, l'autre du XVᵉ siècle, incomplète; publiées d'après les manuscrits français 25.327 et 14.827 de la Bibliothèque Nationale, 109 p. (Paris: Welter).—

This antidotary is a collection of recipes transmitted by Greek and Latin writers to which have been added recipes of Arabic origin. The "Antidotarium" has been translated into many vernaculars and it became the basis of all the later pharmacopoeias. Ms. 25.327 consists of an abridged translation of the "Antidotarium Nicolai", of a series of secrets referring to yeasts and wine, and six medical recipes. The "Antidotarium" comprises 140 sections of which only 85 are translated. The ms. 14.827 is only a small part (12 sections) of a ms. that was complete but of which the main part has been lost. There also exists a Dutch translation by BERG, W. S. v. d., 1917: Eene middelnederlandsche vertaling van het "Antidotarium Nicolai". Met den latijnschen tekst der eerste gedrukte uitgave van het "Antidotarium Nicolai", 278 p. (Leiden: Brill). *Cf.* also: LUTZ, A., 1965: Das "Dispensarium ad aromatarias" des Nicolaus Praepositus (richtig Prepositi) um 1490 und seine Bedeutung für die Geschichte der Pharmazie, 16 p. (Veröffentl. Int. Ges. Gesch. der Pharmazie, N.F., 26: 87-103).

Odo of Meung, *vide* Macer, A., *supra.*

Ortolf von Baierland (fl. *ca.* 1400) — FOLLAN, J., ed., 1963: Das Arzneibuch, 199 p. (Veröffentl. Int. Ges. Gesch. der Pharmazie, N.F., vol. 23) (Stuttgart: Wiss. Verlagsges.).—

Ortolf wrote a book on medicine in German that was very popular in his time and during the whole 15th century. Much of its contents was based upon Salernitan writings; and as to its botanical part, much has been taken from Conrad of Megenberg. The present work is a useful critical edition of the Cologne ms. which in all probability stems from the 14th century.

Peter of Spain (*ca.* 1215-1277) — BERGER, A. M., 1899: Die Ophthalmologie des Pe-

trus Hispanus mit deutscher Uebersetzung und Kommentar. Der von Michel Angelo Buonarroti eigenhändig geschriebenen Augentractat (XVI. Jh.), 23 p. (Munich: Linsbauer).—

Peter of Spain was a Portuguese philosopher, physician, zoologist, psychologist and logician. He wrote many medical works; one of them was the "Liber de morbis oculorum" of which the present book contains a German translation. Concerning his logico-philosophical treatises *cf.* GRABMANN, M., 1936: Handschriftliche Forschungen und Funde zu den philosophischen Schriften des Petrus Hispanus, des späteren Papst Johannes XXI (d. 1277), 137 p. (Sitzber. bayr. Akad. Wiss., phil.-hist. Abt., 1936, pt. 9). Peter also wrote many commentaries on earlier medical works. Famous also are his "Thesaurus pauperum" and his "De anima". As to this last book Sarton (Introd. II (2): 891) writes that it is divided into 13 tractates, of which the last, subdivided into 8 chapters, is a very remarkable history of the evolution of psychological ideas among the Greeks and Muslims. Unfortunately, I have not succeeded in finding reliable translations in one of the Western European languages of these last-mentioned books.

Peter of Ulm (fl. *ca.* 1420-1430) — KEIL, G., 1961: Die "Cirurgia" Peters von Ulm. Untersuchungen zu einem Denkmal altdeutscher Fachprosa mit kritischer Ausgabe des Textes, 518 p. (Diss. Univ. Heidelberg) (Forschungen zur Geschichte der Stadt Ulm, vol. 2).—

Peter of Ulm wrote a "Cirurgia", a manual with many recipes. The present book contains an edition of the text of this book (77 p.) with an extensive commentary, glossaries, a historical review of the mss. and printed editions, an analysis of the sources (*e.g.*, Guy de Chauliac, the Antidotarium Nicolai), and an evaluation of the book within the framework of the developments of mediaeval medicine in Germany.

Petrus Candidus (= Pope Alexander V, *ca.* 1340-1410) — KILLERMANN, S., 1914: Das Tierbuch des Petrus Candidus. Geschrieben 1460, gemalt im 16. Jahrhundert (Codex Vaticanus Urb. lat. 276), 109 p. (Zool. Ann. 6 : 113-221).—

The codex consists of five books, dealing with terrestrial animals, birds, sea animals and fishes, snakes and worms, and with some curiosities respectively. The catalogue has been illustrated beautifully; some

16 photographic reproductions have been included. After a list of animals considered, short descriptions of these animals follow. These descriptions provide a valuable indication of the situation in the zoological sciences during the period between Albertus Magnus and Conrad Gesner.

Petrus de Crescentius (*ca.* 1233 - *ca.* 1320) — SAVASTANO, L., 1922: Contributio allo studio critico degli scrittori agrari italici. Pietro dei Crescenzi, 132 p. (Ann. Staz. Agrum. Frutt. Acireale, vol. 5).—

Petrus de Crescentius wrote a treatise on husbandry entitled "Liber cultus ruris" or "Ruralium commodorum libri XII", of which about 60 Latin editions appeared before 1602, plus translations into Italian, French, German, Polish, and Spanish. The book of Savastano is divided as follows: I: Agriculture in mediaeval times (the Romans, Albertus Magnus, the Circa instans, Avicenna, the compilators, agriculture in Italy in Crescentius' time); II: Analysis of the "Liber cultus ruris" (p. 11-34; a short review of the contents also can be found in Sarton's Introduction III (1): 815); III: Its influence, mss., editions, and translations; IV: History of critical studies devoted to it. Appendix with notes on the authors quoted by Crescentius (*e.g.,* Vincent of Beauvais, Giordano Ruffo), on the medical aspects, the plants mentioned, incunabula and printed editions of the book. Another valuable study treating of Petrus de Crescentius and his work is: ALFONSO, T. R. BOZZELLI, *et al.,* 1933: Pier de 'Crescenzi. Studi e documenti, 377 p. (Bologna: Cappelli). It contains a series of six studies on Crescentius, life and times, five studies on the "Ruralium commodorum", and very elaborate bibliographies of mss. and editions (p. 259-369). Another study, containing beautiful illustrations, is: LINDNER, K., 1957: Das Jagdbuch des Petrus de Crescentius in deutsche Uebersetzungen des 14. und 15. Jahrhunderts, 196 p. + 112 figs. (Quell. Gesch. Jagd, No. 4) (Berlin: de Gruyter).

Philip of Thaon, or Thaun (fl. 1119-1125) — WALBERG, E., 1900: Le bestiaire de Philippe de Thaün. Texte critique publié avec introduction, notes, et glossaire, 144 + 175 p. (Lund: Möller; Paris: Walter).—

Although primarily of a philological character, this study is very useful to the biohistorian as well. Philip wrote the earliest French version of the "Physiologus". It is written *ca.* 1125, and consists of six- and eight-syllabled verses. For a comparison of this bestiary with various other mediaeval bestiaries, *cf.* MANN, M. F., 1884-1886:

Der Physiologus des P. von Thaun und seine Quellen, 94 p. (Anglia 7: 420-468; 9: 391-434; 447-450).

Ramon Lull (*ca.* 1233 - *ca.* 1315) — PEERS, E. A., 1929: Ramon Lull: a biography, 454 p. (London: Society for the Promotion of Christian Knowledge).—

A very readable biography of Ramon Lull, the Catalan logician, philosopher and scientist. He has become famous as inventor of a kind of generalizing or universal logic. Some 6 medical treatises are ascribed to him, but his knowledge in this field was but superficial. According to Sarton the present book is an excellent biography, except that the author has not paid sufficient attention to Lull's logical and scientific works. The book also contains a review of Lullism (p. 376-400) and an elaborate bibliography. In 1946 PEERS published a shorter biographical study of Lull which is largely derived from this book: Fool of Love: the life of Ramon Lull, 127 p. (London: S. C. M. Press). There also exists a French biography of Lull in the form of a novel: GRAUX, L., 1927: le docteur illuminé. Roman, 419 p. (Paris: Fayard). Ramon Lull also published an epos on animals, originally written in the Catalan language, the Libre de Maravelles. *Cf.* PEERS, E. A., 1928: The book of the beasts, 90 p. (London: Burns & Oates). Also in German: HOFFMANN, K., 1871: Ein katalanisches Thierepos von Ramon Lull. (Abh. Kgl. bayr. Akad. Wiss., philos.- philol. Kl. 12, pt. 3: 171-240).

Richard of Wendover (d. 1252) — SUDHOFF, K., 1927: Der "Micrologus". Text der "Anatomia" Richards des Engländers, 20 p. (Arch. Gesch. Med. 19 : 209-239).—

Richard of Wendover, or Ricardus Anglicus, was author of many medical writings, notably the "Micrologus", a brief medical encyclopaedia based on the Greek and Arabic knowledge available in Latin translations. A part of this "Micrologus" formed probably the "Practica". This part has been edited and discussed in two theses of the Sudhoff Institute, *viz.,* those of HELLRIEGEL, H., (1934, 64 p.) and of FRERS, E., (1934, 55 p.). There is also an anatomical treatise attributed to Richard, the so-called Anatomia Ricardi Anglici, but this ascription is not absolutely certain, although Sudhoff in the present study tries to prove that Ricardus Salernitanus must be same person as Ricardus Anglicus (*cf.* CORNER, G. W., 1927, *vide* subsection c).

Robert of Cricklade (2nd half 12th cent.) — RÜCK, K., 1902: Das Exzerpt der Naturalis

Historia des Plinius von Robert von Cricklade, 90 p. (Sitzber. Akad. Wiss. München, philol. Kl.: 195-285).—

This paper opens with a biography of Robert of Cricklade who was prior of a monastery in Oxford. He was interested in natural science and he wrote a collection of extracts from Pliny's natural history, the "De floratio naturalis historiae Plinii Secundi" in 9 books. Although the present study is primarily of a philological character, it nevertheless gives some information of interest to the biohistorian. It contains long extracts and many references to RÜCK's previous work on the mediaeval tradition of Pliny.

Robert Thornton (fl. 1st half 15th cent.) — OGDEN, M. S., 1938: The "Liber de diversis medicinis" in the Thornton manuscript (Ms. Lincoln Cathedral A.5.2.), 160 + 8 p. (London: Early English Text Soc.).—

The "Liber de diversis medicinis" is a compendium of remedies for various ailments. The remedies are arranged according to the part of the body affected, proceeding *a capite ad calcem*. They are for the most part in the form of recipes or prescriptions and vary widely in lenght. There are also passages listing the signs of death and simple surgical treatments in the case of head wounds, and a three-page discussion of the symptoms and treatment of pestilence. The text is in (archaic) English with many Latin passages.

Roger of Salerno (fl. *ca.* 1170) — STÄPS, J., 1938: Die Chirurgie des Roger von Salerno, 89 p. (Diss. Univ. Düsseldorf) (Quakenbrück: Trute).—

Roger was the greatest Salernitan surgeon. He wrote the "Practica chirurgiae", the earliest surgical treatise of the Christian West, containing much of his own experience. The present study contains a German translation of Roger's anatomical treatise. The treatise on the wounds of the head is dealt with at length (p. 4-35); the other pages deal with the treatment of the other parts of the body. In his study "Die Chirurgie des Roger Frugardi von Salern" in: Beitr. zur Geschichte der Chirurgie im Mittelalter II: 148-236, SUDHOFF gives a new edition of the "Practica chirurgiae", followed by various mediaeval commentaries (*vide* subsection c). *Cf.* also: LANGEBARTELS, E., 1919: Zahnheilkunde und Kieferchirurgie in der chirurgischen Literatur von Salerno, und der weiteren Roger-Glosse unter Mitherausgabe der zahnheilkundlichen Roger-Margi

nalien im Codex Amplonianus 62 a, 63 p. (Diss. Sudhoff Inst.); and: PAZZINI, A., 1966: Ruggero di Giovanni Frugardo. Maestro di chirurgia a Parma e l'opera sua, 87 p. (Roma: Ist. Storia Med. dell' Univ. Roma).

Rufinus (2nd half 13th century) — THORNDIKE, L., ed., 1945: The herbal of Rufinus, ed. from the unique manuscript, 43 + 476 p. (Chicago, Ill.: Chicago U.P.).—

A printed edition of the Latin ms. of the Laurenziana of Florence. Rufinus compiled his "De virtutibus herbarum" not long after 1287 and followed in it the Salernitan and Italian medical tradition and incorporated much of the Circa instans. Rufinus added a large amount of new botanical knowledge. There are indexes of herbs, diseases; measures, instruments and utensils; persons and titles of books; places.

Scellinck (fl. 1317-1343) — LEERSUM, E. C. VAN, ed., 1928: The "Book of Surgeries" of Master Thomas Scellinck from Thienen. After the manuscripts of the Royal Library, The Hague, and of the British Museum, London, 44 + 334 p. (Opuscula Selecta Neerlandicorum de Arte Medica, vol. 7) (Amsterdam: Ned. Tijdschrift voor Geneeskunde).—

The "Book of Surgeries" is an original treatise on surgery in Flemish, divided into 4 parts. Part 1 deals mainly with various wounds, part 2 with wounds, skin troubles, swellings of glands, and apostemes, part 3 with the eyes, nose, teeth, mouth, tonsils, ears, lice, fistulae, stones, cramps, *etc.;* and vol. 4 mainly consists of an antidotary. Although Scellinck does not mention the work of his contemporary Jan Yperman, their treatises have much in common, because they made use of the same sources. The present edition contains many footnotes, a very elaborate glossary (p. 287-328), many additional notes (p. 277-286), and a bibliography.

Theobald (1st half 11th cent.) — RENDELL, A. W., 1928: Physiologus: a metrical bestiary of twelve chapters by Bishop Theobald printed in Cologne 1492, 134 p. (London: Bumpus).—

This book contains a facsimile reproduction of the original text. This reproduction is preceded by a foreword containing a short account of the abbey and college of Monte Cassino, of which it is believed

Bishop Theobald was abbot (1022-1035), and containing an attempt to fix the identity of Bishop Theobald and the date of his original ms. The reproduction is followed by an English translation of the Physiologus and in an appendix Rendell compares three Latin versions of the Physiologus, *viz.*, the text printed in Cologne, 1492, the text discovered recently in Codex No. 5 and the text of Migne, Tom. 171, col. 1217-1224.

Theodoric Bourgognoni (1205-1298) — CAMPBELL, E. & J. COLTON, 1955-1960: The surgery of Theodoric, ca. A. D. 1276. Vol. I (1955): 223 p.; Vol. II (1960): 233 p. (New York, N.Y.: Appleton Century, Crofts).—

Theodoric was Dominican friar and bishop of Cervia. This English translation of his "Cirurgia" (based on the 1498 and 1510 editions) gives a useful account of the awakening of modern surgery. The first volume consists of Books I and II of Theodoric, the second volume of Books III and IV. Theodoric is also of importance for the history of veterinary medicine: he wrote a treatise on horse medicine, *cf.* KARL, L., 1928: La chirurgie, le traitement des chevaux et des oiseaux par Théodoric le Catalan, 18 p. (Rev. bibliogr. Sci. nat. Paris, 1928).

Thomas of Cantimpré (*ca.* 1204 - *ca.* 1275) — KAUFMANN, A., 1899: Thomas von Cantimpré, 138 p. (Cologne: Bachem).—

Thomas of Cantimpré was a Flemish encyclopaedist, whose popular encyclopaedia of science, the "De natura rerum", is of interest to our purpose. It consists of 19 books: Bk. 1. deals with the human body (anatomy, physiology, gynaecology), 2. with the soul, 3. with strange human beings, 4. with quadrupeds, 5. with birds, 6. with marine monsters (and herring fisheries), 7. with fishes, 8. with snakes, 9. with worms, amphibians, tortoises, *etc.*, 10-12. with trees, medicinal plants and herbs, and the other books with waters, stones, metals, astronomy, astrology, meteorology and elements. The work as a whole has been based on Aristotle, Pliny, Solinus, Ambrose and Basil, Isidore, Adelard of Bath, and James of Vitry. It has been translated into Flemish by Jacob van Maerlant, and into German by Conrad of Megenberg. Of Thomas' work no complete edition exists (one is in course of preparation at the Latin Institute, University of Utrecht), only parts of it have been translated, *e.g.*, FERCKEL, C., 1912: Die Gynäkologie des Thomas von Brabant. Ein Beitrag zur Kenntnis der mittelalterlichen Gynäkologie und ihre Quellen, 83 p. (Mu-

nich: Kuhn). Facsimile reprint of the original manuscript, partly in colours. After a short introduction containing a historical review of the "De natura rerum" and its existing mss., some parts from the first book are quoted (p. 19-32), to which abundant notes and a critical discussion are added. Another part of the "De natura rerum" of which a modern edition with annotations exists is Book 3: HILKA, A., 1933: Eine altfranzösische moralisierende Bearbeitung des Liber de monstrosis hominibus orientis aus Thomas von Cantimpré, De natura rerum, nach der einzigen Handschrift (Paris: Bibl. nat. franç. 15.106), 73 p. (Abh. Wiss. Ges. Göttingen, phil.-hist. Kl., 3. Folge, No. 7) (Berlin: Weidmann). Although mainly of philological importance, it contains much of interest to the biohistorian as well. Many notes and index of names.

Trotula (fl. *ca.* 1150) — SPITZNER, H. R., 1921: Die salernitanische Gynäkologie und Geburtshilfe unter dem Namen der Trotula, 43 p. (Diss. Sudhoff Inst.) (Leipzig: Zeulenroda).—

The "Trotula" is an obstetrical and gynaecological treatise; Sarton dates its compilation to the first half of the 12th century. Spitzner analyses its 60 chapters on the basis of the printed editions, gives a list of mss., and compares the printed text with that of some mss. The conclusion of Spitzner is that Trotula was a famous Salernitan midwife in whose honour this treatise was named. This conclusion is in contradiction to that of K.C. HURD-MEAD, 1930: Trotula (Isis 14: 349-367) who defends the position that Trotula was a woman physician, wife of John I Platearius.

Ugo Benzi (1376-1439) — LOCKWOOD, D. P., 1951: Ugo Benzi: mediaeval philosopher and physician, 1376-1439, 441 p. (Chicago, Ill.: Chicago U.P.).—

Ugo Benzi (or Hugh of Siena) was one of the most prominent medical philosophers of his time and he can be considered as one of the most enlightened students of the nature of scientific method since antiquity. The author of the present biography tries to give a chronological reconstruction of Ugo's life. In this biography a newly-discovered ms. entitled "Vita Ugonis" and written by Ugo's son Socino, plays an important role. From this ms. the original text and an English translation have been given.

Urso (fl. *ca.* 1163) — CREUTZ, R., ed., 1936: Die medizinisch-naturphilosophischen Aphorismen und Kommentare des Magister

Urso Salernitanus nach Handschriften lateinisch und deutsch herausgegeben, 192 p. (Quell. Gesch. Naturw. 5) (Berlin: Springer).—

The table of contents is as follows: 1. Zur Einführung von Paul Diepgen; 2. Vorbemerkungen des Verfassers; 3. Der lateinische Text der Aphorismen; 4. Urso's Vorrede zu den Glosulae; 5. Der lateinische Text der Glosulae; 6. Die deutsche Uebertragung der Vorrede Urso's; 7. Die deutsche Uebersetzung der Aphorismen und die auszügliche Uebertragung der Glosulae. *Cf.* CREUTZ, R., 1934: Urso, der letzte des Hochsalerno, Arzt, Philosoph, Theologe, 14 p. (Arch. Gesch. Med., Heft 5) (Berlin: Ebering). Recently reprinted, 1968 (New York, N.Y.: Johnson). *Cf.* also: MATTHAES, C., 1918: Urso und seine beiden Schriften "De effectibus qualitatum" und "De effectibus medicinarum", 74 p. (Diss. Sudhoff Inst.) (Borna-Leipzig: Noske).

Vincent of Beauvais (*ca.* 1195 - *ca.* 1264) — BOURGEAT, J. B., 1856: Études sur Vincent de Beauvais. Théologien, philosophe, encyclopédiste, ou spécimen des études théologiques, philosophiques et scientifiques au Moyen-Âge, XIIIe siècle, 1210-1270, 231 p. (Paris: Durand).—

Vincent of Beauvais compiled an immense encyclopaedia, the "Speculum majus", consisting of 32 books, divided into 3,718 chapters in which considerable space was given to plants and animals (5 books deal with zoology). In it Vincent quotes fully and explicitly from a large number of Latin, Greek, Arabic, and Hebrew writings *(ca.* 450), but nowhere has any attempt been made to be up-to-date or to bring in anything new. In an introductory chapter, Bourgeat considers the influence of the church and its philosophy on mediaeval life and science, and in chapters 2 and 3 he gives a review of life and works of Vincent. The 4th chapter deals with the general character of the "Speculum majus" and its subdivisions; chapter 14 deals with natural sciences (incl. botany, zoology, anatomy, physiology, and medicine), chapter 15 with anthropology and the science of Man, and chapter 28 with the origin and creation of Man. For the medical aspects of Vincent, *cf.* RIEUNIER, A., 1892: Quelques mots sur la médecine au Moyen-Âge, d'après le Speculum majus de Vincent de Beauvais, 60 p. (Paris: Ollier-Henry); or CREUTZ, R., 1938: Die Medizin im Speculum maius des Vincentius von Beauvais (Arch. Gesch. Med. 31: 297-313).

Walafrid Strabo (*ca.* 808-849) — LAM-

BERT, R. S., 1924: Hortulus or the little garden, a ninth-century poem, 33 p. (Wembley Hill, Middx.: Stanton Press).—

Walafrid Strabo was a Carolingian educator and botanist who *inter alia* wrote a poem, the "De cultura hortorum" or "Hortulus", which is a description of the various herbs of his monastic garden, with reference to their properties. The introduction contains a brief biography of Wal. Strabo. There also exists a German translation: Des Walahfrid von der Reichenau Hortulus. Gedichte über die Kräuter seines Klostergartens vom Jahre 827, 1926, 24 + 24 p. (Munich: Verlag Münchner Drucke). Contains a facsimile of the first ed., Vienna, 1510, with introduction by K. SUDHOFF (on medical), H. MARZELL (on botanical), and E. WEIL (on typographical aspects). Also in French translation: LECLERC, H., 1933: Le petit jardin (hortulus) de Walahfrid Strabus, abbé du monastère de Reichenau, 108 p. (Paris: Legrand).

——, PAYNE, R., ed., 1966: Hortulus, 91 p. (Hunt Facsimile Ser., No. 2) (Pittsburgh, Pa.: Hunt Botanical Library).—

A facsimile reproduction of the 9th-century manuscript, resulting from cooperation with the Bibliotheca Apostolica Vaticana in Rome. The transcription and English translation appear on facing pages, and the text is accompanied by a biographical account of Strabo by Wilfrid BLUNT. Moreover, this booklet contains a bibliographical study of previous editions, an account of the plants mentioned, a list of references, and 28 lino-cuts of page decorations by Henri EVANS.

Walter Agilon (*ca.* 1250) — DIEPGEN, P., 1911: Gualteri Agilonis Summa medicinalis. Nach den Münchener Codex lat. Nr. 325 und 13124 erstmalig ediert mit einer vergleichenden Betrachtung älterer medizinischer Kompendien des Mittelalters, 232 p. (Leipzig: Barth).—

Walter Agilon was a Salernitan physician living in the middle of the 13th century, and strongly influenced by Giles de Corbeil. After a brief introduction in which the editor places Walter in a historical framework, he gives the original sources of his compendium, *i.e.,* a review of the authors quoted by Walter. A third chapter deals with the general composition of the work; following chapters deal with the pathology, diagnostics and therapy of the compendium and the drugs mentioned (in alphabetical arrangement). Last the (Latin) text itself follows (p. 81-228). Walter's pathology and therapeutics are largely based on uroscopy; this is summarized in his "Compendium urinarum". The text of this "Compendium" has been edited and annotated by: PFEFFER, J., 1891: Das Compendium urinarum des Gualterus Agulinus. (Diss. Univ. Berlin).

Walter of Henley (fl. *ca.* 1250) — LAMOND, E., 1890: Walter of Henley's husbandry together with an anonymous husbandry, seneschausie and Robert Grosseteste's rules, with transcripts, translations and glossary, 44 + 171 p. (London: Longmans, Green).—

Walter wrote a book on husbandry in French, entitled Hosebondrie which remained the leading book on the subject in England until the appearance of Sir Anthony Fitzherbert's Husbandrie (1523). After a long and valuable introduction the author gives the text of Walter both in the original French and in English translation on pages opposing each other. Then he gives the translation of Walter's husbandry, as it is attributed to Robert Grosseteste (in archaic English), followed by the French text and English translation of an anonymous husbandry (p. 59-83) and similarly of the Seneschaucie (The office of Seneschal) (p. 83-119); it closes with a chapter on the rules of St. Robert, also in the original French setting, together with the English translation on pages opposite each other. It contains rules, made up for the Countess of Lincoln to guard and govern her lands and hostel. Glossarial index. *(Cf.* also CRIPPS-DAY, F. H., *vide* subsection b).

Walter of Metz (fl. *ca.* 1246) — PRIOR, O. H., 1913: L'image du monde de maître Gossouin. Rédaction en prose. Texte du ms. de la Bibliothèque nationale, fonds français no. 574, 216 p. (Lausanne: Payot).—

L'image du monde is an encyclopaedia in French, dealing with cosmogony, theology, geography, natural history, meteorology, and astronomy. It has much been based on elements derived from Honorius Inclusus, Alan of Lille, James of Vitry and others, and it deals with such topics as: strange animals in India, the rhinoceros, the tiger, the beaver, the lion, the panther, the mares

of Cappadocia, elephants, strange serpents, the phoenix, amazons and other savage fighting women in India, the pelican, the fishes of India, the whale, the mermaid, the date-palm, bananas, and other trees of India, the early paradise, *etc.* In 1481, Caxton prepared an English version of the "L'image du monde" which has been reprinted by O. H. PRIOR, 1913: Caxton's Mirror of the world, 192 p. (London: Kegan Paul).

William the Clerc (fl. 1208-1226) — REINSCH, R., ed., 1967: Le Bestiaire. Das Thierbuch des normannischen Dichters Guillaume le Clerc, zum ersten Male vollständig nach den Handschriften von London, Paris und Berlin, mit Einleitung und Glossar, 441 p. (Wiesbaden: Sändig).—

A reprint of the 1892 edition (Leipzig). Guillaume le Clerc or le Normand's bestiary is the most artistically composed and the longest (4,174 lines) of the rhymed French bestiaries. There exist some 23 mss. and this bestiary seems to have been rather popular. There also exists an English translation: DRUCE, G. C., ed., 1938: The bestiary of Guillaume le Clerk, originally written in 1210-11. (Ashford, Kent: Headley Bros). This book was printed for private circulation.

William of Saliceto (*ca.* 1210 - *ca.* 1280) — SCHAARSCHMIDT, F. O., 1919: Die Anatomie des Wilhelm von Saliceto, 75 p. (Diss. Sudhoff Inst.) (Borna-Leipzig: Noske).—

William of Saliceto was an Italian physician and surgeon. Except his medical works he published an anatomical treatise, of which Schaarschmidt composed a new edition, followed by an elaborate analysis and bibliography. William's most famous works are the "Cyrurgia" and the "Summa conservationis et curationis". As to the contents of these works *cf.* Sarton's Introd. II (2): 1087. *Cf.* also LOEWY, E., 1897: Beiträge zur Kenntniss und Würdigung des W. Saliceto als Arzt (Diss. Berlin); BASCH, O., 1898: Materialien zur Beurteilung des W. Saliceto als Arzt (Diss. Berlin); und NEUGEBAUER, H. G., 1924: Die chirurgisch-klinische Kasuistik in den beiden Bearbeitungen der Chirurgia des Wilhelm von Saliceto (XIII. Jahrhundert), 38 p. (Diss. Sudhoff Inst.) (Breslau: Schlesische Volkszeitung).

B. HISTORIOGRAPHY OF THE LIFE AND MEDICAL SCIENCES DURING THE RENAISSANCE AND LATER PERIODS, ACCORDING TO SUBJECT (incl. general histories)

1. HISTORY OF THE LIFE SCIENCES IN GENERAL

a. *History of general biology*
(incl. taxonomy)

ALMQUIST, E., 1931: Grosse Biologen. Eine Geschichte der Biologie und ihrer Erforscher, 143 p. (Munich: Lehmann).—

> This history of biology is centred around the immutability of species and the role of hybridization in establishing new stable units. The author considers 23 biologists, viz., Mendel, Schleiden, Schwann, A. Meyer, Virchow, De Bary, Schwendener, Brefeld, Koch, von Baer, Nägeli, Pasteur, Jordan, Gobineau, Harvey, F. Bacon, Mill, Linnaeus, Hansen, Aristotle, de Vries, and T. Smith.

ANKER, J. & S. DAHL, 1938: Werdegang der Biologie, 304 p. (Leipzig: Hiersemann).—

> A popular and very readable introduction to the history of biology, originally published in Danish. Also in Dutch translation: Leven en wetenschap; 3000 jaren biologie, 1944, 268 p. (Zutphen: Thieme). *Cf.* SIRKS, M. J. & C. ZIRKLE, 1964, *vide infra*.

BALLAUF, T., 1954: Die Wissenschaft vom Leben. Vol. I: Eine Geschichte der Biologie vom Altertum bis zur Romantik, 432 p. (Freiburg i. Br.: Alber).—

> This work consists of four parts. The first part is entitled: Aufgabe und Ueberblick über die Problemgeschichte der Biologie in der Antike (p. 1-8). The second part: Die Entfaltung des Lebensproblems in der Antike (p. 9-86), discusses the ideas of Alcmaeon, Heraklitos, and Empedocles, 'the "Peri Sarkon" and the "Peri Diaites I" of the Corpus Hippocraticum, Aristotle, Theophrastos, the Stoa, Galen, and Pliny. The third part (p. 87-118): Biologisches Denken im Mittelalter deals with biology and the Bible, Albertus Magnus, St. Thomas Aquinas, and Konrad of Megenberg. The fourth part (p. 121-392) is entitled: Der Aufbau der biologischen Wissenschaft in der Neuzeit, and deals with such subjects as: herbals and bestiaries, Renaissance anatomy, Paracelsus, van Helmont, Gessner, Fuchs, Spallanzani, Bonnet, Leibniz, Kant, Schelling, German "Naturphilosophie", *etc.* Extensive bibliography, useful biographical register. Vol. II of this series "Die Wissenschaft vom

Leben" is still to be published; Vol. III, dealing with the development of biology during the last decennia has been written by UNGERER, E., 1966, *vide infra*. *Cf.* also: HESSE, P., 1943: Der Lebensbegriff bei den Klassikern der Naturforschung. Seine Entwicklung bei 60 Denkern und Forschern bis zur Goethezeit, 180 p. (Jena: Fischer), a book about which I do not possess any further information; and NORDENSKIÖLD, E., 1928, *vide infra*.

BEAUVERIE, J., 1932: La systématique des formes, les grandes étapes du progrès de la classification naturelle, ses tendances actuelles, 64 p. (Paris: Éd. du Cerf).—

> "This address traces the progress of systematic botany from ancient times to the present. The paper is a concise history of taxonomy and comparative morphology with the minimum of technicality". (From Biol. Abstr. 9: 967). *Cf.* DAUDIN, H., 1926; CROIZAT, L., 1945; and ZUNCK, H. L., 1840, *vide infra*.

BEEBE, W., 1944: The book of naturalists: an anthology of the best natural history, 499 p. (New York, N.Y.: Knopf).—

> A collection of essays, or parts of essays, in English translation, written by famous naturalists. To mention some names: Aristotle, Pliny, Frederick II, C. Gessner, A. v. Leeuwenhoek, Linnaeus, Gilbert White, W. Bartram, A. von Humboldt, Audubon, C. Darwin, A. R. Wallace, L. Agassiz, T. H. Huxley, J. H. Fabre, H. F. Osborn, J. S. Huxley, E. A. Armstrong, R. L. Carson, and some 27 others. *Cf.* PEATTIE, D. C., 1936, *vide infra*.

BODENHEIMER, F. S., 1958: The history of biology: an introduction, 465 p. (London: Dawson).—

> The text is divided into three parts. The first part gives a brief outline of the relations and associations of the history of science with other branches of culture (such as sociology, religion, economics), of a number of methodological problems related to the history of biology (such as analogy and homology in the history of biology), of problems of priority, of the philosophical preparations of the background of biological solutions, and of the uniqueness of Aristotle in the history of biology. The second part gives a short factual history of biology (p.

82-144) and the third part contains sources (in English translation) derived from some 133 authors from Egyptian papyri up to T. H. Morgan. *Cf.* NORDENSKIÖLD, E., 1928, *vide infra.*

BÖHNER, K., 1933-1935: Geschichte der Cecidologie. Ein Beitrag zur Entwicklungsgeschichte naturwissenschaftlicher Forschung und ein Führer durch die Cecidologie der Alten. Mit einer Vorgeschichte zur Cecidologie der klassischen Schriftsteller von Felix VON OEFELE, 2 vols. Vol. I: Allgemeiner Teil, 466 p.; Vol. II: Besonderer Teil, 712 p. (Mittenwald, Bayern: Nemayer).—

A history of cecidology (*i.e.,* the study of the galls produced on plants by insects, mites, or fungi). An introductory chapter (64 p.) dealing with "prehistoric cecidology" has been written in cooperation with F. VON OEFELE. Other chapters of vol. 1 deal with: the concept of galls and the older ideas concerning the formation of galls and their inhabitants up to the days of microscopy; oakgalls described by Theophrastos and Pliny; Albertus Magnus; gallnuts as drugs to the middle of the 13th century; gallnuts as drugs in later mediaeval times; galls in pharmacy and chemistry; galls in the arts and commerce; Clusius and his oakgalls; progress in cecidology in the era of microscopy (p. 275-364); folklore (p. 365-430). A series of appendixes contain apothecary accounts of the 16th-18th centuries and the relevant texts of Clusius, Malpighi, and Réaumur. The second vol. is devoted to the systematic study of individual galls in the order of the plants concerned, but contains much that is of historical interest. Indexes of zoological, botanical, chemical and mineralogical names, of drugs, and of names of persons. A reprint has been announced by Sändig (Wiesbaden).

BUDDENBROCK, W. VON, 1930: Bilder aus der Geschichte der biologischen Grundprobleme, 158 p. (Berlin: Borntraeger).—

The history of biology has been treated in 4 main divisions: 1. Origin of life (spontaneous generation, the fertilization problem, embryogenesis); 2. Organization of life (cell-doctrine, problem of organic fitness); 3. Position of organisms in nature (the energy principle and life, chemistry and life); 4. The maintenance of life and organic evolution (heredity, origin of species). Portraits of famous (mainly German) biologists have been included. A second edition appeared in 1951 under the title: Biologische Grundprobleme und ihre Meister, 161 p. (Berlin: Borntraeger).

BURCKHARDT, R., 1905: Zur Geschichte der biologischen Systematik, 52 p. (Verh. Naturforsch. Ges., Basel 16 : 388-440).—

This is not a history of biological taxonomy, but a historical and critical evaluation of the systematization of those sub-sciences which belong to the science of biology

CALLOT, E., 1951: La renaissance des sciences de la vie au XVIe siècle, 204 p. (Paris: Presses Univ. de France).—

A historical review of biology against the philosophical and cultural background of the period considered. Separate chapters deal with: the methodology of 16th-century naturalists (p. 9-71); the morphology and description of living organisms (p. 72-103); anatomy and the problem of organization (p. 104-123); physiology and the problem of life (p. 124-155); order in nature (p. 156-184). This book also contains much information on: travels and the discovery of new animals and plants; cabinets, herbals, botanical gardens; dissections; cultivation of plants and breeding of animals. Good bibliography. No index.

——, 1966: Histoire de la philosophie biologique par les textes, 436 p. (Paris: Doin).—

In this work the editor aims at illustrating the history of biological methodology by quoting relevant passages from the works of great biologists. After an introductory chapter, explaining the scope of biological philosophy, three sections follow considering the following problems: 1. What is biology? (p. 29-64); 2. The methodology of biology (data and their representation, experiments, classification, causality, *etc);* 3. The epistemology of biology (the essence of life, its manifestations, origin, evolution and future; order and organization; ontogenesis and heredity; *etc.).*

CAULLERY, M., 1966: A history of biology, 158 p. (New York, N.Y.: Walker).—

This is an English translation of "Les étapes de la biologie", originally published in 1941 (128 p., Paris: Presses Univ. de France) and many times reprinted afterwards. The text consists of a short history of biology. Ch. 1 (p. 8-13) deals with Greek science and biology (Hippocrates, Aristotle, Galen); ch. 2 (p. 14-23) with the Renaissance and the revival of the science of antiquity (anatomy, botany, zoology); ch. 3 (p. 24-46) with biology in the 17th and 18th centuries (Descartes, A. v. Leeuwenhoek, Réaumur, Spallanzani, Lavoisier); ch. 5 with the 19th and 20th centuries (considering *e.g.,* morphology, marine zoology, oceanography, palaeontology, cytology, bacteriology, physiology, genetics, evolution theory). *Cf.* also THÉODORIDÈS, *vide infra.*

COLE, F. J., 1926: The history of protozoology: two lectures delivered before the University of London at King's College in May, 1925, 64 p. (London: U.P.).—

> The first lecture deals chiefly with systematic protozoology, the contributions of early scientists (*e.g.,* Clusius, Gessner) of Hooke, and especially of A. v. Leeuwenhoek. The second lecture discusses problems of a more general nature, *e.g.,* the distinction between lower animals and plants, Haeckel's contributions, evolution theory, spontaneous generation (Redi, Joblot, Spallanzani, Pasteur), and the immortality of protozoa.

——, 1930: Early theories of sexual generation, 230 p. (Oxford: Clarendon Press).—

> A critical evaluation of scientific ideas concerning theories of sexual generation. Separate sections deal with such subjects as: the earlier and later history of the discovery of sexual generation; the illustrations and interpretations of the spermatozoa; the first statements and further developments of the preformation doctrine; the origin and further developments of the competing theory of epigenesis; the early theories of fertilization and development. *Cf.* also GASKING, E., 1967, *vide* this section *infra;* and BILIKIEWICZ, T., 1932, *vide* subsection e.

CROIZAT, L., 1945: History and nomenclature of the higher units of classification, 23 p. (Bull. Torrey Bot. Club 72 : 52-75).—

> This short history gives a review of the fundamental literature between the years 1735 and 1789, during which period artificial and natural classification became separated. In this context the works of Linnaeus, Adanson, Lamarck, de Jussieu, Gleditsch, Haller, Necker, Ventenat, Geoffroy St.-Hilaire, and de Candolle have been considered. *Cf.* BEAUVERIE, J., 1932, *vide supra.*

DAUDIN, H., 1926: Études d'histoire des sciences naturelles, 2 vols. Vol. I: De Linné à Jussieu. Méthodes de la classification et idée de série en botanique et en zoologie (1740-1790), 264 p.; Vol. II: Cuvier et Lamarck. Les classes zoologiques et l'idée de série animale (1790-1830), 460 + 338 p. (Paris: Alcan).—

> A history of biological classification and of the role of the Chain of Beings from a philosophical point of view mainly restricted to the period between Linnaeus and Darwin and to the situation as it developed in Paris. The first part may be largely considered as a general introduction to the second part. It deals with aims and methods of classification during and after the time of Linnaeus and the ideas concerning the Chain of Beings during this same period. In the second volume the author makes clear how under Lamarck (Histoire naturelle) and Cuvier (Règne animal), classification came to maturity and the author tries to evaluate the influence of these works on future research. In the last part the author elucidates how both Lamarck and Cuvier arrived at a system of classification, each, however, starting from different points of view, *viz.,* from the existence of a Chain of Beings and from the immutability of existing types. *Cf.* also: GRÜNBERG, F., 1949: Die Verwandtschaft der Lebewesen. Wesen und Geschichte der Systematik in Zoologie und Botanik, 110 p. (Bios, Vol. 5) Vienna: Hollinek); and SPIX, I., 1811: Geschichte und Beurteilung aller Systeme in der Zoologie nach ihrer Entwicklungsfolge von Aristoteles bis auf die gegenwärtige Zeit, 710 p. (Nuremberg: Schrag). Unfortunately I am not able to give further information about these last mentioned books. For a concise historical review, *cf.* BEAUVERIE, J., 1932, *vide supra; vide* also LOVEJOY, A., 1961, *infra.*

DAWES, B., 1952: A hundred years of biology, 429 p. (London: Duckworth).—

> A very readable book holding somewhat the middle between an introductory text and a historical review of some modern branches of biological sciences during the last five or six decades. Valuable and helpful bibliography containing some 1,200 items arranged according to subject. *Cf.* UNGERER, E., 1966, *vide infra.*

FOURNIER, P., 1932: Voyages et découvertes scientifiques des missionaires naturalistes français à travers le monde pendant cinq siècles (XVᵉ à XXᵉ siècles), 108 + 258 p. (Encycl. Biol., Vol. X) (Paris: Lechevalier).—

> The first part (108 p.) deals with the voyageurs-naturalistes of the French clergy prior to the Revolution, a period in which the French clergy were more eminent as explorers than as colonizing missionaries. The second part (258 p.) deals with the contributions of French missionaries to the progress of the natural sciences in the 19th and 20th centuries; it is mainly a biograph-

ical catalogue of the missionary naturalists, giving a total of 400 names, with a bibliography of the scientific contributions of each.

GABRIEL, M. & S. FOGEL, 1955: Great experiments in biology, 317 p. (Englewood Cliffs, N.J.: Prentice Hall).—

A collection of some 63 papers (in English translation) containing first-hand reports of old and more recent "classics" of biological experimentation. Some of them are abridged or excerpted. The book contains the following sections: the cell theory, general physiology (incl. enzymes, hormones, vitamins, metabolism), microbiology, plant physiology (with sections on auxins and on photosynthesis), embryology (incl. germ-cell theory and embryonic differentiation), genetics, evolution. Each section is preceded by a brief chronological review, and a short note indicating the original source.

GAGE, A. T., 1938: A history of the Linnean Society of London, 175 p. (London: Linnean Society).—

This booklet was published on the occasion of the 150th anniversary of the foundation of the Society. It starts with a chapter on the various biological societies which flourished during the period preceding the foundation (1788). The second chapter deals with the period from 1788 to 1802: from foundation to incorporation of the Society. Chapters III - VIII contain much information on, *e.g.*, the purchase of the Linnean Collections (1829), the influence of the publications of the "Origin of species", the creation of botanical and zoological secretaryships, the admission of women, the various homes of the society, the celebrations, the medals presented, and much information concerning some of its famous members *(e.g.,* Bennett, R. Brown, Bentham, Darwin, Wallace, Hooker, *etc.).* Special chapters deal with meetings, papers and publications, collections and the library, members and elections, and finance and special funds.

GARDNER, E. J., 1965: History of biology, ed. 2, 376 p. (Minneapolis, Minn.: Burgess).—

The book is designed for use as a text "for a junior-senior college course that enrolls science majors, premedical and predental students, and individuals interested in broad cultural aspects of science." The first part (p. 1-94) gives in chronological order the significant developments in biology,

from the earliest periods for which evidence is available, to the Renaissance; the second part (p. 95-204) considers the development of methods and approaches to modern biology, with sections on academies, publications, and museums; the microscope; classification of plants and animals; and biological explorations. The third part considers some themes of modern biology, *inter alia,* biogenesis, organization and life processes, development of individual organisms, evolution, genetics and eugenics, and biology of the 20th century. The first edition was published in 1960 under the title: History of life and science. A comparable book is: MOORE, R., 1967: The coil of life: the story of the great discoveries in the life sciences, 418 p. (New York, N.Y.: Knopf). A popular history of the last 200 years. *Cf.* also: SIRKS, M. J. & C. ZIRKLE, 1964, *vide infra.*

GASKING, E., 1967: Investigations into generation 1651-1828, 192 p. (London: Hutchinson; Baltimore, Md.: Johns Hopkins Press).—

This book mainly deals with the theories of generation in the 17th and 18th centuries, from 1651, when Harvey published his "De generatione", to 1828, when von Baer announced his discovery of the mammalian egg. The central problem is the question why so implausible a theory as the theory of preformation could play such an important role. This book contains much that can also be found in the book of COLE, F. J., 1930, *vide supra.*

GEDDA, L., 1961: Twins in history and science, 240 p. (Springfield, Ill.: Thomas).—

For more details, *vide* section Philosophy of the life sciences.

GEISER, S. W., 1937: Naturalists of the frontier, 341 p. (Dallas, Tex.: Southern Methodist U.P.).—

The history of exploration and settlement of Texas during the period 1820-1880. It mainly deals with 10 plant- and animal collectors who worked there, and with their collections as they are still preserved in the great herbaria and museums of the United States. A second ed. appeared in 1948 (296 p.).

GRAUBARD, M., 1964: Circulation and respiration: the evolution of an idea, 278 p. (New York, N.Y.: Harcourt, Brace & World).—

"The purpose of this volume is to trace the full course of development of our scientific conception of the flow of blood in the vertebrate organism and the incipient notion of its role. The task is carried out by the reproduction of significant excerpts from the works of seventeen key contributors, from Aristotle to Borelli, with each text followed by a commentary to highlight the aim, approach, difficulties, and achievements of the scientist." (From the preface). The contributors considered are: Aristotle, Galen, Ibn Nafis, Vesalius, Servetus, Columbus, Caesalpinus, Frabricius, Harvey, Malpighi, A. v. Leeuwenhoek, G. Borelli, R. Hooke, R. Lower, J. Mayow, R. Boyle, and two papers from the Philosophical Transactions. *Cf.* WILLIUS, F. A. & T. J. DRY, 1948, *vide infra.*

GUYÉNOT, E., 1957: Les sciences de la vie aux XVIIe et XVIIIe siècles, 462 p. (Paris: Michel).—

The text has been divided into 4 parts. The first part deals with such subjects as: the classification of plants and animals in a natural system, and nomenclatural problems; the second part with: anatomy and physiology of plants, animals, and Man, speculative and experimental physiology, and with some great naturalists and experimentalists; the third part deals with spontaneous generation, with problems of foetal development, with the ovist-animalculist controversy, with sexuality, fecundation, preformation, epigenesis, and heredity. The fourth part deals with the origin of the ideas concerning transformism and with the precursors of Lamarck. A comparable book, written in Spanish is: PAPP, D. & J. BABINI, 1958: Biología y medicina en los siglos XVII y XVIII, 258 p. (Buenos Aires: Espasa-Calpe Argentina). As to the history of the life sciences in the 17th century, *cf.* PAGEL, W., 1935, *vide infra;* as to the history of the life sciences in the 18th century, *cf.* RITTERBUSH, P. C., 1964; and ROGER, J., 1963, *vide infra.*

HALL, T. S., ed., 1951: A source book in animal biology, 716 p. (New York, N.Y.: McGraw-Hill).—

In this book the editor aims to present the most significant passages from the works of the most important contributors to biology during the last four hundred years. Most of the items are separate papers, single chapters, or sizable excerpts, most of them having been reprinted in their entirety. The excerpts are brought together under the following chapter headings: The organization of animal life: papers relating to comparative and systematic zoology and the organization of the individual (p. 1-96); The activities of the animal organism: contributions to physiology (p. 97-270); The basis of animal behaviour: contributions to physiological and general animal psychology (p. 271-334); The origin and development of the individual (p. 335-428); Cellular biology (p. 429-470); Pathology: contributions to parasitology and to the biological foundations of pathology (p. 471-554); Evolution and heredity (p. 555-682); Zoogeography (p. 683-706). Index. *Cf.* ZUCKERMAN, S., 1960, *vide infra.*

HOENIGER, F. D. & J. F. M., 1969: The growth of natural history in Stuart England from Gerard to the Royal Society, 54 p. (Folger Booklets on Tudor and Stuart Civilization) (Charlottesville, Va.: Univ. Press of Virginia; London: Oxford U.P.).—

The chief figures in the account are T. Browne, Gerard, Grew, Hooke, Leeuwenhoek, Malpighi, Moffet, Parkinson, and Ray. This booklet is published for the Folger Shakespeare Library.

LANHAM, U., 1968: Origins of modern biology, 273 p. (New York, N.Y.: Columbia U.P.).—

"As a series of loosely connected essays on various aspects of biology, the book may serve the function of stimulating biologists to rethink some of the questions faced by their predecessors. But as a history of biology ... it will not bear serious scrutiny." (From a review in Science 163: 64-65). A comparable booklet may be: MAZZEO, J. A., 1967: The design of life: major themes in the development of biological thought, 227 p. (New York, N.Y.: Pantheon Bks.). I could not find further information about this book. *Cf.* also SIRKS, M. J. & C. ZIRKLE, 1964, *vide infra.*

LIPPMANN, E. O. v., 1933: Urzeugung und Lebenskraft. Zur Geschichte dieser Probleme von den ältesten Zeiten an bis zu den Anfängen des 20. Jahrhunderts, 136 p. (Berlin: Springer).—

The book contains much material concerning the history of opinions relative to the origin of life and the nature of the vital force. The author gives the opinions of men of science as well as of speculative philosophers from early antiquity up to the beginning of the 20th century. He concludes that not much has changed during these 25 centuries of thought on these problems, which, according to the author, do not belong to natural (physical) science, but which are problems belonging to the realm of metaphysics.

LOVEJOY, A., 1961: The great chain of beings: a study of the history of an idea, 382 p. (seventh printing) (Cambridge, Mass.: Harvard U.P.).—

This book contains the William James lectures delivered at Harvard University, 1933. The titles of the lectures are as follows: 1. Introduction: the study of the history of ideas; 2. The genesis of the idea in Greek philosophy: the Three Principles; 3. The chain of being and some internal conflicts in medieval thought; 4. The principle of plenitude and the new cosmography; 5. Plenitude and sufficient reason in Leibniz and Spinoza; 6. The chain of beings in 18th-century thought, and man's place and role in nature; 7. The principle of plenitude and 18th-century optimism; 8. The chain of beings and some aspects of 18th-century biology; 9. The temporalizing of the chain of beings; 10. Romanticism and the principle of plenitude; 11. The outcome of the history and its moral. *Cf.* DAUDIN, H., 1926, *vide supra.*

MANN, A. L. & C. VIVIAN, 1963: Famous biologists, 127 p. (London: Museum Press). —

A series of biographies dealing with Aristotle, W. Harvey, M. Malpighi, A. v. Leeuwenhoek, Linnaeus, J. von Liebig, C. Darwin, G. Mendel, L. Pasteur, R. Koch, J. H. Fabre.

MEYER-ABICH, A., 1949: Biologie der Goethezeit. Klassische Abhandlungen über die Grundlagen und Hauptprobleme der Biologie von Goethe und den grossen Naturforschern seiner Zeit, 302 p. (Stuttgart: Hippocrates).—

In this anthology, the author tries to illuminate Goethe's position in science by giving quotations out of the works of his predecessors and contemporaries. The book starts with a selection of Goethe's own writings on general morphology and on the philosophy of morphology. Other authors considered are Forster, A. von Humboldt, L. Oken, C. G. Carus, C. E. von Baer and Joh. Müller. *Cf.* also: WEHNELT, B., 1943. *vide* section History of the plant sciences, subsection History of phytopathology.

NORDENSKIÖLD, E., 1928: The history of biology: a survey, 629 p. (New York, N.Y.: Tudor).—

Perhaps the best one-volume history of the life sciences, stressing the philosophical and medical background. It is based on a course of lectures given at Helsinki University during the academic year 1916/17, and thus its story ends at that year. Originally published in Swedish (3 vols., 1920/24). In 1926 a German translation appeared, entitled: Die Geschichte der Biologie (Jena). An English translation appeared in 1928 which was reprinted in 1932, 1935 and 1946. The subject-matter has been divided as follows: 65 pages have been devoted to antiquity; only 14 to the Middle Ages; 39 to the Renaissance; 180 pages to the 17th and 18th centuries (treated together!); and 316 pages (*i.e.* half of the work) deal with the 19th century. Although the general treatment is as objective as possible, the author's intention is anti-Darwinian. *Cf.* BALLAUF, T., 1954; BODENHEIMER, F. S., 1958, *vide supra;* and SINGER, C., 1959, *vide infra.*

NOWIKOFF, M., 1949: Grundzüge der Geschichte der biologischen Theorien. Werdegang der abendländischen Lebensbegriffe, 222 p. (Munich: Hanser).—

The first part (p. 15-28) deals with antiquity, the second part (p. 29-38) with the Middle Ages, and the remaining part with the 16th century (Gessner, Aldrovandus, Vesalius, Italian anatomists); the 17th century (Harvey, Willis, Malpighi, A. v. Leeuwenhoek, Swammerdam and other Dutch anatomists); the 18th century (the preformist-epigenesis-controversy, modern systematics, descriptive zoology, "Naturphilosophie"); the 19th century (Darwin and his predecessors, Haeckel and monism, the cell-theory, protistology, comparative anatomy, embryology, vital processes, genetics, psychology. A concluding chapter deals with such subjects as: mechanism, iatrochemistry, vitalism, pantheism, holism, agnosticism, *etc. Cf.* RÄDL, E., 1905-1909, *vide infra.*

PAGEL, W., 1935: Religious motives in the medical biology of the seventeenth century, 86 p. (Baltimore, Md.: Johns Hopkins Press).—

This booklet contains the text of a series of papers originally published in the Bull. Inst. Hist. Medicine, Vol. 3: 97-128, 213-221, and 265-312. In a review of this book in Isis 28: 103, J. Needham writes that "the main argument of this book may be conveniently summarized in the following way: the origins of modern science are to be found in the strife between four factors, two on one side and two on the other. In the first place, theological Scholasticism allied with Aristotelian Rationalism. In the second place, theological Mysticism allied with experimental Empirism. Once this cleavage is fully appreciated, much that was formerly inexplicable falls into its place in the history of 17th-century science ... it needs but a slight acquaintance with seventeenth-century biology to realise that all biologists then read the Kabbalah, under the impression that such ancient mystical writings contained concepts of importance for them; or that theologians believed that research into the principles of generation in insects might throw light on the doctrine of original sin in an age of reason." *Cf.* GUYÉNOT, E., 1957, *vide supra.*

PEATTIE, D. C., 1936: Green laurels: the lives and achievements of the great naturalists, 368 p. (New York, N.Y.: Simon & Schuster).—

In this book the author includes biographies of great naturalists. He discusses the herbalists of the Renaissance; the early microscopists (Malpighi, Swammerdam, A. v. Leeuwenhoek); the famous French naturalists of the 18th century (*e.g.,* Buffon, Réaumur); Linnaeus and his school; Cuvier and Lamarck; early plant collectors in America (Bartram, Michaux); birdsmen (Wilson, Audubon); naturalists of the "New Harmony Settlement" (Say, Rafinesque, Lesueur); the romantic nature-philosophers (Rousseau, Goethe, Richard Owen); the originators of the "Origin of species" (Wallace and Darwin). *Cf.* BEEBE, W., 1944, *vide supra.*

RÀDL, E., 1905-1909: Geschichte der biologischen Theorien, 2 vols. Vol. I: 320 p. (revised ed., 1913, 351 p.); Vol. II: Geschichte der Entwicklungstheorien in der Biologie des XIX. Jahrhunderts, 604 p. (Leipzig: Engelmann).—

A well-documented and well-written history of the evolution of biological principles and theories from a (subjective) philosophical point of view (a mixture of Aristotelism, vitalism and romanticism) and the way in which it deals with its subject may best be characterized by Sarton's words: "It is less a history (of biology), than a philosophical discussion of evolving biology". Vol. I considers the period from antiquity, through the Middle Ages, Renaissance, *etc.,* down to the beginnings of the 19th century.

Vol. II largely deals with the 19th century and is strongly anti-Darwinian in its method of treatment. The revised edition of Vol. I together with Vol. II form much more a unity than the first ed. of Vol. I together with Vol II; the author's ideas on the subject apparently have evolved between 1905 and 1909. There also exists an English edition: RÀDL, E., 1930: The history of biological theories, 408 p. (transl. and adapted from the German by E. J. HATFIELD) (New York, N.Y. & London: Oxford U.P.). Roughly speaking this edition is a condensed adaptation of only a part (p. 107-580) of Vol. II of the original work, dealing with the development of biology in the period between Darwin and Driesch.

RAVEN, C. E., 1947: English naturalists from Neckham to Ray: a study of the making of the modern world, 379 p. (Cambridge: U.P.).—

The present work primarily deals with John Ray's predecessors. Starting with two chapters on nature and mediaeval science and art, the author gives the general intellectual background of such men as Neckham, Grosseteste, Bartholomew, and Roger Bacon. These men are taken as a starting-point for the development of natural history in England and Western Europe and with the aid of biographies of such naturalists as W. Turner, J. Caius, T. Penny, T. Mouffet, J. Gerard, E. Topsell, J. Parkinson and T. Johnson, the author illustrates how step by step the mediaeval world-view becomes gradually superseded as a result of empirical investigations which gradually destroyed this definite and static world view.

RITTERBUSH, P. C., 1964: Overtures to biology: the speculations of eighteenth-century naturalists, 287 p. (New Haven, Conn.: Yale U.P.).—

A narrative history of two themes of speculation prominent in the writings in the 18th century, *viz.,* that electricity should be the explanation of life itself, as well as of diverse other phenomena (called the idea of immanence); and that, because of their proximity on a scale of being, plants and animals had analogous capacities for performing vital functions (called the idea of botanical analogy). Separate chapters deal with such subjects as: the discovery of electricity and its influence on biology; analogy as an aid to understanding; plant nutrition and growth, 1660-1727; plant generation, 1676-1830; Linnaeus, analogy, and the Scale of Beings; problematical organisms; E. Darwin, Lamarck, the rejection of analogy; John Hunter, the first of the modern biologists; the romantic protest. Extensive bibliography (p. 211-273) and useful index. The literature considered is mainly English. *Cf.* GUYÉNOT, E., 1957, *vide supra.*

ROGER, J., 1963: Les sciences de la vie dans la pensée française du XVIIIe siècle. La génération des animaux de Descartes à l'Encyclopédie, 842 p. (Paris: Colin).—

A very elaborate treatise. The first part (p. 7-162) deals with the period between 1600 and 1670, the end of the Renaissance (dealing with such subjects as: the medical and scientific spirit of the period, anatomy and physiology, fecundation, conception, embryo, heredity, Harvey's Aristotelism, renaissance of atomism, Descartes). The second part (p. 163-456) deals with the period between 1670 and 1745 (the new physicians, new discoveries in animal generation, ovists and animalculists, preformation and epigenesis, *etc.*). The third part (p. 457-764) deals with the period between 1745 and 1770 (Maupertuis, La Mettrie, de Maillet, Buffon, Diderot and his encyclopaedia, *etc.*). Very elaborate bibliography (containing 877 items) and useful index of names. The book has been written by a literary historian who attempts to characterize French thought of the 18th century by means of an analysis of the role which the ideas concerning the generation of animals played in French cultural life. It gives an accurate and detailed review of the gradual clarification of biological and philosophical ideas prevailing during that period. Considerable portions of the text have been devoted to minor contributors. *Cf.* GUYÉNOT, E., 1957, *vide supra.*

ROOK, A., ed., 1964: The origin and growth of biology, 403 p. (Harmondsworth, Middx.: Penguin Bks.).—

After a general introduction by the editor on the origins of biological thought, selections follow from the writings of 33 great biologists and natural scientists from the 5th century B.C. to the 19th century A.D. The readings are grouped in 7 chronologically-arranged sections, and each section is preceded by an informative commentary. *Cf.* ZUCKERMAN, S., 1960, *vide infra.*

ROSTAND, J., 1958: Aux sources de la biologie, 276 p. (Paris: Gallimard).—

A series of historical studies of biological problems. It contains chapters on such subjects as: the heritability of acquired characters from Hippocrates to recent times;

the idea of human parthenogenesis; Francis Bacon as biologist: the sources of experimental biology; the embryological and genetical work of Réaumur; Isidore Geoffroy Saint-Hilaire and the science of genetics; the possible influence of Colladon on Mendel; tissue and organ transplantation; antibiotics. Separate chapters are devoted to L. Cuénot, F. Caridroit, and E. Bataillon.

——, 1964: Esquisse d'une histoire de la biologie, 247 p. (Coll. Idées, 64) (Paris: Gallimard).—

A thoroughly and attractive historical review of the following three major problems of biology; the formation of living beings, the evolution of species, and the genesis of life. Also in Spanish translation: Introducción a la historia de la biologia, 221 p. (Barcelona: Ediciñs 62). A publication written by the same author, and dealing with the history of ideas concerning spontaneous generation is: La genèse de la vie. Histoire des idées sur la génération spontanée, 203 p. (Paris: Hachette).

RUSSELL, E. S., 1916: Form and function: a contribution to the history of animal biology, 383 p. (London: Murray).—

The author traces the development of animal morphology from Aristotle to the beginning of the present century in a more or less historical way. As one of the main questions the author considers the interrelation between form and function and he tries to illustrate how - in the course of history - at least three currents of morphological thought can be distinguished, *viz.*, the functional or synthetic (*e.g.,* Aristotle, von Baer, Lamarck, Butler), the formal or transcendental (*e.g.,* E. Geoffroy Saint-Hilaire, Owen, and the German transcendentalists), and the materialistic or desintegrative *e.g.,* Schwann, Virchow, Haeckel, Roux, Loeb).

SCHUSTER, J., 1930: Die Anfänge der wissenschaftlichen Erforschung der Geschichte des Lebens durch Cuvier und Geoffroy Saint Hilaire. Eine historisch-kritische Untersuchung, 180 p. (Arch. Gesch. Math., Naturw. u. Technik, Vol. 12, part 3; durch Vorwort und Literaturverzeichnis vermehrte Ausgabe) (Leipzig: Vogel).—

A historical study of the controversy between Cuvier and Etienne Geoffroy Saint-Hilaire. This study tries especially to evaluate Geoffroy's contributions to the development of biology in general and to Darwin's theory in particular. He shows how

Geoffroy's combination of the ideas of analogy, connection, election, and balance, led him to his fundamental idea of the unity of organic structure. A bibliography of Geoffroy Saint-Hilaire's palaeontological writings has been added. Of the contemporaries considered in this book may be mentioned Isidore Geoffroy Saint-Hilaire, Kielmeyer, Lyell, A. von Humboldt, Bronn, Joh. Müller, and A. Braun.

SINGER, C., 1921: Greek biology and its relation to the rise of modern biology, 101 p. (Studies Hist. Method. Sci. 2 : 1-101).—

In this study the author deals *inter alia* with the work of Theophrastos and Nicander, the probable author of the Alexipharmaca and Theriaca, the work of Crateuas and the Julia Anicia ms., the Greek codices of Dioscorides, the naturalistic and the romanesque schools of botanical illustration, the "De Vegetabilibus" of Albertus Magnus, compiled from Nicolas of Damascus, the ms. and early editions of the "Herbarius" and the "Hortus Sanitatus", the increase in knowledge of classification, of generation, and of form and structure.

——, 1956: Discovery of the circulation of the blood, 80 p. (London: Dawson).—

A reprint with a few minor changes and corrections and a revised bibliography of a 1922 edition. The booklet starts with a simple outline of the anatomy of circulation; then the views of Galen, Leonardo da Vinci, Vesalius, Servetus, Columbus, Fabricius, and especially those of Harvey are considered. A book dealing with the same subject is: DOBY, T., 1963: Discoverers of blood circulation: from Aristotle to the times of da Vinci and Harvey, 285 p. (New York, N.Y.: Schuman). According to a review in Isis 55: 379, however, "the errors of factual data detract sufficiently to make the book of dubious value". A short review of the history of this subject, accompanied by very beautiful illustrations is: BOENHEIM, F., 1957: Von Huang-ti bis Harvey. Zur Geschichte der Entwicklung des Blutkreislaufs, 60 p. (incl. 41 full-page photographs) (Jena: Fischer). *Cf.* WILLIUS, F. A. & J. T. DRY, 1948, *vide infra.*

——, 1957: A short history of anatomy and physiology from the Greeks to Harvey, 209 p. (New York, N.Y.: Dover).—

This is a new edition of "The evolution of anatomy: a short history of anatomical and physiological discovery to Harvey, 1925, 209 p. (New York, N.Y.: Knopf; London: Kegan Paul, Trench & Trubner). It is

a brief but authoritative and well-written history. This story ends before chemistry transformed physiology and before the microscope put its stamp on biology. Its contents are as follows: 1. The Greeks to 50 B.C.; II. The Empire and the Dark Ages, 50 B.C. - A.D. 1050; III. The Middle Ages and Renaissance, 1050-1543; IV. Modern times to Harvey, 1543-1628. Many topics have been considered, among them, *e.g.,* the effect of the development of naturalism in art on anatomy.

——, 1959: A history of biology to about the year 1900: a general introduction to the study of living things, ed. 3, 36 + 580 p. (London & New York, N.Y.: Abelard-Schuman).—

One of the best-qualified textbooks of the history of biology, that has proved to be of great use to students of the history of biology. It is well written; up to the Renaissance it treats history in a chronological way, afterwards it discusses the major scientific activities in biology as a whole (*i.e.,* plant and animal sciences not separated). Nearly half of the book deals with biology in the 19th century - a period of rapid development. It is shown how medicine, anatomy, philosophy, geology, chemistry, psychology, each brings its contribution to biology. The first ed. appeared in 1931 (New York, N.Y.: Harrap; Oxford: Clarendon Press), the second ed. in 1950 (New York, N.Y.: Schuman). Also in French translation: Histoire de la biologie, 1934, 613 p. (Paris: Payot), and in Spanish translation: Historia de la biologia, 1947, 550 p. (Buenos Aires: Espasa-Calpe Argentina). *Cf.* NORDENSKIÖLD, E., 1928, *vide supra.*

SIRKS, M. J. & C. ZIRKLE, 1964: The evolution of biology, 376 p. (New York, N.Y.: Ronald Press).—

A survey of the main phases of the development of biology, mainly from the point of view of the geneticist. The forerunner of this book was written by SIRKS and published in Dutch. In this English translation various sections have been enlarged. Good bibliography. *Cf.* ANKER, J. & S. DAHL, 1938; GARDNER, E. J., 1965; and LANHAM, U., 1968, *vide supra.*

SMALLWOOD, W. M., 1941: Natural history and the American mind, 445 p. (In collaboration with M.S.C. SMALLWOOD) (New York, N.Y.: Columbia U.P.).—

A very good historical review of the history of American biology in particular and of the history of American science in general. Its contents can best be made clear from the chapter headings: Early writings on American natural history; Natural history in the colleges, 1640-1790; What Americans studied in European universities; Some early cultural centers; Diffusion of natural history culture; The contribution of publishers, artists, and engravers to the science of natural history; The part played by the microscope; The philosophy of the naturalist; Amos Eaton and the academies; Early teaching of natural history in the colleges; Natural history struggles for academic recognition; The passing of the naturalist. Extensive bibliography (p. 355-424). *Cf.* MEISEL, M., ed., 1924-1929, *vide* section Bibliographies, subsection b.

SNYDER, E. E., 1940: Biology in the making, 539 p. (New York, N.Y.: McGraw Hill).—

A popular history of biology and its applications in medicine, based on biographies of leading investigators. Separate chapters deal with specific fields of biological research. In her preface the author writes: "The purpose of this book is to trace the development of biological discoveries, not as so many facts, but as the product of real men whose lives for one reason or another made them outstanding in their fields."

STERNE, C. (= E. KRAUSE), 1901: Geschichte der biologischen Wissenschaften im neunzehnten Jahrhundert, 171 p. (In: STOCKHAUSEN, G., ed., Das deutsche Jahrhundert, part XII: 563-734) (Berlin: Schneider).—

The aim of this series is to summarize in brief and rather popular form the achievements of German science and culture during the 19th century; this part deals with the biological sciences. The author describes how the biological sciences ascended from an often disparagingly treated and exclusively descriptive science, to a generally accepted natural science, ranking equally with other natural sciences; and although it did not contribute so much to the progress of material wealth, it nevertheless has had a great influence on the cultural image of the century. Short biographies of the biologists mentioned have been added. At the same time a more extensive history of the organic sciences was published: MÜLLER, F. C., 1902: Geschichte der organischen Naturwissenschaften im neunzehnten Jahrhundert, 714 p. (Berlin: Bondi). This book contains the history of botany, zoology, and medicine during the 19th century, particularly in Germany. *Cf.* MEYER-ABICH, A., 1949, *vide supra.*

THÉODORIDÈS, J., 1965: Histoire de la biologie, 124 p. ("Que sais je?" No. 1) (Paris: Presses Univ. de France).—

This booklet essentially contains a completely rewritten text of CAULLERY's Les étapes de la biologie (*vide supra*). Ch. 1 (p. 7-12) deals with prehistory and oriental antiquity; ch. 2 (p. 12-18) with classical antiquity; ch. 3 (p. 19-22) with the Middle Ages in East and West; ch. 4 (p. 23-40) with the 16th and 17th centuries; ch. 5 (p. 41-67) with the 18th century (Linnaeus, Buffon, comparative anatomy, voyageur-naturalists, experimental biology, embryology); ch. 6 (p. 68-111) with the 19th century (Lamarck, Cuvier, Geoffroy Saint-Hilaire, cell-theory, sexuality, Darwin and Darwinism, biochemistry); ch. 7 (p. 112-122) deals with the 20th century (cellular biology, genetics and evolution, microbiology, physiology, and biochemistry). Another short French history of biology is: DELAUNAY, A., 1965: Histoire de la biologie, 112 p. (Lausanne: Rencontre).

THOMSON, J. A., 1932: The great biologists, 173 p. (London: Methuen).—

In this book some 30 biologists are considered, each of them representing a specific field of biological discovery or of evolutionary thought. Among them are: Aristotle, Galen, Harvey, Redi, Spallanzani, Hooke, Mayow, Hales, Linnaeus, Lamarck, Cuvier, Goethe, Jenner, von Baer, Schwann, Schleiden, Müller, Darwin, Bernard, Spencer, Galton, Pasteur, Fabre, Hofmeister, Huxley, Weismann, Haeckel, and Lankester.

UNGERER, E., 1966: Die Wissenschaft vom Leben. Eine Geschichte der Biologie. Vol. 3. Der Wandel der Problemlage der Biologie in den letzten Jahrzehnten, 405 p. (Orbis academicus, Vol. 2, 14) (Freiburg i. Br. & Munich: Alber).—

"Der erste Teil befasst sich mit den naturphilosophischen Deutungen und erkenntnistheoretischen Grundlagen der modernen Biologie, vor allem mit der Diskussion des Lebensproblems. Im zweiten Teil entwickelt der Verfasser die neueren Erkenntnisfortschritte der Biologie im Zusammenhang mit ihren wissenschaftstheoretischen Grundlagen, wobei sich neue Wege der Forschung und der Formulierung ihrer Ergebnisse abzeichnen. Der umfangreiche dritte Teil geht den Auswirkungen der neueren Forschung im Bereich der einzelnen Spezialdisziplinen der Biologie nach. Die Anmerkungen erhalten zugleich eine Einführung in das besonders wichtige Schrifttum." The first volume of this series "Die Wissenschaft vom Leben" was written by T. BALLAUF (1954, *vide supra*), and deals with the history of biological thought from antiquity up to German romanticism at the beginning of the former century. The second vol. is still in preparation. *Cf.* DAWES, B., 1952, *vide supra*.

VON HAGEN, V. W., 1948: The green world of the naturalist, 392 p. (New York, N.Y.: Greenberg).—

    An anthology summarizing five centuries of natural history in South America in the words of explorers (such as von Humboldt, Bates, Darwin, Beebe) and of navigators, courtiers, chroniclers, pirates, engineers, and men of letters (such as Melville, Tomlinson, Hudson). Also in French translation: Le continent vert des naturalistes, 1950, 411 p. (Paris: Durel).

WILLIUS, F. A. & T. J. DRY, 1948: A history of the heart and the circulation, 456 p. (Philadelphia, Pa. & London: Saunders).—

    The period covered in this history ranges from *ca.* 5000 B.C. through the first quarter of the 20th century A.D., and the topics considered are the history of anatomy, physiology, pathology, and treatment of the heart and the circulatory system. A first section of the book contains a chronological presentation of knowledge relating to the heart and the circulation, a second section contains selected biographies of scientists who contributed to our knowledge about these topics, and a third section comprises a summarily presentation of the subjectmatter of the book, containing 18 separate chronologies arranged according to subject. *Cf.* also: WILLIUS, F. A. & T. E. KEYS, 1961: Classics of cardiology: a collection of classic works on the heart and circulation, with comprehensive biographic accounts of the authors, 2 vols., 858 p. (New York, N.Y.: Dover). (Originally published 1941, St. Louis, Mo.: Mosby). An authoritative and beautifully illustrated historical review of the study of the circulation during the 19th and 20th centuries is: FISHMAN, A. P. & D. W. RICHARDS, eds., 1964: Circulation of the blood, men and ideas, 859 p. (New York, N.Y.: Oxford U.P.). It consists of 16 contributions on many specialized subjects such as: the physiology of the heart muscle, electrocardiography, arterial

hypertension, circulation in the kidneys, the liver, the brain, *etc.* As a whole it gives a very good insight into the progress made during the last 150 years. *Cf.* GRAUBART, M., 1964; and SINGER, C., 1956, *vide supra*.

ZUCKERMAN, S., ed., 1960: Classics in biology: a course of selected readings by authorities: with an introductory reading guide, 351 p. (New York, N.Y.: Philosophical Library).—

    Each selection averages about eight pages. 29 selections represent the 20th century, 6 the 19th century, 2 the 18th and 1 the 17th century. Book I is entitled "The unity of life" (11 selections from, *inter alia*, T. H. Huxley, Pasteur, Bernal, Darwin); book II is entitled "The diversity of life" (15 selections from, *inter alia*, Waddington, Mendel, J. Huxley, Ford, Zuckermann, N. Wiener); book III is entitled "Biology and health" (12 selections from, *inter alia*, A. V. Hill, A. Fleming, J. Huxley, D'Arcy Thompson). Included are short transitional commentaries between succeeding selections, biographical notes, introductions to supplementary reading, and an index. A comparable book of which I have no further information at my disposal seems to be: PI SUÑER, A., 1955: Classics of biology, 337 p. (authoritative English translations by C. M. STERN) (New York, N.Y.: Philosophical Library). *Cf.* HALL, T. S., 1951; and ROOK, A., 1964, *vide supra*.

ZUNCK, H. L., 1840: Die natürlichen Pflanzensysteme geschichtlich entwickelt, 208 p. (Leipzig: Hinrich).—

    A history of botanical classification, discussing the classificatory systems of Aristotle, Theophrast, Dioscorides, Pliny, Lobelius, Cesalpin, Tournefort, Ray, Linnaeus, Adanson, Oeder, Gärtner, de Jussieu, de Candolle, Batsch, Oken, Reichenbach, Schweigger, Schultz, Lindley, Bartling, Perleb, Rudolphi, Martius, Unger, Endlicher. There are short reviews concerning the character of natural *vs.* artificial systems and concerning the history of botany. *Cf.* also: ULBRICH, E., 1919-1920: Pflanzenkunde, 2 vols. Vol. I: Geschichte des Pflanzensystems. Die niederen Pflanzen, 445 p.; Vol. II: Die Blütenpflanzen, 460 p. (Leipzig: Reclam). *Cf.* BEAUVERIE, J., 1932, *vide supra*.

b. *History of human biology* (incl. anthropology)

BORK-FELTKAMP, A. J. VAN, 1938: Anthropological research in the Netherlands: a historical study, 166 p. (Verh. Kon. Ned. Akad. Wetensch., Afd. Natuurkunde, 2e sectie, Vol. 37, No. 3) (Amsterdam: Noord-Hollandsche Uitg. Mij.).—

Chronological review of the anthropology of the Netherlands and of the achievements in this field of science by the Dutch, from the 18th century up to 1938, whereby it is made clear that in the older works the term anthropology includes a wide range of subjects. In general no mention is made of the studies of the Dutch investigators on foreign races. Also excluded are studies in which the Dutch population has been used as material for comparison, studies which are based on pathological cases, and studies based on criminal aspects of anthropology.

BREW, J. O., ed., 1968: One hundred years of anthropology, 276 p. (Cambridge, Mass.: Harvard U.P.).—

A series of lectures delivered on the occasion of the 1966-centennial of the foundation of the Peabody Museum of Archaeology and Ethnology. The first paper (by J. O. BREW) contains a biographical sketch of George Peabody, the founding, evolution, *etc.* of the Museum; the second paper (by G. R. WILLEY) deals with the history of American anthropology of the past 100 years; the third (by G. DANIEL) deals with Old World prehistorical techniques; the fourth (by S. L. WASHBURN) discusses biological anthropology and the modern view of Darwinism; the fifth (by F. EGGAN) deals with ethnology and social anthropology in their relation to other disciplines; and the sixth lecture describes the development in anthropological linguistics. Together these papers present a concise review of the history of anthropology during the past century. *Cf.* PENNIMAN, T. K., 1965, *vide infra.*

CHILDE, V. G., 1951: Man makes himself, 192 p. (A Mentor book) (New York, N.Y.: New American Library).—

A very readable introduction, dealing with such subjects as: human and natural history, organic evolution and cultural progress, time scales, food gatherers, the Neolithic revolution, prelude to the second revolution (*i.e.,* the establishment of the city-states), the urban revolution, the revolution in human knowledge, and the acceleration and retardation of progress. Index.

CLARK, W. E. LE GROS, 1959: The antecedents of man: an introduction to the evolution of the Primates, 374 p. (Edinburgh: U.P.).—

A description of the evolutionary history of man; the evidence of his dentition, skull, limbs, brain, special senses, digestive system, reproductive system, *etc.,* is considered.

COON, C. S., 1962/'63: The origin of races, 41 + 724 + 21 p. (New York, N.Y.: Knopf; London: Cape).—

Chapter headings: The problem of racial origin; Evolution through environmental adaptation; Evolution through social adaptation; The order of Primates; Man's place among the Primates; The fossil record: from lemurs to swamp apes; The earliest hominids; An introduction to fossil man; *Pithecanthropus* and the Australoids; *Sinanthropus* and the Mongoloids; The Causasoids; Africa; The dead and the living. Very extensive and useful bibliography. A sequel to this book: COON, C. S. & E. E. HUNT, 1966: The living races of man, 344 p. (London: Cape). *Cf.* also: NESTURKH, M. F., 1963: The races of mankind, 133 p. (Moscow: Progress Publishers). A second printing appeared in 1966.

DAY, M., 1965: Guide to fossil man: a handbook of human palaeontology, 289 p. (London: Cassell).—

The book discusses the environmental, cultural and anatomical evidence relating to the study of fossil man. Part I deals with the Pleistocene period, the geology of the fossil sites, stone tools, and with modern dating methods. Part II deals with the anatomy of fossil man, with anatomical assessment of bones and teeth in terms of normal, sexual and age variation, and Part III describes 40 key sites and specimens, their location, dating, morphology, description of the remains, associated fauna, artifacts, *etc.* 80 photographs, 12 maps.

HADDON, A. C., 1934: History of anthropology, rev. ed., 144 p. (Thinker's Library, No. 42) (London: Watts).—

Short sketch. The table of contents is as follows: 1. The pioneers of physical anthropology; 2. The systematization of physical anthropology; 3. The older anthropological controversies; 4. The unfolding of the antiquity of man; 5. Individual and ethnic psychology; 6. The classification and distribution of man; Cultural anthropology or ethnology; 7. The history of archaeological discovery; 8. Linguistics; 9. The growth of ethnology: comparative sociology; 10. Sociology (including religion). A German historical review covering the whole field of anthropology, especially valuable for the period before 1930 is: MÜHLMANN, W. E., 1948: Geschichte der Anthropologie, 274 p. (Bonn: Universitätsverlag) (ed. 2, 1968, 327 p., Frankfurt a. M. & Bonn: Athenäum), and a French one, of which I am not able to give any further information is: MERCIER, P., 1966: Histoire de l'anthropologie, 222 p. (Paris: Presses Univ. de France).

HARRIS, M., 1968: The rise of anthropological theory: a history of theories of culture, 806 p. (London: Routledge & Kegan Paul).—

    This study traces the development of anthropological thought from its beginnings to the present. The important theories of culture advanced in the past two hundred years are summarized and critically examined. The main purpose of writing this book is, according to its author, "to reassert the methodological priority of the search for the laws of history in the science of Man."

HAYS, H. R., 1959: From ape to angel: an informal history of social anthropology, 461 p. (London: Methuen).—

    This is a popular history of social anthropology by an American who has studied primitive societies for many years. It introduces the reader to this young and vigorous science through the findings of such scholars as, *inter alia,* Sir James Frazer and Bronislaw Malinowski. The development of various schools of ethnological thought is also traced.

HODGEN, M. T., 1964: Early anthropology in the sixteenth and seventeenth centuries, 523 p. (Philadelphia, Pa.: Univ. Pennsylvania Press).—

    This book contains much documentary material and is as such of special importance to historians of anthropology. The authoress demonstrates that the roots of many of the fundamental problems and methodological presuppositions and theoretical schemes of recent anthropology go back to Renaissance and even mediaeval sources.

HOWELLS, W., 1963: Back of history: the story of our own origins, rev. ed., 384 p. (Garden City, N.Y.: Doubleday).—

    The first edition appeared in 1959 under the title: "Mankind in the making:

the story of human evolution". Other comparable publications dealing with the same subjects are: PANNEKOEK, A., 1953: Anthropogenesis: a study of the origin of man, 120 p. (Amsterdam: North-Holland Publ. Co.). Also in Dutch: Anthropogenese. Een studie over het ontstaan van den mensch, 1945, 70 p. (Verh. Kon. Ned. Akad. Wetensch., Afd. Natuurkunde, 2e sectie, Vol. 42, No. 1); NESTURKH, M., 1959: The origin of man, 349 p. (Moscow: Foreign Language Publ. House); PIVETEAU, J., 1962: L'origine de l'homme. L'homme et son passé, 201 p. (Paris: Hachette); GREGOR, A. S., 1966: The adventure of man: his evolution from prehistory to civilization, 192 p. (New York, N.Y.: Macmillan).

MANNERS, R. A. & D. KAPLAN, eds., 1968: Theory in anthropology: a sourcebook, 578 p. (London: Routledge & Kegan Paul).—

    A collection of essays reflecting current theoretical interests of anthropology and including a number of contributions by writers outside the discipline, who have illuminated problems that are of direct concern to anthropological method and theory. Separate sections deal with: explanation in social science; methodology in anthropology; functionalism, evolution, and history; culture and personality; ecology; ideology, language and values; structuralism and formal analysis.

MEAD, M. & R. L. BUNZEL, eds., 1968: The golden age of American anthropology, 630 p. (New York, N.Y.: Braziller).—

    The golden age of American anthropology can be placed between the years 1880, when the Bureau of American Ethnology was established, and 1920, before the post-World War I reorganization of university departments of anthropology. The choice of individual anthropologists is confined to those who were already productive before 1920. The 57 contributions are distributed under the following section headings: 1. Exploring the New World (the beginnings of American anthropology); 2. Trying to cope with the Indians (Aztec beliefs and practices, the Jesuit relations, speculations on the origin of the American Indian); 3. Gaining understanding of the Indians; 4. Preserving the remnants of Indian cultures: the role of the private museums; 5. Building a science of Man in America; 6. New horizons (the aims of anthropological research, the conflict and survival of cultures, the contributions of psychiatry to an understanding of behaviour of society). *Cf.* also: HELM, J., ed., 1966: Pioneers of American anthropology: the uses of biography, 247 p. (Amer. Ethnol. Soc., Monograph No. 43) (Seattle, Wash.: Univ. Washington Press).

OAKLEY, K. P., 1950: Man the toolmaker, ed. 2, 98 p. (London: Brit. Mus. Nat. Hist.).—

A history of cultural evolution and as such a complement to the studies on biological evolution. Materials for tools are discussed under wood, bone, shell, stone, metal. Separate sections deal with such topics as: the evolution of Palaeolithic cultures, implements associated with fossil man, tradition and invention, science and religion, control of environment. At the end of the book a chart is enclosed demonstrating the sequence and interrelationships of the cultural traditions of early man in Europe, Asia, and Africa. Cf. also OAKLEY, K. P., 1964: The problem of man's antiquity. (Brit. Mus. Nat. Hist. Bull.). Reprinted 1966 (New York, N.Y.: Johnson). Cf. CHILDE, V. G., 1951, vide supra.

——, 1966: Frameworks for dating fossil man, ed. 2, 355 p. (London: Weidenfeld & Nicolson).—

First published in 1964. "It provides for the first time in one volume an authoritative and concise account of many of the dating methods used today and of the main cultural successions in the Old World up to the end of Mesolithic times." (Quoted from a publisher's announcement in: Nature 211: XXVIII, September 3, 1966). Cf. ZEUNER, F. E., 1958, vide section Prehistoric and primitive biology and medicine, subsection a.

PENNIMAN, T. K., 1965: A hundred years of anthropology, ed. 3, 397 p. (Duckworth's 100 years series) (London: Duckworth).—

First published in 1935. A classic in the field of the history of anthropology, giving a history of the main trends in all branches of anthropology. Anthropology has been defined by the author as the generic science of man embracing the biological, historical, cultural and social conditions of his existence. The subject matter has been divided as follows: 1. The "Formulary period", from the Greeks to 1835; 2. The "Convergent period" (1835-1859); 3. The "Constructive period" (1859-1900); 4. The "Critical period" (1900-1935); 5. The "Period of Convergence and Consolidation", since 1935. This second edition contains extra chapters on recent developments in physical anthropology by J. S. WEINER and on

Americanist studies by B. BLACKWOOD. Cf. BREW, J. O., 1968, vide supra.

SENET, A., 1955/'56: Man in search of his ancestors: the romance of paleontology, 274 p. (London: Allen & Unwin; New York, N.Y.: McGraw-Hill).—

The book has been translated from the French: L'homme à la recherche de ses encêtres. Roman de la paléontologie, 1954, 384 p. (Paris: Plon). It mainly deals with the pioneers (Casimir Picard, Boucher de Perthes, and Ed. Lartet) of the nineteenth century who opened the way to the scientific basis on which twentieth-century knowledge of anthropogenesis rests.

SLOTKIN, J. S., ed., 1965: Readings in early anthropology, 530 p. (Viking Fund Publ. in Anthropology, No. 40) (Chicago, Ill.: Aldine).—

The book consists of quotations of varying length, classified by date and subject and tied together with brief comments. Its chapters cover the period from the Church Fathers up to and including the 18th century. There are subject headings such as: physical anthropology, archaeology, ethnography, and social anthropology. The text is preceded by an unpublished paper of Slotkin, entitled: "Western anthropology from the 12th to the 18th centuries", and the book closes with an "Analytical guide". The function of the book is described as: "a comprehensive anthology of pre-scientific writings on the nature, origin, history and behaviour of Man."

STOCKING, G. W., 1968: Race, culture, and evolution: essays in the history of anthropology, 380 p. (London & New York, N.Y.: Collier-Macmillan).—

A collection of essays dealing with some of the major ideas in anthropology between 1800 and 1930. Throughout the book the great influence of Franz Boas is evident.

TAX, S., 1960: The evolution of man: man, culture and society, 473 p. (= Vol. II of: Evolution after Darwin; for more details, vide subsection: History of genetics and evolution theory).

c. History of human and animal behaviour

BORING, E. G., 1950: A history of experimental psychology, ed. 2, 777 p. (New York, N.Y.: Appleton-Century-Crofts).—

The main part of this book has been devoted to the rise and development of experimental psychology in Germany, Great Britain, and America during the period 1860-1930. A great deal also is concerned with the origins of modern psychology within philosophy and within science. Little is said about practical psychology (e.g., in education, industry, and therapy). It contains an amount of biographical and bibliographical information. (1st ed. 1929). A valuable discussion of the contributions of the Greeks (especially Aristotle) to psychology is: ESPER, E. A., 1964: A history of psychology, 354 p. (Philadelphia, Pa.: Saunders).

——, & G. LINDZEY, eds., 1930-1967: A history of psychology in autobiography, 5 vols. of approx. 400-450 pages each. (New York, N.Y.: Appleton-Century-Crofts).—

These vols. consist of short autobiographies of prominent psychologists who had been asked by the editors to write their "intellectual histories". Vol. I (1930) consists of the autobiographies of: J. M. Baldwin (1861-1934); M. W. Calkins (1863-1930); E. Claparède (1873-1940); R. Dodge (1871-1942); P. Janet (1859-1947); J. Jastrow (1863-1944); F. Kiesow (1858-1940); W. McDougall (1871-1938); C. E. Seashore (1866-1949); C. Spearman (1863-1945); W. Stern (1871-1938); C. Stumpf (1848-1936); H. C. Warren (1867-1934); T. Ziehen (1862-1950); H. Zwaardemaker (1857-1930); Vol. II (1932) of: B. Bourdon (1860-1943); J. Drever (1873-1950); K. Dunlap (1875-1949); G. C. Ferrari (1869-1932); S. I. Franz (1874-1933); K. Groos (1861-1946); G. Heymans (1857-1930); H. Höffding (1843-1931); C. H. Judd (1873-1946); C. L. Morgan (1852-1936); W. B. Pillsbury (1872-1960); L. M. Terman (1877-1956); M. F. Washburn (1871-1939); R. S. Woodworth (1869-1962); R. M. Yerkes (1876-1956); Vol. III (1936) of: J. R. Angell (1869-1949); F. C. Bartlett (1866-); M. Bentley (1870-1955); H. A. Carr (1873-1954); S. De Sanctis (1862-1935); J. Fröbes (1866-1947); O. Klemm (1884-1939); K. Marbe (1869-1953); C. S. Myers (1873-1946); E. W. Scripture (1864-1945); E. L. Thorndike (1874-1949); J. B. Watson (1878-1958); W. Wirth (1876-1952); Vol. IV (1952) of: W. V. D. Bingham (1880-1952); E. G. Boring (1886-); C. L. Burt (1883-); R. M. Elliott (1887-); A. Gemelli (1878-1959); A. Gesell (1880-1961); C. L. Hull (1884-1952); W. S. Hunter (1889-1954); D. Katz (1884-1953); A. Michotte (1881-1965); J. Piaget (1896-); H. Piéron (1881-1964); C. Thomson (1881-1955); L. L. Thurstone (1887-1955); E. C. Tolman (1886-1959); Vol. V (1967) of: G. W. Allport

(1897-); L. Carmichael (1898-); K. M. Dallenbach (1887-); J. F. Dashiell (1888-); J. J. Gibson (1904-); K. Goldstein (1878-1965); J. P. Guilford (1897-); H. Helson (1898-); W. R. Miles (1885-); G. Murphy (1895-); H. A. Murray (1893-); S. L. Pressey (1888-); C. R. Rogers (1902-); B. F. Skinner (1904-); M. S. Viteles (1898-). Of each of them a photograph has been included.

BRETT, G. S., 1912-1921: A history of psychology, 3 vols., 388 + 394 + 322 p. (London: Allen & Unwin).—

The most complete general history of psychology. Vol. 1 (1912): Ancient and patristic; Vol. 2 (1912): Mediaeval and early modern period; Vol. 3 (1921): Modern psychology. Many bibliographical references. Vol. 3 includes a list of general works consulted. An abridged and modernized version appeared in 1953: PETERS, R. S., 1953: Brett's history of psychology. Abridged, 743 p. (London: Allen & Unwin). Cf. KANTOR, J. R., 1963; SIEBECK, H., 1961: SPEARMAN, C., 1937; and THOMSON, R., 1968, vide infra.

DESSOIR, M., 1964: Geschichte der neueren deutschen Psychologie, 626 p. (Amsterdam: Bonset).—

Reprint. Originally published in 1902 (Berlin: Duncker). A short introductory chapter deals with psychology in antiquity and in the Middle Ages. The first section (p. 33-115) deals inter alia with Leibniz, Thomasius, Wolff and his school, and with German and French eclecticism. The second section (p. 116-356) deals with English and French influences, the general cultural background, empirical, physiological, and analytical psychology, and with association psychology. The third and fourth sections (p. 357-606) deal with the development and the contents of German psychology during the 18th century. Name- and subject-indexes. Bibliography.

FLUGEL, J. C., 1964: A hundred years of psychology, 1833-1933, 394 p. (with an additional part, 1933-1963, by D. J. WEST) (New York, N.Y.: Basic Bks.).—

The text has been divided into four parts. The first part deals with psychology in 1833, when Herbard was striving for the recognition of psychology as a science. The second part sketches the development of psychology by J. S. Mill, Bain, Lotze, Joh. Müller, Helmholtz, Fechner, Weber, Elliotson, Esdaile, and Braid. The third part discusses the influence of the concept of evolution on psychology and the rise of experimental psychology. The fourth part considers the period between 1900 and 1933 and treats of the rise of divergent schools of structural and functional psychology, Freudianism, psychoanalysis, mental tests, *etc.* The book closes with discussions of the relations of psychology to anthropology and sociology and its applications in education and industry. The first edition was published in 1933, and a second edition appeared in 1955. The present ed. is the third ed. of the first 4 parts, and the second ed., with additions, of the additional part.

FOULQUIÉ, P. & G. DELEDALLE, 1951: La psychologie contemporaine, 458 p. (Paris: Presses Univ. de France).—

  This book contains a historical exposition of contemporary psychology from the French point of view and the text has been divided into three parts of nearly equal length. The first part describes the trend towards objectivity and deals with Wundt, Ribot, Binet, Dumas, Piéron, with American experimental psychology and with Behaviorism. The second part deals with the reactions against this trend: James, Bergson, Delacroix; Denkpsychologie, Verstehende Psychologie, Schicksalanalyse and psychoanalysis. The third part tries to give a synthesis: Gestalt psychology; psychobiology (Pradines, Ruyer); "psychology of conduct" (Janet, Lagache); phenomenological psychology (Brentano, Husserl, Heidegger, Sartre, Merleau-Ponty). A very important mine of information concerning non-Anglo-Saxon psychology. *Cf.* NYMAN, A., 1966, *vide infra.*

GARDINER, H. M., R. C. METCALF & J. G. BEEBE-CENTER, 1937: Feeling and emotion: a history of theories, 445 p. (New York, N.Y.: American Book Co.).—

  The first eight chapters and a part of the ninth have been composed by the late H. M. GARDINER. These chapters have been revised by R. C. METCALF, and chapters 10 and 11 have been written by J. G. BEEBE-CENTER. Separate chapters deal with the Greek and Roman periods, the patristic and mediaeval period, the Renaissance, Descartes and Malebranche, Spinoza and Hobbes, the British naturalists and associationists of the 18th century, the French and German psychologists of the 18th century from Rousseau to Kant and Maass, affective psychology of the 19th century (with a lengthy discussion of Darwin's

"Expression of the emotions") and a final chapter dealing with theories of emotions in the 20th century (largely dealing with the views of Cannon, Dumas, and Watson).

GRINDER, R. E., 1967: A history of genetic psychology: the first science of human development, 247 p. (New York, N.Y.: Wiley).—

  A selection of passages from Aristotle, the evolutionists and the early genetic psychologists at Clark University, which traces the main lines of thought preceding the behavioural investigations of our era.

HEARNSHAW, L. S., 1964: A short history of British psychology, 1840-1940, 331 p. (London: Methuen).—

  The author has chosen this period, because in 1840 A. Bain published the first textbook of psychology written in the modern manner, and because after 1940 British psychology became more fully international, and also strongly influenced by the American psychologists. Separate chapters deal with, *e.g.,* Alex. Bain; W. McDougall; the biometric school (Galton, Pearson); psychometrics in the London school (Spearman, Burt); physiological, abnormal, comparative, social, systematic, and experimental psychology; British psychology between the wars; applied psychology; evolution and psychology; developments in neurology and neurophysiology; changes in philosophical climate.

HEHLMANN, W., 1963: Geschichte der Psychologie, 464 p. (Kröners Taschenausgabe, Vol. 200) (Stuttgart: Kröner).—

  A recent German-language history of psychology. Separate sections deal with such subjects as: the concept of the soul in antiquity *(e.g.,* in myths, with Plato, Aristotle, St. Augustine); the Middle Ages *(e.g.,* Bonaventura, Meister Eckart, Albertus Magnus, St. Thomas Aquinas); the beginnings of modern psychology (in the Renaissance, with Paracelsus, Descartes, Leibniz, Hume, Hobbes, Rousseau, *etc.);* Enlightenment (incl. German romanticism: Schelling, Oken, Carus); psychology becomes a science (physiology of the senses: Purkyně, Joh. Müller, Helmholtz, *etc.;* Comte, Mill, Mach, Spencer, Wundt, v. Frisch, Janet, Charcot, Jaspers, *etc.);* psychology in 1900 (Klages, Janet, McDougall, Brentano, Freud, Adler, Jung, Bergson, Dilthey, Jaspers, Husserl, James); psychology in the 20th century (Krueger, Wertheimer, Lewin, Mead, *etc. etc.).* P. 419-453 contain a time-table illustrating the history of psychology, p. 454 a short bibliography, and p. 455-464 a rather complete index. *Cf.* also: PONGRATZ, L. J., 1967: Problemgeschichte der Psychologie, 372 p. (Bern & Munich: Francke), a book about which I do not possess further information. *Cf.* MUELLER, F. L., 1960; SIEBECK, H., 1961; and THOMSON, R., 1968, *vide infra.*

HERRNSTEIN, R. J. & E. G. BORING, eds., 1965/'66: A source book in the history of psychology, 636 p. (Cambridge, Mass.: Harvard U.P.; London: Oxford U.P.).—

This source book contains excerpts from the papers of 84 psychologists who contributed to the development of experimental and quantitative psychology. All excerpts are in English; they are arranged according to topic. *Cf.* WAYNE, D., 1948, *vide infra.*

HOLZNER, B., 1958: Amerikanische und deutsche Psychologie. Eine vergleichende Darstellung, 404 p. (Würzburg: Holzner).—

"The author finds that while German and American psychology were once very similar, different conditions, and especially the differing influences of Locke and Leibniz, led to a gap which still is wide today. The leading psychological trends in both countries today are discussed." (From Isis 51: 396).

KANTOR, J. R., 1963: The scientific evolution of psychology, Vol. I: 369 p. (Chicago, Ill. & Granville, O.: Principia Press).—

After short introductory chapters concerning the concepts used and concerning the evolution of psychology into a scientific discipline, the author discusses such topics as: the development of psychology in ancient Greece (in relation to other sciences), considering especially Socrates, Plato, and Aristotle (the latter is thought to be the culminating point of Greek objective naturalism); the psychology of the Cynics, Sceptics, and Stoics; Lucretius as the starting point of subjective personalism; the psychology of early Christendom (the soul is an image of God); Plotinus and his subjective transcendentalism and his influence on St. Augustine; Arabic influences; St. Augustine and his influence on modern psychology; the transformation of Aristotelian psychology into scholasticism, its relation to other scholastic sciences, and its further development from St. Thomas Aquinas through Descartes, Hobbes, Leibniz, Locke, Kant, Herbart and Fechner to

the behaviourists. This last aspect was to be discussed in more detail in a second volume which seems not have appeared up to now. *Cf.* BRETT, G. S., 1912-1921, *vide supra.*

MATHEWS, W. H., 1922: Mazes and labyrinths: a general account of their history and developments, 254 p. (London: Longmans).—

A historical review of the labyrinth idea and its various developments, together with a few speculations upon its origin.

MUELLER, F. L., 1960: Histoire de la psychologie de l'antiquité à nos jours, 444 p. (Paris: Payot).—

Whereas the notion "psychologia" was not introduced into science before the 16th century, this book breaks up into two distinct parts: a (larger) part which is concerned with pre-scientific psychology, dealing with various concepts of "the soul", and a (lesser) part (p. 347-426), which is concerned with aspects of the development of modern psychology, mainly during the last two centuries. The author approaches his problem basically from the philosophical point of view and the presentation is more illustrative than exhaustive. *Cf.* BRETT, G. S., 1912; and HEHLMANN, W., 1963, *vide supra.*

MÜLLER-FREIENFELS, R., 1935: The evolution of modern psychology, 513 p. (New Haven, Conn.: Yale U.P.).—

A critical evaluation of the several schools of psychological thought, treated in chronological order from the psychology about primitive man up to quite recent times. Parapsychology has been considered in a closing section. Selected bibliography; name- and subject-indexes. *Cf.* THOMSON, R., 1968, *vide infra.*

NYMAN, A., 1966: Die Schulen der neueren Psychologie, 258 p. (Bern & Stuttgart: Huber).—

The contents of this book may be made clear from the chapter headings: 1. Alte und neue Psychologie; 2. Der Behaviorismus oder die Psychologie des äusseren Lebensbildes; 3. Die Gestaltpsychologie oder Feldpsychologie; 4. Die Dimensionspsychologie oder die Lehre von der Einheit der Sinne; 5. Die Faktorenanalyse oder die Psychologie der "Ladungen"; 6. Die Psychoanalyse oder die Tiefenpsychologie; 7.

Die Individualpsychologie oder die Psychologie des persönlichen Lebensstils; 8. Die Charakterologie oder die Typenlehre; 9. Die Massen- und Gruppenpsychologie. Index and bibliography. *Cf.* FOULQUIÉ, P. & G. DELEDALLE, 1951, *vide supra.*

REUCHLIN, M., 1957: Histoire de la psychologie, 127 p. (Que sais-je? No. 732) (Paris: Presses Univ. de France).—

A short history of psychology. Ch. 1 (p. 9-31) deals with experimental psychology; ch. 2 (p. 32-42) with animal psychology; ch. 3 (p. 43-59) with differential psychology; ch. 4 (p. 60-82) with pathological psychology and with clinical methods (Ribot, Janet, Dumas, psychoanalysis); ch. 5 (p. 83-103) with child psychology; and ch. 6 (p. 104-122) with social psychology. Another short history of psychology is: LOYE, P. DE, 1967: History of psychology, 112 p. (London: Leisure Arts); this booklet was originally published in French under the title: Histoire de la psychologie, 1967, 112 p. (Paris: Hachette).

ROBACK, A. A., 1952: History of American psychology, 426 p. (New York, N.Y.: Library Publ.).—

A history of the development of psychology in Canada and the United States. It has been divided into four parts. The first part (118 p.) is entitled "In the dominion of physics and the empire of theology". Its final section deals with the "New psychology" as it was introduced by J. Rush, J. Dewey and G. T. Ladd. The second part deals with the development of laboratory psychology (p. 121-210), and does so in a biographical manner (W. James, Stanley Hall, Cattell, Baldwin, Titchener, Münsterberg). The third part describes ten "schools of psychology" (p. 211-373); and part 4, entitled "Growth of branche: the phenomenal expansion of American psychology", deals with a variety of topics and consists of brief sections on, *e.g.,* educational and developmental psychology, psychometry, abnormal, clinical, applied, social, animal, general, experimental, physiological, systematic and theoretical psychology, the study of personality and character, statistics and psychology, *etc.* Another history of American psychology is: FAY, J. W., 1966: American psychology before William James, 240 p. (New York, N.Y.: Octagon). Reprint.

——, 1961: History of psychology and psychiatry, 422 p. (London: Vision).—

A history of psychology, including its medical aspects. Separate sections deal

with British, French, Italian, Dutch, Belgian, Swiss, Scandinavian, Russian, and American psychologists and psychology. Other sections deal with Graeco-Roman psychopathology; daemonism and many other aspects of abnormal and medical psychology; educational psychology; tests and measurements; collective psychology; and with animal psychology.

SIEBECK, H., 1961: Geschichte der Psychologie. Vol. I, pt. 1: Die Psychologie vor Aristoteles, 284 p.; Vol. I. pt. 2: Die Psychologie von Aristoteles bis zu Thomas von Aquino, 532 p. (Amsterdam: Schippers).—

Originally published 1879-1883. The first part deals with the beginnings of psychology as a philosophical discipline by Socrates and Plato. The second part considers the development of psychology in the works of Aristotle, the influence of Neoplatonism, and the influence of Christianity on Greek psychology during the Middle Ages. *Cf.* BRETT, G. S., 1912-1921; and HEHLMANN, W., 1963, *vide supra.*

SPEARMAN, C., 1937: Psychology down the ages, 2 vols. Vol. I: 454 p.; Vol. II: 355 p. (New York, N.Y.: Macmillan).—

A personal discussion of the chief contributions which have affected the development of psychology. The book contains a critical analysis of psychological formulations, theories, and schools, from earliest days down to the present era, seen from the point of view of one who is chiefly interested in cognition. According to a review in Isis (vol. 29: 542), "it is very clearly written and may be read by the untrained as well as by the student and professed psychologist with pleasure and with profit ... it is a very readable and original history of psychology." *Cf.* BRETT, G. S., 1912-1921, *vide supra.*

THOMSON, R., 1968: The Pelican history of psychology, 464 p. (Harmondsworth, Middx.: Penguin Bks.).—

The first part of this booklet (p. 19-224) deals with the history of psychology from the beginnings to the first World War, treating such subjects as: the emergence of experimental psychology, the influence of the evolutionary doctrine on psychology, the influence of physiology, psychoanalysis and the progress of psychology in Germany, the U.S.A., Great Britain and France during the nineteenth century. The second part (p. 225-398) deals with the history of psychology between the Wars, treating of such subjects as: behaviourism, Gestalt psychology, psycho-analysis, dynamic psychology, physiological psychology, experimental psychology, the development of tests, industrial psychology, child psychology, social psychology, and the study of personality. The third part contains a sketch of post-war developments and deals with the achievements and limitations of psychology. Useful bibliography (p.432-457) arranged according to the subjects considered. Index. *Cf.* also CAPRETTA, P. J., 1967: A history of psychology in outline, 226 p. (New York, N.Y.: Dell). No further information available. *Cf.* BRETT, G. S., 1912-1921; HEHLMANN, W., 1963; MUELLER, F. L., 1960; and MÜLLER-FREIENFELS, R., 1935, *vide supra.*

an unconscious develop soon thereafter, became topical around 1800 and effective around 1900. Freud is rightly seen only as one link in a long chain. Then 100 pages of evidence are given, often poorly chosen as to relevancy and formulation. Still there remains enough startling and valuable material beginning with that found in Cudworth, Norris, Malebranche, Leibniz and surveyed partly before in E. von Hartmann's 'Philosophy of the Unconscious' (1868) to make this book worthy of reading and preserving. The last chapter is again written in a spirit of philosophical prophecy which does not fall into domain of this reviewer." (From Isis 53: 570). A reprint of this book was published in 1967 by Social Science Paperbacks, in association with Tavistock Publications (London).

WATSON, R. I., 1968: The great psychologists: from Aristotle to Freud, ed. 2, 613 p. (Philadelphia, Pa.: Lippincott).—

This is a history of psychology emphasizing the "brilliant steps forward" of the great psychologists of the past. The lives, occupations, motives, families, views on fields of knowledge related to psychology, social, political and economic circumstances of each of these men are considered. Full attention has been paid to the Greeks. The first ed. appeared in 1963, 572 p.

WAYNE, D., ed., 1948: Readings in the history of psychology, 587 p. (New York, N.Y.: Appleton-Century-Crofts).—

A source book for the college student, giving an insight into the development of empirical and experimental psychology. The first article deals with Aristotle, the second with Galileo, 6 excerpts deal with the 17th century, 5 with the 18th, 30 with the 19th, and 18 with the 20th century. Some of them appear in English translation. Each of the excerpts is preceded by a brief note giving the bibliographical data and explaining the particular historical significance. *Cf.* HERRNSTEIN, R. J. & E. G. BORING, *vide supra.*

WHYTE, L. L., 1960/'62: The unconscious before Freud, 219 p. (New York, N.Y.: Basic Bks.; Garden City, N.Y.: Anchor Books, Doubleday).—

"On the first 80 pages the author develops his philosophico-historical thesis that a new self-awareness developed in Western man in the 17th century in the form of a static abstract rationalism. That more adequate process-concepts and concepts of

ZIEGLER, H. E., 1920: Der Begriff des Instinktes einst und jetzt. Eine Studie über die Geschichte und die Grundlagen der Tierpsychologie. Mit einem Anhang: Die Gehirne der Bienen und Ameisen, ed. 3, 211 p. (Jena: Fischer).—

Separate sections deal with: animal psychology in antiquity (Greece and Rome); the concept of instinct and Christian belief; the vitalistic interpretation of instinct; the Darwinian and Lamarckian interpretation; modern animal psychology (Weismann, Ziegler, Lloyd Morgan, Whitman, zur Strassen, Forel, Wasmann, Escherich, *etc.*); the difference between instinctive and conscious activities; consciousness; the histological basis of behaviour; the difference between the soul of man and that of animals. Ind :.

d. *History of Anatomy* (incl. cytology and histology)

ANDREOLI, A., 1961: Zur geschichtlichen Entwicklung der Neuronentheorie, 88 p. (Basler Veröff. Gesch. Med. Biol., No. 10) (Basle & Stuttgart: Schwabe).—

A historical review of the evolution of our present-day knowledge of forms and functions of histological structures in the peripheral and central nervous system of both vertebrates and invertebrates. It also contains much information concerning the neurone theory and biographical sketches of the principal investigators in this field. *Cf.* also: MÜHR, A., 1957: Das Wunder Menschenhirn. Die abenteuerliche Geschichte der Gehirnforschung, 464 p. (Olten & Freiburg i.B.: Walter). According to a review in Sudhoffs Archiv 44: 287, this history is not fully reliable.

ASCHOFF, L., E. KÜSTER & W. J. SCHMIDT, 1938: Hundert Jahre Zellforschung, 285 p. (Berlin: Borntraeger).—

A historical and critical review of the discoveries in the field of the cytology of plants (KÜSTER, p. 1-64), animals (SCHMIDT, p. 65-168), and disease (ASCHOFF, p. 169-267), since the formulation of the cell-theory by Schleiden (1837) and Schwann (1838). The reviews are presented in a topical, rather than in a chronological order and stress has been laid on German contributions. The development of cytological concepts and ideas has been followed through their successive stages of discovery, elaboration, and verification. A discussion of conflicting concepts has been included. Cf. HUGHES, A., 1959; and KLEIN, M., 1936, vide infra.

BOERNER, D., 1952: Wege der Histologie, 36 p. (Acta Anat. 14 : 179-215).—

The development of histology from its first beginnings to the present day is traced in close connection with the development of other branches of science, such as physics (microscope) and chemistry (staining techniques). The present situation in histology has been described and the future possibilities have been outlined. Cf. WATERMANN, R., 1964, vide infra.

CHAINE, J., 1922-1925: Histoire de l'anatomie comparative, 2 vols. Vol. I: 276 p.; Vol. II: 461 p. (Bordeaux: Daguerre).—

Vol. I deals with the position of anatomy in science in general, its methods and its goal, and with anatomico-terminological problems. The second volume deals with pre-Aristotelian anatomy, the anatomy of Aristotle and Galen, the development of anatomy between Galen and the invention of the microscope, with Cuvier, his precursors and contemporaries, with Geoffroy Saint-Hilaire and his philosophy of nature, and with the development of comparative anatomy in the preceding century. Cf. COLE, F. J., 1944, vide infra.

CHOULANT, L., 1962: History and bibliography of anatomic illustration, 435 p. (transl. and annotated by M. FRANK) (New York, N.Y.: Hafner).—

This work was originally written by Choulant in German and published in 1852. According to Choulant the purpose of the book was to give "a presentation of the history and the bibliography of representa-

tions of human anatomy by graphic means". It was translated into English by M. FRANK, and, supplied with many annotations, published in 1917. Frank added a short biography of Choulant (p. 1-21) and supplemented and corrected the original text. In 1945 (reprinted in 1962) a revised edition of Frank's work appeared, including a memorial note on M. Frank (by F. H. GARRISON), together with a bibliography of Frank's works (by J. C. BAY) and a historical introduction considering the beginnings of anatomy (by C. SINGER). As appendixes it contains an essay on sculpture and painting as modes of anatomical illustration (by GARRISON & STREETER, p. 370-402) and another essay on anatomical illustration since the time of Choulant (by GARRISON), containing much bibliographical information. Cf. WEGNER, R. N., 1939; and WOLF-HEIDEGGER, G. & A. M. CETTO, 1967, vide infra. Cf. also: HERRLINGER, R., 1967, vide section History of the medical sciences, subsection α, a.

CLARKE, E. & C. D. O'MALLEY, eds., 1968: The human brain and spinal cord: a historical study illustrated by writings from antiquity to the twentieth century, 926 p. (Berkeley & Los Angeles, Calif.: Univ. California Press; London: Cambridge U.P.).—

An anthology dealing with contributions to the history of neuroanatomy and neurophysiology. The excerpts have been arranged under headings representing the main anatomical structures and basic physiological principles. Each of the selected texts is preceded by a brief account about its author, in which the relation of the work with its predecessors is established. The passages quoted are in English. An introductory chapter deals with antiquity and the Middle Ages, and particularly with ideas concerning the brain as the seat of the soul. An appendix deals with neuroanatomical techniques. Bibliography of 53 pages. Cf. POYNTER, F. N. L., ed., 1958, vide infra, subsection f.

COLE, F. J., 1944: A history of comparative anatomy from Aristotle to the eighteenth century, 524 p. (London: Macmillan).—

A very good account of the works of the masters of comparative anatomy. The subject matter has been divided as follows: I. The contribution of Greece (Aristotle, Galen); II. Zootomy down to the 16th century (scholastic period, da Vinci, Vesalius, Belon, Rondelet); III. The development of craftmanship (Coiter, Ruini, Fabricius, Casserius); IV. Harvey and the encyclopaedists (Severino, Blasius, Collins, Valentini); V. The new comparative anatomy (Malpighi, Tyson, Willis, Lister, Grew); VI. The Dutch school (A. v. Leeuwenhoek, Swammerdam, Ruysch); VII. Academies and societies (*e.g.,* the Royal Society, the private college of Amsterdam, the Academia Naturae Curiosorum, L'Académie Royale des Sciences); VIII. The anatomical museum. Useful appendix containing biographical notes, good bibliography and index. *Cf.* CHAINE, J., 1922-1925, *vide supra.*

COLE, H., 1964: Things for the surgeons: a history of the body-snatchers, 174 p. (London: Heinemann).—

A history of the professional graverobbers, who, in years before the passing of the Anatomy Act, supplied the material for the training of physicians. The story dealing with early 19th-century Britain, is compiled from contemporary pamphlets, newspapers, books and medical journals.

CORNER, G. W., 1964: Anatomy, 82 p. (Clio Medica, No. 3) (New York, N.Y.: Hafner).—

Brief introduction to the history of anatomy, especially valuable to the student of medicine. It is a reprint of the 1930 edition (New York, N.Y.: Hoeber). Another short history of anatomy, containing, *inter alia,* a chronological table of 28 great anatomists from Hippocrates to Robert Knox, is: HUNTER, R. H., 1931: A short history of anatomy, ed. 2, 87 p. (London: Bale). First published 1925, 51 p. (London: Bale). *Cf.* also: RUSSELL, E. S., 1916; and SINGER, C., 1959, *vide* subsection a.

HERRLINGER, R. & F. KUDLIEN, eds., 1967: Frühe Anatomie von Mondino bis Malpighi. Eine Anthologie, 306 p. (Stuttgart: Wiss. Verlagsges.).—

A collection of lectures given at the Kieler Institut für Geschichte der Medizin und Pharmazie. Separate lectures deal with: Mondino, Guy de Chauliac, Arabian anatomy, Leonardo da Vinci and anatomy, Italian anatomy before Vesalius, Canano, Estienne, Vesalius on the anatomy of the heart and blood-vessels, Felix Platter, anatomy in England in the 16th and 17th centuries, Stensen, microscopical anatomy.

HUGHES, A., 1959: A history of cytology, 158 p. (New York, N.Y.: Abelard-Schuman).—

A brief but well-documented history of cytology, describing: the history of microscopical technique; the essential steps leading to the recognition of the cell; the discoveries concerning the nucleus, its division, its role in reproduction and heredity; the changing opinions on cytoplasm and the history of the cellular theory in general biology. *Cf.* ASCHOFF, L., *et al.,* 1938, *vide supra.*

KAJAVA, Y., 1928: Die Geschichte der Anatomie in Finland, 1640-1901. Eine Uebersicht, 137 p. (Acta Soc. Med. fenn. Duodecim, Vol. 10, fasc. 3) (Helsinki: Soc. Med. fenn. Duodecim).—

Within the history of Finnish anatomy, two periods can be distinguished, *viz.,* that of the academy of Turku (Åbo), 1640-1827, and that of the university of Helsinki, from 1828 onwards. The present study deals with organization, development, *etc.,* of both institutes during the period considered, discussing such aspects as: anatomical education, publications, teachers, institutes, and collections. Appendixes deal with anthropological publications published in Finland before the year 1901, and with the various ways by which the anatomists were provided with corpses; another appendix contains a list of names of prosectors, assistants, and lecturers connected with the anatomical institutes of Finland before 1901.

KEVORKIAN, J., 1959: The story of dissection, 80 p. (New York, N.Y.: Philosophical Library).—

An account of the - often peculiar - techniques used in the dissection of the animal and human body in antiquity, classical Greece, Hellenistic Alexandria, Rome, Byzantium, the Middle Ages, the Renaissance, the Baroque period, and the 19th and 20th centuries. A history of the anatomical theatre is to be found in: RICHTER, G., 1936: Das anatomische Theater, 156 p. (Abh. Gesch. Med. Naturwiss., Vol. 16) (Berlin: Ebering). *Cf.* LASSEK, A. M., 1958, *vide infra.*

KLEIN, M., 1936: Histoire des origines de la théorie cellulaire, 72 p. (Actualités scientifiques et industrielles, No. 328) (Paris: Hermann).—

The table of contents is as follows: 1: La découverte de la cellule et les débuts de l'anatomie microscopique végétale; 2. Les théories sur la structure élémentaire des êtres vivants au cours du XVIIIe siècle; 3. Genèse de la théorie cellulaire au cours de la première moitié du XIXe siècle; la philosophie de la nature, l'anatomie microscopique végétale, recherches sur la structure des corps animaux depuis Bichat jusqu'à la publication du livre de Schwann, aperçu sur le développement de la théorie cellulaire, de Schwann à Schultze. Between 1948 and 1955, J. R. BAKER published in the Quart. J. Microsc. Sci., Vols. 89-96 a series of papers containing a critical historical review of the cell-theory. Cf. ASCHOFF, L., et al., 1938, vide supra.

LASSEK, A. M., 1958: Human dissection: its drama and struggle, 310 p. (Springfield, Ill.: Thomas).—

This book contains information, chronologically arranged, concerning the dissection of the human body throughout the centuries. The subject matter has been divided into three sections: the first considers the concept regarding the dead in the various ancient civilizations, the Alexandrian School, Galen, and the Middle Ages. The second section deals with anatomy during the Renaissance with special reference to Vesalius. The third section deals with dissection in Europe, the Asiatic countries, the British Isles, and various parts of the U.S.A. Cf. KEVORKIAN, J., 1959, vide supra.

POTONIÉ, H., 1903: Ein Blick in die Geschichte der botanischen Morphologie und die Pericaulom-Theorie, 45 p. (Jena: Fischer).—

For this author morphology in its proper sense starts with Goethe (or probably with C. F. Wolff), and this science has been developed further on by e.g., E. Meyer, Gaudichaud, Nägeli, A. Braun, etc., and all their theories were based on a Platonic type-idea. In a later phase the problem of the transition and change of one organ into another came into the center of interest, and, according to the author, the transition from leaf to stem in the formation of the higher plants, can best be understood by accepting the pericaulous theory.

RUSSELL, K. F., 1963: British anatomy 1525-1800: a bibliography, 254 p. (Melbourne: U.P.; New York, N.Y. & London: Cambridge U.P.).—

A comprehensive bibliography of 90 items, listing all books on human anatomy written by British authors and published in Britain, America, and on the Continent, in all languages and editions, as well as the

works of continental authors translated into English or published in Britain in their original language. The items are alphabetically arranged by name of author, and contain much additional information concerning the books considered. The introduction (35 p.) contains a condensed history of British anatomy.

WATERMANN, R., 1964: Vom Leben der Gewebe. Ein kleines Geschichtsbuch. Der Weg von der antiken Atomistik über die Zellenlehre bis zur modernen Molekularbiologie, 104 p. (Cologne: Kölner Universitätsverlag).—

A historical review of the evolution of ideas concerning the structure of living matter. Starting from investigations made with the aid of electronic microscopes, the author goes back into history, in order to illustrate how the ideas of modern biologists about the structure of living matter are deeply rooted in history.

WEGNER, R. N., 1939: Das Anatomenbildnis. Seine Entwicklung im Zusammenhang mit der anatomischen Abbildung, 199 p. (Basle: Schwabe).—

"Excellent history of artistic anatomy, with bibliography. More material on the later periods than in Choulant." (From Doe & Marshall: 655). With 105 illustrations. Cf. CHOULANT, L., 1962, vide supra.

WEINDLER, F., 1908: Geschichte der gynäkologisch-anatomischen Abbildung, 186 p. (Dresden: Zahn & Jaensch).—

A beautifully illustrated book (some figures in colour), discussing anatomical illustration in gynaecology. The first part (p. 1-42) deals with antiquity (Hippocrates, Aristotle, Herophilos, Rufus, Soranos, Galen, Moschion) the second part with the period up to 1521 (p. 43-80) (H. de Mondeville, Mundinus, Ketham, da Vinci, Magnus Hundt). The third part deals with the period 1521-1543 (p. 81-116) (Berengario of Carpi, Dryander, Walter Ryff, C. Estienne); the fourth part with the period 1543-1627 (p. 117-148) (Vesalius, J. Rueff, Fabr. ad Aquapendente, Eustachius, Vidus Vidius, Platter); the fifth part with the period 1627-1737 (p. 149-172) (Casserius, J. C. Placentinus, J. Remmelin, Bidloo, Pietro Berrettini, R. de Graaf, J. Swammerdam, Gauthier d'Agoty, Boursier); and the sixth part deals with the period 1737-1778 (B. S. Albinus, von Haller, Hunter, Sömmering). Index of names.

WOLF-HEIDEGGER, G., & A. M. CET-
TO, 1967: Die anatomische Sektion in bild-
licher Darstellung, 612 p. (Basle & New
York, N.Y.: Karger).—

P. 1-120 contain a historical introduction to human anatomical dissection; p. 121-
392 a catalogue of anatomical pictures (in
miniatures, paintings, sculpture, reliefs,
medals, title-pages, vignettes, on portraits of
anatomists in the theatrum anatomicum, in
caricature and satire); p. 393-584 contain
355 very beautiful photographs, mentioned
and described in this catalogue. Another
very beautiful history of anatomical illustration (in Italian) is: PREMUDA, L., 1957:
Storia dell'iconografia anatomica, 235 p.
(Milan: Ed. Martello). Cf. also: GARRI-
SON, F. H., 1926: The principles of anatomic illustration before Vesalius: an inquiry into the rationale of artistic anatomy,
58 p. (New York, N.Y.: Hoeber). Of this
book I do not possess further information.
Cf. also CHOULANT, L., 1962, vide supra.

e. *History of embryology*

BILIKIEWICZ, T., 1932: Die Embryologie
im Zeitalter des Barocks und des Rokokos,
183 p. (Arbeiten Inst. Gesch. Med. Univ.
Leipzig, Vol. 2) (Leipzig: Thieme).—

This book mainly deals with the history of generation and as such it is comparable to the book of COLE, vide supra, subsection a. Among the authors considered
we mention: Harvey, De Graaf, W. Needham, Descartes, Borelli, Willis, Redi, Malpighi, Swammerdam, Malebranche, Leeuwenhoek, Maupertuis, Leibniz, Réaumur,
John Needham, von Haller, Bonnet, Spallanzani. Much attention has been paid to
the strife between ovists and animalculists.

CAULLERY, M., 1939: Les progrès récents
de l'embryologie expérimentale, 236 p. (Paris: Flammarion).—

A critical review of the progress of
experimental embryology during the period
1900-1940. Separate chapters deal with such
subjects as: the use of injected dyes, the
historical development of experimental embryology, merogony, exogastrulation by
lithium, the work of Spemann and his school
on morphogenesis and on grafting, the action of organizers, induction by grafts, mechanism and factors of embryonic induction, experimental embryology of insects,
experimental embryology and monstrosities.
395 illustrations.

MEYER, A. W., 1939: The rise of embryology, 367 p. (Stanford, Cal.: Univ. California Press).—

The book consists of a series of critical essays rather than a presentation of a
chronological history of embryology. The
chapters included primarily deal with the
origin and growth of basic embryological
ideas, such as: aboriginal and early historical ideas of generation, spontaneous generation, epigenesis, preformation, pangenesis, panspermia, malformation, morphogenesis, experimental embryology. Other
chapters have been devoted to the discovery
of the spermatozoon, the search for the
mammalian ovum, the role of the "mule",
and to speculations concerning the nature
of impregnation.

——, 1956: Human generation: conclusions
of Burdach, Döllinger and von Baer, 143 p.
(Stanford, Cal.: Univ. California Press).—

This study on the history of embryology contains: 1. An appreciation of K. F.
Burdach (1776-1846), showing that in this
field of knowledge little news had appeared since Harvey. Included are English translations of Burdach's "De primis
momentis formationis foetus" (1814) and
"De foetas humano adnotationes anatomicae" (1828). 2. A discussion of life and
work of J. J. I. Döllinger (1770-1841), including an English translation of his "Versuch einer Geschichte der menschlichen
Zeugung" (1816). 3. An analysis of life and
work of K. E. von Baer (1792-1878), especially of his connections with German "Naturphilosophie", together with an English
translation of his "Commentar zu der
Schrift: De ovi mammalium et hominis
genesi. Epistola ad Academiam scient. Petropolitanam" (1828).

NEEDHAM, J., 1959: A history of embryology, ed. 2, 304 p. (Rev. with assistance
of A. HUGHES) (Cambridge: U.P.).—

A well-written and well-known account of the history of embryology from
ancient speculations to factual observations
in the 17th and 18th centuries up to about
the year 1800. The interconnections between
embryology and social life (including its
many cultural and philosophical aspects)
during the successive periods have been
considered. A very complete bibliography
(containing many titles of old works) has
been added (p. 241-292).

OPPENHEIMER, J. M., 1967: Essays in the
history of embryology and biology, 374 p.

(Cambridge, Mass.: M.I.T. Press).—

A compilation of essays published in various journals. No attempt has been made to offer a complete history of embryology, but in their totality these essays allow the reader to get an idea what were the principal themes in the development of modern embryology.

SOUÈGES, R., 1934: L'embryologie végétale. Résumé historique. 1ʳᵉ époque: Dès origines à Hanstein (1870), 57 p. (Actualités sci. et industr., 142); 2ᵐᵉ époque: de Hanstein (1870) à nos jours, 59 p. (*Idem,* 175) (Paris: Hermann).—

The author tries to elucidate how new achievements in instruments and techniques fostered embryological research. According to the author two periods in the history of plant embryology can be distinguished, periods differing in observational techniques, in methodology and in metaphysical speculations. In the beginning, embryological investigations were almost exclusively of a morphological character; in a later phase the anatomical method became dominant (microscope!). Both these methods have been considered in the first volume. The second volume (1870-1934) consists of two parts; the first part deals with the histological period (1870-1895) and the second with the cytological period (1895-1934).

WILLIER, B. H. & J. M. OPPENHEIMER, eds., 1964: Foundations of experimental embryology, 225 p. (Englewood Cliffs, N.J.: Prentice-Hall).—

A collection of 11 classical papers in experimental embryology in English translation. The papers are linked together by introductory comments. Papers are included of: Roux, Driesch, Wilson, Boveri, Harrison, Warburg, F. Lillie (2), Child, Spemann & Mangold, and Holtfreter.

f. *History of physiology*

BASTHOLM, E., 1950: The history of muscle physiology from the natural philosophers to Albrecht von Haller: a study of the history of medicine, 257 p. (Acta historica scientiarum naturalium, Vol. VII) (Diss. Univ. Copenhagen) (Copenhagen: Munksgaard).—

A historical analysis and critical appraisal relating to the development of theor-ies concerning the functions of the muscles and the mechanism of their actions. The first four chapters deal with the period from the origin of Greek medicine to Fabricius ab Aquapendente at the end of the 16th century. The fifth and last chapter, comprising about half of the volume, covers only the period from Descartes to Haller.

BROOKS, C. M. & P. F. CRANEFIELD, eds., 1959: The historical development of physiological thought: a symposium, 401 p. (New York, N.Y.: Hafner).—

The general topic of this symposium is to show how basic medical science acquired its concepts; the aim was achieved by discussing "physiological concepts which have contributed to our understanding of the operation of biological systems and the behaviour of living organisms." There are five main divisions: 1. Medicine and basic scientific thought; 2. The basis of integrative function and human behaviour; 3. Humoral transport and integrative function; 4. Mechanistic thought, energetics, and control in biology; 5. The vital process and the disease state.

COMFORT, A., 1964: The biology of senescence, 365 p. (London: Routledge & Kegan Paul).—

A historical review of gerontological research, mainly concerned with the last 50 years. The author tries to give a new synthesis of the conflicting philosophical, medico-biological and social aspects of present gerontology. He summarizes his point of view in the following words: "senescence is typically an undirected process - not a part of the programme, but a weakening of the directive force of the programme." *Cf.* GRMEK, M. D., 1958, *vide* section History of the medical sciences, subsection c (geriatrics).

FOSTER, M., 1901: Lectures on the history of physiology during the sixteenth, seventeenth and eighteenth centuries, 310 p. (Cambridge: U.P.).—

Publication of the "Lane lectures" delivered at the Cooper Medical College in San Francisco in the autumn of 1900, consisting of a series of capita selecta about the following topics: Vesalius' influence; Harvey and the circulation of the blood; Borelli and his "New Physics"; Malpighi and the physiology of glands and tissues; van Helmont and the rise of chemical physiology; Sylvius and the physiology of digestion; the English school of the 17th century on respiration; the physiology of digestion in the 18th century; the rise of modern doctrines of respiration; the older doctrines of the nervous system. Reprinted in 1924.

FRANKLIN, K. J., 1949: A short history of physiology, ed. 2, 147 p. (New York, N.Y.: Staples Press).—

The present volume deals with animal physiology and it intends to show the evolution of the experimental method. Thus it is a chronology of discoveries and inventions, and it also contains a description of the techniques used. The author begins his exposition with Alcmaeon and ends his story about 1900. It is intended to provide students with literature for collateral reading as they learn physiology from their standard texts. First ed. 1933, 122 p. (London: Bale & Danielson). Cf. FULTON, J., 1931, vide infra.

FULTON, J. F., 1931: Physiology, 141 p. (Clio Medica, No. 5) (New York, N.Y.: Hoeber).—

A booklet which offers an authoritative introduction to the medical student wishing to obtain an idea of the historical development of physiology. As an appendix, extracts with translations are offered of Claude Bernard's conception of the term "general physiology". Indexes of personal names and of subjects. Cf. FRANKLIN, K. J., 1949, vide supra.

——, 1966: Selected readings in the history of physiology, ed. 2, 492 p. (Completed by L. G. WILSON) (Springfield, Ill.: Thomas).—

The first ed. was published in 1930. A very useful and interesting selection of texts of classics in the history of physiology. Much attention has been paid to recent developments as they took place before the author's untimely death in 1960. Cf. ROTH-SCHUH, K. E., 1968, vide infra.

GOODFIELD, G. J., 1960: The growth of scientific physiology: physiological method and the mechanist-vitalist controversy, illustrated by the problems of respiration and animal heat, 174 p. (London: Hutchinson).—

During the 18th and 19th centuries the problem of animal heat was a physical as well as a biological problem; and since ancient times the source of the body warmth of animals was one of the central problems of biology and one of the central themes around which the mechanist-vitalist controversy raged. The authoress mainly deals with the emergence of scientific physiology in the 19th century, and as a culminating point she considers Claude Bernard's "Introduction to the study of experimental medicine", in which he states that biological phenomena are determined exactly in the same way as physical and chemical phenomena. Cf. MENDELSOHN, E., 1964: vide infra.

GOTTLIEB, L. S., 1964: A history of respiration, 121 p. (Springfield, Ill.: Thomas).—

"The roster of contributors to the science of respiration includes many of the famous names in medical history. Beginning with antiquity, their achievements are traced through the period of Greco-Roman, Arabic, Medieval, and Renaissance medicine." (Publisher's announcement J. Hist. Med. & Allied Sci. 20: 94). Cf. GRAUBARD, M., 1964, vide subsection a.

GRUMAN, G. J., ed., 1966: A history of ideas about the prolongation of life: the evolution of the prolongevity hypothesis to 1800, 102 p. (Trans. Amer. Phil. Soc., Vol. 56, part 9) (Philadelphia, Pa.: Amer. Phil. Soc.).—

A compendium of quotations on the subject of human attitudes towards long life from the remote past up to recent times and dealing with many cultures and religions.

HARVEY, E. N., 1957: A history of luminescence from the earliest times until 1900, 692 p. (Memoirs Amer. Phil. Soc., Vol. 44) (Philadelphia, Pa.: Amer. Phil. Soc.).—

The text of this book has been divided into three parts: 1. Luminescence through the centuries; 2. Luminescence of non-living material; 3. Bioluminescence. This third part deals with shining fish, flesh and wood; with phosphorescence of the sea; and with animal luminescence. The earliest records of bioluminescence stem from the "Thirteen classics" of China. Because the author is an eminent student of bioluminescence, this study can be taken as authoritative.

IZQUIERDO, J. J., 1934: Balance cuatricentenario de la físiologia en Mexico, 358 p. (México: Ed. Ciencia).—

A well-illustrated account of psysiology and medicine in Mexico from the time of the Spanish conquest onwards. Good index and valuable bibliography.

JENSEN, L. B., 1953: Man's foods: nutrition and environments in food-gathering times and food-producing times, 278 p. (Champaign, Ill.: Garrard Press).—

A compendium of enquiry carried out concerning man's nutritional quest from the oldest known Palaeolithic times to classical antiquity. The first part, entitled "Food-gathering times", deals with eating economy of pre-*Homo sapiens* types, and Mesolithic man. The second part, entitled "Food-producing times", deals with dietary practices of Neolithic man, esp. with the introduction of vegetarian dietary components, such as cereals, products of the orchard and garden, but also with the problem of domesticated animals and the role of meat in his diet. The third part contains various topics concerning food in general, such as the psychology of food habits, food and custom, food taboos, food manners and implements, mode of preparation, food and climate, *etc.*

KEELE, K. D., 1957: Anatomies of pain, 206 p. (Oxford: Blackwell).—

In this book the author traces the progression of our knowledge concerning the nature of pain and the character of pain sensation from the Egyptians and Babylonians, through the Greeks and Arabs up to the 20th century. Special attention has been paid to ideas considering the anatomo-physiological correlate of the pain sensation; the author illustrates how this problem is tied up with that of the seat of the soul.

KEILIN, D., ed., 1966: The history of cell respiration and cytochrome, 416 p. (Cambridge: U.P.).—

The first chapters of this book present a historical survey of the subject of cellular respiration up to the 20th century. Chapters follow in which the history of the problem of circulation and the history of our knowledge concerning the problem of respiration have been traced, and chapters in which the concepts and theories concerning cellular oxidations and reductions have been reviewed. The main part of the book describes Keilin's own work on the discovery of the properties of the cytochromes. The book also includes a summary of studies made by other investigators on the subject.

KOSHTOYANT, K. S., 1964: Essays on the history of physiology in Russia, 321 p.

(transl. by P. BODER, K. HANES and N. O'BRIAN) (Washington, D.C.: American Inst. Biol. Sci.).—

In this history of Russian physiology stress has been laid on the achievements of neurophysiology in Russia, centered around the work and life of Sechenov and Pavlov. Separate chapters also deal with the development of the physiology of digestion, and of circulation, and with developmental and comparative physiology. No index. The author's own field of specialization has been in neurophysiology.

LIDDELL, E. G. T., 1960: The discovery of reflexes, 174 p. (London: Oxford U.P.).—

In this book the author sketches the development of scientific thought leading to a better understanding of the essential features of the structure and the function of the nervous system. The book has been written as a "tribute to the life and work of Charles Sherrington", and accordingly the book has been divided into two parts, the first part dealing with the history of neurophysiology before Sherrington's time and the second part dealing with Sherrington's investigations in the field of neurophysiology. There is a good biographical appendix. A book of similar scope is: CANGUILHEM, G., 1955: La formation du concept de réflexe aux XVIIe et XVIIIe siècles, 208 p. (Paris: Presses Univ. de France). *Cf.* also MARX, E., 1939, *vide infra.*

McCOLLUM, E. V., 1957: A history of nutrition: the sequence of ideas in nutrition investigations, 451 p. (Boston, Mass.: Houghton Mifflin).—

The objective of this book is, in the author's own words, "to trace the story of the observations and speculations of early clinicians by which they sought to discover the effects of foods on the sick and well; that of the physiologists, who sought to understand by what processes of change foods so unlike each other and unlike the body constituents could be so altered by digestion as to be prepared for absorption from the alimentary tract and conversion into blood, and then into body tissues; and finally, that of the reasoning and experimenting by which chemists sought to learn the nature of foods and their transformations, or 'metamorphoses', as they served as nutrients for the body."

MAISEL, A. Q., 1965: The hormone quest, 262 p. (New York, N.Y.: Random House).—

A popular, well-written historical review of the subject. Many workers in the field are mentioned and their contributions pinpointed. Ca. 80% of the text deals with the sex hormones, elucidating such timely subjects as the development of synthetic sex hormones, hormones that prevent conception, those which cure infertility, etc.

MARX, E., 1939: Die Entwicklung der Reflexlehre seit Albrecht von Haller bis in die zweite Hälfte des 19. Jahrhunderts, 126 p. (Sitzb. heidelb. Akad. Wissensch., Math.-naturw. Kl., Jg. 1938) (Heidelberg: Weissche Universitätsbuchhandlung).—

Of this publication, P. Diepgen writes in the Mitt. Gesch. Med. 38: 257: "Man kann diese Studie eher eine philosophische Betrachtung der Problematik der Reflexlehre und der Versuche ihrer Lösung als eine geschichtliche Darstellung ihrer Entwicklung in den 100 Jahren zwischen Haller und Ernst Pflüger nennen. Sie ist in einer schwer verständlichen Sprache geschrieben... der Inhalt der Studie... geht in erster Linie den Philosophen an, der Ergebnisse der Naturwissenschaft verwerten und begrifflich ausdeuten will." Cf. also LIDDELL, E. G. T., 1960, vide supra.

MENDELSOHN, E., 1964: Heat and life: the development of the theory of animal heat, 208 p. (Cambridge, Mass.: Harvard U.P.).—

The author analyses the changes undergone by the theory of animal heat since the speculations of the Greeks, through Harvey's ideas related to the circulation of the blood, to the explanations based on ideas of respiration and combustion. The author himself describes his aim with the following words: "This study, then, had its origins in my desire to find out what elements went into concept formation in the biological sciences and what the relation of this process was to the knowledge and techniques of the physical sciences." Cf. GOODFIELD, G. J., 1960, vide supra.

MITTASCH, A., 1951: Geschichte der Ammoniaksynthese, 196 p. (Weinheim: Verlag Chemie).—

After a description of a century of unsuccessful efforts, the author especially considers the period between 1903 and 1920, the period during which Haber made the first attempts (1903), Nernst applied the third law of thermodynamics (1907) and Mittasch synthesized ammonia in the laboratory (1909). The book is mainly concerned with German research in this field. This volume is supplemented by another one of the same author, viz., Salpetersäure aus Ammoniak. Geschichtliche Entwicklung der Ammoniakoxydation bis 1920, 1953, 136 p. (Weinheim: Verlag Chemie).

NASH, L. K., 1952: Plants and the atmosphere, 122 p. (Harvard Case Histories in Experimental Science, Case 5) (Cambridge, Mass.: Harvard U.P.).—

This book tells the story how van Helmont, Boyle, Hales, Lavoisier, Priestly, Ingen-Housz, Senebier, de Saussure laid the foundation for our knowledge of the "feeding" of plants. It makes clear how botanists, physiologists and chemists together discovered that the plants got their "food" from the air, and that the carbon cycle would be impossible without the green plant. Cf. TRÖNDLE, A., 1925, vide infra.

NEUBURGER, M., 1967: Die historische Entwicklung der experimentellen Gehirn- und Rückenmarksphysiologie vor Flourens, 362 p. (Amsterdam: Bonset).—

A reprint of the 1897 edition. Unfortunately I am not able to give further information about this book. Cf. CLARKE, E. & C. D. O'MALLEY, eds., 1968, vide subsection d.

POYNTER, F. N. L., ed., 1958: The history and philosophy of knowledge of the brain and its functions: an Anglo-American symposium, London, July 15-17, 1957, 272 p. (Oxford: Blackwell; Springfield, Ill.: Thomas).—

The 17 papers published in this volume served as a historical introduction to the First International Congress of Neurological Sciences. One of the central themes is that theories of brain functions at any period depend both on knowledge of the anatomical structure and on current philosophical pre-conceptions. Other topics discussed are: old and new concepts of consciousness and the origin of language; mediaeval, Cartesian, and 17th-century ideas and observations; 19th-century and contemporary theory. Besides its historical aspects, the book contains much that is of value to anyone interested in the development of scientific theory. Cf. CLARKE, E. & C. D. O'MALLEY, eds., 1968, vide supra, subsection d.

PREMUDA, L., 1966: Storia della fisiologia, 326 p. (Udine: Del Bianco Editore).—

> The first history of physiology in the Italian language.

ROTHSCHUH, K. E., 1952: Geschichte der Physiologie, 249 p. (Berlin: Springer).—

> This book gives a survey of the history of physiology from antiquity to the turn of the 20th century and is largely based on a biographical approach. It deals in lively fashion with the great founders of physiological schools during the 18th and 19th centuries (to which the greater part of the book, p. 68-216, has been devoted) and their various influences down to quite recent times. The book mainly deals with German physiologists. The author analyses the evolution, transmission and changes of the concept of physiology.

——, 1968: Physiologie. Der Wandel ihrer Konzepte, Probleme und Methoden vom 16. bis 20. Jahrhundert, 407 p. (Freiburg i.B.: Alber).—

> The text of this book consists of a series of selected quotations, arranged according to the various schools of thought. Each of the quotations given is accompanied by a scholarly introduction or comment. *Cf.* also: ROTHSCHUH, K. E., ed., 1964: Von Boerhaave bis Berger. Die Entwicklung der kontinentalen Physiologie im 18. und 19. Jahrhundert mit besonderer Berücksichtigung der Neurophysiologie, 254 p. (Medizin in Geschichte und Kultur, Vol. 5) (Stuttgart: Fischer).

——, 1969: Physiologie im Werden, 188 p. (Medizin in Geschichte und Kultur, Vol. 9) (Stuttgart: Fischer).—

> A series of essays, dealing with the history of physiology, originally published elsewhere. Separate sections deal with such subjects as: what is important to the history of science?; idea and method and their meaning for the development of physiology; physiology in German Romanticism; the system of physiology of Jean Fernel; the development of the theory of the circulation after Harvey; the conflict between Jean Riolan and P. M. Schlegel concerning Harvey's theory; Descartes and his theory of the phenomena of life; spiritus animalis and nervous activity, animal electricity; origin and changes in physiological ideas during the 19th century. Index of names.

STIRLING, W., 1902: Some apostles of physiology: being an account of their lives and labours, 129 p. (London: Privately published by Waterlow & Sons).—

> A history of physiology in biographies, from Vesalius to T. H. Huxley, with frequent quotations from the works of the authors concerned. No table of contents or index. Fine illustrations.

TRÖNDLE, A., 1925: Geschichte des Atmungs- und Ernährungsproblems bei den Pflanzen, 111 p. (Zurich & Leipzig: Füssli).—

> The author reviews the history of the physiology of respiration and nutrition of plants as it took rise from Priestly, Scheele, Ingen-Housz and Senebier, down to de Saussure, stressing the mutual interrelation between the problems to be solved and the advancement of experimental techniques. *Cf.* NASH, L. K., 1952, *vide supra*.

WEEVERS, T., 1949: Fifty years of plant physiology, 308 p. (Amsterdam: Scheltema & Holkema).—

> For more details, *vide* subsection History of botany in general, *vide infra*.

g. *History of microbiology*

BIGGER, J. W., 1939: Man against microbe, 304 p. (New York, N.Y.: Macmillan).—

> A well-written and authoritative history of microbiology, explaining what bacteria are, what they do and how they are studied; the history of the discovery of micro-organisms, their relationship to disease, and their roles in agriculture and industry. The book can be considered as an introduction to BULLOCH's The history of bacteriology, *vide infra*.

BROCK, T., ed., 1961: Milestones in microbiology, 275 p. (Englewood Cliffs, N.Y.: Prentice Hall).—

> A collection of historically important articles written in or translated into English. The subject matter has been divided into 6 sections: 1. Spontaneous generation and fermentation (16 articles: *e.g.*, Leeuwenhoek, Spallanzani, Pasteur, Buchner); 2. Germ theory of disease (11 papers: *e.g.*, Fracastorius, Lister, Koch, Ehrlich); 3. Im-

munology (7 papers: *e.g.*, Jenner, Pasteur, von Behring, Bordet); 4. Virology (4 papers: Loeffler, Beyerinck, d'Herelle, Stanley); 5. Chemotherapy (5 papers: *e.g.*, Ehrlich, Fleming, Domagk, Woods); 6. General microbiology (12 papers: *e.g.*, Cohn, Gram, Beyerinck, Winogradsky, Kluyver).

BULLOCH, W., 1960: The history of bacteriology, 422 p. (London: Oxford U.P.).—

    This is essentially a history of medical bacteriology. It deals with such subjects as: ancient doctrines of contagion, contagion animatum, spontaneous generation, fermentation, putrefaction, putrid intoxications, surgical sepsis, classification and cultivation of bacteria, Pasteur's work on attenuation of virus, and the history of the doctrines of immunity. Extensive and very complete bibliography and a very accurate and valuable biographical dictionary of workers in and contributors to bacteriology. (First ed. 1938). For an introduction to this book, *cf.* BIGGER, J. W., 1939, *vide supra,* or FORD, W. W., 1939, *vide infra.*

CLARK, P. F., 1961: Pioneer microbiologists of America, 369 p. (Madison, Wis.: Univ. of Wisconsin Press).—

    This book covers the early history of American microbiology and contains much information concerning the way microbiology has contributed to fundamental science, to the control of epidemic diseases, to industrial processes, and to agricultural practice in the United States. The subject matter has been divided into 5 sections: 1. Foundation of early bacteriology (4 chapters); 2. The Atlantic seaboard (8 chapters); 3. The Central Valley (2 chapters); 4. Our western lands (2 chapters); 5. Perspective (2 chapters). Extensive index. Contains much biographical information and photographs of 37 microbiologists.

DOERR, H., 1938: Die Entwicklung der Virusforschung und ihre Problematik. Morphologie der Virusarten. Die Züchtung der Virusarten außerhalb ihrer Wirte. Biochemistry and biophysics of viruses, 546 p. (In: R. DOERR & C. HALLAUER, Handbuch der Virusforschung, 1. Hälfte) (Vienna: Springer).—

    The first part of this well-known manual consists of four chapters. The first contains a historical review of virology and the theories concerning the nature of virus and is the most important one from our

point of view. The second chapter deals with viral morphology, *e.g.,* with the form and sizes of viruses and bacteriophages and the methods for their determination, colouring of viruses, inclusion bodies and their relationship to viruses. Chapter 3 deals with the culture of viruses *in vitro* and their growth-processes, and the fourth chapter deals with the biochemistry and biophysics of viruses.

DOETSCH, R. N., ed., 1960: Microbiology: historical contributions from 1776 to 1908, 233 p. (New Brunswick, N. J.: Rutgers U.P.).—

    An anthology, containing 17 papers selected by the decision to proceed "from the question of the origin of microbes (Spallanzani, Schwann, Tyndall) to their role in fermentations (Schwann, Pasteur) to methods for dealing with them in the laboratory (Koch, Ehrlich) and classifying them (Cohn, Orla-Jensen) to a recognition of their importance as biological entities (Lister, Schloesing, Warington, Winogradsky, Burrill, Smith, Beyerinck)."

DUBOS, R. J., 1962: The unseen world, 112 p. (New York, N.Y.: Rockefeller Inst. Press; Oxford: U.P.).—

    A rather popular historical review. It is a series of lectures which have been converted into 5 essays, entitled: Microscopic cells and giant crystals; Microbes as chemical machines; The germ theory of disease; The domestication of microbial life; Biological partnerships; and a supplementary chapter on: Science as a way of life.

FORD, W. W., 1939: Bacteriology, 207 p. (Clio Medica, No. 22) (New York, N.Y.: Hoeber).—

    This booklet contains the following chapters: 1. Early observations and theories which influenced the development of bacteriology; 2. Development of knowledge concerning magnification; 3. Discovery of the bacteria by Leeuwenhoek; 4. Progress in the 18th century in relation to spontaneous generation, origin of disease and knowledge of bacteria; 5. Progress in the first part of the 19th century up to Henle; 6. Life and work of Pasteur, Lister, and Tyndall; 7. The rise of the German school of bacteriologists under Cohn; 8. Life and work of Robert Koch; 9. Pasteur's work on vaccination against anthrax, swine erysipelas and rabies; 10. Bacterial toxins and antitoxins; 11. Development of the subject of immunology; 12. Later development of bacteriology. Like BIGGER's book *(vide supra)*, this book can be considered as an introduction to BULLOCH's work *(vide supra)*. Reprinted in 1964 (New York, N.Y.: Hafner). A French history of microbiology is: HAUDUROY, P., 1944: Microbes. De la naissance et de la vie de quelques découvertes illustres en microbiologie, 136 p., a book of which I could not find further details.

GRAINGER, T. H., ed., 1958: A guide to the history of bacteriology, 210 p. (New York, N.Y.: Ronald Press).—

    This work is a selective, annotated bibliography from which selections for own reading can be made from original contributors and from various selected comprehensive reviews. It includes sections on medical, dairy, dental, food, industrial, insect, marine, sanitary, soil, sewage, military, and water bacteriology. It has been divided into 4 parts. The first deals with the general literature of bacteriology, the second with the history of bacteriology, and the third and fourth parts deal with relevant biographical materials; the last part contains a guide to the bibliographies of 90 selected bacteriologists arranged alphabetically from Behring to Zinsser.

KNAYSI, G., 1951: Historical approach to bacterial cytology, ed. 2, 375 p. (Ithaca, N.Y.: Comstock).—

    Unfortunately I am unable to give any information as to the contents of this book.

LECHEVALIER, H. A. & M. SOLOTOROVSKY, 1965: Three centuries of microbiology, 536 p. (New York, N.Y.: McGraw-Hill).—

    This history is essentially a collection of biographies of outstanding microbiologists and of other scientists whose work has influenced them. After a historical review ranging from Fracastorius to Pasteur, there are chapters on Pasteur and Koch, bacteria as agents of diseases, cellular and humoral immunology, soil microbiology, viruses and rickettsiae, mycology, protozoology, chemotherapy, and genetics. Each chapter has a very complete list of references, containing many biographies; there is a good index.

h. *History of genetics and evolution theory*

BARTHELMESS, A., 1952: Vererbungswissenschaft, 429 p. (Orbis Academicus II/2) (Freiburg i.B. & Munich: Alber).—

    This book describes the development of the science of genetics from its origin up to recent times, in order to arrive at a critical evaluation of its present-day situation. Separate chapters deal with such subjects as: Hippocrates, Aristotle, and the science of genetics; theories of reproduction and development of Harvey, von Haller, Wolff; the species concept of Linnaeus, Koelreuter, Gärtner; the theories of descent of Erasmus and Charles Darwin, and of Lamarck; Mendel; Haeckel, Weismann, His, the Hertwig brothers, Nägeli, Roux; the hypothesis of heredity: Hering, Spencer, C. Darwin, Galton, de Vries, Weismann, Reinke, Roux, Driesch); experimental genetics, the role of the nucleus, cytoplasm, plastids; phylogenesis; phaenogenetics.

BLACKER, C. P., 1952: Eugenics: Galton and after, 349 p. (Cambridge, Mass.: Harvard U.P.).—

    An account of the views of Galton and of the developments which have taken place in the field of eugenics since his death in 1911. The first part (p. 19-128) deals with the life, scientific interests, personality, religious views, *etc.,* of Galton. The second part (p. 129-322) deals with the generation after Galton, stages in population growth, development in testing procedures, developments in genetics after 1911, and with eugenics to-day. Appendixes contain a review of Galton's views on race, and a list of scientific papers, books and other publications by Galton. Index.

CAIRNS, J., G. S. STENDT & J. D. WATSON, eds., 1966: Phage and the origins of molecular biology, 340 p. (Cold Spring Harbor, N.Y.: Cold Spring Harbor Laboratory of Quantitative Biology).—

    A series of 33 papers, contributed by 35 molecular biologists, which together gives a picture of the historical development of molecular biology. Each of the participants has written - more or less - his own chronicle. *Cf.* WATSON, J. D., 1968, *vide infra.*

CARLSON, E. A., 1966: The gene: a critical history, 301 p. (Philadelphia, Pa.: Saunders).—

    This is not a chronological history, but purely a history of the dominant concepts which together have led to the gene concept (*e.g.,* crossing-over, the presence and absence hypothesis, the genomere hypothesis, position effect, point mutation, allelism, the target theory, the plasmagene theory, the one-gene: one-enzyme hypothesis, the coding problem, *etc.* Elaborate bibliography (323 items) and indexes of authors and subjects.

CARTER, G. S., 1957: A hundred years of evolution, 206 p. (London: Sidgwick & Jackson).—

This booklet gives a short and summary account of the history of evolution-theory during the last hundred years, stressing the really significant episodes. It is an attempt to give an unbiassed view of the standpoint generally accepted to-day. Emphasis is laid on the relation between evolution-theory and the development of non-biological thought during this last century. The book is intended to serve non-specialists in the field of evolution-theory. *Cf.* HEBERER, G. & F. SCHWANITZ, 1960, *vide infra.*

CHOUARD, P., 1951: Éléments de génétique et d'amélioration des plantes. I: Les mécanismes de l'hérédité élémentaire ou factorielle, 137 p. (Paris: Centre de Documentation Universitaire).—

"Historical study of the development of the concept of transmission of parental characters from the parents to the offspring, and critical examination of classical theories of heredity in the light of the experimental dates concerning the impact of physiological phenomena, as influenced by chemical and physical agents, on the cytological material intervening in transmission of heritable characters." (Quoted from Isis 44).

DANIELS, J., ed., 1968: Darwinism comes to America, 137 p. (Waltham, Mass. & London: Blaisdell, Ginn).—

A collection of letters, periodicals, and reports in the United States relating to the publication of Darwin's "Origin of species". Separate sections deal with the correspondence between Darwin and Gray, the public debate between Gray and Agassiz in Boston, religious and scientific arguments in the rejection of Darwin's theory, the neo-Lamarckian compromise, the first stirrings of social Darwinism in the U.S.A. No bibliography or index. A review in Isis 60:261 speaks of "this disappointing little book... of only marginal interest to readers of Isis...".

DOBZHANSKY, T., 1951: Genetics and the origin of species, ed. 3, 364 p. (New York, N.Y.: Columbia U.P.).—

A very well written systematization of the advances in genetics since the appearance of Darwin's "Origin of species", and the application of this theory to the theory of evolution. It discusses the mechanism of the formation of species in terms of the known facts and theories of genetics. It is the most comprehensive book on the subject. Very large bibliography. Comparable books are: SCHMALHAUSEN, I. I., 1949: Factors of evolution, 327 p. (Philadelphia, Pa.: Blakiston); SIMPSON, G. G., 1967: The meaning of evolution, ed. 2, 368 p. (New Haven, Conn.: Yale U.P.); and: DARLINGTON, C. D., 1958: Evolution of genetic systems, ed. 2, 265 p. (New York, N.Y.: Basic Bks.). (1st ed. 1939).

DUNN, L. C., ed., 1951: Genetics in the 20th century: essays on the progress of genetics during its first 50 years, 634 p. (New York, N.Y.: Macmillan).—

The present volume consists of 26 essays presented by distinguished American and European geneticists at a meeting of the Genetics Society of America to celebrate the 50th anniversary of the re-discovery of Mendel's principles. The opening address is by R. GOLDSCHMIDT and reviews the impact of genetics on science. Three historical essays follow: ILTIS, H.: Gregor Mendel's life and heritage (p. 25-34); ZIRKLE, C.: The knowledge of heredity before 1900 (p. 35-38); CASTLE, W. E.: The beginnings of Mendelism in America (p. 59-76). Other essays deal with more or less theoretical problems, with chemical aspects of genetics, the genetics of antigens, bacteria, hybrid corn (maize), population genetics and many other topics.

——, 1966: A short history of genetics, 261 p. (New York, N.Y.: McGraw-Hill).—

A clearly-written historical review of the main lines of thinking prevailing in the science of genetics between 1864 and 1939, written by a competent student of genetics. The book especially deals with the pre-Mendelian and Mendelian phases in the development of genetics. Extensive bibliography. Included are brief biographical sketches of some of those men who made outstanding contributions to the science of genetics. *Cf.* RAVIN, A. W., 1965; STUBBE, H., 1965; and STURTEVANT, A. H., 1965.

EISELEY, L., 1959: Darwin's century: evolution and the men who discovered it, 378 p. (London: Gollancz).—

A very readable account of the history of the discovery of the phenomenon of evolution, especially as it took place during the 19th century. The author points out how, during the history of science, the different pieces, stemming from different fields of knowledge, together formed successively the chart of evolution. The book is largely restricted to the Anglo-Saxon contributions, but many of the pieces considered are not readily to be found in other historical reviews. *Cf.* GREENE, J. C., *vide infra.*

FOTHERGILL, P. G., 1952: Historical aspects of organic evolution, 427 p. (London: Hollis & Carter).—

According to a review in Isis 37: 105-106, the author treats of the theory of evolution from a more or less anti-Darwinian point of view. The treatment of the earlier development of the idea of evolution is rather sketchy and not always fair and accurate in every respect. Much literature up to *ca.* 1941 has been included in this book, but the more recent developments should have been better considered.

GEDDA, L., 1961: Twins in history and science, 240 p. (Springfield, Ill.: Thomas).—

For more details, *vide* section Philosophy of the life sciences.

GLASS, B., O. TEMKIN & W. L. STRAUS, eds., 1959: Forerunners of Darwin: 1745-1859, 471 p. (Baltimore, Md.: Johns Hopkins Press).—

A profound study of the development of the idea that the world as it exists has not always been the same. The essays can be divided into three groups. The first is of an introductory character, and contains two essays, one on fossils and early chronology, the second on the germination of the idea of biological species. The second group deals with 18th-century thought, discussing, *inter alia*, the part played by Maupertuis, Buffon, Diderot, Kant, and Herder. The third group deals with 19th-century pre-Darwinian evolutionists such as Lyell and Falconer. The central theme through the book is the never-ceasing conflict between the increasing amount of facts indicating that the world is subject to changes with the growing insight that species have been evolved one from another on the one side, and religious orthodoxy on the other side. A paperback edition appeared in 1968 (Baltimore, Md.: Johns Hopkins Press). A French book dealing with the same subjects is: QUATREFAGES, A. de, 1892: Darwin et ses précurseurs français. Étude sur le transformisme, ed. 2, 299 p. (Paris: Alcan).

GREENE, J. C., 1959: The death of Adam: evolution and its impact on Western thought, 388 p. (Ames, Iowa: Iowa State U.P.).—

A historical description of the changing concepts concerning the nature of the living world during the period lying between John Ray and Darwin-Wallace, during which period the prevailing world view altered from a static into a dynamic conception of the world. It also describes the growing insistence on the great age of the earth and of life on earth. The book is concerned mainly with speculations about the evolution of man, and in this context the author makes clear that two Darwinian principles, *viz.*, that of natural selection and that of the formation of new varieties by isolation, had been formulated many years before Darwin by W. Wells and J. Pritchard while speculating about the origins of the races of man. The book also contains a more general discussion concerning the evolution of the earth as such, the nature of species, the problem of domestication, *etc. Cf.* EISELEY, L., 1959, *vide supra.*

HEBERER, G. & F. SCHWANITZ, 1960: Hundert Jahre Evolutionsforschung. Das wissenschaftliche Vermächtnis Charles Darwin, 458 p. (Stuttgart: Fischer).—

A hundred years ago Darwin's "Origin of species" appeared, the first attempt to analyse the process of evolution scientifically. After the appearance of that book the image of biology altered fundamentally, influenced as it was by the new vision which permeated into all its diverse aspects. The present book is a German contribution to commemorate the centenary of its publication, and its main purpose is to test the validity of Darwin's theses in comparison with present knowledge and research. It discusses such topics as: the causes of evolution, and the role played by environment; the evolution of cultivated plants and domesticated animals; the present position of the theory of natural selection; the alterations which took place in the fields of geology, palaeontology, anthropogeny, geography, genetics, systematics. A bibliography of the publications of Darwin is included. *Cf.* CARTER, G. S., 1957, *vide supra.*

HOOYKAAS, R., 1963: Natural law and divine miracle: the principle of uniformity in geology, biology and theology, ed. 2, 237 p. (Leiden: Brill).—

The book consists mainly of a historical sketch of the role which the principle of uniformity has played in geology and evolution theory, up to recent times. By the principle of uniformity the author means that scientific method which enables our imagination to go from the present to the past (by reconstruction of this past from relics and by analogical reasoning); that method does not rest exclusively upon observation or experiment, not is it the method applied by the true historical sciences (for it deals with phenomena for which in most cases no human testimony is available). The metaphysical character and philosophical implications of this principle are considered, together with a confrontation with theology.

HUTCHINSON, G. E., 1965: The ecological theater and the evolutionary play, 139 p. (New Haven, Conn.: Yale U.P.).—

"The 6 learned and elegant essays here presented may be read as a unit on esthetic and philosophical aspects of the history of biology; but there are specific subjects of interest to the history of genetics, of biogenesis, of evolution theory." (From: Isis 57: 546).

IRVINE, W., 1955: Apes, angels and Victorians: the story of Darwin, Huxley, and evolution, 399 p. (New York, N.Y.: McGraw-Hill).—

A study of the impact of the evolution theory on 19th-century scientific, religious and political concepts, written by a professor of Victorian literature, and based on many hitherto unpublished letters and papers in the Darwin and Huxley collections. The author especially tries to throw new light on the motives of Darwin and Huxley which forced them to propagate their revolutionizing thoughts.

KŘIŽENECKÝ, J., ed., 1965: Fundamenta genetica: the revised edition of Mendel's classic paper with a collection of 27 original papers published during the rediscovery era. Published for the celebration of the centenary of the publication of Mendel's discoveries in Brno in 1865, 400 p. (Brno: Moravian Museum; Prague: Publishing House of the Czechoslovak Acad. Sci.).—

After an introductory essay of B. Němec, entitled: "Before Mendel", and a commentary of J. Křiženecký, the reprinted text follows of papers of Mendel, de Vries (2), Correns (3), Tschermak (2), Bateson (6),

Cuénot, Castle (2), Boveri (2), Cannon, Sutton, McClung, and Garrod.

MAYR, E., 1963: Animal species and evolution, 797 p. (Cambridge, Mass.: Harvard U.P.).—

The author traces the history of concepts related to the theory of evolution, particularly as they were developed since Darwin laid the foundations of the theory of natural selection. It is of special importance for the history of the last thirty years during which period our ideas about biological evolution underwent major changes as a result of the incorporation of many new genetical achievements into these ideas.

MILLHAUSER, M., 1959: Just before Darwin: Robert Chambers and "Vestiges", 246 p. (Middletown, Conn.: Wesleyan U.P.).—

This book is valuable as a reflection of the intellectual climate of Victorian England. For more particulars about this book, *vide* section Biographies, Chambers, Robert.

OLBY, R. C., 1966: Origins of Mendelism, 204 p. (London: Constable).—

A history of the discovery and rediscovery of the Mendelian laws. The author also considers Mendel's precursors, particularly J. Koelreuter and C. Gärtner who made extensive studies in fertilization and pollination. He also notes that F. Galton in 1875, in a letter to Darwin, summed up almost all the elements of Mendelian genetics, without knowing of Mendel's work, and the author elucidates Bateson's part in the dispersion of the knowledge of Mendelian inheritance.

OSBORN, H. F., 1929: From the Greeks to Darwin: the development of the evolution idea through twenty-four centuries, 398 p. (New York, N.Y. & London: Scribner).—

One of the first (or even the first?) attempts to write a history of the evolution theory, written by a well-known palaeontologist. It was first printed in 1894 and contains a series of lectures delivered at Princeton University in 1890 and 1893. The material has been divided as follows: 1. The anticipation and interpretation of nature (p. 1-38); 2. Among the Greeks (p. 39-102); 3. The evolution idea among the theologians and natural philosophers (p. 103-156); 4. The evolutionists of the 18th century (p. 157-218); 5. From Lamarck to Geoffroy Saint-Hilaire, Goethe and Naudin (p. 219-

300); 6. Darwin (p. 301-348). All authors, periods, publications, *etc.*, have been evaluated as to their importance to evolutionary thought.

OSTOYA, P., 1951: Les théories de l'évolution. Origine et histoire du transformisme et des idées qui s'y rattachent, 319 p. (Paris: Payot).—

In this history especially the French contributions (*e.g.,* of Maupertuis, Diderot, Buffon, Lacepède, Lamarck, Geoffroy Saint-Hilaire, *etc.*) have been considered. According to the author the history of the theory of evolution begins only in the 18th century. The book contains a clear exposition of the development of Neo-Darwinism during the 20th century. A book of similar scope seems to be: ROSTAND, J., 1932: L'évolution des espèces. Histoire des idées transformistes, 203 p. (Paris: Hachette). Unfortunately I have not been able to consult this book.

PERSON, S., ed., 1950: Evolutionary thought in America, 462 p. (New Haven, Conn.: Yale U.P.).—

The eleven authors, contributing to this volume, are distinguished leaders in a number of specialized fields, and each contribution deals with the impact of evolution and the development of evolution theory within the speciality concerned. The following essays are included: R. SCOON: The rise and impact of evolutionary ideas; F. S. C. NORTHROP: Evolution in its relation to the philosophy of nature and the philosophy of culture; T. DOBZHANSKY: The genetic nature of differences among man; R. E. L. FARIS: Evolution and American sociology; E. S. CORWIN: The impact of the idea of evolution on the American political and constitutional tradition; J. J. SPENGLER: Evolution in American economics; E. G. BORING: The influence of evolutionary theory upon American psychological thought; M. COWLEY: Naturalism in American literature; D. D. EGBERT: The idea of organic expression and American architecture; W. F. QUILLIAN: Evolution and moral theory in America; S. PERSONS: Evolution and theology in America.

PETERS, J. A., ed., 1959: Classic papers in genetics, 282 p. (Englewood Cliffs, N.J.: Prentice Hall).—

A selection of 28 papers, which, according to the editor in his preface have been selected "for one or more reasons. It may have served to focus attention on a particular facet of genetics. It may well illustrate the impact the study of genetics has on biology or on social and racial relationships. It may have embodied a particular idea unique at the time of publication that has led to extensive research by other geneticists, in many cases still continuing today. It may provide a brilliant example of the rise of the scientific method. It may furnish a clear-cut, concise illustration of incisive reasoning. One or two have the added virtue of having been written in an entertaining style." Among the papers included are those of: Mendel, Johannsen, Bateson, G. H. Hardy, T. H. Morgan (2), A. H. Sturtevant (3), D. S. Wright, L. C. Dunn, H. J. Muller, C. B. Bridges (2), Lederberg & Tatum, B. McClintock (2), N. B. Zinder, N. H. Horowitz, J. D. Watson & F. H. C. Crick, L. J. Stadler. Each paper included is preceded by a short introduction.

RAVIN, A. W., 1965: The evolution of genetics, 216 p. (New York, N.Y.: Academic Press).—

As stated by the author, the book is written for a "broad audience ... undergraduates ... students who are embarking on graduate studies in biology, professional biologists ... interested in current research on heredity, and laymen who have had some education in biology." In this book the author reviews the history of genetics, especially as it developed during the last 65 years. The larger part of the text even deals with the most modern aspects, *i.e.,* the development of the concepts of molecular genetics. A special chapter deals with the relationship between modern genetics and the unanswered questions of genetics in general. *Cf.* DUNN, L. C., ed., *vide supra*.

ROBERTS, H. F., 1929: Plant hybridization before Mendel, 374 p. (Princeton, N.J.: Princeton U.P.).—

The author traces the development of genetics from antiquity down to 1900. He discusses the work of many early hybridists, and the book contains an attempt to evaluate their relationship to one another and to our (post-Mendelian) knowledge. Only those investigators who have contributed in some essential manner to the theory of fertilization and hybridization in plants have been included; the work of individual breeders upon the improvement of some single species of plant has generally been omitted. Mendel's papers too, have been analysed minutely, in order "to bring Mendel's actual work into its deserved relief." Each chapter is followed by a bibliography. Facsimile reprint published in 1965 (New York, N.Y.: Hafner). *Cf.* ZIRKLE, C., 1935, *vide infra.*

SCHMIDT, H., 1918: Geschichte der Entwicklungslehre, 549 p. (Leipzig: Kröner).—

An exhaustive history of the theory of descent from the Darwinian, or better, Haeckelian, point of view, from the old cosmogonic theories up to Haeckel. The author was a pupil and admirer of Haeckel, and the first director of the Haeckel Museum and Archives (now Ernst-Haeckel-Haus) in Jena. A somewhat older treatise dealing with the same subjects is: DACQUÉ, E., 1903: Der Descendenzgedanke und seine Geschichte vom Altertum bis zur Neuzeit, 119 p. (Munich: Reinhardt).

SCHNEIDER, G., 1951: Die Evolutionstheorie, das Grundproblem der modernen Biologie — Ein Abriss des Entwicklungsgedankens von Kaspar Friedrich Wolff über Darwin bis Lyssenko, ed. 2, 141 p. (Berlin: Deutscher Bauernverlag).—

An elementary history of evolutionary thought from a "Lysenkoist" point of view intended for university students of biology. It consists mainly of contributions concerning C. F. Wolff, Lamarck, Darwin, Haeckel, Timiriazev, Michurin and Lysenko. *Cf.* SEGAL, J., 1951: Mitchourine, Lyssenko, et le problème de l'hérédité, 141 p. (Paris: Éd. français réunis).

STEBBINS, G. L., 1950: Variation and evolution in plants, 643 p. (Biological series, Vol. 16) (New York, N.Y.: Columbia U.P.).—

A clearly-written book on the evolution theory, based on a wealth of facts mainly derived from the vascular plants. It discusses such topics as: the basic role of variation, variation patterns, the role of variation in natural selection, genetic systems, the effects of isolation and of hybridization, polyploidy, apomixis, structural hybridity, fossils, rates of evolution. The bibliography contains about 1300 items.

STUBBE, H., 1965: Kurze Geschichte der Genetik bis zur Wiederentdeckung der Vererbungsregeln Gregor Mendels, ed. 2, 272 p. (Jena: Fischer).—

The present study is intended to serve as a general historical introduction to a series of contributions on the fundamentals, the problems, and the results of general genetics. It has been shown how close a connection exists between the history of genetics and the search for the causes lying behind the phenomena of the living world, and how the study of genetics is closely interwoven with social life (*e.g.*, the domesticated animals and the cultivated plants). The author gives a rather brief review of this history from classical antiquity up to the experimental phase of quite recent times. *Cf.* DUNN, L. C., 1966, *vide supra.*

STURTEVANT, A. H., 1965: A history of genetics, 154 p. (New York, N.Y.: Harper & Row).—

A well-written history of genetics from the days of Aristotle to 1950, and the development of its ideas and techniques. Sturtevant himself has been one of the leading geneticists of the last decades and he can be closely identified with many of its major developments during this period. A brief account of the late 19th-century background of genetics and of its 20th-century development is to be found in: BABCOCK, E. B., 1949: The development of fundamental concepts in the science of genetics, 45 p. (Portugaliae Acta Biologica, ser. A., 1-45; also separate: American Genetic Assn.). *Cf.* DUNN, L. C., 1966, *vide supra.*

TAX, S., ed., 1960: Evolution after Darwin. Vol. I: The evolution of life: its origin, history and future, 629 p.; Vol. II: The evolution of man: man, culture and society, 473 p.; Vol. III: Issues in evolution, 310 p. (with C. CALLENDER) (Chicago, Ill.: Univ. Chicago Press; London: Cambridge U.P.).—

A series of essays serving as the basis for discussion which took place between the writers during the Darwin centennial celebrations at the University of Chicago, 1959. Most of them are designed more for the expert than for the general reader.

UHLMANN, E., 1923: Entwicklungsgedanke und Artbegriff in ihrer geschichtlichen Entstehung und sachlichen Beziehung, 114 p. (Jenaische Z. Naturw. 59 : 1-114).—

A historical review of the interrelation between the concept of species and the theory of evolution. The first attempt to formulate a scientific species-concept was made by Linnaeus, and according to the author, any further attempt to arrive at a more satisfactory definition must inevitably have led to ideas about evolution (as with, *e.g.*, Lamarck, but also with Treviranus, Voigt, Cotta, Schleiden, Carus, Nägeli).

Darwin was the first to found his species-concept on an empirical basis ("The origin of species") and modern genetics shows, according to the author, how genotypic changes can take place by means of recombination and mutation.

WATSON, J. D., 1968: The double helix: a personal account of the discovery of the structure of DNA, 226 p. (New York, N.Y.: Atheneum; London: Weidenfeld & Nicolson).—

This book discusses the people and events leading to the discovery of the molecular structure of deoxyribonucleic acid (DNA). It is a personal memoir. Besides it contains much information about the work of Francis Crick, Linus Pauling, and Maurice Wilkins. *Cf.* CAIRNS, J., G. S. STENDT & J. D. WATSON, eds., 1966, *vide supra.*

ZIMMERMANN, W., 1953: Evolution. Die Geschichte ihrer Probleme und Erkenntnisse, 623 p. (Freiburg i.B. & Munich: Alber).—

A history of the gradual emergence of the concept of evolution. The author's method largely consists of giving (often lengthy) quotations (in German) from the authors considered; between these quotations the author gives some comments. The subject matter has been divided into three parts. The first deals with "Doctrines of descent without a scientific foundation" and embraces the ancient period up to the Middle Ages, and deals especially with Greek and Roman philosophers. The second part deals with "Evolutionary science without evolutionary doctrines", embracing the period from the Renaissance up to the 18th century: pioneers of classification (Cesalpinus, Ray, Linnaeus, *etc.),* the development of the scientific method (Bacon, Descartes, Spinoza, Leibniz, *etc.),* the meaning of fossils. The third part deals with "Conscious evolutionary science", covering the pre-Darwinian period (Lamarck, Geoffroy Saint-Hilaire, Oken, Braun), Darwin, and the post-Darwinian period; separate sections deal with the return to the idealistic point of view (Troll), the rate and causes of evolution, the biogenetic law, speciation, *etc.*

ZIRKLE, C., 1935: The beginnings of plant hybridization, 231 p. (Philadelphia, Pa.: Pennsylvania U.P.).—

The present book can be considered as a revised and enlarged edition of the author's papers in the J. of Heredity, Vols. 23 and 25, and it primarily deals with the records of hybridization and sex in plants before Koelreuter's classic hybridization experiments. The author makes it clear that as early as 1760 much knowledge about hybridization in plants had accumulated. Of the many forerunners considered we may mention C. Mather (1716), T. Fairchild (1717), Richard Bradley (1717), P. Miller (1721), P. Dudley (1724), J. Bartram (1739), J. G. Gmelin (1745), Linnaeus (1760). Because the majority of the publications considered are not readily available, the works have been quoted in full, regardless of their merits, since they are essential for an understanding of scientific standards of the first half of the 18th century. *Cf.* ROBERTS, H. F., 1929, *vide supra.*

——, 1946: The early history of the idea of the inheritance of acquired characters and of pangenesis, 60 p. (Trans. Amer. Phil. Soc. 35 : 91-151).—

In this publication the author makes it clear that both the theory of the inheritance of acquired characters and the theory of pangenesis are much older than either Lamarck or Darwin. With the aid of quotations (in English translation) from older (sometimes much older) sources, he elucidates this statement. In his introduction the author says "Now the doctrine of the inheritance of acquired characters is so intimately connected with the hypothetical mechanism which explained its occurrence that neither idea can be given an adequate historical treatment alone."

h.* *History of palaeontology*

EDWARDS, W. N., 1967: The early history of palaeontology, 58 p. (London: British Museum Nat. Hist.).—

An introductory text, based on the author's "Guide to an exhibition illustrating the early history of palaeontology, 1931. (British Museum Nat. Hist., Special guide No. 8).

FURON, R., 1951: La paléontologie; la science des fossiles, son histoire, ses enseignements, ses curiosités, 291 p. (Paris: Payot).—

This history has been built up mainly by means of biographies. Especially the first part (p. 15-129) deals with the history of palaeontology proper. It tells the story chronologically. The second part deals with the palaeontological history of the different groups of organisms.

GOTHAN, W., 1948: Die Probleme der Paläobotanik und ihre geschichtliche Entwicklung, 92 p. (Berlin: Wiss. Editionsges.).—

The author traces the substance, contents, materials, and history of palaeobotany. Besides he discusses such topics as: the use of fossil plants as stratigraphical indices and their importance for general questions such as: palaeography, plant geography, palaeoclimatology, formation of rocks, the history of forest evolution in post-glacial times, *etc.*

HABER, F. C., 1959: The age of the world: Moses to Darwin, 303 p. (Baltimore, Md.: Johns Hopkins Press).—

A very readable history of the period during which the Mosaic chronology had to give way to the ever-increasing amount of facts indicating that the world was not created at once, but has gradually evolved to its present state. The history extends roughly to 1900. The author gives an account of philosophers, theologians and scientists (many of them are not readily to be found discussed elsewhere); he treats his history mainly from the theological point of view. Stress has been laid on the 18th and the early 19th centuries.

HÖLDER, H., 1960: Geologie und Paläontologie in Texten und ihrer Geschichte, 565 p. (Freiburg i.B. & Munich: Alber).—

In this book the author presents the major problems of geology accompanied by the successive interpretations generated by the consecutive stages of knowledge prevailing at a given time. Among the topics discussed are: basic geological concepts, the nature of observations in the field, their classification and interpretation; mountain building; the evolution of structural geology; the effects of water; the significance of fossils; the dispute between Neptunists and Plutonists; the theory of uniformitarianism. Very extensive bibliography divided into the following major groups: 1. historical literature, 2. biographical literature, 3. literature arranged by subject, 4. a list of introductory works to the major disciplines of geology. A glossary of technical terms is added.

SCHINDEWOLF, O. H., 1948: Wesen und Geschichte der Paläontologie, 108 p. (Berlin: Wiss. Editionsges.).—

A semi-popular introduction to the methods and history of palaeontology.

ZEUNER, F. E., 1958: Dating the past: an introduction to geochronology, ed. 4, 516 p. (New York, N.Y.: Longmans & Green).—

A discussion of this book is to be found in the section: Prehistoric and primitive biology and medicine, subsection a.

ZITTEL, K. A. v., 1901: History of geology and palaeontology to the end of the nineteenth century, 562 p. (London: Scott).—

This is a somewhat curtailed translation of von Zittel's "Geschichte der Geologie und Paläontologie" (Munich: Oldenbourg), published in 1899 (868 p.). For the history of palaeontology two chapters are of special importance, *viz.*, that on the beginnings of palaeontology and geology (p. 11-46), discussing the various opinions about the nature of fossils, hypotheses of the earth's origin and history, and the role of Buffon, and that chapter which contains an analytic palaeontological history of the different groups of plants and animals (p. 363-424). The English translation was reprinted in 1964 (Weinheim: Cramer).

h.** *History of the domestication of animals and plants*

AMES, O., 1939: Economic annuals and human cultures, 153 p. (Cambridge, Mass.: Bot. Museum, Harvard Univ.).—

Angiosperm seeds (and especially those of annual crops) provided the means by which mankind obtained an assured food supply, initiating perhaps the economic evolution of the human race. Whereas (according to AMES) Man had to evolve together with his food plants, because he had to become adapted to them, the origin of economic botany should be one of the most fascinating examples of biological coincidence. Much stress is laid on a clear distinction between the notions agriculture and horticulture (Part V). 28 Full-page drawings, most of a high quality; very good index. Intended for the layman, the botanist, as well as for the anthropologist.

ANDERSON, E., 1967: Plants, man and life, 245 p. (Berkeley, Calif.: Univ. California Press).—

This book consists of 12 essays dealing with the (often obscure) prehistoric origin of some of our cultivated plants and most common weeds, discussing such aspects as: their cultivation, hybridization, and dispersion. As a result this book contains much research material for the study of evolution, and it also contains much that is of interest about our own prehistory. It bears principally upon the origins of wheat, cotton, and maize. Originally published in 1952 (Boston, Mass.: Little, Brown).

BOIS, D., 1927-1937: Les plantes alimentaires chez tous les peuples et à travers les âges. Histoire, utilization, culture, 4 vols. Vol. 1 (1927): Phanérogames légumières, 593 p.; Vol. II (1928): Phanérogames fruitières, 637 p.; Vol. III (1934): Plantes à épices, à aromates, à condiments, 289 p.; Vol. IV (1937): Plantes à boisson, 600 p. (Paris: Lechevallier).—

A survey of the plants which man, the world over, has used for drink and sustenance. It includes descriptions of all the species used and the modes of preparation.

CANDOLLE, A. DE, 1959: Origin of cultivated plants, 468 p. (New York, N.Y.: Hafner).—

A reissue of the second English edition of 1886 of this famous work of de Candolle in which he discusses the discovery of the places of origin of our cultivated plants. This discovery proceeds along the following three main lines: 1. We may assume that a cultigen originated in a region where its wild relatives still are to be found; 2. Philological studies: the name often travels together with the plant; 3. There are some historical records of plant-migrations which actually took place. Because only agriculture could support a stabilized population large enough for the development of cities, agriculture had to precede civilization, and thus has played an essential role in human (social) evolution.

GUILLAUMIN, A., 1946: Les plantes cultivées. Histoire. Économie, 352 p. (Paris: Payot).—

A historical account of the origin of many important economic plants and of the manner in which they are presumed to have been dispersed to the various regions where they are now grown. Separate chapters deal with such subjects as: cereals, legumes and tubers, industrial plants, dyes, insecticides, rubbers, perfumery plants, ornamental plants, poisonous weeds, etc. Comparable books are: GUYOT, L., 1963: Histoire des plantes cultivées, 216 p. (Paris: Collin); and

HAUDRICOURT, A. G. & L. HÉDIN, 1943: L'homme et les plantes cultivées, ed. 8, 234 p. (Paris: Gallimard).

HEHN, V., 1911: Kulturpflanzen und Haustiere in ihrem Übergang aus Asien nach Griechenland und Italien, sowie in das übrige Europa. Historisch-Linguistische Skizzen, ed. 8, 665 p. (Berlin: Borntraeger).—

A classic. It contains much information on early civilizations, on the migration of tribes and their methods of acquiring food, clothes, etc. Also in English translation: Cultivated plants and domestic animals on their migration from Asia to Europe, 1891, 530 p. (ed. by J. S. STALLYBRASS) (London: Sonnenschein). First ed. 1870 (Berlin: Borntraeger).

SCHWANITZ, F., 1966: The origin of cultivated plants, 175 p. (Cambridge, Mass.: Harvard U.P.; London: Oxford U.P.).—

This booklet offers a well-illustrated semi-popular discussion of the history of the improvement of crops by selective breeding. The main problem discussed is the transformation of wild species into cultivated plants (especially food plants), and in what respects these plants differ in their genetic and other mechanisms from wild ones and how these mechanisms arose. Originally published in German: SCHWANITZ, F., 1957: Die Entstehung der Kulturpflanzen, 151 p. (Verständliche Wissenschaft, Vol. 63) (Berlin, Göttingen & Heidelberg: Springer). Cf. also: SCHWANITZ, F., 1967: Die Evolution der Kulturpflanzen, 463 p. (Munich: Bayerischer Landwirtschaftsverlag). A study particularly devoted to the origin of our cereals is: SCHIEMANN, E., 1948: Weizen, Roggen, Gerste. Systematik, Geschichte und Verwendung, 102 p. (Jena: Fischer).

UCKO, P. J. & G. W. DIMBLEBY, eds., 1969: The domestication and exploitation of plants and animals, 581 p. (London: Duckworth).—

This volume contains 47 contributions by 45 authors. They deal with the origins of domestication, methods of investigation, regional and local evidence for domestication, studies of particular taxonomic groups, and with human nutrition. Sections of special interest for our purpose are those dealing with e.g., the ecological background of plant domestication; the weedy ancestors of our bread weeds; early agriculture and the "stable food supply";

animals in Egyptian sculpture, relief and painting; the domestication of bovids; the history and ethnography of manioc, arrowroot, and zamia; origin, variability and spread of the groundnut; and the domestication of the horse.

WEATHERWAX, P., 1954: Indian corn in old America, 253 p. (New York, N.Y.: Macmillan).—

The author has recorded what is known about the early history of corn (maize) as well as the present status of still unsolved problems. Indian corn cannot shed its seeds, and therefore human intervention is necessary to maintain it. It is a creation of the American Indian, but we do not know where it originated. There exist numerous local varieties very well adapted to their local circumstances.

ZEUNER, F. E., 1963: A history of domesticated animals, 560 p. (London: Hutchinson).—

The text has been divided into a general part and a special part. The general part (p. 15-78) deals with the origins and evolution of domestication, the conquest of environment, the origins and stages of domestication, and the effects of domestication on animals. The special part deals with domesticated animals: mammals domesticated in the pre-agricultural phase (cattle, buffalo, pig), mammals domesticated primarily for transport and work (elephants, horse, camel, onager, ass and mule), pestdestroyers (cat, ferret, mongoose), various other mammals (e.g., small rodents), birds, fishes and insects (domestic fowl, pigeon, falcon, goose, duck, cormorant, canary, etc.; carp, goldfish, paradise fish; silk-moths, honeybee). Bibliography and index. Also in German translation: Geschichte der Haustiere, 1967, 448 p. (Munich: Bayerischer Landwirtschaftsverlag). A shorter "adaptation" of Zeuner's book is: DAVIS, P. D. C. & A. A. DENT, 1968: Animals that changed the world, 121 p. (New York, N.Y.: Crowell-Collier).

i. *History of plant and animal geography* (incl. ecology)

ALLEE, W. C. & T. PARK, 1950: The history of ecology, 59 p. (In: W. C. ALLEE, *et al.,* Principles of animal ecology, p. 13-72) (Philadelphia, Pa. & London: Saunders).—

As far as the present author is aware this is the most complete and reliable historical review of (animal) ecology. It forms the contents of the first section of a large manual on animal ecology and consists of two chapters, viz., "Ecological background and growth before 1900" by W. C. ALLEE, reviewing the development of ecology from the Greeks onwards, with short summaries of the development of hydrobiology, oceanography, and limnology) and "First four decades of the twentieth century" (by Thomas PARK). In this chapter the author sums up the most important achievements of each of these decades, and at the end he gives a very useful bibliography of books, journals, review articles, and summarizing articles, representative of one or more of the several fields of ecology, published between 1931 and 1942.

BAKER, J. N. L., 1931: History of geographical discovery and exploration, 544 p. (London: Harrap).—

An elaborate summary of modern exploration. The subject matter is in two parts, the first dealing with the period before the 19th century, the second with the 19th century and after. A more or less popular and lavishly illustrated account of geographical discovery is: DEBENHAM, F., 1968: Discovery and exploration: an atlas-history of man's journeys into the unknown, ed. 2, 272 p. (London: Hamlyn).

ENGLER, A., 1899: Die Entwicklung der Pflanzengeographie in den letzten hundert Jahren und weitere Aufgaben derselben, 247 p. (Berlin: Kühl).—

Review and discussion of the acquisitions of (physical and physiological) plant geography during the nineteenth century and a short explanation of aims and methods of this discipline, as they were considered at the end of the nineteenth century.

HERDMAN, W. A., 1923: Founders of oceanography and their work: an introduction to the science of the sea, 340 p. (London: Arnold).—

The author of this book himself was a well-known oceanographer. Of its 17 chapters, the first seven are historical (the others give introductory information on some of the more interesting aspects of oceanography). Three chapters deal exclusively with the British impact to the science of oceanography; the author distinguished the period of Edw. Forbes (1815-1854), the period of W. Thomson (1830-1882) culminating in the Challenger expedition) and the post-Challenger period of John Murray

(1841-1914). The three following chapters deal respectively with Louis and Alex. Agassiz, Albert of Monaco, and Anton Dorn. The last historical chapter deals with some historical aspects of sea-fisheries, and marine biological stations of research. A more recent publication, seemingly dealing with similar aspects is: Colloque international sur l'histoire de la biologie marine, les grandes expéditions scientifiques et la création des laboratoires maritimes, 1965, 371 p. (Vie et Milieu, Suppl. No. 19) (Banyuls-sur-Mer: Laboratoire Arago; Paris: Masson). Unfortunately I am unable to give more details concerning this publication.

HOFSTEN, N. VON, 1916: Zur älteren Geschichte des Diskontinuitätsproblems in der Biogeographie, 157 p. (Zool. Ann. 7 : 197-353). (Also separate, Würzburg: Kabitzsch).

—

This publication deals with such subjects as: animal and plant geography during Antiquity and the Middle Ages (considering, *e.g.,* Hippocrates, Theophrastos, Aristotle, Pliny, Clemens Alexandrinos, Joh. Philoponos, Isidore of Seville, Albertus Magnus, Bacon, St. Thomas Aquinas, Vincent of Beauvais, and St. Augustine); the influence of the discovery of America on the problem of discontinuity; the voyages of discovery during the 16th and 17th centuries; the ideas of Buffon, Linnaeus, Gmelin, von Haller, Pallas, Forster, and E. A. W. Zimmermann; armchair philosophy about the distribution of plants and animals at the end of the 18th century; new ideas in the 19th century: von Humboldt, Milne Edwards, E. Fries, H. G. Bronn, Louis Agassiz, E. Forbes; the influence of Darwinism *(e.g.,* J. D. Hooker, A. de Candolle); the "Atlantis" theory; the ideas of Darwin and of Wallace; and the problem of the polytopic origin of species.

KEMPER, H., 1968: Kurzgefasste Geschichte der tierischen Schädlinge, der Schädlingskunde und der Schädlingsbekämpfung, 381 p. (Berlin: Duncker & Humblot).—

A history of the growth of our knowledge of injurious animals, and the techniques to combat them. A first (general) part (p. 11-60) shows how the storage of human food-products led to an improvement of the habitat of these animals, how they became dispersed all over the world by our means of transport, how we created favourable conditions in our storage rooms, and how all this leads to a disturbance of the biotic equilibrium. A second part (p. 61-130) discusses the increase of our knowledge concerning some injurious organisms *(e.g.,* fungi, worms, molluscs, insects, spiders, birds, mammals). A third part (p. 131-236) considers the various techniques of destruction employed in the Far East, Egypt, Mesopotamia, in Bible and Talmud, during Classical Antiquity, the Middle Ages, the Renaissance, and during modern times (from Linnaeus onwards). A special section deals with helminthology and nematology. A fourth part (p. 237-332) deals with the history of the battle against these organisms (the greater part deals with the role of chemicals in this battle, p. 274-309). The book contains much biographical information and a useful bibliography (mainly dealing with German literature, p. 347-366), and an index of subjects.

KLAAUW, C. J. VAN DER, 1936: Zur Geschichte der Definitionen der Ökologie, besonders auf Grund der Systeme der zoologischen Disziplinen, 41 p. (Ökologische Studien und Kritiken II) (Sudhoffs Arch. Gesch. Med. u. Naturwiss. 29 : 136-177).—

This study starts with a critical historical analysis of the concept of ecology, especially as it has been coined by Haeckel in his "Generelle Morphologie". Some earlier authors also have been considered, *e.g.,* Isidore Geoffroy Saint-Hilaire, and Bichat. Then the author tries to ascertain what were the exact outlines of the concept of ecology as it was, and is still understood in the practice of biology. This is followed by a methodological analysis, from which the author concludes, that there is a fundamental difference between ecology on the one side and physiology on the other side. In a continuation of this study, the author tries to prove that there also exists a fundamental difference between the study of the ecology of the individual or species and that of a community of living organisms, *cf.* KLAAUW, C. J. VAN DER, 1936: Zur Aufteilung der Ökologie in Autökologie und Synökologie, im Lichte der Ideen als Grundlage der Systematik der zoologischen Disziplinen, 44 p. (Acta Biotheor. 2: 197-241).

2. HISTORY OF THE ANIMAL SCIENCES

a. *History of zoology in general*

BRZEK, G., 1955: Histoire de la zoologie en Pologne jusqu'à 1918. IIIᵉ partie, 455 p. (Ann. Univ. M. Skłodowska-Curie, Sectio C, Suppl. 7).—

The first volume treats of the history of zoology from its origin to the 18th century, and the second volume deals with the history of zoology at the University of Vilna between 1781 and 1918. (Both volumes were published in 1947). The third volume deals with the history of zoology at the University of Warsaw between 1772 and 1918 including the history of the various scientific institutes, societies, museums, *etc.*, and the position of zoology in the agronomical institute in Marymont, the veterinary school and the polytechnical school. This work contains much biographical information. Some other regional histories of zoology, books of which I am unable to give any details, are: SZILADY, Z., 1927: Die Geschichte der Zoologie in Ungarn, 116 p. (Debrecen: Kertesz); and: BROCH, H., 1954: Zoologiens historie i Norge til annen verdenskrig, 158 p. (Oslo: Akademisk Vorlag).

BURCKHARDT, R., 1907: Geschichte der Zoologie, 156 p. (Leipzig: Göschen).—

Separate chapters deal with such subjects as: the systematics of the science of zoology (p. 7-9); the beginnings of zoology: zoology in Asia (p. 9-14); zoology in antiquity: Aristotle, Greek and Roman zoology, Alexandrian anatomy (p. 14-39); zoology during the Middle Ages (p. 40-47); zoology up to the middle of the 18th century: zoogeography, systematics, John Ray, Linnaeus, Pallas (p. 48-81); French zoology: Buffon, Lamarck, Geoffroy Saint-Hilaire, Cuvier (p. 82-101); German zoology: enlightenment, "Naturphilosophie", cell-theory (p. 101-122); English zoology: Darwinism, American zoology; zoogeography (incl. itineraries and marine biology). In 1921 a second edition appeared (not seen) by R. BURCKHARDT & H. EHRHARD, entitled: Geschichte der Zoologie und ihrer wissenschaftlichen Probleme, in 2 vols., 103 + 136 p. (Leipzich: Göschen).

CARUS, J. V., 1872: Geschichte der Zoologie bis auf Johannes Müller und Charles Darwin, 739 p. (Geschichte der Wissenschaften in Deutschland, Neuere Zeit, Vol. XII) (Munich: Oldenbourg).—

According to Carus no history of zoology can be written without knowledge of cultural history, for any history of zoology depends on the way in which man evaluates his own position with respect to the animal world. This is the reason why, according to the author, a third of this book has been devoted to the development of zoology during antiquity and the Middle Ages and why the author makes a first attempt to evaluate the position of the Arabs

in the history of zoology and their role in the continuation of zoological knowledge. The history of zoology during the more recent times has been divided into three periods: 1. that of the establishment of encyclopaedias (*e.g.,* Gessner, Aldrovandi) biblical zoology, and the results of the first voyages (to America, Africa and the East Indies); 2. the period of systematics (Ray, Linnaeus), the advancement of anatomy (Malpighi, Leeuwenhoek, Swammerdam, Redi, P. Camper, von Haller, Spallanzani, Wolff, Hunter, Vicq d'Azyr), foundation of academies, museums and zoological gardens; 3. the period of morphology: German "Naturphilosophie" (Schelling, Oken, Burdach, Carus, Goethe), the rapid development of comparative anatomy (Kielmeyer, Geoffroy Saint-Hilaire, Cuvier, Bichat, Blumenbach, Döllinger, Meckel, Joh. Müller, Owen), embryology (v. Baer, Pander, Rathke), cell-theory (Schwann), scientific expeditions, advances in invertebrate systematics, first thoughts on evolution (Lamarck, Geoffroy. Saint-Hilaire, Darwin). The book ends with Darwin, without trying to evaluate Darwin's position in the light of future developments of zoology. In 1880 a French edition appeared: Histoire de la zoologie depuis l'Antiquité jusqu'au XIXᵉ siècle (Paris: Baillière). By this time still another French history of zoology had appeared, *viz.,* HOEFER, F., 1873: Histoire de la zoologie depuis les temps les plus reculés, 410 p. (Paris: Hachette); this book, however, seems to be far inferior to Carus' history of zoology.

CHALMERS MITCHELL, P., 1929: Centenary history of the Zoological Society of London, 307 p. (London: Zool. Society).—

The Zoological Society is a scientific institution founded in 1829. Its task is twofold: at first: the introduction of "new and curious subjects of the Animal Kingdom", which led to the establishment of Zoological Gardens. Secondly the "advancement of Zoology and Physiology". For this second part of the task it should be noted that a) as formerly the study of physiology was more restricted to the breeding, acclimatization, and influence of the environment on the living animal, much was learned about hygiene in Zoological Gardens; b) museums were provided with material, an extensive library was founded, research in anatomy and taxonomy was stimulated, and the publication of the results was supported. Many beautiful portraits of past officers of the Society have been added. *Cf.* SCHERREN, H., 1905: The Zoological Society of London: a sketch of its foundation and development and the story of its farm, museum, gardens, menagerie and library, 252 p. (London: Cassell).

COLE, F. J., 1926: The history of protozoology, 64 p. (London: Universities Press).—

> For more details about this book, *vide supra,* section History of general biology. *Cf.* also: WICHTERMAN, R., 1953: The biology of Paramecium, 543 p. (New York, N.Y.: Blakiston), a history of knowledge of this species from 1674 up to the present day.

DELAUNAY, P., 1962: La zoologie au seizième siècle, 338 p. (Paris: Hermann).—

> An authoritative history of the period, discussing such subjects as: the use of animals, animals in the arts, the heritage of the mediaeval knowledge of animals, the influence of new geographical discoveries, collections and cabinets, zoological iconography, animal nomenclature, the chain of beings, *etc.*

GOLDSCHMIDT, R. B., 1956: Portraits from memory: recollections of a zoologist, 181 p. (Seattle, Wash.: Univ. Washington Press).—

> A series of sketches recording personal encounters and experiences of the author with leading German zoologists living at the end of the former and the beginning of the present century, *e.g.,* E. Haeckel, O. Bütschli, W. Roux, H. Driesch, O. & R. Hertwig, K. Gegenbaur, T. Boveri, F. Schaudin, C. Herbst, J. von Uexküll, and many others. Also in German translation: Erlebnisse und Begegnungen. Aus der grossen Zeit der Zoologie in Deutschland, 1959, 165 p. (Hamburg: Parey).

KOLLER, G., 1949: Daten zur Geschichte der Zoologie. Zeittafel, Forscherliste, Artentafel, 64 p. (Bonn: Athenäum).—

> For more details, *vide* section Some recommended encyclopaedias, *etc.,* subsection d.

LECLERCQ, J., 1959: Perspectives de la zoologie européenne. Histoire, problèmes contemporains, 162 p. (Gembloux: Éd. Duculot; Paris: Librairie agricole de la Maison Rustique).—

> One of the best short histories of zoology. Brief introduction considering

prehistoric zoology. Chapters follow on zoology in the 15th - 18th centuries, taxonomy, philosophy of nature, Cuvier and the 19th century, the origin and development of the cellular theory, Darwin, Lamarck, the integration of the 20th century. Recently a supplementary vol. appeared: LECLERCQ, J. & P. DAGNELIE, 1966: Perspectives de la zoologie européenne. Un sondage d'opinions des zoologistes, 215 p. (Gembloux: Duculot). This publication is of little historical interest.

LEY, W., 1941: The lungfish and the unicorn: an excursion into romantic zoology, 305 p. (New York, N.Y.: Modern Age).—

> "This is a very readable account of mythical animals, such as the unicorn, the basilisk or the sea serpent; extinct ones, like the urus, wisent, great auk, giant sloth, or dodo; and the so-called living fossils, such as *Limulus* and *Latimeria,* platypus, lung fish, and the remaining fauna of Gondwana." (G. Sarton in Isis 33: 405). For more information, *vide* section Middle Ages in the West, subsection b. *Cf.* also LEY, W., 1968, *vide* section Antiquity in general, subsection b.

MORUS, 1954: Animals, men and myths: a history of the influence of animals on civilization and culture, 374 p. (London: Gollancz; New York, N.Y.: Harper).—

> Morus is the pen-name of the German naturalist R. LEWINSOHN, and the book was first published in German under the title: "Eine Geschichte der Tiere, ihr Einfluss auf Zivilisation und Kultur", 1952, 400 p. (Hamburg: Rowohlt). The book deals with the impact of animals on human culture, not only upon our material needs but also upon every aspect of spiritual life. It deals also with the contrary aspect: the impact of human culture upon animal life. Throughout the book man takes the central position. The treatment is selective, well-documented with plenty of examples, and pleasantly written. It takes its examples from many fields of knowledge, *e.g.,* husbandry (the influence of sheep-rearing and the agricultural revolution, accompanied by social and cultural catastrophes in England); visual arts (Dürer, Potter); literature (fables of La Fontaine); mythology (the role of fabulous animals in antiquity, in the Middle Ages and in the Renaissance); economy (the disappearance of herrings from the Baltic precipitated the downfall of the Hansa); history (the Roman lack of cavalry was one of the main causes of the fall of the Western Empire). Also in Dutch translation.

NISSEN, C., 1951: Schöne Fischbücher. Kurze Geschichte der ichthyologischen Illustration. Bibliographie fischkundlicher Abbildungswerke, 108 p. (Stuttgart: Hempe).—

A historical bibliography of ichthyological illustration, divided into two parts, *viz.,* a bibliography of ichthyological books and a catalogue of works containing ichthyological illustrations. Both parts are arranged alphabetically by author and give abundant bibliographical information, including references to published sources of information about the books and their authors. Index of designers, engravers, lithographers, printers, wood-engravers, and collectors. *Cf.* DEAN, B., ed., 1962, *vide* section Bibliographies, subsection d.

——, 1966: Die zoologische Buchillustration. Ihre Bibliographie und Geschichte. Vol. I: Bibliographie, Fasc. 1: Vorwort, Abkürzungen, Titel Nr. 1-744 (Abbati-Bungartz), 80 p.; Fasc. 2: Titel Nr. 745-1534 (Bungartz-Gerber), p. 81-160. (Stuttgart: Hiersemann).—

A historical bibliography of zoological illustration, covering the illustrations of all groups of animals. The book has been set up somewhat along the lines of the author's "Schöne Fischbücher" *(vide supra)* and of his "Die illustrierten Vögelbücher" *(vide* subsection Ornithology, *infra).* The whole work, about 13 fascicules of *ca.* 80 pages each, will be published in approximately 4 years.

PETIT, G. & J. THÉODORIDÈS, 1962: Histoire de la zoologie dès origines à Linné, 360 p. (Paris: Hermann).—

The notion zoology is used in the French sense, *i.e.,* it means the identification, description, and classification of animals, rather than a collective term for the anatomy, physiology, *etc.,* of the animals. Whereas, from the very beginning of his existence, primitive Man had to deal with animals (for food, protection, *etc.),* zoology is as old as Man himself, and the authors continue the development of this science up to the close of the 17th century. There are many interesting essays considering the zoological knowledge of ancient non-Western people. Brief and instructive bibliographies have been added to each chapter.

SAVORY, T. H., 1961: Spiders, men, and scorpions: being the history of arachnology, 191 p. (London: Universities Press).—

"This excellent summary serves both as a concise reference work and as a very readable account of a subject which has fascinated many remarkable biologists from Aristotle onwards. The illustrations contain portraits of arachnologists and of a few representatives of the group they study. The maps in the text, showing the 'geographical distribution' of arachnologists in their respective countries, are of considerable interest." (From: J. Soc. Biblphy. nat. Hist. 4: 83).

TOPSELL, E. & T. MUFFET, 1967: The history of four-footed beasts and serpents and insects, 3 vols. Vol. 1: The history of four-footed beasts, 620 p.; Vol. 2: The history of serpents, 246 p. by Edward TOPSELL. Vol. 3: The theater of insects, 270 p. by T. MUFFET. (Facsimile reprint of the 1658 (London) edition, with an introduction by Willy LEY) (New York, N.Y.: Da Capo; London: Cass).—

A facsimile edition of the first animal book in English to be printed in Great Britain. The first two vols. (by TOPSELL) are in fact translations of Conrad Gesner's "Historia animalium". The third vol. (by MUFFET) also leans heavily on Gesner, *viz.,* on the manuscript sources derived from Gesner's entomological collections.

USCHMANN, G., 1960: Geschichte der Zoologie und der zoologischen Anstalten in Jena 1779-1919, 249 p. (Jena: Fischer).—

This historical study of the zoological sciences at Jena University starts with the year 1779, because in this year the Walch collection was purchased which gave rise to the foundation of the Zoological Museum. In the year 1919 E. Haeckel died. The Zoological Museum played a world-wide role in the second half of the preceding century, when Gegenbaur and Haeckel guided zoological science at Jena, and as such this history is of far more than only regional importance. The book gives many chronological and biographical details on all zoologists ever connected with Jena during the period considered. A very good bibliography and a complete index to all persons mentioned have been added.

a.* *History of entomology*

BODENHEIMER, F. S., 1928-1929: Materialien zur Geschichte der Entomologie bis Linné, 2 vols. Vol. I: 498 p.; Vol. II: 486 p. (Berlin: Junk).—

This history consists of a collection of materials offering German versions of (or extracts from) entomological works written during the period considered, together with brief biographical and bibliographical notes. The first volume deals with the history of oriental entomology (Far East, Egypt, Mesopotamia, Bible and Talmud), European antiquity (Greeks and Romans), the Middle Ages (incl. the Arabic period) and with modern times, *i.e.*, from Aldrovandi onwards (Aristotelian renaissance, foundation of modern taxonomy and morphology and the bionomic period, 1660-1750). The second volume mainly considers the period 1660-1750 and deals with such topics as: applied entomology, learned societies and academies, increase of knowledge due to explorations, history of the knowledge of cochineals, various efforts and publications of the 17th and 18th centuries, and the history of entomological collections. Valuable series of 43 tables (p. 312-456) constitutes a very clear survey of pre-Linnean entomology.

ESSIG, E. O., 1965: A history of entomology, 1029 p. (New York, N.Y.: Hafner).—

In this history of entomology stress has been laid on the economic aspects and on the situation in the Western part of the U.S.A.; but besides these restrictions it contains much that is of value to the historically-minded biologist. The book starts with a chapter on prehistoric entomology, then it discusses the food habits of native Indians in California who were to a large extent entomophagous. Other chapters deal with: the history of the organization of entomological research and instruction in the Californian Academy of Sciences and other educational centres; the more important orchard mites and insects of California; the history of the growing practice of using predacious and parasitic insects to destroy the insect enemies in crops and fruits; a historical account of the scientific elaboration and commercial development of insecticides; entomological legislation on matters of inspection, quarantine, insecticides, and other sanitary matters. One chapter gives biographies of 114 entomologists, a statement of his most important studies and discoveries, a list of insects named by him and after him, and a list of his most important publications. This book was originally published in 1931 by Macmillan (New York, N.Y.). A shorter historical introduction is: ESSIG, É. O., 1936: A sketch history of entomology, 43 p. (Osiris 2: 80-123).

HORN, W. & J. KAHLE, 1935-1937: Ueber entomologische Sammlungen, Entomologen und entomo-Museologie. Ein Beitrag zur Geschichte der Entomologie, 388 p. (Unter Mitarbeit von R. KORSCHEFSKY) (Entomologische Beihefte aus Berlin-Dahlem, Vol. II (1935) : 1-160; Vol. III (1936) : 161-296; Vol. IV (1937) : 297-388).—

A reissue of a publication by W. HORN in the "Supplementa entomologica", No. 12, 1926, entitled: "Ueber den Verbleib der entomologischen Versammlungen der Welt." It is the best source available concerning the information about disposal and location of entomological collections. In a certain sense this study is a prodromus to a history of entomology; it contains much biographical information, and historical information concerning entomological societies, entomological publications, and museums (London, Leningrad, Vienna, Paris, and Berlin). Extensive index. *Cf.* also: DERKSEN, W. & U. SCHEIDING, eds., 1963→: Index literaturae entomologiae, *vide* section Bibliographies, subsection d.

HOWARD, L. O., 1930: A history of applied entomology (somewhat anecdotal), 564 p. (Smithsonian Misc. Coll., No. 84) (Washington, D.C.: Smithsonian Instn.).—

A history of economic or applied entomology largely based upon personal experience, whereby stress has been laid on the maleficent activities of insects. Actually this history begins in the second half of last century. The main division of this work is geographical and the largest part (182 p.) has been devoted to the U.S.A. It contains some 250 portraits of entomologists.

OSBORN, H., 1937-1946: Fragments of entomological history including some personal recollections of men and events, 2 vols. Vol. I: 393 p.; Vol. II: 232 p. (Columbus, O.: Author).—

The author has been professor of zoology and entomology during 35 years and has played an important role in the building up of the science of entomology in the U.S.A. Both volumes deal especially with the development of the many aspects of entomology during the present century, *i.e.*, with such topics as: Federal service in entomology; state entomologists, inspectors and quarantine officers; experiment station entomology; entomological instruction in colleges; entomological societies; personal sketches (146 pages and 375 portraits); insect collections; research agencies; entomological publications; commemorative events and memorials; buildings and equipment for insect study; insecticides and machinery. Vol. I starts with a brief historical review of the history of entomology in the U.S.A. The same author published a supplementary text to this book: OSBORN, H., 1952: A brief history of entomology, including the time of Demosthenes and Aristotle to modern times with over five hundred portraits, 303 p. (Columbus, O.: Spahr & Glenn).

OUDEMANS, A. C., 1926-1937: Kritisch-historisch overzicht der acarologie. Eerste gedeelte, 850 v. Chr. tot 1758 (1926): 500 p.; Tweede gedeelte, 1759-1804 (1929): 1097 p.; Derde gedeelte, 1805-1850 (1936-1937): 1998 p. (Tijdschrift voor Entomologie, Suppl. vols. 69 and 72) (Leiden: Brill).—

A monumental work containing the material necessary to write a definitive history of acarology. It is a chronological and bibliographical table with critical notes and series of summaries. The first part deals with Acarida from Homer's time to the 10th edition of Linnaeus' "Systema naturae" in 1758. The second part deals with the period between this edition and the publication of Hermann's "Memoire aptérologique" in 1804. The third part has been divided into 4 parts: A. (430 p.) dealing with the Acari in general, with Holothyroidea Reuter 1909, and with Mesostigmata Can. 1891; B. (362 p.) with Ixodides Leach 1815; C. (549 p.) with Tarsonemini Can. & Franz. 1877, Stomatostigmata Oudms. 1906. Elentherengona Oudms. 1909; D (649 p.) with Parasitengona Oudms. V, 1909.

WILSON, H. F. & M. H. DONER, 1937: The historical development of insect classification, 133 p. (Madison, Wisc.: The authors).—

This history of insect classification has not been based on a chronological order, but the arrangement in which the various systems have been considered is in accordance with the dominant quality (-ies) on which the older entomologists based their classificatory system, for which they utilized such characters as: habitat, wings, metamorphosis, embryological characters, segmentation, phylogenesis, etc. In this way the authors demonstrate the various views prevailing in insect classification from Democritos, Aristotle, Pliny, Aldrovandi, Agricola, Swammerdam, Ray, Fabricius, Lamarck, Illiger, Cuvier, and many others up to more recent systems of classification.

a.** *History of ornithology*

ALLEN, E. G., 1951: The history of American ornithology before Audubon, 206 p. (Trans. Amer. Phil. Soc., N.S., 41 : 385-591).—

A reference-work in this field, containing a comprehensive bibliography. It considers the story of the observation, description and classification of birds as they have been studied by ornithologists from Aristotle to Alex. Wilson (the "Father of American ornithology"), immediate predecessor of Audubon. According to a review in Isis 43: 298, the references are not fully reliable.

ANKER, J., 1938: Bird books and bird art: an outline of the literary history and iconography of descriptive ornithology based principally on the collection of books containing plates with figures of birds and their eggs now in the university library at Copenhagen and including a catalogue of these works, 251 p. (Copenhagen: Levin & Munksgaard).—

After an outline of the literary history and iconography of descriptive ornithology, covering 87 pages and 12 beautiful plates, an elaborate catalogue follows, containing 548 illustrated books on birds and their eggs, which in its turn is followed by a bibliography of general and comprehensive bibliographies (nos. 549-590), a bibliography of works relating to the history of art and ornithology (nos. 591-648), and a list of special works in the field of ornithology (nos. 649-918). Rich index of names (34 columns) and geographical index. *Cf.* also NISSEN, C., 1953; and SITWELL, S., *et al.,* 1953, *vide infra.* For more bibliographical information, *vide* section Bibliographies, subsection d, HARTING, J. E.; RONSIL, R.; and STRONG, R. M.

BOUBIER, M., 1932: L'évolution de l'ornithologie, nouv. ed., 308 p. (Paris: Alcan).—

A descriptive history of the different problems related to ornithology, first published in 1925. The first chapter is introductory in character and deals with the earliest achievements by, *e.g.,* Aristotle, J. W. von Caub, Belon, Gesner, Aldrovandi; ch. 2 deals with regional faunal descriptions, and with Buffon's contributions to European ornithology; ch. 3 deals with the ornithological results of the 18th-century expeditions and voyages as they appear from old journals: Magellan, Hernandez, Marcgraaf,

Sloane; ch. 4 with *idem* for the 19th century, *e.g.*, the voyages of Péron to Australia, of Quoy and Gaimard to Tierra del Fuego, and Darwin's voyage with the Beagle; ch. 5 deals with the history of the bird-migration question; ch. 6 with the history of bird nomenclature from Willughby to Schlegel; ch. 7 with the advancement of anatomical and palaeontological knowledge, dissections, and the significance of Volcher Coiter; and ch. 8 with the history of bird classification (esp. the classificatory systems of Aldrovandi and of Willughby-Ray), Helpful index of personal names. *Cf.* STRESEMANN, E., 1951, *vide infra.*

BROUWER, G. A., 1954: Historische gegevens over onze vroegere ornithologen en over de avifauna van Nederland, 226 p. (Diss. Univ. Leiden) (Leiden: Brill).—

A history of ornithology in the Netherlands from the 13th century onwards. Valuable bibliography (p. 188-217) and index of names; together they are invaluable for every study of Dutch ornithology. Index of subjects and of geographical names.

CHAPMAN, F. M. & T. S. PALMER, eds., 1933: Fifty years' progress of American ornithology 1883-1933, 249 p. (Lancaster, Pa.: Amer. Ornithol. Union).—

This volume was published on the occasion of the semi-centennial anniversary of the American Ornithologists' Union. It contains papers on such subjects as: the history of the American ornithologists' Union; American ornithological literature 1883-1933; fifty years of bird migration; bird banding; economic ornithology; collections of birds in the U.S.A. and Canada; history and progress of bird photography, and bird-art; fifty years of bird protection; ornithological education in America; *etc.*

GURNEY, J. H., 1921: Early annals of ornithology, 240 p. (London: Witherby).—

In his preface, the author states that "the idea with which this little volume originated was to collect all the ancient passages about birds, of any special interest, but more particularly those which concerned British birds, and to string them together in order of date." All passages quoted are in English translation. A valuable book to anyone interested in the history of ornithology and the literary aspects of biohistory.

NISSEN, C., 1953: Die illustrierten Vogelbücher, ihre Geschichte und Bibliographie, 223 p. (Stuttgart: Hiersemann).—

A bibliography of the combined fields of natural history and fine art, forming part of a series that is intended to provide a general bibliographical coverage of biological book illustration *(cf.* some other works of NISSEN, *vide* sections: History of zoology in general and History of botany in general). The present book contains 1,025 entries, arranged alphabetically, and ranging from the Upper Palaeolithic to the date of compilation. They include biographical data, short title and imprint, format, number and type of plates, later editions, data on artists, and references. The text is preceded by a historical survey of bird illustration, and is supplemented by indexes of artists, bird species, countries, and authors. *Cf.* also ANKER, J., 1938, *vide supra;* SITWELL, S., *et al., vide infra;* and ZIMMER, J. T., ed., 1962: Catalogue of the Edward E. Ayer ornithological library, *vide* section Bibliographies, subsection d.

SITWELL, S., H. BUCHANAN & J. FISHER, 1953: Fine bird books 1700-1900, 120 p. (New York, N.Y.: Van Nostrand; London: Collins).—

The editors give one, two, or three stars in ascending order of merit, to works they regard as especially notable. The purpose of this book is the same as those of J. ANKER *(vide supra)* and of C. NISSEN *(vide supra),* however, it is less complete.

STRESEMANN, E., 1951: Die Entwicklung der Ornithologie von Aristoteles bis zur Gegenwart, 431 p. (Berlin: Peters).—

A philosophical account of the development of ornithological science. The book starts with an introductory part (p. 1-40) which traces the survey down to 1600. Other parts deal with the development of systematics and the theory of evolution and with biological investigations. In it lively descriptions have been given of 17th-century systematics, the foundation of the natural system in the 18th century, the role of nature philosophy, the significance of Darwinism for the development of ornithology, and the synthesis between systematics and evolution during the 20th century. Special attention has been given to the 20th century. The method employed is primarily biographical; the book includes many quotations from the ornithologists considered. Moreover, a number of special topics have been treated such as: the sub-species problem; problems of nomenclature; bird illustration; museum collections; the importance of bird behaviour, *etc. Cf.* BOUBIER, M., 1932, *vide supra.*

b. *History of veterinary science*

BIERER, B. W., 1955: A short history of veterinary medicine in America, 113 p. (East Lansing, Mich.: Michigan State U.P.).—

The first chapter (p. 1-23) contains an account of the development of the veterinary sciences up to the end of the 18th century and tries to give some idea of the prevailing conditions in America at that time; ch. 2 (p. 24-46) shows how the progress of American agriculture resulted in the development of the veterinary sciences "along agricultural lines", and how this resulted in the establishment in the U.S.A. of a national bureau of animal industry; ch. 3 (p. 47-85) contains a review of the efforts made in controling and eradicating animal plagues; and ch. 4 describes the development of veterinary schools and indicates how the practice of veterinary medicine was regulated by state and provincial examining boards. *Cf.* MERILLAT, L. A. & D. L. CAMPBELL, 1935; and SMITHCORSS, J. F., 1963, *vide infra.*

EICHBAUM, F., 1885: Grundriss der Geschichte der Thierheilkunde. Für Thierärzte und Studirende, 328 p. (Berlin: Parey).—

In this book the history of veterinary science has been studied from a geographical point of view. Special attention has been paid to veterinary schools, veterinary education, organizations, *etc.*, in Italy, Spain, Germany, France, England, and some other countries.

FROEHNER, R., 1952: Kulturgeschichte der Tierheilkunde. Ein Handbuch für Tierärzte und Studierende. Vol. I: Tierkrankheiten, Heilbestrebungen, Tierärzte im Altertum, 187 p.; Vol. II: Geschichte des deutschen Veterinärwesens, 390 p. (Konstanz: Terra-Verlag).—

A history of veterinary science on a regional basis: Western Asia, Arabia, Egypt, Carthage, Persia, India, China, Japan, Greece, Rome, and Germany are considered. Much literature has been incorporated. Many illustrations. The second vol. deals exclusively with the history of veterinary science in Germany from ancient times up to *ca.* 1950. Extensive name- and subject-indexes. *Cf.* KLEE, R., ed., 1901, *vide* section Bibliographies, subsection d.

LECLAINCHE, E., 1936: Histoire de la médecine vétérinaire, 812 p. (Toulouse: Office du Livre).—

For centuries it was believed that animals did not have a soul, and therefore veterinary medicine was left outside the realm of (human) medicine. As a consequence veterinary medicine for a long time has been a much-neglected field of science and its history is still somewhat obscure. The present text deals with its subject in two parts, *viz.,* 1. ancient veterinary science, *i.e.,* the period ending with the establishment of veterinary schools (227 p.), and 2. the history of modern veterinary science, *i.e.,* from *ca.* 1763 onwards (585 p.). Nearly 75% of the text has been devoted to modern veterinary medicine. No illustrations, bibliography, or index. *Cf.* also: BEAUJOUAN, G., *et al.,* 1966, *vide* section Middle Ages in the Latin West, subsection c.

——, 1955-1956: Histoire illustrée de la médecine vétérinaire, présentée par G. RAMON, 2 vols., 250 + 250 p. (Paris: Michel).—

A beautifully-illustrated history of veterinary medicine, which, because it includes so many fine reproductions of paintings of old masters, also has importance from the art-historical point of view. The first vol. deals with antiquity (East Asia, Egypt, Jews, China, India, Greeks and Romans), the Middle Ages (religious aspects, Arab influences, veterinary practice), and the Renaissance (special attention has been paid to Leonardo da Vinci). The second volume deals with veterinary medicine of the 17th and 18th centuries up to the foundation of veterinary schools, and with medical education on these schools.

MERILLAT, L. A. & D. L. CAMPBELL, 1935: Veterinary military history of the United States, 2 vols., 1172 p. (Chicago, Ill.: Veterinary Magazine Corp.).—

A full-scale history of American veterinary science (mainly dealing with horses) from 1792 up to 1935. A very large section has been devoted to the veterinary services of the American Expeditionary Forces, 1916-1920.

POSTOLKA, A., 1885: Geschichte der empirischen Thierheilkunde, 399 p. (Vienna: Beck).—

A history of veterinary science, dealing with *e.g.,* Aesculapius, Hippocrates, Xenophon, Aristotle, Diocles of Caristos, Erasistratos, Cato, Varro, Virgil, Celsus, Pliny, Dioscorides, Columella, Martialis, Apsyrtus, Hierocles, Vegetius Renatus, Theomnestos, Pepagomenos.

PUGH, L. P., 1962: From farriery to veterinary medicine, 1785-1795, 178 p. (Cambridge: Heffer).—

This book contains primarily an accurate historiography of the development of veterinary medicine during the formative period in England. Especially the establishment of the London Veterinary College in 1791 and the difficult period which followed are well described. The study has been based on many newly-discovered documents.

SENET, A., 1953: Histoire de la médecine vétérinaire, 117 p. ("Que sais-je?" No. 584) (Paris: Presses Univ. de France).—

A short history of veterinary science. Separate chapters deal with prehistoric veterinary medicine, oriental sources, Greek hippiatrics, Roman and Byzantine veterinarians, veterinary medicine in antiquity (pathology, therapy, surgery, zootechnique), horse-medicine of the Arabs, Renaissance veterinary science, the foundation of the veterinary school in Lyons, veterinary medicine in the 19th and 20th centuries.

SMITH, F., 1919-1933: The early history of veterinary literature and its British development, 4 vols. Vol. I (1919): 373 p.; Vol. II (1924): 224 p.; Vol. III (1930): 184 p.; Vol. IV (1933): 161 p. (London: Baillière, Tindall & Cox).—

A well-illustrated history of veterinary medicine. The first vol. treats of it from the earliest period to A.D. 1700, and is in two parts. Part 1 (p. 1-122) deals with the period from antiquity up to the 16th century, and is, according to a review in Isis 3: 307, not fully reliable. The second part, however, dealing with the 16th and 17th centuries, is very important. The second vol. deals with the 18th century, a period of remarkable interest, since it witnessed the transfer of the art of veterinary medicine from untrained men to the graduates of the first veterinary school in the U.K. The third vol. deals with the period 1800-1823, and the fourth vol. with the period 1823-1860. These vols. deal with the lives and publications of the leading members of the faculties of the Veterinary Schools of Edinburgh and of London, and of the Royal College of Veterinary Surgeons, and with the history of certain outbreaks of animal plagues. A historical survey of British veterinary science during part of the last century is: Animal health: a centenary, 1865-1965. A century of endeavour to control diseases of animals, 396 p. (London: H.M.S.O.), in which the activities of the State Veterinary Service are described up to 1965 from the formation of a Veterinary Dept. of the Privy Council in 1865.

SMITHCORS, J. F., 1957: Evolution of the veterinary art: a narrative account to 1850, 408 p. (Kansas City, Mo.: Veterinary Med. Publ.).—

A well-written history of veterinary medicine from prehistoric times up to the middle of last century. It contains numerous instructive illustrations, many of them taken from early veterinary books. The author shows how there are many parallels in the development of veterinary and human medicine, and that in ancient times both were held in high esteem. But after the decline of the Byzantine empire the veterinary profession got into a lowly state, which situation was still characteristic for the beginnings of the 19th century when treatment of animals was left to the physician in absence of trained veterinarians.

——, 1963: The American veterinary profession: its background and development, 704 p. (Ames, Iowa: Iowa State U.P.).—

This book deals with such matters as: veterinary public health in colonial America, witchcraft *vs.* animal medicine, early veterinary literature, veterinary medicine in the agricultural press, patent medicines, the USVMA, its organization, constitution, leaders, *etc.*, the (periodical) American veterinary Review, the Bureau of Animal Industry, veterinary economics, *etc.* G. C. CHRISTENSEN wrote a chapter (p. 641-666) on education for the veterinary profession, and E. B. MILLER a chapter (p. 666-684) on military veterinary history. With many illustrations and indexes of subjects and names. *Cf.* BIERER, B. W., 1955; and MERILLAT, L. A. & D. L. CAMPBELL, 1935, *vide supra.*

WEST, G. P., ed., 1961: A history of the overseas veterinary services, Part 1, 143 p. (London: British Veterinary Assn.).—

The veterinary services in India, Burma, Ceylon, Malaya, the Sudan are discussed.

WESTER, J., 1939: Geschiedenis der vee-artsenijkunde, 575 p. (Utrecht: Hoonte).—

A history of the development of veterinary medicine in the Netherlands.

3. HISTORY OF THE PLANT SCIENCES

α. *History of the pure plant sciences*

a. *History of botany in general*

ARBER, A., 1953: Herbals: their origin and evolution. A chapter in the history of botany 1470-1670, ed. 2, 350 p. (Cambridge: U.P.).—

> This is a history of printed (European) herbals from 1470 to 1670, containing many reproductions, nearly all derived from the old herbal woodcuts. After a brief historical introduction and a discussion of the earliest printed herbals (15th cent.), the author arrives at the 16th- and 17th-century herbals with special emphasis upon their taxonomic aspects, to which the greater part of the work has been devoted. Separate chapters deal with the early history of the herbal in England, the evolution of the art of plant description, of plant classification, and of the art of botanical illustration, and with the doctrine of signatures and astrological botany. An appendix contains a chronological list of the principal herbals and related botanical works published between 1470 and 1670. *Cf.* HEILMANN, K. E., 1966; SAINT-LAGER, 1886; SCHMIDT, A., 1939; and SCHREIBER, W. L., 1924, *vide infra.*

BEAUVERIE, J., 1932: La systématique des formes. Les grandes étapes du progrès de la classification naturelle, ses tendances actuelles, 64 p. (Paris: Ed. du Cerf).—

> For more details, *vide* section History of the life sciences, subsection a.

BEHLING, L., 1957: Die Pflanze in der mittelalterlichen Tafelmalerei, 221 p. and many reproductions (Weimar: Böhlau).—

> Whereas the authoress has been trained in both biology and in art history, a very fertile intermingling of two different scientific methods could result, and of this the book is a very fine illustration. It throws a new light on many old problems, and as such it is of great value both to the history of biology and to the history of art. It deals especially with German and Dutch painters living between the 14th and the first half of the 16th century, and much stress has been put on the symbolic value of plants to mediaeval men. Changing views in this symbolic meaning are accompanied by changing representations of plants, and in this context the comparison with old herbals is very in-

teresting. A second ed. appeared in 1967 (Cologne & Graz: Böhlaus).

———, 1964: Die Pflanzenwelt der mittelalterlichen Kathedralen, 227 p. and many illustrations (Cologne & Graz: Böhlau).—

> This study of plant ornaments in (for the greater part) German and French cathedrals has been set up along the same lines as the authoress's "Die Pflanze in der mittelalterlichen Tafelmalerei", *vide supra.* The plants considered have been supplied with fragments of texts of Hildegard of Bingen, Albertus Magnus, and Konrad of Megenberg, which fragments illuminate the symbolic meaning of these plants. Many illustrations (243); most of them are very beautiful photos.

BLUNT, W., 1950: The art of botanical illustration, 304 p. (with the assistance of W. T. STEARN) (London: Collins).—

> This book is of equal interest to the gardener, the artist, the botanist, and the book-lover. It deals with the artist and his products, and contains much biographic details. It is lavishly illustrated; the illustrations serve as samples of artistic, botanical, and technical developments from the early paintings and sculptures of the Egyptians and Cretans down to the work of living artists. The appendix contains eight articles on botanical drawing by W. H. FITCH, originally published in "The Gardener's Chronicle" of 1869. *Cf.* also NISSEN, C., 1951 and TREVIRANUS, L. C., 1949, *vide infra.*

COSTANTIN, J., 1934: Aperçu historique des progrès de la botanique depuis cent ans (1834-1934), 193 p. (Paris: Masson).—

> A review of the achievements in the field of botany as they are reflected in the contents of the "Annales des Sciences naturelles" in the first century of the existence of that periodical. The first section deals with some general problems, such as: spontaneous generation, the distinction between animals and plants, sap circulation, the plant cell, the division of the nucleus; other sections deal with such problems as: systematics, reproduction, fecundation, factors of the environment (plant life on mountains, in glasshouses, on islands, parasitic and carnivorous plants, myrmecophilous plants), normal and pathological plant morphology and physiology, the geography of recent and fossil plants, and applied botany (agricultural-, industrial-, and colonial botany, the origin of cultivated plants). Index of names and subjects.

GREEN, J. R., 1909: A history of botany, 1860-1900: being a continuation of Sachs "History of Botany, 1530-1860", 543 p. (Oxford: Clarendon Press).—

A supplementary volume to SACHS's "History of Botany" (vide infra). The author's approach to the history of botany closely follows the general scheme set up by Sachs in order to show what were - according to the author - the main trends of thought in the different sections distinguished by Sachs (vide etiam) in the period considered. It is of interest to notice that in the present book the first section largely deals with morphology rather than with classification, and that the third section, dealing with plant physiology, is extended considerably in length compared with the same section in Sachs's book. Cf. also WEEVERS, T., 1949, vide infra.

GREENE, E. L., 1909: Landmarks of botanical history: a study of certain epochs in the development of the science of botany. Part I: Prior to 1562 A.D., 330 p. (No other parts have been published) (Smithsonian Misc. Coll., Vol. 54) (Washington, D.C.: Smithsonian Instn.).—

This book is not really a history of botany of the common type; it starts from the philosophical rather than from the industrial point of view. By botany the author means that science which "occupies itself with the contemplation of plant as related to plant, and with the whole vegetable kingdom as viewed philosophically - not economically or commercially - in its relation to the mineral on the one hand, and to the animal on the other", thus excluding agriculture, floriculture, horticulture, forestry and pharmacy. His method of approach is primarily biographical as may be seen from his table of contents: Ch. 2. Theophrastus of Eresus; 3. Greeks and Romans after Theophrastus; 4. Introduction to the 16th-century German fathers; 5. Otto Brunfelsius; 6. L. Fuchsius; 7. H. Tragus; 8. E. Cordus; 9. V. Cordus. Index.

GUÉRIN, L., 1869: Précis de l'histoire de la botanique, 535 p. (Paris: Morgan).—

This book is vol. 17 of the botanical encyclopaedia "Le règne végétal", edited by A. DUPUIS, F. GÉRARD, and O. RÉVEIL (Paris, 1864-1869). It is a rich source of information since it contains long lists of names of botanists and of titles of publications, and as such it has much similarity to PRITZEL's "Thesaurus literaturae botanicae" (vide section Bibliographies, subsection c₁), but it contains more information concerning French botany. Its subject-matter is arranged chronologically and covers the history of botany from antiquity up to the 19th century. Some supplementary maps on plant geography have been included. The index comprises the names of all authors mentioned in the book.

HARVEY-GIBSON, R. I., 1919: Outlines of the history of botany, 274 p. (London: Black).—

This book comprises the substances of a course of lectures given to students during their third year of study and discusses the more important features in the advance of botanical knowledge from the earliest times down to ca. 1919. According to a statement of Singer it "is unquestionably the most satisfactory general history of Botany for students." Only 50 pages have been devoted to the period before Linnaeus, for, as a matter of fact, the later period is more likely to appeal to the average student, because botany before the 17th century was largely merged with medicine and because the study of this older botany is only possible by means of rather difficult methods of research. In 1926 a condensation and rearrangement of this work appeared under the title: A short history of botany, 96 p. (New York, N.Y.: Dutton). Cf. REED, H. S., 1942, vide infra.

HEILMANN, K. E., 1966: Kräuterbücher in Bild und Geschichte, 425 p. (Munich: Kölbl).—

A historical review of mediaeval and Renaissance herbals. The book is profusely illustrated, mainly by means of facsimile reproductions of title-pages, and pages and illustrations derived from the books considered. The book can best be characterized as a pictorial history of herbals; the contents of the present book are mainly based on the private collection of the author. This book also contains much information concerning the printers of the Renaissance and their technique. For the older history of herbals, cf. BUDGE, E. A. W., 1928; and SINGER, C., 1927, vide section Antiquity in general, subsection b. Cf. also: ARBER, A., 1953, vide supra.

JESSEN, K. F. W., 1948: Botanik der Gegenwart und Vorzeit in cultur-historischer Entwicklung. Ein Beitrag zur Geschichte der abendländischen Völker, 495 p. (Pallas, Vol. I) (Waltham, Mass.: Chronica Botanica).—

This "classic" was first published in 1864 (Leipzig: Brockhaus) and is the best extant concise history of botany. If compared with Sachs's "Geschichte der Botanik" (which is of about the same period), this treatise is less nationalistically biassed, and less stress has been laid on the achievements of experimental botany of the 19th century. The history of botany of the 19th century is restricted to a chapter of 63 pages, and within this chapter also much attention has been paid to "Naturphilosophie", morphology, embryology and systematics. This situation is characteristic for the whole treatment. Relatively much space has been devoted to ancient (p. 1-109) and mediaeval (p. 109-166) botany. The cultural implications of botany have been treated well.

KREMPELHUBER, A. v., 1867-1872: Geschichte und Literatur der Lichenologie von den ältesten Zeiten bis zum Schlusse des Jahres 1865, 3 vols. Vol. I (1867): Geschichte und Literatur, 616 p.; Vol. II (1869): Die Flechten-Systeme und Flechten-Spezies, 776 p.; Vol. III (1872): Die Fortschritte und die Literatur der Lichenologie in dem Zeitraume von 1866-1870 incl. nebst Nachträgen zu den früheren Perioden, 216 p. (Munich: Selbstverlag).—

Of this privately-published book, the first vol. is in two parts of which the first part (p. 1-464) contains a comprehensive history of lichenology from antiquity up to 1865, followed by indexes of authors, collectors, etc. The second part consists of a systematical and chronological bibliography of lichenology (of 1412 items), followed by a list of herbals of lichens and the places where they are. The second vol. is in three parts. The first part contains a historical review of the place occupied by the lichens in the various classificatory systems (p. 1-14), the second part contains a historical review of the various genera distinguished by the various lichenologists (p. 15-490), and the third part contains a review of the species of lichens distinguished by botanists living before and after Linnaeus. Extensive indexes of botanical names and of names of persons. The third vol. deals with the same subjects as vols. I and II, but is exclusively restricted to the period of 1866-1870 incl.

LOEW, E., 1895: Einführung in die Blütenbiologie auf historischer Grundlage, 432 p. (Berlin: Dümmler).—

A (pre-Mendelian) historical review on flower biology and on theories of fertilization in plants, from antiquity up to 1882.

The larger part (p. 96-407) is devoted to the Darwinian period and stress has been laid on Darwin's own achievements in these fields.

MEYER, E. H. F., 1854-1857: Geschichte der Botanik, 4 vols. Vol. I (1854): 406 p.; Vol. II (1855): 430 p.; Vol. III (1856): 554 p.; Vol. IV (1857): 451 p. (Königsberg: Borntraeger).—

By far the most authoritative and comprehensive history of pure and applied botany for the period from antiquity to the Renaissance. Vol. I is in four parts, viz., 1. Anfänge der Botanik bei den Griechen (p. 1-78); 2. Blüthe der Botanik bei den Griechen (p. 79-201); 3. Verfall der Botanik unter den Griechen bis zur Gründung der römischen Weltherrschaft (Augustus) (p. 202-333); 4. Botanische Anklänge bei den Römern vor und unter Augustus (p. 334-399). The second vol. also is in 4 parts, viz., 5. Heilmittellehre, Landwirthschaft und mercantilische Waarenkunde, von Augustus bis Nero (p. 1-92); 6. Blüthe und Verfall der Arzneimittellehre als Trägerin der Pflanzenkunde. Von Vespasianus bis zu den Antoninen (69-180 A.D.) (p. 93-176); 7. Kurzer neuer Aufschwung der Medicin und Agronomie unter den Griechen und Römern, bei fortschreitendem Verfall der Wissenschaft überhaupt (180-363 (p. 177-273); 8. Langes Siechthum europäischer Wissenschaft überhaupt. Von Julianus Tode bis gegen die Zeit Karls des Grossen (363- ca. 800) (p. 274-423). Vol. III is in 3 parts, viz., 9. Zur Geschichte der Botanik bei den ältern ostasiatischen Völkern (p. 1-88); 10. Zur Geschichte der Botanik bei den Arabern (p. 89-327); 11. Neue, auch die Botanik berührende Geistesregungen in den christlich-europäischen Ländern, von Kaiser Karl dem Grossen bis zum Mönch Albert dem Grossen (ca. 800-1250) (p. 328-542). Vol IV again is in 4 parts, viz., 12. Die Botanik unter den erneuerten Einfluss der aristotelischen Naturphilosophie (p. 1-106); 13. Neuer von weniger wachen Momenten unterbrochener Schlummer der Botanik (p. 107-206); 14. Rückkehr durch das Studium der klassischen Literatur der Naturbeobachtung (p. 207-288); 15. Entwickelung der Pflanzenkunde über die Grenzen der Heilmittellehre hinaus (p. 289-444). Each volume contains an index of personal names. Reprinted 1965 (Amsterdam: Asher).

MÖBIUS, M., 1937: Geschichte der Botanik von den ersten Anfängen bis zur Gegenwart, 458 p. (Jena: Fischer).—

In this encyclopaedic history of botany stress has been laid on German botany.

The subject matter has been divided into three parts. From these the first part has been divided into 84 sections, of which the first three sections (p. 1-38) deal with botany in the ancient world, the Middle Ages and the beginnings of modern botany. The other sections of this part treat of the history of botany on a topical basis. Thus, sections 4 and 5 deal with artificial and natural systems (p. 38-48); section 6 with the effect of evolutionary aspects on systematics (p. 48-54); sections 7-28 deal with Cryptogamia; 29-33 with Pteridophyta; 34-39 with Gymnosperms; 40-83 with Angiosperms; and section 84 with phytopalaeontology. The second part (p. 383-418) deals with applied botany and the third part (p. 418-440) with aids in botanical research and instruction (botanical gardens, herbals, botanical illustrations, textbooks, *etc.*). Biographical and bibliographical data are restricted to footnotes. Extensive personal index. The main difference as to the books of SACHS (*vide infra*) and GREENE (*vide supra*) is that the book by Möbius includes more information on such topics as: plant geography, palaeontology, morphology, histology, cytology, and applied botany. A second ed. appeared in 1968 as a reprint of the first ed. (Stuttgart: Fischer).

NISSEN, C., 1951: Die botanische Buchillustration. Ihre Geschichte und Bibliographie, 2 vols. Vol. I: 264 p.; Vol. II: 324 p. (Stuttgart: Hiersemann).—

Vol. I contains a history of botanical illustration. It contains chapters on the incunabula, mediaeval manuscripts, the Renaissance, and the Baroque period. For the mid-eighteenth century onwards the author has devoted a separate section to each nation contributing to the history of botanical illustration. Vol. II contains an alphabetically-arranged bibliography of the illustrated botanical literature produced by artists from the beginning of printing to the date of compilation, comprising 2387 entries. It includes books with plates, textbooks and periodical articles. A section on periodicals, anonymous and serial works has been included, together with a list of artists, of plants, of countries, and of editors. In 1966 a second edition appeared as a reprint of vols. 1 and 2 of the first ed., with a supplement (= vol. 3). They were published by Hiersemann in Stuttgart as 3 vols. in one (687 p.). The third vol. lists corrections and additions and is available as a separate publication. A more or less abridged version of "Die botanische Buchillustration" is: NISSEN, C., 1958: Herbals of five centuries: a contribution to medical history and bibliography, 86 p. (Zurich: L'art ancien). Also in German translation: Kräuterbücher aus

fünf Jahrhunderten. Medizinhistorischer und bibliographischer Beitrag, 1966, 83 p. (Zurich: L'art ancien). *Cf.* also the works of NISSEN, mentioned in the sections History of zoology and History of ornithology, and the works of BLUNT, W., 1950, *vide supra* and TREVIRANUS, L. C., 1949, *vide infra*.

PICKERING, C., 1879: Chronological history of plants: Man's record of his own existence illustrated through their names, uses, and companionship, 1222 p. (Boston, Mass.: Little, Brown).—

The author starts this monumental work with the following words: "In the distribution of species over the globe the order of nature has been obscured through the interference of Man. He has transported animals and plants to countries where they were previously unknown; extirpating the forest and cultivating the soil, until at length the face of the globe itself is changed. To ascertain the amount of this interference, displaced species must be distinguished, and traced each to its original home... A list will naturally assume the chronological order, beginning with Egypt, the country that contains the earliest records of the human family; and receding geographically from the same point of reference..." Very extensive and complete indexes to foreign words, to names of persons, and to names of plants.

REED, H. S., 1942: A short history of the plant sciences, 328 p. (Waltham, Mass.: Chronica Botanica).—

A history of botany written for "the average graduate student . . . rather than for the specialist in science or in history", and mainly treated from the physiological point of view. Such topics as taxonomy, phylogeny, palaeobotany, and genetics have been omitted. The first half of the book deals with the history of botany up to the end of the 18th century: gardeners and herbalists of antiquity; the nascent period from the 6th cent. B.C. to the end of the 2nd cent. A.D.; the retrogressive period (200-1200); the renascent period (1200-1600); the 17th and 18th centuries. The second half covers the 19th and 20th centuries and the chapter headings are as follows: plant geography in the 19th century; morphology; cytology; water economy; fixation of carbon; assimilation; fixation and metabolism of nitrogen; plant nutrition; mineral constituents; mycology; plant pathology. Short bibliographies at the end of the chapters.

SACHS, J., 1906: History of botany (1530-1860), ed. 2, 865 p. (Oxford: Clarendon Press).—

　　　This "classic" in the history of botany is an English translation of SACHS, J., 1875: Geschichte der Botanik vom 16. Jahrhundert bis 1860, 612 p. (Geschichte der Wissenschaften in Deutschland, Neuere Zeit, Band XV) (Munich: Oldenbourg). In this book botany has been divided into the following three branches of knowledge: 1. Classification founded on morphology; 2. Vegetable anatomy; 3. Vegetable physiology; according to the author, these three branches differ in their methods of research. The present book gives the main lines of development within these three branches. On the one hand the text has been based on those facts of which can be shown (or, for more recent times, can be supposed) that they have promoted the development of science. On the other hand, it is the author's aim to present a picture of the way in which the first beginnings of scientific studies of the vegetable world in the 16th century made their appearance in alliance with cultural traditions prevailing at that time, and to show how they developed up to 1860, and led to a still deeper insight into the outer form and inner organisation of the plant. The book is unique for the way in which it treats of the development of 19th-century plant physiology. No bibliography. There also exists a French translation: Histoire de la botanique du XVIe siècle à 1860, 1892, 584 p. (Paris: Reinwald). Cf. GREEN, J. R., 1909, vide supra; and WEEVERS, T., 1949, vide infra.

SAINT-LAGER, 1886: Histoire des herbiers, 120 p. (Ann. Soc. Bot. Lyon 13: 1-120).—

　　　The author makes an attempt to trace the history from the ancient herbal to the dried plant collections of the modern botanical museum. It is certain that collections of dried plants existed as early as 1553 and probably even in 1545; a more general application of this technique took place after 1650. Among the oldest collections of dried plants are those of Aldrovandi, Jean Girault, Cesalpino, Rauwolf, and Bauhin; these collections are discussed and mostly provided with lists of plants mentioned. Cf. HEILMANN, K. E., 1966, vide supra.

SCHMID, A., 1939: Ueber alte Kräuterbücher, 85 p. (Berne & Leipzig: Haupt).—

　　　A general introduction to the history of, and genetical relationships between, old herbals. It also contains a schematic genealogical review of all herbals known so far. In order to elucidate the development of the art of plant illustration, pictures of only one plant (viz., of Symphytum officinalis) have been given, in order to exemplify the way in which it was represented in the different herbals. Cf. HEILMANN, K. E., 1966, vide supra.

SCHREIBER, W. L., 1924: Die Kräuterbücher des XV. und XVI. Jahrhunderts und die Hortus Sanitatis, deutsch von Peter Schöffer, Mainz, 1485, 720 + 83 p. + 379 figs. (Munich: Münchener Drucke).—

　　　A facsimile reproduction of the Hortus Sanitatis, followed by 53 pages on which Schreiber gives a review of: Schöffers "Herbarius" (1484), the "Hortus Sanitatis" of Johann von Cube (1485), "Der grosse Hortus Sanitatis" (1491), "Der Gart der Gesundheit" (1492), the Strasbourg herbals, the herbals of Brunfels (1532), Fuchs (1542), Bock (1539), Matthiolus (1554), Ryff and Lonicer (1550), Tabernaemontanus (1588), Thurneisser (1578), and the plant drawings of Gessner.

SPRENGEL, K. P. J., 1817-1818: Geschichte der Botanik, 2 vols. Vol. I: 424 p.; Vol. II: 396 p. (Altenburg & Leipzig: Brockhaus).—

　　　An old but still very valuable history of botany. At about the same time another German history of botany appeared, containing much information concerning botanical gardens, viz., SCHULTES, J. A., 1817: Grundriss einer Geschichte und Literatur der Botanik, von Theophrastos Eresios bis auf die neuesten Zeiten; nebst einer Geschichte der botanischen Gärten, 411 p. (Vienna: Schaumburg).

STEERE, W. C., ed., 1958: Fifty years of botany, 638 p. (New York, N.Y.: McGraw-Hill).—

　　　The book contains a collection of papers written by members of the Botanical Society of America to commemorate the golden anniversary of its foundation. The authors were selected to present contributions delineating the major advances in the various fields of plant sciences during the past fifty years, emphasizing present trends and future problems. Consequently a variety of topics has been discussed, e.g., the recent history of physiology, morphology, taxonomy, microbiology, palaeobotany, mycology, phycology, various aspects of ecology, plant diseases, applied botany, gardening, and botanical gardens.

TREVIRANUS, L. C., 1949: Die Anwendung des Holzschnittes zur bildlichen Darstellung von Pflanzen. Nach Entstehung, Blüthe, Verfall und Restauration, 75 p. (Classics of Natural History, Reprint No. 1) (Utrecht: de Haan; Amsterdam: Asher).—

A reprint from the original edition of 1855. This booklet deals chiefly with the woodcuts employed by 16th and 17th-century herbalists *(e.g.,* Brunfels, Fuchs, Bock, Gessner, Matthiolus, Dodonaeus, M. de Lobel, Clusius, Rauwolf, Camerarius, Bauhin), but also with the restoration of the woodcut by T. Bewick. There is an index of artists, botanists, and printers. *Cf.* also the works of BLUNT, W., 1950 and of NISSEN, C., 1951, *vide supra.*

VON HAGEN, V. W., 1945: South America called them, 322 p. (New York, N.Y.: Knopf).—

A well-written account of the voyages of exploration in South America, undertaken by the great naturalists C. M. de la Condamine, A. von Humboldt, C. Darwin, and R. Spruce. But besides these naturalists, many others have been considered in some detail. The book is well illustrated and contains a good bibliography and a helpful index. In 1946 a Spanish translation appeared: Sudamérica los llamó. Exploraciones de los grandes naturalistas. La Condamine, Humboldt, Darwin, Spruce, 479 p. (México, D. F.: Ed. Nuevo Mundo).

WEEVERS, T., 1949: Fifty years of plant physiology, 308 p. (Amsterdam: Scheltema & Holkema).—

As far as the history of plant physiology is concerned, the book is a logical continuation of both J. SACHS's and J. R. GREENE's histories of botany *(vide etiam),* albeit that - as Went states in his introduction - the title of this book might have been "Textbook of plant physiology on a historical basis". The chapters deal with: respiration, imbibition and movement of water, mineral nutrition (incl. photosynthesis), translocation of organic substances, heterotrophic metabolism, growth, geotropism, differentiation and correlation, movements. Special attention is given to Dutch plant-physiologists working between 1895 and 1945.

WHEELWRIGHT, E. G., 1935: The physick garden, 288 p. (Boston, Mass.: Houghton Mifflin).—

This book deals with such subjects as: aboriginal uses of herbs, the drug plants of Mesopotamia, India, and China, Egyptian records of medicinal plants, drugs in Greek and Roman medicine and in the early Christian era, the first physick gardens at St. Gall in Switzerland, herbals, the increase of interest in botanic gardens in the 16th century with the importance of plants from newly explored lands, English herbals, botanic gardens and gardeners, the use of pharmacopoeias, the medicinal plants of Great Britain, the trade in medicinal herbs, drug farms in Great Britain, *etc.*

WINCKLER, E., 1854: Geschichte der Botanik, 646 p. (Frankfurt a. M.: Literarische Anstalt).—

A review of the main lines of development of (mainly systematic) botany from the earliest times up to *ca.* 1850. The subject matter has been divided into three major sections: I. From antiquity up to 1500 (p. 1-63); II: From 1500 to Antoine de Jussieu dealing with, *inter alia,* Lorenzo de Medici, Bauhin, Tournefort, Linnaeus (p. 64-258); III: From de Jussieu up to *ca.* 1850, dealing with, *inter alia,* Robert Brown, de Candolle, v. Humboldt. Abundant footnotes give additional bibliographical information.

ZUNCK, H. L., 1840: Die natürlichen Pflanzensysteme geschichtlich entwickelt, 208 p. (Leipzig: Hinrich).—

For more details, *vide supra,* subsection History of general biology.

b. *Some regional histories of the pure plant sciences*

b.* *Europe*

Austria

LINSBAUER, K. & L. v. PORTHEIM, 1903: Wiesner und seine Schule. Ein Beitrag zur Geschichte der Botanik, 259 p. (Vienna: Hölder).—

Although published as a Festschrift on the occasion of the thirtieth anniversary of the plant-physiological institute of the university of Vienna, its historical value lies in its bibliographical information. It lists all botanical literature published at this institute between 1873 and 1909. A supplement was published in 1910, 72 p.

MAIWALD, V., 1904: Geschichte der Botanik in Böhmen, 297 p. (Vienna: Fromme).—

> A valuable history of botany, containing very much information concerning the history of botany of Bohemia. It starts with botanical glossaries from the 12th century, existing in ms. in some monastery- and other libraries. It deals with old herbals, the immense influence of Mattioli (1501-1577) on botany, cultivation of plants and herbs, viticulture, the introduction of plants, botanical education, *etc.* It contains much biographical information.

Finland

COLLANDER, R., 1965: The history of botany in Finland 1828-1918, 159 p. (With an appendix on forest science by Yrjö ILVESSALO) (Helsinki: Soc. Sci. Fenn.).—

> This book gives brief historical reviews of the development of the various botanical disciplines between 1828 and 1918, including such disciplines as: systematics (incl. lichenology, bryology, algology, mycology), physiology, plant-ecology and plant-palaeontology. Moreover, it contains much biographical information concerning: C. R. Sahlberg, J. M. af Tengström, J. E. A. Wirzén, J. Fellman, the Nylander brothers, S. O. Lindberg, F. Elfving, P. A. Karsten. Special chapters have been devoted to the history of teaching in botany since 1857, the national herb-garden, the botanical museum, and to Finnish forestry. Very good bibliography.

France

COMBES, R., 1933: Histoire de la biologie végétale en France, 172 p. (Paris: Alcan).—

> A historical review of the development of botany during the period 1830-1930, stressing the achievements of French botanists in the fields of absorption, circulation, transpiration, assimilation, respiration, fecundation, the formation of organs, cellular differentiation, plant geography, and palaeobotany. Contains many biographical details of French botanists who lived during the period considered.

CRESTOIS, P., 1953: Contribution à l'histoire de l'enseignement de la pharmacie: l'enseignement de la botanique au Jardin Royal des Plantes de Paris, 132 p. (Cahors: Coueslant).—

> The first section (p. 13-48) deals with the "Jardin Royal des Plantes médicinales de Paris", considering such subjects as: botany in the beginning of the 17th century, the medical faculty, Guy de la Brosse, Fagon, the development of the botanical garden in the 19th century. The second part (p. 49-88) deals with botanical education in the Royal Botanical Garden, considering such subjects as: courses of lectures, scientific and medical botany, plant-collections, *etc.* The third part (p. 89-121) deals with the professors of botany (emphasizing their activities in pharmacobotany) and the head gardeners of the Garden. This part contains much biographical information (not always reliable). Bibliography.

DAVY DE VIRVILLE, A., ed., 1954: Histoire de la botanique en France, 394 p. (Paris: Soc. d'Ed. d'Enseignement Supérieur).—

> The first part (p. 19-120) traces the history of French botany from the Middle Ages down to the 18th century. This part has been written by Davy de Virville. The second part, dealing with modern botany, has been divided into sections dealing with the history of various specialities - each written by a specialist - as: the history of morphology, anatomy, cytology, phycology, lichenology, phytography, agronomy, forestry, pathology, mycology, palaeobotany, palynology, and botanical voyages and explorations. *Cf.* also LEROY, J., ed., 1957, *vide infra,* subsection Other parts of the world.

FOURNIER, P., 1947-1948: Le livre des plantes médicinales et vénéneuses de France, 3 vols. (Paris: Lechevalier).—

> For more details, *vide* section Some recommended encyclopaedias, subsection c1.

Germany

MARZELL, H., 1937 →: Wörterbuch der deutschen Pflanzennamen. (Leipzig: Hirzel).—

> For more details, *vide* section Some recommended encyclopaedias, subsection c1.

SACHS, J., 1875: Geschichte der Botanik vom 16. Jahrhundert bis 1860, 612 p. (Geschichte der Wissenschaften in Deutschland, neuere Zeit, Vol. XV) (Munich: Oldenbourg).—

> A discussion of this book has been given in the section History of botany in general, *vide supra*. *Cf.* also: URBAN, I., 1881: Geschichte des Königlichen botanischen Gartens und des Königlichen Herbariums zu Berlin, nebst einer Darstellung des augenblicklichen Zustandes dieser Institute, 164 p. (Berlin: Borntraeger); URBAN, I., 1916: Geschichte des Königlichen Botanischen Museums zu Berlin-Dahlem (1815-1913) nebst Aufzählung seiner Sammlungen, 457 p. (Bot. Centralblatt, 1. Abt., 34, Beiheft 2) (Dresden: Heinrich); and FISCHER, H., 1929, *vide* section Middle Ages in the Latin West, subsection b.

Great Britain

BOWER, F. O., 1938: Sixty years of botany in Britain (1875-1935): impression of an eyewitness, 112 p. (London & New York, N.Y.: Macmillan).—

> Besides much biographical information, the book also contains much that is of importance to an understanding of the development of the various aspects of British botany between 1875 and 1935, the period during which the author himself was actively engaged in botanical research. He was a pupil of T. H. Huxley and he knew personally such famous biologists as J. D. Hooker, G. Bentham, D. Oliver Thiselton-Dyer, Marshall Ward, B. Balfour, D. H. Scott and others.

BRITTEN, J., G. S. BOULGER & A. B. RENDLE, 1931: A bibliographical index of deceased British and Irish botanists, 342 p. (London: Taylor & Francis).—

> For more details about this book, *vide* section Biographical dictionaries, subsection b.

CLOKIE, H. N., 1964: An account of the herbaria of the Department of Botany in the University of Oxford, 280 p. (London: Oxford U.P.).—

> Separate sections deal with: Makers of the herbaria (R. Morison, Jacob Bobart, W. Sherard, C. du Bois, J. J. Dillenius, H. & J. Sibthorp, H. B. Fielding, C. G. B. Daubeny, M. A. Lawson, G. C. Druce); Special collections (the Gregorio a Reggio herbarium; the herbaria of Jacob Bobart the younger; the Sherard, du Bois, Dillenian, Fielding, and Druce herbaria); Alphabetical list of collectors' names under the names of areas where they collected; Index of collectors (p. 120-269); Bibliography.

FISHER, R., 1932-1934: The English names of our commonest wild flowers, 2 vols. Vol. I (1932): 249 p.; Vol. II (1934): 344 p. (Arbroath: Buncle).—

> Fore more details, *vide* section Some recommended encyclopaedias, *etc.*, subsection c1.

GILMOUR, J., ed., 1944: British botanists, 48 p. (Britain in Pictures) (London: Collins).—

> Brief accounts with bibliography and fine illustrations of the leading botanists of England from 1550 up to 1900; agriculturists and horticulturists are not included. Among the persons considered are: T. H. Huxley, Darwin, Hooker, Ray, S. Hales, N. Grew, Turner, Parkinson, and Gerard.

GREEN, J. R., 1914: A history of botany in the United Kingdom from the earliest times to the end of the 19th century, 648 p. (London & Toronto: Dent; New York, N.Y.: Dutton).—

> The subject matter has been divided into 8 books. Bk. 1 deals with early botany and the herbalists (Turner, Bulleijn, Penny, Hill, L'Obel, Lyte, Gerard, Johnson, Parkinson, Langham, Bobart, Tradescant, How, Merrett). Bk. 2 deals with the rise of systematics: John Ray, R. Morison, Hooke, Grew; Bk. 3 with the period between Ray and Linnaeus: contemporary botany at Oxford, Cambridge, in Scotland and Ireland, and with the Linnean system; Bk. 4 with the ascendancy of the Linnean system (Martijn, Banks, Dillenius, J. E. Smith); Bk. 5 with the revival of the natural system (R. Brown, J. Lindley, Henslow); Bk. 6 with the period between Lindley and Darwin; Bk. 7 with the influence of Darwin's "Origin of Species", J. D. Hooker, G. Bentham and their influence, and with the coming of the botanical laboratory; Bk. 8 with the more recent and applied aspects of botany, *e.g.*, with morphology, palaeobotany, physiological- and pathological research, and the progress of agriculture. *Cf.* also GUNTHER, R. T., 1922: Early British botanists and their gardens, based on unpublished writings of Goodyer, Tradescant and others, 417 p. (Oxford: U.P.). A special aspect of the history of British botany is considered by: TURRILL, W. B., 1959: The Royal Botanic Gardens, Kew, 256 p. (London: Jenkins).

RAVEN, C. E., 1947: English naturalists from Neckham to Ray: a study of the making of the modern world, 379 p. (Cambridge: U.P.).—

 For more details, *vide supra,* subsection History of biology in general.

ROHDE, E. S., 1922: The old English herbals, 255 p. (London: Longmans, Green).—

 A rather popular and instructive treatise. Ch. 1 deals with Anglo-Saxon herbals and demonstrates that books on herbs were studied as early as the 8th century A.D. Ch. 2 deals with later manuscript herbals and the early printed herbals *(e.g., Barth.* Anglicus's "De proprietatibus rerum", Bancke's "Herbal", and the "Grete Herbal"). Ch. 3 deals with Turner's herbal and the influence of the foreign herbalists *(inter alia,* Gessner, Fuchs, Dodonaeus, Clusius, and Lobelius); ch. 4 with Gerard's "Herball" (1597); ch. 5 with herbals of the new world (chiefly dealing with Nicholas Monardes's "Dos libros", Seville, 1569 and its English translation by J. FRAMPTON). Ch. 6 is devoted to John Parkinson, the last of the great English herbalists (who composed the "Paradisus", 1629 and the "Theatrum Botanicum", 1640) and ch. 7 to the later 17th-century herbals and 16th- and 17th-century still-room books; the latter are commonly associated with cookery. Three appendixes follow: the first contains a list of manuscript herbals kept in English libraries (9th - 15th centuries); the second contains a catalogue of English printed herbals (from 1495 to 1838); the third is a catalogue of the main herbals printed abroad (from 1470 to 1670).

Hungary

KANITZ, A., 1863: Geschichte der Botanik in Ungarn, 199 p. (Pesth).—

 Unfortunately I am unable to give further information about the contents of this book. The Brit. Mus. Catalogue gives: (Skizzen); printed in Hannover, published in Pesth; only 70 copies printed.

Luxemburg

LEFORT, F. L., 1949: Contribution à l'histoire botanique du Luxembourg, 127 p. (Soc. Naturalistes Luxembourgeois, Bull. 1949, N.S., No. 43: 33-160).—

 A historical review of the botanical history of Luxemburg starting with the year

1810, when A. P. de Candolle integrated the flora of Luxemburg into the botanical geography of Europe. Of the botanists considered we mention: Redouté, A. P. de Candolle, Lejeune, Dumortier, Van Hall, Wirtgen, Tinant, Krombach, Crépin, Koltz, Klein, Emberger.

The Netherlands

SIRKS, M. J., 1935: Botany in the Netherlands, 140 p. (Leiden: Brill).—

 This booklet was edited for the organizing committee of the sixth Intl. Bot. Congress. It contains a sketch of the history and present position of botanical science in the Netherlands and their overseas territories, with descriptions of botanical institutes of university colleges in the Netherlands (Leyden, Groningen, Utrecht, Amsterdam, Delft, Wageningen); of autonomous official and semi-official institutions; of societies; and of botanical gardens, experiment stations, *etc.,* of the Netherlands East Indies (now: Indonesia), Surinam and the Antilles. A very complete history of the famous botanical garden of the university of Leyden (including much biographical information concerning its directors) can be found in: VEENDORP, H. & L. G. M. BAAS BECKING, 1938: Hortus Academicus Lugduno Batavus: the development of the gardens of Leyden University, 1587-1937, 218 p. (Haarlem: Enschede). *Cf.* also HONIG, P. & F. VERDOORN, *vide infra,* subsection Other parts of the world.

Russia

ASMOUS, V. C., 1947: Fontes historiae botanicae Rossicae, 31 p. (Chronica botanica XI, No. 2: 87-118).—
 A bibliography of sources pertaining to the history of botany in Russia. It consists of a list of authors and their publications. The titles have been given both in transliteration and in English translation. Some items cited contain sizeable bibliographical lists offering useful material to the historian of Russian plant study. The subject-index is in 3 parts, *viz.,* bibliographies, biographies, and history and progress of botany.

SHETLER, S. G., 1967: The Komarov Botanical Institute: 250 years of Russian research, 240 p. (Washington, D.C.: Smithsonian Instn. Press).—

 The contributions of the Komarov institute and its predecessors in descriptive botany are discussed, and whereas the Komarov institute has always maintained the leading position in this field in Russia, this book mirrors the history of much of Russian botany as a whole.

TRAUTVETTER, E. R., 1837: Grundriss einer Geschichte der Botanik in Bezug auf Russland, 145 p. (Petrograd: Kaiserl. Akad. Wiss.).—

The first section (p. 4-48) contains a sketch of botanical exploration of Russia; the sections 2 and 3 deal with scientific organizations fostering botany in Russia and contain a list of botanical institutes and gardens. The fourth section (p. 55-136) contains a geographically-arranged bibliography of works treating of the flora of Russia or dealing with Russian botanists.

Sweden

FRIES, R. E., 1950: A short history of botany in Sweden, 162 p. (with contributions by K. V. D. Dahlgren, A. Müntzing, A. Åberg & H. Osvald) (Seventh Intl. Bot. Congress, Stockholm, 1950) (Uppsala: Almqvist & Wiksells).—

A short historical review, dealing with the development of many aspects of botany, especially as it took place in Sweden. Special chapters deal with botanical cytology and embryology (by DAHLGREN); botanical genetics (by MÜNTZING) botanical physiology (by ÅBERG), and applied botany (by OSVALD). One of the most interesting aspects of this book is a map, compiled by R. E. FRIES, indicating the journeys undertaken by Linnaeus's disciples.

KROK, T. O. B. N., 1925: Bibliotheca botanica suecana ab antiquissimis temporis ad finem anni MCMXVIII, 799 p. (Uppsala & Stockholm: Almqvist & Wiksells).—

Exemplary bibliography of all publications by Swedish botanists (or by others) about the Swedish flora until 1919. Includes many bibliographical details *(e.g.,* about translation, abstracts, *etc.),* cross-references, *etc.,* not to be found elsewhere; also short biographical notes.

b.** *Other parts of the world*

BOONE, W. W., 1965: A history of botany in West Virginia, 196 p. (Parsons, W. Va.: McClain).—

Unfortunately I am unable to give further information about this book!

CLUTE, W. N., 1942: The common names of plants and their meanings, ed. 2, 164 p. (Indianapolis, Ind.: W. N. Clute).—

For more details, *vide* section Some recommended encyclopaedias, subsection c1.

CONDE, J. A., 1958: Historia de la botánica en Cuba, 353 p. (La Habana: Junta Nac. de Arqueologia y Etnologia).—

Contains very much biographical information; biographies are often accompanied by portraits.

EWAN, J., 1950: Rocky Mountain naturalists, 358 p. (Denver, Col.: Denver U.P.).—

This book contains biographies (p. 1-117) of nine leading naturalists of the Rocky Mountain area (with portraits), *viz.,* E. James, J. C. Fremont, C. C. Parry, E. L. Green, T. C. Porter, H. N. Patterson, M. E. Jones, E. Penard, T. D. A. Cockerell, followed by explanatory notes, a bibliography, a very useful roster of natural history collectors 1682-1932 (p. 138-343), and an index of personal names.

HONIG, P. & F. VERDOORN, eds., 1945: Science and scientists in the Netherlands Indies, 491 p. (New York City, N.Y.: Board for the Netherlands Indies, Surinam and Curaçao).—

The book contains 81 contributions of 75 authors, who primarily deal with botanical research, and as such it contains much that is of a historical interest. Of the subjects considered we may mention: regulation and export of rubber, the history of the Treub Laboratory and Botanic Gardens in Bogor (1884-1934), agricultural history, history of cinchona, forestry, climate and soil, pulpwood supplies, palaeobotanical research, tobacco, the history of the botanical garden in Tjibodas, *etc.* Besides, it contains much information of a more general nature. *Cf.* also SIRKS, M. J., ed., 1935, *vide supra,* subsection Europe and STEENIS-KRUSEMAN, M. J. v., 1950: *vide* section Biographical dictionaries, subsection b.

HUMPHREY, H. B., 1961: Makers of North American botany, 265 p. (Chronica Botanica, No. 21) (New York, N.Y.: Ronald Press).—

This book describes life and work of some 122 North American botanists. The botanists included were selected for their important contributions, for pioneering activities in new areas, for great teaching or administrative ability, or productive research activities. No living persons are included. A book dealing with similar topics seems to be: EIFERT, V. L., 1965: Tall trees and far horizons: adventures and discoveries of early botanists in America, 301 p. (New York, N.Y.: Dodd, Mead). Unfortunately I am unable to give further information.

LEROY, J., ed., 1957: Les botanistes français en Amérique du Nord avant 1850, 360 p. (Coll. Inst. Centre Natl. Rech. Sci. LXIII) (Paris: Centre Natl. Rech. Scient.).—

The record of an international symposium. Among the persons considered are: Rafinesque, A. P. de Candolle, La Galissonière, A. and F. A. Michaux, Trécul, Lamare-Picquot, Bachelot de la Pylaie, Bernard de Jussieu, Prat, Delile, A. Plée, M. Sarrazin, J. F. Gaultier, Linnaeus, Kalm. The book contains much information concerning the introduction of American plants and trees into France in particular, and into Europe in general. For a table of contents, *vide* Isis 49: 203.

REIFSCHNEIDER, O., 1964: Biographies of Nevada botanists, 1844-1963, 165 p. (Reno, Nev.: Univ. Nevada Press).—

A series of biographies of some 47 Nevada botanists, giving together a review of the development of botany in this state. The volume contains a remarkable collection of portraits and is further illustrated with maps and early drawings from historical explorations.

RODGERS, A. D., 1944: American botany, 1873-1892: decades of transition, 340 p. (Princeton, N.J.: Princeton U.P.).—

The book is primarily biographical in character, and only secondarily does it deal with the history of American botany. Among the botanists considered in detail are: Asa Gray, Engelmann (taxonomist) and Lesquereux (palaeobotanist). But besides, it gives much information on such topics as: the botanical exploration of the West, the emergence of horticulture, the establishment of botanical research institutes and agricultural stations, the development of plant morphology and the impact of European influences (especially German) on the development of American botany. A reprint of this ed. appeared in 1968 (New York, N.Y. & London: Hafner).

ROUSSEAU, J., 1937: La botanique canadienne à l'époque de Jacques Cartier, 86 p. (Contrib. Lab. Botanique, Univ. Montréal) (Montréal: Inst. de Botanique de l'Univ.).—

"Excerpts from the original edition of the diaries of Jacques Cartier and other discoverers, containing notes pertaining to Canadian botany, are cited and discussed. Explorers other than Jacques Cartier whose works have been analysed from a botanical viewpoint are: Roberval, Jean Alfonse, André Thévet, Jacques Noël, Jean Cabot, Gaspar Corte-Real, Verrazzano, *etc.* A short chapter is devoted to Norsemen's travel to Vinland. The paper ends with an annotated list of all plants mentioned in the discussion of the discoverers' texts." (Author's abstract in Biol. Abstr., Vol. 16, no. 15730).

TORREY BOTANICAL CLUB, 1969: Index to American botanical literature, 1886-1966, 4 vols. (Boston, Mass.: Hall).—

"This index in book form is an author catalog of botanical books and papers based on materials from North, South and Central America. It includes the taxonomy, phylogeny, and floristics of the fungi, pteridophytes, and spermatophytes; morphology, anatomy, cytology, genetics, physiology, and pathology of the same groups; plant ecology; and general botany, including biography and bibliography. Future issues of the 'Index to American Botanical Literature on Cards' will be published annually by G. K. Hall... A book-form supplement is planned every ten years. Estimated 106,000 cards reproduced in 4 volumes..." (From an announcement in Nature 29: xviii, September 7, 1968).

VERDOORN, F., ed., 1945: Plants and plant science in Latin America, 40 + 384 p. (A new series of plant science books, XVI) (Waltham, Mass.: Chronica Botanica).—

An encyclopaedic work consisting of contributions of some 85 scientists. The editor wrote a general introduction which is of special interest to those interested in the organization of science. It includes three special bibliographies, *viz.*, on travel books of botanical interest, on miscellaneous supplementary references of a botanical interest, and on recent publications of the Office of Foreign Agricultural Relations of the U.S Dept. of Agriculture. Part I begins with some introductory chapters entitled: Problems of tropical agriculture; Phytogeographic sketch; Economic plants; Historical sketch (dealing with the impact of American plants on the Old World). The next 35 chapters are concerned with local floras, plant resources, vegetation and agriculture of the individual Latin American countries. These are followed by 23 chapters of a more general nature, discussing such topics as: climatology, geology, soils, pathology, forestry, *etc.* Part II consists of 20 chapters of regional descriptions followed by a special supplement by the editor, listing plant science institutes, stations, museums, gardens, societies, and commissions in Central and South America. A very detailed table of contents and a complete index of personal names have been added.

β. History of the applied plant sciences

a. *History of agriculture*

BRAUNGART, D., 1911: Die Urheimat der Landwirtschaft aller indogermanischen Völker an der Geschichte der Kulturpflanzen und Ackerbaugeräte in Mittel- und Nordeuropa nachgewiesen, 470 p. (Heidelberg: Winter).—

> The main thesis of this book is that the Indo-German agricultural implements have a common origin. They apparently developed in Central and Northern Europe and from there were distributed to the southern and eastern parts of Europe and to the Middle East and India.

BROWNE, C. A., 1944: A source book of agricultural chemistry, 290 p. (Waltham, Mass.: Chronica Botanica).—

> In this book the author tries to express the relationship of Justus von Liebig's work with that of his predecessors, who "in selected passages give their own accounts of the work selected for description, with no attempts at modernization of language." Beginning with Thales, the ideas and contributions of philosophers and scientists who made suggestions in the field of agricultural chemistry are considered in historical sequence. *Cf.* MOULTON, F. L., 1942, *vide infra.*

CHEVALIER, A., 1946: Révolution en agriculture, 360 p. (Paris: Presses Univ. de France).—

> Survey of the development of agriculture from early times and in various countries.

CURWEN, E. C. & G. HATT, 1953: Plough and pasture: the early history of farming, 329 p. (New York, N.Y.: Schuman).—

> This volume actually consists of two separate books bound together. The first, written by CURWEN, is entitled: "Prehistoric farming of Europe and the Near East"; it had been published under the title: "Plough and pasture", 1946, 122 p. (London: Colbert). The second book (p. 151-308) entitled: "Farming of non-European peoples" has been written by G. HATT and essentially gives a description of present agricultural usages in those parts of the world where European agriculture is not practised.

FRANKLIN, T. B., 1948: A history of agriculture, 239 p. (London: Bell).—

> A rather popular historical review of the development of agriculture from Old Testament times up to the period immediately following the Second World War. The book is especially meant for English readers.

FUSSELL, G. E., 1966: Farming technique from prehistoric to modern times, 269 p. (Oxford: Pergamon).—

> From the table of contents: 1. Prehistoric farming; 2. Graeco-Roman and Mediterranean farming: 500 B.C.-A.D. 500; 3. The Dark Ages: A.D. 500-1000; 4. The Middle Ages: A.D. 1000-1500; 5. 16th century: slow progress; 6. 17th century: age of promise; 7. 18th century: spread of improved farming; 8. 1815-1914: progress *vs.* industry and world competition; 9. 1914...: regulations, mechanization, science. The systems of cropping and the preparation of the soil for sowing the seed, systems of land drainage and reclamations are included. Bibliography and index. The care, maintenance and breeding of livestock form an important part of this work. As to these last aspects, *cf.* also: LORD, R., 1963: The care of the earth: a history of husbandry, 384 p. (New York, N.Y.: New American Library).

GRAND, R. & R. DELATOUCHE, 1940: L'agriculture au moyen âge de la fin de l'empire romain au XVIe siècle, 740 p. (L'agriculture à travers les âges, III) (Paris: Boccard).—

> This is a continuation of the late SAVOY's work (*vide infra*) "l'Agriculture à travers les âges"; for more details about the present vol., *vide* section The Middle Ages in the Latin West, subsection b.

HALE, P. H., 1915: Hale's history of agriculture by dates: a simple record of historical events and victories of peaceful industries, ed. 5, 95 p. (St. Louis, Mo.: Hale).—

> Citation of events in agriculture from 4241 B.C. tot 1910 A.D.

HAUDRICOURT, A. G. & M. J. B. DELAMARRE, 1955: L'homme et la charrue à travers le monde, 506 p. (Paris: Gallimard).—

> The most elaborate study on the subject, tracing the history of the plough as it took place in the different parts of the world from 4000 B.C. onwards. Extensive bibliography. A comparable book seems to be: WERTH, E., 1954: Grabstock, Hacke und Pflug. Versuch einer Entwicklungsgeschichte des Landbaues, 435 p. (Ludwigsburg: Ulmer). Of this book I have no other information at my disposal, than that it contains 231 figures and 25 maps.

LORD, R., 1962: The care of the earth: a history of husbandry, 480 p. (New York, N.Y. & Edinburgh: Nelson).—

> A history of agriculture from earliest times up to the present century. It deals mainly with American circumstances. The first part (p. 19-58) deals with the operation of elements of ecology in the course of time; the second part (p. 59-142) deals with gardeners and farmers; the third part (p. 143-203) with ancient and mediaeval tillage; the fourth part (p. 204-274) with the agricultural transformation of America. In the five closing chapters (p. 273-460), the author tries to sketch "a personal forecast or projection of growths and portents I have seen take form in my country (the U.S.A.) since the second quarter-century of my time."

MOULTON, F. R., ed., 1942: Liebig and after Liebig: a century of progress in agricultural chemistry, 111 p. (Amer. Assn. Adv. Sci., Publ. 16) (Washington, D.C.: Amer. Assn. Adv. Sci.).—

> A collection of papers presented at a symposium in commemoration of the 100th anniversary of the publication of Liebig's "Die organische Chemie in ihrer Anwendung auf Agricultur und Physiologie". After a brief biographical review, the contents are as follows: Liebig's influence on the promotion of agricultural chemical research; L. and the chemistry of proteins; L. and the chemistry of enzymes and fermentation; L. and the chemistry of animal nutrition; L. and the chemistry of the soil; L. and the humus theory; L. and the chemistry of mineral fertilizers; L. and the law of the minimum; mineral requirements of plants as indicated by means of solution cultures. *Cf.* BROWNE, C. A., 1944, *vide supra.*

SAUER, C. O., 1952: Agricultural origins and dispersals, 110 p. (New York, N.Y.: Amer. Geogr. Soc.).—

> The aim of this book can best be explained in the author's own words: Man's "mastery over the organic world began with his employment of and experiments with fire. Sedentary fishing peoples perhaps commenced the cultivation of plants and became the first domesticators of plants and animals. The earliest plant selection was by vegetative reproduction and the early domestic animals were part of the household. Later came plant selection by seed reproduction and the keeping of flocks by seed farmers. I have thought to link these inventions in series, possibly beginning from a common center, and to follow their dispersals and divergences." (p. 103, quoted after J. C. Malin, in Agricult. Hist. 27:34).

SAVOY, E., 1935: L'agriculture à travers les âges. Histoire des faits, des institutions, de la pensée et des doctrines économiques et sociales. Vol. I: Quelques problèmes d'économie sociologique. Prolégomènes, 667 p.; Vol. II: Première période, de Hammourabi à la fin de l'empire romain, 478 p. (Paris: Boccard).—

> A large-scale history of agriculture. The subject matter has been divided by topics, such as: races, lands, dwellings, tools, exchanges, means of communication, money, *etc.* The first volume consists of the following parts: General introduction (p. 1-38); Quelques problèmes d'économie sociologique (p. 39-64); La production (p. 76-236); La répartition (p. 239-339); La circulation des richesses (p. 343-519); La consommation (p. 524-550); L'agriculture dans ses rapports avec la question sociale et la civilisation (p. 554-628). Vol. II consists of the following sections: L'hypothèse économique et le cadre de la première période, de Hammourabi à la fin de l'empire romain (p. 15-120); La production agricole, les faits et les institutions, les facteurs de la production et la pensée et les doctrines économiques et sociales relatives au travail dans l'antiquité (p. 121-405); Le capital (p. 407-478). No index. The third vol. was brought out by R. GRAND & R. DELATOUCHE, 1940 *(vide*

supra) and the fourth volume by E. SO-REAU, 1952 (*vide infra*).

SCHWENDIMANN, J., 1945: Der Bauernstand im Wandel der Jahrtausende, 275 p. (Einsiedeln & Cologne: Benziger).—

The first part deals with the farmer in antiquity (Israel, Egypt, Greece and Rome), the second part, p. 52-94, with the farmer in the Middle Ages, the third part, p. 95-214, with the development of the social status of the farmer since the Renaissance; special attention has been paid to some economic aspects, such as the influence of the industrial development, and to the farmer's customs. The last part of this book deals with such subjects as: the farmer's house, the farmer's ties with the soil on which he lives, his religious constitution, his position in society, his education, *etc.* Many well-chosen illustrations.

SLICHER VAN BATH, B. H., 1963: The agrarian history of Western Europe A.D. 500-1850, 364 p. (London: Arnold).—

As far as the editor is aware this is the only history of West-European agriculture and its mutual influences on a supra-national level. The author discusses many topics, such as: external and internal factors influencing the development of agriculture; feudalism; the manorial system; agriculture and land in the Middle Ages; prices and wages; agriculture and the land in het modern era (1550- *ca.* 1850). Many references. Index. Originally published in Dutch under the title: De agrarische geschiedenis van West-Europa (500-1850), 416 p. (Utrecht & Antwerpen: Aula).

SOREAU, E., 1952: L'agriculture du XVIIᵉ siècle à la fin du XVIIIᵉ, 454 p. (L'agri-culture à travers les âges, IV) (Paris: Boc-card).—

This is a continuation of Savoy's work (*cf* E. SAVOY, 1935, and R. GRAND & R. DELATOUCHE, 1940, *vide supra*). This last volume of the series deals with agriculture as it has developed in various parts of the world. Separate chapters deal with the history of agriculture in Europe as a whole, the history of agriculture in Germany and Austria, Switzerland, the Baltic countries, mediterranean Europe, the Netherlands, Great Britain and Ireland, France, Latin America, North America, Africa, China, Japan, and some large islands. This volume contains a bibliography but no index.

STEENSBERG, A., 1943: Ancient harvesting implements: a study in archaeology and human geography, 296 p. (Nationalmuseets skrifter, Arkaeologisk-historisk raekke I) (Copenhagen).—

Unfortunately I am unable to give further information about this book.

TROW-SMITH, R., 1967: Life from the land, 238 p. (London & New York, N.Y.: Longmans).—

In this book the author traces the main course of western European farming from prehistoric times down to the technical revolution of the present day, incl. such aspects as: social organization, changes in livestock, changes in implements, economics, *etc.*

b. *History of horticulture*

ANDRÉ, E., 1879: L'art des jardins. Traité général de la composition des parcs et jardins, 888 p. (Paris: Masson).—

A very comprehensive reference on the history and technique of landscaping and garden design, illustrated with 11 coloured plates and 520 illustrations in the text.

BALTET, C., 1895: L'horticulture dans les cinq parties du monde, 778 p. (Paris: Soc. Natl. d'Horticulture).—

The author describes development and present state (in 1895) of horticulture of many parts of the world, *e.g.*, Algeria, Germany, Central America, England, Argentina, Australia, Austria, Hungary, Belgium, Brazil, Bulgaria, Canada, Chile, Denmark, Spain, United States, Finland, France, Greece, the Netherlands, Italy, Japan, Mexico, Norway, Poland, Portugal, Rumania, Russia, Sweden, Venezuela. For each country considered he also reviews: horticultural societies, journals dealing with horticulture, botanical gardens, *etc.*, so that this work could also be used as a directory.

BERRALL, J. S., 1966: The garden: an illustrated history from ancient Egypt to the present day, 388 p. (London: Thames & Hudson).—

"The author's research has been thorough and careful, and she has gone out of her way to unearth unfamiliar descriptions of gardens and to give unhackneyed quotations whenever possible. The result is an absorbing and scholarly study of history of the garden, its uses, its development, its national and climatic characteristics, and its relation to historical events and the evolution of ideas." (From a review in The Times Lit. Suppl. of April 20, 1967: 339).

COATS, A. M., 1969: The quest for plants: a history of the horticultural explorers, 400 p. (London: Studio Vista).—

This book deals with those explorers who collected the trees, shrubs, and flowers which today are to be found in our garden, with the plants they discovered, the dangers they encountered, and more especially with their personality. They are treated chronologically, from the Renaissance to the outbreak of the Second World War, within ten geographical areas. This book contains a wealth of information.

DIETRICH, L. F., 1863: Geschichte des Gartenbaus in allen seinen Zweigen von den frühesten Zeiten bis zur Gegenwart, 280 p. (Leipzig: Schäfer).—

A history of gardening from the oldest times up to *ca.* 1860. Separate sections deal with such subjects as: gardening in the ancient Near East, Greece, Rome, during the Middle Ages, gardening in France, England, Scandinavia, Russia, Italy, China, and the history of some cultivated plants such as the rose, tulip, hyacinth, orange, orchids, palms, *etc.*

ERDBERG, E. v., 1936: Chinese influence on European garden structures, 221 p. (Cambridge, Mass.: Harvard U.P.).—

This book deals with the styles and sources of knowledge of Chinese architecture in the 18th century, the Anglo-Chinese garden, designs of garden buildings and their architectural details, and with the evolution, types, and details of the imitative style. Useful bibliography, containing many garden histories.

GOTHEIN, M. L., 1928: A history of garden art from the earliest times to the present day, 2 vols. Vol. I: 458 p.; Vol. II: 486 p. (London & Toronto: Dent; New York, N.Y.: Dutton).—

The first vol. deals with the gardens of ancient Egypt (cultivation of trees, vineyards, vegetables, tomb inscriptions relating to gardens, gardens of kings, consecration to religion, garden songs, *etc.*), of Western Asia (the cedar forests, early pictures of trees, garden temples, hanging gardens, hunting parks, Persian parks, the gardens of the Israelites, trees of Buddha, *etc.*), of ancient Greece (gardens in Homeric poetry, nymph sanctuaries, temple gardens and sacred groves, the academy at Athens, the importance of Delphi and Pergamon in garden history, influence of oriental gardening, gardens in Greek romance, the Geoponica), of the Roman Empire (the hortus, Seneca and Cicero on gardens, description of many gardens, *etc.*), of Byzantine gardens and the countries of Islam (water works, the importance of carpets in Persian garden art, the place of the Arabs in garden art, parks in Spain, Egypt, Persia, Samarkand, *etc.*), of the Middle Ages in the West (cloister gardens, town gardens, Albertus Magnus, Petrus Crescentius, *etc.*), of Italy in the time of the Renaissance and the Baroque style, and with the gardens of Spain, Portugal, France, and England in the time of the Renaissance. The second vol. deals with the garden in Germany and the Netherlands in the time of the Renaissance, the influence of the Louis XIV style on gardening, the influence of the French garden in the other European countries, the gardens of China and Japan, the English landscape garden, tendencies of garden art in the 19th century, modern English gardening, and landscape architecture in North America (U.S.A. and Canada). Short bibliography, but extensive index. The book was reprinted in 1966 (New York, N.Y.: Hacker). Originally published in German: GOTHEIN, M. L., 1914: Geschichte der Gartenkunst, 2 vols. Vol. I: Von Aegypten bis zur Renaissance in Italien, Spanien und Portugal, 453 p.; Vol. II: Von der Renaissance in Frankreich bis zur Gegenwart, 506 p. (Jena: Diederichs). A second German edition appeared in 1926. A comparable book is: CLIFFORD, D., 1963: A history of garden design, new ed., 232 p. (London: Faber & Faber; New York, N.Y.: Praeger). *Cf.* also: WETHERED, H. N., 1933: A short history of gardens, 323 p. (London: Methuen).

HADFIELD, M., 1955: Pioneers in gardening, 240 p. (London: Routledge & Kegan Paul).—

"This work is concerned with the designs of some pioneers, and the astonishing explorations of others; leading from the formal gardens of two and three hundred years ago, to the bandits, hunger and avalanches encountered by explorers in the nineteenth century to gain some of the plants which flower easiliy and commonly in our gardens today." (From the dust cover).

MANGIN, A., 1888: Histoire des jardins anciens et modernes, 400 p. (Tours: Mame).—

    The first part deals with gardens in antiquity (Champs Elysées, paradise of Mahomet, island of Calypso, paradise of Quetzalcoatl, the old gardens of China and India, the garden of the Persians, Babylonians, Hebrews, Greece, Romans, *etc.*). The second part deals with the gardens of the Middle Ages and the Renaissance (monastic gardens, the gardens of Paris, Alhambra, Seville, the gardens of Mexico, of the Incas, floating gardens, Renaissance gardens in France and Italy, *etc.*). The third part deals with French and English gardens and the last part with the gardens of the 19th century.

ROHDE, E. S., 1932: The story of the garden, 326 p. (with a chapter on American gardens by F. KING) (Boston, Mass.: Hale, Cushman & Flint).—

    The various chapters deal with the following subjects: the traditional influence of ancient garden lore, the mediaeval garden, the Tudor age, Stuart times, French and Dutch influences, the Georgian period, the landscape school and the Victorian and Edwardian eras, American gardens, (this last chapter by Mrs. F. KING). Included are a bibliography and an index. The book mainly deals with English situations, as the chapter-headings clearly indicate.

WHITTLE, T., 1970: The plant hunters, being an examination of collecting with an account of the careers and the methods of a number of those who have searched the world for wild plants, 257 p. (London: Heinemann).—

    A book of somewhat "popular" style about hunting for rare and exotic plants from the first recorded expeditions (1482 B.C.) up to the present. Appendixes deal with the principles of plant distribution, the principles of plant classification, and the technique of collecting and preserving plants. There is much in it concerning the history of gardens and gardening.

WRIGHT, R., 1934: The story of gardening: from the hanging gardens of Babylon to the hanging gardens of New York, 475 p. (London: Routledge).—

    The chapter-headings clearly reflect the contents of this book. They are as follows: How gardening began; Down the West Asian road; Gardening in ancient Greece; On Roman roof gardens and country places; Monastic and mediaeval gardens; A cycle of gardening in Cathay; In old Japan; Mohammedan gardens go westward; The garden flowering of the Renaissance and afterward; Two centuries of English gardening; Le Nôtre and the spread of his gardens; Gardening in eighteenth-century England; The rise of gardening in America; The eighteenth century in France and on the continent; Mingled garden advances in the nineteenth century; The threshold of our own times. Bibliography (of *ca.* 600 items) and index. Reprinted 1964 (New York, N.Y.: Dover).

ZANDER, R., 1952: Geschichte des Gärtnertums mit Zeittabellen vom Jahre 30-1935, 120 p. (Stuttgart: Ulmer).—

    For more details, *vide* section Some recommended encyclopaedias ... subsection c_2.

c. *History of forestry*

BOERHAVE BEEKMAN, W., 1949-1955: Hout in alle tijden, 6 vols. Vol. I (1949): Praehistorie en historie tot en met de Iraniërs, 715 p.; Vol. II (1949): Historie van de Grieken tot en met de Byzantijnen; bijzondere toepassingen tot het eind der XIXe eeuw, 776 p.; Vol. III (1951): De voornaamste bostypen en houtsoorten der wereld, 800 p.; Vol. IV (1952): Ontbossing en herbebossing; bomen en hout voor bijzondere doeleinden, 448 p.; Vol. V (1955): I. Chemische houttechnologie. II. Mechanische houttechnologie, 619 p.; Vol. VI (1955): I. Algemene vraagstukken. II. Bijzondere vraagstukken, 439 p. (Deventer: Kluwer).—

    A very beautifully illustrated review of wood, trees, forests, and forestry. It discusses many historical aspects as well as the application of wood in art, crafts, *etc.*, and it also discusses the chemical and mechanical technology of wood industry. The vols. I and II are of a biohistorical character, and discuss such topics as: the development of forests during geological times, the application of wood in Palaeo-, Meso-, and Neolithic culture, the use of wood among the Egyptians, Hebrews, and Iranians, the role of forests, trees, and the application of wood in the Graeco-Roman, Byzantine, and mediaeval cultures, the use of wood in furniture, in buildings, in preparation of instruments of music, statues, *etc.* Vol. IV-VI deal with the technical applications of wood.

FABRICIUS, L., 1905: Geschichte der Naturwissenschaften in der Forstwissenschaft bis zum Jahre 1830, 137 p. (Naturwiss. Ztschr. Land- und Forstwiss., Beih. 2).—

Unfortunately, I am unable to give further information about this book.

FERNOW, B. E., 1913: A brief history of forestry in Europe, the United States and other countries, ed. 3, 506 p. (Washington, D.C.: Amer. Forestry Assn.).—

After an introductory chapter on the forests of the ancients, the author gives a review of the history of forestry in general on a geographical basis. Much information has been given on the situation in Germany, where forest policy has developed furthest. Stress has been laid on the interconnections between forestry on the one hand and the economic and cultural conditions of the country considered on the other hand. It is shown that the idea of a science of forestry originated during the 19th century, especially during the second half.

HESKE, F., 1960: The history of forestry in the world: a short survey, 25 p. (Cah. Hist. mond., 1960, 5 : 748-773).—

The first section deals with forestry from the ethical point of view, considering the purpose of the forest in modern civilization (as source of raw material, socio-economic aspects, conservational aspects, forest policy, *etc.*). The second section contains short reviews considering the contributions of various countries and regions to forestry; in this section many historical notes have been included. The third and last section (two pages only) deals with the necessity for a universal forest policy.

SEIDENSTICKER, A., 1886: Waldgeschichte des Altertums. Ein Handbuch für akademische Vorlesungen, 2 vols. Vol. I: Vor Caesar, 403 p.; Vol. II: Nach Caesar, 460 p. (Frankfurt a.O.: Trowitzsch).—

For more details, *vide* section Antiquity in general, subsection b.

d. *History of phytopathology and mycology*

BRAUN, H., 1965: Geschichte der Phytomedizin, 140 p. (Berlin & Hamburg: Parey).—

This booklet contains the following chapters: 1. Antike; 2. Religion und Kirche im Kampf gegen Pflanzenkrankheiten und -schädlinge; 3. Mittelalter und Neuzeit bis zum Ausgang des 17. Jahrhunderts; 4. J. R. Glauber (1604-1670); 5. Das 18. Jahrhundert; 6. M. Tillet (1714-1791); 7. Die Pathologie der deutschen Romantik; 8. ätiologisch-parasitologische Pflanzenpathologie; 9. Wiedererwachende Konstitutionspathologie und Prädispositionslehre; 10. Bakteriosen in der Phytomedizin; 11. Virosen in der Phytomedizin; 12. Pflanzenschutzdienst. Very valuable bibliography. Index of names and subjects. *Cf.* SAVASTANO, L., 1890/'91, *vide* section Antiquity in general, subsection b.

CAREFOOT, G. L. & E. R. SPROTT, 1967: Famine on the wind: man's battle against plant disease, 231 p. (Skokie, Ill.: Rand McNally).—

A rather popular account, containing the sociological and historical consequences of plant diseases. The examples discussed are: ergot, wheat rust, grain smuts, coffee rust, potato, blight, grape mildew, banana diseases, South American leaf blight of rubber trees. The last two chapters discuss bacterial and viral diseases and some tree diseases. In 1969 an English edition appeared under the title: Famine on the wind: plant diseases and human history, 222 p. (London: Angus & Robertson).

COOK, M. T., 1947: Viruses and virus diseases of plants, 244 p. (Minneapolis, Minn.: Burgess).—

The text leans considerably toward the historical and chronological side of the subject. The book has been written by one of the pioneers of plant pathology. The author has recorded some of the earliest theories and conceptions as to the nature of virus diseases of plants. Bibliography of some 1,400 titles, arranged according to the principles of plant virology and intended as a historical review and guide. Very detailed table of contents.

HOLTON, C. S., ed., 1959: Plant pathology: problems and progress 1908-1958, 588 p. (Madison, Wisc.: Univ. Wisconsin Press).—

The Golden Jubilee volume of the American Phytopathological Society. It contains the text of some 10 symposia, of which only the first one is of biohistorical importance with lectures considering: The role of plant pathology in the scientific and social development of the world (by E. C.

STAKMAN); The beginnings of plant pathology in North America (by J. A. STEVENSON); The American Phytopathological Society: the first fifty years (by S. E. A. MCCALLAN); Landmarks during a century of progress in the use of chemicals to control plant diseases (by G. L. MCNEW).

LARGE, E. C., 1940: The advance of the fungi, 488 p. (New York, N.Y.: Holt; London: Cape).—

A full-scale history of plant pathology. Its author is an English mycologist who has lately specialized in insecticides and fungicides; and he describes his subject against a background of economic, political, and social history. The book is well-written.

LÜTJEHARMS, W. J., 1936: Zur Geschichte der Mykologie. Das XVIII. Jahrhundert, 262 p. (Thesis Univ. Leiden) (Gouda: Koch & Knuttel).—

Also published as Vol. 23 of the "Mededeelingen van de Ned. Mycologische Vereeniging". Besides a fairly complete history of mycology, the book contains a full discussion of the scientific methods involved, and thus it contains much more than the title promises. In the first chapter the necessity of historical investigations has been explained. The second chapter has been devoted to a discussion of scientific methods applied to the history of botany and especially Sachs's (positivistic) method has been severely criticized. The third chapter and the introduction to the fourth chapter deal with methodological problems and the second part of Ch. 4. deals with history of mycology before the 18th century; its development has been traced back to antiquity. Ch. 5 deals with the methods of classification of Fungi during the 18th century and the author makes clear that the methods applied depend on prevailing views as to the nature of Fungi (e.g., whether they are considered to be animals or plants, whether they have a *generatio spontanea* or not, whether they have sexuality or not, *etc.*).

ORLOB, G. B., *ca.* 1965: The concepts of etiology in the history of plant pathology, 82 p. (PflSchutz-Nachr. "Bayer" 1964 (17): 186-268).—

From a review in Isis 56: 525: "This is a small monograph, with a bibliography of 193 items. We are informed that it is available in English, German, French, and Spanish from Bayer AG., Leverkusen."

WEHNELT, B., 1943: Die Pflanzenpathologie der deutschen Romantik als Lehre vom kranken Leben und Bilden der Pflanzen, ihre Ideenwelt und ihre Beziehungen zu Medizin, Biologie und Naturphilosophie historisch-romantischer Zeit, 236 p. (Bonn: Scheur).—

The contents of this book may become clear from the chapter headings, which are as follows: Die vorromantischen Verhältnisse in der deutschen Pflanzenpathologie; Allgemeine Uebersicht über die Literatur zur romantischen Pflanzenpathologie; Die Naturphilosophie; Die Identitätslehre; Naturphilosophie in der Pathologie; Polarität-Dynamik; Die Organismusidee; Konstitution; Lehre von der Stufenfolge; Entwicklungsgedanke; Die Dimensionen; Die naturhistorische Schule; Ontologie; Humoralpathologie; Die Matrix; Die Urzeugung; Lebenskraft und Bildungstrieb; Metamorphose; Afterorganismus; Exanthem; Das Ursache-Folge-Problem; Krankheit als Schuld; Die wichtigsten Pflanzenkrankheiten im Spiegel romantischer Pflanzenpathologie; Romantik.

WHETZEL, H. H., 1918: An outline of the history of phytopathology, 130 p. (Philadelphia, Pa.: Saunders).—

The earlier development of phytopathology is but poorly treated; only two pages have been devoted to the so-called "Dark Ages" (6th-16th cent.). The premodern era (1600 to about 1850) has been divided into 3 periods: 1. Renaissance, a period of the revival of interest in plant diseases amongst agriculturists and gardeners; first laws directed toward plant disease control; 2. Zallingerian period, in which great efforts were taken to name and classify plant diseases based on analogies of human pathology; 3.Ungerian period, the physiologic or autogenetic period; new theories of nutrition and irritability. The modern era (1853 to about 1906) has been divided into 2 periods: 1. The Kühnian period (1853-1883) during which the causal nexus between fungi and rust and smut diseases was found and wherein plant diseases were classified upon an etiological basis; 2. the Millardetian period during which emphasis was put on the economic side of plant pathology and the role of bacteria in the causation of plant diseases.

e. *Some regional histories of the applied plant sciences*

e.* *Europe*

Belgium

DE WILDEMAN, E., 1950: Notes pour l'histoire de la botanique et de l'horticulture en Belgique, 832 p. (Acad. roy. Belgique, Cl. Sci. Mém., 2ᵉ série, Vol. 25: 1-832).—

> The book mainly consists of an enumeration of plants cultivated in Belgium in the 17th century. An older, and probably more general, history of Belgian horticulture is: BALTET, C., 1865: L'horticulture en Belgique, son enseignement, ses institutions, son organisation officielle, 184 p. (Paris: Masson). Unfortunately I am not able to give more information concerning this book.

GOBLET D'ALVIELLA, E. F. A., 1927-1930: Histoire des bois et forêts en Belgique. Dès origines à la fin du régime autrichien, 4 vols. Vol. I: 489 p.; Vol. II: 349 p.; Vol. III: 140 p.; Vol. IV: 448 p. (Paris: Lechevalier; Brussels: Lamertin).—

> Unfortunately I could not consult these vols., nor could I find more details elsewhere.

VAEREN, J. v. d., 1930: Les faits principaux de l'histoire de l'agriculture belge durant un siècle, 1830-1930, 148 p. (Brussels: Dewit).—

> An authoritative historical review of Belgian agricultural history during the period considered, dealing with many topics, such as: the appearance of *Phytophthora infestans* in the potato fields; the food crisis of 1845-1847; the bovine pest of 1865; the organization of scientific agricultural investigations at Louvain; the agricultural crisis of 1878-1880; agriculture during the First World War; the abandonment of the land by the workers; introduction of machinery and commercial fertilizers; legal enactments touching on agricultural matters; *etc.* Also in Dutch translation (Leuven, 1930). An exhaustive history of Belgian agriculture (written in Dutch) is: LINDEMANS, P., 1952: Geschiedenis van de landbouw in België, 2 vols. Vol. I: 472 p.; Vol. II: 541 p. (Antwerpen: De Sikkel).

Czechoslovakia

NOŽIČKA, J., 1956: Z minulosti slezských lesů: nástin jejich vývoje od nejstraršich časů do r. 1914, 129 p. [The history of the Silesian forests: an outline of their development from the most ancient times to 1914] (Opavá: Slezský Studijni Ustav).—

> With indexes of personal and place names.

——, 1957: Přehled vývoje našich lesů, 462 p. [Historical review of the development of the forests of Czechoslovakia] (Lesn. Knihovna, velká Rada).—

> Divides the history into 3 main periods: from prehistoric times to 1754, 1754-1848, and 1848-1914. There is a 5-page English summary, and indexes of proper names, places and subjects. (From: Forestry Abstr. 20: 5394).

Finland

ILVESSALO, L., 1926: Forest research work in Finland: the origins and development of forest research work and a review of the investigations carried out up to date, 92 p. (Acta forest. Fenn., No. 31).—

> Of this publication I cannot give more details. For a brief review of the history of Finnish forestry during the previous century, *cf.* the relevant chapter by Yrjö ILVESSALO in: COLLANDER, R., 1965: The history of botany in Finland 1828-1918, *vide* section History of the plant sciences α, subsection b.

France

BLOCH, M., 1952-1956: Les caractères originaux de l'histoire rurale française, 2 vols. Vol. I: 265 p.; Vol. II: 230 p. (Paris: Colin).—

> A new edition of this history of French agriculture (First ed. 1931, Paris: Les Belles Lettres). The first vol. affords information on the early land tenure, peasantry and feudalism in France. The second vol. has been prepared by R. DAUVERGNE and consists of notes and other addenda to the first edition which M. Bloch himself made between 1931 and 1944, the year he died as a victim of the German occupation. As stated in a review in Agric. Hist. 42(3): 280, this book "Serves as a model for both medieval historians and historians of agriculture in other times and places". In 1966 an English translation of the first volume appeared under the title: French rural history: an essay on its basic characteristics, 34 + 257 p. (Berkeley & Los Angeles, Calif.: Univ. California Press).

BOURDE, A. J., 1953: The influence of England on the French agronomes 1750-

1789, 250 p. (Cambridge & New York, N.Y.: Cambridge U.P.).—

The agronomes were eighteent-century French students of agricultural methods, who played an important role in the agricultural revolution. The first part of this book deals with French agricultural literature before 1750, the second part with old French husbandry, the third part with agrarian repercussions of the "Nouveau Système", the fourth part with the new crops introduced by the new husbandry, and the fifth part with some aspects of the international effect of the agronomic movement, and the problem of how the agronomists obtained their information.

——, 1967: Agronomie et agronomes en France au XVIIIe siècle, 3 vols., 1740 p. Vol. I: p. 1-595; Vol. II: p. 596-1192; Vol. III: p. 1193-1740. (Les Hommes et la Terre, 13) (Paris: S.E.V.P.E.N.).—

In an introductory chapter (p. 35-178), the author deals with the 16th and 17th centuries, considering such subjects as: publications in the fields of agriculture and fruit-growing, garden instructions, the botanical gardens of Montpellier and Paris, legal aspects. The second part (p. 179-456) deals with the agronomical systems as they were developed by Liger in his "Nouvelle maison rustique" (1700), and by d'Ebandi de Fresne in his "Traité d'agriculture" (1788), and with the publications of, *e.g.*, Le Marquis de Turbilly, Noël Chomel, Jethro Tull, Pattullo and some others. The second part (p. 457-1076) deals with such subjects as: the various products cultivated, agricultural techniques, sylviculture, domestic animals, amelioration of the soil, agricultural chemistry, the rural society, *etc.* The third part (p. 1077-1560) deals with some political and administrative aspects of agronomy, with some aspects of "experimental agriculture", and with centres of agronomical research (such as the "Académie des sciences et de l'agronomie" and various provincial academies), journals dealing with agronomy, *etc.* Important bibliography (p. 1657-1730).

DEVÈZE, M., 1961: La vie de la forêt française au XVIe siècle, 2 vols. Vol. I: 325 p.; Vol. II: 473 p. (École pratique des Hautes Études, VIe Section) (Paris: S.E.V.P.E. N.).—

An introductory chapter deals with the history of French forests up to and including the 15th century (p. 39-76). The first vol. is in two parts: the first part deals with the condition of the forest at the beginning of the 16th century (customs in forestry, usage of the forests, legal aspects, industrial applications, p. 77-164); the second part deals with the royal administration. This part contains much information of regional importance. The second vol. also consists of two parts, *viz.*, one dealing with the crises in forestry during the first half of the 16th century (p. 1-174) and the other part with the history of forestry during the era of religious troubles. Valuable index (p. 419-465).

GROMAS, R., 1947: Histoire agricole de la France dès origines à 1939, 304 p. (Mende, Lozère: Author).—

A rather popular history of French agriculture from prehistoric times up to the present. Each chapter contains descriptions of rural life during the period considered. A comparable booklet is: DAUZAT, A., 1950: La vie rurale en France, dès origines à nos jours, ed. 2, 134 p. (Que sais-je? No. 242) (Paris: Presses Univ. de France).

Germany

ALLINGER, G., 1950: Der deutsche Garten. Sein Wesen und seine Schönheit in alter und neuer Zeit, 300 p. (Munich: Bruckmann).—

A beautifully-illustrated treatise of the development of German horticulture and garden design from early times up to the present. The volume is supplied with many excellent illustrations and discusses *e.g.*, representations of well-known pictures of artists to illuminate the ideals of natural landscapes; reconstructions of houses of prehistoric times with their small gardens; monastic gardens and old-town-gardens; the garden culture in Italy, France and England, and their influences on German garden culture, *etc.*

BERTSCH, K., 1940: Geschichte des deutschen Waldes, 120 p. (Jena: Fischer).—

An introduction into the history of Middle-European forests, from the last glacial onwards, particularly based on pollen analysis. It elucidates the influence of weather conditions on the distribution of trees. A second edition appeared in 1949 and a third in 1951. *Cf.* also FIRBAS, F., (1949-1952): Spät- und nacheiszeitliche Waldgeschichte Mitteleuropas nördlich der Alpen, 480 p. (Jena: Fischer); and BERTSCH, K., 1935: Der deutsche Wald im Wechsel der Zeiten. Wald- und Klimageschichte Deutschlands von der Eiszeit bis zum Gegenwart,

91 p. (Biologie in Einzeldarstellungen, 1) (Tübingen: Heine). The most complete history of German forestry is: BERNHARDT, A., 1872-1875: Geschichte des Waldeigenthums, der Waldwirtschaft und Forstwissenschaft in Deutschland, 3 vols. Vol. I (1872): Von den ältesten Zeiten bis zum Jahre 1750, 260 p.; Vol. II (1874): Von 1750-1820, 260 p.; Vol. III (1875): Von 1820-1860, 420 p. (Berlin: Springer). Cf. also: BERG, C. H. E. von, 1966: Geschichte der deutschen Wälder bis zum Schlusse des Mittelalters, 360 p. (Amsterdam: Liberac). Facsimile reprint of the original ed. of 1871 (Dresden: Schönfeld).

FRAAS, C., 1865: Geschichte der Landbau- und Forstwissenschaft. Seit dem sechszehnten Jahrhundert bis zur Gegenwart, 668 p. (Munich: Cotta).—

A thorough study of the history of agriculture (p. 3-480) and of forestry (p. 483-668), mainly restricted to Germany during the period between 1500 and 1865. Also animal husbandry has been briefly considered.

FRANZ, G., ed., 1962 →: Deutsche Agrargeschichte, 5 vols. Vol. I (1969): Vor- und Frühgeschichte. Vom Neolithikum bis zur Völkerwanderungszeit by H. JANKUHN, 300 p.; Vol. II (1962): Geschichte der deutschen Landwirtschaft vom frühen Mittelalter bis zum 19. Jahrhundert by W. ABEL, 333 p. (ed. 2, 1967, 361 p.); Vol. III (1963): Geschichte der deutschen Agrarverfassung vom frühen Mittelalter bis zum 19. Jahrhundert by F. LÜTGE, 269 p. (ed. 2, 1967, 323 p.); Vol. IV (1970): Geschichte des Bauernstandes vom frühen Mittelalter bis zum 19. Jahrhundert by G. FRANZ, 288 p.; Vol. V (1963): Die deutsche Landwirtschaft im technischen Zeitalter by H. HAUSHOFER, 290 p. (Stuttgart: Ulmer).—

The first part of Vol. I deals with prehistory, e.g., the origins of agriculture, agriculture during the Neolithic age, and agriculture before the Romans (p. 13-113). The second part (p. 114-187) deals with agriculture of the Celts, Romans (incl. such aspects as settlement, feeding, traffic, trade, crafts, etc.). Appendixes deal with the development of the cultivated plants in prehistory and Neolithic times (by U. WILLERDING, p. 188-233) and with origin and development of domesticated animals (by E. MAY, p. 234-262), and with some linguistic witnesses of the earliest stages of agriculture (by H.

JANKUHN, p. 263-278). Indexes of authors and subjects. Vol. II continues this history through the Middle Ages, the 16th and 17th centuries up to the 18th century. Vol. III contains the following chapter-headings: Die Agrarverfassung zur Zeit des Tacitus; die Fortentwicklung der Agrarverfassung in der fränkischen Zeit; Die Fortentwicklung der Agrarverfassung vom Ausgang der Karolingerzeit bis zur Konsolidierung des Territorialstaates; Die Fortentwicklung der Agrarverfassung vom 15./16. bis zum 18. Jahrhundert; Die Auflösung der Grund- und Gutsherrschaft; Die Bauernbefreiung. Vol. IV considers the history of the farmer's life and his social position, the interrelation between peasantry and town, etc. Vol. V deals with the most recent developments of German agriculture in all its aspects. Each chapter gives references and suggestions for further reading. Illustrations and very useful indexes. As an introduction to this comprehensive history may be considered: ABEL, W., 1964: Die drei Epochen der deutschen Agrargeschichte, ed. 2, 131 p. (Hannover: Schaper). A study especially dealing with the social position of the German farmer in the course of agrarian history is: GOLDENBAUM, E., 1952: Die deutschen Bauern in Vergangenheit und Gegenwart, ed. 2, 205 p. (Berlin: Deutscher Bauernverlag). (Not seen). Cf. also: KRZYMOWSKI, R., 1951, vide infra.

HENNEBO, D. & A. HOFFMANN, 1962-1965: Geschichte der deutschen Gartenkunst, 3 vols. Vol. I (1962): Garten des Mittelalters, 196 p.; Vol. II (1965): Der architektonische Garten. Renaissance und Barock, 431 p.; Vol. III (1963): Der Landschaftsgarten, 303 p. (Hamburg: Broschek). —

The first vol. has been considered in more detail in the section: Middle Ages in the West, subsection b. The second vol. deals with the period 16-18th centuries. Special attention has been paid to foreign influences, particularly from Italy and Western Europe (accordingly much attention is devoted to the Baroque gardens of Italy, France, and Holland), and to the cultural background in Germany during the period considered (especially the disastrous influence of the Thirty Years War has been considered). Descriptions of a number of German gardens, accompanied by instructive pictures. Extensive bibliography. The third vol. traces the history from 1760 onwards; here special attention has been paid to the distribution of landscape gardens in Germany, a type of gardens very popular in England in those days. This vol. also is supplied with many beautiful illustrations and an extensive bibliography. No indexes. *Cf.* ZANDER, R., 1952, *vide* section Some recommended encyclopaedias, subsection c₂.

KRZYMOWSKI, R., 1951: Geschichte der deutschen Landwirtschaft (bis zum Ausbruch des 2. Weltkrieges 1939) unter besonderer Berücksichtigung der technischen Entwicklung der Landwirtschaft, ed. 2, 372 p. (Stuttgart: Ulmer).—

> A full-scale history of German agricultural history from prehistory up to the beginning of the Second World War. The author has stressed the cultural influences on agriculture. Many theories concerning the agricultural habits of the Germanic peoples have been critically evaluated, and much attention has been paid to agrarian circumstances under feudalism, the period in which the colonization of the eastern German regions took place. P. 190-356 deal with the 19th and 20th centuries, considering such men as Stein and Hardenberg, A. Thaer, Schwerz, Thünen, J. von Liebig, and the various races of cattle, horses, *etc.* bred in Germany. A third ed. appeared in 1961, 441 p. (Berlin: Duncker & Humblot). A book dealing with German agriculture during the Middle Ages is: BELOW, G. von, 1937, *vide* section Middle Ages in the Latin West, subsection b.

Great Britain

ANDERSON, M. L., 1967: A history of Scottish forestry, 2 vols. Vol. I: From the Ice Age to the French Revolution, 662 p.; Vol. II: From the Industrial Revolution to modern times, 654 p. (London & Edinburgh: Nelson).—

> This work has been edited posthumously by C. J. TAYLOR. It is the result of "thirty years" research into archives in old Scots dialect, monastic accounts in Latin, and many newspapers, journals and books. Forest law, flora, fauna, agriculture, geography, history, economics and politics are all covered in an account unique in its scope, from the Ice Age to modern times." Vol. I begins in 12.000 B.C. and deals with the primeval forests of Scotland, the forests in the Palaeolithic, Neolithic, Bronze, and Iron Ages (4250 B.C.-A.D. 81), the Roman period (81-446), the Celtic Kings (446-1097), feudalism (1097-1400), the Stuart dynasty (1400-1603), and the period from the Union of Crowns to the French Revolution (1603-1789). The second vol. deals with the period of colonial expansion and the industrial revolution (1790-1854), the period of inaction and a policy of "Laissez-faire" (1854-1915), and the period of crises and of action by the State (1914-1960). Generally the period

considered in the second vol. is the period in which afforestation seriously damaged the landscape.

CECIL, E., 1910: A history of gardening in England, ed. 3, 393 p. (London: Murray).—

> Of this book the first (1895) and second edition (1896) appeared under the name A. M. T. AMHERST. It is an attempt to make a classification of gardens and to arrange them in a chronological order. The subject matter has been divided as follows: 1. monastic gardening; 2. 13th century; 3. 14th century and 15th century; 4. early garden literature; 5. early Tudor gardens; 6. the Elizabethan flower garden; 7. kitchen gardening under Elizabeth and James I; 8. Elizabethan garden literature; 9. 17th century; 10. gardening under William and Mary; 11. dawn of landscape gardening; 12. landscape gardening; 13. 19th century; 14. modern gardening. Many fine illustrations and extensive bibliography of printed works on English gardening from the earliest recorded date to the year 1837. A much older but still very valuable history of English gardening is: JOHNSON, G. W., 1829: A history of English gardening, chronological, biographical, literary, and critical: tracing the progress of the art in this country from the invasion of the Romans to the present times, 445 p. (London: Baldwin & Cradock and Longman). *Cf.* also COX, E. H. M., 1935: History of gardening in Scotland, 228 p. (London: Chatto & Windus).

ERNLE, L., 1961: English farming: past and present, ed. 6, 165 + 559 p. (ed. by G. E. FUSSELL & O. R. MCGREGOR) (London: Heinemann).—

> The standard work on English agricultural history. In their preface the editors write: "We have not attempted to bring this classic up-to-date by textual exegesis or by amending the appendices. Our aim has been to supply critical and bibliographical introductions in the form of commentaries both upon the sources used by Lord Ernle and upon subsequent writing." Photomechanical reprint, 1966 (London: Cass). There also exists a French translation: Histoire rurale de l'Angleterre 1953, 610 p. (Paris: Gallimard). (Not seen). A minor classic in this field of somewhat older date is: HAGGARD, R., 1902: Rural England, being an account of agricultural and social researches carried out in the years 1901 and 1902, 2 vols. Vol. I: 584 p.; Vol. II: 633 p. (London: Longmans) 2nd ed. 1906; and several later eds. *Cf.* ORWIN, C. S. & E. H. WHETMAN, 1964; and WHITLOCK, R., 1965, *vide infra*.

FLETCHER, H. R., 1969: The story of the Royal Horticultural Society, 1804-1968, 564 p. (London: Oxford U.P. for the Roy. Hort. Soc.).—

An authoritative account of the story of the Society from its foundation by John Wedgwood in 1804 to the present day. It deals with such subjects as: the founders and the foundation, the early meetings, the objects of the society, its headquarters, the garden, plant introduction, the gardens in jeopardy, the Kensington adventure, Chiswick garden, horticultural education, *etc.* The five appendixes contain: 1. Calendar of events, 1804-1968; 2. Original charter of the Horticultural Society of London, 1809; 3. Past and present holders of the Victoria Medal of Honour; 4. Past and present associates of honour; 5. Veitch memorial trust: awards 1922-1967. Many illustrations and extensive index.

FRANKLIN, T. B., 1952: A history of Scottish farming, 149 p. (Edinburgh: Nelson).—

This booklet deals with early farming, serfdom, monastic agriculture, land owners, farmers, craftsmen and farm workers, tenures and rents, arable and stock farming and the introduction of English farming techniques. A more elaborate study is: SYMON, J. A., 1959: Scottish farming past and present, 475 p. (Edinburgh & London: Oliver & Boyd). With very good bibliography and index. *Cf.* also HANDLEY, J. E., 1953, *vide infra.*

FUSSELL, G. E., 1947-1950: The old English farming books from Fitzherbert to Tull, 1523 to 1730, 141 p. and More old English farming books from Tull to the Board of Agriculture, 1731 to 1793, 186 p. (London: Crosby Lockwood).—

The first volume deals with the history of agriculture during Tudor times, during the age of Markham, the age of Hartlib, the age of Worlidge and Houghton, and the age of Richard Bradley. The book begins with Fitzherbert's "Boke of Husbondrye", the first book on farming that has been printed in England. The second book starts with the year 1731 in which Jethro Tull published his "New horse houghing husbandry" which made possible the cultivation of turnips and meant the final break with the ancient three-field system. It ends with the year 1793, the year of the foundation of the first Board of Agriculture which has had a great influence on the further development of English agriculture. A somewhat complementary treatise is: MCDONALD, D., 1908, *vide infra.*

——, 1952: The farmers' tools 1500-1900: the history of British farm implements, tools and machinery before the tractor came, 246 p. (London: Melrose).—

An authoritative, well-documented and well-written treatment of the subject. The book deals with farmers in the field, their tools, machines, and industry, with drainage, preparation of the seed bed, sowing, harvesting, threshing, *etc.* It is well illustrated (117 figures in all, most of them full-page). The history runs from 1500 (since it was only after the invention of printing that ideas could be widely spread) up to 1900 (which year marks the beginning of the transition from horse to tractor). The author summarizes his aim in the following words: "the plan of the book is to follow the seasons throughout the year and to tell the story of the progress made in improving the implements and machines used for each season's work during four centuries." Another beautifully illustrated book dealing with the same topics is: WRIGHT, P. A., 1961: Old farming implements, 95 p. (London: Adam & Black).

—— & K. R. FUSSELL, 1953: The English countrywoman: a farmhouse social history A.D. 1500-1900, 221 p. (London: Melrose).—

This book can be considered as a supplement to FUSSELL's "Farmers' tools" (*cf. supra*) in that it deals with the "internal" aspects of country life, *e.g.*, with food, clothes, cooking, furnishings, wages, servants, social customs, *etc.* Complementary to this book are: FUSSELL, G. E. & K. R. FUSSELL, 1955: English countryman: his life and work, A.D. 1500-1900, 172 p. (London: Melrose); and FUSSELL, G. E., 1966: The English dairy farmer, 1500-1900, 357 p. (London: Cass). This last study covers a period during which dairying was mainly a small-scale industry devoted to the production of butter and cheese, although, in the second half of the 19th century the concentration of liquid milk in big centres was already moving to its present situation.

HANDLEY, J. E., 1953: Scottish farming in the eighteenth century, 314 p. (London: Faber & Faber).—

This book presents a picture of rural life and customs in 18th-century Scotland, at the end of which century the old system of farming was beginning to change. The author describes the land, its roads, means of transport, the arable and pastural systems under which the farmers worked, the choice of crops, tillage methods, farming implements, treatment of livestock, living conditions, *etc.*, and the reforming spirit which entered agricultural conditions at the end of the century. Special attention has been paid to the Highlands and Islands. *Cf.* FRANKLIN, T. B., 1952, *vide supra.*

MCDONALD, D., ed., 1908: Agricultural writers from Sir Walter of Henley to Arthur Young, 1200-1800, 228 p. (London: Cox).—

This book is especially valuable in that it gives many reproductions in facsimile of parts of old manuscripts and old books (esp. title pages and illustrations). Moreover, it gives extracts of these old writings and short biographies of their authors. P. 199-224 contain the literature and bibliography of British agriculture from 1200 up to 1800. The items are chronologically arranged. Reprinted 1967 (New York, N.Y.: Franklin). *Cf.* FUSSELL, G. E., 1947-1950, *vide supra.*

ORWIN, C. S., 1949: A history of English farming, 152 p. (London & Edinburgh: Nelson).—

A very readable and accurate account of English agrarian history from Neolithic times up to the present. Of special interest are those parts in which the author evaluates the influence of the plague epidemics (marking the break up of the old feudal system and the beginning of independent farms) and of the agrarian revolution in the midst of the last century (marking the increase of animal husbandry and the application of mechanical power in agriculture). A more recent book is: WHITLOCK, R., 1965: A short history of farming in Britain, 246 p. (London: Baker).

ORWIN, C. S. & E. H. WHETMAN, 1964: History of British agriculture 1846-1914, 411 p. (London: Longmans).—

In their preface the authors write: "Lord Ernle's 'English farming past and present' is stil the best comprehensive account of the development of agriculture in England over six centuries. But it does not cover Scotland or Wales; and those living in the second half of the twentieth century inevitably have a different attitude towards the events which Ernle lived through but could not see in historical perspective. Modern research has thrown further illumination on the great technical, economic and social changes which occurred both in agriculture and in the British nation between the Repeal of the Corn Laws and the outbreak of the First World War." For some technical changes - particularly those based on adoption of fertilizers and *Trifolium repens* seed into British grassland production - which were taken up mainly after 1890, *cf.* NICOL, H., 1967: The limits of Man: an enquiry into the scientific basis of human population, *vide* section "Philosophy of the life sciences . . ."

PERKINS, W. F., ed., 1939: British and Irish writers on agriculture, ed. 3, 226 p. (Lymington, Hants.: King).—

A bibliography of some 1,500 British and Irish writers on the agriculture of the United Kingdom, from the earliest printed books up to 1900. Included are books on agricultural chemistry, botany, grasses, weeds, drainage, improvements, weights, and measures. Excluded are manuscripts, anonymous British writers on foreign or colonial agriculture, and English translations of foreign writers, serials, journals, herd books, catalogues.

RUSSELL, E. J., 1966: A history of agricultural science in Great Britain, 1620-1954, 493 p. (London: Allen & Unwin).—

This book has been written by a man who was for more than 30 years director of the Rothamsted Experimental Station, which had for long been the only real centre of continuous agricultural research in Great Britain. Separate sections deal with the establishment of the Royal Agricultural Society of England, experimental research at Rothamsted between 1850 and 1900, agricultural chemistry, artificial insemination, institutes for animal nutrition, research in the cultivation of plants and of fruit trees, soil science, herbicides, milk production and -products, *etc.*

SEEBOHM, M. E., 1952: The evolution of the English farm, ed. 2, 365 p. (London: Allen & Unwin).—

This study covers the development of farms and farming in England from Neolithic times to the present century. Many footnotes and bibliography.

THIRSK, J., ed., 1967: The agrarian history of England and Wales, Vol. IV: 1500-1640, 40 + 919 p. (Cambridge & New York, N.Y.: Cambridge U.P.).—

This is the first vol. published of a complete seven-volume social and economic history of rural England and Wales from the beginning of systematic agriculture in the Neolithic period to the present. The term "agrarian history" covers "arable and pastoral husbandry, the marketing of produce, housing, the distribution of land ownership, and the structure of the rural society". The period considered in the present vol. is the turning point between the mediaeval and the modern ways of agriculture. Sections of special interest from our point of view are those dealing with: the various farming regions, farming techniques, landowners (the crown, noblemen, the church), farm labourers, rural housing; two chapters of some 100 pages each deal with the economic aspects (marketing, prices and profits, land-rents, *etc.*). Select bibliography and index.

TROW-SMITH, R., 1951: English husbandry from the earliest times to the present day, 239 p. (London: Faber & Faber).—

A history of British farm practices, farm implements, and farm livestock as they have evolved in the four thousand years since prehistoric man first cultivated the soil of Britain. Useful bibliography and good index. A two-volme study by the same author, more especially dealing with the evolution of breeds of farm animals and of the techniques of animal husbandry, is: A history of British livestock husbandry to 1700, 1957, 286 p. (London: Routledge & Kegan Paul), and *idem*, 1700-1900, 1959, 351 p. (London: Routledge & Kegan Paul). *Cf.* FUSSELL's books, *vide supra*. An economic agrarian history of England in the thirteenth century is: KOSMINSKII, E. A., 1956, *vide* section The Middle Ages in the Latin West, subsection b.

WEBBER, R., 1968: The early horticulturists, 224 p. (Newton Abbot, Devon: David & Charles).—

This book contains 13 brief biographies of those men who played leading parts in the development of British horticulture and gardening between Tudor and Edwardian times. In addition, this book also contains information on such subjects as: commercial horticulture from the early Iron Age until about 1900, a listing indicating where the most familiar plants grown in Great Britain came from, and the history of some famous British gardens.

WHITLOCK, R., 1965: A short history of farming in Britain, 246 p. (London: Baker).—

"The book deals with farming from prehistoric times to today and includes a look at the future. Contents include: subsistence farming; farming for profit; food from overseas; the story of soil; the story of our crops; the story of our livestock; the story of farm implements; the story of our farm buildings; farmer's warfare; money and markets; the future?; bibliography; index. Ralph Whitlock is a well known farmer; broadcaster and writer. He is farming editor of the 'Field'." (From a letter of the publisher). *Cf.* ERNLE, L., 1961, *vide supra*.

Hungary

PACH, Z. P., 1964: Die ungarische Agrarentwicklung im 16.-17. Jahrhundert. Abbiegung vom westeuropäischen Entwicklungsgang, 167 p. (Budapest: Akad. Kiadó).—

A study of Hungarian agricultural history during the transition period from feudalism to capitalism.

Italy

NICCOLI, V., 1902: Saggio storico e bibliografico dell'agricultura italiana dalle origini al 1900, 575 p. (In: ALPE, V. & M. ZECCHINI, eds., Enciclopedia agraria italiano, Disp. 72) (Turin: Unione tipografico).—

Standard work of Italian agricultural bibliography, especially valuable for its historical sections.

Latvia

SCHWABE [= Švābe], **A.**, 1930: Agrarian history of Latvia, 124 p. (Riga: Lamey).—

An abridgement of the author's great scientific work entitled Grundriss der Agrargeschichte Lettlands, 1928, 359 p. (Riga: Lamey), intended for the guidance of English speaking readers. Also in an abridged French version: Courte histoire agraire de la Lettonie, 1926, 63 p. (Riga: Ministère des Affaires étrangères de Lettonie).

The Netherlands

BROUWER, W. D., 1967: Bibliografie van de Nederlandse bosbouwgeschiedenis, 88 p. (Wageningen: Landbouwhogeschool, Afd. Agrarische Geschiedenis).—

A full-scale bibliography of Dutch forestry, indispensable for any study of the history of Dutch forestry.

SANGERS, W. J., 1952: De ontwikkeling van de Nederlandse tuinbouw (tot het jaar 1930), 351 p. (Zwolle: Tjeenk Willink).—

> The only history of Dutch horticulture given in a chronological order. Written in Dutch. It is supplemented by a little volume containing the original sources on which this study has been based, *viz.,* SANGERS, W. J., 1953: Gegevens betreffende de ontwikkeling van de Nederlandse tuinbouw (tot het jaar 1800), 152 p. (Zwolle: Tjeenk Willink).

SNELLER, Z. W., ed., 1951: Geschiedenis van de Nederlandse landbouw 1795-1940, ed. 2, 535 p. (Groningen: Wolters).—

> The only history of Dutch agriculture. It deals with the 19th century. Written in Dutch.

Poland

FRYDE, M. M., 1952: Selected works on Polish agrarian history and agriculture: a bibliographical survey, 87 p. (New York, N.Y.: Mid-European Studies Center).—

> The only source of Polish agricultural history I could find. Unfortunately I know it only by title. *Cf.* also: KOSIEK, Z., 1962: Bibliografia polskich bibliografii gospodarstwa wiejskiego, 119 p. (Warsaw: Pánstw. wydawn. roln. i lésne). A bibliography of Polish agricultural bibliographies, which I have not seen, but which must contain much that is of interest to the historian of Polish agriculture.

MAGER, F., 1960: Der Wald in Altpreussen als Wirtschaftsraum, 2 vols. Vol. I: 391 p.; Vol. II: 328 p. (Cologne/Graz: Böhlau).—

> Most of the contents of this book are of economic importance, but especially the first chapter gives a very complete history of the forests in Altpreussen (an area between the Vistula and the Memel deltas).

VIETINGHOFF-RIESCH, A., 1961: Der Oberlausitzer Wald. Seine Geschichte und seine Struktur bis 1945, 284 p. (Hannover: Schaper).—

> A monograph on this region, now in Poland, covering geography, geology, climate, ownership, species composition and changes therein, silviculture, utilization, game, *etc.*

WIECKO, E., 1960: Lasy i przemysł leśny w Polsce, 436 p. [Forests and the forest industry in Poland] (Warsaw: Pánstw. wydawn. roln. i leśne).—

> A comprehensive survey of forestry, the forest industry, trade, and forest products. It covers the period from feudal times to the Second World War; part II from 1945 onwards.

Switzerland

HAGEN, C., 1960: Die Entwicklung der forstlichen Zustandserfassung in einigen Waldgebieten der Ostschweiz und ihre Beziehung zur allgemeinen Entwicklung. Ein Beitrag zur Geschichte der Forsteinrichtung und Waldwertschätzung, 78 p. (Diss. Eidgenoss. Hochschule, Zurich) (Schweiz. Anstalt für das Forstliche Versuchswesen, Vol. 36, Fasc. 3 : 139-217).—

> A description of the evolution of forest survey. This study has been restricted to Eastern Switzerland and is based on thorough studies of archival documentation. Many parallels with the situation in Southern Germany and France have been outlined. The period studied ranges from the beginnings to the year 1800. In 1964 the Schweiz. Zeitschr. Forstwiss., Vol. 115: 579-700, devoted a special issue to the history of Swiss forestry. Included are articles on such subjects as: Forest legislation in Canton Vaud in the 19th century; Old boundary markings in the forest; The importance of forest history at the time of the foundation of the Swiss confederation; and some other contributions.

U.S.S.R.

BUCHHOLZ, E., 1961: Die Waldwirtschaft und Holzindustrie der Sowietunion, (Munich: Bayer. Landwirtschaftsverl.).—

> After a brief historical review (p. 1-17), chapters follow dealing with: the natural environment of forests and forestry, the influence of the forest on the landscape, nature protection, organization and management of the forests (p. 18-121). The rest of the book deals with economic aspects of forestry *(e.g.,* production, trade, traffic, industry, *etc.).*

VOLIN, L., 1970: A century of Russian agriculture: from Alexander II to Khrushev, 650 p.—

> "This is one of the most thorough studies ever made of Russian agriculture.

Emphasizing the continuity of **problems** and policies too often dichotomized into tsarist and soviet eras, Mr. Vrolin has created a monumental work - a sweeping panorama of the century between the emancipation of the serfs and the present." (From an announcement).

e.** *Other parts of the world*

BIDWELL, P. W. & J. I. FALCONER, 1941: History of agriculture in the Northern United States, 1620-1860, 512 p. (New York, N.Y.: Smith); GRAY, L. C., 1941: History of agriculture in the Southern United States to 1860, 2 vols., 1086 p. (New York, N.Y.: Smith).—

These volumes are primarily of economic rather than of technical historical value. They describe the system of agricultural organization, *e.g.,* land policy and tenure, legal and economic characteristics of slavery and servitude, the mechanism of marketing and credit, *etc.* The volume of BIDWELL & FALCONER contains a critical bibliography (p. 454-473) which is of considerable assistance in finding the widely scattered source-materials on the subject for the area and time indicated in the title of the book. Both books were reprinted in 1966 (Magnolia, Mass.: Smith). A very extensive history of agricultural economics is: TAYLOR, H. C. & A. D., 1952: The story of agricultural economics in the United States, 1840-1932: men-services-ideas, 1121 p. (Ames, Iowa: Iowa State College Press).

CARMAN, H. J., ed., 1939: American husbandry, 61 + 582 p. (New York, N.Y.: Columbia U.P.).—

This book was originally published in 1775 (London: Bew); it still is the most significant source of information concerning American colonial agricultural practices. It treats its subject topographically, incl. the various states now constituting the U.S.A., Canada, Jamaica, Barbados, Leeward Islands, Ceded Islands, and Bahama Islands. Of each of the regions considered, the author discusses such subjects as: soil and climate, agriculture, fishing, lumber, exports, inhabitants, winter food for cattle, management of the plantations, *etc.*

CLARK, W. H., 1945: Farms and farmers: the story of American agriculture, 346 p. (Boston, Mass.: Page).—

The author deals with his subject in a chronological way. After a brief introduc-

tion, sections follow dealing with: 1. Savage America (the forest, the Indian's bequest to the colonists, the English background of the colonial farmer); 2. The Colonial period, 1600-1784 (New England: subsistence and toil; the middle colonies; Virginia: tobacco and luxury; the South: rice, indigo, and silk); 3. The great expansion, 1784-1861 (cotton, land policies); 4. Agriculture comes of age, 1861-1929 (the frontier ends, the tide of discontent, the response of government, regional development, the introduction of machines); 5. Today and tomorrow (conservation and regimentation, chemical fertilizers). The appendix contains an agricultural chronology. Bibliography and index. *Cf.* BIDWELL, P. W. & J. I. FALCONER, 1941, *vide supra.*

COLÓN, E. D., 1930: Datos sobre la historia de la agricultura de Puerto Rico antes de 1898, 302 p. (San Juan, P. R.: Cantero, Fernandez).—

A chronological history of the development of the agricultural industry from the discovery of the island in 1493 up to 1898 when the U.S.A. took possession. The social, political, and agricultural conditions are discussed in their relation to the introduction of the most important crops, *viz.,* sugar cane, coffee, tobacco, and cotton. Already early in the 16th century the first experiment station in the New World was established in the island by King Ferdinand of Spain.

DIES, E. J., 1949: Titans of the soil: great builders of agriculture, 213 p. (Chapel Hill, N.C.: North Carolina U.P.).—

In this book the author presents biographical sketches of 17 American agricultural leaders, *viz.,* George Washington, Thomas Jefferson, E. Watson, Eli Whitney, H. L. Ellsworth, Edm. Ruffin, John Deere, C. H. McCormick, J. S. Morrill, S. W. Johnson, W. O. Atwater, S. A. Knapp, S. M. Babcock, T. Smith, M. A. Carleton, H. W. Wiley, and G. H. Shull. Each biography is six or seven pages long and is accompanied by a portrait and a bibliography. There are also short biographies of A. Lincoln, L. Burbank, D. Fairchild, L. H. Bailey, H. Ford, G. W. Carver, and some others.

EDWARDS, E. E., ed., 1967: A bibliography of the history of agriculture in the United States, 307 p. (Detroit, Mich.: Gale). —

This is a photomechanical reprint of the 1930 edition which was originally published by U.S. Govt. Printing Office (U.S. Dept. Agric. Misc. Publ., No. 84). Subjects discussed which are of special importance for our purpose are, *e.g.,* American histories, scope of the history of American agriculture, bibliographies (p. 1-11); Geographical factors in American history (p. 12-20); Indian contributions (p. 21-31); Colonization, land policy, *etc.* (p. 32-59); History of American agriculture (p. 59-72); Agricultural leaders (p. 218-233); Farmers and political activity since the American Revolution (p. 239-281); Index (p. 283-307). In Agricultural History 42: 391 I found the following commentary: "The Agricultural History Branch of the U.S. Department of Agriculture and the Agricultural History Center at the University of California at Davis have cooperated to compile and distribute sections of an ultimate comprehensive bibliography of American agricultural history. This is intended to revise and update the bibliography compiled by Everett E. Edwards over thirty years ago. 'A list of References for the History of Fruits and Vegetables', compiled by Earl M. Rogers, was distributed by the Agricultural History Branch in 1963, but the supply is exhausted. 'A Preliminary List of References for the History of Agricultural Science and Technology' was compiled by Carroll W. Pursell, Jr., and Earl M. Rogers in 1966; a limited number of copies are available from the Agricultural History Branch, Economic Research Service, U.S. Department of Agriculture, Washington, D.C. 20250. A contribution to the same enterprise was a list of master's theses and doctoral dissertations written in history departments on American agricultural history subjects, and published in the July 1967 number of 'Agricultural History' (Dennis S. Nordin, 'Graduate Studies in American History'). This is available as a current number of the journal ($1.50) from the Periodicals Department, University of California Press, Berkeley, Calif. 94720. 'A Preliminary List of References for the History of Agriculture in California', compiled by James H. Shideler and Lawrence B. Lee, and 'A Preliminary List of References for the History of the Granger Movement', compiled by Dennis S. Nordin, were distributed in 1967. Both of the latter titles are available upon request to the Agricultural History Center, University of California, Davis, Calif. 95616. Forthcoming from the Agricultural History Center are lists on the Pacific Northwest and Alaska, apiculture and sericulture, and agriculture during the New Deal period."

GEISER, S. W., 1945: Horticulture and horticulturists in early Texas, 100 p. (Dallas, Texas: Southern Methodist U.P.).—

"Part I treats of fruit culture in early Texas; census returns for fruit crops in Texas, 1850-1930; wild fruits in early Texas; early Texas horticultural societies, 1870-1896; and some Texas horticultural journals 1868-1907. A bibliography of 28 titles is added. Part II contains a list of 144 Texas horticulturists, 1858-1910, with biographical, horticultural and bibliographical data. The horticultural data include information on the introduction of new varieties, the origination of new strains, services to the fruit industries and other public activities, a county index to horticulturists in early Texas, and a list of over 250 horticultural varieties originated and introduced into Texas. This document is one of permanent value in the history of botanical sciences in America and of the industries dependent thereon." (From Isis 37, 1947, p. 260).

HARDING, T. S., 1947: Two blades of grass: a history of scientific development in the U.S. Department of Agriculture, 352 p. (Norman, Okla.: Oklahoma U.P.).—

This book is a chronicle of progress in American agriculture, presenting in a popular way the more valuable and sensational achievements obtained by the scientists of the Dept. of Agriculture. It contains much information on a variety of topics, such as the introduction of new valuable plants (*e.g.,* Acala cotton, Sudan grass, mosaic-resistant sugar canes, *etc.*); a review of the research that led to the control of cattle tick fever, hookworm, many plant diseases, *etc.,* breeding of hybrid corn; breeding of disease-resistant varieties of plants; contributions to the application of D.D.T., penicillin, fermentation processes, *etc.* The book also contains (brief) biographical and bibliographical information about the more prominent scientists of the Department.

HEDRICK, U. P., 1950: A history of horticulture in America to 1860, 551 p. (New York, N.Y.: Oxford U.P.).—

In his preface, the author makes clear that this book is primarily concerned with gardening, fruit growing and viticulture and not with gardens, orchards or vineyards. The development of American horticulture is a rather complex story for it rests on different pillars: 1. Old Indian horticulture (the Indians were fairly good cultivators of vegetables); 2. The different ethnological groups: Spaniards, French, Dutch, Swedes, Germans, resp., which peopled the U.S.A., each introducing their own plants, techniques, *etc.;* 3. Superimposed on this were British agriculture and horticulture which put its stamp on every aspect. As a result American horticulture strongly depends on wild plants from America as well as upon those from foreign countries; a special chapter has been devoted to botanical explorers and botanic gardens. Other chapters have been devoted to plant breeding, to horticultural literature, and horticultural societies. Much information has been given about the development of horticulture in the different parts of the U.S.A.

JARCHOW, M. E., 1949: The earth brought forth: a history of Minnesota agriculture to 1885, 314 p. (St. Paul, Minn.: Minnesota Historical Soc.).—

A regional history, especially dealing with harvests and markets, transportation, elevators and milling, buildings and agricultural fairs, advance of mechanization, *etc.*, in the American Midwest.

LOEHR, R. C., 1952: Forests for the future: the story of sustained yield as told in the diaries and papers of David T. Mason, 1907-1950, 285 p. (St. Paul, Minn.: Minnesota Historical Soc.).—

The book comprises the personal diaries of D.T. Mason, one of America's best-known foresters, and it gives a good picture of the history of American forestry and forest-product industries during the first half of the present century.

MACEWAN, J. W. G., 1948: The sodbusters, 240 p. (Toronto: Nelson).—

Canadian agricultural history written in a popular style with biographies of Angus MacKay, Pat Burns, Dean Rutherford, J. D. McGregor, Sam Larcombe, Galbraith, John Sanderson, Arch. Wright, Fr. Collicut, K. Brown and some others. *Cf.* also: MACEWAN, J. W. G. & A. H. EWEN, 1936: The science and practice of Canadian animal husbandry, 462 p. (Toronto: Nelson).

MUNNS, E. N., 1940: A selected bibliography of North American forestry, 2 vols., 1142 p. (U.S.D.A. Misc. Publ., 364) (Washington, D.C.: U.S. Dept. Agric.).—

A classified list, including references to material in books, periodicals, government bulletins, *etc.*, published in the United States, Canada and Mexico, prior to 1930. Vol. I deals with general forestry (literature, research, education, history), forest botany (physiology, anatomy, dendrology, phenology, ecology, forest distribution, forest types, geologic history of trees, sylviculture, tree introduction, tree breeding, *etc.),* forest

protection (forest fires, animals and birds, forest pathology, forest entomology, climatic and mechanical injuries, forest mensuration, logging and lumbering). Vol. II deals with: wood technology, forest economics, forest resources, administration, legislation, policy, and with forest influences and forest aesthetics. With author index.

NANO, J. F., 1953: Brief history of forestry in the Philippines, 118 p. (Philipp. J. For. 8(1/4) : 9-127).—

Unfortunately I am unable to give more details about this publication.

NEIDERHEISER, C. M., 1956: Forest history sources of the United States and Canada, 140 p. (St. Paul, Minn.: Forest History Found.).—

A guide to manuscripts pertaining to forestry and the forest industries, contained in public and private archives or collections. It is arranged geographically and is indexed by subject and by names of persons or businesses, *etc.,* whose papers are included.

RANGE, W., 1954: A century of Georgia agriculture 1850-1950, 333 p. (Athens, Ga.: Univ. Georgia Press).—

A historical account of the major developments in Georgia agriculture in which the author emphasizes the political, economic, and educational influences that changed the agricultural pattern in the state. The first part (p. 3-76) describes the period 1850-1865, the end of the Golden Age, and the devastation by the Civil War; the second part (p. 79-168) describes the period 1865-1900, a period of economic depression; the third part (p. 169-286) describes the period 1900-1950, a period in which Georgia agriculture underwent rapid development in mechanization and application of scientific methods. *Cf.* BONNER, J. C., 1964: A history of Georgia agriculture, 242 p. (Athens, Ga.: Univ. Georgia Press).

RASMUSSEN, W. D., ed., 1960: Readings in the history of American agriculture, 340 p. (Urbana, Ill.: Univ. Illinois Press).—

This volume contains 52 selections from literature, highlighting the important landmarks in American agricultural history. Each account is preceded by a note explaining its importance and relating it to the total picture. The subject matter has been divided into eight parts, *viz.*, 1. The beginnings of American agriculture, 1607-1775

(English influences, Indian crops, the English agricultural revolution); 2. Agriculture during the Confederation; 3. Gradual improvements in American agriculture, 1789-1861 (first American agricultural journal, local agricultural societies, introduction of improved cattle, steel plows, commercial fertilizers, *etc.*); 4. The first American agricultural revolution, 1861-1914 (establishment of U.S.D.A., Homestead Act, sugar beet, cattle industry of the Great Plains, State experimental stations, breeding of the first disease-resistant strains of plants, *etc.*); 5. World War I stimulated demands for farm products; 6. Return to normalcy and agricultural depression, 1920-1932; 7. The New Deal; 8. World War II and the second agricultural revolution. Extensive chronology of American agriculture (p. 295-311), bibliography and index. A representative American point of view about American agricultural policy in the 20th century is: MCGOVERN, G., ed., 1967: Agricultural thought in the twentieth century, 55 + 570 p. (Indianapolis, Ind. & New York, N.Y.: Bobbs Merrill). From the table of contents: The golden age of agriculture 1900-1920; Farm depression 1920-1932; The New Deal 1933-1940; World War Two and new horizons 1941-1952; The crisis and the opportunity of abundance 1953-1966.

SLOSSON, E., 1951: Pioneer American gardening, 306 p. (New York, N.Y.: Coward-McCann).—

This is a collection of stories out of America's horticultural history "contributed by the 41 states whose 250,000 federated gardeners constitute the National Council of State Garden Clubs". These stories are presented under the following seven headings: New England region, central Atlantic region, south Atlantic region, central region, south central region, Rocky Mountains region, Pacific coast region.

THOMPSON, J. W., 1942: A history of livestock rising in the United States 1607-1860, 182 p. (Agricultural History Ser., No. 5) (Washington, D.C.: U.S. Dept. Agric.).—

This study deals with such subjects as: the importation of livestock into the American Colonies, stock raising as a factor in frontier economy, the introduction of improved breeds from Europe, shelter and winter conditions of cattle, *etc.*

TRUE, A. C., 1928, 1929: A history of agricultural extension work in the United States 1785-1923, 220 p. (1928); A history of agricultural education in the United States 1785-1925, 436 p. (1929) (Washington, D.C.: U.S. Dept. Agric.).—

Both these works, together with a third one (*vide infra*) give a comprehensive summary of the history of agricultural education, extension, and research in the U.S.A. The first of these books deals with the movement which resulted in the establishment of the U.S. national system of cooperative extension work in agriculture and home economics, and insofar as extension is a part of the system of agricultural education both works are supplementary to each other. The second volume deals with agricultural education and its relation to the general development of science and education and to the background of economic conditions and of the organizations of various kinds for the promotion of agriculture and country life. It tries to evaluate the influence which agricultural colleges have had on agricultural progress through their experiment stations and extension work, as well as the promotion of agricultural instruction in secondary and elementary schools. *Cf.* TERRELL, J. U., 1966: The United States Department of Agriculture: a story of food, farms and forests, 130 p. (New York, N.Y.: Duell, Sloan & Pearce).

——, 1937: A history of agricultural experimentation and research in the United States, 1607-1925: including a history of the United States Department of Agriculture, 321 p. (Washington, D.C.: U.S. Dept. Agric.).—

In this history of agricultural experimentation in the U.S.A., the development of machinery has been emphasized. It gives typical examples of the work of private individuals and organizations in laying the foundation for the establishment of public agencies for agricultural research. The early work of the U.S. Dept. of Agriculture and the State Experiment Stations has been described in some detail. Biographical information regarding the early workers has been included. A bibliography containing 327 items, subject-index, and name-index have been icluded.

WINTERS, R. K., ed., 1950: Fifty years of forestry in the U.S.A., 385 p. (Washington, D.C.: Soc. Amer. Foresters).—

This book deals with the period 1900-1950 and deals with such subjects as: forest protection; forest management, utilization, and influences; silviculture; range and wildlife management; the U.S. Forest Service and other federal agencies; state, industrial and farm forestry; the Society of American

Foresters; education in professional forestry; American and world forestry. One of the three appendixes contains a listing of the schools of forestry in the U.S.A. Biblio-graphy and index. *Cf.* also: AMERICAN FORESTRY: six decades of growth, 319 p., a book published by the Society of American Foresters in 1960.

4. HISTORY OF THE MEDICAL SCIENCES (*incl. therapy*)

α. *History of the medical sciences in general*

a. *General histories of medicine*

ACKERKNECHT, E. H., 1955: A short history of medicine, 258 p. (New York, N.Y.: Ronald Press).—

A well-written basic text in the history of medicine intended for the medical student and the educated layman. The material is presented systematically in 20 short chapters, giving an account of the social and cultural aspects of medical science. The book begins with a consideration of prehistoric medicine, of medicine in Pharaonic Egypt, of medical knowledge of Asia, and of the medical contributions of classical antiquity. History is traced through the Middle Ages, Renaissance, 17th, 18th and 19th centuries, till it terminates in the period of rapid growth of modern medicine. In an appendix a useful list with suggestions for further reading has been included. Also in German translation: Kurze Geschichte der Medizin, 1959, 216 p. (Stuttgart: Enke). *Cf.* SINGER, C. & A. E. UNDERWOOD, 1962, *vide infra.*

ASCHOFF, L., P. DIEPGEN & H. GOERKE, 1960: Kurze Uebersichtstabelle zur Geschichte der Medizin, ed. 7, 85 p. (Heidelberg: Springer).—

For more details, and for other chronologic reference works, *vide* section Some recommended encyclopaedias, subsection e.

ATKINSON, D. T., 1956: Magic, myth and medicine, 320 p. (Cleveland, O. & New York, N.Y.: World Publ.).—

A semi-popular description of the history of medicine from the dawn of science to quite recent times. The book is very readable, combining the wisdom of a scientist and the readiness of a story teller. Much attention has been paid to the influence of naval medicine on the development of late 17th-century European medicine. The book may be of interest to everyone interested in the history of medicine: professional as well as layman. *Cf.* CALDER, R., 1958; and MCMANUS, J. F. A., 1963, *vide infra.*

BARIÉTY, M. & C. COURY, 1963: Histoire de la médecine, 1217 p. (Paris: Fayard).—

A well-written review of the history of medicine from the earliest times up to recent times, intended for reading by students and those non-professional scientists who are interested in medical history. In this respect the appendix (p. 827-928), glossary (p. 1157-1200), biographical index (p. 1051-1155) and synoptic chronology (p. 929-1049) are very helpful. The appendix contains 42 *capita selecta* on specialized subjects in the field of the history of medicine, such as the history of anatomy since the 16th century, surgery during the 17th century, the history of cancer, of virus diseases, of homoeopathy, *etc.* The synoptic chronology consists of a schedule in which the facts belonging to general history (esp. those of a cultural-historical interest) are compared with facts belonging to the history of medicine (incl. geographical aspects, important publications, foundation of hospitals and learned societies, *etc.*). *Cf.* GARRISON, F. H., 1961, *vide infra.*

BOUISSOU, R., 1967: Histoire de la médecine, 382 p. (Paris: Larousse).—

A well-written introductory history of medicine, drawn from standard sources in French and English. The period covered extends from the beginnings of medicine to the present. Appended to the text are tables mentioning the major infectious diseases, their causes, prevention, treatment; and a list of Nobel Prize winners in medicine and physiology. Bibliography and index.

BRABANT, H., 1966: Médecins, malades et maladies de la Renaissance, 294 p. (Bruxelles: La Renaissance du Livre).—

After a brief introduction, the book contains chapters headed as follows: Les grandes maladies de la Renaissance (p. 15-150); La grande bataille des idées médicales (p. 151-208); Grands hommes de la médecine et médecins de grands hommes (barbiers-chirurgiens, chirurgiens-bourreaux et bourreaux-guérisseurs; mages, médecins, médicastres et morticoles) (p. 209-272); bibliography; indexes of names and of subjects.

BUCK, A. H., 1917: The growth of medicine from the earliest times to about 1800, 582 p. (New Haven, Conn.: Yale U.P.; London: Oxford U.P.).—

> The first part deals with ancient medicine (oriental medicine, Greek and Roman medicine, medical authors of the early centuries of the Christian era). The second part deals with mediaeval medicine (medicine at Byzantium, the Arab Renaissance, hospitals and monasteries in the Middle Ages, progress of medicine and surgery in Western Europe during the 13th-15th centuries, brief history of the allied sciences; pharmacy, chemistry and balneotherapeutics). The third part deals with medicine during the Renaissance (founders of human anatomy and physiology, advances in internal medicine, developments in Italy, France, Germany, England, Holland, Switzerland, Spain, Portugal).

——, 1920: The dawn of modern medicine: an account of the revival of the science and art of medicine which took place in Western Europe during the latter half of the eighteenth century and the first part of the nineteenth, 288 p. (New Haven, Conn.: Yale U.P.; London: Oxford U.P.).—

> The contents may be illustrated by a summing up of the chapter headings: 1. T. Renandot, physician, founder of the first French newspaper; 2. State of medicine in W. Europe at the beginning of the 18th century; 3. The Vienna School of medicine; 4. Medicine in Italy; 5. Smallpox, one of the world's greatest scourges; 6. Awakening of the chemists, physiologists and pathologists; 7. Medicine in England; 8. Medicine in France; 9. Medicine at the height of the French revolution; 10. Broussais and Broussaism; 11. The Golden Age of surgery in France; 12. Desgenettes and Larrey, France's most celebrated military surgeons; 13. A few of the important hospitals and their principal organizations in Paris for teaching medicine and midwifery.

CALDER, R., 1958: Medicine and the man: the story of the art and science of healing, 256 p. (New York, N.Y.: New American Library).—

> A well-written popular introduction to the history of medicine, reporting many interesting discoveries in medicine, surgery, anaesthesia, physiology, psychiatry, and public health from shamanism to the discovery of sulpha drugs, antibiotics, and complex surgery of modern times. Cf. ATKINSON, D. T., 1956, vide supra.

CAMAC, C. N. B., ed., 1959: Classics of medicine and surgery, ed. 2, 436 p. (New York, N.Y.: Dover).—

> A paperback edition of the book: Epoch-making contributions to medicine, surgery and the allied sciences; being reprints of those communications which first conveyed epoch-making observations to the scientific world, together with biographical sketches of the observers, 1909, 435 p. (Philadelphia, Pa. & London: Saunders). It contains unabridged texts of writings by Lord Lister (on antisepsis), William Harvey (on motion of the heart and blood), L. Auenbrugger (on percussion of the chest), Laënnec (on auscultation and the stethoscope), E. Jenner (on smallpox), W. Morton (on anaesthesia), J. Y. Simpson (on chloroform), and O. W. Holmes (on puerperal fever). Cf. CLENDENING, L., 1960, vide infra.

CASTIGLIONI, A., 1950: A history of medicine, ed. 2, 1192 + 56 p. (New York, N.Y.: Knopf).—

> Originally published in Italian: the first English edition was published in 1941. A book comparable with GARRISON's (vide infra), but in Castiglioni's book the parts on palaeopathology, the School of Salerno, and on mediaeval and Renaissance Italian medicine are especially valuable. A very good and comprehensive textbook and useful detailed introduction. Cf. GARRISON, F. H., 1961, vide infra.

CLENDENING, L., 1960: Source book of medical history, 685 p. (New York, N.Y.: Dover).—

> First published in 1942: this is a new edition. It includes translated excerpts from outstanding contributions which range from the medical papyri up to 1895. It includes quotations from some 120 authors, including medical passages from lay literature (e.g., from Dickens and Chaucer), thus giving a contemporary view of medical life in various ages. Biographical sketches of the authors considered, a good index, and suggestions for additional reading, are added. Cf. CAMAC, C. N. B., 1959; LEIBBRAND, W., 1954; and LOPES PIÑERO, J. M., 1969, vide infra.

DELAUNAY, P., 1949: L'évolution des théories et la pratique médicales. (Paris: Hippocrate).—

> A collection of essays formerly published in Le Scalpel, especially dealing

with the period 1795-1848 (Dupuytren, Laënnec, Guillotin, Treviranus, Magendie, Ramazzini). Special sections deal with iatrochemistry, the influence of chemistry on medicine (Lavoisier, Fourcroy), philosophical influences (Kant, Schelling), vitalistic influences, and humoral pathology.

DIEPGEN, P., 1949-1955: Geschichte der Medizin. Die historische Entwicklung der Heilkunde und des ärztlichen Lebens. Vol. I: Von den Anfängen der Medizin bis zur Mitte des 18. Jahrhunderts, 355 p.; Vol. II, part 1: Von der Medizin der Aufklärung bis zur Begründung der Zellularpathologie (*ca.* 1740 - *ca.* 1858), 271 p. (ed. 2, 1959); Vol. II, part 2: Die Medizin vom Beginn der Zellularpathologie bis zu den Anfängen der modernen Konstitutionslehre (etwa 1848 - 1900), mit einem Ausblick auf die Entwicklung der Heilkunde in den letzten 50 Jahren, 336 p. (Berlin: de Gruyter).—

A textbook attempting to present the historical development of the science of medicine, not from the more or less chronological-biographical point of view, but aiming at discussing the origin of medical concepts and their role in the development of general medical thought and practice. It deals also with the life of the physician as it has resulted from the interplay of folk-medicine, the scientific art of healing, and theory and practice, on the one hand, and the intellectual and material culture of the various periods of time on the other hand. Achievements of Germans have been emphasized. Vol. I deals with: the beginning of medicine, medicine of the primitive peoples, folk-medicine, medicine of the cultured peoples of the ancient world, in Greece and Rome, and the medical Middle Ages, the turn to modern medicine in the 16th century, and with medicine in the Baroque period. Vol. II, part 1, deals with the development of the natural sciences and their influence on medicine; the biological fundamentals of medicine, the development of the separate medical subsciences, and with the foundation of cellular pathology. Vol. II, part 2, covers the period 1858 to 1900 and also contains a very brief survey of medical history of the last 50 years. Attention has been paid to the relationship between philosophy and natural science, between the exact and the natural sciences, the impact of psychology on the theory and practice of medicine; and special mention must be made of the chapters treating of the history of homoeopathy, diet therapy, psychotherapy in psychosomatic diseases, and with forensic medicine — subjects often neglected in other histories of medicine. *Cf.* GARRISON, F. H., 1961, *vide infra.*

DUMESNIL, R., 1950: Histoire illustrée de la médecine, 195 p. (Paris: Plon).—

The author tries to elucidate the influence of humanism on the development of medical science, and more especially how medical theories and hypotheses have been influenced by current philosophical views during the past centuries. The author starts from the assumption that medicine is not just an exact science, and is not even a science at all, but more a kind of art and that - strictly speaking - there consequently exists not a history of medicine, but only a history of medical men. *Cf.* STAROBINSKI, J., 1964, *vide infra.*

FULTON, J. F., 1951: The great medical bibliographers: a study in humanism, 107 p. (Philadelphia, Pa.: Univ. Pennsylvania Press).—

The present volume contains the text of a series of three lectures. The first deals mainly with the origin of bibliography (Johann Tritheim, 1494), the first medical biography (of Symphorien Champier, 1596), and with the outstanding bibliographer C. Gessner. The second lecture deals with the first medical book sales, with the great medical bibliographer A. von Haller (1708-1777), and with the medical dictionary writers such as N. F. J. Eloy and James Atkinson. The third lecture deals with medical subject-indexes and the contributions of W. G. Ploucquet, J. Forbes, A. C. Callisen and J. S. Billings. At the end of the book details are given about the medical bibliographical works of L. Choulant, W. Osler, and G. Keynes.

GALDSTON, I., 1940: Progress in medicine: a critical review of the last hundred years, 347 p. (New York, N.Y.: Knopf).—

This story is an attempt "to trace the progression of ideas as witnessed in the development of medicine during the last hundred years". This the author illustrates by tracing the developments of the last hundred years in four major fields of medicine, *viz.*, the germ theory of disease (its origin, Pasteur, Lister, Koch), the newer knowledge of nutrition, new discoveries in the fields of physiology and of the internal secretions, and the discovery of sulphanilamide and related compounds. *Cf.* BUCK, A. H., 1920, *vide supra;* and LLOYD, W. E. B., 1968, *vide infra.*

GARRISON, F. H., 1961: An introduction to the history of medicine with medical chronology, suggestions for study and bibliographic data, ed. 4, 996 p. (Philadelphia, Pa. & London: Saunders).—

This is a reprint of the 1929 edition. It has been written primarily for medical students, and, whereas especially 19th-century achievements and investigators are most often quoted to them in their medical literature, emphasis has here been laid on the latest developments in medical history. About the contents of this book: 62 p. have been devoted to primitive medicine, 42 p. to Greek and Graeco-Roman medicine, 72 p. to mediaeval medicine, 52 p. to the Renaissance up to 1600, 65 p. to the 17th century, 97 p. to the 18th century, and 401 p. to the 19th century and after. The appendixes contain a chronology of medicine and public hygiene from earliest times up to 1928 (70 p.), bibliographical notes for collateral reading of histories of medicine, a list of medical biographies (arranged alphabetically according to names of the physicians) and a list of histories of special subjects (arranged according to subject). In 1966 a collection of essays, written by GARRISON, and published in the Bull. New York Acad. Medicine between 1925 and 1935, has been published under the title: Contributions to the history of medicine, 989 p. With introduction (by M. W. CUMMINGS), bibliographies, and index (History of Medicine Series, No. 27) (New York, N.Y.: Hafner). Cf. BARIÉTY, M. & C. COURY, 1963; CASTIGLIONI, A., 1950; DIEPGEN, P., 1949-1955, vide supra; and MAJOR, R. H., 1954/ '55, vide infra.

GORDON, B. L., 1960: Medieval and Renaissance medicine, 243 p. (London: Owen).—

For more details, vide section The Middle Ages in the Latin West, subsection c.

GUTHRIE, D., 1958: A history of medicine, 464 p. (London & Edinburgh: Nelson).—

This is a new and revised edition of a well-known and often-reprinted textbook, first published in 1945. It is a well-written introductory text, especially directed to the medical student. Each chapter is supplemented by a list of "books for further reading". Reprinted in 1960. Also in German translation: Die Entwicklung der Heilkunde. Die Medizin im Wandel der Zeit, 383 p. (Zu-

rich: Büchergilde Gutenberg). Cf. SINGER, C. & A. E. UNDERWOOD, 1962 vide infra.

HAESER, H., 1875-1882: Lehrbuch der Geschichte der Medicin und der epidemischen Krankheiten, ed. 3, 3 vols. Vol. I (1875): Geschichte der Medicin im Alterthum und Mittelalter, 876 + (35) p.; Vol. II (1881): Geschichte der Medicin in der neueren Zeit, 1120 p.; Vol. III (1882): Geschichte der epidemischen Krankheiten, 995 p. (Jena: Fischer).—

According to Garrison-Morton: "The most important German work on the history of medicine and one of the most outstanding contributions." It gives much bibliographical information and it contains excellent summaries of medical achievements in certain periods. There is a detailed table of contents but no subject-index. Vols. I and II give a chronologic history up to the beginning of the 19th century; vol. III consists of a history of epidemics. A comparable work in the French language is: DAREMBERG, C., 1870: Histoire des sciences médicales, comprenant l'anatomie, la physiologie, la médecine, la chirurgie et les doctrines de pathologie générale, 2 vols. Vol. I: Depuis les temps historiques jusqu'à Harvey, 580 p.; Vol. II: Depuis Harvey jusqu'au XIXe siècle, p. 577 (!)-1303. (Paris: Baillière). Cf. NEUBURGER, M. & J. PAGEL, 1902-1905, vide infra.

HAHN, A., P. DUMAÎTRE & J. SAMION-COUTET, eds., 1962: Histoire de la médecine et du livre médical à la lumière des collections de la bibliothèque de la Faculté de Médecine de Paris, 432 p. (Paris: Perrin).—

This book contains the history of medicine and of medical literature from the beginning of printing to the middle of the 19th century. Its subject matter is divided in centuries, and each survey of a century is followed by a review of the development of the printed book as exemplified in the most important medical books of the period. The entire work is mainly based on the rich collections of the library of the Paris Medical Faculty. It contains a wealth of illustrations (263) and a very good bibliography. There are anatomical and surgical plates, engraved frontispieces, title-pages, portraits, and vignettes.

HERRLINGER, R., 1967: Geschichte der medizinischen Abbildung. I. Von der Antike bis um 1600, ed. 2, 180 p. (Munich: Moos).—

A history of medical illustration in general, although the emphasis is upon anatomy. The first part (p. 9-28) deals with the ancient period; the illustrations have been traced back to such mediaeval illustrations as probably had ancient origins. The second part (p. 29-71) deals with the Middle Ages (extending this period to about 1500), and includes such illustrations as: blood-letting figures, uroscopy, wound-men, teratology, medical botany, surgery, religious and astrological woodcuts, *etc.* The last section deals with the 16th century, considering the anatomical drawings of Leonardo da Vinci, Berengario da Carpi, Dryander, Canano, and Vesalius and his successors. According to a publisher's advertisement, a second vol. will be published dealing with medical illustration since 1600. The untimely death of the author leaves me uncertain whether this second vol. will be published. *Cf.* CHOULANT, L., 1962, *vide* section History of biology in general, subsection d.

HURD-MEAD, K. C., 1938: A history of women in medicine from the earliest times to the beginnings of the nineteenth century, 569 p. (Haddam, Conn.: Haddam Press).—

A history of women in medicine. The story is treated century by century from primitive times through Egypt, Greece, Rome, Middle Ages, and Renaissance up to the end of the eighteenth century. A second volume is planned and will complete this history up to modern times. I could not verify, whether this second vol. has appeared. The general scheme of the work is to present for epoch or century its general cultural and scientific background, the medical advances and outstanding contributions, and thence to pass on to a consideration of the medical women of the period. In a review in Isis 29: 477-479, J. B. de C. M. Saunders warns us of the many inaccuracies hidden in this book. *Cf.* LIPINSKA, M., 1930; and SCHÖNFELD, W., 1947, *vide infra.*

INGLIS, B., 1965: A history of medicine, 196 p. (London: Weidenfeld & Nicolson).—

A profusely illustrated (by reproductions of original paintings, drawings and engravings) introductory history of medical treatment from primitive peoples to the present day. Separate chapters deal with medicine and primitive man, medicine in early civilizations, Greece and Rome, Islam (Razes, Avicenna, Cordova), during the Middle Ages (Galenism, Christianity, plague epidemics), during the Renaissance (Paracelsus, Vesalius, Paré), and the 17th century (Sydenham, the new systematics); other chapters deal with preventive medicine, mental illnesses, mesmerism, homoeopathy, diagnosis, and with the history of medicine in modern times (anaesthetics, Pasteur, public health, psychiatry, stress and disease, *etc.*). Short bibliography. Index. Also in German translation: Geschichte der Medizin, 1965, 240 p. (Bern, Munich & Vienna: Schetz).

KEELE, K. D., 1963: The evolution of clinical methods in medicine, 115 p. (London: Pitman).—

The book consists of the FitzPatrick Lectures delivered at the Royal College of Physicians during 1960-1961, and its purpose is to show how medical practice is time-bound. The author traces the changes in clinical methods throughout the centuries, showing how they have reached their present form. The infiltration of the basic sciences (incl. physics and chemistry) into clinical medicine has been elucidated.

KING, L. S., 1958: The medical world of the 18th century, 346 p. (Chicago, Ill.: Chicago U.P.; London: Cambridge U.P.).—

A series of authoritative but personal and loosely-connected essays concerning some aspects of the intellectual, social, economic, moral, and technical problems of the 18th-century physicians, and based mainly on original sources. The book includes *inter alia* a summary review of the controversy between the apothecary and the physician at the beginning of the century, a long and detailed account of Boerhaave, regarded as both a systematist and a scientist, together with an analysis of his theories, methods, and ideas; and a discussion of current homoeopathy, nosology, pathology, medical ethics and practice, *etc. Cf.* RATHER, L. J., 1965, *vide infra.*

——, 1963: The growth of medical thought, 254 p. (Chicago, Ill.: Chicago U.P.).—

This is a history of the methodology of medicine, rather than a history of the science of medicine. The author is concerned with the thoughts lying behind medical procedure that gave rise to medical science rather than with the accumulation of isolated facts. The author distinguished between some different patterns of medical knowledge, *e.g.,* the Hippocratic School where the first generalizations from case-histories by means of induction are to be found; the methodological progress made by Galen; the rather strange mixture of mediaeval alchemy, astrology and magic, and the dynamics of Renaissance ideas of Paracelsus; the origins of modern anatomy and physiology as formulated by *e.g.,* Vesalius and Harvey; the achievements of modern cell-theory, chemical pathology, molecular medicine, *etc.,* and the growth of modern medicine.

KNIPPING, H. W. & H. KENTER, 1961: Heilkunst und Kunstwerk. Probleme zwischen Kunst und Medizin aus ärztlicher Sicht, 152 p. (Stuttgart: Schattauer).—

    Even in the remote past, there always has existed an interconnection between medicine and art. From recent art and from the history of art, much can be learned by any physician about the structure and the essence of Man. On the other side medicine has attracted many artists, because they were touched by sufferings of Man. Also some therapeutic aspects have been considered.

LAIGNEL-LAVASTINE, F., ed., 1939-1949: Histoire générale de la médecine, de la pharmacie, de l'art dentaire et de l'art vétérinaire, 3 vols. Vol. I (1936): 683 p.; Vol. II (1936): 670 p.; Vol. III (1949): 816 p. (Paris: Michel).—

    This history of medicine is especially valuable for its many beautiful illustrations, which are fine products of printing technique. The first volume deals with palaeopathology, Assyrian and Babylonian medicine, Egyptian, Greek, Roman, Indian, Iranian, Arabian, Chinese and Japanese medicine, and with pharmacy and dental and veterinary medicine during antiquity. The second volume deals with the history of medicine during the Middle Ages, the Renaissance and the 17th century, with pre-Columbian medicine, with the history of anatomy, physiology, histology, surgery, dermatology, cancer, venereal diseases, and with the history of dentistry and veterinary science from the Middle Ages up to the end of the 18th century. The third volume deals with the history of surgery from the end of the 18th century onwards, with the history of gynaecology, obstetrics, orthopaedics, epidemiology, infectious diseases, tuberculosis, gout, diabetes, pediatrics, psychiatry, neurology, ophthalmology, oto-rhino-laryngology, urology, cardiology, gastro-enterology, hygiene, pharmacy, homoeopathy, physiotherapy, radiology, the role of weather conditions, gymnastics, and with dental and veterinary medicine from the end of the 18th century onwards. The various chapters differ

in competence. *Cf.* NEUBURGER, M. & J. PAGEL, 1902-1905, *vide infra.*

LAIN ENTRALGO, P., 1963: Historia de la medicina moderna y contemporanea, 773 p. (Madrid & Barcelona: Ed. Científico Médica).—

    According to a book recension by P. Huard and J. Brocas in Arch. int. d'Hist. sci. 10 (No. 40): 279-280, this is an excellent book, written in a lucid style. The author begins his history in 1453 (conquest of Constantinople). For each of the periods considered (Renaissance, 1453-1600; Baroque, 1600-1740; enlightened despotims, 1740-1800; Romanticism, 1800-1848; Positivism, 1848-1914; and the contemporary era, starting 1914-1918), the author gives a general review of its scientific and philosophical climate, including a consideration of national, religious and social factors. The book is of particular interest to historians of medicine because it contains much more information on developments in Spain and South America than the average history of medicine. The same author also wrote an interesting study of the history of the description of diseases, *viz.,* LAIN ENTRALG0, P., 1961: La historia clínica. Historia y teoría del relato patografico, 668 p. (Barcelona: Selvat). A short history of medicine in Spanish is: GRANJEL, L. S., 1968: Manual de historia de la medicina, 195 p. (Salamanca: Univ. de Salamanca, Semenario de Hist. Med. Española).

LEIBBRAND, W., 1954: Heilkunde. Eine Problemgeschichte der Medizin, 437 p. (Munich & Freiburg: Alber).—

    An anthology in which the history of medicine has been described mainly in the words of its makers. All quotations are in German translation, and are elucidated by interconnecting texts. The subject matter has been divided into four parts, *viz.,* medicine in Hellas and Rome, medicine and Christianity, the interrelations between medicine and modern philosophical systems, and a draft of a new anthropology. Many biographical references, good name- and subject-indexes. *Cf.* CLENDENING, L., 1960, *vide supra.*

LEONARDO, R. A., 1946: History of medical thought, 92 p. (New York, N.Y.: Froben).—

    An introduction to the historical development of the fundamental views and approaches in medical theory and practice. The outstanding men of each period are cited and their contributions discussed. The book is intended as a guide to the medical practitioner and the average student of medicine interested in, but unacquainted with, its history.

LIBBY, W., 1922: History of medicine in its salient features, 427 p. (Boston, Mass.: Houghton Mifflin).—

A very readable introductory text. Chapter headings are as follows: 1. The priest-physician of Egypt and Babylonia; 2. Hippocrates the father of medicine; 3. Roman anatomy and surgery; 4. The transmission of medical science by the Arabs; 5. The revival of anatomy and surgery in the 16th century; 6. William Harvey and the revival of physiology; 7. Science and practice: Sydenham, Boerhaave; 8. Comparative anatomy: John Hunter; 9. Morbid anatomy, and histology: Morgagni, Bichat; 10. Local diagnosis: Auenbrugger, Laënnec; 11. Advances in physiology; 12. Embryology and Karl Ernst von Baer; 13. The cell-theory and cellular pathology; 14. The introduction of anaesthetics; 15. The theory of organic evolution; 16. The founders of bacteriology; 17. Antiseptic surgery: Lord Lister; 18. The history of syphilis; 19. Preventive medicine in the tropics; 20. Medical science and modern warfare.

LINDEBOOM, G. A., 1961: Inleiding tot de geschiedenis der geneeskunde, 342 p. (Haarlem: Bohn).—

A well-illustrated and nicely-balanced concise history of medicine. p. 301-335: "Biblio- en biografische aantekeningen" (somewhat along the lines of the "Biographical Addenda" in MAJOR's A history of medicine, *vide infra*).

LIPINSKA, M., 1930: Les femmes et le progrès des sciences médicales, 235 p. (Paris: Masson).—

The first section deals with primitive medicine (p. 1-8); the second section with classical antiquity (p. 9-26) considering the position of the woman priest in sacerdotal medicine, woman magicians, medical women in Rome; the third section deals with the Middle Ages (p. 27-48): Italy (*e.g.*, Salerno, Florence, Venice, Padua, Naples); Germany (Hildegard of Bingen); women healers in France; the fourth section (p. 49-124) deals with the period between the Middle Ages and the 19th century: Spain, women surgeons in France, medical publications by women; the women healers in Switzerland, Holland, Germany, Poland, Italy, and

France; the fifth section (p. 125-231) deals with the 19th and 20th centuries. The 10 chapters treat of the subject matter in a regional way. *Cf.* SCHÖNFELD, W., 1947, *vide infra;* and BAUDOUIN, M., 1906, *vide* section Biographical dictionaries.

LLOYD, W. E. B., 1968: A hundred years of medicine, ed. 2, 352 p. ("Hundred Years Series") (London: Duckworth).—

The book is in three parts, *viz.*, 1. Introductory: the state of medicine early in the last century; 2. Scientific discovery (including developments in pathology, anaesthetics, food chemistry, the germ theory, drugs, radium and the latest surgical advances); 3. Health organization (incl. public health and sanitary legislation, hospital reform, maternity services, factory medicine and mental health). This book has been entirely rewritten since its first appearance in 1936, 344 p. *Cf.* GALDSTON, I., 1940, *vide supra.*

LOPEZ PIÑERO, J. M., 1969: Medicina Historia Sociedad. Antologia de clasicos médicos, 343 p. (Barcelona: Ariel).—

An anthology of classical texts in chronological order derived from nearly one hundred medical authors representative of different historical periods and medical fields, including Greek, Arab, mediaeval and Renaissance authors. The book is of special importance as a source of information about the Spanish authors included. *Cf.* CLENDENING, L., 1960, *vide supra.*

McMANUS, J. F. A., 1963: The fundamental ideas of medicine: a brief history of medicine, 115 p. (Springfield, Ill.: Thomas).—

The purpose of this book is to trace the ways in which modern diagnosis and treatment have evolved. This has been done by considering and describing the basic ideas in medicine. As the publisher states, this booklet is intended to serve as an introduction to the history of medicine for workers in medical fields and for the interested and inquiring non-medical persons. An appendix contains brief biographic notes of over 150 scientists (incl. physicians, scientists and philosophers who have contributed to the development of medical ideas). A comparable booklet: GREEN, J. R., 1968: Medical history for students, 197 p. (Springfield, Ill.: Thomas). *Cf.* ROGERS, F. B., 1962, *vide infra.*

MAJOR, R. H., 1954/'55: A history of medicine, 2 vols. Vol. I: 563 p.; Vol. II: p.

565-1055. (Springfield, Ill.: Thomas; Oxford: Blackwell).—

A well-written and well-illustrated history of medicine intended primarily for students. It describes the history of medicine from prehistoric times up to the introduction of sulpha drugs and antibiotics. Each main section is followed by a few pages of biographical addenda in which the chief personalities and chief events are listed. Useful subject- and author-index, general bibliography, and list of selected references bearing on each chapter have been included. Also in Italian: Storia della medicina, 2 vols., 947 p. (Florence: Sansoni). *Cf.* GARRISON, F. H., 1961, *vide supra.*

METTLER, C. C., 1947: History of medicine: a correlative text arranged according to subjects, 1215 p. (ed. by F. A. METTLER) (Philadelphia, Pa.: Blakiston).—

A useful reference-book on the history of medicine, containing a great number of quotations from original sources translated into English. Each chapter covers the entire evolution and progress of the subject with which it deals. There are 15 chapters dealing with: history of anatomy, physiology, pharmacology, pathology and bacteriology, physical diagnosis, medicine, neurology and psychiatry, venereology, dermatology, pediatrics, surgery, obstetrics and gynaecology, ophthalmology, otology, and laryngology. The humanistic and cultural background of medicine has not been considered. There are many illuminating footnotes, good indexes of subjects and persons, and each chapter is accompanied by a list of selected readings.

MEYER-STEINEGG, T. & K. SUDHOFF, 1950: Geschichte der Medizin im Ueberblick. Mit Abbildungen, ed. 4, 442 p. (Jena: Fischer).—

A very useful introduction into the history of medicine intended especially for students of medicine and for the interested physician. Part I (by MEYER-STEINEGG) deals with primitive medicine, medicine of the ancient east and with medicine of classical antiquity down to Galen (140 p.). Part II (by SUDHOFF) deals with the middle period: from Galen's death to Francis Bacon (159 p.) and part III deals with modern times from Harvey down to our days (125 p.), and has been written by MEYER-STEINEGG. Many (208) fine illustrations. The first edition appeared in 1921, and a 5th edition, ed. by R. HERRLINGER & F. KUDLIEN, in 1965 under the title: Illustrierte Geschichte der Medizin, 349 p. +

227 illus.) Stuttgart: Fischer). *Cf.* SINGER, C. & A. E. UNDERWOOD, 1962, *vide infra.*

NEUBURGER, M. & J. PAGEL, eds., 1902-1905: Handbuch der Geschichte der Medizin, 3 vols. Vol. I (1902): 756 p.; Vol. II (1903): 960 p.; Vol. III (1905): 1128 p. (Jena: Fischer).—

A classic in the field of the history of medicine, initiated by T. PUSCHMANN. Each chapter is written by a competent author. Vol. I gives the history of medicine during the ancient and mediaeval periods; Vols. II and III the history of medicine from the 16th century up to *ca.* 1900. In these last two volumes the history of medicine is treated by means of the history of the separate disciplines. This work is somewhat antiquated, but still very useful because of the vast amount of knowledge it contains. *Cf.* HAESER, H., 1875-1882; and LAIGNEL-LAVASTINE, F., 1939-1949, *vide supra. Cf.* also: NEUBURGER, M., 1910-1925, *vide* section Antiquity in general, subsection c.

OSLER, W., 1921: The evolution of modern medicine, 243 p. (New Haven, Conn.: Yale U.P.).—

According to Garrison-Morton it is one of the most interesting histories of medicine, written in a charming style and perhaps the best book with which to commence the study of medical history. It comprises a series of six lectures, dealing with various phases of oriental medicine, including Hebrew, Chinese and Japanese medicine, with Greek medicine, with mediaeval medicine, with Renaissance medicine, and with the rise of modern medicine and of preventive medicine. Reissued, 1943 (New Haven, Conn.: Yale U.P.).

PETROW, B. D., ed., 1957: Geschichte der Medizin, 255 p. (Berlin: Volk und Gesundheit).—

A history of medicine from the Marxist point of view. This history of medicine has been divided into the following main sections: 1. Medicine during the age of slavery (China, India, Mesopotamia, Egypt, Greece, and Rome); 2. Medicine during the period of feudalism (Byzantium, Tibet, Arabs, and Western Europe); 3. Medicine during the period of capitalism (morphology, physiology, pathology, microbiology, hygiene, preventive medicine, *etc.*). A comparable book: METTE, A. & I. WINTER, 1968: Geschichte der Medizin. Einführung in ihre Grundzüge, 553 p. (Berlin: Volk und Gesundheit).

POYNTER, F. N. L., ed., 1968: Medicine and science in the 1860s, 324 p. (London: Wellcome Inst. Hist. Med.).—

A series of essays, dealing with clinical medicine, cellular pathology, the germ theory, the impact of Darwin's "Origin of species" on medicine and biology, and some other topics.

RATHER, L. J., 1965: Mind and body in eighteenth-century medicine: a study based on Jerome Gaub's De regimine mentis, 274 p. (London: Wellcome Historical Medical Library).—

"Dr Rather has contrived to present us with two works woven into one on the psychosomatic medical ideas of the eighteenth century. The one consists of a very valuable translation of the two Essays of Jerome Gaub on the relation between mind and body; the other, woven into the first, consists of commentaries putting the various views expressed by Gaub into their historical and contemporary context, and comparing them on occasions with the present outlook on psychosomatic problems". (From: Med. Hist. 10: 301-302). *Cf.* KING, L. S., 1958, *vide supra.*

ROBINSON, V., 1943: The story of medicine, new ed., 564 p. (The New Home Library) (New York, N.Y.: Garden City).—

A reliable introductory text, first published in 1931. It is a well-written one-volume history of medicine. This new ed. has a chapter containing brief historical sketches of social problems that are of medical interest, such as: housing, slum clearance, sanitation, child welfare, social work, hospital social service, municipal hygiene, *etc.* Bibliography and index of individuals and subjects. *Cf.* SINGER, C. & E. A. UNDERWOOD, 1962, *vide infra.*

ROGERS, F. B., 1962: A syllabus of medical history, 112 p. (Boston, Mass.: Little, Brown).—

As has been stated in the foreword, this syllabus is a primer on medical history suitable for those who wish to familiarize themselves with the field without wading through detailed and extensive treatises. The book is designed to be of service to college and medical students, busy practitioners, and the general reader interested in health problems. *Cf.* MCMANUS, J. F. A., 1963, *vide supra.*

ROLLESTON, H. D., 1930: Internal medicine, 92 p. (Clio Medica, No. 4) (New York, N.Y.: Hoeber).—

A short history of the subject, giving an account of discoveries in the fundamental medical sciences as far as they are related to internal medicine. Long index of personal names, Subject-index, but not a good bibliography.

ROSEN, G. & B. CASPARI-ROSEN, 1947: 400 years of a doctor's life, 429 p. (New York, N.Y.: Schuman).—

A collection of extracts from medical autobiographies in which we learn medicine from the doctor's point of view. The material has been arranged according to subject as follows: 1. Early years; 2. Schooldays; 3. The medical student; 4. The practice of medicine; 5. Scientist, scholar, teacher; 6. The doctor marries; 7. The doctor as a patient; 8. The doctor goes to war; 9. Writing and politics; 10. Reflections on life and death.

SCHÖNFELD, W., 1947: Frauen in der abendländischen Heilkunde vom klassischen Altertum bis zum Ausgang des 19. Jahrhunderts, 176 p. (Stuttgart: Enke).—

A chronological history of the role of the medical women with many biographical details. Separate sections deal with: the role of women in medicine in Greece; Rome (midwifery, obstetrics, alchemy); the Middle Ages (nuns: Hildegard, Jutta, and others; mulieres salernitanae: Trotta, Sigelgaita, *etc.:* women physicians in Italy, Germany, France, England, Poland); 16th century (dilettantes, *e.g.,* Anna Sophie v. Sachsen, Anna Wecker); 17th century (midwives in France, Germany; women physicians; dilettantes in France, Germany and England); 18th century (midwives in France, Germany, Switzerland, England; women physicians in Italy, Germany, France, England; dilettantes and women quacks in France, Germany, Italy, and England); 19th century (dilettantes, women quacks, midwives, and the first women physicians educated at the university). *Cf.* HURD-MEAD, K. C., 1938; and LIPINSKA, M., 1947, *vide supra.*

SHRYOCK, R. H., 1947: The development of modern medicine, an interpretation of the social and scientific factors involved, new ed., 457 + 15 p. (New York, N.Y.: Knopf).—

This study undertakes to depict certain major developments in the history of medicine against the general background of social and intellectual history, in which the patient deserves a more prominent place than in most older histories of medicine. Also in French translation: Histoire de la médecine moderne, 312 p. (Paris: Colin), and in German translation: Die Entwicklung der modernen Medizin in ihrem Zusammenhang mit dem sozialen Aufbau und den Naturwissenschaften, 1940, 374 p. (Stuttgart: Enke).

SIGERIST, H. E., 1932: Man and medicine: an introduction to medical knowledge, 340 p. (New York, N.Y.: Norton).—

This is a translation of SIGERIST's "Einführung in die Medizin", 1931, 405 p. (Leipzig). This study tries to erect a historical background aiming to be a guide to the beginning medical student. Ch. 1: Man - a brief review of the growth of our knowledge of the body; Ch. 2: The sick Man - the position of the sick in various civilizations; Ch. 3: The signs of disease; Ch. 4: Disease; Ch. 5: Causes of disease. In these chapters the author traces the development of our knowledge of disease, early theories, the great epidemics, *etc.*, and the mutual influences of disease and cultural conditions; Ch. 6: Medical aid - the efforts made to recognize and cure disease; Ch. 7: The physician - especially dealing with the position of the physician in social life. Also in French translation: Introduction à la médecine, 1932, 356 p. (Paris: Payot).

——, 1932: Grosze Aerzte. Eine Geschichte der Heilkunde in Lebensbildern, 310 p. (Munich: Lehmann).—

The individual scientist never works in isolation, and many brains and many hands are needed before a discovery is made. This discovery is often made by a man of genius who synthesizes a wealth of knowledge. Whether a genius succeeds is determined by the structure of the society and the climate of opinion, but once he succeeds, he can at the same time be considered as the representative of a trend, of a school, or of a period. Starting from this thesis the author makes a selection of representative individuals, and with the aid of their biographies he tries to trace the development of medical thought. The 5th ed. appeared in 1965, 494 p. (Munich: Lehmann). There is also an English translation: The great doctors: a biographical history of medicine, ed. 3, 1958, 422 p. (Garden City, N.Y.: Doubleday).

SINGER, C. & E. A. UNDERWOOD, 1962: A short history of medicine, ed. 2, 854 p.

(Oxford: Clarendon Press).—

A standard work on the history of medicine intended for the medical student, teacher and practitioner, the aim of this book being to illustrate the continuous evolution of the subjects which the medical student is compelled to study. The first edition was prepared by C. Singer in 1928 and has had many reprintings. This second edition has been greatly revised by Underwood; it opens with a section on medicine before the age of the Greeks, and the last two-thirds of the original book, dealing with the 19th and 20th centuries, have been entirely rewritten (esp. those parts dealing with physiology, bacteriology, and the history of infectious diseases and preventive medicine), while a discussion of the evolution of some specialities in the clinical field has been included. *Cf.* ACKERKNECHT, E. H., 1955; GUTHRIE, D., 1958; MEYER-STEINEGG, T. & K. SUDHOFF, 1950; ROBINSON, V., 1943; SHRYOCK, R. H., 1947,*vide supra;* and WALKER, K., 1954, *vide infra.*

STAROBINSKI, J., 1964: A history of medicine, 111 p. (The new illustrated library of science and invention, Vol. 12) (New York, N.Y.: Hawthorn Books).—

A beautiful book with about 200 pictures (of which fewer than a dozen are portraits) and a text of about 2000 words. Chronological table but no index. It has been translated from the French: Histoire de la médecine, 1963, 104 p. (La science illustrée, No. 12) (Lausanne: Rencontre); also in German: Geschichte der Medizin, 1963, 104 p. (In Wort und Bild, Vol. 12) (Lausanne: Rencontre). Comparable books are: BETTMAN, O. L., 1962: A pictorial history of medicine, 318 p. (Springfield, Ill.: Thomas); and: LEWIS, P., ed., 1968: An illustrated history of medicine, 319 p. (New York, N.Y.: Golden Press). *Cf.* also DU-MESNIL, R., 1950, *vide supra.*

SUDHOFF, K., 1922: Kurzes Handbuch der Geschichte der Medizin, 534 p. (Berlin: Karger).—

The first (1897) and second (1915) editions of this book appeared under J. PAGEL's name and under the title: "Einführung in die Geschichte der Medizin". The present edition contains a compact history of medicine and is especially valuable for the period before 1800. The book has the character of a manual; it contains a wealth of factual and bibliographical information. This book is well known under the name "Pagel-Sudhoff".

TAUBERT, A., 1964: Die Anfänge der graphischen Darstellung in der Medizin, 75 p. (Kieler Beiträge zur Geschichte der Medizin und Pharmazie, part 1) (Kiel: Inst. Gesch. Med. u. Pharm.).—

"Eine historisch gesehene Zusammenstellung medizinischer Diagramme, gegliedert in einen Abschnitt über Registrierung direkt gewonnener Kurven ... und einem zweiten Abschnitt, der die aus Handzeichnungen resultierenden Graphiken enthält. 37 Abbildungen aus 93 bibliographisch genau ausgeführten Arbeiten sind als Belege beigegeben. Die Studie erweist die vielseitigen Anwendungsmöglichkeiten graphischer Darstellungen." (From: Gesnerus 25: 231-232).

THORNTON, J. L., 1966: Medical books, libraries and collectors: a study of bibliography and the book trade in relation to the medical sciences, 445 p. (Rev. ed.; introd. by G. KEYNES) (London: Deutsch).—

For more details, *vide* section Bibliographies, subsection e.

TISCHNER, R., 1950: Das Werden der Homöopathie. Geschichte der Homöopathie vom Altertum bis zur neuesten Zeit, 211 p. (Stuttgart: Hippocrates).—

This is an abridged version of TISCHNER's standard work on the history of homoeopathy: Geschichte der Homöopathie, 1932-1939, 4 vols., 837 p. (Leipzig: Schwabe). The present text has been divided into 4 parts; the relating subtitles are the same as those of the four volumes of the standard edition, *viz.*, 1. Die Vorläufer der Homöopathie (p. 9-25); 2. Hahnemann (a description of his life and work, p. 26-108); 3. Die Ausbreitung der Homöopathie bis 1850 (p. 109-161); and 4. Die Homöopathie seit 1850 (incl. a short section of 4 pages, dealing with the development of homoeopathy in Italy, France, England, Russia, and the U.S.A.). A publication of much interest to the historian of medicine, especially of homoeopathic medicine, is: PROKOP, O. & L., 1957: Homöopathie und Wissenschaft. Eine Kritik des Systems, 223 p. (Stuttgart: Enke).

WALKER, K., 1954: The story of medicine, 343 p. (London: Hutchinson).—

Its contents can best be made clear by the table of contents: 1. Prehistoric medicine; 2. Greek medicine; 3. The medicine of Alexandria and Rome; 4. The Middle Ages; 5. Mediaeval epidemics; 6. The Renaissance; 7. The 17th century of genius; 8. The period of consolidation (1700-1825); 9. The age of science and specialization; 10. The story of surgery; 11. The conquest of pain; 12. The mastery of wound infection; 13. Man *vs.* the micro-organisms; 14. Man's defences against infection; 15. Tropical diseases; 16. Deficiency diseases; 17. Public health; 18. Diversion on the subject of mind; 19. Illnesses of the mind and their treatment; 20. Quackery. No bibliography; rather short index. Also in French translation: Histoire de la médecine. Des pratiques anciennes aux découvertes les plus modernes, 1962, 378 p. (Verviers: Gérard). *Cf.* SINGER, C. & E. A. UNDERWOOD, 1962, *vide supra.*

WARTHIN, A. S., 1931: The physician of the Dance of Death: a historical study of the evolution of the Dance of Death mythus in art, 142 p. (New York, N.Y.: Hoeber).—

A reprint of a series of articles from the Annals of Medical History, N.S., vols. 2 and 3. It contains a chronological history of the dance macabre, a motive that found wide expression throughout Christian Europe in frescoes, charnel-houses, cloisters, churchyards, paintings, tapestries, clocks, drinking cups, prayer books, and sculptures. In this study the author traces and interprets the representations of the physicians. A book of similar scope is: BLOCK, W., 1966: Der Arzt und der Tod. In Bildern aus sechs Jahrhunderten, 194 p. (Stuttgart: Enke).

WITHINGTON, E. T., 1964: Medical history from the earliest times, 424 p. (London: Holland Press).—

This is a reprint of the 1854 edition and one of the best short histories ever written. Owing to its popularity it now has been reprinted. However, no attempt has been made to bring the book up-to-date, so that the author ends his history with Bichat, and does not deal with medical history of the 19th century.

WOGLOM, W. H., 1949: Discoverers for medicine, 229 p. (New Haven, Conn.: Yale U.P.; London: Oxford U.P.).—

The subject of this book is to present case-histories of scientific discoveries made by "amateurs" that have led to notable advances in medicine, *e.g.*, Stephen Hales and blood pressure; Lavoisier and respiration; Withering and the foxglove; Jenner and vaccination; Garcia and the laryngeal mirror; Guyot and the Eustachian tube; Franklin and the eyeglasses and spectacles; Renucci and the itch; Metchnikoff and phagocytosis; Roentgen and X-rays; Mendel and heredity; Rowe and milk sickness. The author also cites the contributions made by medicine to etching, music, literature, politics and science. Good bibliography and index.

b. *Some regional medical histories of a more general importance*

b.* *Europe*

Austria

BREITNER, B., 1951: Geschichte der Medizin in Oesterreich, 270 p. (Oesterr. Akad. Wiss., phil.-hist. Kl., vol. 226, pt. 5) (Vienna: Rohrer).—

    Among the topics discussed are: the historical development of Austrian folk medicine (of which a very good review has been given), the role of the University of Vienna, the medical schools of Graz and Innsbruck, and the medical achievements of *e.g.,* Billroth, J. P. Frank, A. v. Eiselsberg, I. P. Semmelweiss, Freud, L. v. Auenbrugger, and others.

LESKÝ, E., 1965: Die wiener medizinische Schule im 19. Jahrhundert, 660 p. (Studien zur Geschichte der Universität Wien, Vol. VI) (Graz/Cologne: Böhlau).—

    A detailed history of Vienna's medical school and its teachers during the 19th century (its most famous period) based on original sources such as the various archives of Vienna, and unpublished autobiographies, and also on an enormous bibliographical material. There are one hundred pictures, mainly consisting of portraits of 19th-century Vienna physicians. A somewhat older Viennese medical history written for students and practising physicians, covering a period of six centuries, is: SCHÖNBAUER, L., 1947: Das medizinische Wien. Geschichte. Werden. Würdigung, ed. 2, 484 p. (Vienna: Urban & Schwarzenberg). It contains some 214 illustrations, a bibliography and an index. The first edition of this book appeared in 1944. For a collection of excerpts from diaries, daybooks, travels, and memoirs of visitors to medical Vienna from the days of van Swieten to the Vienna Congress (1815), accompanied by commentaries, *vide:* NEUBURGER, M., 1921: Das alte medizinische Wien in zeitgenössische Schilderungen, 264 p. (Vienna & Leipzig: Perles). *Cf.* also KÜHNEL, H., 1965, *vide* section The Middle Ages in the Latin West, subsection c.

Belgium

FLORKIN, M., 1954: Médecine et médecins au Pays de Liège, 231 p. (Univ. Liège, Travaux du séminaire d'histoire de la médecine, Vol. I) (Liège: Vaillant-Carmanne).—

    A logical history, covering two centuries of medical life in Liège and in the neighbouring town of Spa. The first part of the book is mainly devoted to three 18th-century physicians who were strongly influenced by Boerhaave, *viz.,* le Dran, de Presseux, and de Limbourg. These physicians were unanimous in their belief that the waters of Spa were of remarkable therapeutic efficacy in the treatment of many diseases. The second part of the book deals more particularly with Pierre Hubert Nysten, who became famous as the author of a medical dictionary which remained popular for many decades. Some chapters of this book go far beyond its local interest, because the springs in the neighbourhood of Spa were of major importance in reviving a world-wide interest in baths and mineral springs during the 18th and 19th centuries. Also written by M. FLORKIN: Médecins, libertins et pasquins, 1964, 198 p. (Médecine et médecins au Pays de Liège, Vol. 3) (Liège: Gothier).

RENAUX, E., A. DALCQ & J. GOVAERTS, 1947: Aperçu de l'histoire de la médecine en Belgique, 85 p. (Collection Nationale, No. 84) (Bruxelles: Office de Publicité).—

    Sarton writes about this book in Isis 40: 183 "History of medicine in Belgium divided as follows: I. Anatomy, histology, embryology. II. Surgery. III Medicine and experimental sciences. Indexes of people and subjects. 20 portraits.

SCHWETZ, J., 1946: L'évolution de la médecine au Congo belge, 132 p. (Actualités sociales, nouv. série) (Bruxelles: Office de Publicité).—

    A history of the development of health services in the former Belgian African colony, written for the general reader. From 1908 onwards medical services were gradually organized. More than half of the publication has been devoted to the suppression of sleeping sickness and malaria, a fight in the course of which the colonial government developed a system of social medical services, with stress on prevention rather than cure.

Croatia

GRMEK, M. D., 1955: Hrvatska medicinska bibliografija; opis tiskanih knjiga i članaka s produčja humane i veterinarske medicine i farmacije, koji se odnose na Hrvatsku. Dio I: Knjige Svl: 1470-1875, 230 p. [Croatian medical bibliography. Description of printed books and articles from the area of human and veterinary medicine and pharmacy that bear upon Croatia. Vol. I., part 1: 1470-1875] (Zagreb: Izdavacki Zavod Jugoslavenske Akademije).—

> The book not only contains scientific works from the fields mentioned in the title, but also medico-educational works, descriptions of conditions of health, public medicine, health institutions, curative herbs and waters, considerations of animal husbandry, descriptions of certain epidemics, surveys of the organization of health services, and biographies of distinguished physicians.

France

ACKERKNECHT, E. H., 1967: Medicine at the Paris hospitals 1794-1848, 242 p. (Baltimore, Md.: Johns Hopkins U.P.).—

> Considers such famous men as P. J. G. Cabanis, Pinel, Bichat, Broussais, Corvisart, Bayle, Laënnec, Chomel. Louis, Andral, Trousseau, and many others.

BARUK, H., 1967: La psychiatrie française de Pinel à nos jours, 152 p. (Paris: Presses Univ. de France).—

> A history of French psychiatry since the days of Pinel. Special attention has been paid to Pinel, Magnan, Kraepelin, Seglas, Clérambault, A. L. Bayle, Morel, and Janet.

BRUNET, P., 1926: Les physiciens hollandais et la méthode expérimentale en France au XVIIIème siècle, 154 p. (Paris: Blanchard).—

> A study of Dutch Cartesianism and its influence on medicine via Leeuwenhoek, Boerhaave, 's-Gravensande, P. and J. Musschenbroeck; and its influence on France

(Nollet, du Fay, Deslandes, Sigaud de la Fond, la Mettrie, de Joncourt, Allamand, *etc.*).

COURY, C., 1968: L'enseignement de la médecine en France dès origines à nos jours, 200 p. (Paris: L'expansion scientifique française).—

> A brief history of medical teaching in France from Carolingian times onward. Stress has been laid on increasing formalism in medical education in pre-revolutionary France, and the new approach to clinical medicine after the Revolution and the increasing significance of the hospital in medical teaching. This study also contains much information on such subjects as: medical corporations, extra-mural courses, private teaching, and professional and scientific societies and their publications.

DARNTON, R., 1968: Mesmerism and the end of the Enlightenment in France, 218 p. (Cambridge, Mass.: Harvard U.P.; London: Oxford U.P.).—

> Mesmerism has its origins in the theory that health depended on the harmony between the individual microcosm and the celestial macrocosm, in combination with the application of electricity, a mysterious "fluid" present throughout the universe, affecting the human body. F. A. Mesmer based a system of cure upon this mixture of ideas which was very attractive to his contemporaries. The present book tries to demonstrate the influence of these ideas on the social and political climate from the eve of the French Revolution up to Victor Hugo.

DE FOURMESTRAUX, I., 1934: Histoire de la chirurgie française (1790-1920), 232 p. (Paris: Masson).—

> A history of French surgery from the French Revolution onwards, and ending in 1920.

DELAUNAY, P., 1935: La vie médicale au XVIe, XVIIe et XVIIIe siècles, 556 p. (Paris: Ed. Hippocrate).—

> Deals with students of medicine, especially with the private, professional, corporative, religious, political, social, intellectual, and doctrinal life of the physician during the period considered. A book dealing with 19th-century French medicine is: CARIAGE, J.L., 1965: L'exercice de la médecine en France à la fin du XIXe siècle et au

début du XXe siècle (Honoraires-Syndicats-Éthique médicale), 434 p. (Besançon). Unfortunately I cannot give further information about this book.

LÉVY-VALENSI, J., 1933: La médecine et les médecins français au XVIIe siècle, 668 p. (Paris: Baillière).—

A thorough study of 17th-century French medicine, dealing with the position, contents, *etc.,* of medical science in general (incl. the treatment of various diseases, therapeutics, surgery, *etc.,* p. 1-218), with medical education, public services (incl. hospitals), and with the medical practitioner (physician, surgeon, midwife, barber, apothecary). The last section (p. 487-661) contains 37 biographies of French physicians, some surgeons, and midwives, living during the period considered.

GUIART, J., 1948: Histoire de la médecine française. Son passé, son présent, son avenir, 290 p. (Paris: Nagel).—

This brief chronological survey contains the following chapters: Notre mère de la Grèce (from Hippocrates to Galen); De la préhistoire à la Gaule (magic medicine); La Gaule romaine (Graeco-Roman medicine); Les temps barbares (religious and lay medicine); La naissance des universités (Arabian medicine, the renaissance of the 13th century); La grande renaissance (the century of anatomy); Le XVIIe siècle; le XVIIIe siècle (surgery and the beginnings of pharmacy); Révolution et Empire (organization of surgical and pharmaceutical education); Le XIXe siècle (clinical medicine and the birth of homoeopathy, the triumph of bacteriology); Période contemporaine (triumph of parasitology and tropical medicine); La médecine de demain (the renaissance of Hippocratic medicine). An outline of the history of French medicine is to be found in: LAIGNEL-LAVASTINE, M. & M. R. MOLINERY, 1934: French medicine, 188 p. (Clio Medica, No. 15) (New York, N.Y.: Hoeber). *Cf.* also MACKINNEY, L. C., 1937, *vide* section The Middle Ages in the Latin West, subsection c.

MAURIAC, P., 1956: Libre histoire de la médecine française, 287 p. (Paris: Stock).—

The first part of this book *(ca.* 150 p.) deals with the history of French medicine from the Middle Ages up to the end of last century. The last part considers some aspects of the development of medicine since Pasteur, and mainly deals with the progress of some specialties.

VALLERY-RADOT, P., 1947: Deux siècles d'histoire hospitalière de Henri IV à Louis Philippe, 1602-1863. Paris d'autrefois; ses vieux hôpitaux, 262 p. (Paris: Dupont).—

A history of the Paris hospitals between 1602 and 1836. Of each of the hospitals considered (*e.g.,* Hôtel Dieu, Saint-Louis, La Charité, Bicêtre, La Salpêtrière), he gives a vivid description of its present state and the history of its various components and of the most famous physicians who worked there, *e.g.,* l'Hôtel-Dieu: Bichat, Dupuytren, Trousseau; La Charité: Corvisart, Laënnec; St. Louis: Alibert, Bazin, Fournier; La Pitié: Lasègue, Jaccoud, Babinski; Les Incurables: Mm. de la Sablière, Landouzy; Bicêtre: Pinel; la Salpêtrière: Pinel, Esquirol, Charcot; Necker: Laënnec, Guyon; Cochin: Widal; Beaujon: Robin; Saint-Antoine: Hayem, Hanot, Chauffard; Le Val de Grâce: Larrey, Desgenettes, Vincent; la Maternité; and some others. Continued in: VALLERY-RADOT, P., 1948: Un siècle d'histoire hospitalière de Louis Philippe jusqu'à nos jours, 1837-1949; nos hôpitaux parisiens, 219 p. (Paris: Dupont).

WICKERSHEIMER, E., 1906: La médecine et les médecins en France à l'époque de la Renaissance, 668 p. (Paris: Maloine).—

Deals with such topics as: physicians and society (dress, fees, quacks, *etc.),* the medical schools, the students, courses, examinations, *etc.* in Paris, Montpellier and the other French universities, surgery in Paris and in the country, medical doctrines, anatomy, embryology, physiology, public and personal hygiene, hospitals, pathology, obstetrics and gynaecology, therapeutics, the apothecary, and legal medicine.

Germany

FISCHER, W. & G. GRUBER, 1949: Fünfzig Jahre Pathologie in Deutschland, 334 p. (Stuttgart: Thieme).—

A good history of the development of modern pathology in Germany. Useful bibliography and elaborate index.

GOERKE, H., ed., 1965: Berliner Aerzte. Selbstzeugnissen, 308 p. (Berlin: Berliner Verlag).—

Contains much biographical material in the form of biographies, letters, lectures, and extracts from diaries and publications of, *e.g.,* Virchow, von Graeffe, Leyden, von Bregmann, Koch, and A. Bier.

HABERLING, W. G. M., 1934: German medicine, 160 p. (Clio Medica, No. 13) (New York, N.Y.: Hoeber).—

An attempt to give an account of the development of medicine in Germany and to discuss the role of German medicine in the development of medicine in general. Separate sections deal with German medicine during Antiquity, and during the Middle Ages, with Paracelsus, F. Hoffmann, Stahl, von Haller, van Swieten, natural philosophy, magnetism, homoeopathy, Joh. Müller, T. Schwann, R. Virchow. R. Koch, E. Behring, P. Ehrlich, and with the development of modern specialties.

JETTER, D., 1966: Geschichte des Hospitals. I. Westdeutschland von den Anfängen bis 1850, 271 p. (Sudhoffs Archiv, Beiheft 5) (Wiesbaden: Steiner).—

The story starts with the Roman valetudinaries and ends with the year 1848, because after that date the material available is too abundant to be incorporated in this study. The study is restricted to Western Germany (a study of French hospitals is announced in the preface of this study), and deals with such subjects as: the hospital of the emperor, of bishops and monasteries in the Middle Ages, municipal and university hospitals, houses of correction, madhouses and mental hospitals.

KILLIAN, H. & G. KRÄMER, 1951: Meister der Chirurgie und die Chirurgenschulen im deutschen Raum. Deutschland, Oesterreich, Deutsche-Schweiz, 231 p. (Stuttgart: Thieme).—

This is a history of surgeons and surgical schools. The first 31 pages give a historical introduction to surgery up to about 1860. The other pages contain the surgical history of 35 German-speaking universities, together with a list of all professors of surgery with short accounts of their life and work. This book does not seem to be fully reliable; therefore great caution should be observed.

LEIBBRAND, W., 1956: Die spekulative Medizin der Romantik, 324 p. (Hamburg: Claasen).—

A history of medicine as it occurred in Germany in the first part of the last century. It is an extension of a former work of the same author, entitled: Romantische Medizin, 1938, 210 p. (Hamburg & Leipzig:

Goverts). *Cf.* WEHNELT, B., 1943, *vide* section History of the pure plant sciences, subsection d.

MITSCHERLICH, A. & F. MIELKE, 1949: Doctors of infamy: the story of the Nazi medical crimes. With statements by three American authorities identified with the Nuremberg medical trial: Andrew C. Ivy, Telford Taylor, and Leo Alexander. And a note on medical ethics by Albert Deutsch. (Including the new Hippocratic oath of the World Medical Association), 39 + 172 + 13 p. + 16 p. of photographs. (New York, N.Y.: Schuman).—

In this book the authors recount the evidence presented at the Nuremberg trial of 23 German physicians accused of carrying out experiments on Jews, Poles, Russians, and Catholic priests. The book has been written mainly to inform the German medical profession and the German public of the Nazi criminal activities conducted under medical auspices. It deals especially with the experiments performed to discover the minimal conditions for functional survival of human beings and the extermination programme carried out under medical auspices during the period of Nazism. Originally published in the German language: Das Diktat der Menschenverachtung, eine Dokumentation vom Prozess gegen 23 SS-Aerzte und deutsche Wissenschaftler, 175 p. (Heidelberg: Schneider).

ROHLFS, H., 1875-1880: Geschichte der deutschen Medizin. Die medicinischen Classiker Deutschlands, 2 vols., 1212 p. (Stuttgart: Enke).—

Vol. I considers P. G. W. Werlhof, 1699-1767 (p. 31-81); J. G. Z. von Zimmermann, 1728-1795 (p. 82-134); J. E. W. Wichmann, 1740-1802 (p. 135-175); P. G. H. Hensler, 1733-1805 (p. 176-247); J. S. Stieglitz, 1767-1840 (p. 248-322); K. F. H. Marx, 1796-1877 (p. 323-429); E. L. Heim, 1747-1834 (p. 480-520); P. K. Krukenberg, 1788-1865 (p. 520-556). Unfortunately I have been unable to consult the second vol.

SCHOLZ, W., 1961: 50 Jahre Neuropathologie in Deutschland, 1885-1936, 123 p. (Stuttgart: Thieme).—

Separate chapters deal with Carl Weigert, L. Edinger, F. Nissl, A. Alzheimer, A. Jacob, W. Spielmeyer, Oskar and Cecile Vogt, M. Bielschowsky, K. Brodmann, and E. Kraepelin. Together these biographies give a vivid picture of the development of cellular pathology of the nervous system between 1885 and 1935. *Cf.* KIRCHHOFF, T., 1921: Deutsche Irrenärzte. Einzelbilder ihres Lebens und Wirkens, *vide* section Biographical dictionaries, subsection c.

Great Britain and Ireland

CLARK, G., 1964-1966: A history of the Royal College of Physicians of London, 2 vols. Vol. I (1964): 425 p.; Vol. II (1966): 373 p. (Oxford: Clarendon Press).—

This work, based on original sources, preserved mainly by the College itself, is the first to give a connected account of the College as an institution and of its place in social history. The first vol. deals with the period between 1518 and 1688, a period marked by religious upheaval, wars, plague, fire and famine. It deals with such subjects as: the state of medical care in Britain prior to the foundation of the College; Thomas Linacre, co-founder, first president, and benefactor of the College; the Royal Charter of 23 September 1518 by which the College received licensing powers; the opposition from rival corporations of surgeons and apothecaries; the many quarrels between the members of the College; John Caius, William Harvey. The second vol. covers the history of the College between the Glorious Revolution of 1688 and the Medical Act of 1858. *Cf.* also: WOLSTEN-HOLME, G., ed., 1964: The Royal College of Physicians of London: portraits, 468 p. (Portraits described by D. PIPER) (London: Churchill); and MUNK, W., ed., 1878: The roll of the Royal College of Physicians of London, *vide* section Biographical dictionaries, subsection c.

COMRIE, J. D., 1932: History of Scottish medicine, ed. 2, Vol. I: 396 p.; Vol. II: 441 p. (London: Baillière, Tindall & Cox).—

Vol. I deals with Scottish medicine from its primitive phase up to the establishment of the early medical schools at Aberdeen and King's College. It contains much information concerning medicine during the Roman occupation, folk medicine and cures, ancient lore connected with charms, spells and amulets. Besides it gives interesting biographical information of Highland physicians; and a special chapter deals with early public health enactments and measures against leprosy and syphilis. Vol. II discusses the development of general and of military medicine from the 18th century up to *ca.* 1930. For the history of Scottish psychiatry *cf.* HENDERSON, D. K., 1964, *vide infra.*

COPE, Z., 1959: The Royal College of Surgeons of England: a history, 360 p. (London: Blond).—

The history of the Royal College goes back to 1800. The Royal College was preceded by the Surgeon's Company (1745-1800) (*cf.* WALL, C., 1937: A history of the Surgeon's Company 1745-1800, 255 p., London: Hutchinson), and the United Company of Barber Surgeons, founded in 1540 (*cf.* YOUNG, S., 1890: The annals of the Barber Surgeons of London: compiled from their records and other sources, 623 p., London: Blades, East & Blades). A decisive factor in the establishment of the College was the purchase of the Hunterian Collection, comprising preparations dealing with pathological and anatomical subjects, which collection is allocated to the Hunterian Museum (*cf.* NEGUS, V., 1966: Royal College of Surgeons of England: history of the trustees of the Hunterian Collection, 140 p., Edinburgh & London: Livingstone). This book by Cope covers a very important period in the history of surgery; life and work of many outstanding Fellows of the College have been considered. *Cf.* also: LEFANU, W., ed., 1960: A catalogue of the portraits and other paintings, drawings and sculpture in the Royal College of Surgeons of England; and: PLARR, V. G., ed., 1930: Plarr's lives of the Fellows of the Royal College of Surgeons of England, *vide* section Biographical dictionaries, subsection c.

COPEMAN, W. S. C., 1960: Doctors and disease in Tudor times, 186 p. (London: Dawson).—

A study of the position and influence of the Royal College of Physicians, the Barber Surgeons Company, and the Society of Apothecaries during the period considered. Other subjects discussed are: medical education, the role played by humoral pathology, herbals, astrology, alchemy, magic, *etc.,* the art of diagnosis, the use of drugs, bloodletting, the methods used in surgery and in preventive medicine, *etc.*

DAVIDSON, M., 1955: The Royal Society of Medicine: the realization of an ideal (1805-1955), 201 p. (London: Royal Soc. Medicine).—

A story of the origins and growth of the Royal Society of Medicine of Great Britain. The record was prepared for the celebration of fifty years of amalgamation of the Medical and Chirurgical Society with the Royal Colleges of Medicine and of Surgery and with the special societies to the number of some sixteen, as parts of the Royal Society of Medicine. The greater part of the work has been devoted to the period 1905-1955; the history of the first hundred years was already recorded in the centenary volume of 1905: The Royal Society of Medicine: records of the events and work which led to the formation of that society by the amalgamation of the leading medical societies of London with the Royal Medical and Chirurgical Society. Being extracts from the medico-chirurgical Transactions, 1905-1907. London, 1914.

DEBUS, A. G., 1965: The English Paracelsians, 222 p. (Oldbourne History of Science Library) (London: Oldbourne).—

A book about Paracelsianism in England before 1640. Only two Englishmen can be considered to be direct followers of Paracelsus, *viz.*, Bostocke and Fludd. The author makes clear that English apothecaries accepted the new drugs Paracelsus introduced but generally rejected his mystic theory.

FLEETWOOD, J., 1951: History of medicine in Ireland, 420 p. (Dublin: Browne & Nolan, Richview Press).—

This book contains a wealth of information concerning the development of Irish medicine from prehistory up to recent times. It discusses such topics as: descriptions of diseases occurring in the Bronze Age; pre-Christian medicine in Ireland, a mixture of folklore with pagan and Christian superstitions; the role of the Druidic priests; leper houses; the story of the Trinity College, Dublin; the story of the Royal College of Physicians, the Royal College of Surgeons, the Apothecaries, the Dublin School of Midwifery, the Belfast School, and the story of famous hospitals, medical schools, and professional societies. Re-issued in 1964 (Mystic, Conn.: Verry).

GRAY, J., 1952: History of the Royal Medical Society 1739-1937, 355 p. (Edinburgh: U.P.).—

A readable history of the Royal Medical Society at Edinburgh. Especially the history of its first period has been treated very well. After the author died in 1942, the material was prepared for press by D. GUTHRIE. The study has been based upon the Society's minutes and many printed materials. The study contains much personal information about many a distinguished physician who once has been member of the Society. Good index and an appendix listing the names of the annual presidents (four a year) from 1764 up to 1952.

HENDERSON, D. K., 1964: The evolution of psychiatry in Scotland, 300 p. (Edinburgh & London: Livingstone).—

The first half of the book is concerned with the history of psychiatry in Scotland before Henderson came on the scene, the second half is an account of his own experiences and of the development of modern psychiatry both in Scotland and in England. An evaluation of the Edinburgh School of psychiatry and its influence on the development of psychiatry, especially in Great Britain and France.

JARAMILLO-ARANGO, J., 1953: The British contribution to medicine, 220 p. (Edinburgh & London: Livingstone).—

A historical review of British contributions to quite recent achievements of medicine. The text was primarily designed for the information of physicians, surgeons, and students of medicine in the Latin-American countries. It contains a detailed study of five special subjects in which British investigators achieved major discoveries, *e.g.*, the conquest of typhoid and paratyphoid fevers (Almroth Wright), the conquest of infection (Alex. Fleming, H. Florey, E. Chain), the history of antibiotics (incl. recent work on streptomycin), the conquest of malaria (Patrick Manson, Ronald Ross), vitamins and the conquest of nutritional diseases (F. G. Hopkins, E. Mellanby). A concluding chapter contains an account of the struggle for the conquest of cancer.

LEIGH, D., 1961: The historical development of British psychiatry, Vol. I: Eighteenth and nineteenth centuries, 277 p. (Oxford & New York, N.Y.: Pergamon).—

The contents of this book are focussed upon three major figures, *viz.*, John Haslam (1767-1844), James Cowles Prichard (1786-1848), and John Conolly (1794-1866). The author also discusses the status of mental hospitals, the practice of blood-letting, of cupping and scarifying, and the methods for mechanical restriction of the patients.

MACMICHAEL, W., 1953: The gold-headed cane, ed. 6, 32 + 185 p. (Springfield, Ill.: Thomas).—

This is an "autobiography" of the gold-headed cane which now rests in a glass case in the library of the College of Physicians, London. The owners of the cane were five famous London physicians of the period from 1650 to 1823. The first of them was

John Radcliffe, the others R. Mead, A. Askew, William and David Pitcairn, and M. Baillie. The cane, in delightful autobiographical style, chats about the great medical events of England, and in this way it not only gives much biographical information of its several owners, but it also contains interesting information on the conditions of medicine in England, especially during the 18th century. Its life-history was written down by Wm. Macmichael and was published anonymously in 1827 (London: Murray). A year later, in 1828, a second edition appeared (London: Murray). This second edition has been reprinted in 1932, supplied by explanatory and illustrative notes and an essay on William Macmichael, M. D., his life, his works, and his editors, by H. S. RO-BINSON. It contains the original illustrations of the 1828 edition and hitherto unpublished portraits of the Macmichael family and a reproduction of William Macmichael's handwriting, 31 + 223 p. (New York, N.Y.: Froben). A third edition, ed. by W. MUNK appeared in 1884 (London: Longmans, Green). This edition was reprinted in 1965, 206 p. (London: Johnson). A fourth edition appeared in 1915, ed. by F. R. PACKARD (New York, N.Y.: Hoeber), and a fifth appeared in 1923, with introduction and annotations by G. C. PEACHEY, 195 p. (London: Kimpton). That edition was reprinted in 1930. (New York, N.Y.: Macmillan). A reprint of the original edition was published in 1968 by the Royal College of Physicians, London, 26 + 179 p.

MOORE, N., 1908: The history of the study of medicine in the British Isles, 202 p. (Oxford: Clarendon Press).—

This book contains the text of a series of 4 lectures. The first deals with medical study in London during the Middle Ages and with John Mirfeld, a physician who lived in London in the reign of Richard II. The second lecture deals with the education of physicians in London in the 17th century (*inter alia,* T. Linacre, John Caius, E. Browne), the third and fourth lectures deal with the history of the study of clinical medicine (John Caius, W. Gilbert, W. Harvey, C. Benet, T. Sydenham, W. Heberden, E. Tyson, Hans Sloane, and others), and with the influence of Boerhaave. *Cf.* SILVETTE, H., 1967: The doctor on the stage: medicine and medical men in seventeenth century England, 290 p. (Knoxville, Tenn.: Univ. Tennessee Press).

——, 1918: The history of St. Bartholomew's Hospital, 2 vols. Vol. I: 614 p.; Vol. II: 992 p. (London: Pearson).—

A large-scale history of one of the oldest hospitals in the world, founded in 1123. It includes such aspects as the social life (especially in the City of London), the organization of several parts of the profession of medicine, the growth of medical education, the increase of medical knowledge, and the life of many of those men who have been engaged in the practice and teaching of medicine.

O'MALLEY, C. D., 1965: English medical humanists: Thomas Linacre and John Caius, 54 p. (Logan Clendening lectures on the history and philosophy of medicine, 12th series) (Lawrence, Kans.: Univ. Kansas Press).—

Both humanists, Linacre and Caius, received their medical education in the Univ. of Padua. Both were consistent Galenists; Linacre translated some of Galen's works into Latin from the original Greek, Caius promoted the study of anatomy in Cambridge and London and wrote a famous account of the epidemic of the sweating sickness in England in 1551.

POWER, D'Arcy, 1930: Medicine in the British Isles, 84 p. (Clio Medica, No. 2) (New York, N.Y.: Hoeber).—

An outline, discussing early conditions, medical corporations, the hospitals, medical education, specialism, nursing, medical societies, and some makers of British medicine (John Arderne, Harvey, Sydenham, John Hunter, E. Jenner, Lister, and some others). A study especially dealing with nursing and midwifery in England is: AVELING, J. H., 1967: English midwives: their history and prospects, 186 p. (London: Elliot). This is a reprint of the 1872 edition, with an introduction, a select bibliography of midwifery and a biographical sketch of the author by J. L. THORNTON. *Cf.* also TALBOT, C. H., 1967, *vide* section The Middle Ages in the Latin West, subsection c.

POYNTER, F. N. L., ed., 1964: The evolution of hospitals in Britain, 294 p. (London: Pitman).—

The contents consist of 14 essays entitled: Monastic infirmaries; The Royal hospitals before 1700; The hospital movement of the 18th century; The history of the Dispensary Movement; Materny hospitals; Children's hospitals; Mental hospitals; Naval hospitals; Military hospitals; The rise of specialism and special hospitals; The hospital as a teaching centre; The development of hospital design and planning; The history of hospital finance and administration; The influence of professional nursing on the development of the modern hospital. A more or less anecdotal narrative of the development of hospitals in England from the Middle Ages to the present can be found in: DAINTON, C., 1962: The story of England's hospitals, 184 p. (Springfield, Ill.: Thomas). *Cf.* also: ABEL-SMITH, B & R. PINKER, 1964: The hospitals, 1800-1948: a study in social administration in England and Wales, 514 p. (Cambridge, Mass.: Harvard U.P.; London: Heinemann).

RAACH, J. H., 1962: A directory of English country physicians, 1603-1643, 128 p. (London: Dawsons).—

An alphabetical check-list of 814 licensed physicians who were practising outside London between 1603 (the accession of James I) and 1643 (the abolition of episcopacy). The lists of names are collected in two groups: those appearing in the records of the province of Canterbury, and those of the province of York. Within each group the individuals are firstly arranged alphabetically with their dates, degrees, and places of residence, if these facts are known, and with biographical references, if available. Then comes a listing according to county and town or village. It does not include surgeons.

VAUGHAN, P., 1959: Doctor's commons: a short history of the British Medical Association, 254 p. (London: Heinemann).—

A non-chronological historical review of the various activities performed by the British Medical Assn. *Cf.* LITTLE, E. M., 1932: History of the British Medical Association 1832-1932, 342 p. (London: British Med. Assn.).

WIDDESS, J. D. H., 1963: A history of the Royal College of Physicians of Ireland, 1654-1963, 255 p. (Edinburgh & London: Livingstone).—

Unfortunately all the documents before the 19th century have been lost as a consequence of the fact that the Royal College acquired no permanent home before 1863. This story contains much biographical information.

——, 1967: The Royal College of Surgeons in Ireland and its Medical School, 1784-1966, ed. 2, 152 p. (Edinburgh & London: Livingstone).—

A revision of the first ed., published in 1949. Included are lists of the Presidents

and the Honorary Fellows of the College and its Faculties and a chronological summary of notable events in the history of medicine in Ireland.

Italy

BELLONI, L., ed., 1963: Per la storia della neurologia italiana, 266 p. (Istituto di Storia della Medicina di Milano, Studi e Testi, Vol. 6) (Milan: Università degli Studi).—

This volume records the proceedings of the Intl. Sympos. on the History of Neurology, Varenna, 1961. It contains 19 papers dealing with the contributions of Italians to neurology, but especially to neuro-anatomy and neuro-physiology. Separate studies deal *inter alia* with Leonardo da Vinci, Lombroso, Spallanzani, Fontana, Galvani, Volta, Golgi, and the study of the brain during the Italian Renaissance.

CASTIGLIONI, A., 1932: Italian medicine, 134 p. (Clio Medica, No. 6) (New York, N.Y.: Hoeber).—

A useful historical review of Italian medicine beginning with Empedocles. True Italian medicine began in the 9th century with the founding of the School of Salerno. Among the famous Italian physicians considered are: Leonardo, Berengario, Canano, Vesalius, Falloppio, Colombo, Cesalpino, Fabricius, Spallanzani, Benivieni, Malpighi, Morgagni, Fracastoro, Tagliacozzi. A bibliography, covering the whole field of preclinical and clinical medicine, medical biography and history, and medical institutions is: PAZZINI, A., 1946: Bibliographia di storia della medicina d'Italia, 455 p. (Roma: Tosi). *Cf.* also: TABANELLI, M., 1965, *vide* section The Middle Ages in the Latin West, subsection c.

——, 1934: The Renaissance of medicine in Italy, 91 p. (Publ. Inst. Hist. Med. Johns Hopkins Univ., Ser. 3, No. 1) (Baltimore, Md.: Johns Hopkins U.P.).—

This is the text of a series of two lectures which bear the following titles: 1. The dawn of the renaissance in the life, art and science of Italy; the thought of Leonardo; 2. The flowering of medical studies at the Italian universities from Berengario to Cesalpino; the legacy of scientific renaissance and the main currents of thought from Fracastoro to Galileo. Preface by H. SIGERIST. The author describes how the progress of medicine developed together with trade, exploration, art and letters in one movement of creative thinking; he also considers the relation between Italian Renaissance and the medicine of Classical Antiquity, and the spread of this new Italian knowledge to other parts of Europe.

PITRÉ, G., 1942: Medici, chirurgi, barbieri e speziali antichi in Sicilia. Secoli XIII-XVIII. Curiosità storiche e altri scritti. A cura di Giovanni Gentile, 405 p. (Edizione nazionale, 41) (Firenze: Barbèra).—

> This is vol. 41 of the Opera complete di Giuseppe Pitré. It contains a study of the history of medicine in Sicily from the thirteenth to the eighteenth century. It was first published in Palermo in 1910.

Malta

CASSAR, P., 1965: Medical history of Malta, 586 p. (London: Wellcome Hist. Med. Libr.).—

> This work is especially valuable as to the early history of medicine of Malta. Its importance lies mainly in the fact that the pattern of diseases as it is described in this book is characteristic for most parts of the Mediterranean basin. Special sections deal with the Order of Knights Hospitallers, the development of the Faculty of Medicine of the Royal University, the Infirmary, the evolution of public health, social services, medical education, and with the impact of the two World Wars.

The Netherlands

BAUMANN, E. D., 1951: Uit drie eeuwen Nederlandse geneeskunde, 320 p. (Amsterdam: Meulenhoff).—

> The history of medicine in the Netherlands formally begins with the foundation of the Univ. of Leiden, in 1575. Before that date most physicians and surgeons of the "Low Countries" came from Flanders which now belongs to Belgium. The book starts with a short review of the period immediately preceding the founding of the Leiden University; then chapters follow on: this foundation and the first medical professors in this newly established university (*e.g.,* Pieter van Foreest, Heurnius, Pieter Paauw, Bontius); famous Dutch physicians of the 17th century (*e.g.,* Coster, Tulp, Joh. van Beverwijck, Franciscus de le Boë Sylvius, Joh. de Wale); Dutch achievements in the field of tropical medicine (*cf.* SCHOUTE, *vide infra);* the Leiden School

of iatrochemistry; Dutch anatomy in the 17th century (Joh. van Horne, Fred. Ruysch, Jan Swammerdam, Regnier de Graaf); surgeons of the 17th and 18th centuries; Herman Boerhaave and his pupils (*e.g.,* Gerard van Swieten); Dutch medicine in the 18th century after the death of Boerhaave (*e.g.,* Matth. and Steven Jan van Geuns, Ed. Sandifort, W. van Doeveren, Petrus Camper, *etc.*); a short review of Dutch medicine in the 19th century.

SCHOUTE, D., 1929: De geneeskunde in dienst der Oost-Indische Compagnie in Nederlandsch-Indië, 347 p. (Amsterdam: de Bussy).—

> A history of medicine in the service of the Dutch East-Indian Company in the former Dutch East Indies, primarily dealing with the 17th and 18th centuries. The text is an important contribution to the history of tropical medicine. The medicine introduced was primarily Dutch in origin. A continuation of this work is: SCHOUTE, D., 1936: De geneeskunde in Nederlands-Indië gedurende de negentiende eeuw, 381 p. (Batavia: Kolff).

——, 1937: Occidental therapeutics in the Netherlands East Indies during three centuries of Netherlands settlement (1600-1900), 214 p. (Publ. Netherlands Indies Public Health Service) (Batavia: Kolff).—

> A concise English summary of what the author had published in the two abovementioned volumes (in Dutch). Separate chapters deal with: the establishment of the United Neth. E.I.C., the surgeons on the Company's ships, the accommodation on the ships, mortality during the voyages, difficulties in victualling the ships; supply of drinking-water, scurvy and fevers, Bontius and his work, Dureus as surgeon, the development of therapeutics in India, the hospitals in the N.E.I. during the 17th century, mortality of Europeans at Batavia, vaccination, the struggle against syphilis, the hospitals, the treatment of the insane, *etc.*

Poland

SOKOŁ, S., 1967: Historia chirurgii w Polsce. Cz. 1. Chirurgia okresu cechowego, 262 p. [A history of surgery in Poland. Part 1. Surgery in the Guild Period] (Polish Acad. Sci., Research Centre Hist. Sci. Technol., Monographs Hist. Sci. Technol., Vol. 37) (Wrocław, Warsaw, Kraków: Ossolineum Publ. House).—

An outline history of surgery in Poland from the middle of the 15th century up to the end of the 18th century. During this period the surgeons were organized in guilds, and the author gives an account of the organization of these guilds. The study has been based upon much source material. Summaries in French and English. A short historical review of the history of medicine in Poland is to be found in: SKARZYNSKI, B., 1956: L'histoire de la médecine en Pologne. Aperçu sur son évolution, 23 p. (Warsaw: Ed. médicales de l'État).

Portugal

PINA, L. de, 1935: Histoire de la médecine portugaise. Abrégé, 132 p. (Porto: Enciclopédia portuguesa).—

The subject is divided as follows: 1. Temps préhistoriques jusqu'à 1130 (Foundation of the School of Santa Cruz, Coimbra); 2. De 1130 à 1290: Institution des études gerais (= générales) à Lisboa: Université; 3. De 1290 à 1504: Statuts de l'Hôpital Royal de Todos-os-Santos, à Lisboa; 4. De 1504 à 1772: réforme des études universitaires: Marquis de Pombal; 5. 1772 à 1825 (Foundation of the schools of surgery of Lisboa and Porto); 6. De 1825 jusqu'à 1900. It is of much biographical interest.

Rumania

BARBU, G., G. BRATESCU & V. MANO-LIU, 1957: Aspects du passé de la médecine dans la République Populaire Roumaine: Iconografie, 210 p. (Bucarest: Ministère de la santé et de la prévoyance sociale, Institut de la santé publique et d'histoire de la médecine).—

An interesting collection of plates, including portraits, views of hospitals, title pages of books and of periodicals devoted to medicine and the sciences, medical manuscripts, implements of folk medicine, etc., from Neolithic times up to the present.

Russia

GANTT, W. H., 1937: Russian medicine, 214 p. (Clio medica, No. 20) (New York, N.Y.: Hoeber).—

A historical review. After a general introduction, chapters follow dealing with such subjects as: the period of primitive medicine up to the reign of Peter the Great;

the period of Peter the Great; foreign influences which followed this period; the period of independent Russian medicine; famines and epidemics; the Great War (1914-1918) and the Revolution; Soviet medicine. Included are a bibliography, a comparative chronology, an author-index and a subject-index. The most elaborate work on the history of Russian medicine is: RICHTER, W. M., 1813-1817: Geschichte der Medizin in Russland, 3 vols. Vol. I: 457 p.; Vol. II: 32 + 440 + 178 p.; Vol. III: 32 + 629 p. (Moscow: Vsevolojsky). This book was recently reprinted (1965) by the Zentralantiquariat, Leipzig. (Not seen).

RAVITCH, M. L., 1937: The romance of Russian medicine, 352 p. (New York, N.Y.: Liveright).—

This book deals with about the same topics as GANTT's booklet (vide supra), but it does so in a more extensive way.

SIGERIST, H. E., 1947: Medicine and health in the Soviet Union, 364 p. (New York, N.Y.: Citadel Press).—

After a short historical introduction, giving an account of conditions as they existed in old Russia down to the time of the Revolution, Sigerist gives an elaborate description of Soviet medicine as it existed and functioned shortly after the Second World War.

Spain

GRANJEL, L. S., 1962: Historia de la medicina española, 206 p. (Barcelona: Sayma).—

A short and introductory history of Spanish medicine. A somewhat older but well-written and fairly complete history of Spanish medicine is: GARCIA DEL REAL, E., 1921: Historia de la medicina en España, 1148 p. (Madrid: Reus-Canizares). L. S. GRANJEL also wrote some books dealing with the history of some medical specialities in Spain, viz., Historia de la oftalmologia española, 1964, 150 p.; Historia de la pediatría española, 1965, 111 p.; Cirurgia española del renacimiento, 1968, 84 p. All these books were published in Salamanca by the Seminario de la historia de la medicina española. As to the history of surgery in Spain, cf. also: RIERA, J., 1968: Los textos quirurgicos españoles de la segunda mitad del siglo XVIII, 98 p. (Reprinted from Cuadernos Hist. Med. Espagñola 7:35-133) (Salamanca: Univ. de Salamanca). As to the legal aspects, *cf.* GARRIDO, R. M., 1967: Ejercicio legal de la medicina en España (siglos XV al XVIII), 158 p. (Cuardernos Hist. Med. Espagñola, Monografías VI) (Salamanca: Univ. de Salamanca). A review of laws and decrees relating to the practice of medicine in Spain from the 15th through the 18th centuries.

——, 1965-1966: Bibliografia historica de la medicina española, 2 vols. Vol. I: (1-2000), 188 p.; Vol. II (2001-4000), 185 p. (Salamanca: Univ. Salamanca).—

> A bibliography of the publications related to the history of medicine in Spain and the former South American colonies. Indexes of authors, of persons whose bibliographies have been written, of subjects, and of pathobiographies. An older, alphabetically arranged bibliography of books, monographs and papers relating to the history of medicine of the Spanish-speaking nations, containing 1,521 references, is: GRANJEL, L. S. & M. S. SANTANDER, 1957: Bibliografia española de historia de la medicina, 242 p. (Publ. del Seminario de historia de la medicina de la Universidad de Salamanca, Ser. B, Vol. 1) (Salamanca: Univ. Salamanca). Included are indexes of biographies, of subjects, and of pathobiographies. *Cf.* also MOREJON, A. H., 1967: Historia bibliografica de la medicina española. A facsimile to the Madrid 1842-1845 edition, 7 vols. (New York, N.Y.: Johnson).

——, 1967: Médicos españoles, 374 p. (Estudios de historia de la medicina española, Vol. 1) (Salamanca: Gráficas Cervantes).—

> A reprint of biographical studies on Spanish physicians published by the author over the past twenty years in different Spanish medical journals. Of each of the persons included are given: a short biographical review, a critical examination of his works, and a bibliographic review of his publications and published references. *Cf.* ALVAREZ-SIERRA, J., 1963: Diccionario de autoridades médicas, 593 p. (Madrid: Ed. Nacional); and GUERRERO, R., 1938-1963: Diccionario biographico y bibliografico de autores farmaceuticos españoles, vol. 1, 802 p. (Madrid). Of these last mentioned books, I am unable to give further information. *Cf.* also: LOPEZ PIÑERO, J. M., 1969, *vide supra,* subsection a.

PINERO, J. M. L., ed., 1967: La trepanación en España. Clásicos neuroquirúrgicos españoles, 480 p. (Madrid).—

> This vol. was prepared on the occasion of the third European Congress of

Neurosurgery, Madrid 1967. It is primarily an evaluation of the role of Spain in the development of surgery. Separate sections deal with prehistoric trepanations on the Iberian peninsula, Spanish contributions to neurosurgery in the Middle Ages, the Renaissance, the 17th century and later periods, the development of neurosurgery in Spain during the last decades of the nineteenth and first decades of the twentieth century.

ULLERSPERGER, J. B., 1954: La historia de la psicologia y de la psiquiatria en España desde los más remotos tiempos hasta la actualidad, 206 p. (Notas y apendices por V. PESET) (Madrid: Ed. Alhambra).—

> The present work was originally published in German in 1871: Die Geschichte der Psychologie und der Psychiatrie in Spanien (Würzburg: Strober's Buchhandlung). The first hundred pages of the present book are devoted to the Greek, Roman, and Arabic periods in Spain. The remaining part of the book consists mainly of a collection of biobibliographical sketches in different fields which are of importance for the history of philosophical psychology rather than for the history of clinical psychiatry. Included is a chapter on the history of the most important mental hospitals of Spain. In a long appendix the translator, V. PESET, gave a summary of the development of mental hospitals and of psychiatric thinking in Spain. The translator also wrote an interesting introduction and has added a considerable number of references and notes to bring the work up to date.

Switzerland

BUESS, H., 1945: Schweizer Aerzte als Forscher, Entdecker und Erfinder, 137 p. (Basle: Ciba Aktiengesellschaft).—

> This booklet gives short biographical reviews together with some bibliographical information (restricted to two pages) of 60 Swiss physicians. Many of them were also actively engaged in botanical and/or zoological investigations. Of the scientists considered we mention: Joachim von Watt (Vadian), Paracelsus, C. Gessner; F. Platter, J. and C. Bauhin, J. v. Muralt, J. J. Scheuchzer, A. v. Haller, C. Vogt. R. A. Koelliker, W. His, F. A. and A. H. Forel, H. Binswanger, E. Bleuler, O. Nägeli, and H. Rorschach.

OLIVIER, E., 1961: Médecine dans le Pays de Vaud, dès origines à la fin du XVIIe siècle, 2 vols., 1033 p. (Lausanne: Payot).—

A very complete history of medicine of this area of Switzerland lying to the north of Lake Geneva. Vol. I consists of the following four parts: 1. prehistoric times and the period of Helvetian independence; 2. the Roman period; 3. from the fifth century to 1536; 4. the period from 1536 to 1680. The second volume deals with epidemic diseases and public health measures, the local diet and the economics of Swiss bath houses. Included is a list of 1,261 physicians. This book may be regarded as a supplement to an older book of OLIVIER: Médecine et santé dans le Pays de Vaud au XVIIIᵉ siècle, 1675-1798, 1939, 1349 p. (Lausanne: Ed. La Concorde). Other important Swiss regional medical histories are: GAUTIER, L., 1906: La médecine à Genève jusqu'à la fin du dixhuitième siècle, 696 p. (Geneva: Georg), and: RENNEFAHRT, H. & E. HINTZSCHE, 1954: Sechshundert Jahre Inselspital, 1354-1954, 544 p. (Bern: Huber). *Cf.* also: BRUNNER, C., 1922, *vide* section The Middle Ages in the Latin West, subsection c.

b.** *Other parts of the world*

Australia

BOSTOCK, J., 1968: The dawn of Australian psychiatry, 219 p. (Sydney: Australasian Publ. Co.).—

> A history of Australian psychiatry during the first half of last century. It contains much source-material on the development of psychiatric facilities, particularly of New South Wales.

COHEN, B. C., 1965: A history of medicine in Western Australia, 168 p. (Perth: Paterson Brokensha Pty).—

> Its contents become clear from its subtitle: "Being a biographical and historical account of medical persons and events from the earliest days until the formation of the Western Australian Branch of B.M.A."

GANDEVIA, B., 1955: An annotated bibliography of the history of medicine in Australia, 140 p. (Monographs Federal Council British Med. Assn. in Australia, No. 1) (Glebe, N.S.W.: Australasian Med. Publ. Co.).—

> A very useful key for anyone interested in the history of Australian medicine. This bibliography includes literature on botany, oceanography, the discovery and exploration of Australia, folk medicine, tropical

diseases as they affected Australia, nursing and on the more recent developments of Australian medicine, *e.g.*, preventive medicine, child welfare, medical societies, *etc.* Many biographies are included.

Canada

HEAGERTY, J. J., 1928: Four centuries of medical history in Canada, and a sketch of the medical history of Newfoundland, 2 vols. Vol. I: 395 p.; Vol. II: 374 p. (Bristol: Wright; Toronto: Macmillan).—

> According to Garrison-Morton, this is the authoritative work on the history of medicine in Canada. A comprehensive and detailed study. *Cf.* also KELLY, H. A. & W. L. BURRAGE, *vide infra*, subsection United States.

HOWELL, W. B., 1933: Medicine in Canada, 138 p. (Clio medica, No. 9) (New York, N.Y.: Hoeber).—

> This study consists mainly of biographies of pioneer physicians working in Canada. Separate chapters deal with: Jacques Cartier; Champlain, Hay, Hébert; Giffard, Madry, Sarrazin, Gaulthier; Goudeau, Pouppé, Bouchard, Martinet, Timothée Sylvain; Amoux, Badelart; Abercrombie; Adam Mabane, Latham; Blanchet; J. Douglas; J. Rolph; Schultz; Arch. Menzies; Tolmie; Helmcken. Other sections deal with l'Hôtel-Dieu in Quebec, the hospitals of Montréal, the medical faculty of McGill College, the Toronto General Hospital, and with the physicians working in the rural districts.

Central and South America*

ARCHILA, R., 1955: Bibliografia médica venezolana, ed. 2, 1041 p. (Caracas: Bellas Artes C.A.).—

> This bibliography, written in Spanish, stretches over a century and covers papers published up to 1951. The publications listed are not restricted to medicine, but include some aspects of biological science and subjects as alien to medicine as biographies, essays, chronicles, and speeches delivered in academies or at convocation ceremonies.

Footnote. Only histories of medicine concerning Central and South America published after 1944 have been included in our bibliography; for the older regional histories see: MOLL, A. A., 1944: Aesculapius in Latin America.

The first edition of this bibliography appeared in 1946. An addendum was published in 1960: Bibliografía médica venezolana, 1952-1958, 40 + 494 p. (Caracas: Imprenta Nacional). This bibliography is arranged alphabetically and includes 5,367 medical titles of works published in Venezuela between 1952 and 1958. It also contains a list of physicians who died during the period, and with short biographies, a catalogue of books published in those years with their reviews, and the titles of scientific films produced in Venezuela.

——, 1961: Historia de la medicina en Venezuela: Época colonial, 617 p. (Caracas: Tip. Vargas).——

This work deals with medical history in Venezuela during the 17th and 18th centuries, mainly based upon original documents. A brief introduction covers medical care during the Conquista and early colonial settlement in the 16th century.

——, 1966: Historia de la medicina en Venezuela, 409 p. (Mérida, Venezuela: Universidad de las Andes).——

A compendium, especially suitable for the medical student who takes a course in the history of medicine. One part (13 pages) deals with the aborigines, another part (107 pages) with the colonial period, and still another part (159 pages) describes medical developments during the era of the republic. Other sections deal with medical institutions, modern hospitals, research, and public health.

CHAVEZ, I., 1947: México en la cultura médica, 187 p. (México, D. F.: Ed. de el Colegio Nacional).——

A description of this book has been given in the section "Prehistoric and primitive biology and medicine", subsection d. The most complete history of Mexican medicine is: FLORES, F. A., 1886-1888: Historia de la medicina en México, 3 vols. (México: Of. Tip. de la Secretaría de Fomento). Doe & Marshall write about this book: "Exhaustive and expensive work. No index but detailed table of contents." According to Doe & Marshall, a brief but useful bibliography is: VAN PATTEN, N., 1930: The medical literature of Mexico and Central America, 49 p. (Bibliographical Soc. of America Papers 24: 150-199).

DURÁN, C. M., 1964: Las ciencias médicas en Guatemala: origen y evolución, ed. 3, 710 p. (Guatemala: Ed. Universitaria).——

A history of medicine in Guatemala starting with the medicine of the Maya Indians up to the beginning of the 20th century. There are 161 illustrations, 31 of which deal with Mayan culture. Indexes of historical names, and of medical authors cited, and a useful bibliography have been included. The first edition was published in 1941, 440 p. (Guatemala: Sanchez & De Guise).

FASTLICHT, S., 1954: Bibliografía odontólogia mexicana, 220 p. (México: La médica mexicana).——

This bibliography of mss. and books on Mexican odontology not only contains medical publications, but includes much archaeological material. Lists of theses presented for graduation at the dental schools of Mexico City, Guadalajara, Mérida, Puebla, Monterrey, and some minor dental schools. Contains some 1,635 entries.

LASTRES, J. B., 1951: Historia de la medicina peruana, 3 vols. Vol. I: La medicina Incaica, 352 p.; Vol. II: La medicina en el Virreinato, 386 p.; Vol. III: La medicina de la República, 387 p. (Lima: Univ. of San Marcos).——

This history of medicine is divided into the pre-Inca and Inca periods, the colonial era, and the republic. The first volume is based on old Spanish and Peruvian records and on folklore; it gives a very good picture of magico-religious healing practice, the role of the *mago* or medicine man, the role of the priests, old surgery, anaesthesia, obstetrics, hygiene, psychotherapy, *etc.*, and of the role of the herbalist. The other volumes deal with such topics as: the establishment of the first hospitals, foundation of the university of San Marcos, the epidemics of the 16th and 17th centuries (verruga, smallpox, measles, typhus, *etc.*), military medicine and surgery, magico-religious medicine in the 16th century, the role of the Inquisition, medico-legal autopsies and the study of anatomy in the 17th century, astrology, the history of the medical society, *etc.* This work also gives much biographical information on famous Peruvian physicians.

LAVAL, M. E., 1958: Noticias sobre los médicos en Chile en los siglos XVI, XVII, y XVIII, 137 p. (Santiago: Centro de Investigación de Historia de la Medicina).——

This book contains biographical and bibliographical material of about 158 physicians in Chile up to the close of the 18th century. It also contains much information that is of interest to the medical history of the neighbouring countries. The classic book on the history of Chilean medicine is FERRER, P. L., 1904: Historia general de la medicina en Chile (documentos inéditos, biografias y bibliografia) desde el descubrimiento y conquista de Chile, en 1535, hasta nuestros dias. (Talca: Imp. Talca).

LOUDET, O., 1966: Médicos argentinos, 238 p. (Buenos Aires).—

I was not able to consult this book, nor could I find any secondary information about it; it seems to be a cumulative biography of Argentine physicians.

MADERO, M., 1955: Historia de la medicina en la provincia del Guayas, 283 p. (Guayaquil, Ecuador: Imprenta de la Casa de le Cultura, Núcleo del Guayas).—

In an introductory chapter the author sets out the culture, diseases, food, hygiene, *etc.*, of the native Indians. Then six chapters follow dealing with the colonial period, considering such subjects as: medical problems occasioned by the Spanish conquest, the spread of "verruga" among the Spaniards, the devastating effects of smallpox among the native peoples, early foundation of hospitals, medical books and doctrines imported from Spain; valuable information has been given of Martin de Porres, friar-surgeon, Pedro Guerrero, botanist, and Juan de Nabez (obstetrician). The last five chapters deal with medicine after the year of independence (1820), especially considering the introduction of quinine for the treatment of malaria, epidemics of yellow fever, the establishment of medical schools, new hospitals, and the development of medical specialities.

MOLL, A. A., 1944: Aesculapius in Latin America, 639 p. (Philadelphia, Pa. & London: Saunders).—

A coherent, richly documented and comprehensive account of the development and status of medicine in Latin America. The subject matter has been divided into two parts. Part I deals with the development of medicine during colonial times (1492-1808) and discusses such topics as: Indian medicine, autochthonous diseases, Spain's medical standing, healers and quacks, early physicians, ship's physicians, medical teaching, medical practice and fees, ancient hospitals, surgery. Part II deals with the independent period considering such subjects as: foreign influences on the new surgery

and clinical medicine, teaching reform, pharmacy, botany, dentistry, increasing medical specialization, progress in social medicine, laboratories and institutions, medical history, literature, journals, academies and societies, pan-American co-operation in medical matters. Appended are a chronology of diseases (a list of diseases alphabetically arranged with the date of the first appearance or identification of each and the name of the author first reporting it, when available), together with a medical and general chronology for Latin America (p. 502-581) and a bibliography which is important because it contains many local medical histories. (See note at the beginning of this subsection.) A more recent, Spanish-written, history of the development of medicine in South America during colonial times is: GUERRA, F., 1953: Historiografía de la medicina colonial hispano-americana, 322 p. (México, D.F.: Abastecedora de Impresos).

ROIG DE LEUCHSENRING, E., 1965: Médicos y medicina en Cuba. Historia, biografia, costumbrismo, 269 p. (La Habana: Acad. Ciencias de Cuba, museo histórico de las ciencias médicas "Carlos J. Finlay").—

A collection of essays written by the author and brought out by the Academy of Science of Cuba on the occasion of his 75th birthday. The text is in three parts, *viz.*, History and biography; Finlayism; Contributions to the cultural history of medicine.

SANTOS, L. de C. filho, 1947: Historia da medicina no Brasil (Do seculo XVI ao seculo XIX), 2 vols., 379 and 429 p. (São Paulo: Edit. Brasiliense).—

Doe & Marshall write about this book: "Arranged by subject. With valuable list of hospitals, medical societies, journals, and short biographies of physicians. Bibliography but no index." Of the same author: Perqueñda historia da medicina brasileira, 1966, 150 p. (São Paulo: DESA). Another study dealing with Brazilian medical history is: NAVA, P., 1948-1949: Capitulos da historia da medicina no Brasil, 136 p. (Brasil Medico-Cirurgico, Vol. 10, nos. 4, 5, 8, 10, and 11, and Vol. 11, no. 1).

SANTOVENIA, E. S., 1952: El protomedicato de la Habana, 78 p. (Havana: Ministerio de Salubridad y Asistencia social).—

A review of early royal physicians of Havana. It contains information about the legal background for the establishment of

King's physicians, their care for the health of the Indians, their position in the 19th century, when they had become responsible for the promotion of public health and sanitary measures in order to prevent epidemics. A historical review of Cuban medical history contains: MARTINEZ-FORTUN Y FOYO, J. A., 1947: Cronología médica cubana. Contribución al estudio de la historia de la medicina en Cuba, fasc. 1: 1492-1800 (Havana).

SCHENDEL, G., et al., 1968: Medicine in Mexico: from Aztec herbs to betatrons, 329 p. (Texas Pan-American Series) (Austin, Tex.: Univ. Texas Press).—

Written with the collaboration of J. ALVAREZ AMÉZQUITA and M. E. BUSTAMENTE. Unfortunately I do not possess further details.

SCHIAFFINO, R., 1927-1937: Historia de la medicina en el Uruguay, 2 vols. Vol. I: 563 p.; Vol. II: 610 p. (Montevideo: Imprenta Nacional "Rosgal").—

The first volume consists of five parts dealing with the following subjects: 1. medicine in Spain at the time of the discovery of America (Arabian influences, Galen, Vesalius, hospitals, etc.); 2. the medicine of the Conquistadores (Hernández, J. de Morales, epidemics); 3. the natives (their medical knowledge, agriculture, foods, use of tobacco, knowledge of herbs, of anatomy and of parasites, therapeutical knowledge, etc.); 4. medicine and missionaries (the role of the Jesuits, their botanical, pharmaceutical and veterinary knowledge, the herbals); 5. medicine and literature (in belles letters, in historiography, etc.). The second vol. deals with such subjects as: the position of medicine in Buenos Aires between 1685 and 1748; medicine in the Portuguese colony Sacramento; Francisco Martín; Fermín Cardoso and José Plá; military and naval medicine; popular medicine between 1764 and 1773; the colonial pharmacopoeia; expeditions in the interior and their medical implications; medicine in the colonial era; the medical academy of Montevideo, founded in 1783; hospitals; urban hygiene; Jasé Giró and his influence, etc. In 1952 a third volume seems to have appeared, but of this volume I could not find any detailed information.

South Africa

BURROWS, E. H., 1958: A history of medicine in South Africa to the end of the nineteenth century, 389 p. (Cape Town: Balkema; London: Koston).—

I was not able to consult this book, nor could I find any secondary information about it.

United States

AUSTIN, R. B., ed., 1961: Early American medical imprints: a guide to works printed in the United States 1668-1820, 240 p. (Washington, D.C.: U.S. Dept. of Health, Education and Welfare).—

This bibliography comprises all known medical imprints published up to 1820 in the territory of the present United States. In it 2,106 titles are described; the description of each book includes the location of copies as well as useful bibliographical annotations. The arrangement of the list is alphabetical: by author when the name is known, or by title if no author can be ascribed. No subject-index.

DAVIS, L., 1960: Fellowship of surgeons: a history of the American College of Surgeons, 523 p. (Springfield, Ill.: Thomas).—

The greater part of this book consists of a biography of F. H. Martin, a Chicago surgeon who was very active in the foundation of the American College of Surgeons.

DEUTSCH, A., 1946: The mentally ill in America: a history of their care and treatment from colonial times, 530 p. (New York, N.Y.: Columbia U.P.).—

A history of the care and treatment of mental patients in America during the last one hundred and fifty years. The book consists of 21 chapters, each of which discusses a phase, a period, or a personality. The most famous American pioneer in introducing a humanitarian approach is Benjamin Rush; this also marks the introduction of humanitarian principles in the establishment of institutions for the mentally ill. Scientific investigations of mental disorders gradually extended and led to a steadily increasing acceptance of the claims of the mentally sick, to the organization of suitable institutions, to the evolution of specialized medical personel, and to the introduction of the study of psychiatry into the medical curriculum. The development of the last phase in the evolution of American psychiatry is also to be found in a commemorative volume initiated by the American

Psychiatric Association in 1944: One hundred years of American psychiatry, 649 p. (New York, N.Y.: Columbia U.P.). There exist two books treating the history of psychoanalysis in America, *viz.,* OBERNDORF, C .P., 1953: A history of psychoanalysis in America, 280 p. (New York, N.Y.: Grune & Stratton), and SHERMAN, M. H., ed., 1966: Psychoanalysis in America: historical perspective, 519 p. (Springfield, Ill.: Thomas).

EARLE, A. S., ed., 1965: Surgery in America: from the colonial era to the twentieth century: selected writings, 280 p. (Philadelphia, Pa.: Saunders).—

This collection of selections must, according to its author, be considered as a by-product of another book, still in preparation, on the history of surgery in America. The present book is an anthology, including such men as: R. W. Buck, J. Bard, J. Jones, J. Thacher, S. White, P. S. Physick, J. S. Dorsey, E. McDowell, N. Smith, W. Beaumont, V. Mott, B. W. Dudley, H. H. A. Beach, H. J. Bigelow, J. C. Warren, J. M. Sims, J. S. Billings, H. O. Marcy, R. Matas, C. McBurney, J. B. Murphy, R. C. Kirkpatric, and W. S. Halsted. A short history of surgery, stressing the more recent developments, is: WHIPPLE, A. O., 1963: The evolution of surgery in the United States, 180 p. (Springfield, Ill.: Thomas).

FISHBEIN, M., ed., 1947: A history of the American Medical Association, 1847-1947, 1226 p. (Philadelphia, Pa. & London: Saunders).—

An encyclopaedic history, edited by Fishbein, with contributions of 28 well-informed persons, members of the A. M. A. staff and of the profession. Much attention has been paid to the Journal published by the Association and to the other publications of the Association.

GORDON, M. B., 1949: Aesculapius comes to the colonies: the story of the early days of medicine in the thirteen original colonies, 560 p. (Ventnor, N.J.: Ventnor Publishers).—

A comprehensive history of medicine in the American colonies before they formed the United States. Each of the colonies is treated separately and those without a comprehensive history are treated more extensively than the others. Good sources for further reading and an extensive index containing many personal names. A recently published important medical history of one of the former colonies is: COWEN, D. L., 1964: Medicine and health in New Jersey: a history, 229 p. (Princeton, N. J.: Van Nostrand).

GUERRA, F., 1962: American medical bibliography, 1639-1783, 885 p. (New York, N.Y.: Harper).—

The subtitle of this bibliography is: "a chronological catalogue and critical and bibliographical study of books, pamphlets, broadsides, and articles in periodical publications relating to the medical sciences - medicine, surgery, pharmacy, dentistry, and veterinary medicine - printed in the present territory of the United States of America during British dominion and the revolutionary war." It includes a valuable "Bibliography of bibliographies", indexes of names and subjects. It also contains much that is of interest to the historian of biology *(e.g.,* medical botany, ethnobiology). *Cf.* MILLER, G., ed., 1964, *vide* section Bibliographies, subsection c.

HOLBROOK, S. H., 1959: The golden age of quackery, 302 p. (New York, N.Y.: Macmillan).—

A popular description of American quackery practice as it flourished during the previous century.

HURD-MEAD, K. C., 1933: Medical women of America: a short history of the pioneer medical women of America and of a few of their colleagues in England, 95 p. (New York, N.Y.: Froben).—

About this book G. Sarton writes in Isis 22: 610: "The author of this book has taken great pains to publish as full and fair an account as possible. Her story is followed by a fine series of portraits and is well indexed."

KAGAN, S. R., 1939: Jewish contributions to medicine in America, from colonial times to the present, ed. 2, 792 p. (Boston, Mass.: Boston Med. Publ. Co.).—

The greater part of the work consists of a classification of the various American Jewish contributors to medicine according to their fields of research, such as: internal medicine, surgery, pediatrics, *etc.* Each subject is supplied with a short biography, emphasizing his scientific accomplishments. Illustrated with many portraits. Index of names.

KELLY, H. A. & W. L. BURRAGE, 1920: American medical biographies, 1320 p. (Baltimore, Md.: Norman, Remington Co.).—

Contains 1,948 biographies of medical men who lived from *ca.* 1600 to 1918. It "serves at once to identify, and to give at least the outline facts in the life of, any eminent departed worthy... Our principle of selection has been to include every man who has in any way contributed to the advancement of medicine in the United States or in Canada, or who... has become illustrious in some other field of general science or in literature." Included are homoeopathic physicians and medical women. Special attention has been paid to those physicians who contributed to the natural sciences (incl. botany and zoology). In 1928 the same authors published: Dictionary of American medical biography: lives of eminent physicians of the United States and Canada from the earliest times, 1364 p. (New York, N.Y. & London: Appleton). *Cf.* THACHER, J., 1967, *vide infra.*

KETT, J. F., 1968: The formation of the American medical profession: the role of institutions, 1780-1860, 217 p. (New Haven, Conn. & London: Yale U.P.).—

A study of early American medical organization, licensing, and education. It contains much interesting information about the formative years of American medical institutions. The first part of the book is restricted to the states of Massachusetts, New York, Maryland, South Carolina, and Ohio. Complementary to this book is: SHRYOCK, R. H., 1967: Medical licensing in America, 1650-1965, 124 p. (Baltimore, Md.: Johns Hopkins Press). *Cf.* also NORWOOD, W. F., 1944: Medical education in the United States before the Civil War, 487 p. (Philadelphia, Pa.: Pennsylvania U.P.); and MEANS, R. K., 1962: A history of health education in the United States, 412 p. (Philadelphia, Pa.: Lee & Febiger).

LONG, E. R., 1962: A history of American pathology, 460 p. (Springfield, Ill.: Thomas).—

A richly documented book containing over 1,000 names of American pathologists. The author states that especially after 1875 American pathology developed in its own specific way. Up to 1925 the author illustrates the development and achievements of American pathology with the aid of historiographies of hospitals, universities, and societies; from 1925 onwards achievements have been reviewed under subject

headings. The author also lists specialized journals, and surveys the history of forensic, veterinary, and dental pathology in the U.S.A. Very useful as a reference work.

MILLER, G., ed., 1964: Bibliography of the history of medicine of the United States and Canada (1939-1960), 428 p. (Baltimore, Md.: Johns Hopkins U.P.).—

For more details *vide* section Bibliographies, subsection e. *Cf.* also: GUERRA, F., 1962, *vide supra.*

PACKARD, F. R., 1931: History of medicine in the United States, 2 vols., ed. 2, 1323 p. (New York, N.Y.: Hoeber).—

According to Garrison-Morton this is the authoritative source-book of the history of medicine in the United States. The two volumes are lavishly illustrated and they contain many noteworthy events in the history of American medicine. Chapter headings are as follows: I. Medical events connected with the early history of the English colonies in America; II. Epidemic sickness and mortality in these colonies from its earliest discovery to the year 1800; III. Early medical legislation; IV. The earliest hospitals; V. Medical education before the foundation of medical schools; VI. The earliest medical schools; VII. Pre-revolutionary medical publications; VIII. The medical profession in the War of Independence; IX. The medical department of the army from the close of the revolution to the close of the Spanish-American war; X. History of the medical department of the U.S. navy; XI. Some medical schools founded during the first half of the 19th century; XII. Outlines of the development of medical practice and education in some of the states; XIII. Foreign influences on American medicine; XIV. Some notable events in American medicine and surgery; XV. The beginnings of specialism in America. Very good indexes. Reprinted in 1963 (New York, N.Y.: Hafner). *Cf.* also: ASHBURN, P. M., 1947, *vide* subsection c (pathology).

SHRYOCK, R. H., 1947: American medical research past and present, 350 p. (New York, N.Y.: Commonwealth Fund).—

A well-documented analysis of current medical problems in the light of their evolution, present status and future trends, and against the background of the many social and economic forces which have influenced the development to their present status. Special attention has been paid to the factors responsible for the sudden flowering of American medicine at the turn of this century. A more special study in this field is: YOUNG, J. H., 1961: The toadstool millionaires: a social history of patent medicines in America before federal regulation, 282 p. (Princeton, N. J.: Princeton U.P.).

——, 1960: Medicine and society in America, 1660-1860, 182 p. (New York, N.Y.: New York U.P.).—

The author describes the mutual relationship between medicine and society in America and he elucidates how successively England, France, and Germany were the medical training centres for American physicians. There are four chapters: 1. The origins of the medical profession; 2. Medical thought and practice: 1600-1820; 3. Health and disease: 1660-1820; 4. Medicine and society in transition: 1820-1860. In this last chapter the rise of American medicine has been described. Throughout the book pioneers of American medicine receive particular attention. The same author also published: Medicine in America: historical essays, 346 p. (Baltimore, Md.: Johns Hopkins U.P.), a series of 15 essays reprinted from various journals and originally published between 1930 and 1962, nearly all of them relating to some aspect of American medical history.

SIGERIST, H. E., 1933: Amerika und die Medizin, 352 p. (Leipzig: Thieme).—

Separate sections deal with the following subjects: physical background; colonial times; the United States; pioneers; medical teaching; physician and patient; hospitals; prophylaxis; science. Included are bibliographical guidance for further study, an author- and a subject-index.

THACHER, J., 1967: American medical biography, 2 vols. Vol. I: 436 p.; Vol. II: 280 p. (New York, N.Y.: Da Capo).—

This is a reprint of the 1828 edition. The subtitle of this work is as follows: "Memoirs of eminent physicians who have flourished in America. To which is prefixed a succinct history of medical science in the United States, from the first settlement of the country." The first 85 pages contain a short history of American medicine. Then the biographies follow, most of them accompanied by a portrait of the physician considered. This new edition is accompanied by a new introduction and a bibliography by W. J. BELL. *Cf.* KELLY, H. A. & W. L. BURRAGE, *vide supra.*

THOMS, H., 1962: Chapters in American obstetrics, ed. 2, 158 p. (Springfield, Ill.: Thomas).—

The first edition of this classic appeared in 1933. Separate chapters deal with W. Shippen (the first public teacher of obstetrics in the U.S.A.), Sam. Bard, O. W. Holmes, W. Potts Dewees, Parvin, Platt, H. Miller, Keep Meigs, Hodge, Storer, Richardson. One chapter deals with the colonial era in which the author pays some attention also to the colony of New Amsterdam.

VAN INGEN, P., 1949: The New York Academy of Medicine: its first hundred years, 585 p. (Hist. of medicine series, No. 8) (New York, N.Y.: Columbia U.P.).—

"The growth of the New York Academy of Medicine during its first hundred years of existence. A record of the contributions made by various doctors and the issues under discussion through the changing years."

WARING, J. I., 1964: A history of medicine in South Carolina, 1670-1825, 407 p. (Charleston, S.C.: South Carolina Med. Assn.).—

Contains the history of medicine of South Carolina from the settlement of Carolina to the founding of the medical school in Charleston. It deals with early colonial practice, the epidemics affecting South Carolina, the controversies around inoculation for smallpox, the role of local physicians in the American Revolution, the role of the South Carolina Medical Society, *etc.* It contains much newly-discovered material and a wealth of biographical data.

——, 1967: A history of medicine in South Carolina, 1825-1900, 366 p. (Charleston, S.C.: South Carolina Med. Assn.).—

This second vol. deals with the growth of hospitals, medical education, epidemics, and the medical care of soldiers in the army of the Confederacy. This vol. also contains a series of biographies of distinguished physicians active during the period 1825-1900.

WEINBERGER, B. W., 1948: An introduction to the history of dentistry in America. Washington's need for medical and dental care. Houdon's life-mask versus his portraitures, vol. 2, 408 p. (St. Louis, Mo.: Mosby).—

A description of this book has been included under dentistry, *vide infra*, subsection c.

c. *Histories of some specialties of a more general importance*

(incl. the histories of some diseases)

c1 *allergology*

BRAY, G. W., 1931: Recent advances in allergy (asthma, hay-fever, eczema, migraine, *etc.*), 432 p. (Philadelphia, Pa.: Blakiston).—

A history of all those pathological conditions which arise from reactions of the individual to foreign proteins. The first part treats of allergy in general, including protein skin reactions; the hereditary nervous, endocrine, nasal, toxic, and environmental factors; changes in the blood; biochemical aspects. The second part treats of the individual manifestations of allergy in asthma; hay-fever; cutaneous allergies including eczema, pruritis, ichthyosis, dermatitis venenata, urticaria, and erythrema; cerebral manifestations in migraine and epilepsy; food allergies in muco-membranous colic and purpura; bacterial, physical, and drug allergies; serum reactions; allergic joint, eye reactions, and hypersensitiveness to insects, parasites, moulds, and fungi.

c2 *blood- and cardiovascular diseases*

BURCH, G. E. & N. P. de PASQUALE, 1964: A history of electrocardiography, 309 p. (Chicago, Ill.: Year Book Medical Publ.).—

After an introduction in which the author evaluates the history and present-day status of electrocardiography, a series of short biographies of the "great men" follows. Much attention has been paid to technical developments since 1910 when the instruments came into clinical use. A chronological summary of main events and a bibliography are added.

DREYFUS, C., 1957: Some milestones in the history of hematology, 87 p. (New York, N.Y. & London: Grune & Stratton).—

The first chapter deals with the history of the development of interest in the study of blood; the next three deal with history of certain specific haematological disorders, and the following chapter consists of a biography of Dr. G. Hayem, a man who made important contributions to haematology. Other chapters deal with the growth of knowledge of some blood diseases, *viz.*, chronic haemolytic anaemia, leukaemia, and polycythaemia vera.

HERRICK, J. B., 1942: A short history of cardiology, 258 p. (Springfield, Ill.: Thomas).—

The greater part of the book reviews in chronological order the history of cardiology from Harvey to Virchow, Pasteur and Koch. The rest of the book (55 pages) discusses in brief chapters: inflammation of the heart, affections of the myocardium, syphilis of the heart and aorta, and the coronary artery and its diseases. Stress has been laid on the clinical aspects rather than on the anatomical and/or physiological aspects. The approach is mainly biographical. A more recent study of the history of heart diseases is: EAST, T., 1957: The story of heart disease, 148 p. (London: Dawson). Its contents consist of the FitzPatric lectures for 1956 and 1957. The lectures are entitled: Diagnosis: lessons of the deadhouse; The coronary circulation and its disorders; Failure of the circulation and its treatment.

ROLLESTON, H. D., 1928: Cardio-vascular diseases since Harvey's discovery, 149 p (Cambridge: U.P.).—

There are chapters on anatomical observation, unaided clinical observation, examination of patients with the aid of instruments of precision, and on physiological and pathological experiments. A bibliography is included.

c3 *dentistry*

CAMPBELL, J. M., 1963: Dentistry then and now, ed. 2, 328 p. (Glasgow: Author).—

A well-written authoritative account of the history of dentistry, considering such famous names as: Eleazer Gidney (1797-1876), Barth. Ruspini (1728-1876), John Hunter (1728-1793), P. Fauchard (1678-1761), T. Purland (1805-1881), J. Smith (1825-1910), O. W. Holmes (1809-1894), J. Scott (*ca.* 1770-1828). There are also chapters on such subjects as: sidelights on bygone dental practice, the odonto-chirurgical society of Scotland, nitrous oxide-ether-chloroform, early dental advertisements, dental paintings and prints, early tooth operations, women dentists, early dental journals, tooth-picks and tooth-brushes, *etc.* A study exclusively dealing with images relating to dentistry is: BRUCK, W., 1921: Zahnärztliche Darstellungen aus alter Zeit, 71 p. (Berlin: Berlinische Verlagsanstalt). A first section is devoted to the martyrdom of St. Apollonia (the author collected 160 representations of it); the rest of the material is divided into three sections: before, during, and after the treatment. *Cf.* also PINDBORG, J. J. & L. MARVITZ, 1960: The dentist in art, 144 p. (Chicago, Ill.: Quadrangle Bks.).

GUERINI, V., 1909: A history of dentistry from the most ancient times until the end of the eighteenth century, 355 p. (Philadelphia, Pa.: Lea & Febiger).—

A nicely illustrated and still very valuable history of dentistry published under the auspices of the National Dental Association. Reprinted in 1967 (Amsterdam: Liberac). The book is in three parts. Part 1 (p. 19-120) deals with antiquity (Egyptians, Hebrews, Chinese, Greeks, Etrurians, Romans, and customs relating to the teeth among different primitive peoples). Part 2 (p. 121-160) deals with the Middle Ages (incl. the Arabians), and part 3 deals with modern times (16th, 17th and 18th centuries).

LUFKIN, A. W., 1948: A history of dentistry, ed. 2, 367 p. (Philadelphia, Pa.: Lea & Febiger).—

This book is especially valuable as an introduction to the history of modern dentistry, a subject not included in SUD-HOFF's "Geschichte der Zahnheilkunde" *(vide infra).* The first part of the section, dealing with modern dentistry, treats of dentistry in Italy, France, Germany, Great Britain and the United States, and stress has been laid on dental legislation and education. The second part is devoted to specialities of dentistry, with chapters on: periodontology; oral surgery; operative dentistry; dental prosthesis. Additional chapters are entitled: "The historical sketches in anesthesia" written by H. ARCHER, and "Orthodontics" written by F. M. CASTO. For the older periods Sudhoff's book must be consulted. A comparable book, though more or less restricted to the development of the art of dentistry as it took place in England, is: SMITH, M., 1958: A short history of dentistry, 120 p. (London: Wingate).

PROSKAUER, C. & F. H. WITT, 1962: Pictorial history of dentistry, 220 p. (Cologne: DuMont Schauberg).—

An attempt to reconstruct the history of dentistry by means of pictures. Besides reproductions of works of art, it also contains many technical illustrations. The order of presentation is roughly chronological. A lavishly illustrated history of dental surgery is: ANDRÉ-BONNET, J. L., 1955: Histoire générale de la chirurgie dentale, 252 p. (Lyon: Éd. du Fleuve). This book was first published in 1910 (Paris: Soc. des auteurs modernes); the text is very brief and seems to be inaccurate!

STRÖMGREN, H. L., 1935-1945: Die Zahnheilkunde im achtzehnten Jahrhundert. Ein Stück Kulturgeschichte (1935): 232 p.; Die Zahnheilkunde im neunzehnten Jahrhundert (1945): 274 p. (Copenhagen: Munksgaard).—

Both volumes give a very interesting picture of the development of dentistry during the respective centuries. They contain a large number of extracts from physicians and dentists of that period, reflecting the major achievements and the scientific spirit of the times. Among the subjects considered are: the introduction of anaesthesia, antisepsis and asepsis, the introduction of the foot-type engine, the improvement of the instruments for dental extraction, dental prosthesis, conservation of the teeth, various theories on the origin of caries, professional societies and organizations, dental journalism, *etc.*

SUDHOFF, K., 1926: Geschichte der Zahnheilkunde, ed. 2, 222 p. (Leipzig: Barth).—

This history of dentistry is one of the best available. It traces its history up to the middle of the 19th century. Special chapters have been devoted to prehistoric and primitive dentistry, to dentistry in the Ancient East and in early America, to dentistry during Antiquity, during the Middle Ages (Muslim and Christian), and during the Renaissance. Reprinted 1964 (Hildesheim: Olms). A concise chronological survey of the history of dentistry is to be found in PRINZ, H., 1945, *vide* section Some recommended encyclopaedias, subsection e. *Cf.* also SOULÉ, A., 1913, *vide* section Antiquity in general, subsection c.

WEINBERGER, B. W., 1948: An introduction to the history of dentistry with medical and dental chronology and bibliographic data, 2 vols. Vol. I: 514 p.; Vol. II: 408 p. (St. Louis, Mo.: Mosby).—

The first volume covers the history up to 1800; the second volume deals with the history of American dentistry, especially with its history in the American Colonies and early Republic. G. B. Denton, in a review of this book in the Bull. Hist. Med. 23: 616, writes: "The work, while not to be recommended for indiscriminate reading, is, however, the most comprehensive and up-to-date contribution available to the serious student of early dental history." *Cf.* also: BLACK, A. D., ed., 1921-1939, *vide* section Bibliographies, subsection e.

C4 *dermatology and venereology*

DUJARDIN, B., 1947: L'histoire de la gale et le roman de l'acare, 158 p. (Arch. belges de dermatol. et de syphilographie, juin 1946, novembre 1946 et février 1947) (Bruxelles: Imprimeries médicales et scientifiques).—

Very elaborate study of scabies from ancient times up to the present. The work is well-documented and contains tranlations of early texts relating to the problem concerned. Separate sections deal with: China; Egypt, Israel, India, Greece, Rome, Spain, Congo, Spanish America; Islam; European treatment of scabies from the 13th century to 1668; Bonomo and Cestoni prove the pathogenic action of the itch mite; scabies in the 18th century; the disease continues to be considered as humoral; 19th century: the role of the mite is definitely established; digression on spontaneous generation; history of the etiology of contagious diseases; influence of the discovery of the itch mite on other discoveries concerning parasitic and microbial diseases.

FRIEDMAN, R., 1947: The story of scabies. Vol. I: The prevalence (civil and military), prevention and treatment of scabies, and the biology of *Acarus scabiei,* from the earliest times to the beginning of World War II, 468 p. (New York, N.Y.: Froben).—

A complete and very scholarly history of scabies, summing up nearly all knowledge of this disease, its causing agent, and the remedies used to cure the results of this disease. In fact this volume is a compilation of two other books written by the same author, *viz.,* Scabies civil and military: its prevalence, prevention and treatment, 1941, 288 p. (New York, N.Y.: Froben), and Biology of *Acarus scabiei,* 1942, 183 p. (New York, N.Y.: Froben).

HOLCOMB, R. C., 1937: Who gave the world syphilis? The Haitian myth, 189 p. (New York, N.Y.: Froben).—

In this book the author tries to destroy the "myth" that syphilis in Europe had its origin in Haiti, and that it was imported with the return of Columbus in 1493. He attacks this by a thorough investigation of the original sources; consequently the book contains much valuable information concerning this problem.

JEANSELME, E., 1931: Histoire de la syphilis: son origine, son extension, 432 p. (In E. JEANSELME & E. SCHULMANN, eds., Traité de la syphilis, Vol. I, p. 1-432) (Paris: Doin).—

A very good and carefully documented monograph, and a standard reference work. It contains a very good bibliography but no index or table of contents. A summary review of its contents can be found in Isis 19: 249-250. There is a lengthy discussion of whether or not it is possible to show the presence of syphilis in Europe before the discovery of America. For further particulars concerning this topic, *cf.* HOLCOMB, R.C., 1937 *(vide supra),* and SUDHOFF, K., 1912: Aus der Frühgeschichte der Syphilis. Handschriften- und Inkunabelstudien, epidemiologische Untersuchungen und kritische Gänge, 175 p. (Leipzig: Barth). A somewhat older detailed study of the early history of syphilis is: BLOCH, I., 1901-1911: Der Ursprung der Syphilis. Eine medizinische und kulturgeschichtliche Untersuchung, 2 vols., 765 p. (Jena: Fischer). Good bibliography. *Cf.* also: TRANCH, C. C., 1964: The royal malady, 245 p. (London: Longmans).

PROKSCH, J. K., 1895: Die Geschichte der venerischen Krankheiten, 2 vols. Vol. I: Alterthum und Mittelalter, 424 p.; Vol. II: Neuzeit, 892 p. (Bonn: Hanstein).—

An exhaustive history of the subject. Another very useful history of venereal diseases is STICKER, G., 1931: Entwurf einer Geschichte der ansteckenden Geschlechtskrankheiten, 339 p. (In: J. JADASSOHN, ed., Handbuch der Haut- und Geschlechtskrankheiten, Vol. 23: 264-603) (Berlin: Springer). An invaluable source of bibliographical information is: PROKSCH, J. K., 1889-1900: Die Literatur über die venerischen Krankheiten von den ersten Schriften über Syphilis aus dem Ende des fünfzehnten Jahrhunderts bis zum Jahre 1889. Supplement Band I. Enthält die Literatur von 1889-1899 und Nachträge aus früherer Zeit, 5 vols. (Bonn: Hanstein).

PUSEY, W. A., 1933: The history of dermatology, 223 p. (Springfield, Ill.: Thomas).
—

A chronological history of dermatology. As far as the present editor is aware, it is the only one in English. It traces the history of dermatology from *ca.* 3000 B.C. up to about 1890. There are good biographies of outstanding dermatologists. A historical index of dermatology (33 p.) contains various synonyms and historical data concerning the various dermatoses. Good bibliography and numerous illustrations.

RICHTER, P., 1928: Geschichte der Dermatologie, 252 p. (In: J. JADASSOHN, ed., Handbuch der Haut- und Geschlechtskrankheiten, Vol. 14, part 2) (Berlin: Springer).—

An authoritative history on the subject. Separate chapters deal with: ancient Semitic cultures (p. 1-10); the non-Semitic cultures of Asia (p. 11-19); dermatology of the Greeks (p. 20-57); Byzantine dermatology (p. 58-74); Hellenistic medicine in Rome (p. 75-86); Arabian dermatology (p. 87-113); the Middle Ages in the Latin West (p. 113-140); the Renaissance (in Italy, France, Germany, and England) (p. 140-174); system-builders and dermatology (p. 175-182); dermatology in England (p. 182-200); French dermatology (p. 200-220); German dermatology (p. 220-244); Italian dermatology (p. 245-246); dermatology in the United States (p. 246-247).

SCHÖNFELD, W., 1954: Kurze Geschichte der Dermatologie und Venerologie und ihre kulturgeschichtliche Spiegelung, 150 p. (Heilkunde und Geisteswelt, Vol. 6) (Hannover-Kirchrode: Oppermann).—

A history of dermatology and venereology from the cultural point of view, from antiquity up to recent times. An older study dealing with the same kind of topics is: HELLER, J. & G. STICKER, 1931: Die Haut- und Geschlechtskrankheiten im Staats-, Zivil- und Sozialrecht. Entwurf einer Geschichte der ansteckenden Krankheiten, 642 p. (In: J. JADASSOHN, ed., Handbuch der Haut- und Geschlechtskrankheiten, Vol. 33) (Berlin: Springer).

WAIN, H., 1947: The unconquered plague: a popular story of gonorrhea, 119 p. (New York, N.Y.: Internat. Univ. Press).—

In a popular style the author gives the history, effects, means of transmission, and prophylaxis of gonorrhea. A very readable account.

c5 *endocrinology*

ROLLESTON, H. D., 1936: The endocrine organs in health and disease. With an historical review, 521 p. (London: Oxford U.P.).
—

According to Garrison-Morton: "As a history of the subject this work is unsurpassed in detail and in accuracy". References to all publications of importance are included.

SCHÖNWETTER, H. P., 1968: Zur Vorgeschichte der Endokrinologie, 70 p. (Zürcher Medizingesch. Abh., N.R., No. 61) (Zurich: Juris).—

The author starts his story in 1652, when Thomas Wharton gave expression to his doubt whether all glands have excretory ducts. Special attention has been paid to the contributions of François de le Boë, Nicholas Steno, Marcello Malpighi, John Hunter, Thomas Willis. Johannes Müller was the first who made a distinction between glands without and with an excretory duct, and it was Claude Bernard who introduced the concept of internal secretion. Brown-Séquard, finally was the founder of the first endocrinological theory. Experimental research in the field of endocrinology starts at the beginning of the present century; in this last period the function of the various organs of internal secretion stands at the centre of interest.

c6 *geriatrics*

GRMEK, M. D., 1958: On ageing and old age: basic problems and historic aspects of gerontology and geriatrics, 106 p. (Monographiae biologicae, Vol. V, No. 2) (The Hague: Junk).—

Separate chapters deal with: definitions, the causes and nature of ageing, its phases and symptoms, longevity and rejuvenation, geriatrics in Antiquity and during the Middle Ages, geriatrics in the 19th century, the history of arteriosclerosis, old age as a psychological and social problem, and the modern geriatric movement. Bibliography and index. Useful sourcebook of the historical aspects of growing old; as such it will be of value to the geriatrician and the historian alike. *Cf.* COMFORT, A., 1956, *vide* section History of Biology, subsection f.

LÜTH, P., 1965: Geschichte der Geriatrie. Dreitausend Jahre Physiologie, Pathologie und Therapie des alten Menschen, 271 p. (Stuttgart: Enke).—

A thorough study of the interrelationship between old men and society. Separate sections are devoted to old men in the Palaeolithicum (cannibalism), in Egypt, in the Bible, in China and India, in Hellas (Corpus Hippocraticum, Plato, Aristotle), in Rome (Pliny, Celsus, Galen), during the Middle Ages (Avicenna, Maimonides, Arnald of Villanova, William of Saliceto, *etc.,* Schools of Salerno and Montpellier), during the Renaissance (Leon. da Vinci, Vesalius, Harvey), during the Enlightenment (D'Alembert, Lamettrie, Maupertuis, Voltaire, Kant), during Romanticism (Goethe, Schelling, Hegel, Novalis, *etc.),* during the 19th century (*e.g.,* Hahnemann, Hufeland, Reil, Virchow, Brown-Séquard), and to modern ideas about old people as expressed by *e.g.,* Nietzsche, Kierkegaard, Jaspers, M. Hartmann. The last chapter has been devoted to the situation of geriatrics in Germany, Austria, Switzerland, France, England, Rumania, Bulgaria, Russia, the U.S.A. and Canada.

C7 *hepatology*

FRANKEN, F. H., 1968: Die Leber und ihre Krankheiten. Zweihundert Jahre Hepathologie, 247 p. (Stuttgart: Enke).—

A study of the historical investigations into the development of the ideas on the construction, the function and the pathology of the liver during the last two centuries. Many biographical annotations in an appendix of 28 pages. Extensive bibliography of 997 items and illuminative tables.

MANI, N., 1965-1967: Die historischen Grundlagen der Leberforschung, 2 vols. Vol. I (1965): Die Vorstellungen über Anatomie, Physiologie und Pathologie der Leber in der Antike, 111 p.; Vol. II (1967): Die Geschichte der Leberforschung von Galen bis Claude Bernard, 649 p. (Basler Veröfftl. Gesch. Med. Biol.) (Basle & Stuttgart: Schwabe).—

In the first part of this study, the author considers the mantic meaning of the liver (Babylonia, Assyria, Greece, Etruria, Rome); the meaning of the liver in ratio-empirical aspects of Egyptian and Babylonian medicine; the liver in Greek medicine: pre-Socratic medicine, the Corpus Hippocraticum, Plato, Aristotle, Diocles of Carystos, the School of Alexandria (p. 19-

51); in Roman medicine: Asklepiades, Celsus, Ruphus of Ephesus, Arataios of Cappadocia, and Galen (p. 52-77). The second part of this study starts with Galen and ends with C. Frerichs (1860). This part consists of 404 pages of text, 136 pages of annotations and 50 pages bibliography. Good index. *Cf.* also section Antiquity in general, subsection c; and HAGEN, H., 1961, *vide* section Classical Antiquity α, subsection b.

C8 *neurology and psychiatry* (incl. some aspects of medical psychology)

ACKERKNECHT, E. H., Kurze Geschichte der Psychiatrie, ed. 2, 107 p. (Stuttgart: Enke).—

Also in English translation: A short history of psychiatry, 104 p. (New York, N.Y.: Hafner). A well-written and clear exposition of the history of psychiatry from prehistoric times up to its latest developments, highlighting the major epochs, and including a number of biographies of the great men in psychiatry. Another "factual", unbiased introduction (as the reviewer wrote in Bull. Hist. Med. 35:388) is: SCHNECK, J. M., 1960: A history of psychiatry, 196 p. (Springfield, Ill.: Thomas). Another short history of psychotherapy is: WALKER, N., 1957: A short history of psychotherapy in theory and practice, 185 p. (London: Routledge & Kegan Paul); about this book I possess no further information.

ALEXANDER, F. G. & S. T. SELESNICK, 1966: The history of psychiatry: an evaluation of psychiatric thought and practice from prehistoric times to the present, 487 p. (New York, N.Y.: Harper & Row).—

The subject matter has been divided into three parts. The first considers the pre-Freudian period. According to Ackerknecht in a review in Science 154: 875, this part of the book is not very reliable. The second part deals with the Freudian age, Freud's own evolution, Abraham, Jones, Ferenczi, Adler, Jung, Rank, Bleuler, Piaget, Binet, Rorschach, A. Meyer. The third part deals with the present: learning theory, psychotherapy, social psychiatry, child psychiatry, psychosomatic medicine, *etc.* Also published in London, 1967 (Allen & Unwin). A full-scale German history of psychiatry from classical antiquity up to recent times is: LEIBBRAND, W. & A. WETTLEY, 1961: Der Wahnsinn. Geschichte der abendländischen Psychopathologie, 698 p. (Freiburg/Munich: Alber).

ERNST, F., 1949: Vom Heimweh, 127 p. (Zurich: Fretz & Wasmuth).—

This book on homesickness consists of two parts; the first part deals with the history of the concept of nostalgia; the second part contains an anthology of the most important Latin, German, French and Italian texts on the subject.

FOUCAULT, M., 1965: Madness and civilization: a history of insanity in the Age of Reason, 229 p. (New York, N.Y.: Pantheon Books).—

This is not just a history of psychiatry. According to a review of this book in J. Hist. Med. 21: 333, the contents of this book are "characterized by philosophical complexities and literary subleties". It deals with the following questions: How can the transition from the confinement to the liberation of the mentally ill be explained?, and: What spiritual and cultural movements are at the basis of this substantial change of attitude between the 17th and 18th centuries? According to the reviewer it is "a very important book, written in the style of French rationalism". It is an abridged edition of a French book: Folie et déraison, histoire de la folie à l'âge classique, 1961, 674 p. (Thèse Univ. Paris) (Paris: Plon). Also in an abridged French edition: Histoire de la folie à l'âge classique, 320 p. (Paris: Union générale d'éditions). Cf. also O'BRIEN-MOORE, A., 1924, vide section Antiquity in general, subsection c.

GALDSTON, I., ed., 1967: Historic derivations of modern psychiatry, 241 p. (New York, N.Y.: McGraw-Hill).—

The text of this book consists of the following essays: 1. Psychiatry and ancient medicine (p. 9-18); 2. Psyche and soul: psychiatry in the Middle Ages (p. 19-40); 3. From demonology to the Narrenturm (p. 41-74); 4. The neuropsychologic phase in the history of psychiatric thought (p. 75-138); 5. Neurophysiologic psychiatry: Descartes to Pavlov and after (p. 139-158); 6. The evolution of depth psychology (p. 159-184); 7. Ethology, sensory deprivation, and overload (p. 185-218); 8. Social psychiatry: socioeconomic factors in mental health and disease (p. 219-232). Index of names and subjects.

HARMS, E., 1967: Origins of modern psychiatry, 256 p. (Springfield, Ill.: Thomas).—

The greater part of this book consists of accounts of selected authors, particularly of writings in which they made significant contributions to modern psychiatry. Many of these contributions were originally journal articles.

HORRAX, G., 1952: Neurosurgery: an historical sketch, 135 p. (Springfield, Ill.: Thomas).—

A history of neurosurgery. Separate chapters deal with cranial surgery of prehistoric times, Hippocratic and Galenical writings (with quotations from their writings), mediaeval and renaissance surgeons. A last chapter deals with the development of neurosurgery in modern times (V. Horsley, H. Cushing, Dandy, and others). The most exhaustive account of the subject is: WALKER, A. E., ed., 1951: A history of neurological surgery, 583 p. (Baltimore, Md.: Williams & Wilkins). This book contains a bibliography of nearly 2,400 references. Reprinted in 1967 (New York, N.Y.: Hafner).

HUNTER, R. & I. MACALPINE, 1963: Three hundred years of psychiatry, 1535-1860: a history presented in selected English texts, 1107 p. (London: Oxford U.P.).—

This book reviews the history of theory and practice of psychiatry in a documentary form from its beginnings until its acceptance as an established branch of science. This has been done by the reproduction of excerpts from the works of many writers (physicians as well as psychologists, jurists and philanthropists as well as philosophers, etc.) who from 1535 onwards did increase our knowledge of the insanities, their causes, nature and treatment. German and French excerpts have been translated into English. 5% of the works included deal with the 16th century, 20% with the 17th, 27% with the 18th, and 48% with the 19th century. Each of these excerpts has been prefaced by a critical account and by short biographical details. Moreover, interesting title-pages have been reproduced, and in an essay the authors show how the past may have influenced the development of modern medicine. Cf. CONOLLY, J., 1968: The construction and government of lunatic asylums and hospitals for the insane 37 + 183 p. (London: Dawsons). A reprint of one of the most important documents in the history of psychiatry, originally published in 1847, with informative introduction.

LANGE-EICHBAUM, W., 1956: Genie, Irrsinn und Ruhm, eine Pathologie des Genies, ed. 4, 628 p. (Munich: Reinhardt).—

First ed. 1928. Very useful bibliography containing 2,860 items. Included are 460 pathographies of famous men. The subject-headings of the main parts into which the text has been divided may be quoted in order to make clear the contents of this book: 1. Genie als Problem (historische Entwicklung des Genie-Begriffes, Wertprobleme, der Genieträger als schöpferisch Talent) (p. 27-113); 2. Genie und Ruhm (Das Problem Ruhm, psychologische Voraussetzungen, der Ruhm und sein Schicksal) (p. 114-162); 3. Genie und Irrsinn (Zur Literatur und Historie des Problems, Das Wesen der Krankheit) (p. 163-239); 4. Genie, Irrsinn und Ruhm (p. 240-264); 5. Pathographien. Elaborate indexes of names and subjects.

MCHENRY, L. C., ed., 1969: Garrison's history of neurology, 552 p. (Springfield, Ill.: Thomas).—

A revision of a classic text of the history of neurology. It contains a great amount of factual information and a multitude of references to original works on many subjects. Especially the second half of the book has been brought up to date.

RIESE, W., 1959: A history of neurology, 223 p. (New York, N.Y.: MD Publ.).—

This history of neurology considers the history of neurological ideas rather than that of facts or laboratory techniques. Separate chapters deal with such subjects as: the development of basic neurological concepts; the history of conduction of the nervous impulse; the reflex action from Rhazes to Goldstein; the history of the doctrine of cerebral localization (ca. 45% of the book); pain; diagnosis; prognosis; treatment. Bibliography and a "Neurological chronology" in which neurologists and their main achievements are tabulated in relation to major events in world history. Cf. also: CREUTZ, W., 1934, vide section Antiquity in general, subsection c.

——, 1965: La théorie des passions à la lumière de la pensée médicale du XVIIᵉ siècle, 74 p. (Confinia Psychiatrica, suppl. ad 8).—

A study of the Cartesian theory of emotions followed by an examination of the views of L. de la Forge, Cureau de la Chambre, G. E. Stahl, John Locke, and a 17th-century saint, named Senault.

SACHS, E., 1952: The history and development of neurological surgery, 158 p. (New York, N.Y.: Hoeber).—

A history of neurosurgery written by one of the most famous and experienced neurosurgeons of our days. Roughly one-third of this volume covers the neurological and surgical backgrounds, beginning with the neolithic culture and extending down to the reformations in surgery by Lister. The period of transition from old to new neurosurgery is discussed in a chapter entitled "The Listerian era and the beginnings of neurological surgery". Modern neurological surgery begins, according to the author, with the introduction of ventriculography by Dandy in 1918, by means of which diagnosis was made more definitive than had been the case previously. In his final chapter the author briefly summarizes the scope of work of the neurosurgeon today by discussing the various diversified areas in which he now operates. An autobiography of E. SACHS: Fifty years of neurosurgery: a personal story, 1958, 186 p. (New York, N.Y.: Vantage Press), also gives a very readable account of the development of this discipline.

TEMKIN, O., 1945: The falling sickness: a history of epilepsy from the Greeks to the beginning of modern neurology, 380 p. (Baltimore, Md.: John Hopkins U.P.).—

A well-written and complete survey of the history of epilepsy, a history which shows many points of contact both with the history of neurology and the history of magic. The author shows that epilepsy always has been considered as a disease; frequently it was believed to be a disease of the brain; but there also were many periods during which occult theories of causation influenced medical diagnosis and treatment.

THOMPSON, C. & P. MURRAY, 1956: La psychanalyse. Son évolution, ses développements, 256 p. (Paris: Gallimard).—

A historical and critical study of the development of psychoanalysis since 1885, when the therapeutical applications of hypnosis and the theories of Freud were introduced in medical psychology. The authors distinguish four periods. The first from 1885 up to 1900, characterized by Freud's discovery of the importance of hypnosis as a therapeutic technique, the second from 1900 up to ca. 1915, the period characterized by the theories of sexuality, the third period can be characterized by theories on personality and studies on narcissism and aggressivity, and a fourth period (since *ca.* 1920) can be characterized by its many theories on "eros", and agony and the ideas of Adler, Jung, Rank, Ferenczi, Reich, Sullivan, Horney, Fromm, and others. A popular history of hypnotism is: MARKS, R. W., 1947: The story of hypnotism, 246 p. (New York, N.Y.: Prentice Hall). Another history of psychoanalysis can be found in the first volume of WAELDER, R., 1960: Basic theory of psychoanalysis: the historical development of psychoanalytic thought, 273 p. (New York, N.Y.: Internat. U.P.). A study of its pioneers, containing a wealth of biographical information, is: ALEXANDER, F., S. EINSTEIN & M. GROTJAHN, eds., 1966: Psycho-analytic pioneers, 616 p. (New York, N.Y.: Basic Bks.).

VEITH, I., 1965: Hysteria: the history of a disease, 328 p. (Chicago, Ill.: Chicago U.P.).—

This history of hysteria begins with Egyptian medical papyri, it deals with hysteria in Greek and Roman medicine, in the Far East, and in mediaeval and early modern periods up to the Freudian concept of hysteria, and it deals with the views of such famous physicians as Hippocrates, Galen, Sydenham, Pinel, and Charcot. The authoress shows how this disease often was considered as having its origin in some anatomical or functional malfunction of the uterus, and she makes clear how the explanation of this disease through the centuries was related with the attitudes towards women and marriage of the period considered.

WYSS, D., 1961: Die tiefenpsychologischen Schulen von den Anfängen bis zur Gegenwart. Entwicklung, Probleme, Krisen, 412 p. (Göttingen: Vandenhoeck & Ruprecht).—

The first part (p. 1-222) deals with Freud's conception of psychoanalysis and his school (Karl Abraham, Ferenczi, Fenichel, E. Glover, E. Jones, Anna Freud, Melanie Klein, J. H. Hartmann, E. Kris, R. Loewenstein, R. Spitz, Greenacre, E. H. Erikson, T. Reik, W. Reich, P. Federn, and F. Alexander), and with neopsychoanalysis (Adler, K. Horney, E. Fromm, H. S. Sullivan, H. Schulz-Henke, T. French, S. Radó, and A. Kardiner). The second part deals with the philosophical theories of depth psychology (*e.g.*, Jung, O. Rank, L. Binswanger, von Gebsattel, E. Straus, M. Buber, V. von Weizsäcker, and others). The third part deals with some fundamental problems of psychoanalysis and their possible solution and is not so much of a historical interest. A second ed. appeared in 1966, 445 p. (Same publisher). Also in English translation: Depth psychology: a critical history.

Development, problems, crises, 568 p. (London: Allen & Unwin).

ZILBOORG, G., 1935: The medical man and the witch during the Renaissance, 215 p. (Publ. Inst. Hist. Med., Johns Hopkins Univ., Ser. 3, Vol. 2) (Baltimore, Md.: Johns Hopkins U.P.).—

In this study, witchcraft is seen as the central problem in the development of occidental psychiatry. "In the changing attitude towards witchcraft, modern psychiatry was born as a medical discipline." The book consists of a series of three lectures entitled: The physiological and psychological aspects of the Malleus Maleficarum (The Witch's hammer); Medicine and the witch in the 16th century; Johann Weyer, the founder of modern psychiatry.

——— & G. W. HENRY, 1941: A history of medical psychology, 606 p. (New York, N.Y.: Norton).—

A very readable survey of the history of medical psychology. Good index. *Cf.* also REISMAN, J. M., 1966: The development of clinical psychology, 374 p. (New York, N.Y.: Appleton-Century-Crofts).

c9 *obstetrics and gynaecology*

AUDUREAU, C., 1892: Etude sur l'obstétrique en occident pendant le Moyen Age et la Renaissance, 195 p. (Dyon: Darantière).—

For more details, *vide* section the Middle Ages in the Latin West, subsection c.

CIANFRANI, T., 1960: A short history of obstetrics and gynaecology, 449 p. (Springfield, Ill.: Thomas; Oxford: Blackwell).—

In this history the author elucidates the influence of other medical specialties on the development of obstetrics and gynaecology, while also much attention has been paid to the scientific, religious and political aspects, reproductive habits, and the taboos of the various civilizations considered. Separate chapters deal with, *e.g.*, the customs of primitive people, of Egyptian, Mesopotamian, and Graeco-Roman civilizations (with sidelights on Chinese, Japanese, Hindu and Arabian historical developments), and with the development of obstetrics and gynaecology in Europe from the Renaissance up to modern times. Special chapters are devoted to such topics as *e.g.*, certain aspects of operative gynaecology and obstetrics, to anaesthesia, infections, fistulae, *etc.* Each chapter is followed by a short section entitled: "First occurrences and unusual events" which is a tabular summary of the period considered. A more exhaustive but older history of these specialities is: FASBENDER, H., 1906: Geschichte der Geburtshilfe, 1028 p. (Jena: Fischer). Garrison-Morton write about this book: "Probably the most valuable history of the subject." Reprinted in 1964 (Hildesheim: Olms). Another exhaustive German history of the subject is: SIEBOLD, E. C. J. v., 1901: Versuch einer Geschichte der Geburtshilfe, 3 vols., 1750 p. (Tübingen: Pietzcker). A reprint is announced by Olms (Hildesheim) and will probably appear in 1970. For a more thorough history of gynaecology during antiquity, *cf.* DIEPGEN, P., 1937 and 1963, *vide* section Antiquity in general, subsection c.

JAMESON, E. M., 1962: Gynecology and obstetrics, 170 p. (Clio Medica, No. 17) (New York, N.Y.: Hafner).—

> Paperback reprint of the 1936 edition. A concise survey of the history of obstetrics and gynaecology from early Egyptian times to the present day. A wealth of information has been incorporated; explanations have been reduced to a minimum. Included are brief treatments of the subjects in Egyptian, Greek, Roman, Renaissance and modern times, the development of obstetrical forceps, the understanding of puerperal fever, and evolution and progress in gynaecological surgery. Bibliography, author-, and subject-indexes, and a list of classic works in gynaecology and obstetrics are included.

RICCI, J. V., 1943: The genealogy of gynaecology: history of the development of gynaecology throughout the ages, 2000 B.C. - 1800 A.D., 578 p. (Philadelphia, Pa.: Blakiston).—

> Separate sections of the book deal with the prehistoric period, the ancient epoch (Egypt, Babylonia, Assyria, Hindu, and Biblical literature), the Classic Age, the Byzantine period, the Arabic era, the mediaeval epoch, and the transitional period. The last period, filling almost half of the book, comprises the Renaissance and the 17th and 18th centuries. In a critical review of the book in Bull. Hist. Med. 16: 422-424, O. Temkin warns his readers about the many inaccuracies which deface the first half of the book; the second half, however, gives a fairly reliable account of the development of gynaecology during the 17th and 18th centuries. A second edition appeared in 1950; the text shows evidence of considerable revision in the correction of dates, names, typographical errors, *etc.* and of a thorough verification of quotations. A second ed. appeared in 1950. The development of gynaecology during the 19th century is treated by the same author in another book, *vide infra.*

——, 1945: One hundred years of gynaecology, 1800-1900: a comprehensive review of the specialty during its greatest century, with summaries and case reports of all diseases pertaining to women, 651 p. (Philadelphia, Pa.: Blakiston).—

> This book is a continuation of the former book. It is an encyclopaedic handbook of 19th-century gynaecology, the index of names containing some 8,000 names. The text consists of 33 chapters, each of them for the most part treats of a certain subject, such as: ovarian cysts, ovarian pathology, extra-fundal pregnancy and therapy, *etc.* A valuable reference work. Other books dealing with the development of gynaecology in the previous century are: 1)FEHLING, H., 1925: Entwicklung der Geburtshilfe und Gynäkologie im 19. Jahrhundert, 269 p. (Berlin: Springer): a reliable short history. 2) FISCHER, J., 1928: Historischer Rückblick über die Leistungen des XIX. Jahrhunderts auf dem Gebiete der Geburtshilfe und Gynäkologie, 179 p. (In: J. HALBAN & L. SEITZ, Biologie und Pathologie des Weibes. Ein Handbuch der Frauenheilkunde und der Geburtshilfe, Vol. VIII, pt. 2, Lief. 44: 1343-1522).

SPEERT, H., 1958: Obstetric and gynecologic milestones: essays in eponymy, 700 p. (New York, N.Y.: Macmillan).—

> In this book the author has taken 101 gynaecologists who have given their names to some technique or aspect of gynaecology. The book is composed of 79 independent chapters (some tell of more than one eponym), grouped in 12 sections, each dealing with a different aspect of gynaecology. Each name prompts an essay giving the historical and clinical background to the man's work with extensive quotations from his original description of the phenomenon (in English translation where necessary), and a concise biography of the man himself. Included are 94 portraits, which means that only 7 are missing.

THOMS, H., 1935: Classical contributions to obstetrics and gynecology, 265 p. (Springfield, Ill.: Thomas).—

An anthology, containing quotations of some 57 authors, from the ancients up to the end of the 19th century. To each of the excerpts quoted a short biographical sketch of its author has been added. Good short bibliography of sources. Index.

YOUNG, J. H., 1944: Caesarian section: the history and development of the operation from earliest times, 254 p. (London: Lewis). —

A history of the performance of the Caesarian section in relation to its religious, ethical, legal, as well as its strictly medical aspects. The author shows how important was the relative value placed on the child and on the woman and her rights and place in society in questions of the application of the Caesarian section; decisions were of an ethico-social rather than of a medical character.

C10 *ophthalmology*

ARRINGTON, G. E., 1959: A history of ophthalmology, 174 p. (MD Monographs on Medical History, Vol. 3) (New York, N.Y. MD. Publ.).—

This is not a true history of ophthalmology, but in this booklet the author gives a picture of how ophthalmology came to be, what were its contributions to science and society, and what has been the interest which seeing has stirred in thinking men of all ages. About a third of the text is devoted to prehistory and classical antiquity; one-third to the Renaissance and its aftermath, and the last third part to modern ophthalmology. A handsome short history of ophthalmology in the German language is: SASSE, C. H., 1947: Geschichte der Augenheilkunde in kurzer Zusammenfassung mit mehreren Abbildungen und einer Geschichtstabelle, 60 p. (Stuttgart: Enke). A review in tabular form is printed in the margin.

CHANCE, B., 1962: Ophthalmology, 240 p. (Clio Medica, No. 20) (New York, N.Y.: Hafner).—

Two-thirds of its contents are devoted almost exclusively to the developments that began with the 19th century, and much of this is given to relatively contemporary events, particularly in the U.S.A. It has been written for the busy practitioner, the undergraduate, and the interested layman. A reprint of the 1939 edition.

HIRSCHBERG, J., 1915-1918: Geschichte der Augenheilkunde, 9 parts. (Leipzig: Engelmann).—

According to Garrison-Morton: "This monumental work remains to-day the authoritative history of ophthalmology. Its thoroughness and critical judgment mark it as one of the greatest of all histories of scientific subjects." The second ed. appeared in GRAEFE-SAEMISCH-HESS: Handbuch der gesamten Augenheilkunde, Vol. XIV (1915) (1-4) and XV (1918) (1-2). *Cf.* also MAGNUS, H., 1901, *vide* section Antiquity in general, subsection c.

KOELBING, H. M., 1967: Renaissance der Augenheilkunde 1540-1630, 198 p. (Bern: Huber).—

In a short introductory part of *ca.* 20 pages, the author gives a review of ophthalmology during antiquity and the Middle Ages (Aristotle, Galen, theory of seeing, origin of the spectacles). The main part deals with Renaissance ophthalmology. Separate sections deal with such subjects as: the theory of seeing in humanistic medicine (Joh. Runge, Gesner); the discovery of the function of the retina (*e.g.,* Averroës, Leonardo da Vinci, Vesalius, Platter, Fabricius ab Aquapendente); diseases of the eye (Fabricius Hildanus, Platter, cataract and its treatment, inflammations, tumours, *etc,);* selections from Platters case-histories of diseases; surgery (Pierre Franco, treatment of cataract); ophthalmology and the medical profession. Bibliography and indexes of names and subjects.

SNYDER, C., 1967: Our ophthalmic heritage, 170 p. (London: Churchill).—

A series of 37 historical essays written by the librarian of the Lucien Howe Library of Ophthalmology at Harvard, originally published in the Archives of Ophthalmology. Of particular value for the history of ophthalmology in the United States during the second half of last century.

C11 *orthopaedics*

BICK, E. M., 1948: Source book of orthopaedics, ed. 2, 540 p. (Baltimore, Md.: Williams & Wilkins).—

The first part (p. 1-88) contains a chronologic history throughout the 18th century. The second part deals with contemporary orthopaedic surgery, and with mechanical, physical, manipulative, and drug therapy, and with the rise of orthopaedic hospitals and institutions. In 1968 a reprint-edition was published (New York, N.Y.: Hafner).

RANG, M., 1966: Anthology of orthopaedics, 41 + 243 p. (Edinburgh & London: Livingstone).—

Included is a wide variety of classical papers on orthopaedics, arranged in chapters that deal with the separate aspects of orthopaedics and accompanied by the author's commentaries.

VALENTIN, B., 1961: Geschichte der Orthopädie, 288 p. (Stuttgart: Thieme).—

A general history of orthopaedic surgery. In the first part there are *inter alia* a detailed discussion of club foot and its aetiology and treatment; another (short) section deals with some operations, such as osteotomy and osteoclasis. The second part of the book deals with individual orthopaedic surgeons and institutions in England, France, Germany, the Netherlands, Switzerland, Austria, Scandinavia, Italy, and America. In 1966 the same author published a book on the history of podiatry: VALENTIN, B., 1966: Geschichte der Fusspflege. Pedicurie. Chiropodie. Podologie, 103 p. (Stuttgart: Thieme). In this booklet the evolution from pedicure to what is being called today chiropody, podiatry, or podology, has been given in a well-documented scholarly way.

C12 *oto-, rhino-, laryngology*

KASSEL, K., 1914: Geschichte der Nasen-Heilkunde, 476 p. (Würzburg: Kabitsch).—

"Detailed history with bibliography. Continued through the eighteenth and part of the nineteenth century in articles in Zeitschrift für Laryngologie, Rhinologie, Otologie, 7 (1914-1915) - 11 (1923)." (Doe & Marshall: 480). Reprinted 1967 (Hildesheim: Olms). In a second vol. of the reprint-edition of 182 p., the series of journal articles has been reprinted.

STEVENSON, R. S. & D. GUTHRIE, 1949: A history of oto-laryngology, 155 p. (Edinburgh: Livingstone; Baltimore, Md.: Williams & Wilkins).—

A short history of this discipline from the earliest times up to the present. Separate sections deal with ancient history, Middle Ages and Renaissance, 17th and 18th centuries, otology becoming a separate

discipline, the education of the deaf, and modern history of oto-laryngology. A thorough German history of otology is: POLITZER, A., 1901-1913: Geschichte der Ohrenheilkunde, 2 vols. (Stuttgart: Enke). According to Garrison-Morton this is a masterpiece of historical research.

C13 *paediatrics*

ABT, I. A., ed., 1965: Abt-Garrison history of pediatrics. Reprinted from Pediatrics by various authors, Vol. I, 316 p. (With new chapters on the history of pediatrics in recent times by A. F. ABT) (Philadelphia, Pa.: Saunders).—

This volume contains an unchanged reprint of A. F. ABT & F. H. GARRISON's History of pediatrics, accompanied by an essay of I. A. ABT on "Historic changes and advances in pediatrics during recent times", being a chronicle of 116 pages of some of the important paediatric advances of the last four decades.

PEIPER, A., 1958: Chronik der Kinderheilkunde, ed. 4, 714 p. (Leipzig: Thieme).—

A well-known history of paediatrics with very fine illustrations. The first sections deal with child care in the ancient world; other chapters deal with the physiology of children, vitamin deficiencies, feeding, children's hospitals and with the histories of various child diseases.

——, 1966: Quellen zur Geschichte der Kinderheilkunde, 164 p. (Hubers Klassiker der Geschichte der Medizin und Naturwiss., No. 7) (Bern & Stuttgart: Huber).—

The text consists of a series of 44 extracts (all of them in the German language) on paediatrics, dating from ancient Egypt and classical times up to *ca.* 1850. Included are a table of contents, an index of personal names, a bibliography, and some useful annotations. The author's autobiography also contains much that is of interest for the history of paediatrics, *viz.,* PEIPER, A., 1967: Erinnerungen eines Kinderarztes, 262 p. (Berlin: VEB Volk und Gesundheit).

RUHRÄH, J., 1925: Pediatrics of the past: an anthology, 592 p. (New York, N.Y.: Hoeber).—

An anthology, reproducing early classics *in extenso*. Included are abstracts from the works of Hippocrates, Soranos, Aretaeos, Oribasios, Aetios, Paul of Aegina, Rhazes, Paulus Bagellardus, Bart. Metlinger, Corn. Roelans, Victorius, Phaer, Wuertz, Hyr. Mercurialis, F. Platter, Ballonius, Simon de Vallembert, Grueling, Glisson, Pemell, Sylvius, Wyseman, Sydenham, Mayow, Harris, Tacher, Hoefer, Rosén von Rosenstein, Cadogen, Whytt, Rush, Beardsley, Soemmering, Armstrong, Underwood, Bard, Heberden. Many illustrations.

STILL, G. F., 1931: The history of paediatrics: the progress of the study of diseases of children up to the end of the eighteenth century, 526 p. (London: Oxford U.P.).—

"This work covers the whole field of paediatrics to the end of the 18th century. It is a very readable, interesting and accurate history of the subject." (Garrison-Morton). Reprinted in 1965 (London: Dawson).

C14 *parasitology*

FOSTER, W. D., 1965: A history of parasitology, 202 p. (Edinburgh & Londen: Livingstone).—

This outline history of the medical aspects of parasitology deals only with certain groups of human parasites, *viz.*, helminths and protozoa, and deliberately excludes parasitic fungi and arthropods. The book contains a general survey of medical parasitology from antiquity up to about 1920. Index of authors, but no subject-index. Separate chapters deal with the development of our knowledge of cestodes, trematodes (flukes and schistosomes), nematodes (trichina, hookworm, filariae), and of various groups of pathogenic protozoa (trypanosomes, *Entamoeba histolytica, Babesia,* plasmodia).

HUARD, P. & J. THÉODORIDÈS, 1959: Cinq parasitologistes méconnus, 91 p. (Biologie médicale, 1959).—

A consideration of the parasitological works of scientists of name, but whose parasitological work often is neglected, *viz.*, Réaumur (1683-1757), founder of insect parasitology; Draparnaud (1772-1804) who published in 1803 a fundamental study on medical zoology and human parasites; Laënnec (1781-1826) who made important studies on the larvae of Cestoda; Raspail (1794-1878) who studied human parasitology; and Dujardin (1801-1860) who wrote a manual on helminthology.

WARREN, K. S. & V. A. NEWILL, 1967: Schistosomiasis: a bibliography of the world's literature from 1852 to 1962, 2 vols. Vol. 1: Keyword index, 597 p.; Vol. 2: Author index, 395 p. (Cleveland, O.: Western Reserve U.P.).—

A somewhat older, but still valuable bibliography dealing with the same subject is: KHALIL, M., 1931: The bibliography of schistosomiasis (bilharziasis): zoological, clinical and prophylactic, 506 p. (Publ. Fac. Med. Egypt. Univ. 1931: 1-506). This bibliography is continued in: BOUILLON, A., 1950: Bibliographie des schistosomes et des schistosomiasis (bilharzioses) humaines et animales de 1931 à 1948, 141 p. (Mém. Inst. Colon. Belg. 18(5): 1-141).

C15 *pathology*

ASHBURN, P. M., 1947: The ranks of death: a medical history of the conquest of America, 298 p. (New York, N.Y.: Coward-McCann).—

The book elucidates the profound and specific effect (especially by means of cross-infections) which diseases can have, when different cultures meet each other. This is clearly exemplified by the history of the conquest of America (in those days a real New World with a settled culture) by the white discoverers (coming from the Old World). This situation became still more complicated by the introduction of the black slaves from Africa. With three appendixes (p. 213-286) and index. Among the diseases discussed are: scurvy, eruptive fevers, malaria, yellow jack, respiratory diseases, intestinal infections, parasitic worms, syphilis, leprosy, leishmaniasis, trachoma.

BERGHOFF, E., 1947: Entwicklungsgeschichte des Krankheitsbegriffes, ed. 2, 201 p. (Vienna: Maudrich).—

A historical review of the concept of disease as it developed during human evolution, considered against the philosophical and cultural background of the periods considered. Separate chapters are devoted to pre-historic concepts, pre-Hippocratic theories, Hippocrates and his school, Galen and the Middle Ages, the Renaissance, mesmerism and romanticism, concepts held at the end of the 18th and the beginning of the 19th century, the Vienna school, and to the more modern interpretations of the concept of disease.

BETT, W. R., ed., 1954: The history and conquest of common diseases, 355 p. (Norman, Okla.: Oklahoma U.P.).—

This book is a new edition of an earlier work entitled "A short history of some common diseases", 1934, ed. by W. R. BETT (London: Oxford U.P.). The list of topics discussed is as follows: acute communicable diseases, influenza, pneumonia, rheumatism, arthritis, heart diseases, diseases of tonsils and adenoids, venereal diseases, rickets, diseases of the endocrine glands, gallstones, appendicitis, epilepsy, and cancer. It includes a glossary of medical terms, and indexes of subjects and authors.

FABER, K. H., 1923: Nosography in modern internal medicine, 222 p. (New York, N.Y.: Hoeber).—

A review, showing the steps which have led to a gradual improvement of the description of diseases. It discusses: Sydenham and nosology; François Boissier de Sauvages; the Paris School (Pinel, Bichat, Corvisart, Laënnec); German physiological medicine; bacteriological clino-pathological research (syphilis, tuberculosis); the physiological method (Frerichs and Leyden, Charcot, Kussmaul, Rosenbach, Stokes, *etc.*); constitutional pathology.

FIENNES, R., 1964: Man, nature and disease, 287 p. (London: Weidenfeld & Nicolson; New York, N.Y.: New American Library).—

"This summary treatment of the history and biological nature of disease is an attractive introduction to human ecology, of significance to the general historian and to those seeking an introduction to the entire subject of disease or to a particular historical problem." (From Isis 56: 530).

LONG, E. R., ed., 1961: Selected readings in pathology, ed. 2, 306 p. (Springfield, Ill.: Thomas).—

This volume presents extracts from the writings of famous physicians who have contributed greatly to pathology, starting with Hippocrates. The first ed. appeared in 1929 and considered the period from Hippocrates to Virchow. To this second edition are added new extracts from 30 pathologists, representatives of the many who contributed to pathology during the late 19th and early 20th centuries.

———, 1965: A history of pathology, ed. 2, 199 p. (New York, N.Y.: Dover; London: Constable).—

A paperback edition. The first edition appeared in 1928. For the present edition the author prepared an appendix on recent trends in pathology (1929-1963). The subject is divided as follows: 1. Pathology of antiquity; 2. Galen and the Middle Ages; 3. Pathology of the Renaissance; 4. Seventeenth century; 5. Morgagni and the eighteenth century; 6. The Paris School at the opening of the nineteenth century; 7. Pathology in England in the first half of the nineteenth century; 8. Rokitansky and the new Vienna School; 9. Virchow and the cellular pathology; 10. Pathological histology and the last third of the nineteenth century; 11. Rise of bacteriology and immunology; 12. Experimental and chemical pathology. A history of pathology based on biographies of "great men in pathology" is: KRUMBHAAR, E. B., 1962: Pathology, 206 p. (Clio Medica, No. 19) (New York, N.Y.: Hafner). A very readable history, especially dealing with the clinical aspects is: FOSTER, W. D., 1961: A short history of clinical pathology: with a chapter on the organization of clinical pathology to the present day, by S. C. DYKE, 154 p. (Edinburgh & London: Livingstone).

MAJOR, R. H., 1945: Classic descriptions of disease, ed. 3, 697 p. (Springfield, Ill.: Thomas).—

A collection of original descriptions of most of the important diseases in medicine. Separate chapters deal with particular diseases *(e.g.,* tuberculosis, diphtheria, diabetes, *etc.),* others deal with clinical conditions or syndromes *(e.g.,* heart block, bronchial casts, gallop rhythm, *etc.).* The diseases described are of a somatic nature; in principle no diseases of the mind are included. Biographical sketches of the authors considered have been added, many of them accompanied by portraits.

OLIVER, W. W., 1930: Stalkers of pestilence: the story of man's ideas of infection, 251 p. (New York, N.Y.: Hoeber).—

This booklet contains, in a corrected form, a series of articles originally published in the Amer. J. Surgery, N.S., vol. 7, nos. 3-6, 1929. It is a compendium of basic facts, largely assembled on a biographical pattern. It consists of the following five chapters: prehistoric man to Hippocrates; Arabic medicine; the mediaeval period, and the Renaissance; the 17th and 18th centuries; the 19th century; the 20th century. Bibliography and index of names.

RIESE, W., 1953: The conception of disease, its history, its versions and its nature, 120 p. (New York, N.Y.: Philosophical Library).—

> The topics discussed in this book are *e.g.,* the Stoic conception of disease, the Platonic or cosmological conception, the anthropological, moral, Hippocratic, or historical conception, "Medicina prima (Baglivi) or the natural history of disease", the Galenic or physiological conception, the anatomical (from Leonardo da Vinci to Virchow), the etiological, the social, the psychological, the ontological, and the metaphysical conception of disease. It is not just a historical book, but contains much that is of historical importance.

C15* *avitaminoses*

HARRIS, L. J., 1935: Vitamines and theory in practice, 240 p. (Cambridge: U.P.; New York, N.Y.: Macmillan).—

> This book contains the text of a series of lectures. It contains much information regarding the discovery of vitamins and its discoverer (Casimir Funk, the originator of the "vitamine theory"), and regarding the history of the discovery of the causes of the vitamin diseases. The text is well written and is free from technical details.

beriberi

WILLIAMS, R. R., 1961: Towards the conquest of beriberi, 338 p. (Cambridge, Mass.: Harvard U.P.).—

> This is the history of the discovery and synthesis of thiamine and its role in the fight against the clinical and pathological aspects of beriberi. The author shows that beriberi and thiamine deficiency are essentially the result of a progressing civilization. Besides he also summarizes the various theories which have been proposed in order to describe the phenomena of disease resulting from thiamine malnutrition.

scurvy

HESS, A. F., 1920: Scurvy, past and present, 279 p. (Philadelphia, Pa.: Lippincott).—

> Includes a history and bibliography. The first chapter (p. 1-23) deals with the history of scurvy (outbreaks of scurvy on land and at sea, infantile scurvy, scurvy in the First World War). Other chapters deal with pathogenesis and etiology of scurvy, the antiscorbutic vitamin, scurvy pathology, experimental scurvy, antiscorbutic foods, symptomatology, diagnosis, prognosis, treatment of scurvy, and the relation of scurvy to other diseases. A comparable German publication is: BRÜCK, D., 1935: Zur Geschichte und Klinik des Skorbuts, 105 p. (Diss. Univ. Leipzig).

C15** *diabetes*

PAPASPYROS, N. S., 1952: The history of diabetes mellitus, 100 p. (London: Stockwell).—

> An informative volume, discussing the history of diabetes, the history of diabetes treatment, the discovery of insulin, the surgical treatment of diabetes, and experimental diabetes. Lengthy bibliography. A second edition appeared in 1964, 104 p. (Stuttgart: Thieme). A source of biographical information is: STRIKER, C., ed., 1961: Famous faces in diabetes, 256 p. (Boston, Mass.: Hall), containing many photographs with captions of 25-300 words each. A German history of diabetes is: WOLFF, G., 1955: Zucker, Zuckerkrankheit und Insulin. Eine medizin- und kulturhistorische Studie, 95 p. (Remscheid: Dustri).

C15*** *infectious diseases*
cholera

CHAMBERS, J. S., 1938: The conquest of cholera, America's greatest scourge, 366 p. (New York, N.Y.: Macmillan).—

> A detailed history of cholera in America, chiefly covering the period between 1832 and 1873. A brief chapter concerning epidemics in more recent years and a bibliography have been included. A publication studying the influence of the cholera epidemics from the social point of view rather than from the medical is: ROSENBERG, C. E., 1962: The cholera years: the United States in 1832, 1849, and 1866, 257 p. (Chicago, Ill.: Chicago U.P.). In this study the author analyses public behaviour in terms of religious and social attitudes during the epidemic years and he shows how outlooks shifted with a growing confidence in sanitary reform, combined with a general decline in piety.

CHEVALIER, L., ed., 1958: Le choléra. La première épidémie du XIXᵉ siècle, 188 p. (La Roche-sur-Yon: Imp. Centrale de l'Ouest).—

Ten collaborators discuss the 1831-1832 outbreak of cholera in Paris, Lille, Normandy, Bordeaux, Marseilles, Russia, and England and they do this against a demographical, historical, social and political background. Each section has adequate reference to the literature; maps and charts are included but there is no index. A study concerning the cholera outbreaks in Czarist Russia is: MCGREW, R. E., 1965: Russia and the cholera, 1823-1832, 229 p. (Madison, Wisc.: Wisconsin U.P.). In this study the author follows the cholera outbreaks against the material and ideological structure of society of that period, and the reaction of the medical profession. A detailed history, particularly as it affected the British Isles is: LONGMATE, N., 1966: King cholera, 271 p. (London: Hamish Hamilton).

STICKER, G., 1912: Abhandlungen aus der Seuchengeschichte und Seuchenlehre. Vol. II: Die Cholera, 592 p. (Giessen: Töpelmann).—

After a historical introduction, a detailed and comprehensive review follows of: endemic cholera, infantile cholera, and Indian cholera. Detailed table of contents, but no index. Bibliography is included.

diphteria

BAYEUX, R., 1899: La diphtérie depuis Arétée le Cappadocien jusqu'en 1894 avec les résultats statistiques de la sérumthérapie sur deux cent trente mille cas, 351 p. (Paris: Carré & Naud).—

The text is in three parts, viz., 1. (p. 11-111) a historical part, considering the history of the disease and some great epidemics, and the history of therapy (e.g., Bretonneau and tracheotomy, serum therapy); 2. a statistical part (p. 112-257) containing much quantitative material; 3. a surgical part.

leprosy

WEYMOUTH, A., 1938: Through the lepersquint: a study of leprosy from pre-Christian times to the present day, 286 p. (London: Selwyn & Blount).—

According to Doe & Marshall this is a general history with chronologic tables and bibliography. A detailed study of the subject can be found in: ZAMBACO PACHA, D. A., 1914: La lèpre à travers les siècles et les contrées, 845 p. (Paris: Mas-

son). No index. A sketchy history of leprosy with chronology and illustrations is: MOURITZ, A. A. S. M., 1943: A brief world history of leprosy: Hawaii, U.S. of America, Philippines, Malaya, Fiji, China, India, Europe, ed. 2, 139 p. (Honolulu: Author). A valuable bibliographical tool is: KEFFER, L., 1944-1948: Indice bibliográfico de lepra, 1500-1943, 3 vols. Vol. I (1944): 1500-1944, A-H; Vol. II (1946): 1500-1943, I-P; Vol. III (1948): 1500-1945, Q-Z. (São Paulo: Biblioteca Departemento de profilaxia da lepra do Estado de São Paulo).

malaria

RUSSELL, P. F., 1955: Man's mastery of malaria, 308 p. (London: Oxford U.P.).—

In this book the contents of the Heath Clark lectures, 1953, delivered at the London School of Hygiene and Tropical Medicine, have been published. It is a well-written history of the conquest of malaria, dealing with the discovery by Laveran in 1880 of the etiological agent and its transmission; the speculations about its causes between 1880 and 1897, when R. Ross demonstrated that transmission takes place by means of a mosquito; malaria control: quinine and the new anti-malarials; the conquest of the insect vector; the development of insecticides and the instruction of people in their use of them; international organisations, such as the Malaria Commission of the League of Nations, and the W.H.O. A concluding chapter deals with "Malaria and society", discussing malaria prophylaxis and population-pressure. A more popular book dealing with the same topics is: WARSHAW, L. J., 1949: Malaria: the biography of a killer, 348 p. (New York, N.Y.: Rinehart). Some well-documented regional histories of malaria are: ACKERKNECHT, E. H., 1945: Malaria in the upper Mississippi Valley, 1760-1900, 142 p. (Suppl. Bull. Hist. Med., No. 4) (Baltimore, Md.: Johns Hopkins Press); and CELLI, A., 1933: The history of malaria in the Roman Campagna from ancient times, 226 p. (London: Bale, Sons & Danielsson). This last book comprises a history covering some 25 centuries. The book describes rise and fall of malaria in the pre-Roman, imperial, mediaeval, renaissance and modern time; brief notes on the early 20th century are included. The original Italian edition of this book was published in 1925: Storia della malaria nell' Agro romano... (Mem. R. Accad. Nac. Lincei, cl. fisiche, Ser. 6, Vol. 1, Fasc. 3); also in German translation: Die Malaria in ihrer Bedeutung für die Geschichte Roms und der römischen Campagna, 1929, 118 p. (Leipzig: Thieme).

DURAN-REYNALS, M. L., 1946: The fever bark tree: the pageant of quinine, 275 p. (Garden City, N.Y.: Doubleday).—

A readable story of cinchona from the time of Alexander the Great up to recent times. It deals with the role of the following persons: the Count of Chinchón, the Cardinal de Lugo, Sydenham, Talbor, La Condamine, Joseph de Jussieu, Mutis, Weddell, Laveran, Markham, Spruce, Ledger, Mannel. Separate chapters deal with the Dutch monopoly and with the antimalarials during World War II. Also a French edition: L'arbre de la fièvre, 1949, 264 p. (Paris: Sequana). A study, more particularly dealing with the influence of the Dutch on the production of cinchona is: TAYLOR, N., 1945: Cinchona in Java: the story of quinine, 87 p. (New York, N.Y.: Greenberg): an authoritative and well-written publication, mainly dealing with cinchona in Java, its cultivation, and its medical and socio-economic importance.

plague

BELL, W. G., 1951: The great plague of London 1665, 361 p. (New York, N.Y.: Macmillan).—

This book was first published in 1920; this is a reissue of the revised edition of 1923 (London: Lane). It gives a fascinating and informative description of the Great Plague of London and it provides a very good background for students of the period. An account of this London plague epidemic has been written by the English writer Daniel Defoe (1660-1731) under the title: A journal of the plague year: being observations or memorials, of the most remarkable occurrences, as well public as private, which happened in London during the last great visitation in 1665. Written by a citizen who continued all the while in London, 1722, 287 p. (London: Nutt) Reprinted 1966, 225 p. (London: Penguin Bks.). On the occasion of the third centenary of this outbreak a German translation of this book has been published: DEFOE, D., 1965: Ein Bericht vom Pestjahr London 1665, 359 p. (epilogue by E. G. Jacob) (Bremen: Schünemann). In a postscript, E. G. JACOB gives details of Defoe's life as well as a critical commentary on the "Journal" [of the plague]. The history of plague epidemics of Russia has been written by DÖRBECK, F., 1906: Geschichte der Pestepidemien in Russland von der Gründung des Reiches bis auf die Gegenwart, 220 p. (Abh. Gesch. Med., Heft 18) (Breslau: Kern). A new ed. was published in 1969, 298 p. (London: Oxford U.P.), supplied by useful annotations and an informative introduction by L. LANDA. *Cf.* also: NICHOLSON, W., 1968-1969: The historical sources of Defoe's Journal of the plague year, 182 p. (New York, N.Y.: Kennikat).

CAMPBELL, A. M., 1931: The black death and men of learning, 210 p. (New York, N.Y.: Columbia U.P.; London: Oxford U.P.).—

According to the author: "The object of this study is to treat the Black Death (1347-1350) only as it affected the intellectual classes, and the fields of learning in which they labored. Medicine and education, especially the universities are emphasized, since plague tractates of the period and university records furnish the best source-material."

HIRST, L. F., 1953: The conquest of plague: a study of the evolution of epidemiology, 478 p. (New York, N.Y. & Oxford: Clarendon Press).—

Because plague was so well recognized and so much feared, each step in the knowledge concerning it has been recorded. The author makes it clear that any epidemic of plague is the result of a complex of interactions of a biological (*e.g.,* the proper constellation involving human beings, warm-blooded rodents, cold-blooded arthropods, and virulent bacilli), of a climatological (*e.g.,* the steady elimination of the domestic black rat by the brown wander rat in Europe and the fleas accompanying them) and of a socio-economic (*e.g.,* trade, mode of treatment of patients, quarantine, *etc.*) nature. The author concludes that it is by no means clear which complex of factors actually determined the appearance and disappearance of the great pandemics occurring at long intervals of time. A detailed and comprehensive study describing the plague from the earliest times onwards is: STICKER, G., 1908-1910: Die Pest. Abhandlungen aus der Seuchengeschichte und Seuchenlehre, Vol. I, 542 p. (Giessen: Töpelmann). This book has a good bibliography.

WAKIL, A. W., 1932: The third pandemic of plague in Egypt. Historical and statistical epidemiological remarks on the first thirty-two years of its prevalence, 169 p. (Cairo: Faculty of Medicine, Egyptian Univ.).—

Egypt has always been very important in the spread of infectious diseases throughout the world, and particularly throughout Europe. Egypt always has afforded unique facilities for plague epidemics since its agricultural interests foster rats, its semi-arid conditions favour fleas, the trade from the Orient converged in Egypt, and diverged thence throughout Europe, and sanitary control was absent. These circumstances made of Egypt a perennial source of plagues *(e.g.,* in 542, 7th and 8th centuries, 1010, 1072, 1201, 1296, 1348, 1373, 1443, 1459; between 1783 and 1844, 21 epidemics of plague in Egypt were recorded).

ZIEGLER, P., 1969: The Black Death, 319 p. (London: Collins).—

> A thorough account of the first known pandemic of plague which occurred between 1345 and 1350. Its distribution from Manchuria *via* the Mediterranean seaports has been described (by 1347 it had arrived in Sicily). Thence it spread to the mainland of Europe and by 1348 it reached England, killing supposedly about a third of the population. *Cf.* also: HIRSHLEIFER, J., 1966: Diaster and recovery: the black death in Western Europe, 31 p. (Santa Monica, Calif.: Rand). A book of similar scope is: DEAUX, G., 1969: The Black Death 1347, 229 p. (London: Hamilton).

poliomyelitis

FISHBEIN, M., ed., 1951: A bibliography of infantile paralysis with selected abstracts and annotations compiled by L. HEKTOEN & E. M. SALMONSEN, 1789-1949, ed. 2, 899 p. (Philadelphia, Pa.: Lippincott).—

> A chronological arrangement of 10,367 numbered entries; supplements are planned. Published under the auspices of the National Foundation for Infantile Paralysis. Included are an index of authors, a very good analytical subject-index of almost 100 pages, and selected abstracts and annotations.

FISHER, P. J., 1967: The polio story, 125 p. (London: Heinemann).—

> The first recognizable epidemic of poliomyelitis or infantile paralysis occurred in Sweden in 1887. Since then the world has been faced with a number of epidemics of various degrees of severity. After a general introduction considering the role of bacteria and viruses in the production of diseases, the author gives a readable account of the production of two vaccines, Salk and Sabin, which have been prepared against this disease, and he describes in some detail the controversy which surrounded these two vaccines. A popular narrative of "the for-

ward steps that have been taken since the dawn of the search for a solution of infantile paralysis" is: BERG, L. H., 1948: Polio and its problems, 174 p. (Philadelphia, Pa.: Lippincott); according to a review in the J. Hist. Med. 4: 488, historically this book is not very accurate.

Scabies (vide section Dermatology and venereology)

smallpox

MILLER, G., 1957: The adoption of inoculation for smallpox in England and France, 355 p. (Philadelphia, Pa.: Pennsylvania U.P.).—

> Notwithstanding the geographical limitation mentioned in the title, the present book gives a very useful general history of inoculation from the time the practice began to be adopted in Europe early in the 18th century, until the end of that century, when Jennerian vaccination was introduced. The authoress gives her history against a background of social, political, religious, and intellectual life of the period considered. A German history of smallpox inoculation is: GINS, H., 1963: Krankheit wider den Tod. Schicksal der Pockenschutzimpfung, 376 p. (Stuttgart: Fischer). An exhaustive history of vaccination is: CROOKSHANK, E. M., 1889: History and pathology of vaccination, 2 vols. (Philadelphia, Pa.: Blakiston). Garrison-Morton writes about this book: "This very full history of the subject caused a good deal of controversy, see review of it in Lancet, 1890, 1, p. 470-472".

STEARN, E. W. & A. E., 1945: The effect of smallpox on the destiny of the Amerindian, 153 p. (Boston, Mass.: Humphries).—

> Interesting study of the history of smallpox in America from the 16th to the 20th century. It contains a valuable record of the workings of an epidemic, its rate and manner of spread; much stress has been laid on the social and human aspects. The American Indians were not familiar with smallpox before the white man arrived, and consequently the first encounters with the disease resulted in very high death rates among the Indians.

syphilis (vide section Dermatology and venereology)

tuberculosis

BURKE, R. M., 1955: An historical chronology of tuberculosis, ed. 2, 125 p. (Springfield, Ill.: Thomas).—

The subjectmatter has been divided into 4 chapters. Chapter 1 deals with the period 5000 B.C. to 1600 A.D.; ch. 2 with the period between 1600 and 1800 and the impact of anatomy and physiology upon the study of diseases; ch. 3 with the period between 1800 and 1881, when the techniques of morbid pathology were used; ch. 4 with the period from 1882 to 1955 when bacteriology put its stamp on pathology. An excellent bibliography and an index of names make the book a useful tool for the finding of dates and important personalities concerned with the disease. A monograph containing biographies of the principal contributors to our knowledge of tuberculosis in relation to their times is: CUMMINS, S. L., 1949: Tuberculosis in history from the 17th century to our own times, 205 p. (Baltimore, Md.: Williams & Wilkins); besides it also deals with the schools and their influences on ideas about tuberculosis. An exhaustive history of tuberculosis from the earliest times onwards is: FLICK, L. F., 1925: Development of our knowledge of tuberculosis, 783 p. (Philadelphia, Pa.: Wickersham).

DUBOS, R. J. & J., 1952: The white plague: tuberculosis, man and society, 277 p. (Boston, Mass.: Little, Brown).—

The authors themselves describe their aim as follows: "Tuberculosis is a social disease, and presents problems that transcend the conventional medical approach. On the one hand, its understanding demands that the impact of social and economic factors on the individual be considered as much as the mechanisms by which tubercle bacilli cause damage to the human body. On the other hand, the disease modifies in a particular manner the emotional and intellectual climate of the societies that it attacks. It is the subtle interplay between the social body and the social disease which constitutes the central theme of the present study." The authors make clear how the meaning of the word tuberculosis has changed as our knowledge about the disease and its etiology increased. Special sections have been devoted to the story of developments in the cure and prevention of tuberculosis.

WAKSMAN, S. A., 1964: The conquest of tuberculosis, 241 p. (Berkeley, Cal.: California U.P.).—

A popular book, written by a microbiologist who has much experience of the effectiveness of streptomycin on tuberculosis. A comparable booklet, written by a prominent surgeon, and destined for the layman with no previous technical knowledge of contemporary medical science, is: BANKOFF, G., 1946: The conquest of tuberculosis, 187 p. (London: MacDonald). The historical material is scattered throughout the book.

typhus

ZINSSER, H., 1935: Rats, lice and history: being a study in biography, which, after twelve preliminary chapters indispensable for the preparation of the lay reader, deals with the life history of typhus fever, 301 p. (Boston, Mass.: Little, Brown; London: Routledge).—

A popular but scientifically reliable description of the history of typhus. Also in German translation: Der Roman des Fleckfiebers. Ratten, Läuse, Menschen und Weltgeschichte, 1949, 318 p. (Stuttgart: Calwey); and with the same title: 1948, 257 p. (Vienna: Ring Verlag).

yellow fever

CARTER, H. R., 1931: Yellow fever: an epidemiological and historical study of its place of origin, 308 p. (Baltimore, Md.: Williams & Wilkins).—

In this detailed and comprehensive study, the author describes the epidemiology of yellow fever, and of many other tropical epidemic diseases and he discusses the characteristics which differentiate them, for in the more remote past such diseases as malaria, typhus, relapsing fever, and leptospiral jaundice could hardly be distinguished from yellow fever. After having made clear his medical point of view the author critically discusses the writings of historians and explorers of the African and American tropics, and he defends the theory that the infections came to America through the African slave trade and the activities of the buccaneers. Vivid descriptions of the way the community reacted on a yellow fever epidemic can be found in: POWELL, J. H., 1949: Bring out your dead: the great plague of yellow fever in Philadelphia in 1793, 304 p. (Philadelphia, Pa.: Pennsylvania U.P.); in: SMITH, A., 1951: Yellow fever in Galveston, Republic of Texas, 1839, 135 p. (Austin, Tex.: Texas U.P.); and in: DUFFY, J., 1966: Sword of pestilence: the New Orleans yellow fever epidemic of 1853, 191 p. (Baton Rouge, La.: Louisiana State U.P.).

COPEMAN, W. S. C., 1964: A short history of the gout and the rheumatic diseases, 236 p. (Berkeley/Los Angeles, Cal.: California U.P.).—

A comprehensive history of gout and rheumatic diseases. Chapters 1-7 deal with the history of gout, its clinics, pathology, biochemistry, therapeutics, its role in society, its description in the Corpus Hippocraticum, by Alexander of Tralles, Sydenham, Wollaston, Garrod, *etc.,* and the treatment of gout by colchicum. The last five chapters deal with the history of acute rheumatism, rheumatoid arthritis, ankylosing spondylitis, osteoarthritis, and nonarticular rheumatism.

c17 *tumours*

WOLFF, J., 1907-1929: Die Lehre von der Krebskrankheit von den ältesten Zeiten bis zur Gegenwart, 4 vols. Vol. I, ed. 2 (1929): 753 p.; Vol. II (1911): 1261 p.; Vol. III (1913): 618 p.; Vol. IV (1928): 743 p. (Jena: Fischer).—

An exhaustive and - according to Garrison-Morton - accurate review of all the available information on the subject of cancer. It also is the most important bibliography on the subject. Especially vol. I is of importance to the history of medicine; vol. III deals with the history of cancer in animals and plants. A popular presentation of the history of the problem of malignant tumours, written to interest the public in supporting cancer research, is: BUTLER, F., 1955: Cancer through the ages: the evolution of hope, 147 p. (Fairfax, Va.: Univ. of Virginia Press).

c18 *röntgenology*

DEWING, S., 1962: Modern radiology in historical perspective, 189 p. (Springfield, Ill.: Thomas).—

In this book the author considers the background of radiology before Röntgen's discovery of 1895, and the progress made since, both in technical and in theoretical aspects. Biographical sketches of Röntgen, Becquerel, and the Curies.

GRUBBÉ, E. H., 1949: X-ray treatment: its origin, birth and early history, 154 p. (Saint Paul & Minneapolis, Minn.: Bruce).—

A historical sketch of the early development of the X-ray equipment and X-ray therapy, especially in the U.S.A. Included is a list of pioneers of the X-ray; the author himself belongs to them.

c19 *surgery* (and anaesthesiology)

ARMSTRONG DAVISON, M. H., 1965: The evolution of anaesthesia, 236 p. (Baltimore, Md.: Williams & Wilkins).—

A history of anaesthesiology, in which the author emphasizes that it is not true that man has sought from earliest times to conquer pain - a supposition often held by other historians of medicine and surgery. He shows that it had to be necessary that a certain concern for others and an interest to their welfare must have developed, and that physics and chemistry must be in the position to isolate and synthesize volatile organic compounds, before the science of anaesthesiology could be established. In this way a more or less "objective" history of the evolution of anaesthesia originated, in which the author interprets the events in terms of their contemporary significance. Much attention has been paid to the evolution of various technical and mechanical details of anaesthetic equipment.

BISHOP, W. J., 1959: A history of surgical dressing, 90 p. (Chesterfield: Robinson).—

The book deals with such subjects as: the origin of surgical dressing, dressing among the Berbers and Shawiya, ancient Egypt and the Ebers papyrus, Hindu surgery, Hippocrates, dressings in the mediaeval period, 17th and 18th centuries, antisepsis and asepsis, dressing fabrics, plaster and other fixative dressings, recent developments in surgical dressings. Bibliography included. A book which seems to deal with the same subjects - but of which I am unable to give further information - is: ELLIOT, I. M. & J. R., 1964: A short history of surgical dressing, 118 p. (London: Pharmaceutical Press).

——, 1960: The early history of surgery, 192 p. (London: Hale).—

A semi-popular chronological review of the facts and documents pertaining to the development of surgery from its earliest beginnings to the latter part of the 19th century. The end-point is chosen shortly after the discovery of anaesthesia and the principles of antisepsis. Stress has been laid on the manifold problems confronting surgeons during the preceding centuries and the impact of their discoveries on the future of surgery.

COPE, Z., 1965: A history of the acute abdomen, 123 p. (London: Oxford U.P.).—

This work covers the history of problems and operations related to such diseases as: peritonites, appendicitis, perforated ulcer, intestinal resection and anastomosis, acute cholecystitis, intestinal obstruction, and ruptured ectopic gestation, from the time of Hippocrates to the present.

FAULCONER, A. & T. E. KEYS, 1965: Foundations of anesthesiology, 2 vols., 1337 p. (Springfield, Ill.: Thomas).—

An anthology of 150 papers on anaesthesia and related topics, divided into eight sections, each section being preceded by a short introduction. Translations are in English and for each of the authors included a biographical note is given. The time-span considered extends from the 16th century to 1961.

GURLT, E. J., 1898: Geschichte der Chirurgie und ihrer Ausübung. Volkschirurgie. Alterthum. Mittelalter. Renaissance, 3 vols. Vol. I: 976 p.; Vol. II: 926 p.; Vol. III: 834 p. (Berlin: Hirschwald).—

A classical work dealing with the history of surgery to the end of the 16th century. Vol. I deals with folk surgery as it is and as it has been practised in various parts of the world (p. 1-238), with surgery in Greece (p. 239-313), Rome (p. 314-522), and during the Middle Ages (Byzantium, Arabs, Latin Europe, Italy, School of Salerno, 13th, 14th, and 15th centuries) p. 523-976). Vol. II deals with surgery during the Middle Ages in France, Spain, Belgium, England, Germany, Scandinavia, Hungary, Poland, Russia, and Servia (p. 1-272), and with surgery during the Renaissance in Italy (p. 273-605) and France (p. 606-926). Vol. III deals with surgery during the Renaissance in Germany (p. 1-208); Switzerland; Holland; Belgium; England (p. 340-380); Spain (p. 381-423); Portugal; Denmark; Sweden; and Russia. The last part (p. 459-809) deals with general problems of surgical practice, with fistulae, tumours, wounds, diseases of the skin, arteries, glands, bones, muscles, etc., and with dislocations and injuries, etc., of the skull, ear, nose, mouth, neck, breast, vertebral column, urogenital organs, extremities, etc. Reprinted in 1964, 2816 p. (Hildesheim: Olms). A shorter history of surgery in German has been written by BRUNN, W. von, 1928: Kurze Geschichte der Chirurgie, 339 p. (Berlin: Springer), a useful textbook of which in 1948 an abridged version was published: Geschichte

der Chirurgie, 80 p. (Bonn: Universitätsverlag). Of this abridged version a French translation appeared: Histoire de la chirurgie, 1955, 160 p. (Paris: Lamarre).

HOCHBERG, L. A., 1960: Throacic surgery before the 20th century, 858 p. (New York, N.Y.: Vantage Press).—

This book has been written by a thoracic surgeon. A brief initial chapter deals with early thoracic surgery from prehistory up to the 15th century when this science was limited to the menagement of injuries of the chest and the treatment of empyema. Following chapters deal with a discussion of thoracic anatomy in mediaeval and Renaissance art and medicine, 16th, 17th, and 18th centuries. During this period the progress made was only small: the drainage of suppurations of the lung as well as of the pleural cavity, the removal of foreign bodies from the trachea and oesophagus by instrumentation. Enormous advances were made during the 19th century. Separate and lengthy chapters are devoted to injuries, empyema, pulmonary suppurations, tuberculosis, diaphragmatic hernia, oesophageal surgery, cardiovascular surgery, aspiration of pleural fluid accumulations, thoraxoplasty and pulmonary decortication, pericardial drainage, etc. One chapter deals with nonsurgical contributions to the advancement of thoracic surgery, discussing e.g., percussion, auscultation, antisepsis, anaesthesia, peroral endoscopy and X-rays. Bibliography of 80 pages. For a concise history of chest surgery cf. NISSEN, R. & R. H. L. WILSON, 1960, vide infra. Cf. also MEADE, R., 1961, vide infra.

HUARD, P. & M. D. GRMEK, 1966: Mille ans de chirurgie en Occident: Ve-XVe siècles, 82 p. text + 171 plates and photographs. (Paris: Dacosta).—

For more details, vide section The Middle Ages in the Latin West, subsection c.

——, 1968: La chirurgie moderne. Ses débuts en occident: XVIe, XVIIe, XVIIIe siècles, 253 p. (Paris: Dacosta).—

Not only is the text devoted to the various aspects of general surgery, but much attention has been paid to some of the specialties, such as: anaesthesia, military medicine, odontology, stomatology, neurosurgery, neurology, etc. Much attention has also been paid to the basic sciences which made surgical progress possible, such as: anatomy, physiology, and pathology. "The book is a formidable work, recapitulating important events in the progress of surgical procedures. It brings a very well selected bibliography and brief bio-bibliographies of the great medical men of the three centuries. Understandably, it is predominantly the great French surgeons who are listed." (From a review in: Bull. Hist. Med. 44: 94-95).

HURWITZ, A. & G. A. DEGENSHEIM, 1958: Milestones in modern surgery, 520 p. (London: Cassell).—

This beautifully illustrated book consists of 13 chapters, dealing with: haemostasis; anaesthesia; the milieu intérieur; wound healing and infection; surgery of head and neck, breast, hernia and gastro-intestinal tract; intestinal obstruction; thoracic and cardiovascular surgery; the soul of the surgeon; milestones on the horizon. Each chapter contains prefatory comments, a short biography (with a portrait) of each main builder of the particular milestone and his 'surgical classic', reprinted or translated in full.

LEAKE, C. D., 1947: Letheon: the cadenced story of anesthesia, 128 p. (Austin, Tex.: Texas U.P.).—

The main part of this publication consists of a poem, relating the story of the discovery of anaesthesia. In addition to the poem we are given a chronology of anaesthesia from prehistoric times to 1947, and a bibliography.

LEONARDO, R. A., 1943: History of surgery, 504 p. + 100 plates. (New York, N.Y.: Froben).—

A full-scale history of surgery in English. It deals with primitive, Babylonian, Egyptian, Hebrew, Hindu, Chinese, Japanese, Greek, Alexandrian, Roman, Byzantine, Arabian, Mediaeval and Renaissance surgery, with surgery in the 17th, 18th, and 19th centuries, with surgical obstetrics in the Renaissance and after, with the barber surgeons, and with modern surgery. It has much to say about local developments of surgery in America, England, Switzerland, Italy, France, Germany, Austria, Hungary, Spain, South America, Mexico, and Canada. A book of the same scope seems to be: MEADE, R. H., 1968: An introduction to the history of general surgery, 403 p. (Philadelphia, Pa.: Saunders). (No information available). A well-written introduction to the history of the last achievements of surgery is: CARTWRIGHT, F. F., 1967: The development of modern surgery from 1830, 323 p. (London: Barker).

LERICHE, R., 1944: La chirurgie à l'ordre de la vie, 249 p. (Paris & Aix-les-Bains: la Presse française et étrangère).—

A collection of well-written essays by a famous surgeon dealing with Lister, Cl. Bernard, A. Poncet, A. Lambotte, C. Nicolle, H. Cushing, and W. S. Halsted. In this book the author also develops his idea of a new physiological surgery, *i.e.,* a surgery not as a mere technique but a surgery closely connected with life itself, a surgery in which manual artifices are subordinated to intelligence. A more full-scale French history of surgery is: LECÈNE, P., 1923: L'évolution de la chirurgie, 345 p. (Paris: Flammarion), and a very concise one is: D'ALLAINES, C., 1961: Histoire de la chirurgie, 128 p. (Que Sais-je? No. 935) (Paris: Presses Univ. de France).

MEADE, R., 1961: A history of thoracic surgery, 933 p. (Oxford: Blackwell).—

A very complete history of this speciality going back to 3000 years B.C. The author reviews chronologically the advances in our knowledge of the various pathological lesions and the technique for their treatment. The separate lesions are arranged under separate headings and at the end of each section is an extensive bibliography. For a concise history of chest surgery cf. NISSEN, R. & R. H. L. WILSON, *vide infra.* Cf. also HOCHBERG, L. A., 1960, *vide supra.*

NISSEN, R. & R. H. L. WILSON, 1960: Pages in the history of chest surgery, 166 p. (Springfield, Ill.: Thomas).—

This concise history of thoracic surgery deals with such subjects as: open pneumothorax anaesthesia, pulmonary resection, surgery in pulmonary tuberculosis, surgery of the oesophagus, surgery of the heart, *etc.* It contains many illustrations, comprising photographs or portraits of many of the pioneers of thoracic surgery and reproductions of the title page or first pages of many of the original articles. For more complete histories of chest surgery, cf.: MEADE, R., 1961: and HOCHBERG, L. A., 1960, *vide supra.*

RAPER, H. R., 1945: Man against pain: the epic of anesthesia, 337 p. (New York, N.Y.: Prentice Hall).—

The text has been divided into 4 parts. In the first part, "Background", the author takes us back to the earliest known efforts of man to find some means to deaden pain: the use of anodynes in antiquity and the Middle Ages, the use of such narcotics as mandragora, cannabis, henbane, opium, and alcohol, the role of hypnotism and surgery. The second part deals with the achievements of *e.g.,* Davy, Hickman, Collier, Long, Wells, Morton, Jackson. The third part especially deals with the ether controversy. The fourth part deals with the development of modern anaesthetics and the science of anaesthesiology, with the problem of how anaestetics acted, what the proper times and dosages were, *etc.,* and the development of modern types of anaesthesia. A useful short history of anaesthesiology is: KEYS, T. E., 1945: The history of surgical anaesthesia, 191 p. (New York, N.Y.: Schuman). Reprinted in a paperback edition, 1963 (New York, N.Y.: Dover). Also in German translation: Die Geschichte der chirurgischen Anästhesie, 1968, 230 p. (Berlin: Springer). A book stressing the British contributions to the development of inhalation anaesthesia is: DUNCUM, B. M., 1947: The development of inhalation anesthesia with special reference to the years 1846-1900, 640 p. (London & New York, N.Y.: Oxford U.P.). In this study the author places greater stress on methodology and technique, rather than on biographical details or on the various anaesthetic agents. A very useful bibliographic review on this subject can be found in FULTON, J. F. & M. E. STANTON, 1946: The centennial of surgical anesthesia: an annotated catalogue of books and pamphlets bearing on the early history of surgical anesthesia, 102 p. (New York, N.Y.: Schuman).

THORWALD, J., 1965: Die Geschichte der Chirurgie, 448 p. (Stuttgart: Steingrüben Verlag).—

A popular history of surgery written for a lay public. It is a compilation of the most important parts of two other books of the same author, *viz.,* "Das Jahrhundert der Chirurgen" and "Das Weltreich der Chirurgen". It gives a description of the main events in the history of surgery and of the men who put a stamp on its development *(e.g.,* Warren, Wells, Lister, Simpson, Freud, Porro, Semmelweis, Pasteur, Billroth, Czerny, von Mikulicz, Koch, Bergmann, Langenbuch, Kocher, Bassini, Bier, Schleich, Sauerbruch).

WHIPPLE, A. O., 1963: The story of wound healing and wound repair, 135 p. (Springfield, Ill.: Thomas).—

This publication deals with a series of events which resulted in an advance in

surgical knowledge such as: discoveries in anatomy, physiology, pathology, and bacteriology; the invention of new instruments; war and comparable calamities; economic conditions; the development of anaesthesia; *etc.*

ZIMMERMAN, L. M. & I. VEITH, 1961: Great ideas in the history of surgery, 587 p. (London: Baillière, Tindall & Cox; Baltimore, Md.: Williams & Wilkins).—

The aim of this book is not so much to give a conventional history of surgery, but the authors try "to convey a feeling for the growth of surgery by presenting its leading personalities from the beginning of literary records to the present time" and much attention has been paid to the ideas of the surgeons discussed. As such the book is comparable with SIGERIST's "Great doctors" *vide supra,* section General histories of medicine. Each chapter refers to a particular surgeon, giving an introductory "epigrammatic statement", a biographical sketch giving a general background both in time and space, and a verbatim extract from the writings of the selected surgeon. Reprinted in 1967 (New York, N.Y.: Dover).

C20 *tropical medicine*

OLPP, G., 1932: Hervorragende Tropenaerzte in Wort und Bild, 446 p. (Munich: Gmelin).—

This book contains *ca.* 300 biographies, almost all of them accompanied by a photograph. *Cf.* also OLPP, G., 1936: Characterköpfe der Tropenmedizin, 96 p. (Berlin: Brücke zur Heimat Verlag).

SCOTT, H. H., 1942: A history of tropical medicine, based on the FitzPatrick lectures delivered before the Royal College of Physicians of London 1937-38, 2 vols., 1219 p (London: Arnold).—

A comprehensive history of medical knowledge and practice of tropical diseases, in which their causes, therapeutics, and prevention are discussed, together with their geographical, industrial, and social aspects. The first volume deals with the navy and mercantile marine, the army, the British colonies, protectorates and dominions, with malaria, blackwater fever, yellow fever, trypanosomiasis, leishmaniasis and leprosy. Vol. II deals with cholera, plague, undulant fever, relapsing fever, dengue, amoebic dysentry and hepatitis, ankylostomiasis, and tropical diseases connected with food. It also contains chapters on the Suez and Panama canals and the slave trade in relation to contacts with tropical diseases. Brief biographies are given of: Bontius, Bruce, Carroll, Cruz, Dutton, Finlay, Carcia da Orta, Gorgas, Lazear, Leishman, Lind, Manson, Noguchi, Reed, and Ross.

c21 *urology*

BALLENGER, E. G., ed., 1933: History of urology, 2 vols. Vol. I: 386 p.; Vol. II: 362 p. (Baltimore, Md.: Williams & Wilkins).—

"Every aspect of the subject is covered exhaustively by the various contributors to this collective work; valuable bibliographies are included." A more recent valuable source of information on this subject is: IMMERGUT, M. A., ed., 1967: Classical articles in urology, 329 p. (Springfield, Ill.: Thomas). A collection of 25 classical urological articles. Following each article is a commentary either by the original author or by a contemporary prominent urologist.

d. *History of some social aspects of medicine* ("Community and disease")

d₁. *General aspects*

GILBERT, J. B., 1962: Disease and destiny: a bibliography of medical references to the famous, 535 p. (London: Dawsons).—

A mine of biographical and bibliographical information concerning diseases and deaths, *etc.*, of famous men and women. The names are arranged alphabetically. The kind of information is described as follows: 1. Medical information concerning the person himself; 2. Medical analysis, usually of a psychopathological nature, concerning the works of the person; 3. Biographical or memorabilia; 4. Relations of the person to medicine and doctors; 5. Description of the state or condition of contemporary medicine in the time of the person. *Cf.* STEVENSON, R. S., Famous illnesses in history, 239 p. (London: Eyre & Spottiswoode).

HIMES, N. E., 1963: Medical history of contraception, 53 + 521 p. (New York, N.Y.: Gamut Press).—

A reprint of the 1936 edition, discussing such subjects as: contraceptive techniques before the dawn of written history (*e.g.*, in preliterate societies in Africa, America, *etc.*), contraceptive techniques in Western

antiquity (*e.g.*, Egyptians, in Bible and Talmud, Greek and Roman writers), contraceptive techniques in Eastern cultures (China, India, Japan), *idem* in the West during the Middle Ages and early modern times (*e.g.*, in the Islamic world, in European folk belief, in lay literature, the history of the condom), and with the democratization of contraceptive technique since 1800 (*e.g.*, the early birth-control movement in England and the U.S.A., birth control and mid-19th-century and 20th-century American writers, the probable effect of democratized contraception). A very important study on the subject, especially of interest for the religious aspects, but also containing a wealth of historical information, is: NOONAN, J. T., 1965: Contraception: the history of its treatment by the Catholic theologians and canonists, 561 p. (Harvard, Mass.: U.P.). A short history of contraception, tracing the modes of contraception from the time of the Pharaohs of ancient Egypt to the present, and including much information on recent advances in birth control is to be found in: FINCH, B. E. & H. GREEN, 1963: Contraception through the ages, 174 p. (Springfield, Ill.: Thomas).

SAND, R., 1952: The advance of social medicine, 655 p. (London: Staples).—

The original text, "Vers la médecine sociale", was published in 1948 (Paris: Baillière). It is an encyclopaedic work, divided into 9 parts, *viz.*, history of the medical profession; history of hospitals; history of personal hygiene; history of public hygiene; history of social hygiene; history of industrial medicine; history of welfare work; history of social sciences. Good bibliography and indexes of names, nations, and subjects. An authoritative history. *Cf.* also: DIEPGEN, P., 1934: Geschichte der sozialen Medizin (Leipzig), a book about which I could not find further information.

SIGERIST, H. E., 1943: Civilization and disease, 255 p. (Ithaca, N.Y.: Cornell U.P.).—

The starting point of the author has been that human diseases principally consist of two components, the first being of a purely biological nature, resting on a certain disharmony in the continually changing relationships either between the various parts composing the body, or between the body and the external environment; the second component, however, being of a "social" character, for men can live only in a society. Thus disease should be treated as a socio-biological phenomenon. In the present book, the author consequently seeks to correlate the history of medicine on the one side with the history of civilization (*e.g.,* economics, social life, law, history, religion, philosophy, science, literature, art) on the other side, in order to investigate where they affected and influenced each other. Also in German translation: Krankheit und Zivilisation. Geschichte der Zerstörung der menschlichen Gesundheit, 1952, 264 p. (Frankfurt a. M. & Berlin: Metzner); and in Spanish translation: Civilización y enfermedad, 1946, 287 p. (México, D.C.: Fondo de cultura económica).

———, 1954: Die Heilkunst im Dienste der Menschheit, 116 p. (Stuttgart: Hippocrates).—

> This is a German translation of "Medicine and human welfare", 1941, 148 p. (New Haven, Conn.: Yale U.P.). It contains the text of three lectures delivered in Yale University, entitled I. Disease; II. Health; III. The physician. All chapters try to make clear the changes which have taken place from the old concepts of medicine as a cure of disease, to hygiene as preservation of individual health, and to the broader ideas of preventive and social medicine. It is a very readable book in which the social function of medicine is elucidated with the aid of history.

d2. *History of medical education and the medical profession*

BAAS, J. H., 1896: Die geschichtliche Entwicklung des ärztlichen Standes und der medizinischen Wissenschaften, 492 p. (Berlin: Wreden).—

> Separate sections deal with the position of the physician in the various societies, such as: the preliterate society (the magician, medicine man, priest-physician), the caste-society (caste-medicine in Egypt, India, China), the Greek, Hellenistic, and Roman society (School of Hippocrates, Alexandria, Asclepiades, Galen, the Roman Empire), the mediaeval society in East and West, and in the post-mediaeval society of Western Europe during the Renaissance, and the 17th, 18th, and 19th centuries. *Cf.* FISCHER, I., 1912: Aerztliche Standespflichten und Standesfragen. Eine historische Studie, 190 p. (Vienna & Leipzig: Braumüller).

BULLOUGH, V. L., 1966: The development of medicine as a profession: the contribution of the medieval university to mod-

ern medicine, 125 p. (New York, N.Y.: Hafner).—

> A historical review of the social and economic aspects of the medical profession. Written by a mediaevalist. The first chapter deals with primitive and classical medicine, in which also some attention has been paid to the schools of Dogmatism, Empiricism, Methodism, and Pneumatism. The second chapter deals with the period between the 6th and the 12th century and considers, *e.g.,* Cassiodorus, Paul of Aegina, Isidore of Seville, Gariopontus, Constantine the African, and the influence of monastic medicine in the evolution of the profession. In the last three chapters the author describes the professionalization of medicine, the institutionalization of medical knowledge, interventions of government, and the development of a code of ethics. *Cf.* WATSON, J., 1856, *vide* section Antiquity in general, subsection c.

DELAUNAY, P., 1935: La vie médicale aux XVIe, XVIIe et XVIIIe siècles, 556 p. (Paris: Ed. Hippocrate).—

> This book contains the following chapters: Les étudiants en médecine; La vie privée du médecin; La vie professionnelle; La vie corporative; La vie religieuse; La vie politique; La vie sociale; La vie intellectuelle; La vie doctrinale. It is mainly restricted to French circumstances.

GURLEY, J. E., 1960: The evolution of dental education, 276 p. (Fulton, Mo.: Ovid Bell Press; St. Louis, Mo.: Amer. Coll. Dentistry).—

> The contents of this book may become clear from its full title: The evolution of dental education, including a chronological history of the Dental Educational Council of America, the Dental Faculties of American Universities, the reorganized Dental Educational Council of America; reports of the historian. By the same author: The evolution of professional ethics in dentistry, report of the historian, 1961, 113 p. (St. Louis, Mo.: Amer. Coll. Dentistry). *Cf.* also: GREVE, H. C., 1930: Aphorismen zur Kulturgeschichte der Zahnheilkunde und des zahnärztlichen Standes, 91 p. (Leipzig: Thieme), a book about which I could not find further information.

MARX, C., 1907: Die Entwicklung des aerztlichen Standes seit den ersten Dezennien des 19. Jahrhunderts, 164 p. (Berlin: Struppe & Wickler).—

A history of the development of the medical profession in Germany during the preceding century. Part I is entitled: Der aerztlichen Stand (in the different parts, "Lander", of Germany, the physician's education, specialization, *etc.*). Part II is entitled: Die Einwirkung der Gewerbe- und der sozial-politischen Gesetzgebung auf die rechtliche soziale und wirtschaftliche Lage des aerztlichen Standes; and part III is entitled: Die Organisation des aerztlichen Standes.

NEWMAN, C., 1957: The evolution of medical education in the nineteenth century, 340 p. (London: Oxford U.P.).—

This book traces the evolution of medical education in Great Britain during the former century. The book starts with a review of the medical education and the medical profession in the early years of the 19th century and describes the reforms leading to the Apothecaries Act of 1815 and the Medical Act of 1858. In the last part of the book the author deals with medical education during the second half of the 19th century and the role of the Medical Act of 1886. Bibliography, references, notes, and index. It gives much information concerning the application of the sciences to medicine.

POLLAK, K. & E. A. UNDERWOOD, 1968: The healers: the doctor, then and now, 246 p. (London: Nelson).—

An account of the evolution of the medical practitioner from the Stone Age to the present in the main civilizations of the world, considering the cures prescribed, the punishment if the doctor failed, his fees, clothes, position in society, *etc.* Originally published in German: Die Jünger des Hippocrates. Der Weg des Arztes durch sechs Jahrtausende, 1963 (Düsseldorf & Vienna: Econ). The English edition has been much adapted for the British reader.

PUSCHMANN, T., 1889: Geschichte des medizinischen Unterrichtes von den ältesten Zeiten bis zur Gegenwart, 522 p. (Leipzig: Veit).—

A systematic history of medical teaching from ancient times onwards: India, Egypt, the Jews, the Parsees, the Greeks, the Romans, medical teaching during the Middle Ages, the monastic schools, the School of Salerno, the School of Montpellier, the teaching of medicine in the old universities of Europe, medical teaching in the time of increasing specialization in the different

parts of the world. This edition was reprinted in 1966 (Amsterdam: Israel). There also exists an English translation: History of medical education from the most remote to the most recent times, 1891, 650 p. (London: Lewis). Of this English edition a reprint appeared in 1966 (New York, N.Y.: Hafner) with an introduction by E. H. ACKERKNECHT and supplied with copious footnotes and an index.

TURNER, E. S., 1958: Call the doctor: a social history of medical men, 320 p. (London: Joseph; New York, N.Y.: St. Martin).—

This study deals with the doctor as a member of society from the 14th century to the present time. It deals with the many conflicts which arose between doctors themselves, and between individual physicians and the Royal Colleges or the public (*e.g.*, discussing such themes as body-snatching, man-midwifery, vivisection, control of prostitution, euthanasia, *etc.*), and with many other subjects.

WARTMAN, W. B., 1961: Medical teaching in Western civilization, 307 p. (Chicago, Ill.: Yearbook Med. Publ.).—

This book deals with such subjects as: the Hippocratic reform of priestly medicine, sects and folly in Rome, dogma in the mediaeval university, the birth of modern teaching in the 16th century, the 19th century: observation and analysis in France; English hospital schools, new patterns in 20th-century medicine and its difficulties.

d₃. *History of the care of the sick*

ABLE-SMITH, B., 1960: A history of the nursing profession, 270 p. (London: Heinemann).—

Separate chapters deal with: the untrained nurse, probationers and lady-pupils, paid nurses and pauper nurses, nursing at the turn of the century, acknowledgement of the profession, nursing and parliament, nurse-shortage, nurses' pay.

BAUER, F., 1965: Geschichte der Krankenpflege. Handbuch der Entstehung und Entwicklung der Krankenpflege von Frühzeit bis zur Gegenwart, 384 p. (Kulmbach: Baumann).—

A full-scale German history of all aspects of nursing from prehistory up to and including the period after the second World War. *Cf.* also: STICKER, A., 1960: Die Entstehung der neuzeitlichen Krankenpflege. Deutsche Quellenstücke aus der ersten Hälfte des 19. Jahrhunderts, 382 p. (Stuttgart: Kohlhammer).

CUTTER, I. S. & H. R. VIETS, 1964: A short history of midwifery, 260 p. (Philadelphia, Pa. & London: Saunders).—

> This book deals with the development of clinical midwifery in England, France, Germany and America. Appendixes deal with books on the history of midwifery published since 1933 and a selection of published catalogues of books on midwifery. Index of persons and good index of subjects. A German history of midwifery is: BURCKHARDT, G., 1912: Studien zur Geschichte des Hebammenwesen. I. Die deutschen Hebammenordnungen von ihren ersten Anfängen bis auf die Neuzeit, 258 p. (Leipzig: Engelmann). *Cf.* also: RADCLIFFE, W., 1967, *vide infra*.

DOLAN, J. A., 1963: History of nursing, ed. 11, 360 p. (Philadelphia, Pa.: Saunders).—

> A profusely illustrated history of nursing (293 figures). Separate chapters deal with: Care of the sick among primitive men, care of the sick in ancient cultures, influence of Christianity; early Middle Ages; late Middle Ages; the period of the Renaissance 1500-1700, and with the 18th, 19th and 20th centuries respectively. *Cf.* BULLOUGH, V. L. & B., 1969: The emergence of modern nursing, ed. 2, 277 p. (New York, N.Y.: Macmillan).

FINOT, A., 1958: Notes sur l'histoire de la clinique médicale et de son enseignement, 92 p. (Paris: Legrand).—

> A history of the medical clinic from ancient Egypt up to the beginning of the 19th century. The second half of the book stresses the role of France in the important development of the medical clinic in the 19th century, with names such as: Corvisart, Laënnec, Bretonneau, Trousseau, Bouillaud.

FOUCAULT, U., 1963: Naissance de la clinique. Une archéologie du regard médical, 213 p. ("Galien", Histoire et philosophie de la biologie et de la médecine) (Paris: Presses Univ. de France).—

> Section headings are as follows: 1. Espaces et classes; 2. Une conscience poli-

tique; 3. Le champ libre; 4. Vieillesse de la clinique; 5. La leçon des hôpitaux; 6. Des signes et du cas; 7. Voir; savoir; 8. Ouvrez quelques cadavres; 9. L'invisible visible; 10. La crise des fièvres. "An intensive study of a comparatively brief period (1770-1830) which saw the emergence of an entirely new approach to disease and, literally, the birth of clinical medicine".

HAESER, H., 1966: Geschichte christlicher Kranke-Pflege und Pflegerschaften, 126 p. (Bad Reichenhall: Kleinert).—

> The first section (p. 8-43) deals with Christianity: the nursing houses of the parish, the xenodochia, the hospitals; general equipment of the xenodochia and hospitals. The second section deals with guilds for the care of the sick: guilds of knights, *e.g.*, the Knights of St. John, the German order; the Lazarists; the beguines and beghards; some brotherhoods providing care in sickness; male and women nurses. Originally published 1857 (Berlin: Hertz).

KANNER, L., 1964: A history of the care and study of the mentally retarded, 150 p. (Springfield, Ill.: Thomas).—

> This book has been written by one of the founders of child psychiatry in the U.S.A. An introductory chapter discusses briefly the Latin terminology and the main attitudes toward mental deficiency up to the Enlightenment. This is followed by a chapter in which the first five pioneers are considered extensively, *viz.*, Jacob Pereire, Jean Itard, Johann Guggenbühl, Ed. Séguin, and Samuel Howe. Other sections deal with such subjects as: the expansion of institutions for mental defectives in various countries, the publication of specific journals for mental deficiency, the differentiation of mental deficiency into various groups, *etc.*

NUTTING, M. A. & L. L. DOCK, 1907-1912: A history of nursing, 4 vols. (New York, N.Y.: Putnam).—

> According to Garrison-Morton the authoritative history of the subject. There is an abridged edition of this book: DOCK, L. L. & I. M. STEWART, 1920: A short history of nursing from the earliest times to the present day, 392 p. (New York, N.Y.: Putnam).

RADCLIFFE, W., 1967: Milestones in midwifery, 110 p. (Bristol: Wright).—

> A history of obstetrics from the earliest times up to the 19th century. "Such

a book should have a large circulation. It is very likely to cause the reader to become keen on obstetric history and in any case it is a convenient reference book for one not too deeply involved in medical history." From a book review in Med. Hist. 13: 205. *Cf.* CUTTER, I. S. & H. R. VIETS, 1964, *vide supra.*

RISLEY, M., 1962: The house of healing: the story of the hospital, 208 p. (London: Hale).—

> Unfortunately I am not able to give further information about this book.

ROSEN, G., 1968: Madness in society: chapters in the historical sociology of mental illness, 337 p. (Chicago, Ill.: Univ. Chicago Press; London: Routledge & Kegan Paul).—

> A series of 10 chapters originally published elsewhere. In his preface Rosen writes: "These studies are concerned with the historical sociology of mental illness, not with the history of psychiatry. Their central focus is not the thought and practice of medical men dealing with the phenomena of mental disorder as a medical problem, but rather the place of the mentally ill, however defined, in societies at different historical periods and the factors (social, psychological, cultural) that have determined it."

ROTH, E., 1903: Bibliographie der gesammten Krankenpflege, 878 p. (In: G. LIEBE, P. JACOBSOHN & G. MEIJER, Handbuch der Krankenversorgung und Krankenpflege, Vol. II, pt. 2) (Berlin: Hirschwald).—

> A useful bibliography, including such subjects as: the history of the care of the sick, hospitals and their history, the history of the epidemics *(e.g.,* leprosy, tuberculosis, syphilis), mental diseases, military and naval medicine, *etc.*

SELLEW, G. & C. J. NUESSE, 1946: A history of nursing, 444 p. (St. Louis, Mo.: Mosby).—

> This book is particularly complete and valuable concerning the influence of monasteries on the history of nursing.

SHRYOCK, R. H., 1959: The history of nursing: an interpretation of the social and the medical factors involved, 330 p. (Philadelphia, Pa. & London: Saunders).—

> This book primarily discusses the historical relations between medicine and

nursing, and the author shows that both paths of development run by no means parallel. The author traces his history against a background of political, social, scientific, and religious aspects from pre-Christian times up to the present. He especially deals with the rather complex influences of Christianity on the evolution and growth of both nursing and medicine, and their mutual relations.

STANTON, A. H. & M. S. SCHWARTZ, 1954: The mental hospital, 492 p. (New York, N.Y.: Basic Bks.).—

> A study of the life inside a psychiatric institution as it took place during the last 110 years (in an American mental hospital), based upon participant and non-participant observations. The role of all team members has been described and analysed as well as the "participant role of the psychiatric hospital patient."

d₄. *History of hygiene* (public health, epidemiology, medical geography, and preventive medicine)

d₄*. *History of public health, industrial hygiene, and occupational diseases*

BRAND, J. L., 1966: Doctors and the state: the British medical profession and government action, 307 p. (Baltimore, Md.: Johns Hopkins Press).—

> A detailed history of public health legislation in England, describing, *e.g.,* the activities of the medical department of the Local Government Board, the work of the medical officers of health of the military and colonial medical departments, the Poor Law medical service, the influence of the British Medical Association, and the influence of the medical journals.

BROCKINGTON, C. F., 1966: A short history of public health, ed. 2, 240 p. (London: Churchill).—

> This book mainly deals with the development of public health in England since 1800. The first part, about a third of the book, deals with such topics as: the development of the organization of public health, Poor Law reform, factory legislation, registrations of births and deaths, the formation of the Ministry of Health. The second part deals with such topics as: the different aspects of public health in the latter part of the 19th and the first half of the 20th cen-

tury, maternal and child welfare, mental hygiene, control of tuberculosis and venereal diseases, care for the aged, and the growth of housing. The book is intended as a work of reference for students. First ed. 1956. *Cf.* also BROCKINGTON, C. F., 1965: Public health in the nineteenth century, 287 p. (Edinburgh & London: Livingstone). The central theme of this book is the history of the attempts to set up a national administrative organization to deal with problems of community health in England between 1800 and 1871. A history of English public health during the former century and the first part of the present century is: FRAZER, W. M., 1590: A history of English public health, 1834-1939, 498 p. (London: Baillière, Tindall & Cox), *Cf.* also ECKSTEIN, H., 1958: The English Health Service: its origin, structure, and achievements, 289 p. (Cambridge, Mass.: Harvard U. P.).

CHARLES, J., 1961: Research and public health, 114 p. (London: Oxford U.P.).—

The author tries to elucidate the function of our present health organizations, such as the British Medical Committee and Council, the Health Committee of the League of Nations and the World Health Organization, against a historical background.

EBERSON, F., 1941: The microbe's challenge, 354 p. (Lancaster, Pa.: Cattell).—

This book contains much historical information on all of the major human diseases of bacterial, protozoan, and virus origin, including such diseases as: influenza, plague, tuberculosis, typhoid and typhus fevers. It contains much that is of interest in the history of preventive medicine.

FISCHER, A., 1933: Geschichte des deutschen Gesundheitswesens, 2 vols. Vol. I: 343 p.; Vol. II: 591 p. (Berlin: Herbig).—

The main parts of Vol. I are entitled: Vom Gesundheitswesen der alten Deutschen zur Zeit ihres Anschlusses an die Weltkultur bis zur Wirksamkeit des Stadtarztes Struppius (Die ersten 16 Jahrhunderte unserer Zeitrechnung) (p. 13-208). Einzelgebiete des Gesundheitswesens (p. 209-272); Von Guarinonius bis zum preussischen Medizinaledikt (Das 17. Jahrhundert) (p. 273-334). The main parts of Vol. II are entitled: Von den Anfängen der hygienischen Ortsbeschreibungen bis zu F. A. Mais Entwurf einer umfassenden Gesundheitsgesetzgebung (Das 18. Jahrhundert) (p. 1-284) und Von der Bildung der vaterländischen Gesellschaft der Aerzte und Naturforscher Schwabens (1801)

bis zur Gründung des Reichsgesundheitsamtes (1876). Reprinted in 1965 (Hildesheim: Olms).

HODGKINSON, R. G., 1967: The origins of the National Health Service: the medical services of the New Poor Law 1843-1871, 714 p. (Berkeley/Los Angeles, Cal.: Univ. Calif. Press).—

A history of the various professional, social, and institutional developments in health care, considering such subjects as: the rules and regulations of the New Poor Law, the position and problems of the Poor Law Medical Officer, provision for outdoor medical relief, the rise of workhouse infirmaries, interrelationships between the Poor Law and the public health movement, *etc.*

LESKY, E., 1959: Oesterreichisches Gesundheitswesen im Zeitalter des aufgeklärten Absolutismus, 228 p. (Archiv. für Oesterr. Geschichte, Vol. 122, Pt. 1) (Vienna: Rohrer).—

The text consists of the following chapters: 1. Staatliches und ständisches Gesundheitswesen; 2. Konservatismus und medizinische Polizei; 3. Einzelgebiete des Gesundheitswesens; 4. Drei habsburgische Leibaerzte als Träger des oesterreichischen Protomedikats (van Swieten, A. von Störck, J. A. von Stifft).

LICHT, S., ed., 1948: Occupational therapy source book, 90 p. (Baltimore, Md.: Williams & Wilkins).—

This book contains a compilation of some 10 articles dealing with the development of occupational therapy from the time of Pinel up to 1914, especially dealing with the psychiatric aspects of the subject. In an introduction the editor reviews the history of the idea of occupational therapy from Asclepiades to Barton.

MEYER, K. F., 1962: Disinfected mail, 341 p. (Holton, Kans.: Gossip Printery).—

This book contains a lot of information on such subjects as: postal arrangements, quarantine regulations, disinfection procedures, and epidemic visitations; as such it contains much that is of importance to historians of public health and medicine.

REYNOLDS, R., 1946: Cleanliness and Godliness, 326 p. (Garden City, N.Y.: Doubleday).—

This is a history of sewage disposal, in which the author traces the history of the privy and related matters from Mohenjo Daro and Crete to the present day, and in which he shows how human excreta disposal and sanitation are related to and influenced by factors such as religion and taboo. Its full title reads as follows: "Cleanliness and Godliness or the further metamorphosis. A discussion of the problems of sanitation raised by Sir John Harrington, together with reflections upon further progress recorded since that excellent Knight, by his invention of the metamorphosed Ajax, father of conveniences revolutionized the system of sanitation in this country but raised the same time fresh problems for posterity which are discussed in all their implications, with numerous digressions upon all aspects of cleanliness."

ROSEN, G., 1943: The history of miners' diseases: a medical and social interpretation, 490 p. (New York, N.Y.: Schuman).—

The first part of this book deals with miner's diseases from neolithic times to the end of the 18th century. For Neolithicum, Antiquity, and Middle Ages, these diseases can not be distinguished with certainty, but with Agricola and Paracelsus we come on firmer ground. The second part of the book takes almost two-thirds of its space and has been limited to caol mining and the so-called "collier's lung" and contains a lot of information on the evolution of clinical and pathological knowledge of the "miner's lung" during the 19th century. Besides it gives information on mining conditions, mortality of miners, therapy, prophylaxis, and social and protective legislation.

——, 1958: A history of public health, 551 p. (MD Monographs on Medical History, No 1) (New York, N.Y.: MD Publ.).—

A historical review of public health from prehistory to the present. In each period the author surveys the methods of providing medical care, together with their social implications, the environmental aspects, endemic and epidemic diseases, occupational diseases and public administration. The book also contains a collection of brief notes on "Memorable figures in the history of public health", a selected list of periodicals concerned with public health, a list of public health societies and associations (esp. in the U.S.A.), a list of schools of public health, an author-index and a very useful subject-index.

SIGERIST, H. E., 1956: Landmarks in the history of hygiene, 78 p. (London: Oxford U.P.).—

This work contains the text of five lectures: 1. Galen's "Hygiene"; 2. The "Regimen sanitatis salernitatum" and some of its commentators; 3. The quest for long life in the Renaissance; 4. Johann Peter Frank: a pioneer of social medicine; 5. The changing pattern of medical care. Sigerist describes how - in the course of history - medicine has become less the healing art and more the means of promoting health. He does so by choosing as illustrations certain high points in the history of hygiene. A history of hygiene in the German language is: RUBNER, M., 1911: Die Geschichte der Hygiene, 149 p. (In: M. RUBNER, M. v. GRUBER & M. FICKER, Handbuch der Hygiene, Vol. I: 21-170) (Leipzig: Hirzel).

STERN, B. J., 1946: Medicine in industry, 209 p. (New York, N.Y.: Commonwealth Fund).—

This book contains a broad historical review of the history of medicine in industry. Among the topics discussed we may mention: a critical analysis of the historical development of medical services in industry; the development of knowledge of occupational diseases; the social and legislative developments; the jurisdictional conflicts between labour and health agencies: industrial disability; the problem of the handicapped worker and rehabilitation; medical care and group insurance plans in industry; the status of the industrial physician.

TELEKY, L., 1948: History of factory and mine hygiene, 341 p. (New York, N.Y.: Columbia U.P.).—

This book is not an exhaustive history but rather an outline of a history of industrial hygiene, and it discusses such topics as: organizations and associations co-operating in industrial hygiene, methods of preventing injuries to health, accident-prevention, safety and health education, research in industrial hygiene, progress in toxicology, and the influence of physiology and statistics on industrial hygiene.

——, 1950: Die Entwicklung der Gesundheitsfürsorge: Deutschland, England, Berlin, U.S.A., 142 p. (Berlin: Springer).—

A comparative picture of the evolution of public health during the past hundred years in Germany, England, and the United States. The author traces the history of the development of social hygiene, the distribution of health personnel and facilities, social insurance, tuberculosis control and welfare, venereal disease control, care of mother and child, control of diphtheria and rickets, the health of the school child, nutrition

THOMAS, M. W., 1948: The early factory legislation: a study in legislative and administrative evolution, 470 p. (Leigh-on-Sea, Essex: Thames Bank).—

> A useful history of factory hygiene, especially devoted to its legislative and administrative evolution as it took place in England in the last century. The author shows how the lack of an administrative mechanism hampered the progress of factory legislation. Special attention has been paid to the influence of Benthamism on English history.

WILCOCKS, C., 1965: Medical advance, public health and social evolution, 271 p. (Oxford: Pergamon).—

> This book aims "to illustrate the link between historical advances in medical and public health affairs and the cultural and intellectual climates of various periods and places. Use of drugs and plants, superstitious practices, various concepts of prevention and of treatment, and some highlights of the evolution of public health measures are reviewed... In the 17 chapters are discussed the development of hygiene, the bacteriological era, food, water, and other environmental factors in the transmission of diseases, occupational medicine, degenerative diseases, psychological medicine, statistical methods, and experiments." (From a review in the J. Hist. Med. 23: 125).

WILLIAMS, R. C., 1951: The United States public health service, 1798-1950, 890 p. (Washington, D.C.: Commissioned Officers Assn. of the U.S. Public Health Service).—

> Information is presented concerning the origin, evolution, organization, and activities of the Public Health Service since its establishment in 1798.

d₄**:*History of epidemiology and medical geography*

ACKERKNECHT, E. H., 1965: History and geography of the most important diseases, 224 p. (New York, N.Y.: Hafner).—

> A condensed history, covering some 38 diseases. Symptoms, history, geography, and other details of the diseases considered have been given. This is an English translation of the German original: Geschichte und Geographie der wichtigsten Krankheiten, 1963, 183 p. (Stuttgart: Enke).

COCKBURN. A., 1963: The evolution and eradication of infectious diseases, 255 p. (Baltimore, Md.: Johns Hopkins Press).—

> A history of human diseases, mainly from the epidemiologist's point of view and based on a great personal experience. The story especially deals with smallpox, poliomyelitis, malaria, and tuberculosis. The author treats his subject from an evolutionist's point of view, for, as he states, evolutionary processes lie at the base of the development of the parasite, of the host (and intermediates) and of the environment of both host and parasites.

CREIGHTON, C., 1965: A history of epidemics in Britain: with new introductory material by D. E. C. EVERSLEY, E. A. UNDERWOOD, and L. OVENALL, ed. 2, 2 vols. Vol. I: 120 + 706 p.; Vol. II: 883 p. (London: Cass).—

> First published in 1891 and 1894. The first volume deals with the famine fevers of the Anglo-Saxon period, the plague in mediaeval, Tudor, and Stuart periods, leprosy and the sweating sickness, typhus fever, syphilis, and with smallpox and measles. The second volume considers the period between 1666 and 1893 and deals mainly with typhus, dysentery and continued fevers, influenza, whooping cough, scarlet fever and diphtheria, Asiatic cholera, and again with smallpox and measles. There are recently written essays on "Epidemiology and social history" by D. E. C. EVERSLEY, on "Charles Creighton, the man and his work" by E. A. UNDERWOOD, and "A select bibliography of epidemiological literature since 1894" by L. OVENALL.

HANSSEN, P., 1925: Geschichte der Epidemien bei Menschen und Tiere im Norden. Nach Untersuchungen ausgehend von Schleswig-Holstein, 228 p. (Glückstad: Augustin).—

> A chronological history. The book has been divided as follows: Geschichte der Epidemien (p. 9-11); Allgemeines, Gesundheitswesen, Verordnungen, nicht epidemische Krankheiten; Geburten, Sterbe- und Einwohnerzahlen; Die Epidemien nach Jahren (p. 29-178); elaborate index (p. 188-225).

HARE, R., 1954: Pomp and pestilence: infectious disease: its origins and conquest, 224 p. (London: Gollancz; New York, N.Y.: Philosophical Library).—

A semi-popular and well-written short history of epidemiology written by a bacteriologist. It discusses such topics as: parasites and parasitism, man and his parasites, parasites and pestilence, miasmas or microbes, the reaction of the communtiy, the reaction of the individual, and parasites and populations.

HENSCHEN, F., 1966: The history and geography of disease, 344 p. (New York, N.Y.: Delacorte Press; London: Longmans).—

First published in 1934 in the Swedish language under the title: "Sjukdomarnas historia och geografi". This is a study of geographical pathology. The text is in two parts: one on infectious diseases, another on non-infectious diseases, accompanied with diseases of organs. The author gives a short survey of the history of the progress and distribution of the diseases concerned. Numerous illustrations. By far the most successful book on historical geographical pathology is: HIRSCH, A., 1881-1886: Handbuch der historisch-geographischen Pathologie, ed. 2, 3 vols. Vol. I (1881): Die fections- und Intoxicationskrankheiten, 481 p.; Vol. II (1883): Die chronischen Infections- und Intoxicationskrankheiten, parasitäre Wundkrankheiten und chronische Ernährungs-Anomalien, 467 p.; Vol. III (1886): Die Organkrankheiten, 577 p. (Stuttgart: Enke). This book contains an overwhelming amount of information and literary references. Also in English translation: Handbook of geographical and historical pathology, 3 vols., 1883-1886 (London: New Sydenham Society). This English edition has an excellent index. The German edition will be reprinted by Olms (Hildesheim). A still older history of epidemic diseases is: WEBSTER, N., 1967: Brief history of epidemic and pestilential diseases, ed. 2, 2 vols., 716 p. (New York, N.Y.: Da Capo). This is a reprint of the 1799 edition including the previously unpublished revisions by Webster.

KOLLATH, W., 1951: Die Epidemien in der Geschichte der Menschheit, 99 p. (Wiesbaden: Gericke).—

A historical review of such diseases as: malaria, yellow fever, hookworm, tuberculosis, plague, smallpox, cholera, typhus, diphtheria, venereal diseases, and some others. A comparable booklet seems to be: COLMAT, A., 1937: Les épidémies et l'histoire, 191 p. (Paris: Ed. Hippocrate).

PAVLOVSKY, E. N., 1966: Natural nidality of transmissible diseases. With special reference to the landscape epidemiology of Zooanthroponoses, 261 p. (English translation edited by N. D. LEVINE) (Urbana, Ill.: Univ. Illinois Press).—

The value of this book lies in presenting a synthesis of Russian investigations on zoonoses and epidemiology, as reflected by 174 references to Soviet papers compared with 36 non-Soviet references, of which some are either of an incidental nature or of no historical value.

SCOTT, H. H., 1934: Some notable epidemics, 272 p. (London: Arnold).—

A collection of the histories of 23 epidemics in Great Britain between 1854 and 1923 (cholera, enteric fever, paratyphoid, scarlet fever, streptococcal sore throat, botulism, and dysentery), together with an analysis of their causes and characteristics, elucidated against a background of recent epidemiological findings and principles.

TOP, F. H., 1952: The history of American epidemiology, 190 p. (St. Louis, Mo.: Mosby).—

This book consists of four essays. The colonial era and the first years of the Republic (1607-1799): The pestilence that walketh in darkness; The period of great epidemics in the United States (1800-1875); The bacteriological era (1876-1920); The twentieth century - yesterday, today and tomorrow. A book of a more restricted scope is: DUFFY, J., 1953: Epidemics in colonial America, 274 p. (Baton Rouge, La.: Louisiana U.P.).

WINSLOW, C. E. A., 1943: The conquest of epidemic disease: a chapter in the history of ideas, 411 p. (Princeton, N.J.: Princeton U.P.; London: Oxford U.P.).—

The author gives a harmonious description of how clinical evidence and theoretical thinking together established the science of epidemiology, and how this interaction of theory and practice led to so many medical triumphs. The book deals with primitive supernatural, and animistic conceptions of disease in general and epidemic disease in particular; with Greek medicine as represented by Hippocrates and Galen; with the influence of atmospheric disturbances, individual predisposition, and contagion in the genesis of disease; with the opinions of Fracastorius, Sydenham, Mead, Pettenkofer, Snow, Budd, Panum, and with the great contributions of Pasteur. Reprinted in 1967 (New York, N.Y.: Hafner).

——, 1952: Man and epidemics, 246 p. (Princeton, N.J.: Princeton U.P.).—

Chapter headings are as follows: 1. The evolution of the public health program; 2. Objectives and approaches; 3. The problem of pure water; 4. Disposal of human wastes; 5. Milk supply; 6. Sanitary problems of food supply; 7. Insects and the transmission of disease; 8. Scourges of the past; challenges of the future. There is a good bibliography and an index. The book has been written by an expert in this field, and it gives a very good survey of the fight against epidemic diseases. A book mainly concerning the developments of epidemiology in the last 25 years, during which infectious diseases were almost banished from advanced Western countries is: BURNET, M., 1962: Natural history of infectious diseases, ed. 3, 377 p. (New York, N.Y. & London: Cambridge U.P.).

——, W. G. SMILLIE, J. A. DOULL & J. E. GORDON, 1952: The history of American epidemiology, 190 p. (St. Louis, Mo.: Mosby).—

A series of four essays. The first (by C. E. A. WINSLOW) deals with epidemiology during the colonial era and the first years of the republic; the second essay (by W. G. SMILLIE) contains a survey of the great epidemics which ravaged the U.S. between 1800 and 1875; the third essay (by J. A. DOULL) contains a study of American contributions and activities in the field of bacteriology between 1876 and 1920; the fourth essay (by J. E. GORDON) discusses the development of epidemiology since 1920.

d₄***. *History of preventive medicine, immunization, etc.*

EBERSON, F., 1948: Microbes militant: a challenge to man: the story of modern preventive medicine and control of infectious diseases, 401 p. (New York, N.Y.: Ronald Press).—

A well-written account of the development of preventive medicine and the control of infectious diseases; it first appeared under the title "The microbe's challenge" (1941). The discussion of parasitism, antibiotics, viruses, and epidemics is placed in a historical setting, and the book can be used by the trained physician as well as by the intelligent layman.

MCNEIL, D. R., 1957: The fight for fluoridation, 241 p. (New York, N.Y.: Oxford U.P.).—

A history of the development of fluoridation practice, based on extensive manuscript materials, printed documentary sources and personal interviews. More than half the book is concerned with events since 1950. Special attention has been paid to the often long discussions between adherents and opponents of fluoridation.

MULLETT, C. F., 1956: The bubonic plague and England: an essay in the history of preventive medicine, 401 p. (Lexington, Ky.: Kentucky U.P.).—

For this book the author received the Welch Medal in 1958. As Dr. Mullett states in his preface, he assembled the scattered materials on one central disease for one country in order to illustrate the evolution of concepts of public health and preventive medicine. The author did it so well that the book constitutes an important contribution to the history of preventive medicine in general.

NEWMAN, G., 1932: The rise of preventive medicine, 270 p. (London: Oxford U.P.).—

In his preface the author writes that he is offering "a general and introductory bird's-eye view of the subject of the origins of preventive medicine", *i.e.,* that branch of medicine "which is concerned with the preventive aspects as distinct from the curative function". Separate chapters deal with such subjects as: hygienic customs in primitive society and the importance of general cultural history in the development of medical thought, the laws of hygiene in ancient Egypt; Hippocrates on the prevention of disease; the contributions of the Greeks and Romans in sanitation, water supply, sewage disposal *etc.;* the Middle Ages and the plague epidemics; discoveries in anatomy and physiology in relation to preventive medicine; clinical studies of diseases; modern discoveries in pathology and bacteriology; application of new discoveries; political and economic organization of the community and preventive medicine. An important French history of preventive medicine and hygiene throughout the ages is: TRISCA, P., 1923: Aperçu sur l'histoire de la médecine préventive, 603 p. (Paris: Maloine). *Cf.* also NEWSHOLME, A., 1927: The evolution of preventive medicine, 226 p. (London: Baillière, Tindall & Cox; Baltimore, Md.: Williams & Wilkins), and NEWSHOLME, A., 1929: The story of modern preventive medicine, being a continuation of "The evolution of preventive medicine", 295 p. (Baltimore, Md.: Williams & Wilkins; London: Baillière & Co.).

PARISH, H. J., 1965: A history of immunization, 356 p. (Edinburgh & London: Livingstone).—

After an introductory survey of the whole subject, the author discusses such topics as: prophylactic inoculation against smallpox, the attenuation of viruses and the prevention of anthrax, fowl cholera, swine erysipelas, and rabies, humoral and cellular immunity, the discovery of antitoxins, the standardization of toxins and antitoxins, active and passive immunization, bacteriolysis, haemolysis, agglutination of blood corpuscles, *etc.*

d5. *History of military, naval, and aviation hygiene and medicine*

ADAMS, G. W., 1952: Doctors in blue: the medical history of the Union Army in the Civil War, 253 p. (New York, N.Y.: Schuman).—

A complementary volume is: CUNNINGHAM, H. H., 1958: Doctors in gray: the Confederate medical service, 339 p. (Baton Rouge, La.: Louisiana State U.P.). A good and rather complete historical review of the medical aspects of the Civil War is to be found in: BROOKS, S., 1966: Civil War medicine, 148 p. (Springfield, Ill.: Thomas). The most extensive medical history of the Civil War is: WOODWARD, J. J., C. SMART, G. A. OTIS & D. L. HUNTINGTON, 1870-1888: The medical and surgical history of the War of the Rebellion, 1861-1865, 6 vols. *Cf.* also: STEINER, P. E., 1966: Physician-generals in the Civil War: a study in nineteenth mid-century American medicine, 194 p. (Springfield, Ill.: Thomas).

ALLISON, R. S., 1943: Sea diseases: the story of a great natural experiment in preventive medicine in the Royal Navy, 218 p. (London: Bale Medical Publ.).—

Formerly sea diseases formed a serious obstacle in the way of naval exploration and warfare, for disease was then a far more important cause of death than battle casualties. This booklet is a semi-popular story of the conquest of sea diseases, such as scurvy, yellow jack, typhus, and dysentery, and the role played by fleet physicians, especially those of the 17th and 18th centuries, such as T. Dover, J. Lind, and G. Blane.

BAUER, W., 1958: Geschichte des Marinesanitätswesens bis 1945, 138 p. (Marine Rundschau, Beiheft 4) (Berlin/Frankfurt a.M.: Mitler).—

After an introductory review concerning the activities of the naval surgeon and medicine up to 1848, the greater part of the book deals with the history of German naval medicine between 1848 and the end of the Second World War. Especially the history between the two great wars received much attention, a period not dealt with in LLOYD & COULTER's stury, *vide infra*. Other regional histories concerning the marine hospital service and its evolution are: STRAUS, R., 1950: Medical care for seamen: the origin of public medical service in the United States, 165 p. (New Haven, Conn.: Yale U.P.). In this study the author tries to analyse the historical circumstances that led the United States government to enter the field of medical care in general and that of medical care for seamen in particular. Also: LARSEN, Ø., 1968: Schiff und Seuche 1795-1799. Ein medizinischer Beitrag zur historischen Kenntniss der Gesundheitsverhältnisse an Bord dänisch-norwegischer Kriegsschiffe an den Fahrten nach Dänisch-Westindien. Mit englischer, französischer und russischer Zusammenfassung, 267 p. (Oslo: Universitets Forlaget).

CABANÈS, A., 1918: Chirurgiens et blessés à travers l'histoire. Dès origines à la Croix-Rouge, 624 p. (Paris: Michel).—

A comprehensive treatise, containing 275 illustrations. This book deals with the transport and surgical treatment of the wounded, from earliest times up to about 1900. *Cf.* GURLT, E., 1967: Zur Geschichte der internationalen und freiwilligen Krankenpflege im Kriege, 866 p. (Wiesbaden: Sändig). Reprint of the 1873 edition.

FULTON, J. F., 1948: Aviation medicine in its preventive aspects: an historical survey, 174 p. (London: Oxford U.P.).—

This book contains the text of a series of lectures and it deals with the discovery of oxygen and the history of respiratory physiology, the problems of high altitude, diving, and oxygen poisoning, with decompression sickness, with the genesis of the tissue bubble, with the use of pressurized cabins in aircraft, with the effects of acceleration during a dive, and with problems of safety in flight. Some other histories of aviation medicine about which I can not give further information are: GARSAUX, P. A. V., 1963: Histoire anecdotique de la médecine de l'air, 191 p. (Paris: Ed. du Scorpion); and SERGEYEV, A. A., 1965: Essays on the history of aviation medicine, 413 p. (NASA TT F-176) (Washington, D.C.: Nat. Aeronautics and Space Adm.).

GARRISON, F. H., 1922: Notes on the history of military medicine, 206 p. (Washington, D.C.: Assn. Military Surgeons).—

A history of military hygiene, sanitation, and surgery, of medico-military administration, transport, recruiting, sanitary formations and training, in Antiquity, Greece, Rome, during the Middle Ages, *etc.*, up to the twentieth century, including the first World War. For a history of the British Army nursing service from its beginning up to 1950, *cf.* BEITH, J. H., 1952: One hundred years of army nursing: the story of the British Army Services from the time of Florence Nightingale to the present day, 387 p. (London: Cassell).

KEEVIL, J. J., 1957-1958: Medicine and the navy, 1200-1900. Vol. I (1957): 1200-1649, 255 p.; Vol. II (1958): 1649-1714, 332 p. (Edinburgh & London: Livingstone).—

The first volume is a well-written and informative historical account dealing with naval medicine from 1200 to 1649. It shows that the Laws of Oléron, introduced about 1194, contain the first English formulation of rules for the treatment of the sick and disabled seaman. The origin of these laws lies far back in history but their influence on later regulations of medical customs appeared to be far-reaching. The author has paid special attention to the small hospitals in naval ports where sick and wounded seamen were nursed. Many sidelights have been thrown on medical practice throughout mediaeval and Tudor England and the Barber-Surgeon Company. Vol. II deals with a period of a revolutionary character in politics as well as in science and medicine. It is the period between the establishment of the Commonwealth and the death of Queen Anne; during this period the basis had been laid for a corporate organization of medical care, the Royal Hospital was built at Greenwich, and hospital ships were equipped. For vols. III and IV of this standard work, *cf.* LLOYD & COULTER, *vide infra.*

KÖHLER, A., 1901: Grundriss einer Geschichte der Kriegschirurgie, 138 p. (Berlin: Hirschwald).—

Deals with military medicine of prehistoric peoples, of the Jews, China, India, the Greeks, Homer, Hippocrates, Xenophon, Alexander the Great, the School of Alexandria, Rome, the Arabs, Germans, the 30-Years-War, and with the development of special techniques for wound healing and wound repair, anaesthesiology, blood transfusion, ambulance transport, trepanation, amputation, *etc. Cf.* also GULEKE, N., 1945: Kriegschirurgie und Kriegschirurgen im Wandel der Zeiten, 44 p. (Jena: Fischer).

LLOYD, C., ed., 1965: The health of seamen: selections from the works of Dr. James Lind, Sir Gilbert Blane and Dr. Thomas Trotter, 320 p. (London: Navy Records Soc.).—

Extracts from the works of the three pioneers of naval medicine. The abstracts have been taken from: LIND's "A treatise of the scurvy" (1753) and his "Essay on the most effectual means of preserving the health of seamen in the Royal Navy" (1779), from BLANE's "Observations on the diseases of Seamen" (1789), and his "Select dissertations" (1822), and from TROTTER's "Medicina nautica" (1804).

——, & J. L. S. COULTER, 1961-1963: Medicine and the Navy, 1200-1900. Vol. III (1961): 1714-1815, 402 p.; Vol. IV (1963): 1815-1900, 300 p. (Edinburgh & London: Livingstone).—

Vol. I and II of this work were written by the late J. KEEVIL, *vide supra.* The authors of these last two volumes made a modification in plan: instead of the chronological arrangement of vols. I and II, they treated separate subjects in separate sections. Vol. III deals with, *e.g.,* the medical department, the medical history of the wars of the 18th century, the naval hospitals and their improvement, and with sea diseases and Dr. Lind's work on scurvy. IV gives a review of the administrative chiefs during the period considered, deals with the naval surgeon and the gradual rising of his status, the instruction of the naval surgeon and the naval school at Haslar, the problems of hygiene, ventilation, and the preservation of food on ships; with the story of the convict ships, the work of the surgeon naturalists, naval surgeons in arctic expeditions, naval nursing services, fevers and other diseases, the Royal Naval Hospitals, and with the history of the West African Squadron, which fought a losing battle against the slave-traders.

NIEDNER, O., 1903: Die Kriegsepidemieen des 19. Jahrhunderts und ihre Bekämpfung, 227 p. (Berlin: Hirschwald).—

Of each of the military expeditions having taken place during the 19th century the author describes the outbreaks of cholera, typhoid fevers, dysentery, smallpox, ophthalmia militaris, malaria, and scurvy.

PRINZING, F., 1916: Epidemics resulting from wars, 340 p. (Oxford: Clarendon Press).—

A study of epidemics caused by wars. Special studies have been devoted to the pestilences occurring during the Thirty-Year's-War, the typhus epidemic after Napoleon's Russian Campaign, and the outbreak of smallpox after the Franco-German War of 1870-71. A separate chapter deals with epidemics in besieged strongholds: Mantua (1796-97); Danzig (1813); Torgau (1813); Mainz (1813-14); Paris (1870-71); Port Arthur (1904).

RING, F., 1962: Zur Geschichte der Militärmedizin in Deutschland, 371 p. (Berlin: Deutscher Militärverlag).—

A history of German military medicine from the Middle Ages up to the present time, the development of its technical equipment, organization, etc.

RODDIS, L. H., 1941: A short history of nautical medicine, 359 p. (New York, N.Y.: Hoeber).—

Separate sections deal with such topics as: early nautical medicine, disease and disaster in the old sailing ships, the medical departments of naval vessels, the rise of naval hygiene, naval medicine in the U.S. navy, hospitals for seamen and hospital ships, nautical medicine and the merchant marine, and research in nautical medicine.

SCHLOSSBERGER, H., 1945: Kriegsseuchen. Historischer Ueberblick ueber ihr Auftreten und ihre Bekämpfung, 84 p. (Jena: Fischer).—

1. Allgemeines über das Wesen der Seuchen, sowie über ihr Auftreten und ihre Verbreitung, besonders in Kriegszeiten; 2. Ueber die im Verlauf der letzten 1000 Jahre in Zusammenhang mit Kriegen beobachteten wichtigsten Seuchenausbrüche; 3. Ueber die Bekämpfung der Kriegsseuchen. Bibliography of over 500 items.

β. *History of therapy*
'a. *Works of a more or less general importance*

a1. *History of therapy in general*

BAUER, J., 1966: Geschichte der Aderlässe, 234 p. (Munich: Fritsch).—

Originally published in 1870 (Munich: Gummi). A history of blood letting from the pre-Christian era up to the end of the former century. A large part of the text deals with blood letting in Greek and Hellenistic times (Hippocrates, Galen, *etc.*); other sections deal with the Arabs, the Middle Ages in the Latin West (*e.g.*, Salerno), Vesalius, Paré, Paracelsus, blood letting and the discovery of the circulatory system, Broussais. Very interesting are the author's explanations of the interrelationship between philosophical ideas and the blood letting technique employed.

BRAUCHLE, A., 1951: Die Geschichte der Naturheilkunde in Lebensbildern, 374 p. (Stuttgart: Reclam).—

A first comprehensive history of natural cure, *i.e.*, of those curative methods which are based on experience according to Paracelsus' dictum that the disease as well as its cure both arise from nature. Among the topics discussed are: the art of healing by means of water, dietetic methods, vegetarianism and the use of uncooked food, hygienic gymnastics, and psycho-therapeutical healing methods. The book is intended alike for students of the history of medicine and for sick persons.

BROCKBANK, W., 1954: Ancient therapeutic arts, 162 p. (London: Heinemann).—

This is the text of the FitzPatrick lectures of 1950 and 1951 in which the author, without giving any theoretical backgrounds, treats the story of a number of the older therapeutical procedures which had dominated medicine for centuries, such as: enema administration, cupping and leeching, methods of counter-irritation, intravenous injection of drugs, *etc.* The material has been assembled with the aid of quotations from primary sources.

COULTER, J. S., 1932: Physical therapy, 142 p. (New York, N.Y.: Hoeber).—

A historical introduction to modern physical therapy. The subject matter is presented as follows: I. Physical therapy from ancient times to the Renaissance; II. Massage and exercises; III. Water; IV. Electricity; V. Radiant energy. Good bibliography and index.

GUYOTJEANNIN, C., 1951: Contribution à l'histoire de l'analyse des urines, 104 p. (Créteil: Marest).—

"Ce travail, appuyé sur d'abondantes références, est une fresque d'ensemble permettant d'embrasser d'un seul regard l'histoire de l'analyse des urines depuis les plus lointaines origines jusqu'aux laboratoires actuels de biochemie". (From: Hist. Pharm. 10: 261).

HAAS, H., 1956: Spiegel der Arznei. Ursprung und Idee der Heilmittelkunde, 256 p. (Berlin: Springer).—

A history of therapy and therapeutics from ancient times up to the time of antibiotics and sulphadrugs. It is not a chronological history, but the author reviews the various theories about therapy and therapeutics as they reappear regularly during history, and he correlates these guiding principles with empirism, magic, vitalism, experimentation, chemistry, botany, toxicology, etc.

HAMILTON, M., 1906: Incubation: the cure of disease in pagan temples and Christian churches, 228 p. (St. Andrews: Henderson).—

A historical sketch of the development of the practice of incubation from earliest times up to ca. 1900. The first part (p. 1-108) deals with incubation in the cult of Asclepios (Epidauros, Rome, Lebene, Athens, Cos), with incubation at the oracles of Amphiaraos, Trophonios, Dionysos and with incubation in the cults if Isis and Serapis. Part 2 deals with incubation in Christian churches during the Middle Ages (St. Cosmas and St. Damian, St. Therapon, St. Thekla, St. Michael, St. Cyrus and St. John, St. Julian, St. Martin, St. Maximinus, St. Fides). Part 3 deals with the practice of incubation during modern times (in Italy, Sardinia, Austria, the Greek islands and the mainland of Greece, and with the festival at Tenos).

KREIG, M. B., 1965: Green medicine: the search for plants that heal, 463 p. (London: Harrap; Chicago, Ill.: Rand McNally).—

A description of the explorations which gave us new plants for the treatment of disease (e.g., digitalis, chaulmoogra oil, quinine, curare, sarsaparilla), together with biographical sketches of some of the discoverers.

KROEBER, L., 1947-1949: Das neuzeitliche Kräuterbuch. Die Arzneipflanzen Deutschlands in alter und neuer Betrachtung, 3 vols. Vol. I, ed. 4 (1948): 454 p.; Vol. II, ed. 3 (1947): 336 p.; Vol. III, ed. 2 (1949): 476 p. (Stuttgart: Hippocrates).—

A standard text. The first part contains an introduction, considering old herbals, conservation, dosage and preparation of herbs, followed by a series of plant-monographs (p. 25-415), in which the plants are arranged in alphabetical order, according to their German name. This is followed by short sections dealing with such subjects as: drugs and folk medicine, signature-doctrine, etc., and by indexes of plant names in German and in Latin. The second vol. also contains an alphabetically-arranged series of plant-monographs and indexes of German and Latin plant names. The third volume deals with poisonous plants. In this volume the series of plant monographs (p. 71-448) is preceded by some short sections dealing with the contents of the concept of poison, and with the role of poisonous plants in life and cult of various peoples; it is followed by a short section (p. 448-466) concerning poisonous fungi. Indexes of German and Latin plant names.

MARIE, R., 1955: Contribution à l'histoire des insectes en thérapeutique, 129 p. (Thèse Univ. Strasbourg) (Cahors: Coueslant).—

This work consists of 41 chapters, each of them treating of one or some species of insects used in medicine, either directly, or by means of their derivates. These insects belong to one of the following orders: Archiptera, Orthoptera, Hemiptera, Neuroptera, Coleoptera, Hymenoptera, Lepidoptera, and Diptera. Bibliographical information is scanty. Indexes of: therapeutic properties attributed to insects, illnesses treated, and names of the insects and their products.

PETERSEN, J., 1966: Hauptmomente in der geschichtlichen Entwicklung der medicinischen Therapie, 400 p. (Hildesheim: Olms).—

A reprint of a book first published in 1877 (Copenhagen: Höst). The author distinguished between two controversial systems of thought which were predominant in the history of medicine, viz., the dogmatic and the empirico-rational system of thought, and accordingly the text is in two parts. Pt. 1 is entitled "Dogmatische Richtungen in der Heilkunst" (p. 14-116) and contains the following sections: Mystische Richtungen;

die teleologischen Physiatrie; der Methodismus; die Chemiatrie. Pt. 2 is entitled "Empirische und empirisch-rationelle Richtungen in der Heilkunst" (p. 117-400) and contains the following sections: die empirische Richtung; die Therapie unter Einwirkung der pathologischen Anatomie; die Therapie unter Einwirkung der pathologischen Anatomie und Physiologie; Hauptmomente im therapeutischen Standpunkt unserer Zeit.

WARING, E. J., 1878-1879: Bibliotheca therapeutica, or bibliography of therapeutics, *etc.*, 2 vols., 934 p. (London: New Sydenham Soc.).—

Fore more details, *vide* section Bibliographies, subsection e.

a2. *History of pharmacotherapy*

a2*. *History of pharmacy, pharmacognosy, and the apothecary*

BERENDES, J., 1907: Das Apothekenwesen. Seine Entstehung und geschichtliche Entwicklung bis zum 20. Jahrhundert, 366 p. (Stuttgart: Enke).—

This book essentially is a complement to "Die Pharmazie bei den alten Kulturvölkern" (*vide* section Antiquity in general, subsection c). The first hundred pages trace the history of pharmacy from antiquity (Egypt, Mesopotamia, Far East, *etc.)* down to the Middle Ages. The remaining part of the text deals mainly with the situation of the German apothecary as it developed from the 15th century onward, considering such subjects as: pharmaceutical literature, guilds, legal and fiscal problems, connections with botany and chemistry, trade, the military apothecary, *etc.* Indexes of names and of subjects.

BERMAN, A., ed., 1967: Pharmaceutical historiography, 145 p. (Madison, Wisc.: Amer. Inst. Hist. Pharmacy).—

This book presents the text of the papers from a colloquium sponsored by the American Institute of the History of Pharmacy. The central theme of the colloquium is George Urdang's "Wesen und Bedeutung der Geschichte der Pharmazie", published in 1927. Included is an English summary of that book. The presentations are in two sections, *viz.*, 1. Urdang's concept of the nature and meaning of the history of pharmacy; 2. the history of pharmacy in selected cultural areas (France, Great Britain, and the U.S.A.).

BOUSSEL, P., 1949: Histoire illustrée de la pharmacie, 300 p. + 235 illustrations (Paris: Le Prat).—

A beautifully printed popular history of pharmacy. The text is beautifully illustrated; there are many plates, some of which are coloured. A good popularization. No references to sources, no indexes, no bibliography, and no portraits of famous pharmacists. *Cf.* also: BENDER, G. A., 1966: Great moments in pharmacy: a history of pharmacy in pictures, 238 p. + 40 illus. (Detroit, Mi.: Northwood Inst. Press). This is a compilation of the series "A history of pharmacy in pictures", distributed by Parke, Davis & Co. Stories by G. A. BENDER, paintings by R. A. THON.

COUVREUR, A., 1953: La pharmacie et la thérapeutique au XVIIIe siècle, vues à travers le "Journal Encyclopédique" de Pierre Rousseau à Bouillon, 2 vols., 410 + 490 p. (Paris: Vigot).—

The "Journal encyclopédique" appeared from 1756 up to 1973, containing information concerning the sciences and the arts, and as such it can be considered as a supplement of the "Encyclopédie". The present book is a useful reference work for the development of pharmacy and medicine of the period considered. Much bibliographical information.

DANNER, H., 1951: Leitfaden der Pharmaziegeschichte, 67 p. (Hamburg: Govi).—

Introductory text written for the beginning student and interested layman. A comparable booklet: FABRE, R. & G. DILLEMAN, 1963: Histoire de la pharmacie, 127 p. (Que sais je? No. 1035) (Paris: Presses Univ. de France).

DOYLE, P. A., ed., 1962: Readings in pharmacy, 429 p. (New York, N.Y. & London: Interscience).—

An assembly of texts compiled from a variety of sources of the art and practice of pharmacy. The author has included extracts from established authors who describe their personal reactions to the work of the pharmacist, and from those works which describe the pharmacist in the world of music, literature, theatre, *etc.*

LAWALL, C. H., 1927: Four thousand years of pharmacy: an outline history of pharmacy and allied sciences, 665 p. (Philadelphia, Pa.: Lippincott).—

This book is the product of a course in the Philadelphia College of Pharmacy and Science. The author indicates how the history of pharmacy is closely connected with the history of general science, the history of arts, and especially with the history of the sciences particularly related to pharmacy. The author shows how at the beginning pharmacy was dominated by magic and superstition, in close connection with religion and medicine, how it was influenced by alchemy for more than a thousand years, and how commercialism of the present era puts its stamp on it. There are chapters on ancient pharmacy, pharmacy during the Greek and Roman periods, the Arabs as preservers of the pharmaceutical art, mediaeval pharmacy and its relation to alchemy (2), the new impulses Paracelsus gave to pharmacy in the 16th century, the famous pharmacopoeias of the 17th century and the development of modern chemistry and pharmacy from the 18th century onwards (3). Chronological table (p. 553-584) and extensive index (585-665). For the older periods, cf. BERENDES, J., 1891; and ARTELT, W., 1937, vide section Antiquity in general, subsection c.

PHILLIPPE, A., 1853: Histoire des apothicaires chez les principaux peuples du monde, depuis les temps les plus reculés jusqu'à nos jours. Suivi du tableau de l'état actuel de la pharmacie en Europe, en Asie, en Afrique et en Amérique, 452 p. (Paris: Direction de Publ. Médicale).—

Separate sections deal with such subjects as: the meaning of the words pharmacist and apothecary; the history of pharmacy in ancient China, Egypt, Mesopotamia, Persia, Greece, Rome, Byzantium, etc.; Arabian pharmacists; the French apothecary of the 13th-17th centuries; the clyster and its applications; the conflict between the pharmacist and the physician in the 18th century (mainly restricted to the French situation); royal pharmacists; the foundation of the "Société libre de Pharmacie"; some legal aspects; the pharmaceutical schools of Paris, Montpellier, and Strasbourg; pharmacopoeias of the 19th century; some magical aspects of drugs; some famous pharmacists (p. 344-884); a chronology containing name, date of birth, experiments, discoveries and/ or most important publications (included are many botanists); pharmacist-poets; modern pharmacy in France, China, Persia,

Turkey, Greece, Egypt, Russia, Sweden, Norway, Denmark, Germany, the Netherlands, America, Great Britain, Spain, Italy, Sicily. Extensive index (p. 1086-1122). Also in German translation: PHILLIPPE, A., 1858: Geschichte der Apotheker bei den wichtigsten Völkern der Erde seit den ältesten Zeiten bis auf unsere Tage nebst einer Uebersicht des gegenwärtigen Zustandes der Pharmacie in Europa, Asien, Afrika und Amerika, 1022 p. (Wiesbaden: Sändig). Reprinted, 1966 (Stuttgart: Fischer).

REUTTER DE ROSEMONT, L., 1931-1932: Histoire de la pharmacie à travers les âges. Vol. I: De l'antiquité au XVIe siècle, 605 p.; Vol. II: Du XVIIe siècle à nos jours, 676 p. (Paris: Peyronnet).—

The first volume consists of six parts, viz., 1. The history of pharmacy in antiquity (Israel, Mesopotamia, Egypt, India, Greece, Rome); 2. Idem during the first centuries of the Middle Ages (in East and West); 3. Idem in the 14th century (the apothecary, pharmacy in the university); 4. Idem in the 15th century; 5. Idem in the 16th century (the creation of botanical gardens); 6. Magic and alchemy. The second vol. consists of 4 parts, viz., 7. The history of pharmacy in the 17th century; 8. Idem in the 18th century; 9. Idem in the 19th century; and the last part deals with some 33 drugs. In a review of this book (in Isis 19: 314), I found the following critical statement: "Vaste compilation hétéroclyte, écrite dans un style étrange qui en rend la lecture singulièrement pénible. L'illustration n'a le plus souvent aucun rapport avec le texte dans lequel elle s'insère...". An older history of pharmacy written in the French language is: GILBERT, E., 1892: La pharmacie à travers les siècles (antiquité, moyen-âge, temps modernes), précédée d'un coup d'oeil historique et bibliographique sur les sciences naturelles qui lui sont accessoires, botanique, minéralogie, zoologie, depuis l'antiquité jusqu'au milieu du XVIIIe siècle, 455 p. (Toulouse: Vialelle). Contains the following appendixes: 1. Notes sur la pharmacie dans l'ancienne Rome; 2. L'hydrologie aux XVIIe et XVIIIe siècles; 3. Inventaire d'une pharmacie au XVIIe siècle; 5. Une consultation médicale au Moyen-Âge; 6. Bibliographie et sources principales des matières contenues dans l'ouvrage.

SCHELENZ, H., 1904: Geschichte der Pharmazie, 936 p. (Berlin: Springer).—

A full-scale history of pharmacy from ancient times (Mesopotamia, Egypt, India, etc.) to the present. This work contains much biographical information about those persons who contributed to the development of pharmacy. Much attention has been paid to the position of the pharmacist in cultural life in the various cultural epochs considered *(e.g.,* his social position, education, guilds, trade, *etc.).* Reprinted in 1962 (Hildesheim: Olms).

SCHMITZ, R., 1966: Mörser, Kolben und Phiolen. Aus der Welt der Pharmazie, 208 p. (Stuttgart: Franckh'sche Verlagshandlung). —

A profusely illustrated (nearly half of the pages consist of full-page coloured plates) history of pharmacy, elucidating its cultural, biological and medical implications. Separate sections deal with Galen and pharmacy, pharmacy of the Arabs and of the Schools of Salerno and Toledo, the remedium caeleste, alchemy and magic, the apothecary, drugs, mortars, flasks and phials, pharmaceutical education, and with the position of the pharmacist and apothecary in older historiography.

STERNON, F., 1933: Quelques aspects de l'art pharmaceutique et du médicament à travers les âges, 235 p. (Paris: Masson).—

"The history of the art of pharmacy is outlined and the evolution of pharmacy from primitive times up to the present is discussed". (Biol. Abstr. 10: 1094). A comparable book seems to be: GRIER, J., 1937: A history of pharmacy, 274 p. (London: Pharmaceutical Press), a book about which I could find no further information.

THOMPSON, C. J. S., 1929: The mystery and art of the apothecary, 287 p. (London: Lane).—

A chronologically-arranged short history of pharmacy from the Babylonian and Assyrian herbs, drugs, and preparations, up to the apothecaries of the 18th century.

TREASE, G. E., 1964: Pharmacy in history, 265 p. (London: Baillière, Tindall & Cox).—

A monograph treating of the development of pharmacy in history, dealing with such subjects as: the experience of primitive men with plants, spices and poisons; the association of drugs with magic and religion in primitive people; the influence of folk medicine; Egyptian materia medica; the contributions of Greek civilization (Hippocrates, Theophrastos); Pliny, Celsus, Dioscorides, Galen; Middle Ages and alchemy; the influence of the development of weighing, pottery, ceramic and glass, oils, perfumes and cosmetics, *etc.,* on the development of pharmaceutical preparations, spicery, apothecary and grocery; the long quarrels between apothecaries and physicians, *etc.*

TSCHIRCH, A., 1930-1933: Handbuch der Pharmakognosie, ed. 2, Vol. I: Allgemeine Pharmakognosie, 3 parts, 2015 p. (Leipzig: Tauchnitz).—

From this manual of pharmacognosy, the volumes II and III exclusively deal with special pharmacognosy; vol. I, however, contains much that is of interest to biohistory. The first part (p. 1-583) deals with general pharmacognosy, its object and methodology, the culture, collection and preparation of herbs, drug-traffic, applied pharmacognosy, and with reference works, periodicals, journals, *etc.,* in the field of pharmacognosy. Part 2 (p. 584-1151) deals with pharmaco-botany (incl. systematics, morphology, anatomy, physiology, genetics, pathology), pharmaco-zoology, -chemistry, -physics, -geography, and contains an extensive biographicon (p. 1008-1151). Part 3 (p. 1152-2015) gives a history of pharmacognosy (containing much information concerning old herbals and mediaeval, Arabic, Oriental, and post-Columbian botany), of pharmacoethnology (incl. much information on folkmedicine) and of pharmaco-etymology.

URDANG, G., 1946: Pharmacy's part in society, 93 p. (Madison, Wisc.: Amer. Inst. Hist. Pharmacy).—

This booklet deals with the role played by the pharmacist in society. It discusses such topics as: the evolution of the pharmacist from the alchemist, the separation of medicine and pharmacy, the contribution of pharmacists to botany and to plant chemistry (isolation and alkaloids), the discoveries of pharmacists in other fields of knowledge and techniques, the literary work of some pharmacists, *etc.*

WOOTTON, A. C., 1910: Chronicles of pharmacy, 2 vols. Vol. I: 428 p.; Vol. II: 332 p. (London: Macmillan).—

This is not really a history of pharmacy, but in this work the author shows how kings, quacks, philosophers, priests, men of science, *etc.,* have contributed to the development of pharmacy. The first volume deals *inter alia* with the myths of pharmacy, with pharmacy in the times of the Pharaohs, the Bible, Hippocrates, Galen, and the Arabs, and with pharmacy in Great Britain; with dogmas and delusions, with masters in pharmacy and royal pharmacists, and with medicines from the metals. The second volume deals *inter alia* with animals in pharmacy, familiar medicines, pharmacopoeias, Shakespeare's pharmacy, noted nostrums, poisons in history; one chapter deals with some noted drugs.

a₂** *History of pharmacology and toxicology* (excl. chemotherapy)

BENEDICENTI, A., 1947-1951: Malati, medici e farmaciste. Storia dei rimedi traverso i secoli e delle teorie che ne spiegono l'azione sull'organismo, ed. 2, 2 vols., 1457 p. (Milano: Hoepli).—

A richly illustrated history of drug therapy from earliest times. The book contains a wealth of information and also much that is of interest to the historian of medicine and of chemistry. Many biographical notes. Author- and subject-indexes.

DURAN-REYNALS, M. L., 1946: The fever bark tree: the pageant of quinine, 275 p. (Garden City, N.Y.: Doubleday).—

Vide section History of the medical sciences, subsection c, malaria.

GILG, E. & P. N. SCHÜRHOFF, 1926: Aus dem Reiche der Drogen. Geschichtliche, Kulturgeschichtliche und botanische Betrachtungen über wichtigere Drogen, 272 p. (Dresden: Schwarzeck).—

Chapter headings are as follows: Die Kräuterbücher des Mittelalters; Die Signaturlehre; Die Destillierkunst; Die Gewürzkriege; Der Anbau der Drogen in Deutschland; Die Chinarinde; Das Süssholz; Die tropeïnhaltigen Nachtschattengewächse; Strophanthus; Giftige und unschädliche Strychnosarten; Der Holunder; Indischer Hanf; Die Yohimberinde; Das Gujakholz; Die Sarsaparillwurzel; Das Hirtentäschel; Der "deutsche" Rhabarber; Der Eisenhut; Das Opium; Die Canthariden. *Cf.* SCHMIDT, A., 1924, *vide* section Antiquity in general, subsection c.

HOLMSTEDT, B. & G. LILJESTRAND, 1963: Readings in pharmacology, 395 p. (Oxford: Pergamon).—

A collection of anthologies of outstanding achievements in literature from different times and countries, in order to illustrate in this way some of the more remarkable steps in the growth of pharmacology from a purely empirical part of medicine to a modern science. It contains the following chapters: 1. Glimpses of the development of pharmacology until the end of the 18th century (Egyptian and Graeco-Roman medicine, Byzantine and Arabian medicine, the School of Salerno, the Renaissance, discoveries of effective therapeutics from the 16th to the 18th centuries); 2. The rise of experimental pharmacology; 3. Volatile anaesthetics, hypnotics, alcohol, theory of narcosis; 4. Local anaesthesia; 5. Pharmacology of the autonomic nervous system; 6. Psychopharmacology; 7. Some technical advances; 8. Some chemical aspects; 9. Chemotherapy (quinine, organic arsenicals, the sulphonamides, antibiotics); 10. Vitamins and hormones; 11. Varia (chemoreceptors, the revolution of two ancient oriental drugs: ephedrine, reserpine); 12. Toxicology. Name- and subject-index.

LELEUX, C., 1923: Le poison à travers les âges, 320 p. (Paris: Lemerre).—

"Histoire du poison et des empoisonneurs célèbres dans l'ancien Orient, la Grèce, à Rome, en Italie (époque des Borgia), et en France; un chapitre sur l'emploi des gaz asphyxiants pendant la guerre." (From Isis 6: 234).

LEWIN, L., 1962: Die Gifte in der Weltgeschichte. Toxikologische, allgemein-verständliche Untersuchungen der historischen Quellen, ed. 5, 1087 p. (Ulm: Haug).—

This book (first published in 1920, 596 p., Berlin: Springer) contains an encyclopaedic history of poisonings from the most ancient times to the present century. It deals with: development, diffusion and application of toxicological knowledge in ancient times (poisons and magic, love potions, abortives, *etc.*); poisonings from the pathological point of view (poisons simulating diseases, causing mental disorders, *etc.);* toxicological therapeutics in ancient times (antidotes, emetics, *etc.*); laws concerning poisonings; poisonings by means of drugs; poisoning caused by indirect means (*e.g.,* by means of perfumes, scented flowers, poisoning of wounds, nails and weapons, *etc.);* suicide by poisoning; antiquity and significance of arsenical compounds as poisons; prominent men who were the perpetrators or victims of poisonings; poisonings perpetrated by women; priests who were the authors or victims of poisonings, poisons in warfare. A completion of this study of the malicious use of poisons throughout the ages is: LEWIN, L., 1923:

Die Pfeilgifte nach eigenen toxikologischen und ethnologischen Untersuchungen, 517 p. (Leipzig: Barth). *Cf.* also: SCHMIDT, A., 1924, *vide* section Antiquity in general, subsection c.

REKO, V. A., 1949: Magische Gifte. Rausch- und Betäubungsmittel der Neuen Welt, ed. 3, 175 p. (Stuttgart: Enke).—

In this booklet the author considers some 15 drugs (*viz.,* ololiuqui, peyotl, marihuana, chicalote, ayahuasca, toloachi, colorines, sinicuichi, coztic-zapote, nanácatl, xomil-xihuite, minapatli, hierbas locas, camotillo, cohombrillo). For each of the drugs considered the author gives many details concerning the plants producing the substance, its action and application (pharmacologically as well as sociologically), and the role it plays in manners and customs of the natives.

SHUSTER, L., ed., 1962: Readings in pharmacology, 294 p. (Boston, Mass.: Little, Brown).—

An anthology consisting of some 19 (English) papers representing a sampling of approaches and techniques that have been applied to some of the basic problems in pharmacology. These papers are published under the following section headings: 1. Autonomic pharmacology (papers of H. H. Dale, 1914; Langley & Dickinson, 1889; D. A. Robertson, 1863; C. Bernard, 1856; Rall, Sutherland & Berthet 1956; Wilson & Ginsburg, 1955); 2. Cardiovascular drugs (papers of W. Withering, 1785; T. L. Brunton, 1867; Carlsson, Rosengren, Bertler & Nilsson, 1957); 3. Pharmacology of the central nervous system (papers of Fischer & von Mehring, 1903; H. W. Haggard, 1924; Gasser & Erlanger, 1929; Brodie & Shore, 1957); 4. Chemotherapy (papers of J. Lister, 1867; P. Ehrlich, 1906; A. Fleming, 1929; Park & Strominger, 1957; Bueding & Mansour, 1956; Stocken & Thompson, 1946).

TAYLOR, N., 1949: Flight from reality, 237 p. (New York, N.Y.: Duell, Sloan & Pearce).—

Botanical sources, history, and use of narcotic, stimulating and euphoric drugs. A book dealing with the same topics is: LEWIN, L., 1964:Phantastica; narcotic and stimulating drugs, their use and abuse, 335 p. (Transl. from the 2nd German ed.) (New York, N.Y.: Dutton). First published in English in 1931.

THOMAS, K. B., 1963: Curare: its history and usage, 144 p. (Philadelphia, Pa.: Lippincott; London: Pitman).—

A description of the first searches for the drug and its botanical identification, the interest contributed by such famous men as: W. Raleigh, A. von Humboldt, Tennyson, Virchow, C. Bernard; the myoneural junction; curare in diseases and in anaestesiology; and other recent pharmacological and clinical applications of curare. An older study, dealing with the same kind of problems is: MCINTYRE, A. R., 1947: Curare: its history, nature, and clinical use, 240 p. (Chicago, Ill.: U.P.) *Cf.* also: VELLARD, J., 1965: Histoire du curare. Les poisons de chasse en Amérique du Sud, 215 p. (Paris: Gallimard).

WATSON, G., 1966: Theriac and mithridatium: a study in therapeutics, 165 p. (Publications of the Wellcome Historical Medical Library, N.S., Vol. IX) (London: Wellcome Hist. Med. Library).—

A very readable history of two miracle-drugs which had a great influence in the history of therapeutics, *viz.,* Theriaca (the working of which was described by Nicander of Colophon, *ca.* 150 B.C., in a poem against the effects of the bites of venomous beasts), and Mithridatium (a drug ascribed to Mithridates Eupator, King of Pontus, 164-121 B.C.). The first two chapters deal with the origins of theriac and mithridatium and their early history; the third and last chapter deals with their later history, especially during the Middle Ages and their use in England. Both therapeutics were still included in a French pharmacopoeia as late as 1884. Good index.

a₂***. *History of chemotherapy* (esp. of antibiotics)

BALDRY, P. E., 1965: The battle against bacteria: a history of the development of antibacterial drugs, for the general reader, 102 p. (Cambridge: U.P.).—

An introductory history of man's battle against epidemic diseases, starting with A. van Leeuwenhoek's discovery of microbes in 1676. The major part of the book is devoted to an account of the discovery of defensive measures, especially chemotherapeutic agents and antibiotics.

BÖTTCHER, H. M., 1959: Wunderdrogen. Die abenteuerliche Geschichte der Heilpilze, 555 p. (Cologne & Berlin: Kiepenheuer & Witsch).—

In his introduction, the author gives definitions of the concepts used. In the first section (p. 31-134) he considers the usage of antibiotics in primitive cultures (Egypt, Mesopotamia, Israel, India, East Asia, and South America). The second section (p. 135-182) deals with antibiotics used in Greece and Rome, and with more or less magical therapeutic techniques applied during the Middle Ages. The third section (p. 183-432) deals with the modern antibiotics: penicillin, streptomycin, aureomycin, and terramycin; the fourth section (p. 433-500) deals with plants possessing antibiotic properties; the last section considers the effect of antibiotics upon modern society. Bibliography and index.

EPSTEIN, S. & B. WILLIAMS, 1946: Miracles from microbes: the road to streptomycin, 155 p. (New Brunswick, N.J.: Rutgers U.P.).—

A popular historical review of the discovery of antibiotics. The authors start their story with a historical review of our ideas concerning the nature and causes of infectious diseases, and the role played by such men as: Paracelsus, Fracastorius, Leeuwenhoek, Spallanzani, Needham, Henle, Pasteur, Cohn, Koch, Lister, Ehrlich, Waksman, Dubos, Fleming, Florey, and some others, in the discovery of the therapy of these diseases.

GALDSTON, I., 1943: Behind the sulfadrugs: a short history of chemotherapy, 174 p. (New York, N.Y.: Appleton-Century Co.).—

A popular, but historically reliable, survey of the destructions of specific infectious organisms causing diseases in Man and animals, by means of specific chemicals. The book deals with the history of chemotherapy from Paracelsus to Pasteur, Koch, Ehrlich and Domagk, and the author gives a clear review of the mechanism of the sulphonamides and of their significance in modern medicine. A comparable text is: TAYLOR, F. S., 1942: The conquest of bacteria: from salvarsan to sulphapyridine, 175 p. (New York, N.Y.: Philos. Library).

GOLDSMITH, M., 1946: The road to penicillin: a history of chemotherapy, 174 p. (London: Drummond).—

A short history of the treatment of diseases by chemical agencies from earliest times up to the discovery of penicillin. A very readable book, discussing the work of *e.g.,* Fracastorius, Paracelsus, Leeuwenhoek, Jenner, Perkin, Lister, Pasteur, Koch, Ehrlich, Fleming, and Florey. Comparable books are: RATCLIFF, J. D., 1945: Yellow magic: the story of penicillin, 173 p. (New York, N.Y.: Random House), and MASTERS, D., 1946: Miracle drugs: the inner history of penicillin, 191 p. (London: Eyre & Spottiswoode).

HARE, R., 1970: The birth of penicillin and the disarming of microbes, 236 p. (London: Allen & Unwin).—

A description of the discoveries which have led to our present knowledge to cure or prevent infectious diseases. The book has been written by one of the leading participants in the search for and discovery of antibiotics; as a result it contains many personal experiences, and new additions to existing histories of the discovery of penicillin.

PODOLSKY, E., 1947: Doctors, drugs and steel: the story of medicine's battle against death, 384 p. (London & New York, N.Y.: Medical Publications).—

The story of penicillin, the sulpha drugs, hormones, and other recent medical discoveries by which it is hoped to lengthen Man's life span. Popular.

SOKOLOFF, B., 1949: The miracle drugs, 308 p. (New York, N.Y. & Chicago, Ill.: Ziff Davis).—

A semi-popular history giving much information about preliminary steps leading to the discovery of the various anti-infective agents. Four chapters have been devoted to penicillin; all other antibiotics are treated in the remaining two chapters. Important features of the manufacture of the antibiotics considered are also included.

b. *Some works of a regional importance*

b.* *Europe*

Austria

ZEKERT, O. & K. GANZINGER, 1961: Beiträge zur Geschichte der Pharmazie in Oesterreich, 125 p. (Vienna: Oesterr. Ges. Gesch. der Pharmazie).—

A collection of contributions: ZE-KERT deals with L. Winckler, founder of the Society for the History of Pharmacy in the German-speaking countries; K. SCHADELBAUER with remedies against plague according to a ms. of Vintler; E. HOLZMAIR discusses some numismatic aspects of the Brettauer collection; K. GANZINGER discusses the evolution of the Austrian pharmacopoeia between 1812 and 1836; E. LESKY the role of M. Ehrmann in the pharmaceutical reform of 1848; A. BREIT the introduction of pharmaceutical specialities in Austria; F. CZEIKE the sources of a pharmaceutical history of Vienna; O. NOWSTNY discusses the history of some apothecaries in the town of Steyr, during the second half of the 16th century.

France

ANDRÉ-PONTIER, L., 1900: Histoire de la pharmacie. Origines, Moyen Âge, temps modernes, 730 p. (Paris: Doin).—

This book is essentially a history of pharmacy in France. The introduction contains a review of the study of pharmacy in France (about 1900!) and a biobibliography of some highly qualified pharmacists. Ch. 1 deals with the history of pharmacy in the different regions of France between 1340 and 1803, and also deals briefly with the history of pharmacy of the Egyptians, Greeks, Romans and Arabs. Ch. 2 deals with the history of pharmacy in Paris; ch. 3 with the history of pharmacy since 1803. Other chapters deal with the development of military and naval pharmacy in France (and some other important countries of Europe); with the "Union scientifique des pharmaciens de France"; and with the situation of pharmacy in the monasteries. The last chapter deals with the situation of pharmacy in some other countries. Bibliography and name- and subject-indexes.

ANONYMOUS, 1953: Figures pharmaceutiques françaises. Notes historiques et portraits, 1803-1953, 276 p. + 38 pls. (Paris: Masson).—

This book has been written on the occasion of the 150th anniversary of the "enseignement pharmaceutique" in France. It contains autobiographies of 38 great French pharmacists who contributed greatly to the development of pharmacy in general; among the persons included are: Parmentier, Pelletier, Bussy, Soubeiran, Chatin, Dorvault, Berthelot, Limousin, Vigier, Milne-Edwards, Choay, Poulenc, Fourneau, Tiffeneau. Of all the persons considered, por-

traits are added. *Cf.* also TOUYA, R., 1962: Pharmaciens françiens de la marine et de l'outre-mer, 130 p. (Marseille: Author).

BOUVET, M., 1937: Histoire de la pharmacie en France dès origines à nos jours, 445 p. (Paris: Occitania).—

This history is provided with numerous plates and illustrations of which 6 plates in colour, showing contemporary prints, caricatures, *etc.*, relative to pharmacy, old pharmacy jars, labels, envelopes, *etc.* A shorter history of French pharmacy is: PERCHERON, M. & M. LE ROUX, 1955: Petite histoire de la pharmacie, 224 p. (Avignon: Aubanel). *Cf.* also LE POLLÈS, M. Gruget, 1957: Contribution à l'histoire de la pharmacie à Nantes: l'enseignement de la pharmacie dès origines à l'installation de la Faculté, 243 p. (Thèse Univ. Nantes). [Dactylographed.]

——, 1957: Les travaux d'histoire locale de la pharmacie en France dès origines à ce jour. Répertoire bibliographique, 43 p. (Paris: Soc. de la Pharmacie).—

A list of publications of histories on the national, regional, and local levels. This booklet appeared as a supplement to the Revue d'Histoire de la Pharmacie.

Germany

ADLUNG, A. & G. URDANG, 1935: Grundriss der Geschichte der deutschen Pharmazie, 647 p. (Berlin: Springer).—

Chapter headings are as follows: Die Vorgeschichte der Pharmazie bis zum Entstehen der Apotheken im heutigen Sinne; Das Apothekergewerbe; Der Arzneischatz der Apotheken; Die pharmazeutische Technik; Pharmazeutische Kulturgeschichte; Pharmazeutisch-Biographisches; Die deutsche Apotheke im Wandel der Zeit. In 1954 appeared an abridged edition under the title: Einführung in die Geschichte der deutschen Pharmazie, 142 p. (Frankfurt: Govi), written by G. URDANG & H. DIECKMANN. An illustrated history of the German apothecary is to be found in HEIN, W. H., 1960: Die deutsche Apotheke. Bilder aus ihrer Geschichte, 231 p. (Stuttgart: Deutscher Apothekerverlag). With 110 beautiful illustrations. *Cf.* also: VESTER, H., 1953 and 1956-1961, *vide* section Bibliographies, subsection e; and VALENTIN, H., 1950, *vide* section Some recommended encyclopaedias, subsection e.

LINDNER, J., 1957: Zeittafeln zur Geschichte der pharmakologischen Institute des deutschen Sprachgebietes, 167 p. (Aulendorf: Cantor).—

For more details, *vide* section Some recommended encyclopaedias, subsection e.

SCHNABEL, R., 1965: Pharmazie in Wissenschaft und Praxis. Dargestellt an der Geschichte der Klosterapotheken Altbayerns vom Jahre 800 bis 1800, 201 p. (Veröffentl. Inst. für Pharmazie der Ludwig-Maximilians Univ., München, Pharmaziegeschichtliche Abt.) (Munich: Moos).—

A beautifully printed and very readable history of the apothecaries of the monasteries of Bavaria from 800-1800. 9 full-page coloured plates, and many beautiful photographs.

Great Britain

COPEMAN, W. S. C., 1967: The Worshipful Society of Apothecaries of London: a history 1617-1967, 112 p. (Oxford & New York, N.Y.: Pergamon).—

This book deals with the origin and growth of the apothecaries, especially in England. The first chapter deals with the evolution of medicine prior to 1617, when a Royal Charter was granted to the Society of Apothecaries. Other chapters deal with the Chelsea Physick Garden, the troubles with the physicians, the establishment of the apothecary, the development of medical education, some eminent apothecaries, the refusal of Parliament to grant the monopoly of retail drug trading in 1748, the Apothecaries' Act of 1815 and the introduction of qualifying examinations, the Medical Act of 1858, *etc.* This study was published to mark the celebrations of the 350th anniversary of the Society's Charter. For an extensive history, supplemented by copious notes and additions, *cf.* UNDERWOOD, E. A., ed., 1963: A history of the Worshipful Society of Apothecaries of London. Vol. I: 1617-1815, 450 p. (Abstracted and arranged from the manuscript notes of the late Cecil WALL by the late H. Charles CAMERON) (Publ. Wellcome Historical Medical Museum, N.S., Vol. 8) (London & New York, N.Y.: Oxford U.P.).

MATTHEWS, L. G., 1962: History of pharmacy in Britain, 427 p. (Edinburgh & London: Livingstone).—

This book covers the history of pharmacy in Great Britain from the time

of the Roman occupation to the present. It discusses the professional, educational, legal, scientific, technical, commercial, and industrial aspects of pharmacy. Special attention has been paid to the Commonwealth countries. It contains much information concerning many companies and individual scientists. A collection of papers on the development of British pharmacy, read at the Fourth British Congress on the History of Medicine and Pharmacy, held at the Univ. of Nottingham in September 1963 is to be found in: POYNTER, F. N. L., ed., 1965: The evolution of pharmacy in Britain, 240 p. (London: Pitman; Springfield, Ill.: Thomas).

——, 1967: The Royal apothecaries, 191 p. (London: Wellcome Hist. Med. Library).—

A complete account of those pharmaceutical (and medical) practitioners who have provided an essential service for the kings and queens of England from the early 13th century to the present time. The major part of the book deals with individual royal apothecaries in chronological order. Many references and notes. Valuable index.

Yugoslavia

TARTALJA, H., 1957: L'histoire de la pharmacie en Yougoslavie et sa situation actuelle (Thèse Univ. Paris).—

Unfortunately I have not been able to provide further information about this publication. The only thing I know is that Tartalja generally is considered as belonging to the leading pharmaceutical historians of his country.

b**. *America* (North and South)

COWEN, D. L., 1961: America's pre-pharmacopoeial literature, 40 p. (Madison, Wisc.: Amer. Inst. Hist. Pharmacy).—

A description of European pharmacopoeias and dispensatories imported into and printed in America, and the works prepared in America, which were used by American physicians and apothecaries, prior to the appearance of the first United States Pharmacopoeia in 1820.

MUNOZ, J. E., 1952: Apuntes para la historia de la farmacia en el Ecuador, 216 p. (Quito: Ed. Rumiñahui).—

"Abondamment documenté, présenté avec toute la clarté désirable, cet historique de la pharmacie équatorienne s'avère d'autant plus précieux pour nous qu'il nous éclaire du même coup sur le passé professionel de tous les États de l'Amérique centrale et méridionale". (From: Rev. Hist. Pharm. 11: 60). A valuable complement to this book is: CIGNOLI, F., 1953: Historia de la farmacia argentina, 406 p. (Rosario: Ruiz). *Cf.* also: DA SILVA ARAUJO, 1954: Figuras e factos na historia da farmacia no Brasil portugues, 88 p. (Lisbonne: Ed. Imperio).

SONNEDECKER, G., ed., 1964: Kremer's and Urdang's history of pharmacy, ed. 3, 464 p. (Philadelphia, Pa. & Montreal: Lippincott; London: Pitman).—

A well-known history of pharmacy in which stress has been laid on its development in the U.S.A. The book has been divided into four parts. Part I (31 p.) deals with the early backgrounds of pharmacy in the Old World and gives a summary review of the early history of pharmacy from Antiquity through the Middle Ages. Part II (87 p.) deals with the rise of theories and materia medica and the development in Italy, France, Germany and England. Both parts serve as a general introduction to part III (199 p.): Pharmacy in the United States in which the history of pharmacy has been traced topically. In this part the history of the apothecary from the earliest colonial settlements through the Revolution and the period of pioneer expansion has been considered, together with the history of the growth of associations, the rise of legislative regulation, the development of education, the establishment of literature and a review of economic structure. Part IV (30 p.) deals with discoveries, inventions and other contributions to society by pharmacists. A bibliography (29 p.), a chronology, a glossary, and an index have been included. This 3rd edition has been carefully rewritten, and contains many additions in comparison with the 1st (1940) or 2nd (1951) editions, written by E. KREMERS & G. URDANG. Two other books dealing with the history of pharmacy in America are: LLOYD, J. U. & C. G., 1930-1931: Drugs and medicines of North America: a publication devoted to the historical and scientific discussion of the botany, pharmacy, chemistry and therapeutics of the medical plants of North America, their constituents, products and sophistications (1884-1887), 2 vols. Vol. I: 304 p.; Vol. II: 162 p. (Cincinati, O.: Bull. Lloyd Library of Botany, Pharmacy and Materia Medica, No. 29, 30, 31); and LYMAN, R. A., 1951: American pharmacy, Vol. I, ed. 3, 505 p. (Philadelphia, Pa.: Lippincott). Unfortunately I am not able to give further information about these books.

YOUNG, J. H., 1961: The toadstool millionaires: a social history of patent medicines in America before federal regulation, 282 p. (Princeton, N.J.: Princeton U.P.); YOUNG, J. H., 1967: The medical messiahs: a social history of health quackery in twentieth-century America, 460 p. (Princeton, N.J.: Princeton: U.P.).—

Both volumes together review the history of quackery and patent medicines in the U.S.A.

CHAPTER III: A SELECTED LIST OF BIOGRAPHIES, BIBLIOGRAPHIES, *ETC.*, OF FAMOUS BIOLOGISTS, MEDICAL MEN, *ETC,* INCLUDING SOME MODERN REISSUES OF THEIR PUBLICATIONS

Adanson, Michel (1727-1806) — LAWRENCE, G. H. M., ed., 1963-1964: Adanson: the bicentennial of Michel Adanson's "Familles des plantes", 2 vols. Vol. I (1963): 391 p.; Vol. II (1964): p. 393-640. (Hunt Monograph Series, Nos. 1 and 2) (Pittsburgh, Pa.: Hunt Botanical Library).—

When, during 1961, the Adanson collection was acquired by the Hunt Botanical Library, it became apparent that - because of the many new facts now available - a new biography of Adanson, the great 18th-century French naturalist, had to be written. This has been done by J. P. NICOLAS (p. 1-121). Moreover, a new concept of values and priorities of events had to be written, and F. A. STAFLEU undertook this part of the work, giving a review of French botany during the 18th century, in order to elucidate Adanson's position against that background (p. 123-264). W. D. MARGADANT (p. 265-368) gives a description of the Adanson collection of botanical books and manuscripts as it is in the possession of the Hunt Botanical Library. The second vol. contains the following essays: Adanson et le mouvement colonial (by J. P. NICOLAS); Les dessinateurs d'histoire naturelle en France au XVIIIe siècle (by G. DUPRAT); Mathematics and classification, from Adanson to the present (by P. H. A. SNEATH); l'Oeuvre zoologique d'Adanson (by T. MONOD); Adanson's sources, references, and abbreviations (by F. A. STAFLEU); The Adanson medal (by F. SEITZ, W. J. BLENKO, & R. HEIM); Franco-American activities in botany (by R. DE VILMORIN). Index.

Agassiz, Louis Jean Rodolphé (1807-1873) — AGASSIZ, E. C., ed., 1885-1886: Louis Agassiz: his life and correspondence, 2 vols. Vol. I (1886): 400 p.; Vol. II (1885): p. 401-794. (Boston, Mass.: Houghton, Mifflin).—

This book has been edited by Agassiz's second wife and is especially important for the inclusion of many letters to and from eminent men of science.

——, COOPER, L., 1917: Louis Agassiz as a teacher: illustrative extracts on his method of instruction, 74 p. (Ithaca, N. Y.: Comstock).—

A book dealing with the form of instruction employed by Louis Agassiz. A more recent publication which seems to deal with the same kind of subject, but of which I am unable to give details is: DAVENPORT, G., ed., 1963: The intelligence of Louis Agassiz: a specimen book of scientific writings, 237 p. (Boston, Mass.: Beacon).

——, LURIE, E., 1960: Louis Agassiz: a life in science, 449 p. (Chicago, Ill.: Univ. Chicago Press).—

L. Agassiz, a Swiss naturalist and scholar of Cuvier, founder of the Museum of Comparative Zoology at Harvard College, arrived in America in 1846. Because of his great enthusiasm and organizing talents, he had a great influence on the American public and he became mentor in matters of natural history. This book gives a sound historical biography of his life. Especially his strong opposition to Darwin's theory has been described, and it is shown how his religious faith set him against acceptance of any evolutionary theory. As a consequence, he became the last strong defender of the static world view. Reprinted 1966 (Chicago, Ill.: Univ. Chicago Press). A very readable biography, written with much enthusiasm and sympathy, including a bibliography and a chronology of the life of Louis Agassiz is: ROBINSON, M. L., 1939: Runner of the mountain tops: the life of Louis Agassiz, 290 p. (New York, N.Y.: Random House). Also in German translation: Louis Agassiz (1807-1873), 1941, 334 p. (Zürich: Rascher). *Cf.* also: THARP, L. H., 1959: Adventurous alliance: the story of the Agassiz family of Boston, 354 p. (Boston, Mass.: Little, Brown).

—— ——, ed., 1962: Louis Agassiz: essay on classification, 34 + 268 p. (Cambridge, Mass.: Harvard U.P.).—

Agassiz was an active promoter of the study of natural history of the New World. This "Essay" originally was intended to serve as an introduction to his "Contributions to the natural history of the United States", which began to appear in 1857. This "Essay" was printed separately in 1859 in London. The present text is an annotated reissue of that edition. The "Essay" itself contains much documentation concerning classificatory problems and the study of natural history as practiced in the first half of the 19th century in the U.S.A. For Agassiz the study of nature is an attempt to analyse the thoughts of the Creator, for these thoughts should be reflected by the constitution of nature. Within this frame of thought it is understandable that Agassiz has belonged to the most ardent opponents of Darwin's theories.

——, MARCOU, J., 1896: Life, letters and works of Louis Agassiz, 2 vols. Vol. I: 302 p. Vol. II: 318 p. (New York, N.Y. & London: Macmillan).—

This is a valuable biography, especially for the range and accuracy of details. It has been supplemented by 3 appendixes. The first of them contains a list of biographies with short annotations (46 items); the second a list of Agassiz's portraits, engravings, photographs, busts, medals, and tablets; and the third a list of his papers and works arranged chronologically (425 items).

Agricola, Georgius (1494-1555) — WILSDORF, H., 1955-1956: Georg Agricola und seine Zeit, 2 vols. Vol. I: 335 p.; Vol. II: 380 p. (Berlin: Deutscher Verlag der Wissenschaften).—

Agricola is not only the founder of the science of mining, but like so many other humanists of the beginning of the 16th century he also worked in many other fields of knowledge, incl. natural science and medicine. The whole work under consideration will be published in 6 parts, but only parts I and II are of a biohistorical interest. Part I gives many (partly newly published) biographical data, and a listing of the works published by Agricola, incl. those which have been lost. The second part considers, *inter alia,* Agricola as a physician and the position of medical science of those days. This part is supplemented by an extensive review of the literary sources used by Agricola (p. 200-245), and an author-index which gives many biographical details (p. 258-329). *Cf.* also: LEHMANN, E., 1806-1812: Georg Agricola's mineralogische Schriften (De ortu et causis subterraneorum - De natura eorum quae effuunt e terra - De natura fossilium, übersetzt und mit erläuternden Anmerkungen und Excursionen begleitet, 3 vols. (Freyberg). De natura fossilium also exists in an English translation: BANDY, M. C. & J. A., eds., 1955: Georgius Agricola: De natura fossilium. Transl. from the first Latin edition of 1546, 240 p. (Special paper, No. 63, Geological Soc. America) (Boulder, Colo.: Geological Soc. America).

Aldrovandi, Ulisse (1522-1605) — LIND, L. R., ed., 1963: Aldrovandi on chickens: the ornithology of Ulisse Aldrovandi (1600), Vol. II, Bk. XIV, 36 + 447 p. (Norman, Okla.: Univ. Oklahoma Press).—

This is a translation of those parts of Aldrovandi's "Ornithologia" which are concerned with chickens, their anatomy, sex, song, rearing, feeding, habits, *etc.* Besides these biological aspects, Aldrovandi was also interested in the role chickens play in such matters as: proverbs, apologues, emblems, dreams, riddles, secret signs, fables, apophthegms, and especially in their role in medicine. In this way Aldrovandi summarized all that he has been able to learn about chickens in the great collection of books at his disposal and from his own observations. The introduction contains a brief biography. This edition contains beautiful illustrations, a bibliography and an index.

Aschoff, Ludwig (1866-1942) — ASCHOFF, L., 1966: Ein Gelehrtenleben in Briefen an die Familie, 480 p. (Freiburg i.B.: Schulz).—

Ludwig Aschoff was one of the most distinguished pathologists of his age and, moreover, also contributed to the history of medicine, for he wrote a very interesting historical account of the cell-theory in pathology *(vide* section History of anatomy). In the present book some of his other medical historical studies are also considered; it also contains much biographical information on Aschoff's life and medical activities and those of some of his contemporaries.

Audubon, John James Laforest (1780-1851) — ADAMS, A. B., 1967: John James Audubon: a biography, 510 p. (London: Gollancz).—

"This book gives a straightforward account of Audubon's life, but it is far too long, especially because there is no appraisal of Audubon's artistic output, or of the way in which he drew and painted, or of wild nature as it then existed in the United States. Further, the social milieu of the places in which Audubon lived could have been enlarged upon." (From a review of this book in Nature 214: 1171). Bibliography p. 475-486. There also exists a French biography of Audubon: CONSTANTIN-WEYER, M., 1950: Dans les pas du naturaliste, 231 p. (Les livres de nature, No. 77) (Paris: Stock).

——, FORD, A. E., 1964: John James Audubon, 488 p. (Norman, Okla.: Univ. Oklahoma Press).—

"... the present volume, reflecting more than ten years of research into previous inaccessible personal collections of records, documents, and letters, resolves many of the unanswered questions about the great American naturalist and portrays his life and work with new depth and understanding." The authoress is an art historian and artist biographer; she is a well-known authority on Audubon. Other books on Audubon published by her: FORD, A., ed., 1957: The bird biographies of John James Audubon: a selection, 282 p. (New York, N.Y.: Macmillan); and: FORD, A., ed., 1967: The 1826 journal of John James Audubon, 409 p. (Norman, Okla.: Univ. Oklahoma Press). Transcribed with an introduction and notes by A. Ford from the original in the collection of Henry Bradley Martin. *Cf.* also: AUDUBON, M. R., ed., 1960: Audubon and his journals, 2 vols. Vol. I: 532 p.; Vol. II: 554 p. (New York, N.Y.: Dover).

———, HERRICK, F. H., 1938: Audubon the naturalist: a history of his life and time, ed. 2, 2 vols. Vol. I: 451 p.; Vol. II: 500 p. (New York, N.Y. & London: Appleton-Century).—

A full-scale biography of the famous ornithologist, animal painter, and writer. Many fine illustrations. Extensive bibliography and index. An appendix contains 21 original documents, and another appendix gives a review of his drawings and of the collections in which they are now. A reprint edition appeared in 1968 (New York, N.Y.: Dover). *Cf.* also: REILLY, E. M., 1968: The Audubon illustrated handbook of American birds, 524 p. (New York, N.Y.: McGraw-Hill).

Auenbrugger, Leopold (1722-1809) — NEUBURGER, M., ed., 1966: Inventum novum: a facsimile of the first edition with CORVISART's French translation (1803), FORBES' English translation (1824), UNGAR's German translation (1843), 95 + 51 + 36 + 55 + 72 p. (With a biographical account by M. NEUBURGER (London: Dawson).—

This is an English translation of: NEUBURGER, M., 1922: Leopold Auenbrugger's Inventum novum, *etc.*, 51 + 36 + 72 p. (Vienna & Leipzig: Šafár). It is a reprint of that famous publication, first published in Vienna in 1761, in which Auenbrugger introduced the technique of percussion, *i.e.*, the action of striking or tapping with the finger (or with a small hammer)

upon a part of the body, in order to ascertain the condition of some organ by the sound produced. *Cf.* FOSSEL, V., 1912: Leopold Auenbruggers neue Erfindung, mittels des Anschlagens an den Brustkorb als eines Zeichens verborgene Brustkrankheiten zu entdecken (1761), 44 p. (Sudhoffs Klassiker der Medizin, vol. 15) (Leipzig: Barth).

Baer, Karl Ernst von (1792-1876) — HAACKE, W., 1905: Karl Ernst von Baer, 175 p. (Leipzig: Thomas).—

A biography of von Bear, considering his youth, studies, travels, scientific activities, teachings, *etc.* (p. 1-50). The second part deals more especially with his philosophical outlook and with his publications (p. 51-172). The book ends with a chronological bibliography. A new biography of von Baer is in course of preparation; it will be published by the Acad. Leopoldina, Halle/Saale (D.D.R.).

———, O'MALLEY, C. D., ed., 1956: On the genesis of the ovum of mammals and of Man. (Cambridge, Mass.: History of Science Soc.).—

This is a reprint and English translation of von Baer's "De ovi mammalium et hominis genesi epistolam ad Academiam Imperialem Scientiarum Petropolitanam", 40 p. (Lipsiae), the letter von Baer wrote to the Imperial Academy of St. Petersburg in 1827, in which he announced the discovery of the human ovum.

Bailey, Liberty Hyde (1858-1954) — RODGERS, A. D., 1949: Liberty Hyde Bailey: a story of American plant sciences, 506 p. (Princeton, N.J.: Princeton U.P.).—

L. H. Bailey was an all-round botanist. He was especially well acquainted with cultivated plants, and he established the famous Bailey Hortorium, a collection of 200,000 specimens, still the standard for the identification of cultivated plants. A valuable biography based on much source-material. Reprinted 1965 (New York, N.Y.: Hafner).

Banks, Joseph (1743-1820) — CAMERON, H. C., 1952: Sir Joseph Banks: the autocrat of the philosophers, 341 p. (London: Batchworth).—

Compared with SMITH's biography, *vide infra*, this book is more a (fully annotated) monograph of Banks' life-activities, containing much new manuscript material not used in Smith's biography. The book also gives detailed information concerning the (widely scattered) letters and other manuscript documents of Banks and gives much information on Banks' voyages, his botanical explorations (Tahiti, New Zealand, Australia), his interference in affairs of the Kew Gardens, the voyages he sponsored, and his position as president of the Royal Society wherein he acted as a protector of science. Reprinted 1966 (London: Angus & Robertson). *Cf.* also: DAWSON, W. R., ed., 1958: The Banks letters: a calendar of the manuscript correspondence of Sir Joseph Banks preserved in the British Museum, the British Museum, Natural History, and other collections in Great Britain, 42 + 964 p. (London: British Museum).

——, MACKANESS, G., 1936: Sir Joseph Banks: his relations with Australia, 146 p. (Sydney: Angus & Robertson).—

Banks, the companion of Cook on his first voyage in which he visited the shores of Australia, became advisor to the British Government on all matters of colonization, exploration, and administration of this new continent. The present book, although concerned primarily with the relations of Banks with Australia, reveals many scientific activities of Banks, concerning, *e.g.*, the introduction of valuable fruits and vegetables, advice to gardeners how to care for plants in transit, the maintenance of collections of the local fauna and flora, his collections of Australian plants and of marsupials, *etc.* A somewhat older book dealing with the relationship of Banks with Australia is: MAIDEN, J. H., 1909: Sir Joseph Banks: the "father of Australia", 244 p. (Sydney: Gullick; London: Kegan Paul). The chapter headings are as follows: Banks as traveller; Banks' botanical activities; The botanical protégés of Banks; Banks, the president of the Royal Society, and friend of Australia; The works and memorials of Banks. This last chapter contains a section devoted to works written, edited by, or concerning, Banks, *Cf.* MORRELL, W. P., ed., 1958: Sir Joseph Banks in New Zealand: from his journal, 159 p. (Wellington: Reed).

——, SMITH, E., 1911: The life of Sir Joseph Banks, president of the Royal Society with some notices of his friends and contemporaries, 348 p. (London & New York, N.Y.: Lane).—

An autobiographic study, together with an attempt to present some aspects of 18th-century science. For more particulars concerning his voyage with Captain Cook,

cf.: HOOKER, J. D., ed., 1896: Journal of the right hon. Sir Joseph Banks during Captain Cook's first voyage in H.M.S. "Endeavour" in 1768-71 to Terra del Fuego, Otahite, New Zealand, Australia, the Dutch East Indies, *etc.*, 51 + 466 p. (London & New York, N.Y.: Mcmillan). *Cf.* also: BEAGLEHOLE, J. C., ed., 1962: The Endeavour Journal of Joseph Banks, 1768-1771, 2 vols. (Sydney: Trustees of the Public Library of N.S. Wales; London: Angus & Robertson).

Banting, Frederick Grant (1891-1941) — STEVENSON, L., 1946: Sir Frederick Banting, 446 p. (Toronto: Ryerson; Springfield, Ill.: Thomas).—

Sir Frederick Banting was the discoverer of insulin. This is a very complete biography based upon records, notebooks, interviews, *etc.* A more popular biography is: HARRIS, S., 1946: Banting's miracle: the story of the discoverer of insulin, 245 p. (Philadelphia, Pa.: Lippincott).

Barcroft, Joseph (1872-1947) — FRANKLIN, K. J., 1953: Joseph Barcroft 1872-1947, 381 p. (Oxford: Blackwell).—

An authoritative biography of the great British physiologist Sir Joseph Barcroft, written by a friend of the family and his successor in the chair of physiology at St. Bartholomew's Hospital in London. Sir Joseph was particulary engaged in the study of respiratory problems, *e.g.*, general physiology of respiration, mammalian foetal respiration, physiology of haemoglobin and the blood gases, high-altitude physiology, acclimatization. His most famous book was "The respiratory function of the blood", published in 1914. Included are a chronological list of Barcroft's publications and an index.

Bartholin, Thomas (1616-1680) — O'MALLEY, C. D., ed., 1961: On the burning of his library, and on medical travel, 101 p. (Lawrence, Kans.: Univ. Kansas Libraries). —

The book comprises English translations of two of the smaller works of the well-known Danish anatomist Thomas Bartholin. Both books were originally written in Latin. The first book "On the burning of his library" was first published in 1670, and in it the author describes the tragedy of the destruction of his library by fire, together with descriptions of other libraries destroyed by fire, and details of his personal book-collection. In the second book, "On medical travel", he describes his travels in France and Italy between 1640 and 1645; this work was first printed in 1674. It contains information concerning places to visit, advice on health, food and drink. Both booklets give a picture of 17th-century life and thought. *Cf.* also the publication of GARBOE, A., 1950: Thomas Bartholin. Et bidrag til Dansk natur- og laegevidenskabs historie i det 17 aarhundrede (A contribution to the history of Danish natural and medical science in he 17th century), 203 p. (Acta Hist. Sci. Nat. et Med., Vol. 5) (Copenhagen: Munksgaard). English summary p. 188-196.

Bartram, John (1699-1777) and William (1739-1823) — EARNEST, E., 1940: John and William Bartram: botanists and explorers, 187 p. (Philadelphia, Pa.: Univ. Pennsylvania Press).—

　　Linnaeus once referred to John Bartram as "the greatest natural botanist in the world", and William, his son, extended his father's explorations and collections in such a way that his work has achieved a prominent place in the development of natural history in the U.S.A. *Cf.* CRUICKS-HANK, H. G., ed., 1957: John and William Bartram's America: selections from the writings of the Philadelphia naturalists, 418 p. (New York, N.Y.: Devin-Adair).

——, DARLINGTON, W., 1849: Memorials of John Bartram and Humphry Marshall with notices of their botanical contemporaries, 585 p. (Philadelphia, Pa.: Lindsay & Blakiston).—

　　A short biographical sketch and a collection of letters from and to John Bartram, who planned a famous garden near Philadelphia which still forms a part of Philadelphia's park system, and still contains many giant trees planted by John Bartram himself.

——, EWAN, J., ed., 1968: William Bartram: botanical and zoological drawings, 1756-1788, 180 p. (Memoirs Amer. Philos. Soc., Vol. 74) (Philadelphia, Pa.: Amer. Philos. Soc.).—

　　An account of Bartram's life and career. It contains 59 plates, reproduced from the Fothergill Album in the British Museum (Nat. Hist.). The editor has named the subjects pictured by Bartram (as far as possible) and has tried to place them in apparent chronological order to illustrate the progress in the artistic development of Bartram.

——, FAGIN, N. B., 1933: William Bartram: interpreter of the American landscape, 229 p. (Baltimore, Md.: Johns Hopkins Press).—

　　William Bartram is especially known for his "Travels" (1791) through the Carolinas, Georgia and Florida. The present book is in three parts, *viz.*, a biographical part, a part in which the author analyses the elements of Bartram's landscape description, and a part in which he gives a survey of Bartram's influence on literature. Included are a bibliography and an index. A fully annotated and indexed edition of Bartram's "Travels" is: HARPER, F., 1958: The travels of William Bartram, naturalist's edition, 727 p. (New Haven, Conn.: Yale U.P.).

Bates, Henry Walter (1825-1892) — BATES, H. W., 1892: The naturalist on the River Amazons, 84 + 389 p. (With a memoir of the author by E. CLODD) (London: Murray).—

　　Originally published in 1863 in 2 vols. (London: Murray). The contents of this book become clear from its sub-title: "A record of adventures, habits of animals, sketches of Brazilian and Indian life, and aspects of nature under the equator, during eleven years of travel". In 1962 a reprint of this second ed. appeared with a foreword by R. L. USINGER, 465 p. (Berkeley, Calif.: Univ. California Press). In 1873 a slightly abridged ed. appeared, 394 p. (London: Murray); reprinted 1910.

——, WOODCOCK, G., 1969: Henry Walter Bates: naturalist of the Amazons, 269 p. (London: Faber).—

　　Bates was one of the great explorer-naturalists of Victorian England; the mass of data he collected during his stay in South America, was freely used by Darwin in his "Origin of species". The present biography has been written by a traveller; it is based on a good deal of hitherto unpublished material, including letters, journals and other contemporary material. The author describes Bates' meticulous observations of insects, his ideas concerning mimicry, *etc.* Less has been said about Bates' life after his return to England, where he became one of the secretaries of the Royal Geographical Society (for 27 years) and one of the friends of Darwin.

Bateson, William (1861-1926) — BATESON, B., 1928: William Bateson, F. R. S., naturalist: his essays and addresses together with a short account of his life, 473 p. (Cambridge: U.P.).—

> The present volume contains a rather brief biography of Bateson (p. 1-160) and the reproduction of a number of papers, scientific as well as educational. The book was written by his widow. *Cf.* also: PUNNETT, R. C., ed., 1928: Scientific papers of William Bateson, 2 vols. (Cambridge: U.P.).

Bauhin, Joannus (1541-1613) and Caspar (1560-1624) — LEGRÉ, L., 1904: La botanique en Provence au XVI⁰ siècle. Les deux Bauhin, 117 p. (Marseilles: Aubertin & Rolle).—

> Jean Bauhin was a famous botanist and physician, pupil of Leonhart Fuchs (*vide infra*). His most famous work is the "Historia plantarum universalis nova et absolutissima" (1650/'51). For a bibliography of his works *cf.* GAUTIER, L., 1906: La médecine à Genève jusqu'à la fin du dix-huitième siècle, p. 508-510. Caspar Bauhin was his younger brother, the first professor of botany in Basle, and afterwards successor of Felix Platter in the chair of anatomy in this university. He made a first attempt to classify the plants according to a natural system and developed a classification and nomenclature based on a distinction between genus and species. His most famous publication is the "Pinax theatri botanici" (Basle, 1623), a complete list of synonyms of plant-names as they existed in his time. For bibliographical information, *cf.* BURCKHARDT, A., 1917: Geschichte der medizinischen Fakultät zu Basel, p. 95-123. Other botanists considered in some detail in this book are Jean Henri Cherler and Valerand Dourez.

Beaumont, William (1785-1853) — BEAUMONT, W., 1960: Experiments and observations on the gastric juice and the physiology of digestion. With a biographical essay "A pioneer American physiologist" by W. OSLER, 40 + 280 p. (New York, N.Y.: Dover).—

> This is a facsimile reproduction (originally published in 1929, Cambridge, Mass.: Harvard U.P.) of the first edition of Beaumont's "Experiments" (1833). Beaumont was an American army surgeon who accidentally observed, then employed, the permanent gastric fistula. The present edition is identical with that especially prepared for the XIIIth Intern. Physiol. Congr. (1929), when

Beaumont and Pavlov were honoured for their scientific contributions. The text is preceded by an essay written by W. OSLER, giving a sketch of Beaumont's career and work. The text of this essay was originally delivered by Osler before the St. Louis Med. Soc. in 1902. For more biographical details, *cf.* MYER, J. S., 1912: Life and letters of Dr. William Beaumont, 317 p. (St. Louis, Mo.: Mosby). (Reprinted 1939, London: Kimpton); and MILLER, G., 1946: Wm. Beaumont's formative years: two early notebooks, 1811-1821, 87 p. (With annotations and an introductory essay) (New York, N.Y.: Schuman). *Cf.* also CASSIDY, P. A. & R. S. SOKOL, 1968: Index to the Wm. Beaumont, M. D. (1785-1853) manuscript collection, 165 p. (St. Louis, Mo.: Univ. Washington School Med.).

Bell, Charles (1774-1842) — TAYLOR, G. G. & E. W. WALLS, 1958: Sir Charles Bell: his life and times, 288 p. (London & Edinburgh: Livingstone).—

> This is a biography of the famous Scottish anatomist, physiologist, surgeon, artist and philosopher C. Bell, put against the background of his contemporary environment, throwing sidelights on other famous men of the period. Besides some minor advances (made by, *inter alia*, Borell, Glisson, and von Haller), up to the days of Bell, neurology was still mainly based on Galenic doctrines. Anyhow Bell was the first to discover (almost simultaneously with, but apparently independent of, Magendie), that definite nerves have a definite course from the brain to the periphery, and that different nerves have different functions. There are also interesting accounts of the foundation of the Middlesex Hospital Medical School to which Bell was appointed surgeon in 1825; this school owed much to him.

Belon, Pierre (1517-1564) — DELAUNAY, P., 1926: Pierre Belon naturaliste, 271 p. (Le Mans: Monnoyer).—

> Separate chapters deal with: Belon and the philosophy of the natural sciences, Belon as geologist, botanist, mammalogist, ornithologist, herpetologist, ichthyologist, and with Belon and the invertebrates. Supplementary to this volume is: DELAUNY, P., 1926: L'aventureuse existence de Pierre Belon, 180 p. (Paris: Champion). A description of his voyages in Greece, Asia, Judea, Egypt, and Arabia, based upon an unedited ms. of Belon.

Benivieni, Antonio (? 1443-1502) — SINGER, C., ed., 1954: De abditis nonnullis ac mirandis morborum et sanationum causis. The hidden causes of diseases, 46 + 217 p. (Springfield, Ill.: Thomas).—

An English translation of the main work of one of the founders of pathological anatomy. The present book contains a selection of 111 case records. It was first printed in 1507 in Florence. A biographical account was written by E. R. LONG; the translation is by C. SINGER.

Bentham, George (1800-1884) — JACKSON, B. D., 1906: George Bentham, 292 p. (London: Dent; New York, N.Y.: Dutton).—

A biography mainly based on letters written to and by George Bentham, formerly secretary of the Horticultural Society (1829-1840) and president of the Linnean Society (1861-1874). His most famous works are "Handbook to the British Flora" (1858); "Flora Australiensis" (7 vols., 1863-1878); "Genera Plantarum" (7 vols., 1863-1878).

Berengarius, Jacobus (= Berengario da Carpi, Giacomo) (ca. 1470-1530) — LIND, L. R. & P. G. ROOFE, eds., 1959: A short introduction to anatomy (Isagogae breves), 228 p. (Chicago, Ill.: Chicago U.P.).—

Berengario da Carpi was for many years professor of surgery and anatomy at Bologna, and can be considered to be one of the most important forerunners of Vesalius. His major contribution to anatomy was his "Commentaria", containing criticisms and emendations on the "Anatomia mundini" (cf. section Middle Ages in the West, subsection d, Mondino de Luzzi). In 1522 Berengario published a briefer version of this work, and the present work is a translation (by L. R. LIND) of its first edition (although later editions are known). This translation is accompanied by historical notes (by L. R. LIND), by anatomical notes (by P. G. ROOFE) and by an introduction (by L. R. LIND). Cf. also: PUTTI, V., 1937: Berengario da Carpi. Saggio biografico e bibliografico seguito dalla traduzione del "De fractura calvae sive cranai", 352 p. (Bologna: Capelli). This seems to be a very complete and elaborate study of this anatomist, accompanied by beautiful illustrations. Cf. LARKEY, S. V. & L. TUM SUDEN, eds., 1934: Jackson's English translation of Berengarius of Carpi's "Isagogae breves", 1660 and 1664 in Isis 21: 57-70.

Bernard, Claude (1813-1876) — BERNARD, C., 1963: Introduction à l'étude de la médecine expérimentale, 372 p. (Paris: Nouvel Office d'Édition).—

A reissue of Bernard's most famous book originally published in 1865 in which he has analysed the role of thought, ideas, and hypotheses in experimental medicine. A classic in the history of the organic sciences. Also in a paperback edition, ed. by L. BINET, 374 p. (Paris: Nouvel Office d'Editions). An authoritative German translation appeared in 1960: Claude Bernard. Einführung in das Studium der experimentellen Medizin, 359 p. (Sudhoffs Klassiker der Medizin, No. 35) (Leipzig: Barth). The text of this German translation (by P. SZENDRÖ) contains a biographical introduction and useful annotations, both prepared by K. E. ROTHSCHUH and a complete bibliography of all Bernard's works, prepared by R. ZAUNICK: "Zur Bibliographie des Schrifttums von und über Claude Bernard". An unabridged English translation appeared in 1957: GREENE, H. C., ed., 1957: An introduction to the study of experimental medicine, 226 p. (New York, N.Y.: Dover). This translation was first printed in 1927 (New York, N.Y.: Macmillan), reprinted in 1949 (New York, N.Y.: Schuman); it contains an introduction by L. J. HENDERSON. A Spanish translation: Introducción al estudio de la medicina experimental, 1960, 418 p. (México City: Univ. Nac. Autónoma de México). An anastatic reissue of the original (1865) edition appeared in Brussels (Éd. Culture et Civilisation).

——, 1966: Leçons sur les phénomènes de la vie communs aux animaux et aux végétaux, 404 p. (Intr. by G. CANGUILHEM) (Paris: Vrin).—

This book is of great interest, both for the history of philosophical ideas in biology and for the history of physiology.

——, DELHOUME, L., ed., 1947: Claude Bernard. Principes de médecine expérimentale, 48 + 308 p. (Bibliothèque de philosophie contemporaine) (Paris: Presses Univ. de France).—

Sarton (in Isis 39: 256) writes about this book "... the first edition of the 'Principes de médecine expérimentale' on the basis of MSS. preserved by d'Arsonval. The notes ad hoc were written by Bernard between 1862 and 1877, that is almost until the time of his death in 1878. They are not complete, but such as they are, their interest can hardly be exaggerated." The text is preceded by a valuable introduction and is accompanied by notes, all prepared by the editor who is perfectly equipped for this task.

——, GRMEK, M. D., ed., 1965: Claude Bernard. Cahier de notes, 1850-1860. Édition intégrale du "Cahier Rouge", 315 p. (Paris: Gallimard).—

The "Cahier Rouge" is an unpublished notebook covering the period 1850-1860 and dealing with a wide variety of experimental and philosophical problems. Almost simultaneously published in English: GRANDE, F. & M. B. VISSCHER, eds., 1967: Claude Bernard and experimental medicine. Collected papers from a symposium, commemorating the centenary of the publication of "An introduction to the study of experimental medicine", Minneapolis, April 1965, and an English translation of Bernard's "Cahier Rouge", 2 vols. in one, 210 + 120 p. (Cambridge, Mass.: Schenkman).

—— ——, 1967: Catalogue des manuscrits de Claude Bernard avec la bibliographie de ses travaux imprimés et des études sur son oeuvre, 419 p. (Paris: Masson).—

This is a catalogue of the substantial archival collections of material relating to Claude Bernard in the possession of the Collège de France. This extensive bibliography is an invaluable tool to anyone interested in the life and work of Bernard.

——, MANI, N., ed., 1966: Claude Bernard. Ausgewählte physiologische Schriften, 133 p. (Hubers Klassiker der Medizin und der Naturwissenschaften, Vol. 8) (Bern: Huber).—

After a brief introduction (p. 8-20), translations follow of four selected works of Bernard, collected and annotated by the editor. The titles of the selected papers are (in English translation): 1. On pancreatic juice and its role in alimentary digestion; 2. On the physiological mechanism of liver glycogenesis; 3. On the influence of two types of nerve, whereby the colour changes of venous blood in glandular organs is evoked; 4. Physiological studies on some American cases of curare poisoning.

——, OLMSTED, J. M. D. & E. H., 1952: Claude Bernard and the experimental method in medicine, 277 p. (New York, N.Y.: Schuman).—

This volume is supplementary to OLMSTED's standard biography: Claude **Bernard**: physiologist, 1938, 272 p. (New **York**, N.Y.: Harper). In the present volume much new biographical material has been added, derived from the Raffalovich letters and from the ms. material in the care of L.

Delhoume (*vide supra*). Bernard's famous researches on the function of pancreatic secretion, on the liver as a source of sugar, on muscle contraction and the action of curare, his discovery of vasomotor nerves, the development of the theory of glycogenesis, his views on asphyxia, anaesthesia and drug toxicity, and his philosophical reflections, have been considered.

——, SCHILLER, J., 1967: Claude Bernard et les problèmes scientifiques de son temps, 230 p. (Paris: Éditions du Cèdre).—

An attempt to elucidate the interrelation between Claude Bernard the scientist and Claude Bernard the philosopher; as such this book can be considered as a scientific biography. Among the problems discussed are: vivisection, structure and function, the concept of evolution, materialism, idealism, mechanism, vitalism.

——, VIRTANEN, R., 1960: Claude Bernard and his place in the history of ideas, 156 p. (Lincoln, Nebr.: Univ. Nebraska Press).—

In this book Bernard is treated not as a physiologist, but rather as a philosopher. Bernard fought against vitalism in biology, and worked for the acknowledgement of physiology as a scientific discipline. He stressed that living organisms conform to the laws of physics and chemistry, and that this fact is of high medical interest. From this starting-point Bernard considered philosophy of science and nature in a more general way, and that aspect is given special prominence by the present author. He shows the philosophical relationship between Bernard and Bacon, Descartes, Pascal, Leibniz and Kant on the one side, and between Bernard and his contemporaries (Comte, Darwin) and his successors (Bergson) on the other side. A consideration of Claude Bernard from the Marxian point of view is: KAHANE, E., ed., 1961: Claude Bernard. Pages choisies, 200 p. (Paris: Éd. Sociales), with introduction and notes by the editor. Also in English translation: The thought of Claude Bernard, 1966. (Transl. and introd. by H. CHORNICK & P. M. PREBUS) (New York, N.Y.: Amer. Inst. for Marxist studies). Another selection: CLARKE, R., 1961: Claude Bernard. Choix de textes, 222 p. (Paris: Seghers).

——, WOLFF, E., *et al.*, 1967: Philosophie et méthodologie scientifiques de Claude Bernard. An international symposium, Paris, June-July 1965, 170 p. (Paris: Masson).—

The text of a series of papers, read at a symposium held on the occasion of the centenary of the publication of the "Introduction à l'étude de la médecine expérimentale". The papers deal with such problems as: Bernard's influence on English and American physiology, Bernard and the beginnings of biochemistry, the idea of integration and stability of fuctions in the organism as understood by Bernard, Bernard's theory and technique of experimentation, Bernard and the scientific milieu of his day, Bernard's negative attitude toward Darwin's evolution theory, Bernard and clinical medicine, the development of Bernard's concept of the "milieu intérieur". This last topic was the central theme of another symposium held at this same occasion, *viz.,* HEIM, R., ed., 1967: Les concepts de Claude Bernard sur le milieu intérieur, 423 p. (An international symposium, Paris, June-July, 1965) (Paris: Masson). The papers included deal with problems concerning osmoregulation, thermal regulation, and regulation of blood pressure.

Bernardin de St. Pierre, *vide* Saint-Pierre.

Bernouilli, Daniel (1700-1782) — HUBER, F., 1959: Daniel Bernouilli (1700-1782) als Physiologe und Statistiker, 104 p. (Basler Veröffentl. Gesch. Med. Biol., Vol. 8) (Basle & Stuttgart: Schwabe).—

    This study is based upon primary and secondary literature and on unpublished mss. of Bernouilli himself. Bernouilli occupied himself with the physiology of respiration from a physical point of view, with muscle contraction, the function of the heart, haemodynamics, inoculation against small-pox, and in a later phase of his life with medico-statistical questions. Huber critically evaluates these activities against the background of 18th-century medicine.

Beijerinck, Martinus Willem (1851-1931) — ITERSON, G. VAN, L. E. DEN DOOREN DE JONG & A. J. KLUYVER, 1940: Martinus Willem Beijerinck: his life and his work, 193 p. (The Hague: Nijhoff).—

    Beijerinck was a famous Dutch botanist and bacteriologist. This publication consists of three parts, *viz.,* 1. a well-illustrated biography by L. E. DEN DOOREN DE JONG; 2. an evaluation of Beijerinck as a botanist by G. VAN ITERSON, considering, *e.g.,* his studies on phyllotaxis, cross-breeding, colloid chemistry, bacterial root nodules, studies of algae and of galls; 3. an appreciation of Beijerinck's main contributions to microbiology by A. J. KLUYVER, considering, *e.g.,* his studies on luminous bacteria, yeasts, lactic acid bacteria,

acetic acid bacteria, sulphate reduction, denitrification, nitrogen-fixation, urea-decomposition, his investigations of *Bacillus radicicola* and *B. oligocarbophilus, Aerobacter, Sarcina ventriculi,* his contribution to the virus concept, and his studies on microbial variation. His collected writings were published in six volumes (this publication forms the last part of vol. 6, which also contains full indexes to all six volumes).

Bichat, Marie François Xavier (1771-1802) — SOLOVINE, M., ed., 1955: Recherches physiologiques sur la vie et la mort. Facsimile of the edition of 1800, 372 p. (Paris: Gauthier-Villars).—

    Bichat was one of the greatest physiologists, anatomists and surgeons of his age. The "Recherches physiologiques sur la vie et la mort" is a book dealing with organ pathology in which Bichat made serious attempts to correlate symptoms of disease in life with *post mortem* findings. Although the text mentions that this book is a reprint of the 1800 edition (the 2nd ed.), the text actually is a reprint of the third ed. of 1805. *Cf.* also: KERVELLA, E. J., 1931: La vie et l'oeuvre de Bichat, 1771-1802, 85 p. (Paris); and MONTEIL, J., 1964: Le cours d'anatomie pathologique de Bichat. Un nouveau manuscrit, 47 p. (Grenoble: Guirimand).

Billings, John Shaw (1838-1913) — ROGERS, F. B., ed., 1965: Selected papers of John Shaw Billings, 300 p. (Chicago, Ill.: Med. Library Assn.).—

    This volume contains 24 papers. Billings was the principal founder of the Library of the Surgeon-General's Office. He was a distinguished army surgeon in the Civil War. In 1880 he issued the first vol. of the Index Catalogue of the library (assisted by R. FLETCHER, of Bristol, England), the most exhaustive piece of medical bibliography. *Cf.* John Shaw Billings centennial: addresses presented 17 June 1965 in commemoration of the 100th anniversary of Dr. Billing's appointment to head of the library of the Surgeon General's Office, U.S. Army, 70 p. (Bethesda, Md.: Nat. Library Med.).

Boas, Franz (1858-1942) — HERSKOVITS, M. J., 1953: Franz Boas: the science of man in the making, 131 p. (New York, N.Y.: Scribner).—

    An authoritative and well-written biography of the founder, leader and systematizer of anthropology in the U.S.A. Boas himself worked in almost every branch of anthropology. One of his most famous books is "The mind of primitive man", published in 1911 and rewritten in 1932.

Bock, Hieronymus (1498-1554) — BOCK, H., 1964: Kreütterbuch darin underscheidt Namen vnd Würckung der Kreütter, Stauden/Hecken vnnd Beumen/sampt ihren Früchten/so inn Teutschen Landen wachsen ... Item von den vier Elementen/zamen vnd wilden Thieren ... Jetzund auffs new mit allem fleiss vbersehen ... durch den Hochgelehrten Melchiorem Sebizium. Gedruckt zu Strassburg durch Josiam Rihel 1577, 450 p. + 1285 woodcut illustrations (Munich: Köbl).—

Bock's chief claim to remembrance rests on his admirable descriptions of the plants included in his "Kreütterbuch", first published in 1539, written in the vernacular and without illustrations. He also gives much information as to the localities of the plants. In a later edition (1546) woodcuts were added; these woodcuts cannot compete with those in the herbals of Brunfels (1530) or Fuchs (1543), his descriptions, however, are much better. (For Brunfels and Fuchs, *vide infra*). The present book is a very beautiful reprint of the illustrated edition of 1577. A thorough study of Bock's "Kreütterbuch" is: HOPPE, B., 1969: Das Kräuterbuch des Hieronymous Bock. Wissenschaftshistorische Untersuchung mit einem Verzeichnis samtlicher Pflanzen des Werkes, der literarischen Quellen der Heilanzeigen und der Anwendungen der Pflanzen, 421 p. (Stuttgart: Hiersemann). With very valuable introduction (p. 1-89).

Bodenheimer, Fritz Shimon (1897-1959) — BODENHEIMER, F. S., 1959: A biologist in Israel: a book of reminiscences, 492 p. (Jerusalem: Biological Studies Publ.).—

This book is a kind of autobiography, completed shortly before the death of the author. Bodenheimer was one of the former presidents of the Academy for the History of Science, and was very active in the organization of the 1953 congress of this Academy which took place at Jerusalem. Besides his historical activities, Bodenheimer was engaged in many research projects, *e.g.*, in the fields of agricultural entomology, animal ecology, and the study of the fauna of Israel. A bibliography of his writings (419 items) has been added.

Boerhaave, Herman (1668-1738) — Memoralia Herman Boerhaave, 1939, 133 p. (Haarlem: Bohn).—

A collection of contributions delivered by an international group of medical historians in connection with commemorative celebrations held at Leiden and Harderwijk. On the occasion of the 250th anniversary of Boerhaave's birth, in 1918, a commemorative volume of the journal Janus has been published (Vol. 23: 193-369), containing a collection of essays concerning Boerhaave and his influence on the development of medicine and the natural sciences, and two essays concerning some portraits of Boerhaave.

——, LINDEBOOM, G. A., ed., 1962-1964: Boerhaave's correspondence, 2 parts. Part 1 (1962): 241 p.; part 2 (1964): 418 p. (Analecta Boerhaaviana, Vols. 3 and 5) (Leiden: Brill).—

The first part contains letters by and to some English correspondents, *viz.*, Cox Macro (18), Sherard (73), Hans Sloane (27), Mortimer (8), Richard Mead, (5), C. Alston (2), J. Arbuthnot (2), and some others from whom there is only one letter. The second vol. presents a variety of letters to or from correspondents in different countries of Europe. Of particular importance is the correspondence with the Italian physicians Morgagni and Micheli and with the Austrian courtphysician J. B. Bassand. All letters appear in the Latin original and in English translation. In his preface the editor notices that with these two volumes the epistolary sources for the knowledge of Boerhaave's person and life are by no means exhausted, as nearly all existing correspondence with his countrymen remains to be published.

—— ——, 1968: Herman Boerhaave: the man and his work, 452 p. (London: Methuen).—

The first part of this book (p. 1-246) contains a chronological account of Boerhaave's life, considering such subjects as: childhood, university studies, lector in medicine, professorship, illnesses, publishing activities, orations, *etc.* The second part deals with his personality, religious life, philosophical and theoretical medical views (considering, *e.g.*, his relationship to Spinoza, Descartes, Newton, his ideas on materialism, final causes, mind and body, pathology, *etc.*), his clinical teachings, activities as a family doctor and his attitudes toward his patients, activities as a botanist and as director of the botanical garden, his activities in the field of chemistry and his attitude toward alchemy, *etc.* There are three appendixes, a bibliography, beautiful illustrations, an index of persons, and a subject-index. The same author also published a bibliography of Boerhaaviana: LINDE-

BOOM, G. A., 1959: Bibliographia Boerhaaviana: list of publications written or provided by H. Boerhaave or based upon his works and teaching, 108 p. (Leiden: Brill). According to a review in Isis 53: 610 this bibliography is not fully reliable. *Cf.* also: BOERHAAVE, H., 1964: Atrocis, nec descripti prius, morbi historia, 1724. Facsimile of the first edition and of the first French translation, 11 + 60 + 47 p. (Introd. by G. A. LINDEBOOM) (Dutch classics on history of science, No. 9) (Nieuwkoop, The Netherlands: de Graaf). For a survey of the existing portraits of Boerhaave: LINDEBOOM, G. A., ed., 1963: Iconographia Boerhaavii, 9 + 31 p. + 40 plates (Analecta Boerhaaviana, Vol. 4) (Leiden: Brill).

——, SCHULTE, B. P. M., 1959: Hermanni Boerhaave praelectiones de morbis nervorum 1730-1735. Een medisch historische studie van Boerhaave's manuscript over zenuwziekten, 438 p. (Leiden: Brill).—

This book gives a historical introduction into the development of the knowledge of the central nervous system before Boerhaave and a review of the influence of Boerhaave's teachings on the further development of the pathology of the nervous system. The book has been written in the Dutch language. The larger part of the book (p. 47-363) is devoted to the complete text of the lectures of Boerhaave given between 1730 and 1735 on the pathology of the nervous system: the text is given in Latin as well as in Dutch translation. The book is supplemented by English and Russian summaries and a list of Boerhaaviana present in the library of the S. M. Kirov Academy, Leningrad.

Bonnet, Charles (1720-1793) — SAVIOZ, R., 1948: Mémoires autobiographiques de Charles Bonnet de Genève, 414 p. (Paris: Vrin).—

Charles Bonnet was a Swiss naturalist and philosophical writer. In his youth he made some astonishing discoveries. Thus, in 1740, he communicated to the Academy of Sciences in Paris a paper containing a series of experiments establishing what is now termed parthenogenesis in aphids. In 1741 he began to study reproduction by fusion and the regeneration of lost parts in the freshwater hydra and other animals and he discovered that the respiration of caterpillars and butterflies is performed by pores (stigmata). However, eye troubles began to handicap him and he became almost blind. As a consequence he devoted the later part of his life to philosophical meditations. The present autobiographical matters have here

been published for the first time. They were dictated by Bonnet between 1775 and 1791, and the story which they tell ends in 1782. For a short account of his life and work, *cf.:* ROSTAND, J., 1966: Un grand biologiste: Charles Bonnet, expérimentateur et théoricien, 39 p. (Paris: Univ. de Paris).

—— ——, 1948: La philosophie de Charles Bonnet de Genève, 393 p. (Paris: Vrin).—

Especially during the later part of his life, Bonnet devoted himself to philosophical meditations. He was deeply influenced by Descartes, Locke, Malebranche and above all by Leibniz. He was particularly engaged in the struggle between ovists and animalculists; and in the controversy between preformation and epigenesis, he adhered the epigenetic point of view. The present book has been divided into 6 parts: 1. Sources; 2. Natural philosophy; 3. Metaphysics; 4. Psychology; 5. Ethics, logic, paedagogics; 6. The influence of Bonnet's writings (in Germany, France, Italy, Switzerland, Denmark, Holland, and England). Bibliography and index.

Bonpland, Aimé Jacques Alexandre Goujaud (1773-1858) — BOUVIER, R. & E. MAYNIAL, 1950: Aimé Bonpland, explorateur de l'Amazonie, botaniste de la Malmaison, planteur en Argentine (1773-1858), 193 p. (Paris: Soc. d'Édition d'Enseignement supérieur).—

A biography of Aimé Bonpland, especially dealing with his travels in South America. Bonpland was the French traveller and botanist who accompanied A. von Humboldt during five years of travel in Mexico, Colombia, and the districts bordering on the Orinoco and Amazon. In these explorations he collected and classified about 6,000 plants, described in his "Plantes équinoxiales . . ." (Paris, 1808-1816). After his return to France he became superintendent of the gardens at Malmaison. Afterwards he left for Argentina and made travels in the central part of South America. Also in German translation: BOUVIER, E. & E. MAYNIAL, 1948: Der Botaniker von Malmaison, Aimé Bonpland, ein Freund Alexander von Humboldts, 287 p. (Neuwied: Lancelot). A study especially dealing with the last phase of his life (in Argentina, Paraguay - where he was imprisoned from 1820 to 1831 - and Brasilia, where he died in Santa Aña) are described in: SCHULZ, W., 1960: Aimé Bonpland. Alexander von Humboldts Begleiter auf der Amerikareise 1799-1804. Sein Leben und Werken, besonders nach 1817 in Argentinien, 53 p. (Akad. Wiss. Lit. Mainz, Abt. Math.-naturwiss. Klasse, Jg. 1960, No. 9) (Wiesbaden: Steiner).

Boring, Edwin Garrigues (1886—   ) —
BORING, E. G., 1961: Psychologist at large: an autobiography and selected essays, 371 p. (New York, N.Y.: Basic Bks.).—

The first 83 pages comprise an autobiography of the famous American psychological experimentalist, teacher, theorist, expositor, and editor, E. G. Boring. This part is followed by a series of selected essays most of them dealing with the psychology of history, the history of psychology, necrologies, and other subjects of biohistorical importance. There are also 35 pages of letters written by Boring.

Boveri, Theodor (1862-1915) — BALTZER, F., 1967: Theodor Boveri: the life and work of a great biologist 1862-1915, 165 p. (Berkeley, Calif.: Univ. California Press).—

The author was a student and colleague of Boveri. In this study Boveri's work is examined and placed in its historical setting, elucidating the ingenuity of his experimental technique, and making clear how Boveri discovered the cytological basis of Mendelian phenomena. In fact, Boveri combined those disciplines which now belong to the realm of cell-biology. The author especially makes clear the essential relationship between Boveri's artistic temperament and his scientific achievements. Included are a bibliography of Boveri's publications, a glossary and an index. Originally published in German in 1962: Theodor Boveri. Leben und Werk eines grossen Biologen, 1862-1915, 194 p. (Grosse Naturforscher, Vol. 25) (Stuttgart: Wiss. Verlagsges.).

Boyle, Robert (1627-1691) — FULTON, J. F., 1961: A bibliography of the honourable Robert Boyle, fellow of the Royal Society, ed. 2, 217 p. (Oxford: Clarendon Press).—

Boyle was one of the leading founders of the Royal Society, therefore this work has been published during the celebration of the tercentenary of that Society. Boyle's writings give a cross-section of science, philosophy and religious thought during the second half of the 17th century and are as such also of a great biohistorical interest. Fulton gives explanatory introductions to most of the works included, together with many biographical details, and many illustrations of title-pages of old prints. First ed. 1932 (London: Oxford U.P.).

——, HALL, M. B., 1965: Robert Boyle on natural philosophy: an essay with selections from his writings, 406 p. (Bloomington, Ind.: Indiana U.P.).—

This publication contains a lengthy introductory essay (of 113 pages) considering Boyle's life and work. The last 270 pages contain selections from his works, especially dealing with his views on chemistry, pneumatics, and philosophy, illustrating his position in relation to Aristotle, and the application of his philosophy to the physical and chemical properties of matter.

Braun, Alexander Heinrich (1805-1877) — METTENIUS, C., 1882: Alexander Braun's Leben nach seinem handschriftlichen Nachlass, 706 p. (Berlin: Reimer).—

A full-scale biography of the famous German plant-morphologist, well-known as a student of the phenomenon of phyllotaxis. As a morphologist he was a representative of the idealistic point of view. Braun took an active part in the development of botanical cell morphology and plant anatomy and he was an active student of cryptogamic botany. The present biography contains many letters from and to contemporary German botanists, and as such it is a contribution to 19th-century German idealistic plant morphology.

Brentano, Franz (1838-1917) — RANCURELLO, A. C., 1968: A study of Franz Brentano: his psychological standpoint and his significance in the history of psychology, 178 p. (New York, N.Y.: Academic Press).
—

Franz Brentano, an Italian by birth, spent the greater part of his life in Germany and Austria. He became one of the founders of modern psychology. Brentano was especially interested in the interrelations between psychology and philosophy, and whereas Husserl belonged to his most enthusiastic pupils, Brentano also had a share in the foundations of phenomenology.

Bright, Timothy (1550-1615) — KEYNES, G., 1962: Dr. Timothie Bright (1550-1615): a survey of his life with a bibliography of his writings, 47 p. (London: Wellcome Hist. Med. Library).—

Bright was one of the physicians of St. Bartholomew's Hospital; he published his famous book, "A treatise of melancholy", in 1586. Other important books were his "English Medicines" (1580) and his "Book of Martyrs" (1589). Apart from his medical interest and his theological studies, he was a pioneer of modern shorthand. The present publication contains the text of the 1961 Gideon de Laune lecture, given by the author. A complete bibliography of Bright's works with illustrations of many of their title-pages and an index have been added. In 1940 a reproduction appeared of the 1586 edition of "A treatise of melancholy", 285 p. (Facsimile Text Soc., No. 50) (New York, N.Y.: Columbia U.P.). With an introduction by H. CRAIGH, 22 p. For a more extensive biography, *cf.* CARLTON, W. J., 1911: Timothe Bright doctor of phisicke: a memoir of "The Father of modern shorthand", 205 p. (London: Stock).

Brown-Séquard, Charles Édouard (1817-1894) — OLMSTED, J. M. D., 1946: Charles Édouard Brown-Séquard: a nineteenth century neurologist and endocrinologist, 253 p. (Baltimore, Md.: Johns Hopkins Press).—

Brown-Séquard was a French physiologist and neurologist, but long periods of his life were spent in England and in America. He formulated a general theory of internal secretion, which in the main still holds good. Besides much biographical information, the present biographer gives a critical appraisal of Brown-Séquard's positive contributions to physiology and medicine; this belongs to the most interesting and useful parts of the biography.

Browne, Thomas (1605-1682) — FINCH, J. S., 1950: Sir Thomas Browne: a doctor's life of science and faith, 319 p. (New York, N.Y.: Schuman).—

Browne was a medical man and an amateur natural philosopher. This biography places him in the setting of 17th-century science and medicine. The book can best be characterized by the words used by G. K. Chalmers in Isis 42: 249: "The value of this able book lies in its grasp of Browne scholarship of the past three decades, its understanding of the scientific as well as bibliographical history of Browne's times, and its readability". *Cf.* also: DENONAIN, J. J., 1959: La personnalité de Sir Thomas Browne. Essai d'application de la caractérologie à la critique et l'histoire littéraires, 143 p. (Publ. Fac. Lettres et Sciences Humaines d'Alger, No. 33).

——, HUNTLEY, F. L., 1962: Sir Thomas Browne: a bibliographical and critical study, 283 p. (Ann Arbor, Mich.: Univ. Michigan Press).—

T. Browne was an English physician who wrote some books on religious and cultural matters. His most famous books are the "Religio medici" (1642), of which a new edition was prepared by G. KEYNES, 1939 *(vide infra),* and the "Pseudodoxia epidemica" in which Browne published a series of experiments. Both books give a very good picture of the man and the time in which he lived, and they are the main topics considered in this biography, which is supplemented by many particulars concerning his teachers, friends, books, political activities, *etc.* For more bibliographical details *cf.* KEYNES, 1924 *(vide infra).*

——, KEYNES, G., 1924: A bibliography of Sir Thomas Browne, 255 p. (Cambridge: U.P.).—

A bibliography of the works published by Browne, of collections and selections of his works, the sale catalogue of his library, list of libraries with copies recorded, list of printers, booksellers and publishers 1624-1923. A revised and augmented second ed. appeared in 1968, 293 p. (London: Oxford U.P.).

—— ——, ed., 1939: T. Browne: Religio medici, 113 p. (Eugene, Ore.: Univ. Oregon Press).—

The "Religio medici" was written in 1635 as an essay in self-revelation, and was for the first time (anonymously) printed in 1642. During the centuries that followed, many editions were called for, and many translations circulated on the European continent. According to the editor the present text should be as complete and as accurate as it can be made. The value of the work can best be illustrated by the fact that William Osler commended a close study of this book to all students of medicine and young doctors with the following words: "Mastery of self, conscientious devotion to duty, deep human interest in human beings. These are some of the lessons which may be gleaned from the life and writings of Sir Thomas Browne." (From the introduction, p. xiii). Another edition: WINNEY, J., ed., 1963: Religio medici, 34 + 153 p. (Cambridge: U.P.). *Cf.* also: MARTIN, L. C., ed., 1964: Religio medici and other works, 383 p. (Oxford: Clarendon Press). Contains: Religio medici; Hydriotaphia; The garden of Cyrus; A letter to a friend; Christian morals.

—— ——, ed., 1968: Sir Thomas Browne: selected writings, 416 p. (London: Faber & Faber).—

This single-volume selection includes familiar short works in full, with samples from lesser-known ones and specimens of Browne's miscellaneous writings and letters. It is drawn from Keynes' complete edition of Browne's works: KEYNES, G., ed., 1964: The works of Sir Thomas Browne, new ed., 4 vols. (London: Faber & Faber).

Brunfels, Otto (d. 1534) — BRUNFELS, O., 1964: Contrafayt Kreüterbuch 1532 nach vollkommen Art/vormals in deutscher Sprach nye gesehen, 580 p. + 510 woodcut-illustrations (Munich: Kölbl.).—

This herbal was first published in Latin under the title: "Herbarum vivae eicones" (1530) by Schott of Strasbourg. It initiated a new era in the history of botany, because its illustrations were true representations of the plants as they grew in nature, and not in the conventionalised way as they were reproduced before. Hans Weiditz was responsible for these beautiful woodcut-illustrations, which were incomparably better than the text. In 1532 appeared a German translation of this herbal (also published by Schott of Strasbourg); of this German translation the book under consideration is a re-issue. An authoritative study of Brunfels' herbal is: SPRAGUE, T. A., 1928: The herbal of Otto Brunfels, 45 p. (J. Linn. Soc. 48: 79-124).

Buffon, Georges Louis Leclerc, Comte de (1707-1788) — BERTIN, L., et al., 1953: Buffon, 244 p. (Collection des "Grands Naturalistes français") (Paris: Muséum d'Hist. Nat.).—

In the preface R. HEIM gives a very sound review of life and work of Buffon. The various scientific activities are described in a section written by F. BOURDIER; his economic activities in a section by L. BERTIN. Other sections deal with: Buffon and the Jardin du Roi (by Y. FRANÇOIS), his ideas about religious matters (by J. PIVETEAU), and with some of his (up to now unpublished) letters. Various portraits of Buffon, useful bibliography.

——, HANKS, L., 1966: Buffon avant l'"Histoire naturelle", 324 p. (Publ. Fac. des Lettres et Sciences humaines de Paris, Série "Recherches", Vol. XXIV) (Paris: Presses Univ. de France).—

A detailed study of Buffon's life and studies up to the time of his writing the "Histoire naturelle" (1739). The author gives a critical review of Buffon's activities in the fields of mathematics and forestry.

Special appendixes are devoted to some of his earlier works and translations. Valuable index of names.

——, ROGER, J., ed., 1962: Buffon, les "Époques de la nature". Édition critique avec le manuscrit, une introduction et des notes, 152 + 343 p. (Mém. Muséum d'Hist. Nat., N.S., Sér. C, Vol. X) (Paris: Muséum d'Hist. Nat.).—

This is a critical edition of Buffon's "Les époques de la nature", based on an incomplete ms. which included two drafts of several parts of "Les époques", thus elucidating the growth of Buffon's scientific thought. In a lucid introduction, Roger describes the evolution of Buffon's cosmology and his position in 18th-century thought. Many valuable notes, a bibliography, an index of proper names and a lexicon of scientific terms.

——, ROULE, L., 1924: Buffon et la description de la nature, 248 p. (Paris: Flammarion).—

Buffon was one of the greatest scientists of his age. His "Histoire naturelle...", published between 1749 and 1804 in 44 vols., was the first work to present the previous isolated and apparently disconnected facts of natural history in a popular and generally intelligible form. Moreover, he founded the "Muséum d'Histoire Naturelle", and became the intendant of the Garden of medicinal plants. Under his guidance, this garden underwent a great expansion and transformation and it became the "Jardin des Plantes". For a study of Buffon's activities in a broader historical setting, cf.: MORNET, D., 1911: Les sciences de la nature en France, au XVIIIe siècle. Un chapitre de l'histoire des idées, 291 p. (Paris: Colin).

Burbank, Luther (1849-1926) — HARWOOD, W. S., 1941: New creations in plant life: an authoritative account of the life and work of Luther Burbank, 430 p. (New York, N.Y.: Macmillan).—

A popular biography, first published in 1905. There also exists an autobiography, viz., An architect of nature: being the autobiography of Luther Burbank, 1939, 139 p. (With biographical sketch by W. HALL) (London: Watts). Other biographical information has been published by his sister E. BEESON, 1927: The early life and letters of Luther Burbank, 155 p. (San Francisco, Calif.: Wagner). Cf. also BURBANK, L. & W. HALL, 1926: The harvest of the years:

an autobiography, with a biographical sketch by W. HALL, 296 p. (Boston, Mass. & New York, N.Y.: Houghton Mifflin).

———, HOWARD, W. L., 1945: Luther Burbank: a victim of hero worship, 207 p. (Chronica Botanica IX, 5/6: 299-506).—

> During 50 years of working on the improvement of economic plants, Burbank sent out over 800 new varieties of fruits, flowers, and vegetables, many of them turning out to be of permanent value. In a thorough study the author tries to evaluate Burbank's scientific achievements in an objective way. He also gives much information concerning his scientific background, his character, the admiration and detraction he gave rise to, *etc.*, and he gives a summing-up of Burbank's products. The same author also wrote a short account of Burbank's life and works, including a listing of the varieties of plants he is reputed to have created, *viz.,* HOWARD, W. L., 1945: Luther Burbank's plant contributions, 110 p. (Univ. Calif. Agric. Experim. Stat. Bull., No. 691) (Berkeley, Calif.: Univ. California Press).

Butler, Samuel (1835-1902) — STILLMAN, C. G., 1932: Samuel Butler: a mid-Victorian modern, 319 p. (New York, N.Y.: Viking Press).—

> Samuel Butler was an English author, who made some contributions to the theory of evolution; he especially tried to give a theory explaining the origin of variations. His theory, however, had strong vitalistic components, for according to this theory variations should be directed by unconscious memory. The Butler-Darwin controversy is here elucidated. This last problem also has been tackled by RATTRAY, R. F., 1935: Samuel Butler: a chronicle and an introduction, 216 p. (London: Duckworth). This study especially elucidates Butler's views on evolution; it has been based upon some of his books, scientific and popular publications, and upon his correspondence. For more biographical details, *cf.* KEYNES, G. & B. HILL, eds., n.d., Samuel Butler's notebooks: selections, 327 p. (New York, N.Y.: Dutton).

Caius, John (1510-1573) — MALLOCH, A., ed., 1937: A book or counseill against the disease called the sweate (1522): introduction and facsimile reprint, 19 + 39 p. (New York, N.Y.: Scholar's Facsimiles & Reprints).—

> John Caius studied under Vesalius at Padua. After having taken his degree in

physic he returned to England, where he became physician to Queen Mary. He stimulated human dissection in England and was an important pioneer in advancing the science of anatomy. The text is preceded by an introduction of 19 pages, written by A. MALLOCH. The epidemic variously called sweating sickness, sudor anglicus, English or Picardy sweat, cannot be determined by any certainty, but epidemics of this disease occurred in 1485, 1508, 1517, 1529 (on the Continent) and 1551 (these details from Isis 34: 429). *Cf.* ROBERTS, E. S., ed., 1912: The works of John Caius, M. D., second founder of Gonville and Caius College and Master of the College, 1559-1573, 9 pts. (With A. FLEMING's translation of "De canibus britannicis") (Cambridge: U.P.).

Calmette, Léon Charles Albert (1863-1933) — BERNARD, N. & L. NÈGRE, 1939: Albert Calmette. Sa vie. Son oeuvre scientifique, 271 p. (Paris: Masson).—

> The first part of this book (p. 5-118) contains a full biography of Calmette. The second part has been devoted to his scientific activities, considering such aspects as: his research in antivenomous serotherapy, his researches in the domain of hygiene, his struggle against miner's anaemia and tuberculosis, his discoveries, researches, *etc.,* concerning vaccination against tuberculosis by means of B.C.G. The last chapter deals with the developments of antituberculosus vaccination by means of B.C.G. after the death of Calmette. Bibliography of publications of Calmette. In 1961 BERNARD, N., published another book on Calmette, *viz.,* La vie et l'oeuvre d'Albert Calmette (1863-1933), 313 p. (Paris: Michel). *Cf.* also: KERVAN, R., 1962: Albert Calmette et le B.C.G., 222 p. (Paris: Hachette). These last-mentioned books I was unable to consult, nor could I find any supplementary information.

Camper, Peter (1722-1789) — NUYENS, B. W. T., ed., 1939: Petri Camperi itinera in Angliam, 1748-1785, 59 + 264 p. (Opuscula selecta neerlandicorum de arte medica, Vol. 15) (Amsterdam: Ned. Tijdschr. Geneesk.).—

> A publication of Camper's diaries, as far as they are related to his experiences on three journeys he undertook to England. "When in 1748 as a young doctor, in 1752 as a youthful professor at Franeker's university he went to England, he did this to improve his skill in the medical science, preferable in midwifery. When, 37 years later, in 1785 he revisited England, he went

as a scientific man of mature experience, to communicate to his English collaegues his self-assured ideas of obstetrics, the fruits of regular investigations and a long practice." The three diaries are edited in their original language, Dutch or Latin, and translated into English. P. 221-264 contain biographical notes concerning the men mentioned in the text. An interesting publication concerning Camper's activities in the field of surgery is: DOETS, C. J., 1948: De heelkunde van Petrus Camper, 300 p. (Diss. Univ. Leiden) (Leiden: Ydo). In Dutch. *Cf.* also: DOESSCHATE, G. TEN, ed., 1962: Petrus Camper: optical dissertation on vision, 1746. Facsimile of the original Latin text with a complete translation and an introduction, 29 + 25 + 31 p. (Dutch classics on history of science, Vol. 3) (Nieuwkoop, The Netherlands: de Graaf).

Candolle, Augustin Pyramus de (1778-1841) — CANDOLLE, A. P. de, 1862: Mémoires et souvenirs d'Augustin-Pyramus de Candolle écrits par lui même et publiés par son fils, 599 p. (Geneva & Paris: Cherbuliez).—

De Candolle was a Swiss botanist. He planned to publish his "Regni vegetabilis systema naturale", a "natural" system of botanic classification, of which he completed only 2 vols. In 1824 he started to publish his "Prodromus systematis naturalis regni vegetabilis", of which he finished only seven vols. (Anastatic reprint, ed. by BUEK, H. W., 1967, 1570 p., New York, N.Y.: Stechert-Hafner). The table of contents consists of the following parts: I. De ma naissance jusqu'à mon établissement à Paris (1778 à 1798). Enfance et adolescence; II. Jeunesse. Séjour à Paris (1798 à 1808); III. Âge viril. Séjour à Montpellier (1808 à 1816); IV. Âge mûr. Séjour à Genève depuis mon arrivée jusqu'à ma démission de fonction de professeur (1816 à 1834); V. Vieillesse. Genève (1835 à 1841). Pièces justificatives et notes additionnelles.

Cardano, Girolamo (1501-1576) — ECKMAN, J., 1946: Jerome Cardan, 120 p. (Suppl. Bull. Hist. Med., No. 7) (Baltimore, Md.: Johns Hopkins Press).—

A biography of this famous physician and mathematician. His interests in botany and anatomy are also the subject of brief memoirs.

——, STONER, J., ed., 1962: The book of my life (De vita propria liber), 331 p. (New York, N.Y.: Dover).—

Jerome Cardan wrote this autobiography in 1575. The present book is a reprint of the first English translation, published in 1930 (New York, N.Y.: Dutton). It is remarkable that for the first time in history an autobiography came about based on introspective psychological self-analysis. The substance of the book consists only of noteworthy experiences, not of tumultuous events, and was written by a scientist who was deeply interested in the psycho-physical interrelation of his own life. As such this work stands at the beginning of the modern era, and has had much influence on later autobiographies.

Cárdenas, Juan de (1563-1609) — DEUCHLER, W., 1930: Juan de Cárdenas. Ein Beitrag zur Geschichte der spanischen Naturbetrachtung und Medizin in Mexiko während des 16. Jahrhunderts, 127 p. (Bern & Leipzig: Haupt).—

This publication mainly deals with a book entitled: "Problemas y secretos maravillosos de las Indias", written by Cárdenas in 1591 and reprinted in 1913 in Mexico. It deals with the many intellectual conflicts of this 16th-century scientist, educated in scholasticism who had to face the many new circumstances and problems of the New World; altogether, problems which had never been encountered by the old Greek philosophers. The whole book can be considered as one attempt to reconcile his new experiences with the Aristotelian point of view. The author has added a chapter dealing with Spanish medicine in the 16th century.

Carus, Carl Gustav (1789-1869) — ARNIM, S. VON, 1930: Carl Gustav Carus. Sein Leben und Wirken, 115 p. (Dresden: Zahn & Jaensch).—

Carus was a German physiologist and psychologist, who had studied medicine in Leipzig. He was a representative of German "Naturphilosophie". Another biography of Carus: KERN, H., 1942: Carl Gustav Carus: Persönlichkeit und Werk, 204 p. (Berlin: Windukind). For a bibliography of his publications: KEIPER, W., 1934: Ein gesamtverzeichnis der Werke von Carl Gustav Carus, 16 p. (Sonder-Katalog, No. 50) (Berlin: Keiper). *Cf.* also: ZAUNICK, R., 1930: Carl Gustav Carus. Eine historisch-kritische Literaturschau mit zwei Bibliographiën, 39 p. (Dresden: Author); and ZAUNICK, R., ed., 1931: C. G. Carus. Lebenserinnerungen und Denkwürdigkeiten, vol. 5, 221 p. (Dresden: Jess). The first four vols. of his "Lebenserinnerungen" were already published in 1865 (Vols. 1 and 2, 325 + 423 p.) and 1866 (vols. 3 and 4, 511 p.) (Leipzig: Brockhaus).

——, KLEINE-NATROP, H. E., ed., 1969: C. G. Carus in mortis centenarium. Denkschrift und Ausstellungskatalog zum 100. Todestag von Carl Gustav Carus, 48 p. + 40 photographs (Schriftenreihe der Medizinischen Akademie Dresden, Vol. 8) (Dresden: Carus-Akademie).—

This commemorative volume contains a chronology of the life and works of Carus, an essay dealing with Carus as a scientist and man of arts, an essay treating of his artistic development, and a bibliography. This text is followed by short descriptions of 79 paintings produced by Carus and exhibited on the occasion of the centenary of his death; reproductions of 40 of those paintings have been included. For a short, recently published biography of Carus, cf. KLOPPE, W., 1969: Erinnerungen an Carl Gustav Carus, 1789-1869, 38 p. (Berlin: Medicus).

Carver, George Washington (1864-1943) — HOLT, R., 1943: George Washington Carver: an American biography, 342 p. (New York, N.Y.: Doubleday).—

A biography of the American Negro botanist, born of slave parents, and teacher of the backward Negro farmer in using better and more scientific methods of agriculture. He became head of the Agricultural and Dairy Department of Tuskegee, a Negro institute in Alabama, where he remained the rest of his life. In 1935 he was appointed collaborator of the U.S. Dept. of Agriculture, Bureau of Plant Industry, division of mycology and disease survey. Another recent popular biography is: ELLIOT, L., 1966: George Washington Carver: the man who overcame, 256 p. (Englewood Cliffs, N. J.: Prentice Hall).

Cesalpino, Andrea (1524-1603) — DOROLLE, M., ed., 1929: Questions péripatéticiennes, 242 p. (Paris: Alcan).—

Cesalpino was a rigid Aristotelian as becomes clear from the passages translated in this book, which contains fragments in French translation from the 1593 edition of the "Questionum peripateticarum libri quinque" (originally published in 1571). Most of these fragments deal with theoretical aspects of biology. Cesalpino was professor of medicine at Pisa and is by some historians regarded as a discoverer of the circulation of the blood before Harvey. As to this aspect, cf. ARCIERI, J. P., 1945: The circulation of the blood and Andrea Cesalpino of Arezzo, 193 p. (New York, N.Y.: Vanno). This book, however, is strongly biassed! (Cf. review by Singer in Bull. Hist. Med. 19: 122). Moreover, Cesalpino taught botany at Pisa, and was in charge of the botanical garden founded there in 1543. He collected plants from all over Europe and classified them according to their fruits. In 1583 he published his treatise "De plantis libri XVI", of which in 1967 a reprint appeared, 672 p. (Farnborough, Hants.: Gregg).

Chambers, Robert (1802-1871) — MILLHAUSER, M., 1959: Just before Darwin: Robert Chambers and Vestiges, 246 p. (Middletown, Conn.: Wesleyan U.P.).—

This book is valuable as a reflection of the intellectual climate of early Victorian England. The main value of the book lies in chapters V and VI, which describe the public reception of the Vestiges (first published anonymously, 1844); its influence on literary circles has also been discussed. It is shown how the Vestiges helped to prepare public opinion for a more tolerant reception of Darwin's theory. Chapter IV gives a summary review of the contents of the Vestiges but no comparison has been made either with Lamarck's or with Darwin's work. The first chapters contain some introductory historical information; however, they are not very complete. Chambers's book was reprinted recently: CHAMBERS, R., 1969: Vestiges of the natural history of creation, 38 + 390 p. (Leicester: U.P.). With an introduction by G. DE BEER.

Chamisso, Adelbert von (1781-1838) — SCHMID, G., 1942: Chamisso als Naturforscher. Eine Bibliographie, 176 p. (Leipzig: Koehler).—

Chamisso was a German poet and botanist, whose most famous work has been his prose narrative "Peter Schlemihl". In 1815 Chamisso was appointed botanist to the Russian ship "Rurik" (under the command of Otto von Kotzebue) on a scientific voyage round the world. On his return he was made keeper of the botanical gardens in Berlin. The book under consideration contains a complete bibliography of all publications written by Chamisso (whether or not jointly with other authors) and of publications dealing with Chamisso as a scientist. This publication contains much biographical information and a listing of plants and animals named after Chamisso (some 48) and a listing of names of Chamisso's contemporaries mentioned in the text (with short biographical information). A bibliography of his "Peter Schlemihl" can be found in: RATH, P., 1919: Bibliotheca schlemihliana. Ein Verzeichnis der Ausgaben und Uebersetzungen des Peter Schlemihl, nebst neun unveröffentlichten Briefen Chamissos, 96 p. (Berlin: Breslauer). A narrative of his voyage with the "Rurik" is: MAHR, A. C., 1932: The visit of the "Rurik" to San Francisco in 1816, 194 p. (Stanford Univ. Publ., Hist., Economics and Political Science, Vol. II, No. 2) (Stanford, Calif.: Stanford U.P.).

Charcot, Jean Martin (1825-1893) — GUILLAIN, G., 1955: J. M. Charcot (1825-1893). Sa vie, son oeuvre, 188 p. (Paris: Masson).—

Charcot was the founder of modern clinical neurology. Besides the extensive biographical information concerning his character, his habits of work, his routine in daily living, *etc.*, the book contains much information concerning his scientific achievements and his contacts with other famous scientists such as: Freud, Janet, Babinski, and others. In 1962 a reissue appeared of Charcot's "Lectures on the diseases of the nervous system", second series, 399 p. (Hist. of Med. Series, No. 19) (New York, N.Y.: Hafner), a facsimile of the 1881 edition.

Cheselden, William (1688-1752) — COPE, Z., 1953: William Cheselden, 1688-1752, 112 p. (Edinburgh: Livingstone).—

An evaluation of Cheselden's work as anatomist, lithotomist, ophthalmological and general surgeon, teacher, writer, architect, and hospital administrator. It also contains much fresh biographical information.

Clayton, John (1694-1773/'74) — BERKELEY, E. & D. S., 1963: John Clayton: pioneer of American botany, 236 p. (Chapel Hill, N.C.: Univ. North Carolina Press).—

Clayton was one of the most important botanists of the 18th century; he was in correspondence with such famous naturalists as C. Linnaeus, M. Catesby, J. Bartram, P. Kalm, H. Boerhaave, and J. F. Gronovius. He ought to be honoured for his invaluable "Flora Virginia", compiled by J. F. Gronovius, from plants and descriptions supplied by Clayton. His scientific publications have been edited by: BERKELEY, E. & D. S., 1965: The reverend John Clayton: a person with a scientific mind. His scientific writings and other related papers, 244 p.

(Charlottesville, Va.: Univ. Virginia Press). Accompanied by a biographical sketch, a bibliography and an index.

Clusius, Carolus (= Charles de l'Escluse) (1526-1609) — HUNGER, F. W. T., 1927-1942: Charles de l'Escluse (Carolus Clusius). Nederlandsch kruidkundige, 1526-1609, 2 vols. Vol. I (1927): 445 p.; Vol. II (1942): 466 p. (The Hague: Nijhoff).—

Vol. I contains a complete chronologically-arranged biography of one of the most famous botanists of the 16th century. Clusius travelled much in Germany, France, Spain, Portugal, Austria, and England, and he spent the end of his life in Leiden where he became horti praefectus in 1592. He was one of the pioneers in describing plants and local floras; moreover, he edited or translated the works of others. In this vol. are beautiful illustrations (portraits, hand-writting, title-pages, *etc.*), and an index of names. Vol. II contains the text of 195 letters written by Clusius to Joachim Camerarius, belonging to the Trew Collection, library of the Univ. of Erlangen. The text of chapters 2 up to and including 7 (p. 29-206) have been written in German. Indexes of names of persons and of geographical names. Together these two vols. contain much information concerning the history of 16th-century botany. A popular biography of Clusius, largely derived form this standard work, is: THEUNISZ, J., 1939: Carolus Clusius. Het merkwaardige leven van een pionier der wetenschap, 178 p. (Amsterdam: van Kampen). Included is a listing of the works written, edited, or translated by Clusius. For a short biographical review in French, *vide:* MORREN, E., 1875: Charles de l'Escluse, sa vie et ses oeuvres, 1526-1609, 59 p. (Liège: Boverie). (Also in: Bull. Fédération des Soc. d'Horticulture de Belgique, 1875).

——, JONG, M. DE & D. A. WITTOP KONING, eds., 1963: Aromatum, et simplicium aliquot medicamentorum apud Indos nascentium historia (Antwerpiae, ex off. Ch. Plantini, 1567), 64 + 262 p. (Dutch classics of natural science, No. 6) (Nieuwkoop, The Netherlands: de Graaf).—

The main part of this publication consists of a Latin translation (with certain adaptations) of Garcia da Orta's Portuguese account in dialogue form of medicinal plants of India. It was originally published in 1567 by Plantijn at Antwerp. The introduction describes how the economic expansion initiated by the Portuguese opened new fields of natural science and a new approach to matters of medicine; it illustrates the role of the humanists in distributing this knowledge. Moreover, the introduction contains much biographical and bibliographical information concerning Garcia da Orta as well as Clusius, together with translations of relevant documents and extracts from da Orta's original work.

Coiter, Volcher (1534-1576) — HERRLINGER, R., 1952: Volcher Coiter, 1534-1576, 147 p. (Nuremberg: Edelmann).—

A detailed bio-bibliography illuminating the man, his life and works, the circles in which he moved, his place as physician, anatomist, zoologist, and embryologist. It includes much original information. Fine illustrations, and good index.

——, NUYENS, B. W. T. & A. SCHIERBEEK, eds., 1955: (1) Tables of the principal external and internal parts of the human body (1572); (2) Lectures by Gabriel Fallopius on the corresponding parts of the human body, collected with the utmost accuracy from various manuscripts by Volcher Coiter (1575), 79 + 263 p. (Opuscula selecta neerlandicorum de arte medica, Vol. XVIII) (Haarlem: Bohn).—

Volcher Coiter, although not well-known, was one of the most eminent post-Vesalian anatomists, and (according to Cole) was the first to elevate the study of comparative anatomy to the rank of an independent branch of biology. The text mainly consists of a selection of treatises taken from his "Externarum et internarum principalium humani corporis partium tabulae" (Nürnberg, 1572) and his "Lectiones Gabrielis Faloppii de partibus similaribus humani corporis" (Nürnberg, 1575). There are three introductory essays: one containing a detailed biography, one an attempt to evaluate Coiter as a physician, one an evaluation of Coiter as a comparative anatomist, physiologist, and embryologist. In an appendix some newly-discovered documents concerning the life and works of Coiter have been included.

Cook, James (1728-1779) — CARRINGTON, H., 1939: Life of Captain Cook, 324 p. (London: Sidgwick & Jackson).—

An authoritative biography based on much original source-material and on a thorough study of the circumstances in which Cook's voyages must have taken place, e.g., the state of knowledge about the Pacific Ocean, and the essential characteristics of the Polynesian races which inhabited the islands of that ocean. The reaction of the natives to the arrival of the white men is described with regard to their social and religious conceptions, and not from the point of view of the whites as so often has been done. A book of the same rank of excellence - though somewhat older - is: KITSON, A., 1907: Captain James Cook "the circumnavigator", 525 p. (London: Murray).

——, HOLMES, M., 1952: Captain James Cook: a bibliographical excursion, 103 p. (London: Edwards).—

The book begins with brief biographical notes on the more notable people who sailed with Cook. The bibliographical part has been divided into two sections. The first deals with titles, collations, notes, etc., of the first editions of the most important books and pamphlets, and they are, for the most part, the work of Cook's contemporaries. The second section contains a highly selective list of less important or of more modern books and pamphlets with brief notes on their subject-matter. Excluded are all reprints, later editions, collected editions, abridgements of original editions, foreign translations, and contemporary Continental literature other than accounts of the voyages. Where such publications were translated into English, the first edition has been described. Cf. WHITEHEAD, P. J. P., 1968: Forty drawings made by artists who accompanied Captain Cook on his three voyages to the Pacific, 1768-'71; 1772-'75; 1776-'80, some being used by authors in the description of new species, 31 p. + 36 plates. (London: Brit. Museum Natl. Hist.).

——, MERRILL, E. D., 1954: The botany of Cook's voyages, and its unexpected significance in relation to anthropology, biogeography and history, 219 p. (Chronica Botanica, Vol. 14, 5/6) (Waltham, Mass.: Chronica Botanica).—

The author pays particular attention to the introduction of cultivated plants and weeds, mainly of the material collected by Banks and Solander on Cook's first voyage and by the two Forsters on the second voyage. Indexes of plant names and of authors. Cf. also titles relating to BANKS, Joseph, vide supra.

Cooper, Astley Paston (1768-1841) — BROCK, R. C., 1952: The life and work of

Astley Cooper, 176 p. (Edinburgh & London: Livingstone).—

> One of the most famous surgeons the world has ever known. This book is especially valuable as an account of Cooper's work. Stress has been laid on Cooper's research and practice in relation to hernia, arterial surgery, and orthopaedics. Useful bibliography and index. *Cf.* also: KEYNES, G. L., 1922: The life and works of Sir Astley Cooper, 27 p. (St. Bartholomew's Hospital Reports, Vol. 55: 9-36) (London: Murray).

Cope, Edward Drinker (1840-1897) — OSBORN, H. F., 1931: Cope: master naturalist. The life and letters of Edward Drinker Cope, with a bibliography of his writings classified by subject. A study of the pioneer and foundation periods of vertebrate palaeontology in America, 740 p. (Princeton, N.J.: Princeton U.P.).—

> Cope was an American palaeontologist who made very interesting contributions to the theory of evolution of the vertebrates. Much information has been based upon Cope's extensive correspondence. Special attention has been paid to Cope's part in the study of the evolution of the rhinoceroses, horses, mastodons, camels, and carnivores of the Upper Miocene, to his activities as a herpetologist of world fame, and to his ichthyological studies. As an evolutionist, Cope was a confirmed Lamarckian. Included is a classified bibliography of Cope's principal papers (p. 595-740).

Cordes, Valerius (1515-1544) — SPRAGUE, T. A., 1939: The herbal of Valerius Cordes, 113 p. (J. Linn. Soc. 52 : 1-113).—

> Valerius Cordus was a German botanist. His "Historia stirpium" (1561) is especially distinguished by the excellence of its descriptions which belong to the best of 16th-century botany. The present study deals with scope and characteristics of this herbal, previous identifications of the plants described and figured, the systematic conspectus of plants described and figured and enumeration of them and an index of their accepted scientific names. Included is a short biography of Valerius Cordes.

Corvisart-Desmarets, Jean Nicolas (1755-1821) — GATES, J., ed., 1962: An essay on the organic diseases and lesions of the heart and great vessels, 358 p. (History of Medicine Series, No. 16) (New York, N.Y.: Hafner).—

> Corvisart was one of the great clinicians of the Paris school of the early 19th century and personal physician of Napoleon. In this book he attempted to classify diseases of the heart according to their underlying physical or physiological abnormalities. Included are a series of case histories and *post mortem* comparisons. From these findings Corvisart tried to give some general principles of diagnosis, treatment and prognosis of heart diseases. The book was originally published in 1806: "Essai sur les maladies du coeur et des gros vaisseaux" (Paris). In 1812 an English translation was prepared by J. GATES, of which this book is a reprint.

Coulter, John Merle (1851-1928) — RODGERS, A. D., 1944: John Merle Coulter: missionary in science, 321 p. (Princeton, N.J.: Princeton U.P.).—

> Interestingly-written biography of J. M. Coulter, scientist and administrator, who contributed greatly to the advancement of botany in America. Coulter was for a time professor of botany and president of the Univ. of Indiana, and president of Lake Forest College. In 1896 he went to Chicago where he became professor and chairman of the dept. of botany (till 1925), and after his retirement he became chief adviser of the Thompson Foundation, which established the Boyce Thompson Institute for Plant Research. He is well known as founder (1875) and editor of the "Botanical Gazette".

Curtis, William (1746-1799) — CURTIS, W. H., 1941: William Curtis, 1746-1799, fellow of the Linnean Society: botanist and entomologist. With some notes on his son-in-law Samuel Curtis, 142 p. (Winchester, Hants.: Warren).—

> William Curtis translated Linnaeus' "Fundamenta Entomologiae" (1772), published the "Flora Londinensis" (1777) in six fasciculi and in 1781 he founded the "Botanical Magazine". He organised three botanical gardens near London (Bermondsey, Lambeth Marsh, Brompton). As editor and proprietor of the "Botanical Magazine" he was succeeded by his son-in-law, Samuel Curtis (1779-1860). This book gives a complete biography together with a list of W. Curtis' publications.

Cushing, Harvey William (1869-1939) — CUSHING, H., 1939: A bibliography of the writings of Harvey Cushing. Prepared on the occasion of his seventieth birthday, April 8, 1939, by the Harvey Cushing Society, 108 p. (Springfield, Ill.: Thomas).—

The first section (p. 3-10) deals with life, degrees and honours of Harvey Cushing; the second section (p. 11-20) with book and monographs; the third (p. 21-60) with addresses, papers in journals and reports; and the fourth (p. 61-92) with papers from Cushing's clinics and laboratories. An appendix deals with such subjects as: Cushing's assistants, the Harvey Cushing Society. Subject-index. A short-title catalogue of Harvey Cushing's own collection of books and mss., bequeathed to the Medical School of Yale University: The Harvey Cushing collection of books and manuscripts, 207 p. (Yale Med. Library, Hist. library, Publ. No. 1) (New York, N.Y.: Schuman). A useful companion to the "Bibliotheca Osleriana", *vide* OSLER, section Bibliographies, subsection e. *Cf.* also: MATSON, D. D., W. J. GERMAN, *et al.*, eds., 1969: Harvey Cushing: selected papers on neurosurgery, 704 p. (New Haven, Conn.: Yale U.P.).

——, FULTON, J. F., 1946: Harvey Cushing: a biography, 754 p. (Springfield, Ill.: Thomas).—

A well-written and very valuable biography of one of the foremost surgeons of the world, prepared by a famous physician and physiologist. Many illustrations.

——, THOMSON, E. H., 1950: Harvey Cushing, surgeon, author, artist, 347 p. (New York, N.Y.: Schuman).—

A welcome supplement to FULTON's biography *(vide supra)*, giving many particulars of his private life, the influence of his wife on his career, *etc*. The author was able to use much new material (if compared with Fulton) including scrapbooks, notebooks, diaries, annual reports of hospitals, and correspondence files.

Cuvier, Georges Léopold Chrétien Frédéric Dagobert, Baron (1769-1832) — COLEMAN, W., 1964: Georges Cuvier zoologist: a study in the history of evolution theory, 212 p. (Cambridge, Mass.: Harvard U.P.).—

In this well-written book, the author tries to elucidate the philosophical background of Cuvier as it can be deduced from his scientific writings. He illustrates the essential role of the concepts of the conditions of existence, the correlation of the parts and the subordination of the parts, and he makes clear that this did not prevent him from composing a rather pragmatic system, and actually led him to a static conception of nature, in which no room was left either for the idea of the transformation of the species or for the idea of the chain of beings. The author devotes special attention to the role which religion and Aristotelian philosophy have played in the shaping of the above-mentioned concepts.

——, ROULE, L., 1933: Cuvier et la science de la nature, 246 p. (Collection des "Grands naturalistes français", No. III) (Paris: Flammarion).—

A biography, consisting of three parts, considering life, writings, and basic ideas of this great French naturalist and anatomist. Special attention has been paid to Cuvier's organizing activities as Director of the "Musée d'Histoire naturelle". *Cf.* also DEHÉRAN, H., 1908: Catalogue des manuscrits du fonds Cuvier. Travaux et correspondence scientifiques, conservés à la bibliothèque de l'Institut de France, 154 p. (Paris: Champion). Also published in Revue des Bibliothèques, 1907-1908. Some of Cuvier's most famous and fundamental works are recently reprinted, *viz.*, CUVIER, G. L. C. F. D. & F. VALENCIENNES, 1965: Histoire naturelle des poissons, 25 vols. (Amsterdam: Asher). (Originally published in Paris and Strasbourg, between 1828 and 1849); CUVIER, G., 1966: Histoire des sciences naturelles, depuis leur origine jusqu'à nos jours, 5 vols., 2160 p. (Farnborough, Hants.: Gregg); and CUVIER, C., 1970: Rapport historique sur les progrès des sciences naturelles depuis 1789, et sur leur état actuel, (XVI, 394 p.) (Amsterdam: Israel).

Darwin, Charles (1809-1882) — ANONYMOUS, 1960: Handlist of Darwin papers at the University of Cambridge, 72 p. (Cambridge: U.P.).—

A guide to the personal papers of Charles Darwin in the Cambridge University Library. It includes notebooks and diaries kept by Darwin during the voyage of the Beagle, the original mss. of his books, and many letters written to him.

——, BARLOW, N., ed., 1933: Charles Darwin's diary of the voyage of H.M.S. "Beagle", 451 p. (Cambridge: U.P.; New York, N.Y.: Macmillan).—

There exist 18 pocket-books in which Darwin made the first rough pencil notes of his observations and impressions during his five years of travel; these form the text of the present book. From this ms. *ca.* one-third was omitted in the different versions of the "Journal of research" and the 1st and 2nd eds. of the "Voyage". This publication is a welcome addition to both these books.

—— ——, ed., 1945/'46: Charles Darwin and the voyage of the Beagle, 279 p. (London: Pilot Press; New York, N.Y.: Philosophical Library).—

A series of 36 letters written by Darwin to his family during his voyage with the "Beagle". They are "the most intimate record we can have of the emotional and intellectual reactions ... during ... a voyage which (Darwin) himself termed 'by far the most important event of my life'".

—— ——, ed., 1958: The autobiography of Charles Darwin, 1809-1882, with original omissions restored, edited with appendix and notes by his granddaughter, 253 p. (London: Collins).—

This version of Darwin's autobiography, edited by his granddaughter (Lady Nora Barlow), is an accurate transcription from the original manuscript, in which the omissions from the original edition of his autobiography published in 1887 are restored. Lady Nora Barlow has added a great deal of unpublished material in her notes and appendix. A re-publication, without alteration or abridgement of "Charles Darwin, his life told in an autobiographical chapter and in a selected series of his published letters" is: DARWIN, F., ed., 1958: The autobiography of Charles Darwin and selected letters, 365 p. (New York, N.Y.: Dover).

——, BARNETT, S. A., ed., 1958: A century of Darwin, 376 p. (London: Heinemann; Cambridge, Mass.: Harvard U.P.).—

Fifteen authors give up-to-date reviews of Darwin's influence on various biological and other scientific outlooks. The chapters are as follows: 1. Theories of evolution; 2. Species after Darwin; 3. The third stage in genetics; 4. Darwin and animal breeding; 5. Darwin and classification; 6. Darwin and the fossil record; 7. Darwin and embryology; 8. The study of man's descent; 9. The "Expression of the emotions"; 10. Sexual selection; 11. Darwin and the coral reefs; 12. Darwin as a botanist; 13. Darwinism and the social sciences; 14. Natural selection and biological progress; 15. Darwinism and ethics.

——, BATES, M. & P. S. HUMPHREY, eds., 1965: The Darwin reader, 470 p. (New York, N.Y.: Scribner).—

An anthology, containing selections from the Autobiography, The voyage of the Beagle, The origin of species (including the preliminary statement by Darwin and Wallace of 1858), The descent of Man, The expression of the emotions and some short selections grouped together under the title "Plants and Worms". Editorial comments have been limited to the absolute minimum. Good bibliography and good index. Another series of selections from the works of Darwin has been published by: LOEWENBERG, B. J., ed., 1959: Charles Darwin: evolution and natural selection: an anthology of the writings of Charles Darwin, 438 p. (Boston, Mass.: Bacon). *Cf.* also WYSS, W. von, 1965, and HYMAN, S. E., 1963, *vide infra*.

——, BELL, P. R., *et al.*, 1959: Darwin's biological work: some aspects reconsidered, 343 p. (Cambridge: U.P.).—

This book consists of 6 essays written by different authors. WILKIE relates Darwin's work to earlier work by Buffon and Lamarck; CHALLINOR considers one of the problems of the 'Origin', *viz.*, the discrepancy between some fossil evidence and Darwin's theory; the other essays start from one of Darwin's discoveries, and give a review of later work done in the same fields. Thus HALDANE discusses the validity of the theory of evolution by means of natural selection in the light of subsequent research; BELL is concerned with the movements of plants in response to light; MARLER with communication between animals; WHITE-HOUSE with cross- and self-fertilization in plants.

——, CLARK, R. E. D., 1958: Darwin: before and after. An examination and assessment, 192 p. (London: Paternoster).—

A well-written historical outline of evolutionary theories concerning the origin of Man, from Anaximander to the present day; in this setting the author makes clear the significance of Charles Darwin. The ethical relevance of Darwin's work and its effect on social and political life is also reviewed, and much stress has been laid on the religious consequences of the Darwinian theory. In 1948 this book was published under the title: Darwin: before and after. The story of evolution, 192 p. (London: Paternoster).

——, DARWIN, C., 1964: On the origin of species: a facsimile of the first edition, 502 p. (with introduction by E. MAYR) (Cambridge, Mass.: Harvard U.P.).—

It is a great advantage that the first edition (in unaltered pagination) is available again. Most recent reprints are based on the sixth edition of 1872, which was greatly modified as compared with the first edition. These modifications are clearly elucidated by E. MAYR in his introduction to this reissue. A handsome reissue of the 6th ed. is: DARWIN, C., 1958/'61: The origin of species by means of natural selection or the preservation of favoured races in the struggle for life: a reprint of the sixth edition, 592 p. (The world's classics, No. 11) (London: Oxford U.P.; Garden City, N.J.: Doubleday). This sixth ed. is also available as a paperback in the series "Penguin Classics", ed. by J. W. BURROW, 1968, 477 p. (Harmondsworth, Middx.: Penguin Bks.). Cf. also: PECKHAM, M., ed., 1959, vide infra; this last book presents in systematic order the many variations in the text of the six original editions of "The origin of species".

—— ——, 1952: Journal of researches into the geology and natural history of the various countries visited by H.M.S. Beagle: facsimile reprint of the first edition, 615 p. (New York, N.Y.: Hafner).—

This is the second volume in the series edited by Frans Verdoorn called: "Pallas: a collection of offset reprints of out-of-print and classic scientific works". This reprint is based on the London edition of 1839. Cf. also BARLOW, N., ed., 1933, vide supra.

—— ——, 1955: The expression of the emotions in man and animals, 372 p. (New York, N.Y.: Philosophical Library).—

A facsimile reprint of the 1872 edition. With an introduction by M. MEAD, in which Darwin's work has been considered from the modern point of view of the new science of kinaesthetics. Again reprinted 1965 (Chicago, Ill.: Chicago U.P.).

—— ——, 1966: The power of movement in plants, 592 p. (New York, N.Y.: Da Capo).—

A reproduction of the first American edition of 1881. In an introduction B. G. PICKARD discusses Darwin's work from the point of view of modern plant physiology.

—— —— & A. R. WALLACE, 1958: Evolution by natural selection, 288 p. (Cambridge: U.P.).—

In his foreword, Sir Gavin DE BEER traces the evolution of theories of evolution from Darwin's predecessors to the present day. This is followed by an introduction to the "Sketch" of 1842 and the "Essay" of 1844 as it was written by Sir Francis Darwin in 1901. Then reprints follow from the "Sketch" and the "Essay". The book closes with the joint paper of Darwin and Wallace communicated in 1858 to the Journal of the Linnean Society which is entitled: "On the tendency of species to form varieties: and on the perpetuation of varieties and species by natural means of selection". For a German version, cf.: HEBERER, G., ed., 1959: C. Darwin und A. Wallace. Dokumente zur Begründung der Abstammungslehre vor 100 Jahren, 1858/59 - 1958/59, 72 p. (Stuttgart: Fischer). Cf. also: LOEWENBERG, B. J., 1959: Darwin, Wallace, and the theory of natural selection, 80 p. (New York, N.Y.: Taplinger).

——, DARWIN, F., ed., 1887: The life and letters of Charles Darwin, 3 vols. Vol. I: 395 p.; Vol. II: 393 p.; Vol. III: 418 p. (London: Murray); and DARWIN, F. & A. C. SEWARD, eds., 1903: More letters of Charles Darwin: a record of his work in a series of hitherto unpublished letters, 2 vols. Vol. I: 494 p.; Vol. II: 508 p. (London: Murray).—

"The life and letters" contains a relatively short biography together with a selection of letters from C. Darwin and some letters addressed to him. It has been the aim of the editor that they should illustrate C. Darwin's personal character. In appendixes are given a list of works by C. Darwin, a list of existing portraits, and a summing-up of honours, degrees, societies, etc. Reprinted 1969 (New York, N.Y.: Johnson). Also in a French edition: La vie et la correspondance de Charles Darwin avec un chapitre autobiographique, publié par son fils M. Francis DARWIN, 2 vols., 1888, Vol. I: 701 p.; Vol. II: 794 p. The second collection of letters consists of a series of additional letters which were received after the publication of the first series. Of special importance is the correspondence with Hooker, Lyell, Müller, Huxley, Wallace, and Gray. Cf. also BARLOW, N., ed., 1967: Darwin and Henslow: letters, 1831-1860, 251 p. (London: Murray).

——, DE BEER, G. R., 1963: Charles Darwin: evolution by natural selection, 290 p. (London: Nelson).—

A well-written and valuable survey of Darwin's life and scientific work, based on the most recent monographic studies. Special topics considered are: contemporary influences on Darwin (Lyell, Paley, Malthus); Darwin's influence on science and society; the opposition to Darwin; a discussion of Darwin's scientific work after the publication of the "Origin". There is a 1965 edition, 295 p. (Garden City, N.Y.: Doubleday, in cooperation with the American Museum of Natural History).

——, ELLEGÅRD, A., 1958: Darwin and the general reader: the reception of Darwin's theory of evolution in the British periodical press, 1859-1872, 394 p. (Göteborgs Universitets Årsskrift, LXIV) (Stockholm: Almqvist & Wiksell).—

According to the author, the purpose of this book is to describe and to analyse the impact of Darwin's theory of evolution on the British public during the first dozen years after the publication of the "Origin of species". The study is based on 107 British periodicals (which is *ca.* one-third of the total newspaper circulation). Each journal is classified according to political and religious affiliations, its circulation, the educational group to which it appealed, the amount of its coverage of evolution and natural selection, and its attitude to those points. At he end (p. 338-367) statistical tables have been given, which contain much exact information concerning the influence of Darwinism on social life.

——, FREEMAN, R. B., 1965: The works of Charles Darwin: an annotated bibliographical handlist, 81 p. (London: Dawson).—

This book contains a full list of all editions and issues of books written by Darwin that contain original material and have been printed in Britain up to 1965. A preliminary list of foreign editions has been included. It also contains a general bibliographical account of the most important works.

——, GHISELIN, M. T., 1969: The triumph of the Darwinian method, 287 p. (Berkeley, Calif.: Univ. California Press).—

A critical examination of Darwin's published works and the critical commentaries published on the occasion of the centenary in 1959 of the publication of the "Origin". This has been done from a logical and methodological point of view. The author's main theses are, that Darwin operated as a basis for his reasoning from a "selective-retention" model, and that the value of the "Origin" lies in the questions asked rather than in the answers given.

——, GREENE, J. C., 1961: Darwin and the modern worldview, 141 p. (Baton Rouge, La.: Louisiana State U.P.).—

In this study the author places Darwin's work within the framework of scientific, philosophical, economic, and religious thought of his own time and he analyses Darwin's influence on the development of these fields. This booklet can be considered as a continuation of the author's: The death of Adam: evolution and its impact on western thought, 382 p. (New York, N.Y.: Mentor Bks.). Originally published 1959 (Ames, Iowa: Iowa State U.P.).

——, HIMMELFARB, G., 1959: Darwin and the Darwinian revolution, 422 p. (London: Chatto & Windus).—

This book is a biography of Darwin, based on much unpublished material. Why was it given to Darwin, less ambitious, less imaginative and less learned than many of his colleagues, to discover the theory sought after by others so assiduously? To these and many other questions this book tries to give an answer. The book is written essentially from an anti-Darwinian point of view, and according to the authoress Darwin has to be seen as a collector of already existing knowledge rather than as an innovator of biological science, and therefore his generalizations should have caused a shock of recognition in broad sections of the community.

——, HUXLEY, J. & H. B. D. KETTLEWELL, 1965: Charles Darwin and his world, 144 p. (New York, N.Y.: Viking).—

A lavishly illustrated survey of Darwin's life and work. Stress has been laid on the originality of Darwin's researches after he had published his "Origin". Intended to be read by students.

——, HYMAN, S. E., ed., 1963: Darwin for today: the essence of his works, 435 p. (New York, N.Y.: Viking).—

This is a one-volume collection of some of the most important passages of

Darwin's writings, *viz.,* his "Essay" of 1844, containing the substance of the later "Origin of species", his "Autobiography" in its original version (*cf.* BARLOW, N., ed., 1933, *vide supra),* his "Voyage of the Beagle", "Descent of Man", "Expression of the emotions", "Insectivorous plants", "Formation of vegetable mould", and of his "Letters" (to Joseph Hooker and to Charles Lyell). Included are an introduction and a chronology of life and works of C. Darwin. *Cf.* also BATES, M. & P. S. HUMPHREY, 1965, *vide supra,* and WYSS, W. VON, 1965, *vide infra.*

——, KEITH, A., 1955: Darwin revalued, 294 p. (London: Watts).——

In his preface Keith writes: "For more than twenty years I have been living under the shadow of Darwin's old home, Down House, near Farnborough, in Kent. During this time I have become familiar with Darwin's haunts, surroundings, and mode of life, as well as with his works and writings, and I think I have succeeded in building up a mental picture of the day-to-day life led by the great naturalist, and from these various sources has come a knowledge of what he did and thought year by year." .. "The book falls into two parts. Part I (chapters 1-16) is a narrative of Darwin's life told in a particular way; part II, occupying the remainder, is devoted to a re-examination of the way in which his books, his doctrines, and his ideas have stood the test of time. I myself believe that his future will be greater thans his past."

——, LEROY, J. F., 1966: Charles Darwin et la théorie moderne de l'évolution, 209 p. (Collection savants du monde entier, No. 29) (Paris: Seghers).——

An essayistic introduction to the life and work of Charles Darwin. "The book is written in an erudite yet pleasing way, with a definite flair for the literary approach and a feeling for the essentials. As an introduction to Darwin: excellent; as a refresher of one's sometimes too stereotype ideas on the birth of the theories of evolution and their consequences: wellcome; as an assessment of Darwin's place in modern evolutionary thinking: clear." (From: Taxon 16: 335).

——, MOORE, R., 1955: Charles Darwin: a great life in brief, 206 p. (New York, N.Y.: Knopf).——

A well-written biography in which the major aspects of the Darwinian theory

of evolution have been elucidated and in which the main events of the life of C. Darwin have been described.

——, NACHTWEY, R., 1959: Der Irrweg des Darwinismus, 303 p. (Berlin: Morus).——

A critical study of Darwinism in general and of the theory of natural selection in particular. The author also discusses the social implications of Darwinism. One chapter is entitled: "Darwin-Nietzsche-Hitler", and another "Die Raubtier-Ethik Oswald Spenglers".

——, PECKHAM, M., ed., 1959: The origin of species: a variorum text, 816 p. (Philadelphia, Pa.: Univ. Pennsylvania Press).——

This book presents in systematic order the many variations in the text of the six original editions of "The origin of species" that appeared between 1859 and 1872. In the introduction the author gives the publishing history of the subsequent editions and the 13 British reprints of the 6th edition. Starting point in his comparisons is the first edition, each of the sentences of which has been serially numbered chapter by chapter. Immediately following each first-edition sentence is an indication of the changes and deletions occurring in that sentence in each of the subsequent editions. This is followed by the insertion of such sentences as were added and each of these is treated for subsequent changes, deletions, and added sentences.

——, WICHLER, G., 1961: Charles Darwin: the founder of the theory of evolution and natural selection, 228 p. (Oxford: Pergamon).——

The aim of the author is to show "how we owe to Darwin and to him alone, the positive proof of the theory of descent as well as that of the theory of natural selection". In the first part of this study the author reviews those predecessors who made a conscious and critically-evaluated contribution to the idea of evolution. The second part covers the development of Darwin's thought on evolution and natural selection; the third part contains biographical information about Darwin.

——, WEST, G., 1938: Charles Darwin: the fragmentary man, 352 p. (London: Dawson).——

Certainly one of the best biographies of Darwin: well-written and well-documented. A well-written and interesting French biography is: ROSTAND, J., 1947: Charles Darwin, 242 p. (Paris: Gallimard). A short English biography is: OLBY, R. C., 1967: Charles Darwin, 64 p. (The Clarendon biographies, No. 16) (London: Oxford U.P.).

——, WYSS, W. VON, 1959: Charles Darwin. Ein Forscherleben, 355 p. (Zurich: Artemis).—

A valuable biography in German of life and work of Charles Darwin.

—— ——, ed., 1965: Charles Darwin. Eine Auswahl aus seinem Werk, 155 p. (Hubers Klassiker der Medizin u. d. Naturwissenschaften, Vol. V) (Bern & Stuttgart: Huber).—

One of the best general introductions to Darwin's work, particularly useful for the beginning student of biology. It mainly consists of a selection of quotations from the original text in German translation; the quotations are linked up by an informative interconnecting text. *Cf.* also: BATES, M. & P. S. HUMPHREY, eds., 1965; also HYMAN, S. E., 1963, *vide supra*. A short review of Darwin's life and work (p. 1-12), a consideration of his philosophy (p. 13-64), and extracts from his main works (p. 65-100) in French is: CRESSON, A., 1956: Darwin. Sa vie, son oeuvre. Avec un exposé de sa philosophie, 101 p. (Paris: Presses Univ. de France).

Darwin, Erasmus (1731-1802) — KING-HELE, D. G., 1963: Erasmus Darwin, 183 p. (London: Macmillan; New York, N.Y.: St. Martin).—

E. Darwin was a man of science, physician, poet and prolific inventor, a man of great social energy, and founder of three societies. He contributed to such fields as: geology, meteorology, agricultural chemistry, plant physiology, and general biology; he propounded a theory of evolution which anticipated the theory of his grandson Charles. As a poet he wrote the "Botanic garden" which reflects his general scientific enthusiasm, and the "Temple of nature" in which he traces the evolution of life from its origin in primeaval seas to its present culmination. These are the subjects dealt with in this book. A thorough discussion of the "Temple of nature" can be found in: BRANDL, L., 1902: Erasmus Darwin's Temple of nature, 203 p. (Wiener Beiträge zur englischen Philologie, Vol. XVI) (Vienna & Leipzig: Braumüller).

—— ——, ed., 1968: The essential writings of Erasmus Darwin, 223 p. (London: MacGibbon & Kee; New York, N.Y.: Hillary House).—

In this beautifully-illustrated book, the editor tries to show that E. Darwin was one of the most influential men, both in science and literature, of the 18th century. He does so by choosing illuminative passages from the works of E. Darwin and supplementing these pasages with commentaries. Although the author presents an exaggerated picture of his subject, the book nevertheless is a lucid introduction in the main publications of E. Darwin, *viz.*, "The botanic garden", "Zoonomia", "Phytologia", and the "Temple of nature".

——, PEARSON, H., 1930: Doctor Darwin, 242 p. (London & Toronto: Dent).—

E. Darwin was the grandfather of Charles Darwin by his first marriage, and of Sir Francis Galton by his second. He founded the Lunar Society, a remarkable group of thinkers and inventors in the 18th century. Furthermore, he was a philosopher, famous physician and poet, a humanitarian and reformer, and one of the most famous citizens of his time. He is of special importance for his ideas on the evolutionary aspects of the organic world. Of all these various activities, this biography gives accounts. Also in a paperback edition, 1943, 143 p. (Harmondsworth, Mddx.: Penguin Bks.).

Daubenton, Louis Jean Marie (1716-1800) — ROULE, L., 1925: Daubenton et l'exploitation de la nature, 246 p. (Grands naturalistes du Muséum d'Hist. Nat., No. 2) (Paris: Flammarion).—

Daubenton was a French naturalist. He assisted Buffon, *q.v.*, by providing the anatomical descriptions for his grand treatise on natural history (*vide supra*). He was actively engaged in building up the anatomical collections of the Muséum d'Hist. Nat. In his later years he became also professor of mineralogy at the Jardin du Roy.

Da Vinci, Leonardo (1452-1519) — BRAUNFELS-ESCHE, S., 1961: Leonardo da Vinci. Das anatomische Werk. Mit kritischem Katalog und 175 Abbildungen, 176 p. (Stuttgart: Schattauer).—

The author traces the development of Leonardo's anatomical activities from 1487 onwards, and shows how these activities gradually developed from an artistic curiosity to serious investigations, marked by a shift of interest from the outer anatomy to the anatomy of the internal organs and by a concern with questions of function and of general biology. A series of supplements deal with such problems as: Leonardo's various plans for an anatomical treatise, his "comparative anatomy", the significance of mechanics in his anatomical investigations, and with later judgements of Leonardo's anatomical studies. It also contains a catalogue of drawings, reproductions, and comparative illustrations from mediaeval sources and from Vesalius. A book in English dealing with the same subject is: BELT, E., 1955: Leonardo the anatomist, 76 p. (Lawrence, Kans.: Kansas U.P.), being the fourth series of the Logan Clendening Lectures.

——, HUARD, P., 1961: Léonardo da Vinci. Dessins anatomiques, 208 p. (Paris: Dacosta).——

A selection of 80 drawings, mainly from the Windsor collection.

——, KEELE, K. D., 1952: Leonardo da Vinci on movement of the heart and blood, 142 p. (Philadelphia, Pa.: Lippincott).——

This is an attempt to evaluate Leonardo's anatomical writings and drawings by means of a thorough re-examination of his anatomical work, notably of the cardiovascular system, and to make clear the influences of Galen, Avicenna and Mundinus on the one hand, and of his striving for explanations in terms of mechanics on the other hand.

——, McMURRICH, J. P., 1930: Leonardo da Vinci the anatomist, 265 p. (Baltimore, Md.: Williams & Wilkins).——

An attempt to illustrate how many elements of mediaeval thought and tradition Leonardo assimilated. Thus the first three chapters deal with the history of anatomy from Galen through the Middle Ages, and the author shows that Leonardo's anatomical drawings cannot be understood without knowledge of the late-mediaeval Galen-tradition. It has been shown that Leonardo never denied mediaeval anatomical prejudices (he actually made a picture of the non-existent pores in the cardiac septum); but as soon as he restricted himself to keen observation, he nevertheless enriched anatomical knowledge, especially in those fields which were not subject to mediaeval bias.

——, O'MALLEY, C. D. & J. B. de C. M. SAUNDERS, 1952: Leonardo da Vinci on the human body: the anatomical, physiological, and embryological drawings of Leonardo da Vinci, with translations, emendations and a biographical introduction, 506 p. (New York, N.Y.: Schuman).——

In the introduction, information has been given concerning Leonardo's life, the techniques of anatomical illustration anterior to him, his mss., *etc.* All 215 drawings and English translations of the texts belonging to them which have been grouped in systematic order *(e.g.,* skeleton, muscles, *etc.).* Scientific commentaries have been added.

——, PAZZINI, A., ed., 1962-1965: Leonardo da Vinci: Il trattato della anatomia, 3 vols. Vol. I: 391 p.; Vol. II: 383 p.; Vol. III: 142 p. (Rome: Istituto di Storia della Medicina dell'Università di Roma).——

The purpose of this book is to collect the many fragments of Leonardo's anatomical work and to present them as an integrated picture. This has been done in a modern fashion, *viz.,* the material has been arranged according to the various systems of the body. Each anatomical section is prefaced by a brief introduction, followed by a section on the anatomy of the system concerned and a section discussing its physiology. The first vol. mainly deals with the muscular and cardio-vascular systems; the second vol. mainly with neurology and the anatomy of the special senses. In the third vol. R. CIANCHI provides a chronological bibliography of writings on Leonardo's anatomical and related notes from 1550 to 1963.

——, ZUBOV, V. P., 1968: Leonardo da Vinci, 335 p. (Translated from the Russian edition (1962) by D. H. KRAUS) (Cambridge, Mass.: Harvard U.P.).——

An attempt to interpret Leonardo in terms of his own epoch, tracing the main events of his life and work. In a chapter devoted to his scientific achievements, the author considers such subjects as mechanics, planetary motion, and anatomy. A special chapter deals with the nature of the human eye and the science of optics.

Descartes, René, (1596-1650) — DIJK-STERHUIS, E. J., *et al.,* 1950: Descartes et le cartésianisme hollandais. Études et documents, 309 p. (Paris: Presses Univ. de France).—

A series of essays dealing with the influence of Cartesianism in the Netherlands. None of these essays deals with the influence of Descartes on the organic natural sciences in particular. These aspects have been considered in another study, about which I am not able to give any further details, *viz.,* CHAUVOIS, L., 1966: Descartes. Sa méthode et ses erreurs en physiologie, 155 p. (Paris: Ed. du Cèdre). *Cf.* also: CRAPULLI, G. C., ed., 1966: Regulae ad directionem ingenii. Texte critique avec la version hollandaise du XVIIième siècle, 120 p. (Arch. Intl. Hist. des Idées, vol. 12) (The Hague: Nijhoff); and WATSON, R. A., 1966: The downfall of Cartesianism 1673-1712: a study of epistemological issues in late 17th century Cartesianism, 158 p. *(Idem,* Vol. 11) (The Hague: Nijhoff).

——, SEBBA, G., 1964: Bibliographia Cartesiana: a critical guide to the Descartes literature, 1800-1960, 510 p. (The Hague: Nijhoff).—

This book presents the literature of the past 160 years in alphabetical order, combined with a systematic analytical survey and a detailed topical index to the whole. The first part, entitled "Introduction to Descartes studies", lists nearly 600 works on Descartes, each being accompanied by a brief summary of the contents. The "Alphabetical bibliography" lists some 3.000 works. This is followed by a systematic index, in which every aspect of Descartes' work is listed in an appropriate index. Exhaustive analytical index of nearly 60 papers.

——, SMITH, N. K., 1953: New studies in the philosophy of Descartes: Descartes as pioneer, 369 p. and: Descartes' philosophical writings, 317 p. (London: Macmillan; New York, N.Y.: St. Martin).—

The first volume gives a comprehensive account of the development of Descartes' thought and is as such of great value to every student of the history of science. The second volume contains full texts in English translation of Descartes' "Regulae", his "Discours", "Meditationes" and "Les passions de l'âme" and excerpts from the "Dioptrique" *(i.e.,* the physiological basis of vision), the "Objections" *(i.e.,* the mind-body relationship) and his "Recherches de la verité".

Diderot, Denis (1713-1784) — MAYERM, J., ed., 1964: Denis Diderot. Éléments de physiologie, 81 + 387 p. (Paris: Didier).—

A critical edition, with introduction and notes. Unfortunately I am unable to give any further information about this book.

Dodonaeus, Rembertus (= Rembert Dodoens) (1517-1585) — MEERBEECK, P. J. van, 1841: Recherches historiques et critiques sur la vie et les ouvrages de Rembert Dodoens (Dodonaeus), 340 p. (Malines: Hanicq).—

The work has been divided into the following parts: 1. Biographie de Rembert Dodoens; 2. Aperçu du traité de cosmographie de Dodoens; 3. Appréciation des ouvrages de botanique de Dodoens; 4. Revue de la correspondance botanique de Dodoens; 5. Résumé de la lettre de Dodoens sur l'élan; 6. Analyse des ouvrages de médecine de Dodoens; 7. Jugement motivé sur le caractère et les talents de Dodoens; 8. Bibliographie raisonnée des ouvrages de Dodoens; 9. Liste des ouvrages consultés; 10. Appendix (Contains a table of modern names of the plants described by Dodoens). On the occasion of the fourth centenary of his birth, a special issue of the periodical Janus (Vol. 22: 141-204) has been devoted to Dodonaeus. This issue consists of an introduction (by C. E. VAN LEERSUM) and the following essays: Dodoens comme botaniste (by F. W. T. HUNGER); Dodoens and his influence on Flemish and Dutch folk medicine (by M. A. VAN ANDEL); Les portraits de Dodoens (by J. G. DE LINT); and l'Herbier flamand de Dodoens (by M. J. SIRKS).

Dohrn, Felix Anton (1840-1909) — HEUSS, T., 1940: Anton Dohrn in Naepel, 319 p. (Berlin & Zurich: Atlantis).—

A full-scale biography of the German zoologist and founder of the Zoological Station in Naples. This study is based upon much unpublished material, notebooks, letters, *etc.* Much attention has been paid to the activities of the Zoological Station. In 1948 a second edition appeared, 448 p. (Stuttgart & Tübingen: Leins). *Cf.* also: BOVERI, T., 1910: Anton Dohrn. Gedächtnisrede gehalten auf dem Internationalen Zoologen-Kongress in Graz am 18. August 1910, 43 p. (Leipzig: Hirzel).

Driesch, Hans (1867-1941) — WENZL, A., ed., 1951: Hans Driesch. Persönlichkeit und

Bedeutung für Biologie und Philosophie von heute, 221 p. (Basle: Reinhardt).—

This work consists of the following contributions: 1. Das Leben von Hans Driesch (p. 7-20), a biographical review written by his widow; 2. G. v. NATZMER: Die Problemstellung der Biologie durch Driesch und ihre weitere Entwicklung (p. 21-44), an exposition of Driesch's biological points of view compared with those of his contemporaries, *e.g.,* Haeckel, Weismann, W. Roux, *etc.;* 3. U. SCHÖNDORFER: Hans Driesch's philosophisches Werk (p. 45-64), discussing his works on the mind-body problem; 4. A. WENZL: Driesch's Neuvitalismus und der philosophische Stand des Lebensproblems heute (p. 65-179), a confrontation of Driesch's philosophy with modern philosophy; 5. A. MITTASCH: Briefwechsel mit Hans Driesch (1935-1941) (p. 181-207), especially concerning the notions causality and entelechy. Pp. 209-221 contain a chronological list of Driesch's publications from 1889 to 1941. A very good and well-written autobiography exists, *viz.,* DRIESCH, H., 1951: Lebenserinnerungen. Aufzeichnungen eines Forschers und Denkers in entscheidender Zeit, 311 p. (Basle: Reinhardt).

Duchenne, Guillaume Benjamin Armand (1806-1875) — DUCHENNE, G. B., 1949: Physiology of motion, 612 p. (Transl. and edit. by E. B. KAPLAN) (Philadelphia, Pa.: Lippincott).—

Duchenne was a French physician. In 1867 he published his "Physiologie des mouvements" which is considered to be his masterpiece, of which this is the first complete English translation. In this book Duchenne demonstrated the function of the muscles of the human body in health and disease by means of electrical stimulation. This work exerted a great influence upon his contemporaries, and upon the further development of the science of physiology. Reissued 1959 (Philadelphia, Pa. & London: Saunders).

Dupuytren, Guillaume, Baron (1777-1835) — MONDOR, H., 1945: Dupuytren, 312 p. (Paris: Gallimard).—

Deals especially with Dupuytren as a surgeon. The author tries to integrate the biographical facts with Dupuytren's surgical accomplishments, his time, and his character. A somewhat older, however, very complete biography of Dupuytren was written by: DELHOUME, L., 1935: Dupuytren, ed. 3, 494 p. (Publié sous les auspices de la Société archéologique et historique de Li-

mousin) (Paris: Baillière). Also published in the Bull. Soc. Archéol. et Hist. de Limousin, Vol. 76.

Eaton, Amos (1776-1842) — McALLISTER, E. M., 1941: Amos Eaton: scientist and educator, 1776-1842, 587 p. (Philadelphia, Pa.: Univ. Pennsylvania Press).—

Eaton was a great inspirer of botanical studies, author of the first popular manual for the identification of American plants, and is still honoured as founder of the Rensselaer Polytechnic Institute. An inscription on a bronze tablet in Amos Eaton Hall, at Rensselaer, sums up his life in the following words: "Pioneer, as student, teacher, and author, in agriculture, botany, chemistry, and zoology. Promoter of field work and laboratory practice. Father of American geology. One of the great figures in the history of science in the United States. He directed the destinies of Rensselaer School from its inception until the year of his death".

Edwardes, David (*ca.* 1502-1542) — O'MALLEY, C. D. & K. F. RUSSELL, eds., 1961: David Edwardes, introduction to anatomy 1532: a facsimile reproduction with English translation and an introductory essay on anatomical studies in Tudor England, 64 p. (London: Oxford U.P.; Stanford, Calif.: Stanford U.P.).—

A beautifully reproduced reissue of the first English anatomical book (De indiciis et praecognitionibus) which is still mediaeval in style and contents. The reissue is accompanied by a translation in modern English, together with clear interpretations, giving a lucid insight into the history of anatomy and medical education in England of those days.

Ehrlich, Paul (1854-1915) — MARQUARDT, M., 1949/1951: Paul Ehrlich, 255 p. (London: Heinemann; New York, N.Y.: Schuman).—

A biography of the life and achievements of the famous inaugurator of chemotherapy, Paul Ehrlich. Miss Marquardt served him as a personal secretary for thirteen years. Originally published in German: MARQUARDT, M., 1924: Paul Ehrlich als Mensch und Arbeiter. Erinnerungen aus dreizehn Jahren seines Lebens, 1902-1915, 112 p. (Stuttgart). Another German biographical study is: LOEWE, H., 1950: Paul Ehrlich, Schöpfer der Chemotherapie, 255 p. (Grosse Naturforscher, Vol. 8) (Stuttgart: Wiss. Verlagsges.). *Cf.* also HIMMELWEIT, F., ed., 1956: The collected papers of Paul Ehrlich, 4 vols. (London & New York, N.Y.: Pergamon). Vol. 1 deals with histology, biochemistry and pathology; vol. 2 with immunology and cancer research; vol. 3 with chemotherapy; and vol. 4 contains an index and a bibliography. Vol. 1 contains a complete biography.

Ellis, Henry Havelock (1859-1939) — MARSHALL, A. C., 1959: Havelock Ellis: a biography, 292 p. (London: Hart-Davis).—

Henry Havelock Ellis devoted his life to the study of the physiology, psychology, and pathology of sex (his *magnum opus:* Studies in the psychology of sex, 7 vols., 1900-1928, Philadelphia, Pa.: Davis; reissued, 1936, in 4 vols., New York, N.Y.: Random House). This biography is an outstanding contribution to the history of sexology as well. A bibliography, a short list of books about Ellis and an index have been included.

Errera, Léo (1858-1905) — ERRERA, L., 1908: Recueil d'oeuvres de Léo Errera, 4 vols. Vol. I: 318 p.; Vol. II: 341 p.; Vol. III: 336 p.; Vol. IV: 222 p. (Bruxelles: Lamertin).—

The first two vols. deal with the botanical writings of the Belgian plant physiologist Errera. The division is according to subject. Vol. I. deals with structure of the flower and mode of fecundation (p. 31-236); heterostyly (p. 237-268); systematic botany (p. 269-288); protection of plants against animals, and with some other minor fields of research. Vol. II deals with the scientific basis of agriculture (p. 31-62); the descriptive text belonging to the plates concerning botanical physiology (p. 67-156); and the text of a lecture on Darwinism (p. 163-270). Vol. III contains some publications of Errera concerning the position of the laboratory in modern science and a report concerning the organization of a botanical room in the "Palais du Peuple" in Brussels. Moreover, this vol. contains some 10 biographical essays dealing with, *inter alia,* Schleiden, Nägeli, J. E. Bommer, François Crépin, L. Pasteur and É. Laurent. The fourth vol. contains some poems and short essays of literary value.

Escherich, Karl (1871-1951) — ESCHERICH, K., 1944: Leben und Forschen. Kampf um eine Wissenschaft, 277 p. (Berlin: Parey).—

An autobiography of one of the leading entomologists of the first half of this century. Escherich was especially interested in the ecological aspects of entomology and was one of the pioneers of applied entomology. This autobiography contains much information of interest to any historian of the more recent aspects of entomology.

Eustachius, Bartholomaeus (*ca.* 1520-1574) — LANCISIUS, J. M., ed., 1969: Tabulae anatomicae: with Latin notes. (Modena: Ed. Parnaso).—

A full-sized photo-offset reproduction of a beautiful anatomical atlas published in Rome in 1714 with the text entirely in Latin. Eustachius himself managed to publish only the first eight plates in a monograph on the kidney. More than 150 years later the other plates were found in the possession of a descendant of one of Eustachius' disciples and they were published in 1714 accompanied by notes written by the physician of Pope Clement XI.

Eykman, Christiaan (1858-1930) — JANSEN, B. C. P., 1959: Het levenswerk van Christiaan Eykman 1858-1930, 206 p. (Haarlem: Bohn).—

A biography of the famous Dutch physician, who specialized in tropical hygiene and medicine, and discovered the cause of beriberi. Included is a list of his publications.

Fabre, Jean Henri Casimir (1823-1915) — LEGROS, G. V., 1924: La vie de J. H. Fabre, naturaliste, suivi du répertoire général analytique des "Souvenirs entomologiques", 439 p. (Paris: Delagrave).—

A well-written biography based upon personal observation, conversation, and correspondence with Fabre. It also provides a good exposition of Fabre's scientific achievements. A popular booklet, written for young people is: DOORLY, E., 1949: The insect man, 169 p. (Harmondsworth, Mddx.: Penguin Bks.). This booklet describes how an English family set out in a car to discover something about Fabre, the place where he was born, the fields of his investigations, *etc.* A more recent biography is: REVEL, E., 1952: J. H. Fabre, l'homme des insectes, 228 p. (Paris: Delagrave); unfortunately I am unable to give more information about this book. A somewhat older biography in English translation is: FABRE, A., 1921: Fabre, the entomologist, 299 p. (London: Hodder & Stoughton). Also published in the

U.S.A., 1921, 398 p. (New York, N.Y.: Dodd-Mead). (Originally published in French, 1910). *Cf.* also: FABRE, A., 1921: Sur les sommets. Les dernières années de Jean-Henri Fabre, l'entomologiste, 1910-1915, 62 p.

——, TEALE, E. W., ed., 1949: The insect world of J. Henri Fabre in the translation of Alexander Teixeira de Mattos, with introduction and interpretive comments, 333 p. (10th printing) (New York, N.Y.: Dodd-Mead).—

> In this vol. the most famous of Fabre's studies are brought together in one volume in English translation. Each of the 40 sections included is preceded by an introduction. The selection is taken from A. Teixeira de Mattos' English translation of the "Souvenirs entomologique", 1912, 492 p., published by Hodder & Stoughton, London; a new edition of Teale's book appeared in 1956: TEALE, E. W., ed., 1956: The fascinating insect world of J. Henri Fabre, new ed. (New York, N.Y.: Fawcett). An anthology of Fabre's writings in German translation can be found in: GUGGEN-HEIM, K. & A. PORTMANN, eds., 1961: J. H. Fabre. Das offenbare Geheimnis. Aus dem Lebenswerk des Insektenforschers, 325 p. (Zurich & Stuttgart: Atemis).

Fabricius, Hieronymus (1537-1619) — ADELMANN, H. B., ed., 1942: The embryological treatises of Hieronymus Fabricius of Aquapendente. The formation of the egg of the chick (De formatione ovi et pulli). The formed fetus (De formato foetu). A facsimile edition, with an introduction, a translation and a commentary, 883 p. (Ithaca, N.Y.: Cornell U.P.).—

> A splendid facsimile edition of these two treatises of Fabricius, accompanied by an, according to Sigerist, very beautiful translation. In the introduction the editor gives a historical background, including a sketch of the situation in embryology before Fabricius. Bibliography and index (of 71 pages). Reprinted in 1967.

——, FRANKLIN, K. J., ed., 1933: De venarum ostiolis (1603) of Hieronymus Fabricius of Aquapendente (1533?-1619). Facsimile edition with introduction, translation and notes, 98 p. (Springfield, Ill.: Thomas).—

> This book contains a biographical sketch, a chapter discussing the early history

of the work on venous valves, and another chapter containing a description of the amphitheatre in the school of anatomy of Padua. Then a facsimile reproduction of the text follows together with a translation.

Fabry von Hilden, Wilhelm (= Fabricius Hildanus) (1560-1634) — HINTZSCHE, E., ed., 1965: Wilhelm Fabry von Hilden. Gründlicher Bericht vom heissen und kalten Brand, welcher Gangraena et Sphacelus oder S. Antonii- und Martialis-Feuer genannt wird. Nach der 1603 publizierten zweiten deutschen Ausgabe bearbeitet und herausgegeben, 180 p. (Hubers Klassiker der Medizin und der Naturwissenschaften, Vol. 4) (Bern & Stuttgart: Huber).—

> In the introduction the editor has collected all biographical material available. Then he discusses the various editions of "Vom heissen und kalten Brand", the pioneer account of ergotism, first published in 1593. The work is concluded by brief notes, a bibliography of writings dealing with Fabry, and an index of persons and places.

——, QUERVAIN, F. de & H. BLOESCH, eds., 1936: Von der Fürtrefflichkeit und Nutz der Anatomy, 203 p. (Leipzig: Sauerländer).—

> Fabricius Hildanus is known as the "Father of German surgery". The present issue of the "Kurze Beschreibung der Fürtrefflichkeit und Nutz der Anatomy" represents the intended second and revised edition which Fabry had prepared during the last years of his life. The contents of the book is a sound popular introduction to medical science, pointing out the necessary basis of anatomy, and the role of the physician and the surgeon in the maintenance of health.

Fairchild, David Grandison (1869-1954) — FAIRCHILD, D., 1938: The world was my garden. Travels of a plant explorer, 494 p. (Assisted by E. and A. KAY) (New York, N.Y.: Scribner).—

> According to a review by G. Sarton in Isis 31: 200, this is an extremely interesting biography. A popular biography of this famous botanist and plant explorer who brought more than 200,000 species of plants into the U.S.A. and established what is now the New Crops Research Branch of the U.S. Dept. of Agriculture, is: WILLIAMS, B & S. EPSTEIN, 1961: Plant explorer David Fairchild, 192 p. (New York, N.Y.: Messner).

Falloppio, Gabriello (1523-1562) — FAVA-RO, G., 1928: Gabrielle Falloppia, Modenese (MDXXIII-MDLXII). Studio biografico (con ritratto e figure), 254 p. (Modena: Tip. Ed. Immacolata Concezione).—

Falloppius held the chairs of anatomy, surgery and botany at the university of Padua, and became superintendent of the newly-established botanical gardens. The present book is a very elaborate biography of this great anatomist, in which the author has collected all documents which could throw any light on his life. Included are some of his letters, a list in chronological order of all the letters extant, and a chronology of all the known facts of Falloppius' life.

Fauchard, Pierre (*ca.* 1698-1761) — FAU-CHARD, P., 1946: The surgeon dentist, or treatise on the teeth, 184 + 128 p. (Transl. from the 2nd ed., 1746, by L. LINDSAY) (London: Butterworth).—

The writer of this book is the "father of dentistry"; this is the first time that his work has been published in English translation. The full title of the book is: "The surgeon dentist, or treatise on the teeth, in which is seen the means used to keep them clean and healthy, of beautifying them, of repairing their loss and remedies for their diseases and those of the gums and for accidents which may befall the other parts in their vicinity, with observations and reflexions on several special cases." The book contains many case-histories which give a lucid picture of dental practice in mid 18th-century Paris. A monograph on Fauchard has been written by: WEINBERGER, B. W., 1941: Pierre Fauchard: surgeon-dentist, 102 p. (Minneapolis, Minn.: Pierre Fauchard Academy). A facsimile reproduction of the original French second ed. was published in 1961: Le chirurgien dentiste, ou traité des dents, 2 vols. Vol. 1: 494 p.; Vol. II: 425 p. (Paris: Prélat).

Fechner, Gustav Theodor (1801-1887) — ADLER, H. R., ed., 1966: Elements of psychophysics, Vol. 1: 320 p. (Translated from the German edition (1860) by H. R. ADLER, D. H. HOWES and E. G. BO-RING) (New York, N.Y.: Holt, Rinehart & Winston).—

Fechner has been well known as a physiologist, doctor of medicine, poet, aestheticist, satirist and above all as a philosopher. He wrote this book as a contribution to philosophy; its main subject is the relationship between mind and body. The concepts and (quantitative) methods developed in this book have remained central to the problems of the study of sensation and perception. Originally published under the title: "Elemente der Psychophysik", 1860, 2 vols., 336 + 572 p. (Leipzig: Breitkopf & Härtel).

Fernel, Jean François (= Fernelius Joannes) (1497-1558) — CAPITAINE, P. A., 1925: Un grand médecin du XVIe siècle: Jean Fernel, 104 p. (Thèse Univ. Paris) (Paris: Le François).—

After a biographical account, a review follows of Fernel's mathematical treatises. Then a section follows dealing with his anatomo-physiological studies, his pathology, and his therapy. A special section treats of Fernel's treatise on venereal diseases. Included are a bibliography of the works written by Fernel and a bibliography of works consulted. *Cf.* also: HERPIN, A., 1950: Jean Fernel, médecin et philosophe, 85 p. (Paris: Vrin); and ROGER, J., 1960: Jean Fernel et les problèmes de la médecine de la Renaissance, 27 p. (Paris: Libr. du Palais de la Découverte). I am not able to give further information about these books.

——, SHERRINGTON, C., 1946: The endeavour of Jean Fernel: with a list of the editions of his writings, 223 p. (Cambridge: U.P.; New York, N.Y.: Macmillan).—

Fernel was a Renaissance physician and mathematician, a contemporary of Vesalius; according to Sherrington, however, Fernel's thought was far ahead of Vesalius, for "Fernel's view of the body . . . is not a merely static one like that of Vesalius - just a gross shape in frozen time. The living body is expounded by Fernel as a dynamism, but it is a spirit-dynamism - so spiritist that it leaves little or nothing for chemistry and physics to do. Today physiology *is* chemistry and physics." (Quotation from J. Hist. Med. 2: 131). *Cf.* a series of papers published from 1947 onwards by EKEHORN, G.: Sherrington's "Endeavour of Jean Fernel" and "Man on his nature", published in Acta Medica Scandinavica, suppl. 187, 199, 203, 231, *etc.*

Fernow, Bernhard Eduard (1851-1921) — RODGERS, A. D., 1951: Bernhard Eduard Fernow: a story of North American forestry, 623 p. (Princeton, N.J.: Princeton U.P.).—

Fernow came to the United States in 1876 and helped to build up American forestry research, education, and legislation. In 1886 he became chief of the Division of Forestry of the U.S. Dept. of Agriculture and in 1898 he was appointed Director of New York State College of Forestry of Syracuse University, and from 1907-1919 he was Dean of the Faculty of Forestry of Toronto University.

Finlay, Carlos Juan (1833-1915) — FINLAY, C. J., 1965: Papeles de Finlay. Edición commémorativa del cincuentenario de su muerte, 294 p. (Cuadernos de Historia de la Salud Pública, Vol. 29) (Havana: Ministerio de Salud Publica).—

> This volume of "Papers of Finlay" contains much that is of interest to the history of infectious diseases, especially of the discovery of the transmission of yellow fever. It contains much biographical and bibliographical information about one of the pioneers in this field, Carlos J. Finlay, former Director of Health of Cuba 1902-1909. Cf. also: FINLAY, C. J., 1965-1967: Obras completas, 3 vols. Vol. I: 468 p.; Vol. 2: 266 p.; Vol. 3: 587 p. (Havana: Acad. de Ciencias de Cuba, Museo histórico de las ciencias médicas Carlos J. Finlay). Some papers (among them the most important) are in English or French. Vol. 1 contains 46 papers published between 1886 and 1899; vol. 2 contains 32 papers published between 1887 and 1899; vol. 3 contains most of Finlay's published articles and speeches from 1901 forward, and reports dating from 1863 on his less well-known investigations into goiter, cholera, the nature of gravity, and methods of removing cateracts.

Fleming, Alexander (1881-1955) — MAUROIS, A., 1959: The life of Sir Alexander Fleming: discoverer of penicillin, 293 p. (London: Cape; New York, N.Y.: Dutton).
—

> A well-written and very informative biography of the greatest medical discoverer of recent times. Originally published in French: MAUROIS, A., 1959: La vie de Sir Alexander Fleming, 317 p. (Paris: Hachette). Special sections have been devoted to his teacher Almroth Wright and his influence on Fleming, the discovery of lysozyme, his discovery that *Penicillium Notatum* excreted an antibiotic substance (which he called penicillin), the discovery of the sulphonamides by Domagk, and to the stimulus of this discovery which induced Florey and Chain to a biochemical analysis of penicillin. A paperback edition appeared in 1963 (Harmondsworth, Mddx.: Penguin Bks.). Another (more or less popular) biography is:

LUDOVICI, L. J., 1955: Fleming: discoverer of penicillin, 223 p. (Bloomington, Ind.: Indiana U.P.).

Forel, August Henri (1848-1931) — FOREL, A., 1937: Out of my life and work, 352 p. (London: Allen & Unwin; New York, N.Y.: Norton).—

> Although the contents of this autobiography are somewhat disappointing because Forel wrote it during the decline of his powers, the autobiography is nevertheless of great importance, for it gives an insight into the activities of this great psychologist, social reformer, neurologist, brain anatomist, and entomologist. Also in German: FOREL, A. H., 1935: Rückblick auf mein Leben, 295 p. (Zurich: Europa Verlag). Cf. also: WETTLEY, A., 1953: August Forel (1848-1931). Ein Arztleben im Zwiespalt seiner Zeit, 223 p. (Salzburg: Müller), a biography written by one of his pupils. It gives a picture of Forel and his world view against the background of his time.

Forster, Johann Reinhold (1729-1798) and Johann Georg Adam (1754-1794) — STEINER, G. & M. HAECKEL, 1952: Forster. Ein Lesebuch für unsere Zeit, 506 p. (Weimar: Thüringer Volksverlag).—

> Georg Forster and his father Johann Reinhold Forster participated in the first voyage of Captain Cook around the world. Besides, Georg Forster became a famous scientist, philosopher, and notable revolutionary in his country. A popular biography of Georg Forster is: THOMA, F. M., 1954: Georg Forster. Weltreisender, Forscher, Revolutionär, 199 p. (Berlin: Neues Leben). A study dealing with his philosophical publications is: STEINER, G., ed., 1958: Georg Forster. Philosophische Schriften, 257 p. (Mit Einführung und Erläuterungen) (Berlin: Akademie Verlag).

Fothergill, John (1712-1780) — FOX, R. H., 1919: Dr. John Fothergill and his friends: chapters in eighteenth century life, 434 p. (London: Macmillan).—

> Dr. John Fothergill was a London physician, a man of science, Quaker and philanthropist; this book contains an extensive biography. Chapters of special interest for our purpose have been devoted to: his recognition of diphtheria in England (as it is described in his "Account of the sore throat attended with ulcers" (1748); the rise of medical societies in England; botany in the eighteenth century (Collison, Bartram);

his garden, kept up at Upton, Essex (one of the finest botanical gardens of Europe), and the plants introduced by him.

Fracastoro, Girolamo (1483(?)-1553) — BAUMGARTNER, L. & J. F. FULTON, eds., 1935: A bibliography of the poem Syphilis sive morbus gallicus by Girolamo Fracastoro of Verona, 157 p. (New Haven, Conn.: Yale U.P.; London: Oxford U.P.).—

> The editors list more than 100 editions of this poem (66 Latin, 29 Italian, 13 English, 9 French, 6 German, 1 Spanish, and 1 Portuguese). A very good edition of this poem in English is WYNNE-FINCH, H., 1935: Fracastoro: Syphilis or the French disease: a poem in Latin hexameters, with translation, notes, and appendix, 253 p. (London: Heinemann). Another translation in modern English from a more or less literary point of view is: WYCK, W. van, 1934: The sinister shepherd: a translation of Girolamo Fracastoro's Syphilidis sive de morbo gallico libri tres, 88 p. (Los Angeles, Calif.: Primavera). A German translation: SECKENDORF, E. A., ed., 1960: Girolamo Fracastoro. Syphilidis sive morbi gallici libri tres, 90 p. (Schriftenreihe der Nordwestdeutschen Dermatologischen Gesellschaft, Vol. VI) (Kiel: Lipsius & Tischler). This German translation is in trochees and hence much more pleasant to read than the hexameters of the original and of the usual verse translations.

——, WRIGHT, W. C., ed., 1930: Hieronymi Fracastorii De contagione et contagiosis morbis et eorum curatione, libri III. Translation and notes, 57 + 356 p. (N.Y. Acad. of Medicine, Hist. of Med. Series, No. 11) (New York, N.Y. & London: Putnam).—

> A skilful translation of Fracastoro's text accompanied by a valuable bio-bibliographical introduction and by copious notes. This book has been of great importance for the development of medicine; its text contains a philosophical discussion of the concept of contagion, its contents, signs, differentiation, *etc.,* and a summing-up of contagious diseases known by Fracastoro *(e.g.,* poxes, measles, pestilent fevers, typhus, leprosy, scabies, *etc.),* their treatment, specific character, recognition, *etc.*

Frank, Johann Peter (1745-1821) — FRANK, J. P., 1960: Akademische Rede vom Volkselend als der Mutter der Krankheiten (Pavia 1790), 64 p. (Eingeleitet, ins Deutsche übertragen und mit Erklärungen versehen von E. LESKY) (Sudhoffs Klassiker der Medizin, No. 34) (Leipzig: Barth).—

> This lecture meant a turning point in the prevailing ideas about disease. Before Frank's time people generally believed that disease was sent by God; in this lecture Frank spoke the words: "Der grösste Teil der Leiden, die uns bedrücken, kommt vom Menschen selbst".

——, LESKY, E., ed., 1969: Johann Peter Frank. Seine Selbstbiographie, 166 p. (Hubers Klassiker der Med. u. d. Naturwiss., Vol. 12) (Bern & Stuttgart: Huber).—

> Frank started his life as a poor waif, and later on he became one of the greatest medical teachers and practitioners of his time. Between 1777 and 1788 he published his "System einer vollständigen medicinischen Polizey" in 4 vols. (Mannheim: Schwann), which publication can be considered as the foundation of modern public hygiene. The present study contains an evaluation of Frank as a reformer of medical education; the larger part (p. 25-160) contains his autobiography. Bibliography and index. *Cf.* also: DOLL, K., 1909: Dr. Johann Peter Frank, 1745-1821. Der Begründer der Medizinalpolizei und der Hygiene als Wissenschaften. Ein Lebensbild, 85 p. (Karlsruhe: Braun).

Fréypolizeicq, Léon (1854-1935) — FLORKIN, M., 1943: Léon Fréydericq et les débuts de la physiologie en Belgique, 104 p. (Collection nationale, 3me série, No. 36) (Brussels: Office de publicité).—

> Léon Fréypolizeicq, sometime professor of physiology in the University of Liege, has been one of the leading physiologists of his time. This well-written biography contains much information concerning other Belgian physiologists as well; as such it is a valuable historical review of the situation of Belgian physiology from *ca.* 1875 up to 1943. Included is a bibliography of Fréypolizeicq's papers published between 1875 and 1943. *Cf.* also: Un pionnier de la physiologie, Léon Fréypolizeicq. Volume publié à l'occasion du centenaire de sa naissance. Oeuvres choisies, 233 p. (Liège: Sciences et Lettres; Paris: Masson).

Freud, Sigmund (1856-1939) — ANDERSSON, O., 1962: Studies in the prehistory of psychoanalysis: the etiology of psychoneuroses and some related themes in Sigmund Freud's scientific writings and letters 1886-1896, 237 p. (Studia Scientiae Pedagogicae Upsaliensia, Vol. 3) (Uppsala: Norstedts).—

According to the author's own words, it is his aim "to contribute to the knowledge of the development of Sigmund Freud's ideas regarding the etiology of the psychoneuroses", and "to contribute to the knowledge of the development of Sigmund Freud's ideas regarding the psychoneuroses", and he does so by studying the period between 1886, when Freud became acquainted with Charcot's ideas about hysteria, and 1896, when the term "Psychoanalysis" was used for the first time in order to describe Freud's method of research and treatment.

——, BINSWANGER, L., 1956: Erinnerungen an Sigmund Freud, 120 p. (Bern: Francke).—

This book consists essentially of letters exchanged between Freud and Binswanger.

——, COSTIGAN, G., 1965: Sigmund Freud, a short biography, 306 p. (New York, N.Y.: Macmillan).—

A popular and very readable account of Freud's life. Another short biography is: KLAGSBRUN, F., 1967: Sigmund Freud, 160 p. (Immortals of Science Series) (New York, N.Y.: Watts).

——, FREUD, E. L., ed., 1961: Letters of Sigmund Freud 1873-1939, 464 p. (London: Hogarth).—

This series of over 300 letters of Sigmund Freud has been edited by his son. The letters cover a very wide field; there are 102 letters written to his wife, but also letters written to such men as: Karl Abraham, Ferenczi, E. Jones, C. G. Jung, Einstein, Th. Mann, Schnitzler, A. and St. Zweig, H. G. Wells, and R. Rolland.

——, FREUD, S., 1952: An autobiographical study, 141 p. (New York, N.Y.: Norton).—

This work was originally published in 1925; in 1927 it appeared in English translation. This is mainly a new edition of the English translation with footnotes and annotations.

——, JONES, E., 1953-1957: The life and work of Sigmund Freud. Vol. I (1953): The formative years and the great discoveries, 1856-1900, 428 p.; Vol. II (1955): Years of maturity, 1901-1919, 512 p.; Vol. III (1957): The last phase, 1919-1939, 537 p. (New York, N.Y.: Basic Bks.; London: Hogarth).—

An authoritative and well-written biography of Sigmund Freud, including much material from the Freud family archives (especially letters written by Freud). Vol. II starts with the period during which the author was close to Freud, and deals with such topics as: the controversy between Freud and Jung; the technique, theory and applications of psychoanalysis; Freud's way of life and way of working; his character and personality. Vol. III, p. 1-250 are of a biographical character, the rest consists of a historical review of Freud's work: clinical contributions, metapsychology, lay analysis, biology, anthropology, sociology, religion, occultism, art, and literature.

——, ROBERT, M., 1966: The psychoanalytic revolution: Sigmund Freud's life and achievements, 396 p. (Transl. from the French edition, Paris, 1964, by K. MORGAN) (New York, N.Y.: Harcourt, Brace, & World).—

A biographical study mainly based upon the Fliess-Freud correspondence, uncovering some new aspects of Freud's character. A translation of: ROBERT, M., 1964: La révolution psychoanalytique. La vie et l'oeuvre de Sigmund Freud, 2 vols., 256 + 286 p. (Paris: Payot).

Frisch, Karl von (1886-   ) — FRISCH, K. VON, 1967: A biologist remembers, 200 p. (Monographs in History and Philosophy of Science, Vol. 1) (Oxford & New York, N.Y.: Pergamon).—

Von Frisch has been one of the foremost students of animal behaviour, and is well known for his discoveries on the language, behaviour, and senses of the honey bees and for his work on the behaviour of fishes. This is a well-written autobiography in English translation. Originally published in German: Erinnerungen eines Biologen, 172 p. (Berlin, Göttingen & Heidelberg: Springer).

Fuchs, Leonhart (1501-1566) — MARZELL, H., ed., 1938: Leonhart Fuchs. New

Kreüterbuch. Faksimildruck der ersten deutschen Ausgabe (1543) vermehrt durch einen wissenschaftlichen Anhang, 444 + 81 p. + 518 woodcut-illustrations. (Leipzig: Koehler).—

This herbal was originally published in 1542 under the title: "De historia stirpium", dealing with about four hundred native German, and one hundred foreign plants. A year later a German edition followed of which this book is a facsimile reprint. This herbal is of special importance for its beautiful illustrations. H. MARZELL wrote an appendix (of 81 pages) in which all that is known about Fuchs and his work has been brought together, in which the various editions of this herbal have been considered and its contents are analysed in relation to other Renaissance herbals. Moreover, Marzell identifies all plants mentioned by Fuchs and discusses their medical applications, then and now. Extensive indexes. *Cf.* also: BERNUS, A. VON & H. FRANKE, 1935: Von Kraft und Wirkung der Kräuter. Nach dem New Kräuterbüchlein des Leonhart Fuchs, 143 p. (Heilbronn: Salzer).

——, SPRAGUE, T. A. & E. NELMES, 1931: The herbal of Leonhart Fuchs, 97 p. (J. Linn. Soc., London, Bot. section, 48: 545-642).—

This publication gives a short biographical review, and discusses preparation and general characteristics of the herbal, bibliographical sources of the herbal, Fuchs' taxonomy and nomenclature, the scientific value of the herbal, Fuchs' place in the history of botany, and it contains a systematic conceptus of the plants figured, and an identification of these figures.

——, STÜBLER, E., 1928: Leonhart Fuchs. Leben und Werk, 135 p. (Münchener Beitr. Gesch. u. Lit. Naturw. u. Medizin) (Munich: Verlag der Münchner Drucke).—

An evaluation of Fuchs' botanical achievements. In order to complete his picture, the author also discusses Fuchs' other scientific activities, *viz.,* his activities as translator and commentator of the books of Hippocrates and Galen, his interest for the medical problems of his time, and his activities as compiler of medical textbooks written from an anti-Arabic point of view.

Gall, Franz Joseph (1758-1828) — ACKERKNECHT, E. & H. VALLOIS, 1956: Franz Joseph Gall, inventor of phrenology and his

collection, 86 p. (Madison, Wisc.: Univ. Wisconsin Medical School).—

An attempt to place Gall's contributions to the science of medicine in a historical perspective and an attempt to illustrate the importance of Gall's ideas for the development of the concept of cerebral localization. Besides, it contains much biographical information and a description of Gall's collection of skulls, casts of heads, and casts of brains, presently located in the Muséum d'Histoire Naturelle of Paris. Originally published in French: François Joseph Gall et sa collection, 92 p. (Mém. Muséum nat. d'Hist. Nat., série A, Zoologie, Vol. X, fasc. 1: 1-92). *Cf.* also: RITTER, W., ed., 1958: Essays published in honour of the discoverer of the physiology of the brain, Fr. J. Gall, 1758-1958. (London: Lauriston Literature & Art Society). Unfortunately I am not able to give more details about the contents of this book.

——, LANTÉRI-LAURA, G., 1970: Histoire de la phrénologie. L'homme et son cerveau selon F. J. Gall, 263 p. (Paris: Presses Univ. de France).—

The text consists of five chapters, *viz.,* Le cerveau et le crâne, objets d'investigation scientifique au XVIIIe siècle; L'oeuvre et la pensée de F. J. Gall (sources, anatomical and physiological work, knowledge of phrenology); L'expansion de la phrénologie (the influence of Gall); Le declin; L'ombre de la phrénologie sur la culture contemporaine. Valuable bibliography (p. 239-262) including the works published by Gall and by Spurzheim; literature dealing with the anatomy, physiology, and pathology of the brain; studies on phrenology.

Galton, Francis (1822-1911) — PEARSON, K., 1914-1930: The life, letters and labours of Francis Galton, 3 vols. Vol. I (1914): Birth 1822 to marriage 1853, 248 p.; Vol. II (1921): Researches of middle life, 425 p.; Vol. IIIA (1930): Correlation, personal identification and eugenics, 441 p.; Vol. IIIB (1930): Characterization, especially by letters. Index, 673 p. (Cambridge: U.P.).—

This probably is one of the most elaborate biographies ever devoted to a man of science. A large part of the first vol. is devoted to a study of Galton's ancestry; then elaborate accounts follow of his childhood, boyhood, and medical and mathematical studies. In the second vol. the author analyses and discusses every work of Galton. Vol. IIIA consists of three parts, *viz.,*

Correlation and the application of statistics to the problems of heredity; Personal identification and description (*i.e.*, finger-prints); and Eugenics as a creed and the last decade of Galton's life. Vol. IIIB is mainly a collection of letters and documents covering the whole of Galton's life.

Galvani, Luigi (1737-1798) — GALVANI, L., 1954: Commentary on the effect of electricity on muscular motion (transl. by M. G. FOLEY, with notes and introduction by I. B. COHEN), together with a facsimile of Galvani's "De viribus electricitatis in motu musculari commentarius" (1791), and a bibliography of the editions and translations of Galvani's books (prepared by J. F. FULTON & M. E. STANTON), 176 p. (Norwalk, Conn.: Burndy Library).—

In this book Galvani's work has been considered apart from the conclusions Volta drew from it. The book starts with an introduction to Galvani's book, in which the results of Galvani's experiments have been treated in the light of his own time. Cohen gives in connection an exposition of the state reached by the science of electricity in the middle of the 18th century. The effect of the publication of Galvani's book is briefly considered. The translation follows on p. 45-91; it is written in the kind of English that Galvani himself might have used had he been writing in English; it is followed by the original Latin text of 1791 (p. 101-156). Many (some copious) footnotes containing a mass of biographical, bibliographical and explanatory information and a bibliography of 20 pages of Galvani's writings on animal electricity have been added. One year previously, another English translation of Galvani's treatise was published by GREEN, R. M., ed., 1953: A translation of Luigi Galvani's "De viribus electricitatis . . .", 97 p. (Cambridge, Mass.: Licht). In 1889 a German translation appeared, prepared by A. J. VON OETTINGEN, in: Ostwalds Klassiker der exakten Wissenschaften, No. 52, 76 p., under the title: "Abhandlung über die Kräfte der Electricität bei der Muskelbewegung" (Leipzig: Engelmann).

Garrison, Fielding Hudson (1870-1937) — KAGAN, S., 1948: Fielding H. Garrison: a biography, 104 p. (Boston, Mass.: Medico-Historical Press).—

A chronological description of life and work of the well-known medical historian F. H. Garrison, for the greater part illustrated by letters written by him. The same author also published: Life and letters of Fielding H. Garrison, 1938, 287 p. (Boston, Mass.: Medico-Historical Press); with the text of the letters, plates, including portraits, and a bibliography.

Geddes, Patrick (1854-1932) — BOARDMAN, P., 1944: Patrick Geddes: maker of the future, 504 p. (Chapel Hill, N.C.: Univ. North Carolina Press).—

A very readable introduction to the life and work of P. Geddes, professor of botany at Dundee, who was so actively engaged in many aspects of social life. Geddes was among the first to recognize the fallaciousness of the "struggle for existence"-hypotheses and to emphasize the phenomena of cooperation and altruism in nature, which factors would also have played an important role in the evolution of Man. He was actively engaged in many sociological projects (*e.g.*, the establishment of the "first sociological laboratory in the world", the foundation of a student hotel in Scotland), always acting to make the world a happier place in which to live. Besides these (social and biological) activities he was engaged in town planning and was the designer and builder of the Hebrew University of Jerusalem. A French biography is: BOARDMAN, P. L., 1936: Esquisse de l'oeuvre éducative de Patrick Geddes, suivie de trois listes bibliographiques, 203 p. (Montpellier: Imp. de la Charité). *Cf.* TYRWHITT, J., ed., 1947: Patrick Geddes in India: extracts from official reports on Indian cities in 1915-1919, 103 p. (London: Humphries).

Geminus, Thomas (fl. 1540-1560) — GEMINUS, T., 1959: Compendiosa totius anatomie delineatio: a facsimile of the first English edition of 1553 in the version of Nicholas Udall, 39 + 200 p. (Introd. by C. D. O'MALLEY) (London: Dawson).—

For the better education of the barber-surgeons in England a simple and relatively brief manual or guide to dissection was needed. Geminus had prepared copperengraved illustrations, derived from Vesalius' works. With the aid of royal participation, these engravings became the basis of such a guide, and probably Vesalius' text has been used, because this suited the available engravings so well. In this way the "Compendious anatomy" was born, and although it has nothing to offer to the knowledge of anatomy, it played a very great role in the dissemination of Vesalius' achievements in England and elsewhere. The introduction contains much biographical information concerning Geminus and discusses other cases of plagiarism of Vesalius' works. This introduction is followed by a photo-litho offset reproduction of the "Compendious anatomy". *Cf.* LARKEY, S. V., 1933: The Vesalian compendium of Geminus and Nicholas Udall's translation: their relation to Vesalius, Caius, Vicary, and De Mondeville. (Trans. Bibl. Soc.).

Geoffroy Saint-Hilaire, Étienne (1772-1844) — CAHN, T., 1962: La vie et l'oeuvre d'Étienne Geoffroy Saint-Hilaire, 318 p. (Paris: Presses Univ. de France).—

A discussion of the work of the great French naturalist É. Geoffroy Saint-Hilaire within the framework of his time and in its relation with his contemporaries, esp. Goethe and the biologists of German Romanticism. The author follows the trend of thought of Isidore Geoffroy Saint-Hilaire's biography of his father but adds much new information, factual as well as philosophical. Of especial importance is the discussion between É. Geoffroy Saint-Hilaire and Cuvier.

Gerard, John (1545-1612) — WOOD-WARD, M., ed., 1927: Gerard's Herball: the essence thereof distilled by M. Woodward, from the edition of Th. Johnson, 1636, 303 p. (London: Howe).—

In 1597 Gerard's "Herball" was published, which appeared to be an adaptation, mainly of the "Stirpium historiae pemptades" of Dodoens published in 1583 *(cf.* DODONAEUS, *vide supra).* A second edition of this "Herball" with considerable improvements and additions was brought out by Thomas Johnson, a London apothecary, in 1633 and reprinted in 1636. The present work is an abridgement of Johnson's edition of 1636, illustrated with reproductions of the original woodcuts. The introduction contains some biographical information. Reprinted 1964 (London: Spring Bks.). *Cf.* also: WOODWARD, M., 1931: Leaves from Gerard's Herball, 305 p. (London: Howe). With 130 illustrations after the original woodcuts.

Gesner, Konrad (1516-1565) — FRETZ, D., 1948: Konrad Gessner als Gärtner, 312 p. (Zurich: Atlantis).—

The largest part (p. 133-312) deals with the plants Gesner cultivated in his garden. Besides, the book contains much biographical information especially about his activities in and publications on gardening. Other special studies of Gesner are: GÜNTHER, H., 1933: Konrad Gessner als Tier-

arzt, 61 p. (Diss. Univ. Leipzig) (Leipzig: Edelmann); and THÉODORIDÈS, J., 1966: Conrad Gesner et la zoologie: les invertébrés (Gesnerus 23: 230-237).

——, LEY, W., 1929: Konrad Gesner. Leben und Werk, 154 p. (Münchener Beitr. Gesch. u. Lit. Naturwiss. u. Medizin, 15/16) (Munich: Verlag der Münchener Drucke).—

Separate chapters deal with such subjects as: Gesner's life (p. 3-40), his zoological (p. 115-121) achievements, his knowledge of fossils (p. 122-131), Gesner as a physician (p. 137-150), and his publications (p. 151-154). There exists a more recent publication which seems to contain much supplementary biographical information, but unfortunately I have not been able to consult it: FISCHER, H., *et al.,* 1967: Conrad Gesner 1516-1565. Universalgelehrter, Naturforscher, Arzt, 239 p. (Zurich: Orell Füssli).

Goethe, Johann Wolfgang von (1749-1832) — ARBER, A., 1946: Goethe's botany, 61 p. (Chronica Botanica 10: 63-124) (Also separate: Waltham, Mass.: Chronica Botanica).—

This publication mainly consists of English translations of Goethe's "Versuch die Metamorphose der Pflanzen zu erklären", and of the fragment afterwards known as "Die Natur". Both translations are preceded by informative introductions.

——, CARUS, C. G., 1948: Goethe. Zu dessen näherem Verständnis, und Briefe über Goethes Faust, 287 p. (Mit Einl. hrsg. von E. MERIAN-GENAST) (Zurich: Rotapfel).—

A very beautiful reprint (with portraits) of the original text, first published in 1843. Carus was a contemporary of Goethe and a distinguished biologist, physician, natural philosopher, and psychologist *(vide supra).* Carus gives much first-hand biographical information, based on a rather extensive correspondence and on personal contact, including some particulars concerning Goethe's illnesses and personality structure. There also exists a pocket edition, 1948, 216 p. (Herford: Die Arche).

——, FISCHER, H., 1950: Goethes Naturwissenschaft, 94 p. (Zurich: Artemis).—

A short account of Goethe's researches in natural science, discussing his studies in physiognomy, morphology, metamorphosis of plants, comparative anatomy, chemistry, geology, and colour theory. He relates this information to Goethe's general approach to nature and science, and he gives his interpretation against the background of scientific research and philosophy of the time. A pocket-edition of Goethe's publications on zoology, anatomy and physiognomy is: GOETHE, J. W. von, 1962: Schriften zur vergleichenden Anatomie, zur Zoologie und Physiognomik, 227 p. (Munich: Deutscher Taschenbuch Verlag). *Cf.* also: RITTERSBACHER, K., ed., 1968: Der Naturforscher Goethe in Selbstzeugnissen. Ein Beitrag zur Erkenntnis seiner Naturanschauung, 292 p. (Freiburg i.B.: Verlag die Kommenden). In 1947 the "Akademie der Naturforscher (Leopoldina)" (Halle/Saale, DDR) began the publication of all Goethe's works in the field of the (natural) sciences (under the editorship of R. MATTHAEI, G. SCHMIDT, W. TROLL and K. L. WOLF. All volumes to be published (12 in all) will be accompanied by annotations and commentaries. They are published by Böhlau (Weimar). I could trace the following vols.: Abteilung I (Texts): Vol. I (1947): Schriften zur Geologie und Mineralogie 1770-1810, 393 p. (ed. by G. SCHMIDT). Reprinted in 1956 and 1968; Vol. 3 (1951): Beiträge zur Optik und Anfänge der Farbenlehre 1790-1808, 539 p. (ed. by R. MATTHAEI); Vol. 4 (1955): Zur Farbenlehre, 266 p. (ed. by R. MATTHAEI); Vol. 5 (1958): Zur Farbenlehre. Polemischer Teil, 195 p. (ed. by R. MATTHAEI); Vol. 6 (1957): Zur Farbenlehre. Historischer Teil, 450 p. (ed. by D. KUHN); Vol. 7 (1957?) Zur Farbenlehre. Anzeige und Uebersicht, statt des supplementaren Teils und Erklärung der Tafeln, 135 p. + 24 figs. (ed. by R. MATTHAEI); Vol. 8 (1963): Naturwissenschaftliche Hefte, 427 p. (ed. by D. KUHN); Vol. 9 (1954): Morphologische Hefte, 389 p. (ed. by D. KUHN); Vol. 10 (1964): Aufsätze, Fragmente, Studien zur Morphologie, 408 p. (ed. by D. KUHN). Abteilung II, Vol. 3 (1961): Beiträge zur Optik und Anfänge der Farbenlehre. Ergänzungen und Erläuterungen, 52 + 453 p. (ed. by R. MATTHAEI & D. KUHN); Vol. 6 (1959): Ergebnisse und Erläuterungen zu Band 6: Zur Farbenlehre, historischer Teil, 640 p. (ed. by R. MATTHAEI & D. KUHN).

——, MAGNUS, R., 1949: Goethe as a scientist, 259 p. (New York, N.Y.: Schuman).——

An English translation of the original German edition which has been based on a series of lectures delivered at the University of Heidelberg in 1906. The author tries to evaluate the entirety of Goethe's scientific efforts, and the book actually is a profound defense of the scientific prominence and importance of Goethe. Original German edition: MAGNUS, R., 1906: Goethe als Naturforscher, 336 p. (Leipzig: Barth).

——, MUELLER, B., ed., 1952: Goethe's botanical writings, 258 p. (Honolulu, Hawaii: Univ. Hawaii Press).——

This is a collection of Goethe's major and minor writings on botanical subjects. Most of the material translated in this vol. is taken from notes and essays which Goethe published from 1817 to 1824 in journal form. The subjects are grouped as follows: "On morphology", "On his plant studies", and "On general theory". *Cf.* also TROLL, W., ed., n.d., Goethe's morphologische Schriften, 487 p. (Jena: Diederichs).

——, SCHMIDT, G., 1940: Goethe und die Naturwissenschaften. Eine Bibliographie, 620 p. (Halle/Saale: Leopoldinisch-Carolinisch Deutsche Akademie der Naturforscher).——

A magnificent and very complete bibliography, containing the literature from and on Goethe published before 1940, comprising 4,554 items. It consists of 3 parts: I: Works in the field of the natural sciences, published by Goethe himself (with many bibliophilous details); II: Literature concerning Goethe and the natural sciences (arranged according to subject); III: Goethe's contacts with individual natural scientists and physicians (arranged alphabetically). Purely literary works have been excluded for reasons of economy. This bibliography is intended for students of the history of the natural sciences, but is also addressed to specialists in the field of the history of (German) literature, bibliophilists, *etc.* A new bibliography started in 1955, ed. by H. PYRITZ, and was continued by H. NICOLAI, published in fascicules by Winter (Heidelberg).

——, URDANG, G., 1949: Goethe and pharmacy, 76 p. (Madison, Wisc.: Amer. Inst. Hist. Pharmacy).——

Sarton writes about this booklet: "This handsome volume contains all the facts concerning Goethe's interest in pharmacy, and many portraits of the pharmacists with whom he was in contact, either as an individual, or as a Weimar administrator."

——, VIËTOR, K., 1949: Goethe. Dichtung, Wissenschaft, Weltbild, 600 p. (Bern: Francke).——

The text has been divided into 3 parts: I: Der Dichter; II: Der Naturforscher; III: Der Denker. The second part contains a comprehensive survey of Goethe's scientific activities and writings and the development of Goethe's concept of nature. There are chapters on: Goethe's mode of cognition, on the question as to whether or not Goethe can be considered as a predecessor of Darwin, on the discovery of the human os maxillare, on his theory of colour, his geology and meteorology. An English edition appeared in two volumes: Goethe the poet, 1949, 341 p.; and Goethe the thinker, 1950, 212 p. (Cambridge, Mass.: Harvard U.P.).

Goldschmidt, Richard Benedikt (1878-1959) — GOLDSCHMIDT, R. B., 1960: In and out of the ivory tower: the autobiography of Richard B. Goldschmidt, 352 p. (Seattle, Wash.: Univ. Washington Press).—

In this autobiography the author describes his own (important) scientific activities in an appendix of less than 15 pages, excluding the bibliography which contains nearly 300 entries. This book, the last which the author completed just before his death, deals with many different subjects, for Goldschmidt not only was a geneticist or zoologist, but also a world traveller and a connoisseur of art and of men, so that this book gives a lively description of the life of the author outside the research laboratory. Much information concerning famous biologists can be found in it.

Gosse, Philip Henry (1810-1888) — STAGEMAN, P., 1955: A bibliography of the first editions of Philip Henry Gosse, F.R.S., 87 p. (Cambridge: The Golden Head).—

P. H. Gosse was an English naturalist who wrote a number of books on natural history which were very popular in Victorian England, especially his books dealing with marine animals. This bibliography of the first editions of his books (p. 25-77) is preceded by a short biographical note, a list of works in order of publication, an alphabetical list of titles, and two short essays dealing with illustrations and scientific works of Gosse. The bibliography is followed by a list of contributions to periodicals and a list of pamphlets and tracts of which no copies have been traced.

Graaf, Reinier de (1641-1673) — GRAAF, R. de, 1965: De mulierum organis generationi inservientibus, 1672, 334 p. (Facsimile with an introduction by J. A. VAN DON-

GEN) (Dutch Classics on History of Science, Vol. 13) (Nieuwkoop, The Netherlands: de Graaf).—

This work contains the first coherent presentation of the female reproductive tract. It presents, in addition to the original text and illustrations, a concise biographical note (of 26 pages), a bibliography, and iconography. There also exists a reprint of chapters 1 to 7 (out of 11), together with a Dutch translation of his "Tractatus anatomico-medicus de succi pancreati natura et usu", originally published as a thesis in Leiden in 1664. This translation was first printed in 1686 and was reprinted in 1927 in the Opuscula selecta Neerlandicorum de arte medica, fasc. sextus, p. 182-293. (Amsterdam: Nederlandsch Tijdschr. Geneeskunde). Cf. BARGE, J. A. J., 1942: Reinier de Graaf, 1641-1941, 26 p. (Med. Kon. Ned. Akad. Wetensch., afd. Letterk., N. R., Vol. 5, No. 5).

Gray, Asa (1810-1888) — DUPREE, A. H., 1959: Asa Gray, 1810-1888, 505 p. (Harvard, Mass.: Harvard U.P.).—

Asa Gray was the leading American botanist of the 19th century who greatly stimulated botanical exploration and who was the most effective protagonist in America of Charles Darwin's views. He became a friend of Darwin and collaborated with Darwin in the field of botany until the end of Darwin's life. The present book is a full-scale biography of Asa Gray, based on original sources, mainly letters.

——— ——— ed., 1963: Darwiniana by Asa Gray, 327 p. (Cambridge, Mass.: Harvard U.P.).—

This is a reprint of a collection of Gray's pieces on Darwinism, first published in 1876. The articles included are: 1. The origin of species by means of natural selection; 2. Design versus necessity - a discussion; 3. Natural selection not inconsistent with natural theology; 4. Species as to variation, geographical distribution, and succession; 5. Sequoia and its history: the relations of North American to the Northeast Asian and to Tertiary vegetation; 6. The attitude of working naturalists toward Darwinism; 7. Evolution and theology; 8. "What is Darwinism?"; 9. Charles Darwin: a sketch accompanying a portrait in "Nature"; 10. Insectivorous plants; 11. Insectivorous and climbing plants; 12. Duration and origination of race and species; 13. Evolutionary teleology.

——, GRAY, J. L., ed., 1893: Letters of Asa Gray, 2 vols., 838 p. (London: Macmillan).—

It is the aim of the editor to show, as far as possible in his own words, the life and occupations of Asa Gray, the famous American botanist who did so much to introduce Darwin's theory into America. Those parts of his letters have been given which contain something of the personality of the man and of his many interests. These letters are preceded by a brief sketch of his early life, which is a fragment of an autobiography as it had been planned by Gray himself. Vol. I deals with the period 1810-1850, Vol. II with the period 1850-1888.

——, SARGENT, C. S., 1889: Scientific papers of Asa Gray. Vol. I: Reviews of works on botany and related subjects 1834-1887, 397 p.; Vol. II: Essays; biographical sketches 1841-1886, 503 p. (London: Macmillan).—

Vol. I contains reviews of books of: Lindley, de Candolle, Endlicher, Harvey, von Siebold, Moquin-Tandon, Agassiz, von Mohl, Ward, Hooker & Thomson, Henfrey, Naudin, Weddell, Radlkofer, Boussingault, Bentham, de Vilmorin, Engelmann, Curtis, Darwin, Watson, Decaisne, Ruskin, Emerson, Henslow, Ball. Vol. II contains 14 essays and biographical sketches of: Brown, von Humboldt, de Candolle, Greene, Short, Boott, Hooker, Lindley, Harvey, Sartwell, Dewey, Ward, Curtis, von Mohl, Wight, Welwitsch, Torrey, Sullivant, Wyman, Hanbury, von Braun, Pickering, Fries, Bigelow, Carey, James, Lowell, Darwin, Decaisne, Engelmann, Heer, Bentham, Fendler, Wright, Clinton, Boissier, Roeper, Agassiz, Tuckerman.

Grew, Nehemiah (1641-1712) — GREW, N., 1965: The anatomy of plants with an idea of a philosophical history of plants and several other lectures read before the Royal Society, 323 p. (Facsimile of the 1682 edition) (Sources of Science, No. 11) (New York, N.Y.: Johnson).—

Grew's "Anatomy of plants" is a botanical classic. Grew began his observations on the anatomy of plants in 1664 and in 1670 his essay "The anatomy of vegetables begun" was communicated to the Royal Society. In 1672 publication followed. This is a facsimile of the 1682 edition, preceded by an introduction by C. ZIRKLE. *Cf*. also: HOSKIN, M. A., ed., 1963: Experiments in

consort of the luctation arising from the affusion of several menstruums upon all sorts of bodies, exhibited to the Royal Society, April 13 and June 1, 1676, 118 p. (A facsimile of the edition of 1678) (Cambridge: Heffer).

Griesinger, Wilhelm (1817-1868) — GRIESINGER, W., 1965: Mental pathology and therapeutics, 530 p. (Library New York Acad. Med., Hist. Med. Series, No. 26) (New York, N.Y.: Hafner).—

Griesinger has to be remembered for his statement that mental disorders are diseases of the brain. The present book is a facsimile of the English translation (1867) of the second German ed. (1861) of Griesinger's textbook. Introduction by E. H. ACKERKNECHT.

Haeckel, Ernst (1834-1919) — DE GROOD, D. H., 1965: Haeckel's theory of the unity of nature: a monograph in the history of philosophy, 98 p. (Boston, Mass.: Christopher).—

The subjects dealt with in this monograph which are of special value to the historian of biology are: the place of naturalism in the 19th century, the making of Haeckel's philosophy, monism and evolution, the unity of nature and the riddles of the universe, Haeckel's antagonists (Oliver Lodge, Friedrich Paulsen, Ralph Barton Perry), evaluation of Haeckel's work. Bibliography.

——, HEBERER, G., 1968: Der gerechtfertigte Haeckel. Einblicke in seine Schriften aus Anlass des Erscheinens seines Hauptwerkes "Generelle Morphologie der Organismen" vor 100 Jahren, 588 p. (Stuttgart: Fischer).—

The larger part of this book consists of a selection from Haeckel's writings, mainly derived from his "Generelle Morphologie" (p. 45-490). Included are some fragments derived from his journals prepared during his many voyages and some fragments from his works dealing with his monistic philosophy. Extensive Index.

——, SCHMIDT, H., 1934: Ernst Haeckel. Denkmal eines grossen Lebens, 118 p. (Jena: Frommann).—

This biography has been published on the occasion of the centenary of Haeckel's birthday (Feb. 16, 1834). It contains much information concerning his ancestry, family, life, education, scientific achievements, his attitudes as a Darwinist and as a monist, his activities as a teacher, artist, and nationalist. Included are a description of his mental characteristics and some family and personal portraits. More recent biographical studies are: HEMLEBEN, J., 1964: Ernst Haeckel in Selbstzeugnissen und Bilddokumenten, 160 p. (Rowohlts Monographien, No. 99) (Reinbek bei Hamburg: Rowohlt); and: KLEMM, P., 1966: Ernst Haeckel. Der Ketzer von Jena. Ein Leben in Berichten, Briefen und Bildern, 247 p. (Jena: Urania).

———, USCHMANN, G., 1954: Ernst Haeckel. Forscher, Künstler, Mensch, 244 p. (Jena: Urania).—

> With the aid of letters written by Haeckel, the author gives a picture of life, education, travels, scientific and artistic activities, *etc.,* of E. Haeckel. 8 coloured plates of paintings prepared by Haeckel have been included. His youthful correspondence has been edited and translated by GIFFORD, G. B., 1923: The story of the development of a youth by Ernst Haeckel: letters to his parents 1852-1856, 420 p. (New York, N.Y. & London: Harper). Another work containing much biographical information, of which, however, I have not been able to find further information is: FRANZ, V., 1943-1944: Ernst Haeckel. Sein Leben, Denken und Wirken. Eine Schriftenfolge für seine zahlreichen Freunde und Anhänger, 2 Vols. (Jena & Leipzig).

Hahnemann, Samuel (1775-1843) — HAEHL, R., 1922: Samuel Hahnemann. Sein Leben und Schaffen auf Grund neu aufgefundener Akten, Urkunden, Briefe, Krankenberichte und unter Benützung der gesamten in- und ausländischen homöopathischen Literatur, 2 vols. Vol. I. 508 p.; Vol. II: 527 p. (Unter Mitw. von K. SCHMIDT-BUHL) (Leipzig: Schwabe).—

> Extensive biography of Samuel Hahnemann, the famous German homoeopathic physician. Also included are many biographical notes concerning his pupils and contemporaries, both living in Germany as well as abroad, particularly in the United States, and a review of hospitals working according to the homoeopathic method. The second volume is supplementary, containing original documents, such as: letters, reports, bibliographical notes, *etc.* Also in English translation: Samuel Hahnemann: his life and work, 1931, 2 vols. (Ed. by J. H. CLARKE

& F. J. WHEELER) (London: Homoeopathic Publ. Comp.). Some popular biographies of Hahnemann are: HOBHOUSE, R. W., 1933: Life of Christian Samuel Hahnemann, founder of homoeopathy, 288 p. (London: Daniel), largely derived from the biography of the late Richard Haehl; GUMPERT, M., 1945: Hahnemann: the adventurous career of a medical rebel, 251 p. (New York, N.Y.: Fischer), a well-written, but rather idealized, portrait of Hahnemann, originally published in German; LARNANDIE, R., 1954: La vie prodigieuse de Christian-Samuel Hahnemann inventeur de l'homéopathie, 270 p. (Paris: Bonne). A popular biography in the French language.

Haldane, John Burdon Sanderson (1892-1964) — CLARK, R. W., 1968: J. B. S.: the life and work of J. B. S. Haldane, 286 p. (London: Hodder and Stoughton; New York, N.Y.: Coward-McCann).—

> A biography of one of the stormiest, most controversial and most brilliant biologists of our time. Haldane has been reader in biochemistry (Cambridge) and successor of Bateson at the John Innes Horticultural Institution and chairman of the editorial board of the (Communist) "Daily Worker". The last part of his life was spent in India. Haldane's greatest scientific achievements lay in the application of mathematics to evolution. In 1966 a paperback edition of one of his biological masterpieces appeared, *viz.,* HALDANE, J. B. S., 1966: The causes of evolution, 235 p. (Cornell paperback, No. 36) (Ithaca, N.Y.: Cornell U.P.). Originally published in 1932. A study containing much autobiographical information is: HALDANE, J. B. S., 1940: Adventures of a biologist, 281 p. (New York, N.Y.: Harper). An evaluation of Haldane's achievements in and importance for modern biology: DRONAMRAJU, K. R., ed., 1968: Haldane and modern biology, 333 p. (Baltimore, Md.: Johns Hopkins Press; London: Oxford U.P.). An appraisal of Haldane's work, written by 30 of his colleagues.

———, HALDANE, J. B. S., 1968: Science and life: essays of a rationalist, 213 p. (Introd. by J. Maynard SMITH) (London: Pemberton Publishing Company in association with Barry and Rockliff).—

> This book may be considered as the scientific testament of J. B. S. Haldane and consists of essays that were published in the Rationalist Annual between 1929 and 1965. These deal with a wide field of subjects ranging from science to philosophy and religion.

Hales, Stephen (1677-1761) — KENNEDY, A. E. C., 1929: Stephen Hales, D. D., F.R.S.: an eighteenth-century biography, 256 p. (Cambridge: U.P.; New York, N.Y.: Macmillan).—

A biography of this well-known English physiologist, chemist and inventor. Hales applied Newtonian physics to the solution of physiological problems; famous are his experiments on transpiration, capillarity and root pressure in plants and on blood pressure, cardiac output and blood flow in animals, and, according to his biographer, he also discovered the spinal reflexes in frogs. His most famous publication is his "Statical essays". The first vol. "Vegetable staticks" (1727) contains an account of numerous experiments in plant physiology, and the second vol. "Haemostaticks" (1733) contains experiments on the "force of the blood" in various animals. These works have recently been re-published (1964) by Hafner (New York, N.Y.). Of KENNEDY's biography a reprint appeared in 1965 (Ridgewood, N. J.: Gregg).

Haller, Albrecht von (1708-1777) — KING, L. S., ed., 1966: First lines of physiology. Translated from the correct Latin ed. printed under the inspection of William Cullen and compared with the edition published by H. A. Wisberg, 2 vols. in one (Sources of Science, No. 32) (New York, N.Y.: Johnson).—

A reprint of the 1786 edition. In his introduction, the editor places the "First lines" within the framework of 18th-century philosophical debate of biological method. The book was first published in 1749 as a textbook for students; it introduced the medical student to the major functions of the body (e.g., respiration, muscular motion, the senses, digestion, reproduction, etc.), and to the generally accepted ideas on the solids (e.g., fibers, vessels, cellular substances) and humours (blood, secretions).

——, IRSAY, S. d', 1930: Albrecht von Haller. Eine Studie zur Geistesgeschichte der Aufklärung, 98 p. (Arb. Inst. Gesch. Med. Univ. Leipzig, Vol. 1) (Leipzig: Thieme).—

A first attempt to give an account of von Haller's scientific activities. After a short biographical introduction chapters follow on: the scientific aspects of Enlightenment, the philosophical conflict between Voltaire and von Haller, anatomia animata, irritability, medicine, botany and pharmacognosy, von Haller's influence, and bibliographical annotations. A useful alphabetically-arranged bibliography, containing some 720 items, is: LUNDSGAARD-HANSEN-VON FISCHER, S., 1959: Verzeichnis der gedruckten Schriften Albrecht von Hallers, 87 p. (Berner Beitr. Gesch. Med. Naturwiss., No. 18) (Bern: Haupt). Cf. also: VOSS, I., 1937: Das pathologisch-anatomische Werk Albrecht von Hallers in Göttingen, 35 p. (Vorarbeiten zur Geschichte der Göttinger Universität und Bibliothek, Vol. 25); and: ZOLLER, H., 1958: Albrecht von Hallers Pflanzensammlungen in Göttingen. Sein botanisches Werk und sein Verhältniss zu Carl von Linné. (Nachr. der Akad. der Wiss., Göttingen, II. Math.-physikalische Klasse, Jg. 1958, No. 10).

——, SUDHOFF, K., ed., 1922: Von den empfindlichen und reizbaren Teilen des menschlichen Körpers, 58 p. (Sudhoffs Klassiker der Medizin, No. 27) (Leipzig: Barth).—

A German translation of von Haller's "De partibus corporis humani sensibilus et irratibilibus", two lectures delivered by him in 1752 before the Gesellschaft der Wissenschaften of Göttingen. In this study von Haller proved that irritability was an essential property of every muscular tissue. The German translation was made by von Haller in 1772. The study contains a historical review of previous ideas on irritability.

——, ZANETTI, C. & U. WIMMER-AESCHLIMANN, 1968: Eine Geschichte der Anatomie und Physiologie von Albrecht von Haller, 157 p. (Berner Beitr. Gesch. Med. Naturwiss., N.F., Vol. I) (Bern & Stuttgart: Huber).—

The text of this booklet consists of two parts, viz., an anatomical part (p. 11-82), containing a historical account of von Haller's anatomical activities, and a physiological part (p. 83-150), containing a historical account of von Haller's physiological investigations. Both parts place von Haller within the framework of his time.

——, TOELLNER, R., 1969: Albrecht von Haller. Ueber die Einheit im Denken des letzten Universalgelehrten, 180 p. (Sudhoffs Archiv, Beiheft 10) (Wiesbaden: Steiner).—

An attempt has been made to analyse both von Haller's poetical works as well as his scientific works in order to investigate whether a discord could be detected between the poet and the scientist, or between his religion and science. As such the present book may also be considered as a useful contribution to the cultural climate of the 18th century.

Halsted, William Stewart (1852-1922) — CROWE, S. J., 1957: Halsted of Johns Hopkins: the man and his men, 247 p. (Springfield, Ill.: Thomas).—

Halsted was one of the greatest surgeons America has produced. He took a leading part in the introduction in the U.S.A. of the discoveries of Pasteur and their applications by Lister, and he was particularly interested in the processes of the healing of wounds. The present biography has been written by one of his students, and later colleague, at Johns Hopkins. It also contains biographical sketches of some leading members of the "Halsted School", to which, *inter alia*, Harvey Cushing has belonged, *vide supra*. A somewhat older biography of Halsted is: MACCALLUM, W. G., 1930: William Stewart Halsted, surgeon, 241 p. (Baltimore, Md.: Johns Hopkins Press). This book contains a number of portraits of Halsted, a chronological list of his surgical achievements, and a bibliography of publications dealing with his life and work.

Harvey, William (1578-1657) — BRUNN, W. L. von, 1967: Kreislauffunktion in William Harveys Schriften, 161 p. (Berlin: Springer).—

In this booklet the author discusses such problems as: Can Harvey be called a physiologist in the modern sense of the word?; the heart as centre of heat; function of the heart and vessels according to Galen; heat and motion in "De motu cordis et sanguinis"; production and action of the innate heat; blood is its own mover; method of physiology; and the symbolism of circular motion. 46 pages of notes and bibliography.

——, CHAUVOIS, L., 1961: William Harvey. His life and times: his discoveries; his methods, 271 p. (London: Hutchinson).—

A lifelike portrait of Harvey the man and the scientist, an enthusiastic and well-written biography with up-to-date information. Harvey is regarded as the inaugurator of a new era, by giving rise to modern physiology and biological science. Also in a French edition: William Harvey, 1578-1657, sa vie et son temps, ses découvertes, sa méthode, 251 p. (Paris: Soc. d'Éd. d'Enseignement Supérieur).

——, FRANKLIN, K. J., ed., 1957: Movement of the heart and blood in animals: an anatomical essay by William Harvey, 209 p. (Transl. from the original Latin by K. J. FRANKLIN) (Oxford: Blackwell).—

In this translation Franklin tries to bring us closer to Harvey as a person, by preparing a text, which, he supposes, Harvey himself might have written if he were alive in our own century. The Latin text has also been included. The book is very well produced and contains the coloured reproduction of the Janssen portrait of Harvey. *Cf.* WILLIS, R., 1965: *vide infra*.

—— ——, ed., 1958: The circulation of the blood: two anatomical essays by William Harvey, together with nine letters written by him, 184 p. (Oxford: Blackwell).—

This book closely resembles FRANKLIN's "Movement of the heart and blood in animals" *(vide supra)*. To some extent it might be considered to be an appendix to that book, for it summarizes the clinical and experimental observations made since 1628. "De circulatione sanguinis" was first published in 1649, when Harvey published two essays in which he refuted the criticism by Jean Riolan (Paris) of his theories concerning the movement of the heart and circulation. The present edition is preceded by an introductory preface and a short biographical sketch. These are followed by the letters and essays, with short explanatory notes. The Latin version, a short epilogue and selected references complete the volume. There also exists a French translation: La circulation du sang, 1962, 229 p. (Transl. by C. RICHET) (Geneva-Paris-Brussels: Alliance Culturelle du Livre).

—— ——, 1961: William Harvey: Englishman, 133 p. (London: MacGibbon & Kee).—

An authoritative biographical essay full of informative detail and comment. After giving a brief summary of the work of Harvey's predecessors, it proceeds with a biographical description of Harvey's life. Especially his major opus "De motu cordis" is analysed chapter by chapter and its repercussions in Europe are considered. For a complete biography *cf.* KEYNES, G., 1966, *vide infra*.

——, KEELE, K. D., 1965: William Harvey: the man, the physician, and the scientist, 244 p. (British Men of Science, No. 8) (London: Nelson).—

The author tries to put the discovery of the circulation of the blood against the background of Harvey's other activities as a physician or as a scientific researcher, and he tries to elucidate the effect of his discovery on medicine, both at that time and thereafter.

——, KEYNES, G., 1953: A bibliography of the writings of Dr. William Harvey 1578-1657, ed. 2, 79 p. (Cambridge: U.P.).—

An annotated re-publication of the edition of 1928 which was published on the occasion of the 300th anniversary of the publication of Harvey's first and greatest work, "De motu cordis". This bibliography gives full information concerning the works written by Harvey.

—— ——, 1966: The life of William Harvey, 483 p. (Oxford: Clarendon Press).—

An extensive biography of William Harvey, containing a well-documented account of his relations with his colleagues, the College of Physicians, and with St. Bartholomew's Hospital. It also contains a detailed discussion of Harvey's writings. Much attention also has been paid to Harvey's relationship with his contemporaries (e.g., King James, King Charles, Francis Bacon, the Earl of Arundel, Thomas Hobbes, etc.), and to his travels.

——, MEYER, A. W., 1936: An analysis of the "De generatione animalium" of William Harvey, 167 p. (Stanford, Calif.: Stanford U.P.).—

This is the first detailed study of Harvey's embryological treatise "De generatione" (1651). The author places Harvey's work in its historical setting, and discusses Harvey's predecessors and contemporaries in embryology. He also discusses Harvey's philosophical preconceptions and his ideas about spontaneous generation, and on fertilization, his studies on the generation of the chick and the development in mammals. A special chapter has been devoted to his dictum "Ex ovo omnia". Bibliography and index.

——, O'MALLEY, C. D., F. N. L. POYNTER & K. F. RUSSELL, 1961: William Harvey, lectures on the whole of anatomy: an annotated translation of "Prelectiones anatomiae universalis", 239 p. (Berkeley & Los Angeles, Calif.: Univ. California Press).—

The facsimile of the manuscript containing the text of the lectures, together with the transcription made by E. SCOTT, was published under the auspices of the Royal College of Physicians in 1886. The present publication is an improved version of this edition with a multitude of annotations in the text and corrections in many places. The introduction gives a review of the history of anatomical lectures in England. As to the contents of the "Prelectiones", cf. the annotated edition of WHITTERIDGE, 1964, vide infra.

——, PAGEL, W., 1967: William Harvey's biological ideas: selected aspects and historical background, 394 p. (Basle & New York, N.Y.: Karger).—

Separate sections deal with: Harvey and European thought in the 17th century; his "De motu cordis"; his scientific approach and qualification; his circular symbolism; circular symbolism, heart and blood before Harvey; Harvey's predecessors (Galen, Servetus, Realdus Columbus, Vesalius' influence, Cesalpino); Harvey on generation and epigenesis; Harvey's vitalistic criticism of ancient materialism. An appendix deals with Marcus MARCI's "Idea of operative ideas" and Harvey's embryological speculation (p. 285-326). A very useful study.

——, WHITTERIDGE, G., ed., 1959: De motu locali animalium 1627, 163 p. (Cambridge: U.P.).—

This book was published during the commemoration of the tercentenary of the Royal College of Physicians. It gives a good idea of the book on animal movement that Harvey intended to write, but which never was published during his lifetime. A new transcription of the Latin text of the ms. has been made, from which an English translation has been prepared, both published on pages facing each other. Many useful and appropriate editorial annotations have been added in the form of footnotes.

—— ——, ed., 1964: The anatomical lectures of William Harvey: Prelectiones anatomiae universalis; De musculus, 64 + 504 p. (Edinburgh & London: Livingstone).—

Whereas "De musculus" is here printed for the first time, this volume is a great addition to our knowledge of the works of Harvey. The "Prelectiones" (1616) contains general introductory remarks on the subject of anatomy, a discussion of the parts of the body and their classification, a description of the outer parts of the body, a description of the lower belly and the viscera, the middle belly or chest, heart and lungs, and the third belly or head and brain. "De musculus" contains descriptions of the muscles, veins, arteries and nerves of arms and legs, with some account of the muscles of the chest and back. A new transcription of the Latin text has been made, from which a new English translation has been prepared, both published on pages facing each other. *Cf.* also O'MALLEY, *et al.,* 1961, *vide supra.*

——, WILLIS, R., ed., 1965: The works of William Harvey, M. D., 96 + 624 p. (Translated from the Latin with a life of the author) (Sources of Science, No. 13) (New York, N.Y.: Johnson).—

This is a reprint of the 1847 edition. According to KEYNES in his biography of William Harvey *(vide supra),* this is the best translation of the "De motu cordis", and according to a review in J. Hist. Med. 21: 82, FRANKLIN's translation *(vide supra)* is not quite as accurate as is Willis's.

Hastings, Charles (1794-1866) — MC-MENEMEY, W. H., 1959: The life and times of Sir Charles Hastings, founder of the British Medical Association, 516 p. (Edinburgh: Livingstone).—

Charles Hastings, formerly president of the Worcester Medical and Surgical Society, was the most prominent founder of the British Medical Association in 1855. Besides much biographical material concerning the life and activities of Hastings, the author also gives much information about his professional colleagues; and so the book gives an interesting picture of the organization of the medical profession in Britain during the first half of the 19th century.

Heberden, William (1710-1801) — HEBERDEN, W., 1962: Commentaries on the history and cure of diseases, 483 p. (Facsimile of the London 1802 edition, with preface by P. KLEMPERER) (History of Medicine Series, No. 18) (New York, N.Y.: Hafner).—

William Heberden was an English physician of the "Old School". He kept careful notes of his clinical experiences, and it was on the basis of these notes that he composed the "Commentaries" in 1782. A year after his death they were published by his son. In these commentaries were recorded Heberden's descriptions of various diseases, many of them being original accounts *(e.g.,* his famous account of angina pectoris, and

his classic description of the nodules occurring in the fingers in osteo-arthritis). This book is a paperback reproduction in facsimile of the 1802 edition. *Cf.* also: BULLER, A. C., 1879: The life and works of Heberden, 46 p. (London: Bradbury, Agnew).

Helmholtz, Hermann Ludwig Ferdinand von (1821-1894) — KOENIGSBERGER, L., 1902-1903: Hermann von Helmholtz, 3 vols. Vol. I: 375 p.; Vol. II: 383 p.; Vol. III: 142 p. (Braunschweig: Vieweg).—

An extensive biography of this famous German scientist, written by one of his companions during many years of research. Von Helmholtz started his university career as a professor of physiology (1849-1871) at the universities of Königsberg, Bonn and Heidelberg successively. From 1871 until 1888 he was professor of physics at the university of Berlin, and afterwards president of the "Physikalisch-technischer Reichsanstalt". The scientific papers published by von Helmholtz in so many fields of natural science are discussed on the basis of this biography. Also in a popular edition: KOENIGSBERGER, L., 1911: Hermann von Helmholtz. Gekürzte Volksausgabe, 356 p. (Braunschweig: Vieweg). Of this shorter version of Koenigsberger's book an English translation has been prepared, of which a reprint appeared in 1965: KOENIGSBERGER, L., 1965: Hermann von Helmholtz, 440 p. (Transl. by F. A. WELBY) (New York, N.Y.: Dover). A short, modern, semipopular biography is: EBERT, H., 1949: Hermann von Helmholtz, 199 p. (Grosse Naturforscher, Vol. 5) (Stuttgart: Wiss. Verlagsgesells.).

——, WARREN, R. M. & R. P., eds., 1968: Helmholtz on perception: its physiology and development, 277 p. (New York, N.Y.: Wiley).—

This book is meant as an introduction to von Helmholtz. It presents a collection of six of his shorter survey articles, accompanied by comments of the editors. Modern reprints of some of his books: HELMHOLTZ, H. v., 1962: Treatise on physiological optics, 3 vols. in 2, 961 and 734 p. (New York, N.Y.: Dover); again reprinted in 1966 (Magnolia, Mass.: Smith). This is a translation of the 1924 edition of the "Handbuch der physiologischen Optik" (first published 1867). HELMHOLTZ, H. v., 1954: On the sensation of tone as a physiological basis for the theory of music, 576 p. (New York, N.Y.: Dover). *Cf.* also: ATKINSON, E., ed., 1873: Popular lectures on scientific subjects by H. Helmholtz, 397 p. (London: Longmans, Green); and ELLIS, A. J., 1875: On the sensation of tone as a physiological basis for the theory of music, 824 p. (London: Longmans, Green).

Helmont, Johan Baptist van (1577-1644) — DE WAELE, H., n.d.: J. B. van Helmont, 82 p. (Collection Nationale, No. 78) (Brussels: Office de Publicité).—

A semi-popular biography, containing excerpts from van Helmont's treatises in the original Latin or Flemish, together with French translation.

——, PAGEL, W., 1930: Jo. Bapt. van Helmont. Einführung in die philosophische Medizin des Barocks, 224 p. (Berlin: Springer).—

In the introduction, Pagel places van Helmont within the framework of the period and discusses his treatises dealing with catarrh and asthma (p. 1-14). Thorough descriptions follow of the "Catarrhi deliramenta" and the treatise on asthma, together with a discussion of van Helmont's position in relation to his predecessors.

——, 1944: The religious and philosophical aspects of van Helmont's science and medicine, 44 p. (Suppl. Bull. Hist. Med., No. 2) (Baltimore, Md.: Johns Hopkins Press).—

In this publication, the author discusses such matters as: van Helmont's methods (illuminism, empiricism, pyrotechnica), religious motives, relationship to Paracelsus, opinion concerning the interrelation between body and soul, his ideas on matter and its immanent biological impulses, and on biological specificity, his monadology, ideas about the origin of diseases, and his ideas on biological time and theology. *Cf.* also a somewhat older study by the same author, PAGEL, W., 1930, *vide supra*.

His, Wilhelm (1831-1904) — HIS, W., 1931: Wilhelm His der Anatom. Ein Lebensbild, 79 p. (Berlin: Urban & Schwarzenberg).—

A biography of the great German anatomist, with portrait and bibliography, written by his son. A systematic bibliography, containing some 179 items is: FICK, R., 1904, in: Anat. Anz. 25: 161-208.

—— ——, 1965: His der Aeltere. Lebenserinnerungen und ausgewählte Schriften, 139 p. (Hubers Klassiker der Medizin und der

Naturwiss., Vol. VI) (Bern: Huber).—

After a brief introduction, some "Lebenserinnerungen" follow, written by himself. Thereafter his inaugural oration at Leipzig follows and some parts from the "Briefen über unsere Körperform". They together give an idea of his way of thinking.

Hofmeister, Wilhelm (1824-1877) — GOEBEL, K. von, 1924: Wilhelm Hofmeister. Arbeit und Leben eines Botanikers des 19. Jahrhunderts. Mit biographischer Ergänzung von Frau Professor GANZENMÜLLER geb. HOFMEISTER, 177 p. (Grosse Männer, Vol. 8) (Leipzig: Akad. Verlagsgesells.).—

Separate sections deal with: botany at the time of Hofmeister's first publications; his works on the fertilization and seed-formation of the angiosperms; his comparative researches on the germination, development and fruit-formaton of the higher cryptogams and the seed-formation of the conifers; developmental history of the lower cryptogams; Hofmeister and causal morphology; the cell-doctrine; his experimental-physiological works; and Hofmeister as teacher. Also in English translation: Wilhelm Hofmeister: the work and life of a nineteenth-century botanist, with biographical supplement, 1926, 202 p. (London: Ray Society).

Holmes, Oliver Wendell (1809-1894) — TILTON, E. M., 1947: Amiable autocrat: a biography of Dr. Oliver Wendell Holmes, 470 p. (New York, N.Y.: Schuman).—

A chronological biography of this American writer and physician, based on student notebooks, diaries, casebooks, college records, and on manuscripts and newspaper evidence. Holmes' letters were published in 1896 by J. T. MORSE in two volumes. A bibliography has been published by CURRIER, T. F. & E. M. TILTON, 1953: A bibliography of Oliver Wendell Holmes, 708 p. (New York, N.Y.: U.P.). *Cf.* also: RUTMAN, A. & L. T. CLARK, eds., 1960: A checklist of printed and manuscript works of Oliver Wendell Holmes in the library of the Univ. of Virginia, 109 p. (Charlottesville, Va.: Univ. Virginia Library).

Hooke, Robert (1635-1703) — 'ESPINASSE, M., 1956: Robert Hooke, 192 p. (Berkeley & Los Angeles, Calif.: Univ. California Press; London: Heinemann).—

This is the first full-scale biography of Robert Hooke; it gives a very good picture of the life, character, and scientific achievements of this first professional scientist among the amateurs. The central thesis of the book is the controversy between Hooke and Newton, and according to Mrs. 'Espinasse, Newton's personal enmity was largely due to Hooke's frustrated and melancholic behaviour. Much information can be found in: ROBINSON, A. W. & W. ADAMS, 1935: The diary of Robert Hooke, 1672-1708, 527 p. (London: Taylor & Francis).

——, HOOKE, R., 1961: Micrographia or some physiological descriptions of minute bodies made by magnifying glasses with observations and inquiries thereupon, 273 p. (New York, N.Y.: Dover).—

A facsimile reproduction of the Royal Society edition of 1665 (London: Martyn & Allestry), with an index from the editions of 1745 and 1780 and a 1938 preface and supplementary index, prepared by R. T. GUNTHER. In 1966 another reprint appeared, 35 + 256 p. (Brussels: Éd. Culture et Civilisation).

——, KEYNES, G., 1960: A bibliography of Dr. Robert Hooke, 115 p. (Oxford: Clarendon Press).—

Because Hooke's 'Micrographia' was one of the earliest of the books to be published under the aegis of the Royal Society, and because Hooke - the first 'curator of experiments' of the Royal Society - achieved the reputation of being the greatest inventive genius in the field of physics that had ever lived, this bibliography has been compiled during the celebration of the tercentenary of this Society. Hooke's works are herein subjected to full bibliographical investigation for the first time. This bibliography is preceded by a biographical introduction in which Hooke's personality and achievements are described. A list of Hooke's manuscript-papers and letters, a list of printed letters, and a section "Biography and criticism" have been added.

Hooker, William Jackson (1785-1865) and Joseph Dalton (1817-1911) — ALLAN, M., 1967: The Hookers of Kew, 273 p. (London: Michael Joseph).—

An authoritative biography of the father and son Hooker. William Hooker may be regarded as the father of Kew Gardens in their present form, for it was he who became the first director when the gardens were established on their present basis. Sir Joseph's expeditions to the Antarctic and to the Sikkim Himalayas are described and also his position as director of the Gardens in which position he succeeded his father. Besides much biographical information, the book contains much that is of interest to the history of Kew Gardens .

——, HUXLEY, L., 1918: Life and letters of Sir Joseph Dalton Hooker based on materials collected and arranged by Lady Hooker, 2 vols. Vol. I: 546 p.; Vol. II: 569 p. (London: Murray).—

J. D. Hooker was a prolific writer who has written a vast number of letters, e.g., there exist some 700 sheets copied from his letters to Darwin and some 800 typewritten pages of Darwin's letters to Hooker. Besides, there remained more letters to other famous scientists of that period (e.g., Bentham, Harvey, Anderson, Duthtie, T. H. Huxley). All these letters together are a mine of information about the scientific interests of the period and of the many personal relationships of some of its scientific leaders. Vol. I deals with the period up to 1860; Vol. II from 1860 up to his death (1911).

——, TURRILL, W. B., 1963: Joseph Dalton Hooker: botanist, explorer, and administrator, 228 p. (London & Edinburgh: Nelson).—

J. D. Hooker was a famous English botanist, sometime director of the Royal Botanical Gardens, Kew, a great friend of Darwin, and one of the editors of the well-known "Genera Plantarum". Hooker described and classified thousands of plant specimens and made significant contributions to fossil botany, and was an authority on gardening practice.

Humboldt, Friedrich Heinrich Alexander, Baron von (1769-1859) — BANSE, E., 1953: Alexander von Humboldt. Erschliesser einer neuen Welt, 146 p. (Grosse Naturforscher, Vol. 14) (Stuttgart: Wiss. Verlagsges.).—

A short authentic biography of A. von Humboldt, written by a professional geographer. The author suggests that von Humboldt was the last Universal Man, living at the turning point of universal science toward specialization. An authoritative semi-popular biography, stressing von Humboldt's importance for biology is: JAHN, I., 1969:

Dem Leben auf der Spur. Die biologischen Forschungen Alexander von Humboldts, 212 p. (Leipzig: Urania). Another biography, written in a popular style is: SCURLA, H., 1955: Alexander von Humboldt. Sein Leben und Wirken, 386 p. (Berlin: Verlag der Nation). A biography-in-letters is: BORCH, R., 1948: Alexander von Humboldt. Sein Leben in Selbstzeugnissen, Briefen und Berichten, 386 p. (Berlin: Tempelhof). *Cf.* also DE TERRA, 1955, *vide infra.*

——, BECK, H., 1959: Gespräche Alexander von Humboldts. Hrsg. im Auftrage der Alexander von Humboldt-Kommission der deutschen Akademie der Wissenschaften zu Berlin, 492 p. (Berlin: Akademie Verlag).—

This book contains a great amount of source-material by means of which we obtain a clear picture of von Humboldt's personality, especially of his many different social contacts. Most letters and documents deal with the later part of his life. A very complete index of persons rounds off this work of great biographical interest.

—— ——, 1959-1961: Alexander von Humboldt. Vol. I (1959): Von der Bildungsreise zur Forschungsreise 1769-1804, 303 p.; Vol. II (1961): Vom Reisewerk zum Kosmos, 409 p. (Stuttgart: Steiner).—

A magnificent biography of the many-sided naturalist, explorer, statesman, *etc.,* A. von Humboldt, one of the most famous men of his time. The first vol. deals with von Humboldt's family, social background, studies, and the period in which he prepared the grand enterprise of his travels of exploration in South America. The second vol. starts with the period spent in Paris, afterwards in Berlin at the Prussian Court, and elucidates his social activities and his attempts to organize national and international scientific co-operation. The author made use of many new documents, so that this book is an essential tool for those interested in A. von Humboldt and the period in which he lived. An extensive bibliography has been added. *Cf.* also: BIERMANN, K. R., I. JAHN & F. G. LANGE, 1968: Alexander von Humboldt. Chronologische Uebersicht über wichtige Daten seines Lebens, 86 p. (Berlin: Akademie Verlag). A bibliography of his works published in German is: Bibliographie seiner ab 1860 in deutscher Sprache herausgegebenen Werke und der seit 1900 erschienenen Veröffentlichungen über ihn, 45 p. (Sonderbibliographien der deutschen Bücherei, No. 16) (Leipzig: Deutsche Bücherei). *Cf.* also: SUCHOVA, N. G., 1960: Alexander von Humboldt in der rus-

sischen Literatur, 96 p. (Leipzig: Verlag für Buch- und Bibliothekwesen). This booklet contains much biographical and bibliographical information. Included are Russian translations of his works and literature dealing with his voyage through Russia. For the older literature, *cf.* BRUHNS, *vide infra. Cf.* also: DITTRICH, M., 1959: Ideen zu einer Physiognomik der Gewächse, 46 p. (Ostwalds Klassiker der exakten Wiss., No. 247) (Leipzig: Geest & Portig); and: DITTRICH, M., 1960: Ideen zu einer Geographie der Pflanzen. Mit einem Titelbildnis und einer pflanzengeographischen Karte, 180 p. *(Idem,* No. 248) (Leipzig: Geest & Portig).

——, BRUHNS, K., 1873: Life of Alexander von Humboldt, 2 vols. Vol. I: 412 p.; Vol. II: 447 p. (London: Longmans, Green).—

This is an English translation of Bruhn's "Alexander von Humboldt, eine wissenschaftliche Biographie" in 3 volumes (481 + 552 + 314 p.), published in 1872 (Leipzig: Brockhaus). In this English translation the third volume, devoted to a critical investigation of von Humboldt's scientific labours, has been omitted, together with the last section of the second volume of the original German publication which consists of an elaborate catalogue of his voluminous works. This biography is somewhat obsolete. The catalogue of von Humboldt's works has been reprinted quite recently: LÖWENBERG, J., ed., 1960: Alexander von Humboldt. Bibliographische Uebersicht seiner Werke, Schriften und zerstreuten Abhandlungen, 68 p. (Stuttgart: Brockhaus). This is an unaltered reprint of the relevant part of the 1872 edition of "Alexander von Humboldt, eine wissenschaftliche Biographie", ed. by K. BRUHNS. For a more recent biography, *cf.* BECK, H., 1959-1961, *vide supra.*

——, DE TERRA, H., 1955: Humboldt: the life and times of Alexander von Humboldt, 1769-1859, 386 p. (New York, N.Y.: Knopf).—

A more or less popular biography of the famous German explorer, naturalist, humanist, and founder of scientific geography who was so widely honoured during his lifetime. De Terra, himself a distinguished geologist and explorer, gives very good summaries of von Humboldt's expeditions. The great mass of von Humboldt's scientific activities, however, have been left out. The book is well illustrated and is provided with a good index. Another biography is: KELLNER, C., 1963: Alexander von Humboldt, 247 p. (London: Oxford U.P.). *Cf.* also BANSE, E., 1953, *vide supra.*

Hunter, William (1718-1783) and John (1728-1793) — DOBSON, J., 1969: John Hunter, 361 p. (Edinburgh & London: Livingstone).—

A full-scale account of Hunter's life and scientific achievements, as far as possible in Hunter's own words, together with a useful chronological list of his writings, with full titles and references. Much attention has been paid to his collections, still kept in the Hunterian Museum of the Royal College of Surgeons of England, of which Miss Dobson is curator. Much valuable information has been given of John Hunter's activities in the field of natural history.

——, ILLINGWORTH, C., 1967: The story of William Hunter, 134 p. (Edinburgh & London: Livingstone).—

William Hunter was a British physiologist and physician, the first great teacher of anatomy in England. He was an elder brother of John Hunter, *q.v., infra.* In this book the author describes W. Hunter's great contributions to medicine and the collection of books and objects he bequeathed to Glasgow University. This book has been written by a professor of surgery at Glasgow University.

——, KOBLER, J., 1960: The reluctant surgeon: a biography of John Hunter, 359 p. (Garden City, N.Y.: Doubleday).—

A popular biography, well-written and fairly accurate. Another popular biography is: GLOYNE, S. R., 1951: John Hunter, 104 p. (Baltimore, Md.: Williams & Wilkins; Edinburgh & London: Livingstone).

——, OPPENHEIMER, J. M., 1946: New aspects of John and William Hunter. I. Everard Home and the destruction of the John Hunter manuscripts. II. William Hunter and his contemporaries, 188 p. (New York, N.Y.: Schuman).—

This study seeks "to supplement what is published of these men *(i.e.,* John and William Hunter, and Sir Everard Home, their brother-in-law), by interpreting their characters in the light of their relationship with their contemporaries."

Huxley, Julian (1887-   ) — HUXLEY, J., 1970: Memories, 296 p. (London: Allen & Unwin).—

The autobiography of one of the most famous biologists of the present era. Huxley has been active in many fields, such as: the popularization of science, education, nature conservancy and the UNESCO. In this autobiography he describes his youth, his studies at Eton and Oxford, his studies of bird behaviour, his teaching and research activities at Houston and Oxford, his visits to Africa and Russia, *etc.*

Huxley, Thomas Henry (1825-1895) — BIBBY, C., 1959: T. H. Huxley: scientist, humanist and educator, 330 p. (London: Watts; New York, N.Y.: Horizon Press).—

This book does not attempt to give a new biography of T. H. Huxley, for the author limits himself to describing Huxley's place in education in 19th-century Britain. *Cf.* also: DAWSON, W. R., 1946: The Huxley papers: a descriptive catalogue of the correspondence, manuscripts and miscellaneous papers of the Rt. Hon. Thomas Henry Huxley, P. C., D. C. L., F. R. S., preserved in the Imperial College of Science and Technology, London, 201 p. (London: Macmillan).

—— ——, ed., 1967: The essence of T. H. Huxley: selections from his writings edited with several brief interpretative essays, 246 p. (London: Macmillan; New York, N.Y.: St. Martin).—

A selection from Huxley's essays and addresses dealing with such matters as scientific method, philosophy, evolution, and education. The various texts have been connected by interpretative essays. A selection of addresses, most of them directed to an academic audience, has been edited by: WINICK, C., 1964: Science and education, 383 p. (Science Classics Library) (New York, N.Y.: Philosophical Library). In 1868 Huxley delivered one of his most famous lectures, for the workingmen of the city, during the meeting of the Brit. Assn. for the Advancement of Science. Starting from a piece of chalk Huxley described the age-long process by which chalk was laid down beneath the sea, *etc.* This lecture was re-issued in 1967: On a piece of chalk, 90 p. (With introduction and notes by L. EISELEY) (New York, N.Y.: Scribner).

——, CHALMERS MITCHELL, P., 1901: Thomas Henry Huxley: a sketch of his life and work, 297 p. (New York, N.Y. & London: Putnam).—

This book attempts to give an outline of the life of T. H. Huxley, with an account of his contributions to biology, educational and social problems, and to philosophy and metaphysics. *Cf.* also: CLODD, E., 1902: Thomas Henry Huxley, 226 p. (Edinburgh & London: Blackwood). Chronological list of works; and assessment of Huxley as philosopher, interpreter and controversialist.

———, CLARK, R. W., 1968: The Huxleys, 398 p. (London: Heinemann; New York, N.Y.: McGraw-Hill).—

A story of the Huxley family, giving many details about the life and work of Thomas Henry and Julian Huxley (and many other members of the family). This study has been written with the help and co-operation of many members of the family and has been based upon much source-material. With bibliography, family tree and index.

———, FOSTER, M. & E. R. LANKESTER, eds., 1898-1902: The scientific memoirs of Thomas Henry Huxley, 4 vols. Vol. I (1898): 606 p.; Vol. II (1899): 612 p.; Vol. III (1901): 622 p.; Vol. IV (1902): 689 p. (London: Macmillan).—

Re-publication in a collected form of the papers T. H. Huxley contributed to scientific societies and scientific periodicals, and as such a very important bibliographical source. The editors excluded the memoir on "The oceanic Hydrozoa", published by the Ray Society in 1859, because of its size and character. Vol. I contains 50 memoirs originally published between 1847 and 1858, Vol. II 37 (1857-1864), Vol. III 38 (1864-1872) and Vol. IV 38 (1871-1894). One of his most famous books has been re-issued recently, *viz.,* On the origin of species: or, the causes of the phenomena of organic nature, 144 p. (Introd. by A. MONTAGU) (Ann Arbor, Mich.: Univ. Michigan Press; London: Cresset). *Cf.* also: HUXLEY, T. H., 1893/94: Collected essays, 9 vols., 3668 p. Gregg (Farnborough, Hants), announced a reprint of this edition.

———, HUXLEY, L., 1901: Life and letters of Thomas Henry Huxley, 2 vols. Vol. I: 539 p.; Vol. II: 541 p. (New York, N.Y.: Appleton).—

The author (a son of T. H. Huxley), endeavours to give a picture of the life of the man himself, of his character and temperament, and the various circumstances under which his various works were begun and completed. He does so in a chronolog-

ical order, making use of letters and extracts of T. H. Huxley and stressing his interest in human life.

———, MACBRIDE, E. W., 1934: Huxley, 143 p. (Great lives, No. 34) (London: Duckworth).—

An analysis of T. H. Huxley's personal characteristics in relation with his intellectual achievements and public activities, critically evaluating his zoological investigations. *Cf.* also: PETERSEN, H., 1932: Huxley, prophet of science, 338 p. (London: Longmans, Green).

Ingenhousz, Jan (1730-1799) — REED, H. S., 1949: Jan Ingenhousz: plant physiologist. With a history of the discovery of photosynthesis, 111 p. (Chronica Botanica 11, 5/6: 285-396) (Also separate: Waltham, Mass.: Chronica Botanica).—

Ingenhousz can be considered as one of the founders of plant physiology, for he discovered the action of light on green cells of plants and appreciated its importance in the economy of nature. After a brief biographical sketch, showing how Ingenhousz's work was a product of his time, and a review of the conditions of science during his lifetime, a re-issue of the text of the English edition of 1779, with a few interpolations from the French edition of 1787, has been given of the classical work in which he expounded his ideas for the first time. The protocol of the numerous experiments which occupies considerable space in the original publication has not been included. In order to give an insight into the influence of Ingenhousz on various developments in modern research, comments have been added to different sections. For more biographical details, *cf.* WIESNER, J., 1905: Jan Ingen-Housz. Sein Leben und sein Wirken als Naturforscher und Arzt, 252 p. (Unter Mitwirkung von T. ESCHERICH, E. MACH, R. v. TÖPLI and R. WEGSCHNEIDER) (Vienna: Konegen).

Jefferson, Thomas (1743-1826) — BETTS, E. M., 1944: Thomas Jefferson's garden book 1766-1824: with relevant abstracts from his other writings, 704 p. (Memoirs Amer. Philos. Soc., Vol. XXII) (Philadelphia, Pa.: American Philosophical Soc.).—

Jefferson began this book as a diary of his garden. It consists of 158 pages only, 33 of which are filled with Jefferson's notes. The items deal with such topics as: the dates at which some flowers came into bloom, his contacts with overseers, plans for building fish ponds, dates when vegetables were planted, *etc.,* and it gives an insight into his interest in introducing new plants, improving agricultural and horticultural techniques, his introduction of dry rice and the olive tree in South Carolina, *etc.* Moreover, in many of his letters he expresses his theories on agriculture and gardening, he ordered plants, seeds, recorded what he was planting, *etc.* From both these sources, the author made a starting-point to write a major contribution both to our knowledge of Jefferson and to the history of American agriculture of the late 18th and early 19th century.

——— ———, ed., 1953: Thomas Jefferson's farm book: with commentary and relevant extracts from other writings, 176 + 552 p. (Memoirs Amer. Philos. Soc., Vol. XXII) (Princeton, N.J.: Princeton U.P.).—

The original "Farm book" has been reproduced in facsimile (176 p.); it is a plantation account book, chiefly concerned with agricultural economics. In the present book the author collected as much information as he could find in Jefferson's writings which bears upon the economics of the plantation system. As a result the book gives an interesting picture of plantation economics and the efforts of Jefferson (and other plantation owners) to establish a firm plantation economy, and as such it contains much information concerning social life during the age of slavery.

——, BOORSTIN, D. J., 1948: The lost world of Thomas Jefferson, 306 p. (New York, N.Y.: Holt).—

An attempt to reconstruct the leading and pervasive ideas of the Jeffersonian view of the world in its total texture, *i.e.,* to reconstruct the relationship which should exist between God, nature, equality, toleration, education, and government. Especially ch. II (The economy of nature) and ch. III (The equality of the human species) are of biohistorical interest.

——, EDWARDS, E. E., 1943: Jefferson and agriculture, 92 p. (Agricultural History Series, No. 7) (Washington, D.C.: U.S. Dept. of Agriculture).—

Part I of this booklet consists of a laudatory address by H. A. WALLACE, entitled "Thomas Jefferson: farmer, educator and democrat", and an essay by M. L. WILSON, entitled "Thomas Jefferson: farmer". Part II contains selections from Jefferson's writings, systematically arranged. The chief divisions are: 1. Jefferson's view on the nature of national economy; 2. his observations on agriculture in Europe and the United States; 3. his farming activities; and 4. his contributions to the advancement of agriculture.

——, MARTIN, E. T., 1952: Thomas Jefferson: scientist, 289 p. (New York, N.Y.: Schuman).—

In this book the author gives a review of Jefferson's interest in science and his contributions to it. It has been made clear that Jefferson's faith in science and his encouragements of its development were more important than his own discoveries. *Cf.* also BROWNE, C. A., 1934: Thomas Jefferson and the scientific trends of his time, 63 p. (Chronica Botanica, Vol. 8) (Waltham, Mass.: Chronica Botanica). An interesting study with beautiful illustrations and an extensive bibliography.

Jenner, Edward (1749-1823) — FISK, D., 1959: Doctor Jenner of Berkeley, 288 p. (London: Heinemann).—

A popular biography of the country doctor, naturalist and discoverer of vaccination, Edward Jenner. It describes all his many activities and gives a good picture of the many sides of his character and the controversies he met with during the last part of his life. *Cf.* also: EBERLE, I., 1963: Edward Jenner and smallpox vaccination, 153 p. (London: Chatto & Windus).

——, LE FANU, W., 1951: A bio-bibliography of Edward Jenner, 1749-1823, 176 p. (Philadelphia, Pa.: Lippincott).—

This bio-bibliography of the naturalist-physician Jenner contains much biographical information, particularly derived from the correspondence between Jenner and Hunter. A special section has been devoted to listing Jenner's letters and to describing his collections.

Jung, Carl Gustav (1875-1961) — JAFFÉ, A., ed., 1963: Memories, dreams, reflections by C. G. Jung, 398 p. (New York, N.Y.: Pantheon).—

"When he was eighty-one years old, C. G. Jung undertook the telling of his life story. At regular intervals he had conversations with his colleague and friend, Aniela Jaffé, and collaborated with her in the preparation of the text. On occasion, he was moved to write entire chapters of the book in his own hand ...". Separate sections deal with his psychiatric activities, his travels, visions, and his relationship to Freud. An appendix contains letters from Freud to Jung, from Jung to his wife Emma and to Richard Wilhelm. A glossary covers the collected works of Jung.

Jussieu de, family (1712-1853) — LACROIX, A., 1938: Notice historique sur les cinq de Jussieu, membres de l'Académie des sciences (1712-1853). Leur rôle d'animateurs des recherches d'histoire naturelle dans les colonies françaises. Leurs principaux correspondants, 97 p. (Paris: Gauthier-Villars).—

Biographical sketches of five members of a French family distinguished for the botanists is produced, *viz.*, Antoine (1686-1758), successor of Tournefort in Paris; his brother Bernard (1699-1777), successor of Vaillant in Paris; Joseph (1704-1779), another brother of Antoine, traveller; Antoine Laurent (1748-1836), a nephew of the three preceding, published in 1789 his "Genera plantarum ...", a book which formed the basis of modern plant-classification; and his son Adrien Laurent Henri (1797-1853), author of many valuable contributions to botanical literature. The "Genera plantarum" was re-issued in 1964, 48 + 24, 72 + 498 p. (Historiae naturalis classica, Vol. 35) (Weinheim: Cramer; New York, N.Y.: Stechert-Hafner). Introduction by F. A. STAFLEU.

Keith, Arthur (1866-1953) — KEITH, A., 1950: An autobiography, 721 p. (New York, N.Y.: Philosophical Library).—

An autobiography of Sir Arthur Keith, written at the age of 83. Keith was a famous authority on the origin and evolution of Man and author of many books of which at least two have become classics, *viz.*, "The antiquity of Man" and "Human embryology and morphology" both of which have gone through many editions. Because during his long life, Keith was acquainted with many of the great natural scientists and medical men of the preceding 75 years, the book has to be valued not only for its own sake, but also for the information it contains concerning these other men of science.

—— ——, 1952: Menders of the maimed, 335 p. (Philadelphia, Pa.: Lippincott).—

This book first appeared in 1919; its chapters are based on a series of lectures given at the Royal College of Surgeons of England in 1917-1918. Its contents are high-

ly interesting from the medico-historical point of view, especially for the orthopaedic surgeon.

Kerner von Marilaun, Anton (1831-1898) — KRONFELD, E. M., 1908: Anton Kerner von Marilaun. Leben und Arbeit eines deutschen Naturforschers, 392 p. (Geleitwort von R. VON WETTSTEIN) (Leipzig: Tauchnitz).—

A complete biography of the famous Austrian plant biologist, ecologist, geographer and systematist. A special chapter has been devoted to his "Pflanzenleben". Also in English translation: The natural history of plants; their forms, growth, reproduction and distribution (1894). Included are some 40 letters to and from Kerner, a bibliography of his publications (152 in all), a nomenclator Kernerianus, but no index.

Kieser, Dietrich Georg (1779-1862) — BREDNOW, W., 1970: Dietrich Georg Kieser. Sein Leben und Werk, 176 p. (Sudhoffs Archiv, Beiheft 12) (Wiesbaden: Steiner).—

A full biography of one of the most characteristic representatives of German Romanticism. Kieser was a physician (especially interested in balneology). In collaboration with L. Oken, he published the "Beiträge zur vergleichenden Zoologie, Anatomie und Physiologie". He also was active in the field of botany: in 1808 he published his "Aphorismen aus der Physiologie der Pflanzen" and in 1812 he published his "Mémoire sur l'organisation des plantes". During his professorship of special pathology and therapy in the University of Jena, he also lectured on the history of medicine. Of special importance is his initiative towards the publication of the Archiv für thierisches Magnetismus (1817-1824). Later on Kieser became director of the psychiatric clinic and president of the Academia Leopoldina.

Kisch, Bruno (1890-1966) — KISCH, B., 1966: Wanderungen und Wandlungen. Geschichte eines Arztes im 20. Jahrhundert, 360 p. (Cologne: Greven).—

Kisch was one of the foremost physiologists of his age, and, moreover, an enthusiastic student of the history of medicine. This book contains much that is of interest to the history of physiology, both in Europe and the U.S.A., during the twentieth century.

Kluyver, Albert Jan (1886-1956) — KAMP, A. F., J. W. M. LE RIVIÈRE & W. VER-

HOEVEN, eds., 1959: Albert Jan Kluyver: his life and work, 567 p. (Amsterdam: North-Holland Publ. Comp.; New York, N.Y.: Interscience).—

This book was prepared as a tribute to the famous Dutch microbiologist, A. J. Kluyver. It contains reprinted papers on microbiological subjects, articles of a general nature, and texts of several lectures. The book includes a long biographical memoir and a well-documented assessment of Kluyver's scientific achievements. A bibliography has been added, which lists all of Kluyver's publications, a record of doctor's dissertations prepared under his guidance, and all papers issued from his laboratory during his directorate.

Koch, Robert (1843-1910) — BOCHALLI, R., 1954: Robert Koch, der Schöpfer der modernen Bakteriologie, 216 p. (Grosse Naturforscher, Vol. 15) (Stuttgart: Wiss. Verlagsges.).—

A readable biography written for the new generation, concerning life and scientific achievements of Robert Koch. A French biography is: LAGRANGE, E., 1939: R. Koch, sa vie et son oeuvre, 90 p. (Paris: Legrand). A new biography was prepared by HARMS, R., 1966: Robert Koch. Arzt und Forscher. Ein biographischer Roman, 318 p. (Hamburg: Mosaik Verlag) (No further information). The most complete biography is: HEYMANN, B., 1932: Robert Koch. I. Teil: 1843-1882, 352 p. (Leipzig: Akad. Verlagsges.). Unfortunately no further vols. have appeared. An English translation of the original paper announcing the discovery of the tubercle bacillus, read before the Physiological Society in Berlin, March 24, 1882, and published in the Berliner Klinische Wochenschrift 19, p. 221, 1882, was published in the Amer. Rev. of Tuberculosis, March 1932, 48 p., under the title "The aetiology of tuberculosis". This translation was preceded by a well-illustrated and thoughtful introduction.

Kützing, Friedrich Traugott (1807-1893) — MÜLLER, R. H. W. & R. ZAUNICK, eds., 1960: Friedrich Traugott Kützing, 1807-1893. Aufzeichnungen und Erinnerungen, 300 p. (Lebensdarstellungen deutscher Naturforscher, hrsg. Akad. Leopoldina, Halle/Saale, DDR, No. 8) (Leipzig: Barth).—

A biography of the most famous German algologist of the former century. Of

special importance are the annotations and indexes which give much information to anyone interested in the history of botany of the 19th century.

Lacépède, Bernard Germain Étienne de la Ville sur Illon, Comte de (1756-1825) — ROULE, L., 1932: Lacépède et la sociologie humanitaire selon la nature, 244 p. (L'histoire de la nature vivante d'après l'oeuvre des grands naturalistes français, Vol. VI) (Paris: Flammarion).—

Lacépède was one of the collaborators of Buffon, working on reptiles and fishes. Moreover, he frequently used his great political influence to develop the Jardin des Plantes and the Muséum d'Histoire naturelle and its menagerie.

Laënnec, René Théophile Hyacinthe (1781-1826) — KERVRAN, R., 1960: Laënnec: his life and times, 213 p. (London: Pergamon).—

A well-written biography of this most distinguished physician of the early 19th century in France. Besides having many other achievements to his credit, he invented the stethoscope about 1816 and founded a new clinical method of auscultation. His investigations on the lungs and the breath-sounds were of great importance for the development of diagnostics. In 1819 he published what is probably the most important treatise on diseases of the thoracic organs, viz., the "De l'auscultation médiate ou traité du diagnostic des maladies des poumons et du coeur". The most important passages have been translated into English: Translations of selected passages from "De l'auscultation médiate" (first ed.), 1923, 193 p. (With a biography by Sir William HALE-WHITE) (London: Bale & Danielson). Cf. also FORBES, J., ed., 1962: A treatise on the diseases of the chest, 43 + 438 p. (History of Medicine Series, No. 17) (New York, N.Y.: Hafner). A popular biography is: CORBIE, A. de, 1950: La vie ardente de Laënnec, 187 p. (Paris: Spes).

Lamarck, Jean Baptiste Pierre Antoine de Monet, Chevalier de (1744-1829) — PACKARD, A. S., 1901: Lamarck: the founder of evolution, his life and work with translations of his writings on organic evolution, 451 p. (New York, N.Y. & London: Longmans, Green).—

An elaborate sketch of the life and theoretical views of Lamarck, as well as of his works as a philosophical biologist. The author starts with a biographical review (p. 1-63). A discussion follows of his works in meteorology, physical science, geology, invertebrate palaeontology, general physiology, botany, and zoology. The evolutionary views held by Buffon, Geoffroy Saint-Hilaire, and E. Darwin have been considered, as well as the development of Lamarck's ideas on evolution before he published his "Philosophie zoologique"; this is followed by an analysis of the thoughts expressed in this work. Separate chapters have been devoted to an attempt to evaluate Lamarck's position in his own time; to Lamarcks's opinion about the evolution of Man; to his thoughts on morals, and on the relation between science and religion; to the relations between Lamarckism and Darwinism.

——, ROULE, L., 1927: Lamarck et l'interprétation de la nature, 249 p. L'histoire de la nature vivante d'après l'oeuvre des grands naturalistes français, Vol. IV) (Paris: Flammarion).—

A review of the works of this great French champion of transformism in the fields of zoology, botany, general biology, and philosophy. The author shows how Lamarck's emphasis upon the role of the environment in causing progression in the organic world, was in accordance with the dominant social philosophy of the pre-revolutionary and the revolutionary periods in France. Cf. also: BELTRÀN, E., 1945: Lamarck: interprete de la naturaleza, 161 p. (México, D. F.: Soc. Mex. de Historia Natural); and: BRUNELLE, L., ed., 1957: J. B. Lamarck. Pages choisies, 144 p. (Paris: Éd. Sociales). With introduction, notes and commentaries.

——, TSCHULOK, S., 1937: Lamarck. Eine kritisch-historische Studie, 190 p. (Zurich & Leipzig: Niehaus).—

A very valuable critical study of Lamarck's philosophical ideas. The "Philosophie zoologique" has been considered within the framework of Lamarck's scientific and philosophical views in general.

La Mettrie, Julien Offroy de (1709-1751) — VARTANIAN, A., ed., 1960: La Mettrie's l'homme machine: a study in the origins of an idea. Critical edition with an introductory monograph and notes, 264 p. (Princeton, N.J.: Princeton U.P.).—

This is a critical edition of La Mettrie's "l'Homme machine", together with a monograph considering recent works dealing with the Enlightenment. It mainly deals with the vitalist-mechanist controversy, and Vartanian makes clear that La Mettrie offered a biological foundation for mental phenomena, and that his primary task was "to vitalize the Cartesian 'dead mechanism'-approach to biology, in order to lift the homme machine beyond the reach of animistic criticism". Cf. also: BOISSIER, R., 1931: La Mettrie. Médicin, pamphlétaire et philosophe (1709-1751), 184 p. (Paris: Les Belles Lettres). Of this book I am unable to give more information.

Lancisi, Giovanni Maria (1654-1720) — WRIGHT, W. C., ed., 1952: Giovanni Maria Lancisi (1654-1720). De aneurysmatibus. Opus posthumum. Aneurysms. The Latin text of Rome, 1754, rev. with translation and notes, 35 + 362 p. (New York, N.Y.: Macmillan).—

In this edition the Latin text is printed opposite the English. The treatise itself mainly deals with dilatation of the heart and its various causes. Lancisi was the first to describe cardiac syphilis. Abundant notes, historical as well as medical, have been added at the end of the book. Cf. HOFFMANN, M., 1935: Die Lehre vom plötzlichen Tod in Lancisis Werk "De subtaneis mortibus", 60 p. (Abh. zur Gesch. der Medizin, Vol. 6) (Berlin: Ebering).

Lavoisier, Antoine Laurent (1743-1794) — DUVEEN, D. J. & H. S. KLICKSTEIN, eds., 1954: A bibliography of the works of Antoine Laurent Lavoisier 1743-1794, 493 p. (London: Dawson & Weil).—

A personalized bibliography of the great French chemist, administrator, economist, agriculturist, and sociologist. The text consists of various sections, viz., A. contributions to periodical works, arranged in chronological order; B. Lavoisier's four major works; C. his minor separate works and contributions to separate works; D. miscellaneous works containing material written by Lavoisier; E. a group of works with print reports on them submitted to the "Académie" by Lavoisier or by him in collaboration with others; F. collected works devoted to Lavoisier. A supplementary volume appeared in 1965, edited by D. J. DUVEEN, 177 p. (London: Dawson). The most complete biography is: GRIMAUX, E., 1888: Lavoisier 1743-1794, d'après sa correspondance, ses manuscrits, ses papiers de famille et d'autres documents inédits, 399 p. (Paris: Alcan). Éd. 2, 1896, 404 p.; éd. 3, 1899, 404 p.

Leeuwenhoek, Antoni van (1632-1723) —
ANONYMI, 1939→: The collected letters
of Antoni van Leeuwenhoek, 8 vols. Vol. I
(1939): 454 p., 39 tables; Vol. II (1941):
506 p., 29 tables; Vol. III (1948): 566 p., 48
tables; Vol. IV (1952): 384 p., 16 tables;
Vol. V (1957): 457 p., 36 tables; Vol. VI
(1961): 425 p., 32 tables; Vol. VII (1964):
427 p., 33 tables; Vol. VIII (1967): 383 p.,
15 tables. (To be continued) (Amsterdam:
Swets & Zeitlinger).—

In 1931 the Royal Netherlands Academy of Sciences made arrangements for the
publication of all Leeuwenhoek's extant letters, alongside accurate English translations
and pertinent, authoritative comments. The
translation of the first two volumes was
mainly based on the existing old translation
in the Philosophical Transactions; the translation of the later volumes is completely
modern. The letters are (as far as possible)
printed from the original autographs. Vol. I
contains a general introduction, together
with the 21 earliest letters, dating from April
23, 1673 to February 22, 1676; Vol. II letters 22-42 incl., from April 21st 1676 to
February 21st 1679; Vol. III letters 43-69
incl., from April 25th 1679 to July 28th
1682, to which two brief articles have been
added: the first written by G. VAN ITER-
SON on Leeuwenhoek's drawings of wood,
the second by E. J. DIJKSTERHUIS, discussing Leeuwenhoek's arithmetical methods; Vol. IV letters 70-81 incl., written in the
years 1683 and 1684, together with an article
by W. P. C. ZEEMAN on Leeuwenhoek
and ophthalmology and an article by J. I. H.
MENDELS on Leeuwenhoek's language and
style and its meaning for our study of Dutch
philology; Vol. V letters 82-89 incl., written
during the year 1685 and the beginning of
1686; Vol. VI letters 90-101 incl., written
between April 2nd 1686 and July 11th 1687,
to which two essays have been added, written by A. SCHIERBEEK on the history of
the investigation into the genesis of gallnuts and their importance for the manufacture of ink, and on Leeuwenhoek as sur-
veyor and wine-gauger; Vol. VII letters 102-
109 incl., written between 6th August 1687
and 24th August 1688; Vol. VIII letters 110-
119 incl., written between 7th September
1688 and 7th March 1692, incl. a letter from
Richard Waller, secretary of the Royal
Society, and dated 2nd February 1692.

——, DOBELL, C., 1932: Anthony van
Leeuwenhoek and his "Little Animals": being some account of the father of protozoology and bacteriology and his multi-
farious discoveries in these disciplines collected, translated, and edited, from his
printed works, unpublished manuscripts, and
contemporary records. Published on the
300th anniversary of his birth, 435 p. (London: Bale; New York, N.Y.: Harcourt).—

A well-written book, giving an interesting picture of the life and work of the
famous Dutch microscopist A. van Leeuwenhoek. The book gives an up-to-date interpretation of the many discoveries van
Leeuwenhoek has made, and is written by
an author who is himself familiar with the
organisms concerned. There are many fine
English translations, prepared by the author,
of those parts of van Leeuwenhoek's works
which deal with Protozoa and bacteria. The
completeness of Dobell's treatise is shown
in his "Elucidations and annotations" which
cover such subjects as: van Leeuwenhoek's
name, language, microscopes and methods,
dwelling, draughtsmen, portraits and seals.
This book was re-issued in 1958 (New York,
N.Y.: Russell & Russell), with a foreword
by C. B. VAN NIEL. Also a paperbound
edition, 1960, 465 p., published by Dover
(New York, N.Y.). Cf. also SCHIERBEEK,
A., 1959: Measuring the invisible: the life
and works of Antoni van Leeuwenhoek F.
R. S., 223 + 28 p. (Life Science Library,
Vol. 37). According to a review in Isis 52:
120-122, this book is less reliable than Dobell's book.

Leibnitz, Gottfried Wilhelm (1646-1716) —
MEYER, R. W., 1952: Leibnitz and the
seventeenth-century revolution, 227 p. (Chicago, Ill.: Regnery).—

From Isis 46, p. 74: "The bias of
Leibnitz's thinking, political, philosophical,
as well as religious, was towards the renew-
al of a Europe torn and shattered by revolution, a condition of things not unlike
that prevailing today." Originally published
in German. Another biographical study is:
SAW, R. L., 1954: Leibniz, 240 p. (Pelican
Bks., A 305) (Harmondsworth, Mddx.: Penguin Bks.). Cf. also: ROBINET, A., 1954:
Principes de la nature et de la grâce fondées
en raison. Principe de la philosophie, ou
monadologie. Publiés intégralement d'après
les manuscrits d'Hannovre, Vienne et Paris,
et presentés d'après des lettres inédites, 148
p. (Paris: Presses Univ. de France); and:
TOTOK, W. & C. HAASE, eds., 1966: Leibniz. Sein Leben. Sein Wirken. Seine Welt,
552 p. (Hannover: Verlag für Literatur und
Zeitgeschehen). This book contains 20 essays, elucidating the various aspects of Leibniz's life and scientific activities. Cf. also
RAVIER, C. G., 1937: Bibliographie des
oeuvres de Leibniz, 703 p. (Paris: Alcan).

Liebig, Justus von (1803-1873) — DECH-END, H. VON, ed., 1953: Justus von Liebig in eigenen Zeugnissen und solchen seiner Zeitgenossen, 141 p. (Weinheim: Verlag Chemie).—

The volume was prepared to commemorate the 150th anniversary of Liebig's birth. It tries to give a biographical portrait with the aid of excerpts of his letters and publications and those of his contemporaries. The editor has placed Liebig's words on the left-hand pages and those of his contemporaries on the right-hand pages. The volume closes with a bibliography of Liebig's papers and a series of explanatory notes. A second edition appeared in 1963 (158 p.).

——, HOLMES, F. L., ed., 1964: Animal chemistry or organic chemistry in its application to physiology and pathology: a facsimile of the Cambridge edition of 1842, 116 + 40 + 347 p. (Sources of Science, No. 4) (New York, N.Y.: Johnson).—

The first publication of this book in 1842 (ed. by W. GREGORY) demarcates a milestone in the history of chemical physiology. In his introduction, the editor describes the interest of chemists in physiological processes, Liebig's movement from pure organic chemistry to physiological chemistry, and the reception and influence of his "Animal chemistry". In this introduction he shows how Liebig in this book had brought together for the first time a great amount of scientific material, on which he based the new science of physiological chemistry. Original title: Die Thier-Chemie oder die organische Chemie in ihrer Anwendung auf Physiologie und Pathologie (Braunschweig: Vieweg).

Linné, Carl von (= Linnaeus) (1707-1778) — GOERKE, H., 1966: Carl von Linné. Arzt, Naturforscher, Systematiker 1707-1778, 232 p. (Grosse Naturforscher, Vol. 31) (Stuttgart: Wiss. Verlagsges.).—

A biography of Linnaeus, of which ten chapters deal with his life and six with his work. In an introduction the author gives a description of life in Sweden in Linnaeus' time.

——, GOURLIE, N., 1953: The prince of botanists: Carl Linnaeus, 292 p. (London: Witherby).—

A well-informed biography based on many documents. Much attention has been paid to his travels. An appendix deals with the Linnean Society, London. Extensive index.

——, HAGBERG, K., 1952: Carl Linnaeus, 264 p. (London: Cape).—

An informative and well-written biography of Linnaeus, describing his intellectual surroundings, his reactions to external circumstances, the structure of his character, and what he thought about the major scientific and philosophical issues of his time.

——, HJELT, O. E. A., et al., 1909: Carl von Linné's Bedeutung als Naturforscher und Arzt. Schilderungen herausgegeben von der Königl. Schwedischen Akademie der Wissenschaften, anlässlich der 200. jährigen Wiederkehr des Geburtstages Linné's, 168 + 48 + 43 + 188 + 86 + 42 p. (Jena: Fischer).—

This book consists of the following six contributions: Carl von Linné als Arzt und medizinischer Schriftsteller, by O. E. A. HJELT (168 p.); Carl von Linné und die Lehre von den Wirbeltieren, by E. LÖNNBERG (48 p.); Carl von Linné als Entomolog, by C. AURIVILLIUS (43 p.); Carl von Linné als botanischer Forscher und Schriftsteller, by C. A. M. LINDMAN (188 p.); Carl von Linné als Geolog, by A. G. NATHORST (86 p.); Carl von Linné als Mineralog, by H. SJÖGREN (42 p.). Reprinted in 1967 (Wiesbaden: Sändig).

——, LINNAEUS, C., 1957: A catalogue of the works of Linnaeus issued in commemoration of the 250th anniversary of the birthday of Carolus Linnaeus, 1707-78, 180 p. (Stockholm: Sandbergs Bokhandel).—

This catalogue has been founded on the splendid Linnaean collection of A. Liljedahl of Göteborg. With its many bibliographical notes and references, it forms a valuable companion to the work of HJELT, et al., 1909, vide supra. There are three indexes: to the works of Linnaeus, to authors prior to 1850, and to selected subjects respectively. Cf. also: A catalogue of the works of Linnaeus (and publications more immediately relating thereto) preserved in the libraries of the British Museum (Bloomsbury) and the British Museum (Natural History), South Kensington, ed. 2, 1933, 246 + 68 p. (London: British Museum).

—— ——, 1957-1959: Species plantarum: a facsimile of the first edition, 1753. Vol. I

(1957): 176 + 560 p. (With an introduction by W. T. STEARN); Vol. 2 (1959): 839 p. (London: Ray Society).—

In an introduction of 176 pages, W. T. STEARN has assembled much historical and bibliographical information about the botanical works of Linnaeus. The second vol. has an appendix by W. T. STEARN and a key (by J. L. HELLER) to the often very obscure abbreviations of works cited by Linnaeus. Of his "Critica botanica" also a recently published re-issue exists, translated by A. HORT, revised by M. L. GREEN, and published by Quaritch, London, 1938, 239 p. (Ray Soc. Series, No. 124).

—— ——, 1968: Hortus cliffortianus. Plantas exhibens quas in hortis tam vivis quam siccis, Hartecampi in Hollandia, coluit vir nobilissimus & generosissimus Georgius Clifford juris utriusque doctor, reductis carietatibus ad species, speciebus ad genera, generibus ad classes, adjectis locis plantarum notalibus differentiisque specierum. Cum tabulis aeneis, Amsterdam 1737. (Historiae naturalis classica, Vol. 63) (Lehre: Cramer).—

A description of the plants present in one of the richest gardens of the Netherlands in the 18th century, the Hartecamp, owned by G. Clifford, burgomaster of Amsterdam.

Lister, Joseph (1827-1912) — GUTHRIE, D., 1949: Lord Lister: his life and doctrine, 128 p. (Edinburgh: Livingstone; Baltimore, Md.: Williams & Wilkins).—

"In this book there is so much material in addition to the story of Lord Lister that the title might well have been 'The development of safe surgery'. The author has given us an interestingly written and informative volume." (From a review in Bull. Hist. Med. 24: 591). The most complete biography of Lister is: GODLEE, R. J., 1924: Lord Lister, ed. 3, 686 p. (Oxford: Clarendon Press); also in German: Lord Lister, 1925, 351 p. (Transl. from the 3rd ed., 1924) (Leipzig: Vogel). Cf. also LE FANU, W. R., 1965: A list of the original writings of Joseph, Lord Lister, O. M., 20 p. (Edinburgh: Livingstone).

——, THOMPSON, C. J. S., 1934: Lord Lister, the discoverer of antiseptic surgery, 99 p. (London: Bale, Sons & Danielson).—

In this short biography, such subjects have been considered as: Lister's surgical use of the spray, gauze and catgut ligature, a list of instruments invented by him, a list of his honours, his letter to Pasteur, and Lister's relationship to the renaissance of surgery. It also contains a guide to the Lister exhibits in the Museum of the Royal College of Surgeons.

——, TRUAX, R., 1944: Joseph Lister, father of modern surgery, 287 p. (Indianapolis, Ind. & New York, N.Y.: Bobbs-Merrill).—

A popular biography of which the aim is "to describe Lister's work, the birth of modern surgery and its rapid development during his long and active life; in addition, it attempts to tell the personal story of Joseph Lister, the story of a man and of the woman he so deeply loved." Two other popular biographies are: CAMERON, H. C., 1948: Joseph Lister: the friend of man, 180 p. (London: Heinemann); and WALKER, K. M., 1956: Joseph Lister, 195 p. (London: Hutchinson).

——, TURNER, A. L., ed., 1927: Joseph, Baron Lister, Centenary Volume 1827-1927, 184 p. (Edinburgh & London: Oliver & Boyd).—

This volume, edited for the Lister Centenary Committee of the British Medical Assn., includes a biographical sketch, and essays on Lister as physiologist and the influence of Lister's work on surgery. His lecture on the causes of putrefaction and fermentation and his address on the effects of the antiseptic treatment upon the general salubrity of surgical hospitals have been reprinted.

Locke, John (1632-1704) — DEWHURST, K., 1963: John Locke (1632-1704) physician and philosopher: a medical biography with an edition of the medical notes in his journals, 331 p. (London: Wellcome Hist. Med. Library).—

The book has been based on the Lovelace Collection of Locke's papers, acquired by the Bodleian Library and consisting of sixteen medical notebooks, 3000 letters, 1000 miscellaneous papers and 10 volumes of his journal. From this wealth of material, the author has extracted a medical biography of Locke, who, besides his philosophical activities, must also have been an experienced and skilful physician. The book gives a good insight into 17th-century medicine, the more so, since Locke was acquainted with many famous physicians of England, France and Holland.

Loeb, Jacques (1859-1924) — FLEMING, D., ed., 1964: The mechanistic conception of life, 42 + 216 p. (Cambridge, Mass.: Harvard U.P.).—

> This is a re-issue of the 1912 edition of a series of 10 popular essays, written by one of the pioneers of modern experimental biology. In an introductory essay, the editor situates Loeb and his work among his contemporaries. The text itself deals with the mechanistic attitude in biology, which Loeb considered as a principle of economy in scientific explanation.

Ludwig, Carl (1816-1895) — SCHRÖER, H., 1967: Carl Ludwig. Begründer der messenden Experimentalphysiologie 1816-1895, 340 p. (Grosse Naturforscher, Vol. 33) (Stuttgart: Wiss. Verlagsges.).—

> In this biography Carl Ludwig has been considered as one of the initiators of quantitative physiology. The first part describes Ludwig as a scientist until his settlement in Leipzig where he founded a famous institute of physiology and where he accomplished his fundamental work in physiology during some thirty years. The second part is devoted to his scientific discoveries.

Lyell, Charles (1797-1875) — BAILEY, E., 1962: Charles Lyell, 214 p. (London & Edinburgh: Nelson).—

> In opposition to those geologists who believed that the changes which took place at the surface of the earth had been brought about by tremendous catastrophes, Lyell attempted to explain these changes by reference to causes operating at the present day. This point of view has been applied to organic nature by C. Darwin, therefore Lyell's scientific position is also of much importance to the history of biology. Cf. also: NORTH, F. J., 1965: Sir Charles Lyell, interpreter of the principles of geology, 128 p. (London: Barker).

Lyonet, Pierre (1706-1789) — SETERS, W. H. VAN, 1962: Pierre Lyonet, 1706-1789, sa vie, ses collections de coquillages et de tableaux, ses recherches entomologiques, 227 p. (The Hague: Nijhoff).—

> In this book Lyonet has been considered as a son of his time. In his leisure he became an amateur natural scientist. He became known through his studies on insect life and became a member of many learned societies, among these the Royal Society. Cf. also: HUBLARD, E., 1910: Le naturaliste hollandais Pierre Lyonet. Sa vie et ses oeuvres (1706-1789) d'après des lettres inédites, 159 p. (Mém. Soc. des Sciences, des Arts et des Lettres du Hainaut, vol. 61) (Brussels: Labèque).

Magendie, François (1783-1855) — OLMSTED, J. M. D., 1945: François Magendie, pioneer in experimental physiology and scientific medicine in XIXth-century France, 290 p. (New York, N.Y.: Schuman).—

> An exhaustive study of the famous French pioneer in experimental physiology and founder of experimental pharmacology. He took an active part in the French revolution, and afterwards became one of the leading experimental scientists in the fields of biology and medicine.

Malpighi, Marcello (1628-1694) — ADELMANN, H. B., 1965: Marcello Malpighi and the evolution of embryology, 5 vols. Vol. I: 750 p.; Vol. II: 316 p.; Vol. III: 524 p.; Vol. IV: 550 p.; Vol. V: 427 p. (Ithaca, N.Y.: Cornell U.P.).—

> A monumental work containing a full biography of the Italian physiologist Malpighi who has been one of the first to apply the microscope to the study of animal and vegetable structure; his discoveries were so important that he may be considered to be the founder of microscopic anatomy. This work also contains translations of his works, e.g., of his dissertations on the development of the chick, an account of early embryological thought, elucidating Malpighi's contributions in this field; its also contains a historical review of embryological thought before Malpighi's time, and English translations of long extracts from the works of Gassendi, von Haller, C. F. Wolff, and C. E. von Bear. Cf. BELLONI, L., 1967: Marcello Malpighi: opera scelte, 649 p. (Torino: Unione Tipografico-Editrice Torinese). A new edition of Malpighi's work in Italian.

Manson, Patrick (1844-1922) — MANSONBAHR, P., 1962: Patrick Manson: the father of tropical medicine, 192 p. (London & Edinburgh: Nelson).—

> A rather popular description of the life and work of P. Manson, who evolved a new and original conception of the nature of insect-borne diseases which became one of the main factors in the understanding,

treatment, and prevention of the main tropical diseases. This made European settlement in the tropics possible and led to an improvement in the health of native inhabitants. Manson also founded the College of Medicine at Hong Kong.

Marsh, Othniel Charles (1831-1899) — SCHUCHERT, C. & C. M. LEVENE, 1940: O. C. Marsh: pioneer in paleontology, 541 p. (New Haven, Conn.: Yale U.P.).—

Marsh was one of the most famous palaeontologists the world ever has known, and the first professor of palaeontology in the Americas. Well-known are his discoveries of fossils in Wyoming and other regions of America, and is also well-known for his supporting the theory of natural selection. He was aided by a private fortune from his uncle, George Peabody, whom he induced to establish the Peabody Museum of Natural History. For this museum he accumulated the largest and most valuable collection of fossil vertebrates made in his time.

Mather, Cotton (1663?-1728) — BEAL, O. T. & R. H. SHRYOCK, 1954: Cotton Mather: first significant figure in American medicine, 241 p. (Baltimore, Md.: Johns Hopkins Press).—

The book consists of a long introductory essay on Cotton Mather as a medical scientist, plus selected chapters from a manuscript treatise on medicine written by him. The role of Mather in the inoculation controversy and his commitment to the animalcular hypothesis of disease have been considered and stress has been laid on his importance in the field of empirical experimentation with artificial immunity. *Cf.* also: MURDOCK, K. B., ed., 1961: Selections from Cotton Mather, 63 + 377 p. (New York, N.Y.: Hafner).

——, HOLMES, T. J., 1940: Cotton Mather: a bibliography of his works, 3 vols., 36 + 1395 p. (Cambridge, Mass.: Harvard U.P.).—

Sarton writes in Isis 33, p. 260: "This bibliography is truly exemplary. Each item is completely described and beautifully illustrated. Abundant footnotes answer every query the most inquisitive reader could think of asking about the persons mentioned or the subjects dealt with. Finally, the wealth of materials offered to us in such pleasant manner is made fully available by elaborate indices (p. 1321-95). In fact, this is far more than a bibliography, or catalogue raisonné; it is a biographical dictionary".

Mattioli, Petrus Andreas (1501-1577) — KRUTCH, J. W., 1965: Herbal, 255 p. (New York, N.Y.: Putnam).—

"In this unique book, Joseph Wood Krutch, talented naturalist-writer, has successfully reproduced beautiful woodcuts of one hundred plants and six creatures from Mattioli's Commentaries on the Six Books of Dioscorides, issued in Prague in 1563 and in Venice in 1565. A delightful commentary, with appropriate quotations from old herbalists and others, appears on the page facing each illustration". (From: The Garden Journal 16: 77). *Cf.* STANNARD, J., 1969: P. A. Mattioli: Sixteenth century commentator of Dioscorides. Bibliographical Contributions, Univ. Kansas Libraries, Vol. 1: 60-81).

Maupertuis, Pierre Louis Moreau de (1698-1759) — BOAS, S. B., ed., 1966: The earthly Venus (Venus physique), 32 + 86 p. (translation, with notes and introduction) (Sources of Science, Vol. 29) (New York, N.Y.: Johnson).—

Maupertuis was a French mathematician, geographer, biologist, and philosopher. In this book Maupertuis deals, *inter alia,* with fertilization, the preformation theory, hereditary malformations, *etc.* There is much in it that recalls modern points of view.

Meckel, Johann Friedrich (1781-1833) — BENEKE, R., 1934: Johann Friedrich Meckel der Jüngere, 159 p. (Beiträge Gesch. Univ. Halle, No. 3) (Halle: Niemeyer).—

Unfortunately I am unable to give further information about this book.

Mendel, Gregor Johann (1822-1884) — BENNETT, J. H., ed., 1965: Experiments in plant hybridisation, 95 p. (Edinburgh & London: Oliver & Boyd).—

A translation into English of Mendel's famous paper read originally at meetings of the Brno Natural History Society on February 8 and March 8, 1865, and originally published under the title "Versuche über Pflanzenhybriden" in the "Verhandlungen des Naturforsch. Vereins in Brno" in 1866. It is a modified version of BATESON's translation, published in his book "Mendel's principles of heredity" (1909). The present book also includes a reprint of W. Bateson's biographical notice of Mendel, some introductory notes, and comments and assessment by the late R. A. FISHER (*Cf.* also STERN & SHERWOOD, *infra*).

——, ILTIS, H., 1966: Life of Mendel, 336 p. (London: Allen & Unwin).—

This is the most complete biography of Mendel still existing. It is an English translation of: Gregor Johann Mendel. Leben, Werk und Wirkung, 1924 (Berlin: Springer) and a reprint of the first English edition of 1932. It provides a picture not only of the man, but also of his labours and their setting. *Cf.* OREL, V., ed., 1965: Gregor Mendel, zakladatel genetiky: populǎr ně vědecký sbornik, 206 p. [Gregor Mendel, founder of genetics: popular scientific almanac] (Brno: Blok).

——, JAKUBÍČEK, M. & J. KUBÍČEK, 1965: Bibliographia mendeliana, 74 p. (Brno: Universtní knihovna v Brně).—

A bibliography considering the most important publications dealing with the life and work of Mendel, and the re-discovery of the Mendelian laws. Included are 361 items. *Cf.* also: Iconographia mendeliana, 73 p. (Brno: Moravian Museum). Published to the memory of Gregor Johann Mendel for the centenary of the publication of his discovery of the principle of heredity.

——, KŘÍŽENECKÝ, J., 1965: Gregor Johann Mendel (1822-1884). Texte und Quellen zu seinem Wirken und Leben, 198 p. (Lebensdarstellungen deutscher Naturforscher, No. 11) (Festgabe der deutschen Akademie der Naturforscher Leopoldina zum Mendel Memorial Symposium 1865-1965, August 1965 in Brünn) (Leipzig: Barth).—

Contains much biographical information published for the first time, and 24 photographs of Mendel, his birthplace, school, cloister-garden, *etc. Cf.* Mendel memorial symposium, 1865-1965: proceedings of a symposium held in Brno, August 1965, 311 p. (Prague: Czechoslovak Acad. Sci.); published in 1966.

—— ——, & B. NĚMEC, eds., 1965: Fundamenta genetica: the revised edition of Mendel's classic paper with a collection of 27 original papers published during the rediscovery era, 400 p. (Prague: Czechoslovak Akad. of Sciences).—

In this volume a collection of original papers by the pioneers of Mendelism in the early years following the rediscovery are assembled (*e.g.,* of de Vries, Correns, Tschermak, Bateson, Castle, Cuénot, Garrod, Boveri, Wilson, Sutton, Cannon, McClung), in the original languages and with the original pagination indicated.

——, KRUMBIEGEL, I., 1957: Gregor Mendel und das Schicksal seiner Vererbungsgesetze, 144 p. (Grosse Naturforscher, Vol. 22) (Stuttgart: Wiss. Verlagsges.).—

A semi-popular biography of Mendel. It opens with a short exposition of the laws of heredity and of the early history of the subject, and then it deals with Mendel's personality, his life, botanical researches, and his duties as priest. A second ed. appeared in 1967 (160 p.).

——, STERN, C. & E. R. SHERWOOD, eds., 1966: The origin of genetics: a Mendel source book, 179 p. (San Francisco, Calif.: Freeman).—

This book contains a collection of papers and letters, among them 10 letters (in English translation) which Mendel wrote to Carl Nägeli, the foremost authority on plant hybrids of those days, and R. A. FISHER's famous statistical analysis of Mendel's numerical data of the segregation ratios in the pea crosses (commented upon by S. WRIGHT).

Mesmer, Franz Anton (1734-1815) — FRANKAU, G., 1948: Mesmerism by doctor Mesmer (1779): being the first translation of Mesmer's historic "Mémoire sur la découverte du magnétisme animal" to appear in English, 63 p. (London: Macdonald).—

Mesmer was an Austrian physician who believed that the stars exerted an influence on beings living on the earth. He identified the supposed force first with electricity and then with magnetism. From this supposition Mesmer concluded that stroking diseased bodies with magnets might effect a cure. Mesmer's "Mémoire" was first published in Geneva in 1779. To this English translation, the editor has added a brief introduction.

——, GOLDSMITH, M., 1934: Franz Anton Mesmer: the history of an idea, 282 p. (London: Barker).—

General account, in which the author traces the sources of Mesmer's thought and the continuation of his influence after his death. A well-documented study, considering Mesmer, his followers and his opponents is: VINCHON, J., 1936: Mesmer et son secret, 121 p. (Paris: Legrand). Two German biographies, giving much information concerning Mesmer and his influence on his contemporaries, are: BITTEL, K., 1940: Der berühmte Hr. Doct. Mesmer am Bodensee, ed. 2, 108 p. (Friedrichshafen am B.: See-Verlag), and TISCHNER, R., 1928: Franz Anton Mesmer. Leben, Werk und Wirkungen. Mit Bibliographie alter Ausgaben seiner Schriften, 176 p. (Munich: Verlag Münchner Drucke).

——, MILT, B., 1953: Franz Anton Mesmer und seine Beziehungen zur Schweiz. Magie und Heilkunde zu Lavaters Zeit, 139 p. (Mitt. Antiquarischen Ges. Zurich, 38, Heft 1).—

> An evaluation of Mesmer in his relationship to Switzerland, describing his life in that country from 1803 until his death in 1815 and the reception of his theory of animal magnetism by the Swiss.

——, WALMSLEY, D. M., 1967: Anton Mesmer, 192 p. (London: Hale).—

> A well-documented biography, written by a physician long interested in the therapeutic use of hypnotism. According to this biographer, Mesmer was a man of scientific integrity and methodical training.

Metchnikov, Elias (1845-1916) — METCHNIKOFF, O., 1920: Vie d'Élie Metchnikoff (1845-1916), 272 p. (Paris: Hachette).—

> A well-written biography, compiled by his widow. A work more particularly dealing with his scientific achievements, and as such a useful supplement is: BESREDKA, A., 1921: Histoire d'une idée. L'oeuvre de Metchnikoff, 135 p. (Paris: Masson). This work has been written by one of his collaborators. A recent study is: METCHNIKOV, É., 1959: Souvenirs. Recueil d'articles autobiographiques, 327 p. (Moscow: Éd. en langues étrangères). Contains much information concerning Metchnikov's contacts with contemporary scientists. Cf. also: LÉPINE, P., 1966: Metchnikoff, 192 p. (Paris: Seghers).

——, ZEISS, H., 1932: Elias Metschnikow, Leben und Werk. Uebersetzt und bearbeitet nach der von Frau Olga Metschnikowa geschriebenen Biographie, dem Quellenmaterial des Moskauer Metschnikow-Museums

und eigenen Nachforschungen, 196 p. (Jena: Fischer).—

> In this book a considerable volume of additional source material and certain introductory generalizations have been added, if compared with Olga METCHNIKOV's biography (vide supra). Especially his work in zoology (e.g., his basic contributions to the extension of the germ layer theory, to the invertebrates, and his contributions to phagocytosis) has been elucidated, as well as his philosophical ideas about renascence, death, and sex. In 1968 two of Metchnikov's books appeared in English translation, viz., his Lectures on the comparative pathology of inflammation; and his Immunity in infectious diseases (591 p.). Both vols. published by Dover (New York, N.Y.).

Michelangelo (1475-1564) — SCHMIDT, H. & H. SCHADEWALDT, 1965: Michelangelo und die Medizin seiner Zeit, 160 p. (Stuttgart: Schattauer).—

> In the introduction, Schmidt gives a review of life and work of Michelangelo. This is followed by a chapter on Michelangelo's occupation with anatomy and psychology (by SCHMIDT) and by a chapter (by SCHADEWALDT) measuring Michelangelo's influence on the medicine of his time. This is followed by 66 photographs, a bibliography of 98 items and an index.

Michurin, Ivan Vladimirovich (1855-1935) — MICHURIN, I. V., 1949: Selected works, 496 p. (Moscow: Foreign Language Publ. House).—

> This book contains biographical information about Michurin and gives a review of his work on the improvement of fruit culture in Russia. Also in a German edition: HOEPPNER, W., ed., 1951: I. W. Mitchurin. Ausgewählte Schriften, 717 p. (Sowjetwissenschaft, Beiheft 7) (Berlin: Kultur und Fortschritt).

Molisch, Hans (1856-1937) — MOLISCH, H., 1934: Erinnerungen und Welteindrücke eines Naturforschers, 232 p. (Vienna & Leipzig: Haim).—

> An autobiography, describing the author's scientific activities in Vienna, Graz, Prague, and again in Vienna as a professor in plant pathology, and describing his travels around the world, during which travels the author visited many biological (esp. botanical) institutes all over the world.

Morgagni, Giovanni Battista (1682-1771) — MICHLER, M., ed., 1967: Sitz und Ursachen der Krankheiten. Aufgespürt durch die Kunst der Anatomie (Venedig 1761), 195 p. (Hubers Klassiker der Medizin und der Naturwiss., Vol. 10) (Bern: Huber).—

Morgagni's "De sedibus et causis morborum" first appeared in Latin in 1761, and there were several later editions. The present selection begins with a relatively brief historical introduction, including a short biographical sketch and a discussion of Morgagni's significance in his era. The actual selections translated into German include part of the introduction and the dedicatory portions of the "De sedibus", together with excerpts from 26 letters. An appendix contains biographical notes on the authors mentioned in the text. A selected bibliography of 30 pages, compiled by L. PREMUDA. A facsimile reprint of the original text, together with a new English translation, was published in 1960 by Hafner (New York, N.Y.), in conjunction with the New York Academy of Medicine under the title: The seats and causes of diseases investigated by anatomy, in 3 vols. With introduction and preface by P. KLEMPERER.

Müller, Johannes Peter (1801-1858) — EBBECKE, U., ed., 1951: Johannes Müller, der grosse rheinische Physiologe. Mit einem Neudruck von Johannes Müllers Schrift "Ueber die phantastischen Gesichtserscheinungen", 192 p. (Hannover: Schmorl & v. Seefeld).—

A reprint of Joh. Müller's "Ueber die phantastischen Gesichtserscheinungen", published originally in Coblenz in 1826. This is accompanied by an introduction (of 73 pages), in which the editor discusses the work and personality of Müller, and also gives much bibliographical information.

——, KOLLER, G., 1958: Das Leben des Biologen Johannes Müller, 1801-1858, 268 p. (Grosse Naturforscher, Vol. 23) (Stuttgart: Wiss. Verlagsges.).—

A short biography of the famous German biologist Johannes Müller who is best known as a physiologist, but was in reality much more than that. In his youth he worked on experimental physiology, in later years, however, he also worked on human and animal histology, anatomy and pathology, on embryology and systematics, and even on palaeontology. Stress is laid on the fact that the notion "physiology" in those days meant the science of life, *i.e.*, the science of the forms and the activities together constituting the phenomenon of life, rather than the science of the processes taking place on and within the organic body. For an authorized biography *cf.* HABERLING, W., 1924: Johannes Müller. Das Leben des rheinischen Naturforschers. Auf Grund neuer Quellen und seiner Briefe dargestellt, 501 p. (Leipzig: Akad. Verlagsges.). This biography has been based on many letters written by Müller to his wife, his friends, and some of his colleagues.

Müller, Otto Friderich (1730-1784) — ANKER, J., 1950: Otto Friderich Müller's Zoologia danica, 108 p. (Library Research Monographs, No. 1) (Copenhagen: Munksgaard).—

An elaborate study of this illustrious Danish naturalist, or more exactly of one of his works, the "Zoologia danica", the prodromus of which and first two parts appeared within his lifetime (Copenhagen, 1776, 1777, 1780); parts 3 and 4 appeared posthumously (1789, 1806). (After Sarton, Isis 42: 331).

Neuburger, Max (1868-1955) — BERGHOFF, E., 1948: Max Neuburger. Werden und Wirken eines österreichischen Gelehrten, 144 p. (Wiener Beitr. Gesch. Med., Vol. 3) (Vienna: Maudrich).—

A very readable biography of one of the most famous historians of medicine, and founder of the Vienna Institute of Medical History. *Cf.* also: Wiener Beitr. Gesch. Med., Vol. II: "Festschrift zum 80. Geburtstag Max Neuburgers", 1948, 491 p., with 91 contributions in the field of the history of medicine.

Nightingale, Florence (1820-1910) — BISHOP, W. J. & S. GOLDIE, eds., 1962: A biobibliography of Florence Nightingale, 160 p. (London: Dawson).—

A complete guide to Miss Nightingale's work, including books, pamphlets, periodical articles and memoranda, *e.g.*, on army hygiene, sanitation, hospital administration, *etc.* Separate chapters deal with: nursing, the army, India and colonial welfare, hospitals, statistics, sociology, memoirs and tributes, religion and philosophy, and miscellaneous works.

——, WOODHAM-SMITH, C., 1950: Florence Nightingale, 1820-1910, 615 p. (London: Constable).—

A very useful study of Florence Nightingale, containing much original information based on family papers consisting of notes of Florence Nightingale, diaries, letters, reports, *etc.* A shorter ed. was published in 1951 under the title Lonely crusader: the life of Florence Nightingale 1820-1910, 255 p. (New York, N.Y.: McGraw-Hill). Some additional information can be found in: COPE, Z., 1958: Florence Nightingale and the doctors, 163 p. (London: Museum Press), and in: O'MALLEY, J. B., 1931: Florence Nightingale, 1820-1856: a study of her life down to the end of the Crimean War, 416 p. (London: Butterworth). A book which has given an enormous stimulus to the study of nursing, especially in England, is her "Notes on nursing", first published in 1860. Of this first edition a facsimile edition was published in 1946 by Appleton (New York, N.Y., 140 p.), with a foreword by V. M. DUNBAR.

Nuttall, Thomas (1786-1859) — GRAUSTEIN, J. E., 1967: Thomas Nuttall, naturalist: explorations in America, 1808-1841, 481 p. (Cambridge, Mass.: Harvard U.P.).—

A full-length biography of the brilliant English naturalist Thomas Nuttall whose pioneering scientific explorations in the South and Far West have never been equalled, and who made valuable contributions to the fields of botany, zoology, ornithology, geology, mineralogy, and horticulture. This biography contains many vivid descriptions of his encounters with such individuals as Daniel Boone and Audubon, of his travels and living conditions, and of the character of settlers and Indians at the frontier.

Ormerod, Eleanor Anne (1828-1901) — WALLACE, R., ed., 1904: Eleanor Ormerod LL.D. Economic entomologist. Autobiography and correspondence, 348 p. (London: Murray).—

An outstanding woman and entomologist who may fairly be called a pioneer of agricultural entomology. She worked mainly in England but also in South America and South Africa (on insect pests of cattle); for the English Board of Agriculture she wrote voluminous accounts of pests of field crops, orchard and soft fruits that were the first of their kind in Britain. Among her publications in book form were: Guide to methods of insect life, and prevention and remedy of insect ravage, 1884, 167 p. (London: Simpkin Marshall); second ed. published as: A text-book of agricultural entomology, 1892, 238 p. (London: Simpkin Marshall).

Osler, William (1849-1919) — ABBOTT, M.E., 1939: Classified and annotated bibliography of Sir William Osler's publications, 163 p. (Montreal: Medical Museum, McGill Univ.).—

Originally published in the Sir William Osler memorial volume of the Int. Assn. of Med. Museums, Bull. No. IX, 1926, p. 473-605. The subject-matter has been arranged under the following headings: natural science; comparative and human pathology; clinical medicine; literary papers, history, biography, and bibliography; medical education, medical societies, medical profession; public welfare activities; volumes published. Included are a portrait and a detailed and very valuable index.

——, BETT, W. R., 1951: Osler: the man and the legend, 125 p. (London: Heinemann).—

A readable biography in which separate chapters are devoted to one of his many valuable activities. Of course, the greater part is devoted to Osler's strictly medical activities. *Cf.* also: FRANKLIN, A. W., ed., 1958: A way of life and other selected writings of William Osler, 278 p. (New York, N.Y.: Dover). Originally published in 1951. This book contains a collection of interesting contributions of Osler, for the greater part essays, illustrating his historical, philosophical, and bibliographical activities, especially valuable to the student and younger members of the profession. *Cf.* also: MCGHEE, H. A. & V. A. MCKUSICK, eds., 1967: Osler's textbook revisited: reprint of selected sections with commentaries, 361 p. (New York, N.Y.: Appleton-Century-Crofts), and OSLER, W., 1961: Aphorisms from his bedside teachings and writings, ed. 2, 160 p. (Collected by R. B. BEAN, ed. by W. B. BEAN) (Springfield, Ill.: Thomas). Originally published in 1950 (New York, N.Y.: Schuman).

——, CUSHING, H., 1940: The life of Sir William Osler, 2 vols. Vol. I: 685 p.; Vol. II: 732 p. (London, New York, N.Y. & Toronto: Oxford U.P.).—

One of the foremost biographies existing in the field of medicine, dedicated to medical students. Cushing and Osler were on terms of the closest intimacy for nearly twenty-five years. Originally published in 1925.

Paracelsus (= Philippus Theophrastus Bombast of Hohenheim) (*ca.* 1490-1541) — DE-

BUS, A. G., 1965: The English Paracelsians, 222 p. (London: Oldbourne).—

> For more details, *vide* section History of the medical sciences, subsection b (Great Britain).

——, EIS, G., 1965: Vor und nach Paracelsus. Untersuchungen über Hohenheims Traditionsverbundenheit und Nachrichten über seine Anhänger, 183 p. (Medizin in Geschichte und Kultur, Vol. VIII) (Stuttgart: Fischer).—

> A collection of 17 papers, containing new and important manuscript material, for the greater part dealing with the period immediately preceding Paracelsus, for, as the author makes clear, Paracelsus is in many respects not as original as is generally believed.

——, GOLDAMMER, K., ed., 1955: Theophrast von Hohenheim, genannt Paracelsus: Die Kaerntner Schriften. Ausgabe des Landes Kaernten, 396 p.

> A revised and annotated text of the "Carinthian trilogy" of Paracelsus, comprising three classical treatises: the "Seven defensiones", the "Labyrinth of erring physicians", and the "Book on diseases due to tartar". Besides there are chapters on the origin, fate, and characteristics of the Carinthian trilogy (with bibliography), the social and mystical traits in the life and work of Paracelsus, and the synthesis of medicine and the magic world of Paracelsus. *Cf.* also: GOLDAMMER, K., 1953: Paracelsus. Natur und Offenbarung, 115 p. (Heilkunde und Geisteswelt, Vol. 5) (Hannover: Oppermann).

——, HARTMANN, F., n.d.: The life of Philippus Theophrastus Bombast of Hohenheim, known by the name of Paracelsus, ed. 2, 311 p. (London: Kegan Paul, Trench, Trübner).—

> Its sub-title: "The substance of his teachings concerning cosmology, anthropology, pneumatology, magic and sorcery, medicine, alchemy and astrology, philosophy and theosophy extracted and translated from his rare and extensive works and from some unpublished manuscripts", explains the contents of this book very well.

——, LEIDECKER, K. F., 1949: Volumen medicinae paramirum of Theophrastus von Hohenheim called Paracelsus, 69 p. (Bull. Hist. Med., Suppl. No. 11) (Baltimore, Md.: Johns Hopkins Press).—

> The "Volumen paramirum" deals with disease and health, was originally published *ca.* 1520, and was meant as an introduction to a treatise on practical medicine which is lost. It mainly treats of the causes of diseases. The present English translation contains many annotations and useful indexes; it has been based upon the Achelis edition: ACHELIS, J. D., 1928: Paracelsus. Volumen paramirum (Von Krankheit und gesundem Leben), 170 p. (Jena: Diederichs). This German edition is preceded by an introduction (of 45 pages) and by a commentary (of 55 pages).

——, PACHTER, H. M., 1951: Paracelsus: magic into science, 360 p. (New York, N.Y.: Schuman).—

> A very readable and well-documented biography of Paracelsus, accompanied by many notes at the end of the book. The author tries to show how magic and scientific elements together form a well-integrated whole in Paracelsus' teachings, and that Paracelsus can be considered as a turning point from magic into science. *Cf.* PEUCKERT, W. E., 1967, *vide* section Prehistoric and primitive biology and medicine, subsection a.

——, PAGEL, W., 1958: Paracelsus: an introduction to philosophical medicine in the era of the Renaissance, 368 p. (Basle & New York, N.Y.: Karger).—

> Whereas most of Paracelsus' work has been published in German, and whereas it is not easy to read his work because of its seemingly contradictory statements, Pagel makes an attempt to give a review of the range of ideas expounded by Paracelsus, of their influence on his contemporaries and his 17th-century followers and of their place in the history of science and philosophy, in order to make them accessible to further objective study for English speaking people as well. As such it is a standard work in English on Paracelsus. In the first part Paracelsus is considered as a figure of the Renaissance. It gives much biographical information, together with a general exposition of his ideas, his interpretation of truth and nature, and his thoughts on the position of Man in the cosmos. The second part deals with his innovations in medicine and the third part discusses the ancient, mediaeval, and contemporary sources.

————, 1962: Das medizinische Weltbild des Paracelsus. Seine Zusammenhänge mit Neuplatonismus und Gnosis, 136 p. (Wiesbaden: Steiner).—

The author makes a comparison between the complex "Weltanschauung" (view of life) of Paracelsus on the one hand, and the philosophy of the Gnostics, Stoics and Neoplatonists, both in their classical exposition and in the renaissance revival by Christian humanists, on the other hand. The first part of the book gives a lucid introduction to the Paracelsean way of thought. The second part particularly deals with Paracelsian concepts in which the author compares these concepts with those of earlier 'cosmosophies', thereby elucidating the meaning of occult powers and their 'signature'.

————, PEUCKERT, W. E., ed., 1965-1969: Paracelsus' Werke. Studienausgabe in 5 Bde. Vol. I (1965): Medizinische Schriften, 584 p.; Vol. II (1965): Medizinische Schriften (Forsetzung), 544 p.; Vol. III (1967): Philosophische Schriften, 508 p.; Vol. IV (1967): Theologische, religionsphilosophische und sozialpolitische Schriften, 402 p.; Vol. V (1969): Pansophische, magische und gabalische Schriften, 426 p. (Basle & Stuttgart: Schwabe).—

This is an attempt to translate the relevant passages from Paracelsus's works into modern German. The first two vols. deal with medical, the third vol. with philosophical problems. Throughout the work, stress has been laid on the philosophical aspects of Paracelsus's works. In short introductions preceding the translated passages, the editor elucidates the interconnections between medicine, alchemy, philosophy, and theology. An anthology, limited to the ethical parts of Paracelsus's teachings is: JACOBI, J., ed., 1951: Paracelsus: selected writings, 347 p. (Bollingen Series, No. 28) (New York, N.Y.: Pantheon Bks.). The chapter headings are: Credo (autobiographical); man and the created world; man and his body; man and works; man and ethics; man and spirit; man and fate. Originally published in German: Lebendiges Erbe. Eine Auslese aus seinen sämtlichen Schriften mit 150 zeitgenössischen Illustrationen. Wegweisendes und Besinnliches für den Menschen der Gegenwart, 1942, 315 p. (Zurich: Rascher). A French selection: GORCEIX, B., 1968: Oeuvres médicales. Paracelse. Choisies, traduites et présentées, 261 p. (Galien; Histoire et Philosophie de la Biologie et de la Médicine) (Paris: Presses Univ. de France).

————, STREBEL, J., ed., 1944-1949: Theophrastus von Hohenheim genannt Paracelsus. Sämtliche Werke in zeitgemässer Kürzung, 8 vols. (St. Gallen: Zollikofer).—

A (partly grossly) abbreviated text in modern German. Vols. VI-VIII deal with the clinical, surgical, hygienic, epidemiological, pharmacological, and macrobiotic treatises. The last volume contains chronological tables and an index of Paracelsian terms. The most complete version of all Paracelsus's works has been published by SUDHOFF, K., ed., 1929-1933: Theophrast von Hohenheim genannt Paracelsus. Sämtliche Werke, 14 vols. (Munich & Berlin: Oldenbourg). In 1960 an index to this collection of works was published: MÜLLER, M., 1960: Registerband zu Sudhoffs Paracelsus-Gesamtausgabe. Erste Abteilung: Medizinische, naturwissenschaftliche und philosophische Schriften, 281 p. (Nova Acta Paracelsica, Suppl. 1960) (Basle: Karger). This index seems to be very complete; it gives thousands of entries.

————, SUDHOFF, K., 1958: Bibliographia Paracelsica. Besprechung der unter Hohenheims Namen 1527-1893 erschienenen Druckschriften, 722 p. (Graz: Akad. Druck- und Verlagsanst.).—

In 1894 Sudhoff published the first volume of his planned trilogy "Versuch einer Kritik der Echtheit der Paracelsischen Schriften" of which the first volume contained a catalogue and discussion of the printed works of Paracelsus. The present book is a reprint of this volume and is still up-to-date. It contains 518 items, each minutely described with a list of the libraries where it can be found and extensive notes in which its value for final reading of the text and its tradition have been discussed. (Cf. also WEIMANN's Paracelsus-Bibliographie, infra).

————, VOGT, A., 1956: Theophrastus Paracelsus als Arzt und Philosoph, 212 p. (Stuttgart: Hippocrates).—

A semi-popular introduction to Paracelsus and his work for the general reader and medical practitioner. His medical work is considered in relation to his theosophical and anthropological speculations. It gives a clear picture of Paracelsus's views on chemistry, surgery, pathology, and therapy. A comparable useful introduction which gives information in Paracelsus's own words is: BITTEL, K., ed., 1961: Leben und Lebensweisheit in Selbstzeugnissen, ed. 4, 160 p. (Reclams Universal-Bibliothek, No. 7567/68)

(Leipzig: Reclam). Another semi-popular attempt to make Paracelsus understandable for the modern reader is: KERNER, D., 1965: Paracelsus. Leben und Werk, 160 p. (Stuttgart: Schattauer).

——, WEIMANN, K. H., 1963: Paracelsus-Bibliographie, 1932-1960. Mit einem Verzeichnis neu entdeckter Paracelsus-Handschriften (1900-1960), 100 p. (Wiesbaden: Steiner).—

> This bibliography can be considered as a continuation of SUDHOFF's "Nachweise zur Paracelsus-Literatur", published in Acta Paracelsica, Suppl., 1932, 68 p. It gives a documented list containing 1180 items. (N.B. Sudhoff's "Nachweise" contains 1,089 items). Moreover, the book includes a list of Paracelsus-manuscripts which have come to light since 1900 and a survey of the Paracelsus Societies. Good indexes have been included. (Cf. also SUDHOFF's Bibliographia Paracelsica, supra).

——, ZEKERT, O., 1968: Paracelsus. Europäer im 16. Jahrhundert, 184 p. (Stuttgart: Kohlhammer).—

> A chronological biography, based on much newly-discovered material. This publication is of much interest for its many pharmaco-historical details. Valuable bibliography which includes much that has been omitted in Sudhoff's bibliography.

Paré, Ambroise (1510-1590) — DOE, J., 1937: A bibliography of the works of Ambroise Paré, premier chirurgien et conseiller du roy, 266 p. (Chicago, Ill.: Univ. Chicago Press).—

> Each title is followed by the name of the bibliographer, biographical and historical notes on the book, and its relation to other editions and works of Paré, and includes detailed information as to typography, paginations, contents, and errata. The location of copies of each work examined by the author and the copies held in public and private libraries throughout the world are listed. Appendixes with a key to owners of Paré's books, a chronological list of his works, and a catalogue of authors consulted.

——, HAMBY, W. B., ed., 1965: Surgery and Ambroise Paré, 32 + 436 p. (Norman, Okla.: Univ. Oklahoma Press).—

> This is an English translation of J. F. MALGAIGNE's introduction to Paré's "Oeuvres complètes", published in 1840-1841 (Paris: Baillière). It comprises a history of western surgery from the sixth to the sixteenth century and a bibliography of Paré's works. HAMBY also prepared an English translation of another part of Paré's work, viz., The case reports and autopsy records of Ambroise Paré, 1960, 214 p. (Springfield, Ill.: Thomas; Oxford: Blackwell). A new French text of Paré's treatise on gunshot wounds has been prepared by SIGERIST, H. E., 1923: Die Behandlung der Schusswunden (1545), 87 p. (Leipzig: Barth). This new German text has been based upon the original edition "La methode de traicter les playes faictes par hacquebutes et aultres bastons à feu..." and is accompanied by a German translation and a brief introduction (of 9 pages). Cf. also: BOUSSEL, P., ed., 1964: Ambroise Paré. Des monstres, des prodiges, des voyages, 360 p. (Paris: Livre-club du librarie); and: HAMBY, W. B., 1967: Ambroise Paré: surgeon of the Renaissance, 251 p. (St. Louis, Mo.: Green).

——, KEYNES, G., ed., 1952: The Apologie and treatise, containing the Voyages made into divers places; with many of his writings upon surgery, 33 + 227 p. (Chicago, Ill.: Chicago U.P.; London: Falcon).—

> This is a new edition of Paré's most characteristic writing, the "Apologie" together with selections from his surgical writings, containing a general description of surgery, of aneurysms, hernia, wounds in general and by gunshot, amputations, fractures, dislocations, cataracts, stone, and some other topics. Brief but useful annotations. The book starts with a useful introduction containing much information about Paré and his work. Of the "Apologie" a German translation also exists: PARÉ, A., 1963: Rechtfertigung und Bericht über meine Reisen in verschiedene Orte, 125 p. (Hubers Klassiker der Medizin und der Naturwissens., Vol. 2) (Bern: Huber). Also in French: Apologie et traicté contenant les voyages faicts en divers lieux (1585, Paris), inséré dans le 4e édition de ses "Oeuvres".

——, PACKARD, F. R., 1921: Life and times of Ambroise Paré (1510-1590). With a new translation of his Apology and an account of his Journeys in divers places, 297 p. (New York, N.Y.: Hoeber).—

> A well-written account of the life of A. Paré. Packard also discusses the question whether Paré was a Huguenot or not. Many beautiful illustrations. Some other biographies of Paré are: MICHELET, L., 1930: La vie d'Ambroise Paré, chirurgien du Roy,

écrivain, 160 p. (Paris: Librairie Le Fran-çois); and ROBERT, A., 1929: Ambroise Paré, médecin-légiste, 180 p. (Thèse de la Faculté de Médecine, Univ. de Paris) (Paris). *Cf.* also DELAUNAY, P., 1926: Ambroise Paré naturaliste, 70 p. (Paris: Laval).

——, SINGER, D. W., 1924: Selection from the works of Ambroise Paré, with short biography and explanatory and bibliographical notes, 246 p. (London: Bale).—

This selection contains the Epistle dedicatory to Henry III; extracts from Of wounds made by gunshot, *etc.;* Apologie and treatise of voyages into divers places; surgical aphorisms and rules. They are preceded by an introduction of 47 pages. A collection of some 50 excerpts can be found in: DELARUELLE, L. & M. SEN-DRAIL, eds., 1953: Textes choisis d'Ambroise Paré, 292 p. (Paris: Les Belles Lettres). *Cf.* also: PAEPKE, K.: Zahnärztliches aus den Werken von Ambroise Paré, 24 p. (Inaugural Diss., Univ. Leipzig).

Pascal, Blaise (1623-1662) — SCHOLTENS, M., 1963: Pascal. Études médico-psychologiques, 196 p. (Assen, The Netherlands: van Gorcum).—

The contents of this book consist of two parts. The first part (p. 28-95) deals with medico-historical matters, especially with the diseases Pascal suffered from. Moreover, this part contains much biographical information concerning Pascal and his family. The second part deals with medico-psychological problems and contains, *inter alia,* an analysis of Pascal's character and his feelings of anxiety.

Pasteur, Louis (1822-1895) — BLARIN-GHEM, L., 1923: Pasteur et le transformisme, 241 p. (Paris: Masson).—

The present book deals with such subjects as: the species concept (in biology as well as in chemistry); variations of form, more especially in crystals; heredity, hybridization and mutation; the role of microorganisms, their environment, migration and adaptation; modifications of the individual: plasticity, reciprocal adaptations, the struggle for life, selection and acquired characters.

——, DUBOS, R. J., 1952: Louis Pasteur, free lance of science, 418 p. (Boston, Mass.: Little, Brown).—

A biography of life and works of Pasteur in which the author states, that although Pasteur's basic aim was to devote himself to theoretical and fundamental studies such as the structure of crystals and the origin of life, he continually was drawn away from these topics in order to work on practical applications, such as: the mechanism of fermentation, the study of vitiation of beer and wine, the silk-worm disease, and his studies on animal and human pathology which initiated the germ theory of disease and led him to discover the principles of immunity. Also in French: Louis Pasteur, franc-tireur de la science, 435 p. (Paris: Presses Univ. de France). *Cf.* CHANLAINE, P., 1966: Pasteur et ses découvertes, 160 p. (Paris: Nathan).

——, NICOLLE, J., 1953: Un maître de l'enquête scientifique, Louis Pasteur, 224 p. (Paris: Vieux-Colombier).—

In this book the author seeks to demonstrate the logic of the mode of reasoning behind the experiments Pasteur conducted. Chapters are entitled: 1. L'affaire de l'acide tartrique; 2. L'affaire des fermentations; 3. L'affaire des générations dites spontanées; 4. L'affaire du vinaigre; 5. L'affaire des vins; 6. L'affaire des vers à soie; 7. L'affaire de la bière; 8. L'affaire du charbon; 9. L'affaire du choléra des poules; 10. L'affaire de la rage. Also in English translation: Louis Pasteur: a master of scientific inquiry, 1961, 196 p. (London: Hutchinson). A well-written short biography with portraits is: MONDOR, H., 1945: Pasteur, 189 p. (Paris: Correa). An evaluation of the importance of Pasteur in the long line of biological discoveries: MANN, J., 1966: Louis Pasteur, 163 p. (London: Pan Bks.).

——, PASTEUR, L., 1922-1939: Oeuvres rassemblées et classées par ordre chronologique avec des pages inédites et des notes par Pasteur VALLERY-RADOT, 7 vols. Vol. I (1922): 480 p.; Vol. II (1922): 688 p.; Vol. III (1924): 519 p.; Vol. IV (1926): 762 p.; Vol. V (1928): 376 p.; Vol. VI (1933): 918 p.; Vol. VII (1939): 412 p. (Paris: Masson).—

The volumes appeared under the following titles: Vol. I: Dissymétrie moléculaire; Vol. II: Fermentations et générations dites spontanées; Vol. III: Études sur le vinaigre et le vin; Vol. IV: Études sur la maladie des vers à soie; Vol. V: Études sur la bière, avec une théorie nouvelle de la fermentation; Vol. VI: Maladies virulentes, virus-vaccins et prophylaxie de la rage; Vol.

VII: Notes scientifiques diverses; discours; articles; correspondance; table des noms cités; table chronologique des publications de Pasteur, et une table analytique générale. *Cf.* KAHANE, E., ed., 1957: Louis Pasteur. Pages choisies, 128 p. (Avec introduction, notes et commentaires) (Paris: Éd. Sociales); and CUNY, H., 1963: Louis Pasteur. Choix de textes, bibliographie, portraits, fac-similés, 223 p. (Paris: Seghers). Also in English: CUNY, H., 1965: Louis Pasteur: the man and his theories. With plates, including portraits and a facsimile, 190 p. (London: Souvenir Press).

———, VALLERY-RADOT, P., 1958: Louis Pasteur: a great life in brief, 199 p. (New York, N.Y.: Knopf).—

This is a short but well-written account of the famous French scientist, composed by his grandson. The booklet is especially written for the interested layman and the medical student and it gives a clear picture of some of the most ingenious experiments of the whole history of science and of the way in which Pasteur subjected his results to rigid controls. Of the same author appeared: VALLERY-RADOT, P., 1947: Pasteur. Images de sa vie suivies de quelques épisodes dramatiques de sa carrière scientifique, 104 p. (Paris: Flammarion). This is an album of portraits of Pasteur and members of his family, followed by accounts of a few dramatic episodes of his life, such as his anxiety when he inoculated the vaccine of rabies into the body of the nine-year-old boy. Pasteur's correspondence also has been published by his grandson: VALLERY-RADOT, P., ed., 1951: Pasteur Correspondance, réunie et annotée, 4 vols. (Paris: Flammarion).

———, VALLERY-RADOT, R., 1900: La vie de Pasteur, 632 p. (Paris: Flammarion).—

The standard biography of Pasteur. Also in English translation: The life of Pasteur, ed. 12, 1960, 484 p. (New York, N.Y.: Dover). The English translation was first published in two vols. in 1901. Also in German translation: Louis Pasteur. Sein Leben und Werk (Freudenstadt).

———, TOMCSIK, J., ed., 1964: Pasteur und die Generatio spontanea. Aus den Werken von Pasteur, 170 p. (Hubers Klassiker der Medizin u. der Naturwiss., Vol. III) (Bern & Stuttgart: Huber).—

A collection of some 9 fragments derived from Pasteur's publications dealing with the problem of generatio spontanea, published between 1860 and 1864.

Patin, Guy (1601-1672) — PACKARD, F. R., 1925: Guy Patin and the medical profession in Paris in the XVIIIth century, 334 p. (New York, N.Y.: Hoeber).—

Patin was a typical representative of the (conservative) medical profession of the Paris university during the 17th century. The present study discusses such subjects as: Patin's youth and education at the university of Paris, his home life and literary interests, his relationship with his students and with his sons, his opinions and contributions, the situation in the Paris Faculty of Medicine. With bibliographical notes and index. *Cf.* also: PIC, P., 1911: Guy Patin, 301 p. (Paris: Steinheil). With 74 portraits and containing many documents.

Pavlov, Ivan Petrovich (1849-1936) — DUBE, W., ed., 1953: Iwan Petrowitch Pawlow. Bibliographie der Veröffentlichungen über sein Lebenswerk in deutscher Sprache, 74 p. (Leipzig: Harrassowitz).—

This bibliography contains 502 issues published in the German language (incl. translations) of works dealing with conditioned reflexes and the physiology of digestion. The material is classified as follows: 1. General (incl. biographies, commemorations, necrologies); 2. medicine (incl. physiology, psychiatry, neurology, paediatrics, internal medicine, surgery, obstetrics, hygiene, bacteriology, pharmacy, therapeutics and biology); 3. psychology and education; 4. philosophy; 5. popular publications. Excluded are articles in newspapers. Author- and subject-indexes have been added.

———, FROLOV, Y. P., 1937: Pavlov and his school, 291 p. (London: Kegan Paul).—

An exposition of the origin, development, and achievement of Pavlov and his school in the special field of the physiology of the nervous system. Included are some criticisms by Pavlov of certain of the doctrines of psycho-analysis, and Pavlov's demonstrations of the inadequacy of Kretschmer's mind-body typology. For a biography in English: BABKIN, B. P., 1951: Pavlov: a biography, 365 p. (London: Gollancz).

———, KAPLAN, M., ed., 1966: Essential works of Pavlov, 406 p. (New York, N.Y.: Bantam Bks.).—

Another selection: GIBBONS, J., ed., 1955: I. P. Pavlov: selected works, 654 p. (Transl. by S. BELSKY; supervision by K. S. KOSHTOYANTS) (Moscow: Foreign

Language Publ. House). A reprint of one of Pavlov's most famous books in English translation: PAVLOV, I. P., 1960: Conditioned reflexes: an investigation of the physiological activity of the cerebral cortex, 430 p. (New York, N.Y.: Dover). A collection of Pavlov's publications: PAVLOV, I. P., 1953-1956: Sämtliche Werke und Mittwoch-Kolloquien, 12 vols., 4713 p., published by the Academy of Sciences of the U.S.S.R. A reprint edition has been announced by Zeller (Osnabrück).

——, WELLS, H. K., 1956: Ivan P. Pavlov: toward a scientific psychology and psychiatry, 224 p. (Pavlov and Freud, I) (London: Lawrence & Wishart).—

Basing himself on Pavlov's works and on those of Asratyan, Bykov, and Ivanov-Smolensky, the author gives an account of Pavlov's contributions to psychology and psychiatry and of the development of Pavlov's ideas in the Soviet Union. Cf. also: GANTT, W. H., ed., 1964: Lectures on conditioned reflexes: twenty-five years of objective study on the higher nervous activity-behaviour of animals, 2 vols. (London: Lawrence & Wishart).

Pavlovski, Evgeny Nikanorovich (1884-1965) — BORCHERT, A., 1959: J. N. Pawlowski. Leben und Werk, 178 p. (Berlin: Deutscher Verlag der Wissenschaften).—

A short biography of this Russian zoologist and parasitologist (p. 7-35) and a complete bibliography of his numerous publications (1204 entries). Cf. PAVLOVSKY, Y. N., ed., 1964: Human diseases with natural foci, 345 p. (Moscow: Foreign Language Publ. House).

Pettenkofer, Max von (1818-1901) — KISSKALT, K., 1948: Max von Pettenkofer, 135 p. (Grosse Naturforscher, Vol. 4) (Stuttgart: Wiss. Verlagsges.).—

Max von Pettenkofer has been the founder of experimental hygiene, a pupil of Liebig, and professor of hygiene, Munich University (1853), where he founded the first Hygienic Institute. He did much original research in the fields of physiological chemistry, metabolism, epidemiology, experimental hygiene, and metabolism in respiration. Cf. also: HUME, E. E., 1927: Max von Pettenkofer: his theory on the etiology of cholera, typhoid fever and other intestinal diseases. A review of his arguments and evidence. (New York, N.Y.: Hoeber).

Pinchot, Gifford (1865-1946) — MACGEARY, M. N., 1960: Gifford Pinchot, forester-politician, 481 p. (Princeton, N.J.: Princeton U.P.).—

After studying forestry in Europe, Pinchot became the leader of forestry and of timber conservation in the U.S.A. The present biography gives a very clear picture of Pinchot's activities both as forester and as politician. An autobiography, completed by its author just before his death, is: PINCHOT, G., 1947: Breaking new ground, 522 p. (New York, N.Y.: Harcourt, Brace).

Pinel, Philippe (1745-1826) — LECHLER, W. H., 1959: Philippe Pinel, seine Familie, seine Jugend- und Studienjahre, 1745-1778, 292 p. (Diss. Univ. Munich) (Munich: Universitätsinst. Gesch. Med.).—

The first reliable biography of this great French physician whose life history is so interwoven with legend. Lechler attempted to reconstruct the social, political and cultural atmosphere in which Pinel grew up. Interesting descriptions of medical education at Montpellier. This is the first volume and other volumes are promised; together they aim to give a complete biography. The present volume ends with the year 1778 when Pinel left Montpellier to go to Paris.

——, PINEL, P., 1962: A treatise on insanity, 55 + 288 p. (History of Medicine Series, No. 14) (New York, N.Y.: Hafner).—

A facsimile reprint of the 1801 English translation of Pinel's classic, in which the author expresses his disagreement with the common medical treatment of the mentally ill in his day.

Platter, Felix (1536-1614) — BUESS, H., ed., 1963: Observationes. Krankheitsbeobachtungen in drei Büchern. Buch I: Funktionelle Störungen des Sinnes und der Bewegung, 198 p. (Hubers Klassiker der Medizin und der Naturwiss., Vol. I) (Bern & Stuttgart: Huber).—

This is a German translation of the first part of Platter's "Observationes", dealing with functional disorders of the mind and of moving, discussing such topics as: epilepsy in children, catalepsy, inborn mental defect, melancholia, hypochondriasis and stupor following the use of opium. Included are many notes in the text, a list of pharmaceutical drugs, a full bibliography of Platter's publications, a table of contents, and an index. Books II and III will be published later.

——, JENNETT, S., 1961: Beloved son Felix: the journal of Felix Platter, a medical student in Montpellier in the sixteenth century, 158 p. (London: Muller).—

Platter stayed from 1552 to 1557 in Montpellier where he studied under Belon. He wrote an autobiography, first published by A. FECHTER in 1840. From this autobiography a French translation was prepared from that part that dealt with his journey from Basle to Montpellier and back and with his stay in Montpellier. This book provides in its turn an English translation of this French translation. It gives, as the translator says in his introduction "the immediate impression of an inhabitant of Montpellier in the middle of the sixteenth century... life of a period in Montpellier that is not otherwise well supplied with documents, and illustrates something of the manner and the system of medical education."

——, KARCHER, J., 1949: Felix Platter. Lebensbild eines basler Stadtarztes, 1536-1614, 112 p. (Basle: Helbing & Lichtenhahn).—

Platter was an adherent of Vesalius. He wrote the "Praxis medica", a textbook of pathology and therapy. He divided diseases according to their conspicuous features; psychical diseases were ascribed to natural causes. He also possessed a famous herbal. An elaborate study dealing with Platter's botanical activities is: RYTZ, W., 1932-1933: Das Herbarium Felix Platters. Ein Beitrag zur Geschichte der Botanik des 16. Jahrhunderts, 222 p. (Verhandl. naturforsch. Gesellsch. Basel, Vol. 44: 1-122). A bibliography of Platter's publications contains: BURCKHARDT, A., 1917: Geschichte der medizinischen Fakultät zu Basel 1460-1900, 495 p. (esp. p. 72-83) (Basle: Reinhardt).

Pol, Nicolaus (*ca.* 1470-1532) — FISCH, M. H., 1947: Nicolaus Pol Doctor 1494. With a critical text of his Guaiae Tract, 246 p. (New York, N.Y.: Reichner).—

Nicolaus Pol was a humanist, physician, and a great collector of books. The present book is a catalogue listing 467 books, 30 mss., 251 incunabula, and 186 books printed in the early 16th century. It gives full descriptions of the American holdings. Introductory chapters give a good picture of Pol and his collection. It also contains a critical edition and English translation of Pol's "Libellus de cura morbi Gallici per lignum Guaycanum".

Porta, Giovanni Battista della (1545-1615) — PRICE, D. J., 1957: Natural magick, 409 +6 p. (New York, N.Y.: Basic Bks.).—

This is an English version of the 1658 edition of Porta's "Magia naturalis". It contains a description of natural magic as it flourished during the 15th and 16th centuries, and it elucidates the magico-experimental approach to nature. The original text was intended for the interested layman and deals with such subjects as: magnetism, optics, pneumatics, monsters, strange animals, medicine, cookery, cosmetics, hawking and hunting, *etc.*

Purkyně, Jan Evangelista (1787-1869) — JOHN, H. J., 1959: Jan Evangelista Purkyně: Czech scientist and patriot 1787-1869, 94 p. (Mem. Amer. Philos. Soc., Vol. 49) (Philadelphia, Pa.: Amer. Philos. Soc.).—

The only biography of this Czech physiologist in the English language. Very fine illustrations but no index. Some further information as to the meaning and the achievements of Purkyně can be found in ZAUNICK, R., ed., 1961: Purkyně-Symposion der deutschen Akademie der Naturforscher Leopoldina, in Gemeinschaft mit der tschechoslowakischen Akademie der Wissenschaften am 31. Oktober und 1. November 1959 in Halle/Saale, 230 p. (Nova Acta Leopoldina, N. F., 24, 151) (Leipzig: Barth).

——, KRUTA, V., 1964: Počátkúm Vědecké Dráhy J. E. Purkynje. Beginnings of the scientific career of J. E. Purkyně, 207 p. (Brno: Acta Facultatis Medicae Univ. Brunensis).—

In this book the editor has transcribed a great number of letters to, from, and about Purkyně, especially those belonging to the early years of Purkyně's scientific career. Introduction in Czech with English summary. Most letters are in German. Valuable index of names.

—— ——, & M. TEICH, 1962: Jan Evangelista Purkyne, 153 p. (Prague: Staatsverlag für medizinische Literatur).—

Purkyně was one of the founders of modern physiology and contributed with many important discoveries and inventions to the fields of physiology, histology and anatomy. Many eponyms remind us of his achievements. Moreover, he contributed basically to the renaissance of the Czech people and to the development of a scientific Czech language. These are the topics discussed in this book. *Cf.* also: STUDNIČKA, F. K., 1927: Joh. Ev. Purkinjes und seiner Schule Verdienste um die Entdeckung tierischer Zellen und um die Aufstellung der "Zellen-Theorie", 70 p. (Acta Soc. Sci. Nat. Moravicae, Vol. 4: 98-168).

Rafinesque, Constantine Samuel (1783-1840) — RAFINESQUE, C. S., 1944: A life of travels: being a verbatim and literatim reprint of the original and only edition (Philadelphia, 1836), 68 p. (Chronica Botanica VIII, No. 2).—

This work, the full title of which is "A life of travels and researches in North America and South Europe, or outlines of the life, travels and researches of C. S. Rafinesque", can be considered as a brief autobiographical review, for Rafinesque himself states "a short account of all my travels will be also a narrative of my whole life..." In his foreword E. D. MERRILL gives a short review of Rafinesque's life and work and a brief evaluation of his achievements. *Cf.* also: MERRILL, E. D., 1949: Index Rafinesquianus. The plant names published by C. S. Rafinesque with reductions, and a consideration of his methods, objectives and attainments, 296 p. (Jamaica Plain, Mass.: Arnold Arboretum).

——, FITZPATRICK, T. J., 1911: Rafinesque: a sketch of his life with bibliography, 241 p. (Des Moines, Iowa: Hist. Dept. of Iowa).—

After a biographical sketch (p. 11-62), the author gives a very detailed bibliography containing 941 items covering rather thoroughly the published books and papers of Rafinesque (p. 65-216). The writings of Rafinesque are varied and widely scattered. Data concerning his unpublished manuscripts have been included (p. 216-219). The Bibliotheca Rafinesquiana (p. 223-239) lists 134 titles containing data regarding Rafinesque, published by others.

Ramazzini, Bernardino (1633-1714) — WRIGHT, W. C., ed., 1940: Bernardino Ramazzini (1633-1714). De morbis artificum Bernardini Ramazzini diatriba. Diseases of workers. The Latin text of 1713, revised with translation and notes, 48 + 549 p. (History of Medicine Series, No. 7) (Chicago, Ill.: Chicago U.P.).—

The first treatise ever published on occupational diseases (1700, Modena). A

second revised edition appeared in 1713 (Padua). This is the first complete English version of this treatise, accompanied by many instructive notes. Sarton writes about this book: "The book contains a wealth of materials not only of medical, but also of cultural interest. It should be included in any library for the study of eighteenth-century thought." (From Isis 33: 261). *Cf.* KOELSCH, F., 1912: Bernardino Ramazzini, der Vater der Gewerbehygiene (1633-1714). Sein Leben und seine Werke, 35 p. (Stuttgart: Enke).

Ramón y Cajal, Santiago (1852-1934) — CANNON, D. F., 1949: Explorer of the human brain: the life of Santiago Ramón y Cajal (1852-1934) with a memoir by Sir Charles SHERRINGTON, 303 p. (New York, N.Y.: Schuman).—

A well-documented and vividly-written biography of the famous Spanish neurologist. There are many references to one of his most famous works of which the following English translation exists: Degeneration and regeneration of the nervous system, 2 vols., 1928 (London: Oxford U.P.). *Cf.* CRAIGIE, E. H. & W. C. GIBSON, 1968: The world of Ramón y Cajal with selections from his nonscientific writings, 295 p. (A monograph in the Bannerstone Division of American Lectures in Hist. of Med. and Science, No. 718) (Springfield, Ill.: Thomas). Unfortunately I am not able to give further details about this book.

——, RAMÓN Y CAJAL, S., 1966: Recollections of my life, 638 p. (Cambridge, Mass.: M.I.T. Press).—

Ramón y Cajal was a pioneer in the field of neurology; he specialized in the histology of the brain and nerves and fundamentally contributed to our knowledge of the structure and connections of nerve cells, and of the structure of the neuron. The first part of this autobiography deals with boyhood, education and early training in the medical profession; the second part offers a discussion of his early work in neurology and contains many descriptions of his experiments which ultimately led to his professorship in Normal Histology and Pathological Anatomy at Madrid University. This translation has been prepared from the third Spanish edition (1923), and has been reprinted from the Memoirs of the Amer. Philos. Soc., Vol. 8, 1937.

Raspail, François (1794-1878) — WEINER, D. B., 1968: Raspail: scientist and reformer,

336 p. (With a chapter by S. RASPAIL) (New York, N.Y.: Columbia U.P.).—

A full-scale biography of the French scientist and politician. Raspail is the founder of histochemistry. He did much work in the fields of physiology (animal as well as plant) and medicine (where he rediscovered *Acarus scabiei*) especially concerning its social implications.

Rauwolf, Leonhard (*ca.* 1535-1596) — DANNENFELDT, K. H., 1968: Leonhard Rauwolf: sixteenth-century physician, botanist, and traveller, 322 p. (Cambridge, Mass.: Harvard U.P.).—

Rauwolf, a Bavarian physician, was the first modern botanist to collect and describe the flora of the Near East. He visited that part of the world during his voyages between 1573 and 1575, an account of which he published in 1582. Besides, this book contains much that is of interest to the history of the Near East of the period considered and to our knowledge of other Renaissance travellers.

Ray, John (1627-1705) — KEYNES, G., 1961: John Ray: a bibliography, 163 p. (London: Faber & Faber).—

Stimulated by Raven's biography, *vide infra,* Keynes compiled a full-scale bibliography. Each work has been treated separately, and a full description and collation of the several editions has been presented. Each work is introduced by a short discussion of the book, containing information about its composition, printings and/or revisions. As a result this bibliography contains much additional biographical information and may serve as a valuable pendant to RAVEN's biography.

——, RAVEN, C. E., 1942: John Ray: naturalist. His life and works, 502 p. (Cambridge: U.P.).—

An authoritative and detailed biography of the famous English field naturalist who worked in such diverse fields of natural history as botany, zoology, and geology, and was also an eminent Latinist and theologian. His botanical work culminated in his "Historia plantarum" (1686-1704) which was intended to include all botanical knowledge of the time; as such it is a great compilation. His zoological "Synopsis animalium quadrupedum et serpentini generis" (1693) exercised a considerable influence in his time, and the interrelation of his biological achie-

vements and his religious beliefs he summed up in his "The wisdom of God manifested in the work of the creation", in which he maintained a physicotheological point of view. A second edition was published in 1950, 506 p. (Cambridge: U.P.).

Réaumur, René Antoine Ferchault de (1683-1757) — TORLAIS, J., 1961: Réaumur: le biologiste, l'entomologiste, l'inventeur, le métallurgiste, le naturaliste, le physicien, 475 p. (Paris: Blanchard).—

A slightly enlarged reprinting of the edition of 1936: TORLAIS, J., 1936: Réaumur (1683-1757). Un esprit encyclopédique en dehors de l'Encyclopédie d'après des documents inédits, 448 p. (Paris: Desclée de Brouwer). Réaumur's scientific papers deal with nearly all branches of science. He wrote much on natural history. His greatest work is the "Mémoires pour servir à l'histoire des insectes", 6 vols., with 267 plates, published in Amsterdam, 1734-1742. It describes the appearance, habits, and locality of all the known insects except the beetles. Torlais' book contains an account of the life and scientific activities of Réaumur based upon documents and manuscripts present in the Academy of Science and the University Library at Geneva. *Cf.* also: WHEELER, W. M., 1926: The natural history of ants. From an unpublished manuscript in the archives of the Academy of Sciences of Paris, 280 p. (New York, N.Y.: Knopf).

Reil, Johann Christian (1759-1813) — ZAUNICK, R., ed., 1960: Johann Christian Reil, 1759-1813, 159 p. (Nova Acta Leopoldina XXII, No. 144) (Leipzig: Barth).—

On the occasion of the celebration of the two-hundredth anniversary of the birthday of Reil, the Academy of Natural Sciences and the Faculty of Medicine of the University of Halle organized a symposium, at which four orations were delivered, the text of which has been published in the present volume. The first oration gives a short biography and a complete bibliography of Reil's writings, of dissertations presented by his pupils and of articles about him or relevant to his scientific achievements. The second oration deals with his anatomical studies (especially of the brain), the third with his psychiatric writings and the fourth gives a review of Reil's services to Halle as Municipal Physician.

Röntgen, Wilhelm Conrad (1845-1923) — GLASSER, O., 1958: Dr. W. C. Röntgen, ed. 2, 169 p. (Springfield, Ill.: Thomas; Oxford: Blackwell).—

Revision of the first edition (1945) including recent information. A very useful biography. A list of his scientific papers, a chronology of his life and a bibliography of source-material are given in the appendixes. A second German ed. appeared in 1959: Wilhelm Röntgen und die Geschichte der Röntgenstrahlen. Mit einem Beitrag: Persönliches über W. C. Röntgen von M. BOVERI, 381 p. (Berlin: Springer). A more popular biography is: NICOLLE, J., 1965: Wilhelm Röntgen et l'ère des rayons X, 192 p. (Paris: Seghers).

Rokitansky, Carl von (1804-1878) — RO-KITANSKY, C. VON, 1960: Selbstbiographie und Antrittsrede, 111 p. (Eingeleitet, herausgegeben und mit Erläuterungen versehen von E. LESKY) (Oesterr. Akad. der Wiss., phil.-hist. Kl., Sitzber. 234, No. 3) (Vienna: Bohlaus).—

Rokitansky can be considered to be the founder of the Vienna School of pathological anatomy; his name is associated with the second great period of the medical school of Vienna. Besides much autobiographical material, this book gives much information concerning medical life in Vienna in the middle of the last century. This biography was written between 1876 and 1878.

Roux, Paul Émile (1853-1933) — LA-GRANGE, E., 1955: Monsieur Roux, 251 p. (Brussels: Goemaere).—

Roux worked with Pasteur on the etiology and treatment of various infectious diseases. From 1904 up to 1918 he was director of the Pasteur Institute. Besides being a valuable biography, this book is also a good introduction to the history of bacteriology of the periods of Roux and Pasteur.

Rumphius, Georgius Everhardus (1628-1702) — WIT, H. C. D. DE, ed., 1959: Rumphius memorial volume, 462 p. (Baarn, The Netherlands: Hollandia).—

Rumphius spent an important part of his life on the island of Amboina in the Moluccas. The present memorial volume aims at elucidating his manysided contributions to science, considering *e.g.,* his activities as a mammalogist, ornithologist, ichthyologist, entomologist, malacologist, phycologist, and economic botanist, and his contributions to our knowledge of pre-Linnean carcinology, and to our knowledge of echinoderms, corals, and algae. A special chapter deals with his "Herbarium Amboinense"; it includes a checklist to that herbal.

Rush, Benjamin (1746-1813) — BINGER, C., 1966: Revolutionary doctor: Benjamin Rush, 1746-1813, 326 p. (New York, N.Y.: Norton).—

In fact, Rush was the first great American physician. This is a readable biography. Because the author had access to new sources, this biography makes an advance over Goodman's hitherto standard work: GOODMAN, N. G., 1934: Benjamin Rush: physician and citizen 1746-1813, 421 p. (Philadelphia, Pa.: Univ. Pennsylvania Press). A reprint of his most famous book: RUSH, B., 1962: Medical inquiries and observations upon the diseases of the mind, 369 p. (History of Medicine Series, Vol. 15) (New York, N.Y.: Hafner).

——, BUTTERFIELD, L. H., ed., 1951: Letters of Benjamin Rush, 2 vols. Vol. I: 1761-1792; Vol. II: 1793-1813, 87 + 1295 p. (Memoirs Amer. Philos. Soc., Vol. 30) (Princeton, N.J.: Princeton U.P.).—

This is an indispensable source of information, making possible a satisfactory interpretation and evaluation of the man and his work. There are many annotations, and many biographical details have been given relating to the persons mentioned in these letters. The location of the replies to Rush's letters has been included and sometimes even a summary review of the contents of these letters has been added.

——, CORNER, G. W., ed., 1948: The autobiography of Benjamin Rush. His "Travels through life" together with his Commonplace Book for 1789-1813, 399 p. (Princeton, N.J.: Princeton U.P.).—

A well-edited volume with abundant footnotes. This autobiography has been printed in full from the original in possession of the Amer. Philos. Soc. and the Library Company of Philadelphia. Appendixes deal with Rush's medical theories, with the background of the speculation mania of 1791-92 and with the children of Benjamin and Julia Rush.

Ruysch, Frederik (1638-1731) — LUYEN-DIJK-ELSHOUT, A. M., ed., 1964: Dilucidatio valvularum in vasis lymphaticis et lacteis, 49 + 94 p. (Dutch classics in history of science, Vol. 9) (Nieuwkoop, The Netherlands: De Graaf).—

Facsimile of the first ed. of 1665. Ruysch has been professor of anatomy and botany in the Athenaeum Illustre of Amsterdam. In the introduction the editor summarizes the various views on the significance of the lymphatic vessels existing in the early 17th century. Ruysch was the first who could demonstrate the valves in the lymphatic vessels and he also gives his meaning about the form and the function of these valves.

Sachs, Julius (1832-1897) — PRINGSHEIM, E. G., 1932: Julius Sachs, der Begründer der neueren Pflanzenphysiologie, 1832-1897, 302 p. (Jena: Fischer).—

A very useful biography of this famous German plant physiologist in which stress has been laid on his scientific achievements, his position in relation to contemporary ideas and theories, his educational abilities, his published works, *etc.* Valuable indexes of subjects, personal names, and plant names.

Saint-Pierre, Jacques Henri Bernardin de (1737-1814) — ROULE, L., 1930: Bernardin de Saint-Pierre et l'harmonie de la nature, 242 p. (Paris: Flammarion).—

Bernardin de St. Pierre was a man of letters, an engineer, moralist, aesthete, and biologist. According to the author of this biography, the interpretations of Bernardin - although anthropocentric in character - anticipated many modern generalizations in the field of biology. Thus his observations in natural history are pervaded by the idea that all organisms are interdependent; he perceived the idea of adaptation and such phenomena as mimicry, symbiosis, *etc.* His "Études de la nature" (3 vols., 1784) was an attempt to prove the existence of God from the wonders of nature; he was in a philosophical sense strongly opposed to the Encyclopaedists. After his death a complete edition of his works in 18 vols. was published. (Paris, 1818-1820), in 1826 increased by seven vols. of correspondence and memoirs (ed. by A. MARTIN).

Sarton, George Alfred Léon (1884-1956) — VAN OYE, P., 1965: George Sarton. De mens en zijn werk uit brieven aan vrienden en kennissen, 166 p. (Verh. Kon. Vlaamse Acad. Wetensch., Letteren en Schone Kunsten van België, Kl. Wetensch., Jg. XXVII, No. 82) (Brussels: Paleis der Academiën).—

A collection of letters, mainly in French or English. These letters are accompanied by a preface, an introduction, bio-

graphical details, and an interpretation of and comments on the letters (in Flemish). The letters range from early 1905 to 1955. *Cf.* STIMSON, D., ed., 1962: Sarton on the history of science: selected essays by G. Sarton, 383 p. (Cambridge, Mass.: Harvard U.P.).

Scheuchzer, Johann Jacob (1672-1733) — STEIGER, R., 1933: Verzeichnis des wissenschaftlichen Nachlasses von Joh. Jak. Scheuchzer (1672-1733), 75 p. (Vjschr. Naturforsch. Ges.. Zürich, Vol. LXXVIII, Beiheft No. 21, p. 1-75).—

Scheuchzer took his degree of doctor in medicine at the University of Utrecht; afterwards he became town physician in Zurich. The more important part of his published writings relate to his journeys in which he gives fine descriptions, many of which are of importance to the history of biology. The present publication contains dates of his life, a bibliography of his printed writings (173 items), his manuscripts (203 items), his correspondence (58 items), and a list containing the names of 750 correspondents.

Schiller, Johann Christoph Friedrich von (1759-1805) — THEOPOLD, W., 1964: Schiller. Sein Leben und die Medizin im 18. Jahrhundert, 252 p. (Medizin in Geschichte und Kultur, Vol. 6) (Stuttgart: Fischer).—

A well-written and beautifully-illustrated account of medical and literary activities during Schiller's life-time in their mutual relation. This book contains much that is of interest to any study of medical and/or cultural life in Germany in Schiller's time. Bibliography of 241 items.

Schleiden, Matthias Jacob (1804-1881) — MÖBIUS, M., 1904: Matthias Jacob Schleiden. Zu seinem 100. Geburtstage, 106 p. (Leipzig: Engelmann).—

Schleiden was the first to prove that a nucleated cell is the only original constituent of the plant embryo, and that the development of all vegetable tissues must be referred to such cells. He also became famous by publishing his Grundzüge der wissenschaftlichen Botanik, nebst einer methodologischen Einleitung als Anleitung zum Studium der Pflanze, 2 vols., 1842-1843. Vol. I: Methodologische Einleitung. Vegetabilische Stofflehre. Die Lehre von der Pflanzenzelle, 289 p.; Vol. II: Morphologie, 564 p. (Leipzig: Engelmann) - a book that went through several editions and introduced improved technical methods into the science of botany. The present biography also includes a chronologically-arranged bibliography of Schleiden's publications.

Schwann, Theodor (1810-1882) — FLOR-KIN, M., 1961: Lettres de Théodore Schwann, 274 p. (Liège: Soc. Roy. Sci. de Liège).—

Schwann was a German physiologist and professor at the universities of Louvain and Liège. In this book Florkin publishes a collection of letters to and from Schwann. Most of these letters are addressed to his friends and colleagues, amongst them those directed to Van Beneden and Joh. Müller are the most important. They give the best biographical picture of the older Schwann. Letters written in German are given both in the original language and in French translation. This book is a valuable complement to Florkin's monograph of T. Schwann: FLORKIN, M., 1960: Naissance et déviation de la théorie cellulaire dans l'oeuvre de Théodore Schwann, 236 p. (Paris: Hermann). *Cf.* also: FLORKIN, M., 1956: Théodore Schwann et les débuts de la médecine scientifique, 23 p. (Conf. du Palais de la Découverte, ser. D, No. 43) (Paris: Palais de la Découverte); and: STEUDEL, J., L. MÜNSTER, W. MÜLLER & R. WATERMANN, 1964: Theodor Schwann zum Gedenken. Vier Vorträge, gehalten in Neuss, anlässlich des 150. Geburtstages des Anatomen und Physiologen Theodor Schwann, 78 p. (Cologne: Universitätsverlag).

——, WATERMANN, R., 1960: Theodor Schwann. Leben und Werk, 364 p. (Düsseldorf: Schwann).—

The author stresses the great discoveries of Schwann, such as: the discovery of pepsin (1836), the 'muscular law' (1837), the discovery of the microbial origin of fermentation and his refutation of the "spontaneous generation" idea (1837), and formulation of the cell theory (1838). This last publication appeared in an English translation: SCHWANN, T., 1847: Microscopic researches into the accordance in the structure and growth of animals and plants, 268 p. (ed. by H. SMITH) (London: Sydenham Soc.).

Schweitzer, Albert (1875-1965) — SEAVER, G., 1947: Albert Schweitzer: the man and his mind, 346 p. (New York, N.Y.: Harper).—

This biography gives a vivid picture of the man and his work and deals especially with his accomplishments in the fields of philosophy, theology, and history. More documentation concerning his life and work in the Lambarene Hospital can be found in JOY, C. R. & M. ARNOLD, 1948: The Africa of Albert Schweitzer (New York, N.Y.: Harper), or in: HAGEDOORN, H., 1947: Prophet in the wilderness: the story of Albert Schweitzer, 221 p. (New York, N.Y.: Macmillan).

Sechenov, Ivan Mikhailovitch (1829-1905) — SECHENOV, I. M., 1965: Autobiographical notes, 174 p. (Washington, D.C.: Amer. Inst. Biol. Sci.).—

This is a valuable addition to our knowledge of the development of Russian physiology. It contains a portrait of Sechenov's life against the background of scientific developments in Russia during the second half of the 19th century. Sechenov can be considered as a forerunner of Pavlov's work on the physiology of behaviour. Besides, Sechenov conducted many studies in the fields of gas absorption in salt solutions, and of muscular fatigue and recovery. *Cf.* also: SECHENOV, I., 1962: Selected physiological and psychological works, 607 p. (Moscow: Foreign Languages Publ. House; London: Central Bks.). Also in French translation: Oeuvres philosophiques et psychologiques choisies, 598 p. (Moscow: Éd. en langues étrangères). *Cf.* also KOSHTOYANTS, K., ed., 1965: Reflexes of the brain, 149 p. (Cambridge, Mass.: M.I.T. Press).

Semmelweiss, Ignaz Philipp (1818-1865) — SLAUGHTER, F. G., 1950: Immortal Magyar: Semmelweis, conqueror of childbed fever, 211 p. (New York, N.Y.: Schuman).—

This book tells the story of Semmelweis's discovery of the causation of puerperal fever, and how he fought in vain against the opposition which refused to accept the significance of his discovery. A study, more especially dealing with his life in Vienna, is: LESKY, E., 1964: Ignaz Philipp Semmelweiss und die Wiener medizinische Schule, 93 p. (Sitzber. Oesterr. Akad. Wiss., phil.-hist. Kl., Vol. 245, pt. 3) (Vienna: Böhlaus). *Cf.* also: MURPHY, F. P., 1946: Ignaz Philipp Semmelweis (1818-1865): an annotated bibliography, 54 p. (Bull. Hist. Med. 20: 653-707). A modern reprint of his classical work: SEMMELWEIS, I. P., 1965: Die Aetiologie, der Begriff und die Prophylaxis des Kindbettfiebers, 544 p. (New York, N.Y.: Johnson). A reprint of the 1861 edition. His collected works are reprinted in 1966, 604 p. (Wiesbaden: Sändig).

Servetus, Michael (1511-1553) — BAIN-TON, R. H., 1953: Michel Servet, hérétique et martyr, 1553-1953, 150 p. (Travaux d'Humanisme et Renaissance, Vol. 6) (Geneva: Droz).—

A very readable biography of the man who became a martyr of intolerance some 400 years ago. The struggle between Calvin and Servetus is described as a struggle between one of the last great figures of the mediaeval world (Calvin) and the man of the Renaissance (Servetus), theologian, physician, botanist, astrologer, geographer, the man who chose martyrdom above escape. An American edition appeared simultaneously under the title: Hunted heretic: the life and death of Michael Servetus, 1953, 270 p. (Boston, Mass.: Bacon Press). This American edition contains a bibliography of works of Servetus and of works dealing with Servetus.

——, O'MALLEY, C. D., 1953: Michael Servetus: a translation of his geographical, medical and astrological writings, with introduction and notes, 208 p. (Mem. Amer. Philos. Soc., Vol. 34) (Philadelphia, Pa.: Amer. Philos. Soc.).—

This volume is an English translation and contains the most interesting contributions of Servetus. Each of these selections (Ptolemy's geography; The apology against Fuchs; The syrups; The discourse in favour of astrology; The second edition of Ptolemy's geography; The Christianismi Restitutio and the description of the lesser circulation) is preceded by a short commentary in which O'Malley sets forth the conditions under which the work has been written, and the nature of the work itself. Details of the books translated can be found in Fulton's bibliography: FULTON, J. F., 1953: Michael Servetus: humanist and martyr, 98 p. (With a bibliography of his works and census of known copies by M. E. STANTON) (New York, N.Y.: Reichner).

Sherrington, Charles Scott (1857-1952) — COHEN OF BIRKENHEAD, Lord, 1958: Sherrington: physiologist, philosopher, and poet, 108 p. (Liverpool: U.P.).—

This booklet contains the text of three lectures delivered at the University of Liverpool. The first lecture deals with Sherrington's career and achievements in physiology, the second with the historical position of some of his contributions to our knowledge of neuro-physiology, and the third

with Sherrington as a philosopher and a poet. A bibliography of Sherrington's works has been added. Cf. SHERRINGTON, C., 1951: Man on his nature, ed. 2, 300 p. (Cambridge: U.P.). This is essentially a philosophical treatise on the relation of mind, brain, and matter, and the origin of life, written by one of the greatest biologists of the present century.

——, GRANIT, R., 1967: Charles Scott Sherrington: an appraisal, 188 p. (Garden City, N.Y.: Doubleday; London: Nelson).—

A biography of probably the greatest of all British neurophysiologists, written by one of Sherrington's pupils, himself a distinguished physiologist. Only the first chapter contains purely biographical information. In the remainder of the book its author discusses the many remarkable contributions of Sherrington to the physiology of the nervous system and some of the basic concepts introduced by Sherrington in this science. The final chapter deals with Sherrington's literary activities.

Shippen, William (1736-1808) — CORNER, B. C., 1951: William Shippen, Jr., pioneer in American medical education: a bibliographical essay. With notes, and the original text of Shippen's student diary, London, 1759-1760; together with a translation of his Edinburgh dissertation, 1761, 161 p. (Philadelphia, Pa.: Amer. Philos. Soc.).—

This is a biography of W. Shippen, professor of anatomy and surgery in America's first medical school, founded in 1765 at the College of Philadelphia. The book is based on Shippen's student diary, London 1759-1760, and includes a translation of his doctoral thesis on the connection of the placenta with the uterus. This book is a family achievement, because Mrs. B. C. Corner was helped by her husband (an anatomist) and her son (an obstetrician). (After Sarton in Isis 42: 332).

Sigerist, Henri Ernst (1891-1957) — MARTI-IBAÑEZ, F., ed., 1960: Henry E. Sigerist on the history of medicine, 313 p. (Foreword by J. F. FULTON) (New York, N.Y.: MD Publications).—

Henry Sigerist has been one of the greatest historians of science, especially of the science of medicine. This book contains a collection of 27 miscellaneous writings, constituting Sigerist's opera omnia minora in the field of the history of medicine. They cover the period from the beginnings of medical practice up to recent times. Those essays originally written in German or French have been translated into English. *Cf.* also: ROEMER, M. E., ed., 1960: Henry E. Sigerist on the sociology of medicine, 399 p. (New York, N.Y.: MD Publications). In this work Sigerist's views and concepts on medical sociology are clearly presented, and his concern for the future of medicine and of mankind are comprehensively exhibited.

——, MILLER, G., ed., 1966: A bibliography of the writings of Henry E. Sigerist, 112 p. (Montreal: McGill U.P.).—

This bibliography contains 520 items and is a complete list of Sigerist's published works. They are grouped in four sections: books and monographs; edited works, translations, and facsimiles; papers, addresses, prefaces, reports and reviews; editorial work. The index is a guide both to the material in the bibliography and to the subjects discussed in Sigerist's publications.

——, SIGERIST-BEESON, N., 1966: Henry E. Sigerist: autobiographical writings, 247 p. (Montreal: McGill U.P.).—

These autobiographical writings are arranged and preceded by a foreword by his daughter. The first 50 pages of this book present the beginning of the autobiography which Sigerist started but never finished; the rest of the book is pieced together from various earlier sources.

Sloane, Hans (1660-1753) — BROOKS, E. S. J., 1954: Sir Hans Sloane: the great collector and his circle, 234 p. (London: Batchworth).—

An important biography based on much source-material, describing Sloane's collecting activities (of birds, beasts, insects, objects of art and antiquity, jewellery, coins, manuscripts, *etc.*); his vast collection became the nucleus of the British Museum. Special attention has been paid to Sloane as a naturalist.

——, DE BEER, G. R., 1953: Sir Hans Sloane and the British Museum, 192 p. (London: Oxford U.P.).—

The first complete biography of Sloane, bringing together the facts of his life, his education, and his professional career. Of particular interest is his friendship with

Boyle and Ray. Sloane was a great plant collector; the collection of natural history which he built up during his voyage in the West Indies became the nucleus of the British Museum. The relationship between Sloane and the foundation of this museum has been stressed. Sloane succeeded Newton as president of the Royal Society, which he remained for 14 years. A study especially dealing with Sloane's herbal is: DANDY, J. E., ed., 1958: The Sloane herbarium: an annotated list of the Horti sicci composing it; with biographical accounts of the principal contributions, 246 p. (London: British Museum). With 96 illustrations.

Solander, Daniel Carl (1733-1782) — RAUSCHENBERG, R. A., 1968: Daniel Carl Solander: naturalist on the "Endeavour", 65 p. (Trans. Amer. Philos. Soc., N.S., Vol. 59, pt. 8) (Philadelphia, Pa.: Amer. Philos. Soc.).—

This is a well-documented biographical study of Solander who accompanied Cook and Banks on the voyage around the world by the "Endeavour" in 1768-1771. Solander was a pupil of Linnaeus. Solander described many plants collected during the voyage; unfortunately, these descriptions remained in ms. and were not published before 1900-1905. Extensive bibliography.

Spallanzani, Lazzaro (1729-1799)—BIAGI, B., ed., 1958-1964: Epistolario, 5 vols. (Florence: Sansoni).—

A collection of 1,475 letters of Spallanzani, addressed to 174 correspondents, among them *e.g.,* Bonnet, von Haller, Voltaire, Nollet, Needham, A. Vallisnieri, Caldani and J. Senebier, Approximately 85% of the letters presented here have been published for the first time, they are marked by an asterisk. Many useful footnotes. Indexes of letters and of persons and institutions, but no subject index.

——, PRANDI, D., 1951: Bibliografia della opera di Lazzaro Spallanzani, delle traduzioni e degli scritti su di lui, 171 p. (Florence: Sansoni Antiquariato).—

This bibliography consists of three parts: 1. Spallanzani's works; 2. translations into French, German and English; 3. writings on Spallanzani. Excellent index and list of facsimiles. *Cf.* SENEBIER, J., ed., 1956: Expériences sur la digestion de l'homme et de différentes espèces d'animaux, 337 p. (Paris: Gauthier Villars). Translation of the 1787 edition.

——, ROSTAND, J., 1951: Les origines de la biologie expérimentale et l'Abbé Spallanzani, 284 p. (Paris: Fasquelle).——

A useful biography of one of the greatest biologists of all times, well-known for the "ovist" position which he took in the ovist-animalculist controversy. The author also gives a review of Spallanzani's studies on animal digestion, circulation of the blood, respiration, reproduction and regeneration. Included are a useful bibliography of works of and dealing with Spallanzani and index of personal names. This study also contains much information concerning some contemporaries, such as: Réaumur, von Haller, Bonnet, Trembley, Needham, Buffon, and Voltaire. An elaborate biography in Italian is: CAPPARONI, P., 1948: Spallanzani, 311 p. (I grandi italiani, No. 23) (Torino: U.T.E.T.).

Spemann, Hans (1869-1941) — MANGOLD, O., 1953: Hans Spemann. Ein Meister der Entwicklungsphysiologie. Sein Leben und sein Werk, 264 p. (Grosse Naturforscher, Vol. 11) (Stuttgart: Wiss. Verlagsgesells.).——

An authoritative biography of Spemann written by one of his former pupils, the man who eventually succeeded him. The greater part of the book combines an account of Spemann's scientific achievements and a historical review of that new discipline to which Spemann contributed so much *(viz.,* causal developmental physiology).

Spencer, Herbert (1820-1903) — SPENCER, H., 1904: An autobiography, 2 vols. Vol. I: 556 p.; Vol. II: 542 p. (London: Williams & Norgate).——

Herbert Spencer played an important role in the development of British, especially English, philosophy during the second half of last century. Owing to his friendship with men like T. H. Huxley and C. Darwin, his influence on biology was considerable. He tried to give a sound philosophical basis to the idea of progress which pervaded his time; to the more biological fields of science his "Principles of biology" and his "Principles of psychology" are valuable contributions. Consequently there is much in these vols. that is of interest to the historian of biology.

Stahl, Georg Ernst (1660-1734) — GOTTLIEB, B. J., ed., 1961: Georg Ernst Stahl. Ueber den mannigfaltigen Einfluss von Ge-

mütsbewegungen auf den menschlichen Körper (Halle, 1695) und drei weitere Arbeiten, 88 p. (Sudhoffs Klassiker der Medizin, Vol. 36) (Leipzig: Barth.)——

Stahl is still known for his introduction of the concept of the soul into medicine and for his adherence to the phlogiston theory. His concept of the soul was both naive and dualistic, but nevertheless it greatly influenced the development of medicine, for it helped to distinguish between an organism and a mechanism, and some of his theses seem rather modern. The subjects of the three minor works are: the significance of the synergy principle in medicine (1695), the difference between organism and mechanism (1714); and on medical ethics (1703). *Cf.* VAN DE VELDE, A. J. J., 1947: Georg Ernst Stahl, 1660-1734. Het phlogiston en het vitalisme. (Verh. Kon. Vlaamse Akad., Kl. Wetensch., Jg. 9, No. 22).

Stensen, Niels (= Nicolaus Steno, 1638-1686) — SCHERZ, G., 1963: Pionier der Wissenschaft: Niels Stensen in seinen Schriften, 348 p. (Acta Hist. Sci. Nat. Med., Vol. 18) (Copenhagen: Munksgaard).——

A description of Steno's life and works. The main part of the book consists of a German translation of extracts from Steno's scientific and theological works, provided with numerous illustrations. No critical comparisons with contemporaries. More biographical information can be found in another book of the same author: SCHERZ, G., 1956: Vom Wege Niels Stensens, 248 p. (Acta Hist. Sci. Nat. Med., Vol. 14) (Copenhagen: Munksgaard), which also contains a list of his works.

—— ——, 1964: Niels Stensen. Denker und Forscher im Barock, 1638-1686, 275 p. (Grosse Naturforscher, Vol. 28) (Stuttgart: Wiss. Verlagsges.).——

Nicolaus Steno was distinguished as anatomist, geologist, and theologian. The first part of the present biography (p. 11-148) deals more particularly with Steno's theological activities; the second part more particularly with his scientific activities as a biologist (he made, *inter alia,* important contributions to glandular secretion, to the anatomy and physiology of muscle, and discovered that the heart was a muscle), a palaeontologist (he compared fossil with living organisms), and as a geologist (he distinguished, *inter alia,* marine and fluviatile formations). *Cf.* also: BIERBAUM, M.,

1959: Niels Stensen. Von der Anatomie zur Theologie, 159 p. (Münster: Aschendorf).

——, STENO, N., 1950: A dissertation on the anatomy of the brain. Read in the assembly held in M. Thévenot's house in the year 1665, 60 + 50 p. (Copenhagen: Busck).—

> The original text was presented in French at the assembly held in the home of M. Thévenot in 1665. In it Steno criticizes the theory of animal spirits, marvels at the complexities of fibres in the brain, and recommends experiments to determine the function of the brain. (Cf. STENO, N., 1965, infra). There also exists a facsimile reproduction of the "De glandulus oculorum", originally published in Leiden in 1662: STENO, N., 1951: Anatomical observations of the glands of the eye and their new vessels thereby revealing the true sources of tears, 27 p. (Copenhagen: Busck).

——— ———, 1965: Lecture on the anatomy of the brain, 208 p. (Introd. by G. SCHERZ) (Copenhagen: Busck).—

> A fascimile of the 1665 (French) text of a lecture read by Stensen to an assembly of scholars in Paris. This is followed by an introduction by SCHERZ in which he discusses the historical background of the "Discours". Then follow notes to the "Discours" and a new English and a new German translation and a glossary of modern anatomical terms to the structures depicted in two of the brain drawings belonging to the original text. The "Discours" itself is a brief critical review of mid-seventeenth-century knowledge of the form and function of the brain and to start a new programm of research. Cf. STENO, N., 1950, supra; and SCHERZ, G., 1968: Steno and brain research in the seventeenth century, 302 p. (Proc. of the Intl. Hist. Symposium on Nicolaus Steno and brain research in the 17th century held in Copenhagen, 18-20 Aug. 1965) (Analecta medico-historica, Vol. 3) (London: Pergamon).

Swammerdam, Jan (1637-1680) — SCHIERBEEK, A., 1967: Jan Swammerdam (12 February 1637-17 February 1680): his life and works, 202 p. (Amsterdam: Swets & Zeitlinger).—

> This book about the famous Dutch anatomist and entomologist Jan Swammerdam has been translated from the Dutch (1947) (Lochem: De Tijdstroom). The first chapter (p. 1-43) gives a brief biographical account of the life of Swammerdam and his relationship with such men as Thévenot and Niels Stensen (q.v.) and the influence of the religious fanatic Antoinette Bourignon. Other chapters deal with such subjects as: Swammerdam as preparator and collector, as physiologist, as student of human anatomy, as student of the anatomy of the lower animals, as embryologist, and as entomologist, and Swammerdam as botanist. Extensive bibliography of works written by Swammerdam, of books and periodicals with contributions by Swammerdam, of manuscripts of Swammerdam, and with the principle works on Swammerdam.

Swedenborg, Emanuel (1688-1772) — STROH, A. H. & G. EKELÖF, 1910: An abridged chronological list of works of Emanuel Swedenborg. Including manuscripts, original editions and translations prior to 1772, 54 p. (Uppsala: Almqvist & Wiksell).—

> For a complete list of Swedenborg's publications, vide: HYDE, J., 1906: Bibliography of the works of Emanuel Swedenborg, 743 p. (London: Swedenborg Society). Contains 3,500 items.

——, TOKSVIG, S., 1948: Emanuel Swedenborg: scientist and mystic, 389 p. (New Haven, Conn.: Yale U.P.).—

> Swedenborg was chiefly interested in the problem of discovering the nature of soul and spirit by means of anatomical studies. He had, for his days, a thorough knowledge of neuro-anatomical and neurophysiological matters, as can be seen from his work on the cerebrum, of which quite recently an English translatoin appeared from the original ms. written in 1738, viz., ACTON, A., ed., 1938: Three transactions on the cerebrum, 33 + 731 p. + additional vol. of anatomical plates, 89 p. (Philadelphia, Pa.: New Church Book Center). This book contains many quotations from other anatomists of those days. For more biographical information, cf.: ACTON, A., ed., 1948-1955: The letters and memorials of Emanuel Swedenborg, 2 vols. Vol. I (1948): p. 1-508; Vol. II (1955): p. 509-803. (Bryn Athyn, Pa.: Swedenborg Scientific Assn.). A German biography is: BENZ, E., 1948: Emanuel Swedenborg. Naturforscher und Seher, 588 p. (Munich: Rinn).

Sydenham, Thomas (1624-1689) — DEWHURST, K., 1966: Dr. Thomas Sydenham (1624-1689): his life and original writings, 180 p. (London: Wellcome Hist. Med. Library; Berkeley, Calif.: Univ. California Press.).—

According to the author, Thomas Sydenham was "the greatest physician this country (England) has ever produced." The present volume consists of a biographical introduction (of 70 pages) and of a selection of Sydenham's original writings, nearly all hitherto unpublished. *Cf.* also: COMRIE, J. D., 1922: Selected works of Thomas Sydenham 1624-89, 153 p. (London: Bale).

Sylvius, Franciscus (= François de le Boë = François de la Bois, 1614-1672) — BAUMANN, E. D., 1949: François de le Boë, Sylvius, 242 p. (Leiden: Brill).—

A thorough study of Sylvius, placed within the framework of his time. Separate chapters deal with Sylvius's relationship to the University of Leiden, with his activities in anatomy, chemistry, physiology, general pathology, and therapy, and with his "Idea nova", his "Short treatises" and with his "Dissertation on the plague, the cough, and venereal diseases".

Tagliacozzi, Gaspare (1545-1599) — GNUDI, M. T. & J. P. WEBSTER, 1950: The life and times of Gaspare Tagliacozzi, surgeon of Bologna, 1545-1599, with a documented study of the scientific and cultural life of Bologna in the sixteenth century, 538 p. (New York, N.Y.: Reichner).—

A biography based on primary sources, describing Tagliacozzi's family origin, his circumstances, education, patients, friends, patrons, *etc.* The authors place him against the background of scientific and cultural life in Bologna of those days. Tagliacozzi can be considered as the first physician to establish plastic surgery on a scientific basis; in this book the authors trace the history of plastic surgery from ancient times up to quite recent times, and as a result this book gives a fairly complete history of plastic surgery up to the 19th century. The various editions of Tagliacozzi's "De curtorum chirurgia" have been considered, and translations, notes, and other valuable documents have been included.

✓ Teilhard de Chardin, Pierre (1881-1955) — SPEAIGHT, R., 1967: Teilhard de Chardin: a biography, 360 p. (London: Collins).—

According to a review in the Times Litt. Suppl. 66: 874 (Sept. 20, 1967), this is a distinguished biography of the French philosopher and palaeontologist Teilhard de Chardin. "Its clarity and readability will recommend it to everyone who desires to know Teilhard's life and the background of his thought," writes the reviewer. *Cf.* also: GRENET, P., 1966: Teilhard de Chardin: the man and his theories, 176 p. (New York, N.Y.: Eriksson). The most complete biography is: CUÉNOT, C., 1958: Pierre Teilhard de Chardin. Les grandes étapes de son évolution, 58 + 490 p. (Paris: Plon). Also in English translation: CUÉNOT, C., 1965: Teilhard de Chardin: a biographical study, 492 p. (Transl. by V. COLINMORE, ed. by R. HAGUE) (Baltimore, Md.: Helicon). Also in a shorter French edition: CUÉNOT, C., 1962: Teilhard de Chardin, 192 p. (Paris: Éd. du Seuil). *Cf.* also: POLGÁR, L., 1965: Internationale Teilhard Bibliographie, 1955-1965, 93 p. (Freiburg i.B.: Alber).

Thackrah, Charles Turner (1795-1833) — MEIKLEJOHN, A., 1957: The life, work and times of Charles Turner Thackrah, surgeon and apothecary of Leeds (1795-1833), 50 + 238 p. (Edinburgh & London: Livingstone).—

This book contains a facsimile reproduction of the second edition of Thackrah's famous tract entitled "The effects of the arts, trades, and professions, and of civic states and habits of living, on health and longevity: with suggestions for the removal of many of the agents which produce disease, and shorten the duration of life", published in 1832. Thackrah was an anatomist, experimental physiologist, clinician, teacher, pioneer in preventive medicine, and humanitarian, who founded the Leeds Medical School. The book includes a biographical essay, aphorisms of Thackrah's writings, and a selected bibliography.

Thompson, D'Arcy Wentworth (1860-1948) — THOMPSON, D'Arcy, R., 1958: D'Arcy Wentworth Thompson: the scholar-naturalist, 1860-1948, 244 p. (London: Oxford U.P.).—

A biography of the famous English classical scholar and zoologist, written by his daughter. This work is also of great interest for the history of classical biology.

Thudichum, Johann Ludwig Wilhelm (1829-1901) — DRABKIN, D. L., 1958: Thudichum: chemist of the brain, 309 p. (Philadelphia, Pa.: Pennsylvania U.P.).—

Thudichum was a distinguished pioneer of biochemical research who worked on the isolation and characterization of chemical constituents of animal tissues, especially of the brain (he discovered, *inter alia,* cephalin, sphingomyelin, and the cerebrosides phrenosin and kerasin) and he examined pigments of blood, bile, urine, and the corpus luteum. Thudichum did also much research in oto-laringology. He published numerous books, of which his "Treatise on the chemical constitution of the brain" (1884) was the most important. This book was re-issued in 1962, 262 p. (Hamden, Conn.: Archon). This re-issue has been accompanied by a historical introduction by D. L. DRABKIN.

Tissot, Simon André (1728-1797) — BUCHER, H. W., 1958: Tissot und sein Traité des nerfs, 62 p. (Zurich: Juris).—

The "Traité des nerfs" was first published in 1778, and forms the chief contents of the book under consideration. It includes sections dealing with the anatomy and physiology of the nervous system, apoplexy, paralysis, epilepsy, catalepsy, migraine, and insanity. Tissot's descriptions and beliefs are discussed in the light of preceding and contemporary knowledge of the structure and function of the nervous system and its diseases. Besides its interest for the history of neuropsychiatry, the book also contains biographical information about Tissot.

Torrey, John (1796-1873) — RODGERS, A. D., 1942: John Torrey: a story of North American botany, 352 p. (Princeton, N.J.: Princeton U.P.; London: Oxford U.P.).—

An authoritative and detailed biography of the outstanding American chemist and pioneering taxonomic botanist John Torrey, whose life roughly corresponds with a synoptic review of the botanical exploration of North America. Torrey was a taxonomist of great fame, founder of the Torrey Herbarium, and his pupils founded the Torrey Botanical Club. He held very firm and orthodox religious views and he considered species as fixed and unchangeable units. A special chapter has been devoted to his connections with his former student Asa Gray *(q.v.)*. Reprinted 1965 (New York, N.Y.: Hafner).

Tournefort, Joseph Pitton de (1656-1708) — BECKER, G., *et al.,* 1957: Tournefort, 324 p. (Collection "Les grands naturalists français") (Paris: Mus. Natl. Hist. Nat.).—

A co-operative work on various aspects of the life and work of the French botanist Joseph Pitton de Tournefort. Essays on his life, family, and birthplace, his botanical achievements (in Aix, Montpellier, the Pyrenees, the Levant), his medical and

zoological studies, and his classificatory system in botany (which entitles him to be considered a worthy forerunner of Linnaeus). It also contains a translation of his "Isagoge in rem herbariam".

Trembley, Abraham (1710-1784) — BAKER, J. R., 1952: Abraham Trembley of Geneva: scientist and philosopher, 259 p. (London: Arnold).—

A well-written biography of the discoverer of artificial multiplication and a-sexual reproduction by budding of an animal, *viz.,* of a hydra, an event which has had great influence on current biology and even philosophy. Besides, more of Trembley's achievements are mentioned: his numerous important contributions to zoology and microbiology, his researches on grafting of animal tissues, his description of the main physical properties of protoplasm, the use of vital-staining in micro-technique, the discovery of the animal nature of polyps, the first description of multiplication in Protozoa, and the first observation of true cell-division in a single-celled alga. The concluding chapters deal with Trembley's interest and publications in education, politics, religion, and moral philosophy.

Treub, Melchior (1851-1910) — ZEYLSTRA, H. H., 1959: Melchior Treub: pioneer of a new era in the history of the Malay Archipelago, 129 p. (Amsterdam: Kon. Inst. Tropen).—

This biography contains much biographical information and considers such subjects as: Treub's early years and university training, his arrival at 's Lands Plantentuin at Buitenzorg (Bogor), his activities in promoting scientific research in the Netherlands Indies (now Indonesia), his merits in the development of agriculture, his activities as (the first) director of the Dept. of Agriculture in the Netherlands Indies, *etc.* Special chapters deal with Treub's personality and with a pedigree of the family Treub. Included is a chronological list of scientists who during Treub's directorate stayed as guests at s' Lands Plantentuin and made use of its laboratories.

Turner, William (*ca.* 1508-1568) — TURNER, W., 1965: Libellus de re herbaria 1538. The names of herbes 1548. Facsimiles with introductory matter, 275 p. (London: Ray Society).—

Turner was a clergyman, physician, herbalist and naturalist, and was the author of the first two printed books relating to British plants that have any claim to originality; this book contains facsimile reproductions from them. The originals of both books are very rare, owing to the fact that Turner has been among the banned authors. W. STEARN gives a general review of the contents and importance of the book; B. D. JACKSON gives a short biography. A transcription follows the facsimile text. Very good indexes.

Tyson, Edward (1650-1708) — MONTAGU, A. M. F., 1943: Edward Tyson, M.D., F.R.S., 1650-1708, and the rise of the human and comparative anatomy in England, 488 p. (Mem. Amer. Philos. Soc., Vol. 20) (Philadelphia, Pa.: Amer. Philos. Soc.).—

Tyson is amongst the foremost scientific benefactors of all times and is regarded as the founder of human and comparative anatomy in England. He demonstrated for the first time the fact that the anthropoid ape occupies the nearest place to Man in the Great Chain of Beings. This book is a full-length study of Tyson and his contributions, not only in the fields of medicine and science, but also in those of the humanities. Cf. MONTAGU, A. M. F., ed., 1966: Orang-outang, sive Homo Sylvestris: or, The anatomy of a pygmie compared with that of a monkey, an ape, and a man, 1699, 194 p. (London: Dawsons). A facsimile with introduction and notes.

Uexküll, Jakob Johann Baron von (1864-1944) — UEXKÜLL, G. von, 1964: Jacob von Uexküll, seine Welt und seine Umwelt. Eine Biographie, 266 p. (Hamburg: Wegner).—

A biography of one of the most famous German theoretical biologists of this century, written by his widow. Von Uexküll is the initiator of the Umwelt-concept.

Vadian (= Joachim von Watt) (1484-1551) — NINCK, J., 1936: Arzt und Reformator Vadian. Ein Charakterbild aus grosser Zeit, 256 p. (St. Gallen: Fehr).—

A biography of the famous Swiss humanist and physician, friend of Zwingli, and supporter of Luther. Vadian's medical (and other) scientific publications mainly consist of commentaries on older sources of knowledge. (Well-known is his "Pomponius mala", the second edition of which has been accompanied by his "Loca aliquot"). The present biography includes a complete

review of these sources, together with a very good bibliography. Vadian was an opponent of Paracelsus. Another very good bibliography: NÄF, W., 1944: Vadian und seine Vaterstadt St. Gallen. Erster Band bis 1518. Humanist in Wien, 382 p. (St. Gallen: Fehr). Cf. also: MILT, B., 1959: Vadian als Arzt, 148 p. (St. Gallen: Fehr).

Vavilov, Nikolai Ivanovich (1887- ca. 1942) — VAVILOV, N.I., 1949/50: The origin, variation, immunity and breeding of cultivated plants, 364 p. (Chronica Botanica, Vol. 13) (Waltham, Mass.: Chronica Botanica).—

Vavilov has been one of the most outstanding of geneticists and plant breeders. The present book contains the English text of some of his classics in the field of botanico-agricultural literature, publications which existed only in Russian. Its subject matter has been arranged under the following headings: Plant breeding as a science (p. 1-14); Phytogeographic basis of plant breeding (p. 14-55); The law of homologous series in the inheritance of variability (p. 56-95); Study of immunity of plants from infectious diseases (p. 96-169); Scientific basis of wheat breeding (p. 170-314); Selected bibliography of the basic world literature on breeding and genetics of wheat (p. 315-352). Author-index and index of plant names.

Vesalius, Andreas (1514-1564) — BAKELANTS, L., ed., 1961: Préface d'André Vesale à ses livres sur l'anatomie, suivie d'une lettre à Jean Oporinus, son imprimeur. With introduction and annotations, 87 p. (Brussels: Arscia).—

This booklet contains the original Latin text of the preface of the second edition of the "Fabrica", together with a French translation on facing pages. This text has been accompanied by an introduction and by informative commentaries. According to the editor, this preface is an important source of medical historical information, throwing much light on some valid principles of medicine. Comparisons have been made between the first and the second editions of this preface.

——, CUSHING, H., 1962: A bio-bibliography of Andreas Vesalius, ed. 2, 38+264 p. (Hamden, Conn. & London: Archon Bks.).—

The first edition of this book was published in 1943; it is a posthumous contribution of Cushing to the celebration commemorating the publication of Vesalius's immortal work "De humani corporis fabrica" in 1543. This bio-bibliography is largely based on material collected by Cushing during his lifetime. The circumstances in which the publication of Vesalius's several works (and those of his pupils and imitators) took place have been elucidated and in the appropriate places bibliographical details of the various editions have been added. In addition to a facsimile reprint of his first edition, the present edition contains corrigenda and addenda in order to give up-to-date information (up to 1961). That this procedure was necessary may be illustrated by the fact that the added Vesaliana consist of nearly 300 new items, the greater part having been published between 1943 and 1961. *Cf.* O'MALLEY, C. D., 1965: A review of Vesalian literature (Hist. Sci., 1965 (4): 1-14).

——, ERIKSSON, R., ed., 1959: Andreas Vesalius' first public anatomy at Bologna, 1540: an eyewitness report, together with his notes on Matthaeus Curtius' lectures on Anatomia Mundini, 343 p. (Edited, with an introduction, translation into English, and notes) (Uppsala: Almqvist & Wiksells).——

This is a translation of the notes prepared by one of his students, Baldasar Heseler, who attended Vesalius's anatomical course during January, 1540 at Bologna. It gives an interesting picture of Vesalius's scientific development away from the traditional Galenic point of view (presented by Curtius) toward the method of science based on experience. The book gives many new biographical details, it documents many questionable points, and the text contains many valuable annotations.

——, O'MALLEY, C. D., 1964: Andreas Vesalius of Brussels 1514-1564, 480 p. (Berkeley & Los Angeles, Calif.: Univ. California Press).——

A monumental biography of the life and works of Vesalius, giving much detail concerning Vesalius's ancestors, youth, his studies, his persecution by the Inquisition, his life at the courts of Charles V and Philip II, *etc.* Much prominence has been given to the "De humani corporis fabrica" (1543), owing to its importance for understanding Vesalius and his time. O'Malley's book starts with a summary of pre-Vesalian anatomy; then the author explains how Vesalius, after studying carefully Galen's works on anatomy, came to reject many of Galen's interpretations in the light of his own thorough anatomical observations of the human body, and that Vesalius was bold enough to attack the old mediaeval system of teaching anatomy - equipped as he was with knowledge of both the ancient and the new learning.

——, ROTH, M., 1892: Andreas Vesalius Bruxellensis, 500 p. (Berlin: Reimer).——

The standard biography of Vesalius. It considerably revived interest in the life and work of Vesalius. The author was also very well acquainted with the publications of Vesalius's contemporaries. Together with the works of CUSHING and O'MALLEY (both *supra*), this book gives a very complete picture of Vesalius and his influence on the science of anatomy. Reprinted in 1965. (Amsterdam: Asher).

——, SAUNDERS, J. B. de C. M. & C. D. O'MALLEY, 1950: The illustrations from the works of Andreas Vesalius of Brussels: with annotations and translations, a discussion of the plates and their background, authorship and influence, and a biographical sketch of Vesalius, 252 p. (Cleveland, O. & New York, N.Y.: World Publ. Co.).——

Vesalius's works remain among the most magnificent works in the history of printing, and especially his woodcuts were of etxraordinary beauty; they proved, incidentally, that illustrations could help in the advancement of science. In the present work the illustrations (derived from the "Icones Anatomicae", New York, N.Y. & Munich, 1934) from Vesalius's "Fabrica" and "Epitome", "Venesection letter" and "Tabulae sex", as they were prepared by Titian (1477-1576), have been reproduced, in order to make them available to the general reader, and to students of art, science, and medicine. The title pages of the primary editions of the "Fabrica" have been included. Many explanatory notes, and an introduction containing a brief account of Vesalius and his work, complete this edition.

——, SINGER, C., 1952: Vesalius on the human brain, 151 p. (London: Oxford U.P.).——

This is an authoritative translation of the seventh book of the "Fabrica" which deals with the anatomy and physiology of the human brain. From this book the chapters 13 to 17 inclusive (on the organs of special sense; they contain little of interest) and 19 (the final chapter, the contents of which have little to do with the nervous system and of which translations are readily available) have been omitted. Singer has chosen this book because it illustrates so well the (new) Vesalian anatomical method. Extensive notes have been added.

Virchow, Rudolf (1821-1902) — ACKER-KNECHT, E. H., 1953: Rudolf Virchow, doctor, statesman, anthropologist, 304 p. (Madison, Wisc.: Wisconsin U.P.).—

Virchow was the leading German physician of the second half of the 19th century and is well-remembered for the contributions he made to pathology, of which his studies on thrombosis, embolism, cellular pathology, and metaplasia are the greatest. But in addition, he was an anthropologist of world renown, a liberal statesman, a medical historian and brilliant writer. In the present thorough biography, Ackerknecht gives a history of this busy life of Virchow and presents us with a critical discussion of Virchow's medical achievements in pathological anatomy and physiology, in epidemiology and public health, in social medicine and medical history. A German translation: ACKERKNECHT, E., 1957: Rudolf Virchow. Arzt, Politiker, Anthropologe, 245 p. (Stuttgart: Enke). Two other German biographies are: MEYER, E., 1956: Rudolf Virchow, 203 p. (Wiesbaden: Limes), and BOEHHEIM, F., 1957: Virchow. Werk und Wirkung, 392 p. (Berlin: Rütten & Loenig). A valuable Virchow-bibliography is: SCHWALBE, J., ed., 1901: Virchow-Bibliographie, 1843-1901. Coll. by W. BECHER, J. PAGEL, J. SCHWALBE, C. STRAUCH, and T. WEYL, 183 p. (Berlin: Reimer). With extensive index, p. 119-183.

——, RATHER, L. J., ed., 1958: Rudolf Virchow. Disease, life and man: selected essays, 273 p. (Stanford Studies in the Medical Sciences, Vol. 9) (Stanford, Calif.: Stanford U.P.).—

The editor has selected and translated ten essays by Virchow, together giving a good picture of the man and his work. Including notes, German titles, and sources of articles.

Wallace, Alfred Russel (1823-1913) — GEORGE, W., 1964: Biologist philosopher: a study of the life and writings of Alfred Russel Wallace, 320 p. (New York, N.Y.: Schuman).—

The greater part of this book deals with Wallace's work, his travels in South America and Malaya, the discovery of nat-

ural selection, speciation, mimicry, sexual selection, and language. Special attention has been paid to his role in formulating the evolutionary doctrine, and his collaboration and differences with Darwin have been considered.

——, WALLACE, A. R., 1905: My life: a record of events and opinions, 2 vols. Vol. I: 435 p.; Vol. II: 464 p. (New York, N.Y.: Dodd, Mead.).—

An autobiography of A. R. Wallace who originated independently the theory of natural selection. The first accounts of this theory were published by Wallace and Darwin in a joint paper given before the Linnean Society of London in 1858. Reprint is announced (Farnborough: Gregg). Other reprints: WALLACE, A. R., 1968: Natural selection and tropical nature: essays on descriptive and theoretical biology, 504 p. (Reprint of the 1891 edition); and WALLACE, A. R., 1968: The wonderful century: its successes and its failures, 412 p. (Reprint of the 1898 edition). Both were published by Gregg (Farnborough).

Weismann, August (1834-1914) — GAUPP, E., 1917: August Weismann. Sein Leben und Werk, 297 p. (Jena: Fischer).—

August Weismann was a German biologist who started as a zoologist, and afterwards became one of the most active supporters of Darwinism in Germany. His name is best known as that of author of the germ-plasm theory of heredity, by which he denied the transmission of acquired characters. After a brief biographical introduction, the present text deals especially with Weismann's relationship to Darwin, and with his germ-plasm theory and his ideas on fecundation, selection, and variation.

Welch, William Henry (1850-1934) — FLEMING, D., 1954: William H. Welch and the rise of modern medicine, 216 p. (ed. by O. HANDLIN) (Boston, Mass.: Little, Brown).—

This book is supplementary to FLEXNER's *(vide infra)* in that the points of interaction between society and Dr. Welch's activities have been emphasized. Political, cultural, social, and economic factors played a great role, so that stress has been laid on what Dr. Welch did, rather than on what he was. The author has concluded that Welch was "by far the greatest Influential that the biological sciences had yet known in America".

——, FLEXNER, S. & J. T., 1941: William Henry Welch and the heroic age of American medicine, 539 p. (New York, N.Y.: Viking).—

Welch has been one of the foremost leaders in tracing the new line of the 20th-century medicine in the U.S.A. This book deals with the story of his life and achievements, calling to mind his activities in the foundation of the Rockefeller Institute for Medical Research and the Johns Hopkins Medical School; his efforts on behalf of public health and the reform of medical education; and his appointment to a professorship in the history of medicine. Of particular interest is a chapter on the origin of the Institute of Medical History and the Welch Memorial Library. (Cf. FLEMING's biography, vide supra).

Wesley, John (1703-1791) — HILL, A. W., 1958: John Wesley among the physicians: a study of eighteenth-century medicine, 135 p. (London: Epworth).—

This book sketches the medical background from two medical works of John Wesley, viz., "Primitive physick" and "The desideratum". "Primitive physick" was very popular during Wesley's lifetime (it went through 23 editions, and 9 further editions after his death). It gives rules for the preservation of health. In 1760 he published his "The desideratum" in which he described the results of his application of electricity in medicine.

White, Gilbert (1720-1793) — HOLT-WHITE, R., ed., 1901: The life and letters of Gilbert White of Selborne, 2 vols., Vol. I: 330 p.; Vol. II: 300 p. (London: Murray).—

Gilbert White was a famous English writer on natural history. His "Natural history and antiquities of Selborne" (1789) remains a well-known book; it is a parish natural history. The present work, written by his great-grand-nephew, contains a full biography based upon a great collection of letters written by and to Gilbert White. Cf. also: MARTIN, E. H., 1934: A bibliography of Gilbert White, the naturalist and antiquarian of Selborne: with a biography and a descriptive account of the village of Selborne, 193 p. (London: Halton).

——, JOHNSON, W., 1928: Gilbert White: pioneer, poet, and stylist, 340 p. (London: Murray).—

This book contains an evaluation or White's activities as a writer and observer of natural objects.

———, ed., 1931: Journals of Gilbert White, 48 + 463 p. (London: Routledge).—

During his working life Gilbert White filled up a "Journal" day by day. A great deal of the matter in these notes was used in writing his "Natural history of Selborne" (1789). In the present volume the editor has attempted to select all those passages not already used by White in his "Natural history" that have scientific value.

Willis, Thomas (1621-1675) — FEINDEL, W., ed. The anatomy of the brain and nerves, 2 vols. Vol. I: Introduction with a note on Pordage's English translation, 104 p.; Vol. II: Facsimile of the 'Anatomy of the brain and description and use of the nerves', 192 p. (Montreal: McGill U.P.).—

Willis was a famous physician and anatomist. His "Cerebri anatome nervorumque descriptio et usus" was first published in 1664 and was a landmark in the history of science. Willis was the first to use the term "neurology". The present vols. contain descriptions of new methods of dissection of the brain stem, the cerebellum, the basal ganglia, etc., and a discussion of the functions of the various parts of the brain.

——, ISLER, H., 1968: Thomas Willis, 1621-1675. Doctor and scientist, 235 p. (New York, N.Y.: Hafner).—

"In the present investigation I have attempted to outline how Willis lived, what he wrote, what he achieved, why his fame vanished." An instructive discussion of Willis the medical chemist, the physician and the anatomist. Originally published in German as an M.D. thesis, Univ. Zürich: ISLER, H., 1965: Thomas Willis. Ein Wegbereiter der modernen Medizin, 212 p. (Grosse Naturforscher, Vol. 29) (Stuttgart: Wiss. Verlagsges.).

Willstätter, Richard (1872-1942) — WILLSTÄTTER, R., 1949: Aus meinem Leben. Von Arbeit, Musse und Freunden, 453 p. (Weinheim: Verlag Chemie).—

A useful and interesting autobiography of the famous plant physiologist, edited by his pupil, and afterwards co-worker, A. STOLL. In addition, it contains much information concerning Willstätter's contemporaries, such as: Haber, Le Rossignol, Polanyi, Bonhoeffer, Paul Ehrlich, E. Fischer, A. von Baeyer and many others. This autobiography also contains much that is of value to any historian of the science of botany, because Willstätter was famous for his work on synthesis of chlorophyll, *ca.* 1920. Also in English translation: From my life. the memoirs of Richard Willstätter, 1965, 461 p. (New York, N.Y.: Benjamin).

Winogradski, Sergei Nikolaevitch (1856-1953) — WAKSMAN, S. A., 1953: Sergei N. Winogradsky, his life and work: the story of a great bacteriologist, 150 p. (New Brunswick, N.J.: Rutgers U.P.).—

The book consists of a biography (p. 1-86), a selection of correspondence, and a bibliography (p. 87-150), of the great Russian bacteriologist, who is well-known for his work on the autotrophic bacteria, the free-living bacteria which fix nitrogen, and the sulphur bacteria. The author of this biography is himself a distinguished bacteriologist.

Withering, William (1741-1799) — PECK, T. W. & K. D. WILKINSON, 1950: William Withering of Birmingham, M.D., F.R.S., F.L.S., 239 p. (Bristol: Wright; London: Marshall; Baltimore, Md.: Williams & Wilkins).—

This is the first biography since 1822 of this famous English provincial physician, who besides his medical works, wrote a well-known book on British botany ("Botanical arrangement of British plants"). Withering seems to have been the first physician to make use of the foxglove *(Digitalis)* in the treatment of heart diseases. There is also some correspondence with T. A. Knight, containing descriptions of some experiments on growing peas, reminiscent of those of Mendel.

Wolff, Caspar Friedrich (1733-1794) — HERRLINGER, R., ed., 1966: Caspar Friedrich Wolff. Theorie von der Generation in zwei Abhandlungen erklärt und bewiesen. Theoria Generationis, 471 p. (Hildesheim: Olms).—

Wolff can be considered to be the founder of modern embryology. He graduated in medicine at Halle in 1759, his thesis being his famous "Theoria generationis". In this publication Wolff tried to establish the epigenetic theory of embryogenesis. Wolff later published in German an updated and much longer version of this thesis. The present edition contains the text of Wolff's dissertation, together with the longer version in German; both texts are preceded by an introduction by R. HERRLINGER.

Young, Thomas (1773-1829) — WOOD, A., 1954: Thomas Young, natural philosopher, 1773-1829, 355 p. (Completed by F. OLDHAM, with a memoir of A. WOOD by C. E. RAVEN) (Cambridge: U.P.).—

The first 10 chapters were written by A. WOOD before his death, and the work has been completed by F. OLDHAM, who wrote the last 5 chapters. Although Young was a professional physician, his fame was partly due to his establishment of the undulatory theory of light and the interpretation of the Egyptian hieroglyphics on the Rosetta stone. In connection with his discoveries on the nature of light, he did much study of the mechanisms of the eye; he explained accommodation and described astigmatism.

INDEX OF PERSONAL NAMES

1038

1040

Perkins Agricultural Library, see Perkins, W. F.
Catalogue of the Books, etc., of the British Museum (Natl. Hist.), see British Museum (Natl. Hist.)
Catalogue Peabody Museum of archaeology and ethnology, Harvard University, 184
Catalogue of Scientific Papers of the Royal Society of London, 37
Catesby, M., 897
Cato the Censor, 165, 330, 338, 339, 385, 386, 392, 397, 652
Cato, Marcus Porcius, see Cato the Censor
Caton, R., 344
Cattell, J., 80, 593
Caub, J. W. von, 648
Caullery, M., 562, 578, 603
Caxton, 558
Cecil, E., 698
Celli, A., 802
Celsius, A., 76
Celsus, Aurelius Cornelius, 22, 160, 165, 171, 172, 174, 176, 197, 330, 339, 343, 345, 347, 359, 392, 397, 398, 652, 781, 782, 849
Cesalpino, A., 26, 81, 149, 567, 580, 629, 663, 752, 895, 952
Cesalpinus, see Cesalpino, A.
Cestoni, G., 777
Cetto, A. M., 598, 603
Chadwick, J., 360
Chaignet, A. E., 328
Chain, E., 748, 927
Chaine, J., 597, 599
Chakraberty, C., 268, 269
Challinor, J., 906
Chalmers Mitchell, P., 640, 962
Chambers's Dictionary of Scientists, see Howard, A. V.
Chambers's world gazetteer ... etc. see Collocott, T. C.
Chambers, J. S., 800
Chambers, Robert, 18, 624, 896
Chamfrault, A., 297, 301
Chamisso, A. von, 896
Champier, S., 720
Champion, H., 272
Champlain, 760
Chance, B., 791
Chang-Chung-ching, 304, 310
Chang Hui-Chien, 293, 298, 304
Chang Kwang-chih, 281
Chanlaine, P., 998
Chapman, F. M., 649
Charaha, see Caraha
Charaf Ed-Din, 476
Charcot, J. M., 590, 742, 787, 797, 897, 931
Charlemagne, 162, 493, 529, 660
Charles, J., 827
Chassinat, E., 250

Chatin, G. A., 857
Chatton, M. J., 63
Chaucer, Geoffrey, 529
Chauffard, P. E., 742
Chauret, S., 202
Chauvois, L., 917, 949
Chavez, I., 217, 219, 761
Chéhadé, A. K., 465
Chen-Nong, 302
Cheselden, W., 897
Chevalier, A., 677
Chevauer, L., 800
Chevalier, U., 158, 159, 160
Chia-Ssu-hsieh, 296
Child, C. M., 605
Childe, V. G., 151, 581, 585
Chittenden, F. J., 120
Choay, E., 857
Choisy, M., 141
Chomel, A. F., 739
Cholmeley, H. P., 541
Chomel, N., 693
Chopra, I. C., 269
Chopra, R. N., 269
Chornick, H., 878
Chouard, P., 121, 619
Choulant, L., 32, 64, 70, 173, 597, 602, 603, 720, 723
Chou Ting-wang, 294
Christensen, G. C., 654
Christian, P., 184
Christofer, J. B., 9
Chuong Van-Vinh, 297, 298
Cianchi, R., 916
Cianfrani, T., 788
Cicero, Marcus Tullius, 153, 165, 329, 330, 335, 337, 338, 398, 399, 684
Ciferri, R., 47
Cignoli, F., 861
Civil, M., 260
Clagett, M., 10, 160, 328
Clairville, A. L., 143, 146
Claparède, E., 587
Clapham, J. H., 166, 489, 490, 493, 494, 497
Clark, A. S., 142
Clark, G., 5, 184, 186, 745
Clark, J., 189
Clark, J. G. D., 183, 209
Clark, L. T., 956
Clark, P. F., 135, 142, 615
Clark, R. E. D., 906
Clark, R. W., 946, 963
Clark, W. E. Le Gros, 581
Clark, W. H., 707
Clark-Kennedy, A. E.
Clarke, E., 598, 612
Clarke, J. H., 945
Clarke, R., 878
Clarkianus, 424
Clausen, L. W., 193
Clay, R. M., 502, 509, 514
Clayton, J., 897
Clemens Alexandrinos, see Clement of Alexandria

Clement of Alexandria, 427, 637
Clément-Mullet, J. J., 484
Clements, F. E., 202
Clendening, L., 718, 726, 728
Clérambault, G. G. de, 739
Cleve, F. M., 369
Cleveland Public Library, Catalog of folk lore, see Catalog of folk lore and folk songs
Clifford, D., 684
Clifford, G., 977
Clinton, G. W., 943
Clodd, E., 872, 963
Clokie, H. N., 669
Clusius, C., 561, 563, 665, 671, 898, 899
Clute, W. N., 112, 113, 674
Coats, A. M., 683
Cocchi, A., 396
Cockayne, T. O., 503, 504, 505, 514, 517
Cockburn, A., 832
Cockerell, T. D. A., 674
Cohen, B. C., 759
Cohen, I. B., 18, 935
Cohen, M. R., 328, 381
Cohen of Birkenhead, Lord, 1015
Cohn, F., 615, 616, 855
Cohn-Haft, L., 342
Cohnheim, J., 86
Coiter, V., 598, 649, 899
Cole, F. J., 54, 563, 566, 597, 598, 603, 641
Cole, H., 599
Coleman, W., 903
Colin, G., 459, 461
Colin, G. S., 446, 449
Colinmore, V., 1024
Collander, R., 667, 692
Collicut, F., 711
Collier, J. S., 815
Collingwood, R. G., 2, 10
Collins, S., 599
Collocott, T. C., 91, 100
Colmat, A., 833
Colombo, see Columbus, Realdus
Colón, E. D., 708
Colton, J., 553
Columbus, Realdus, 567, 575, 752, 952
Columella, Lucius Junius Moderatus, 338, 339, 385, 386, 388, 399, 652
Colvin, E. M., 48
Combes, R., 667
Comfort, A., 606, 780
Comrie, J. D., 745, 1023
Comte, A., 3, 4, 10, 590, 878
Condamine, C. M. de la, 665, 803
Conde, J. A., 674
Condorcet, M. J. A. N. de Caritat, Marquis de, 3
Conolly, J., 748, 784
Conrad Heingarter, see Heingar-

1043

1044

Davy de Virville, A., 668
Dawes, B., 564, 579
Dawson, O. L., 290
Dawson, W. R., 174, 185, 504, 514, 869, 962
Day, M., 582
Dayton, W. A., 124
Dean, B., 53, 59, 643
Deaux, G., 805
D'Ebandi de Fresne, 693
De Bary, T., 263, 559
De Beer, G. R., 896, 908, 1017
Debenham, F., 636
Debus, A. G., 73, 747, 990
Decaisne, J., 943
De Candolle, A. P., 13, 149, 157, 563, 580, 633, 637, 666, 672, 675, 893, 943
Dechambre, A., 136
Dechend, H. von, 975
Decker, A., 427
Découflé, P., 181
Deere, J., 708
De Fourmestraux, I., 740
De Francesco, G., 202
Defrasse, A., 342, 344
Defoe, D., 803
De Geer, C., see Geer, C. de
Degensheim, G. A., 813
De Grood, D. H., 944
Dehéran, H., 904
Deichgräber, K., 345, 360, 389
Deines, H. von, 244
De Jussieu, A. L., 81, 563, 580, 666
De Jussieu, B., 81, 580, 675
De Jussieu, family, 967
De Jussieu, J., 803
De la Brosse, G., 668
Delacroix, H., 589
De la Forge, L., 785
Delamare, V., 137
Delamarre, M. J. B., 679
Delaruelle, L., 997
Delatouche, R., 489, 493, 678, 680, 681
Delatte, A., 194, 197
Delaunay, A., 578
Delaunay, P., 641, 718, 740, 820, 874, 997
Delebecque, E., 375, 381
Deledalle, G., 589, 593
Delhoume, L., 876, 878, 919
De Lignamine, J. P., see Lignamine, J. P. de
Delile, A., 675
De Limbourg, 738
Delitzsch, F., 256, 258
Delorme, J., 92
De Loye, P., see Loye, P. de
Del Prozo, Efrén, C., 219
Demetrios, 174
Democedes of Crotona, 182, 348, 357
Democritos of Abdera, 153, 164, 335, 347, 348, 350, 352, 353,

357, 358, 647
Demosthenes Philalethes, 172, 351, 647
De Morsier, G., 14
Dooren de Jong, L. E., den, 879
Dengler, R. E., 379
Denis, E. de St., 413
Dennefeld, L., 253
Denonain, J. J., 887
Dent, A. A., 635
Derenbourg, H., 483, 484
Derksen, W., 54, 55, 646
De Sacy, S., 458
De Sanctis, S., 587
De Santillana, G., 333
Desault, J., 87
Descartes R., 8, 14, 17, 27, 73, 75, 154, 562, 573, 589, 590, 591, 603, 606, 613, 629, 783, 785, 878, 882, 884, 916, 917
Deschamps, P. C. E., 92
Desmond, R., 80
Des Étangs, A., 398
Desgenettes, R. N. D., 717, 742
Deslandes, L., 740
Dessoir, M., 588
De Terra, H., 959, 960
Deubner, O., 342
Deuchler, W., 894
Deutsch, A., 744, 766
Deutsche Zahn-, Mund-, und Kieferheilkunde, 70
Devaux, P., 14
Devèze, M., 693
De Vilmorin, R., 863, 943
De Vries, L., 103, 559, 618, 623, 984
De Waele, H., 955
Dewey, J., 593, 943
Dewhurst, K., 978, 1022
De Wildeman, E., 691
Dewing, S., 809
Dexippos of Cos, 346
d'Harcourt, R., 218
Dhorme, E., 256, 314
Dicaearchos of Messina, 335, 418
Dick, E. A., 111, 117
Dickinson, W. L., 853
Dickson, A., 385
Dictionary of Horticulture, see Elsevier's Dictionary of Horticulture
Dictionary catalogue of the Blacker-Wood Library of zoology and ornithology, see Wood, C. A.
Dictionary catalog... Massachusetts Horticultural Society, 51
Dictionary catalogue of the Yale Forestry Library, 51
Dictionary of national biography, 74, 80
Dictionnaire de biographie française, 74
Didymos of Alexandria, 423, 499
Dieckmann, H., 858

Diels, H., 348, 349, 354, 408
Diepgen, P., 85, 134, 174, 209, 422, 504, 526, 555, 556, 715, 719, 721, 789, 818
Dierbach, J. H., 336, 337, 356, 361
Dies, E. J., 708
Dietrich, A., 447, 448
Diderot, D., 573, 621, 625, 918
Dietrich, L. F., 683
Dikaerchos, see Dicaerchos of Messina
Dilleman, G., 846
Dillenius, J. J., 669, 670
Diller, H., 361
Dillon, H., 251
Dilthey, W., 590
Dimbleby, G. W., 194, 634
Dinanah, T., 460
Dingler, H., 14
Dingwall, E. J., 199
Diocles of Carystos, 166, 170, 176, 337, 343, 346, 356, 359, 373, 374, 379, 652, 781
Diodoros of Sicily, 341
Diogenes of Apollonia, 335, 348, 350, 352, 357, 358, 374
Dionysios, 172
Diophanes of Nicaea, 423
Dioscorides of Anazarbos, Pedanios, 22, 74, 166, 169, 170, 172, 197, 313, 331, 339, 394, 400, 401, 418, 430, 433, 445, 446, 457, 459, 467, 469, 475, 477, 492, 522, 529, 541, 543, 575, 580, 652, 849, 982
Directory, the Naturalists' see Naturalists' Directory
Ditler, R., 92
Dittrich, M., 960
Dobell, C., 973, 974
Dobrovici, A., 378
Dobson, J., 103, 110, 961
Dobson, J. F., 407
Doby, T., 575
Dobzhansky, T., 152, 619, 625
Dock, L. L., 824
Dodge, R., 587
Dodonaeus, R., 22, 665, 671, 937
Dodwell, H. H., 265
Doe, J., 62, 64, 995
Dörbeck, F., 803
Doerr, H., 615
Doerr, R., 615
Doesburgh, J. van, 494
Doesschate, G. ten, 893
Doets, C. J., 893
Doetsch, R. N., 616
Doeveren, W. van, 754
Dohr, H., 385
Dohrn, F. A., 637, 918
Dolan, J. A., 823
Doll, K., 930
Döllinger, J. J. I., 604, 640
Domagk, G., 77, 615, 855, 927
Dominic Gundisalvo, 488

1045

1048

George, W., 1031
Georgiadès, N., 240
Gerald the Welshman, 494
Gerard of Cremona, 452, 475, 477, 488, 510, 536
Gerard the Falconer, 498, 499
Gérard, F., 657
Gerard, J., 81, 568, 572, 670, 671, 937
Gerardus Falconarius, see Gerard the Falconer
Gereke, A., 332
German, W. J., 903
Gershon ben Shlomoh d'Arles, 323, 324
Gerste, A., 217, 219
Gerstein, M. J., 106
Gerth van Wijk, H. L., 114
Gervais, A., 303
Gervaise, 496
Gesamtkatalog der Wiegedrucke, 34
Gesell, A., 587
Gesner, C., 22, 81, 559, 560, 563, 570, 640, 644, 648, 664, 665, 671, 720, 758, 792, 937, 938
Gessmann, G. W., 195
Geuns, M. & S. J. van, 754
Geurts, P. M. M., 339, 355
Geyer, B., 27, 523
Geyer, R., 458
Geyl, P., 3, 4
Ghalioungui, P., 243
Ghatrif, 447
Ghinopoulo, S., 343
Ghiselin, M. T., 909
Gibbons, J., 1000
Giboin, L. M., 269
Gibson, J. J., 588
Gibson, W. C., 85, 1006
Gidney, E., 774
Giebel, C. G., 58
Gifford, G. B., 945
Gigon, O., 349
Gilbert the Englishman, see Gilbertus Anglicus
Gilbertus Anglicus, 163, 514, 533, 534, 541
Gilbert, E., 848
Gilbert, J. B., 67, 817
Gilbert, W., 749
Gildas (the Briton), 23
Giles of Corbeil, 515, 534, 541, 556
Gilg, E., 851
Gillispie, C. C., 15, 16
Gilmour, J., 670
Gilmour, J. S. L., 48
Gimlette, J. D., 227, 228
Gins, H., 806
Ginsburg, S., 853
Giordano Ruffo, 549
Giovanni of Arcoli, 516
Giovanni da Ketham, see Joannes de Ketham Alemanus
Girard, P., 342

Girault, J., 663
Giró, J., 765
Giuffre, L., 532
Glass, B., 621
Glasser, O., 1008
Glauber, J. R., 688
Gleditsch, J. G., 563
Glisson, F., 795, 874
Glover, E., 787
Gloyne, S. R., 961
Gmelin, J. G., 630, 637
Gnudi, M. T., 1023
Gobineau, Count, 559
Goblet d'Alviella, E. F. A., 691
Gode von Aesch, A., 16
Godlee, R. J., 977
Goebel, K. von, 956
Goerke, H., 134, 715, 742, 975
Goethe, J. W. von, 23, 24, 149, 569, 571, 578, 601, 640, 781, 937, 938, 939, 940, 941
Goetz, A., 410
Goldammer, K., 991
Goldenbaum, E., 696
Goldie, S., 988
Goldie, W. H., 228
Goldschmidt, R. B., 620, 641, 941
Goldsmith, M., 855, 984
Goldstein, K., 153, 588
Goldstein, M., 243
Golgi, C., 77, 752
Gompertz, M., 236
Gomperz, T., 349, 363
Goodall, G., 94
Goodfield, G. J., 607, 611
Goodman, N. G., 1010
Goodrich, L. C., 284
Goodyer, J., 400, 401, 670
Gorce, M., 17
Gorceix, B., 993
Gordon, B. L., 176, 505, 721
Gordon, C. A., 408
Gordon, H. L., 324
Gordon, J. E., 835
Gordon, M. B., 767
Gorgani, see Ismā'il ibn Ḥasan al Jurjānī
Gorgias, W. C., 817
Gorgias, 358
Gorlin, M., 325
Gosse, P. H., 941
Gossen, H., 394, 396
Gosset, M., 73
Gothan, W., 631
Gothein, M. L., 167, 683, 684
Gottheil, R. J. C., 433
Gottlieb, B. J., 1019
Gottlieb, L. S., 608
Gould Medical Dictionary, 137
Gourlie, N., 975
Govaerts, J., 738
Gow, A. S. F., 411
Graaf, R. de, 602, 603, 754, 941
Grabmann, M., 548
Grabner, E., 203, 206, 208
Graeffe, A. von, 742, 956

Graesse, J. G. T., 31, 33, 92
Graham, T. F., 516
Grainger, T. H., 617
Gram, C., 615
Grand, R., 489, 493, 678, 680, 681
Grande, F., 877
Granit, R., 1016
Granjel, L. S., 726, 756, 757
Granqvist, H., 440, 468
Grant, R. M., 161
Grapow, H., 243, 244
Gratarolo, Guglielmo (=William Gratarolus), 26
Gratius, 338
Grattan, J. H. G., 503, 505, 514
Graubard, M., 566, 580, 608
Graustein, J. E., 989
Graux, L., 550
's-Gravensande, P., 739
Grawinkel, C. J., 181
Gray, A., 25, 619, 675, 908, 942, 943, 1025
Gray, J., 747
Gray, J. L., 943
Gray, L. C., 707
Gray, P., 102, 105
Grazioso, P., 185, 186
Green, C. E., 122, 123
Green, H., 818
Green, J. R., 657, 663, 670, 728
Green, M. L., 977
Green, M. M., 108
Green, R. M., 395, 401, 403, 935
Greenacre, P., 787
Greenblatt, R. B., 322
Greene, E. L., 657, 661, 665, 674
Greene, H., 876
Greene, J. C., 10, 621, 622, 910, 943
Greene, M., 371
Greenway, P. J., 228
Gregor, A. S., 584
Gregorius Abu'l-Farag, see Bar-Hebraeus
Gregory I, the Great, pope, 26
Gregory of Nyssa, 515
Gregory, N., 98
Gregory, W., 94, 98, 975
Grene, M., 153
Grenet, P., 1024
Grensemann, H., 363, 379
Greve, H. C., 820
Grew, N., 8, 81, 568, 599, 670, 943
Grier, J., 849
Griesinger, W., 944
Grieve, M., 112
Griffith, F. L., 244
Griffith, G. T., 384
Grīghōr (Abu al-Faraj), see Bar-Hebraeus
Grimal, P., 386
Grimaux, E., 972
Grim(m), H. N., 229
Grinder, R. E., 590
Grmek, M. D., 56, 218, 222, 224,

300, 476, 506, 509, 513, 606, 739, 780, 812, 877
Gromas, R., 694
Gronovius, J. F., 897
Groos, K., 587
Gross, S. D., 86
Grosseteste, R., *see* Robertus Grosseteste
Grotjahn, M., 83, 787
Grousset, R., 305
Grove, A. R., 217
Grubbé, E. H., 809
Gruber, G., 742
Gruber, M. v., 830
Grueling, P. G., 795
Grünberg, F., 564
Grumach, E., 371
Gruman, G. J., 608
Grunebaum, G. E. von, 441
Gruner, O. C., 471
Guaineri, Ant., 26
Gualterus Agulinus, *see* Walter Agilon
Gudger, E. W., 53
Günther, H., 937
Günther, K., 542
Guérin, L., 657
Guerini, V., 775
Guerlac, H., 17
Guerra, F., 764, 768, 770
Guerrero, P., 763
Guerrero, R., 757
Guggenbühl, J., 824
Guggenheim, K., 923
Guiard, E., 203
Guiart, J., 741
Guido de Vigevano, 546
Guigues, P., 473, 476, 481
Guilford, J. P., 588
Guillain, G., 897
Guillaume le Clerc, *see* William the Clerck
Guillaume de Moerbeke, 428
Guillaumin, A., 633
Guillelmus Falconarius, *see* William the Falconer
Guillotin, J. J., 719
Guinochet, M., 114
Guitard, E. H., 67, 73
Guleke, N., 840
Gulik, H. v., 290
Gummerus, H., 390
Gumpert, C. G., 395, 396
Gumpert, M., 946
Gunst, P., 51
Gunther, R. T., 394, 400, 670, 957
Gupta, A. K., 176
Gupta, H. N., 274
Gupta, K. V. N. S., 275
Gurley, J. E., 820
Gurlt, E. J., 811, 838
Gurney, J. H., 649
Guthrie, D., 721, 747, 793, 977
Guthrie, W. K. C., 350
Gutschmidt, A. von, 463

Guttmacher, A. F., 418
Guy de Chauliac, 26, 87, 163, 476, 501, 513, 516, 534, 535, 548, 599
Guyénot, E., 567, 571, 573
Guyon, F., 742
Guyot, L., 633, 737
Guyotjeanin, C., 843

Haacke, W., 868
Haas, H., 843
Haase, C., 974
Haber, F., 611, 1035
Haber, F. C., 631
Haberkamp, G., 122, 126
Haberling, W. G., 743, 988
Hadas, M., 383
Haddon, A. C., 582
Hadfield, M., 684
Hadzsits, G. D., 334, 408
Haeckel, E., 157, 563, 570, 574, 578, 618, 627, 638, 641, 644, 919, 944, 945
Haeckel, M., 928
Haedike, W., 339
Haehl, R., 945, 946
Haensch, G., 122, 126
Haeser, H., 722, 730, 824
Haffner, A., 458
Haffner, E. A., 399
Hagberg, K., 976
Hagedoorn, H., 1014
Hagen, C., 706
Hagen, H., 337, 782
Hagen, H. A., 54, 55
Haggard, H. W., 853
Haggard, R., 698
Hague, R., 1024
Hahn, A., 722
Hahnemann, S., 735, 781, 945
Hain, L., 34
Halban, J., 790
Haldane, J. B. S., 906, 946
Halde, J. B. du, *see* Du Halde, J. B.
Hale, P. H., 122, 679
Hale-White, W., 970
Hales, S., 8, 578, 612, 670, 736, 947
Ḥalifa al Ḥalabi, 450, 451
Hall, A. R., 7, 17, 18
Hall, C. van, 672
Hall, M. B., 18, 885
Hall, S., 593
Hall, T. S., 567, 580
Hall, W., 890, 891
Hallauer, C., 615
Haller, A. von, 24, 69, 75, 563, 602, 603, 605, 606, 611, 618, 637, 640, 720, 743, 758, 874, 947, 948, 980, 1018, 1019
Halliday, W. R., 330
Halsted, W. S., 767, 814, 949
Hamarneh, S., 449, 475

Hamby, W. B., 995, 996
Ḥamdullah al Mustaufi al-Qazwīnī, *see* Al-Kazwīnī
Hamer, G. T., 318
Hamilton, M., 843
Hammond, E. A., 514
Hampp, I., 204
Hanbury, D., 943
Handerson, H. E., 533
Handley, J., 699, 700
Handlin, O., 1032
Hanes, K., 610
Haniff, M., 226, 228
Hanks, L., 889
Hanot, V. C., 742
Hans Suff von Göppingen, 513
Hansen, E. C., 559
Hansmann, L., 183, 186, 190, 192
Hanssen, P., 832
Hanstein, J. L. E. R., 605
Harada, J., 291, 295
Hardenberg, *see* Stein
Hardin, G., 152, 153
Harding, T. S., 710
Hardy, G. H., 626
Hare, R., 173, 832, 856
Haring, F., 125
Harington, J., 519
Harkins, P. W., 404
Harley, G. W., 229, 231
Harms, E., 783
Harms, R., 969
Harper Encyclopedia of Sience, *see* Newman, J. R.
Harper, F., 872
Harriman, P. L., 94, 96, 100
Harrington, J., 829
Harris, L. J., 795, 799
Harris, M., 583
Harris, S., 870
Harrison, F., 485
Harrison, R. G., 605
Harrison, R. J., 104
Harting, J. E., 55, 648
Hartlib, S., 699
Hartman, L. F., 253, 257
Hartmann, E. von, 152, 596
Hartmann, F., 237, 519, 520, 542, 991
Hartmann, J. H., 787
Hartmann, M., 77, 149, 153, 781
Hartner, W., 29, 300, 302
Harvard University, Peabody Museum, *see* Catalogue Peabody Museum of Archaeology and Ethnology
Harvey, E. N., 608, 611, 613, 618
Harvey, W., 8, 24, 27, 75, 152, 559, 566, 567, 569, 570, 573, 575, 576, 578, 598, 603, 606, 718, 725, 727, 729, 745, 749, 750, 774, 781, 896, 943, 949, 950, 951, 952, 953, 958
Harvey-Gibson, R. J., 18, 658
Harwood, W. S., 890
Hasenrück, E., 124

1050

Haskins, C. H., 485
Haslam, J., 748
Hastings, C., 953
Hatfield, E. J., 572
Hatt, G., 678
Hauber, D. E. D., 33
Haudicourt, A. G., 634, 679
Hauduroy, P., 617
Hauer, J. W., 264, 282
Hauger, A., 386, 387, 389
Hauke, E., 404
Haupt, J., 528
Haupt, M., 430
Haushofer, H., 695
Hausmann, U., 343
Haussig, H. W., 161
Haussleiter, J., 327
Hawkes, J., 187
Hawley, R. C., 123, 127
Hay, S., 263, 760
Hayem, G., 742, 774
Haymaker, W., 86
Hays, H. R., 583
Heagerty, J. J., 760
Heaney, H. J., 498
Hearnshaw, L. S., 590
Heberden, W., 749, 795, 953, 954
Heberer, G., 619, 622, 908, 944
Heckel, M., 125
Hecker, J. F. C., 505
Hédin, L., 634
Hedin, S., 76
Hedrick, U. P., 710
Heer, O., 943
Hegel, G. W. F., 3, 4, 781
Hehlman, W., 590, 591, 594, 595
Hehn, V., 634
Heidegger, M., 589
Heilmann, K. E., 492, 655, 658, 663, 664
Heim, E. L., 744
Heim, R., 863, 879, 889
Heinecke, W., 412
Heingarter, Conrad, 26
Heinrich Louffenberg, 512
Heinrich von Pfalzpeunt, 513
Heinrich Steinhöwel, 513
Heitland, W. E., 337, 385
Heizer, R. F., 187
Hektoen, L., 805
Heliodoros the Surgeon, 393
Heller, J. L., 779, 977
Hellriegel, H., 550
Helmholtz, H. L. F. von, 588, 590, 954
Helmont, J. B. van, 8, 27, 74, 197, 559, 606, 612, 955
Helson, H., 588
Hemleben, J., 945
Henderson, D. K., 745, 748
Henderson, I. F., 102, 105
Henderson, L. J., 876
Henderson, M. J., 49
Henderson, W. D., 102, 105
Henfrey, A., 943
Henle, J., 86, 616, 855

Henn, A. W., 53
Hennebo, D., 493, 696
Hennefrund, H. E., 196
Henri of Mondeville, 163, 512, 513, 515, 535, 602, 937
Henricus Breyell, 536
Henry, G. W., 788
Henschel, T., 520
Henschen, F., 833
Hensler, P. G. H., 744
Henslow, G., 494, 670, 908, 943
Heraclitos of Ephesos, 332, 335, 347, 348, 349, 350, 351, 353, 354, 357, 358, 365, 374, 375, 559
Herakleides von Tarent, 390
Herbart, J. F., 23, 588, 591
Herbst, C., 641
Herder, J. G. von, 3, 23, 621
Herdman, W. A., 636
Herelle, F. d', 615
Hering, E., 82, 618
Hermann, F., 647
Hernández, F., 765
Herndon, T., 508
Herodikos of Selymbria, 358
Herodotos of Halicarnassos, 337, 338, 372, 375, 393
Heron, F. G., 546
Heron-Allen, E., 494
Herophilos of Chalcedon, 172, 174, 337, 347, 392, 407, 602
Heros Iatros, 343
Herpin, A., 926
Herrad of Landsberg, 536
Herrick, F. H., 867
Herrick, J. B., 774
Herrlinger, R., 110, 598, 599, 722, 729, 899, 1036
Herrnstein, R. J., 591, 595
Herskovits, M. J., 880
Hertwig, the brothers, 618, 641
Hertwig's Jahresbericht, 56
Hervey-Saint-Denys, L., 291, 292
Herzfeld, E., 436
Herzog, R., 342, 344
Heseler, B., 1029
Hesiod, 171, 329, 337, 347, 349, 351, 352, 353, 357, 375, 423
Heske, F., 687
Hess, A. F., 799
Hess, W. R., 77
Hesse, P., 560
Hett, W. S., 370
Heurne, J. van, see Heurnius, J.
Heurnius, J., 753
Heuss, T., 918
Hewat, M. L., 231
Heymann, B., 969
Heymans, G., 587
Heyne, R., 392
Hiärne, U., 76
Hickman, C. J., 101, 815
Hierocles, 652
Hieronymous Brunschwig, 512, 513. 536, 537

Hiersemann, C., 520
Hildegard of Bingen, 23, 26, 162, 169, 437, 492, 504, 522, 537, 538, 656, 727, 732
Hilgenberg, L., 281
Hilka, A., 554
Hill, A. V., 77, 580, 670
Hill, A. W., 1033
Hill, B., 891
Hill, R. H., 69
Hill, W. W., 219, 221
Himes, N. E., 817
Himmelfarb, G., 910
Himmelweit, F., 921
Hintzsche, E., 759, 924
Hippias of Elis, 348
Hippocrates of Cos, 22, 74, 153, 155, 171, 172, 175, 176, 180, 182, 313, 333, 336, 337, 339, 341, 343, 345, 346, 347, 353, 354, 356, 358, 359, 360, 361, 362, 363, 364, 365, 366, 367, 368, 373, 375, 378, 379, 380, 398, 403, 404, 416, 418, 419, 431, 444, 448, 467, 469, 470, 472, 507, 529, 535, 541, 544, 546, 559, 562, 573, 602, 618, 637, 652, 724, 727, 781, 784, 787, 795, 796, 797, 798, 799, 809, 810, 819, 834, 836, 840, 842, 849, 850, 933
Hippon, 348, 357
Hirsch, A., 85, 86, 833
Hirsch, G. C., 106
Hirsch-Schweigger, E., 133
Hirschberg, J., 241, 245, 424, 450, 451, 466, 471, 792
Hirschberg, P. S. von, see Pankratius S. von Hirschberg
Hirshleifer, J., 805
Hirst, L. F., 804
His, W., 618, 758, 955
Hitti, P. K., 483
Hjelt, O. E. A., 976
Hobbes, T., 14, 589, 590, 591, 951
Hobhouse, R. W., 946
Hochberg, L. A., 812, 814
Hocking, G. M., 137
Hodes, F., 30
Hodge, P., 225, 773
Hodgen, M. T., 583
Hodgkinson, R. G., 828
Hoefer, F., 640, 795
Höffding, H., 587
Höfler, M., 137, 210
Hölder, H., 631
Hönger, F., 522
Hoeniger, F. D., 568
Hoeppli, R., 300
Hoeppner, W., 986
Hoernlé, A. F. R., 275, 276
Hoerr, N. L., 135, 137
Hoff, H. E., 324
Hoffman, M., 972
Hoffmann, A., 696

1052

1053

1061

1066

1067

Wells, W., 15, 622, 815
Weltforstatlas, 127
Welwitsch, F. M. J., 943
Weniger, L., 336, 357
Wenzl, A., 918, 919
Werlhof, P. G. W., 744
Werner, C. F., 106
Werner, K., 499
Werth, E., 679
Wertheimer, M., 590
Wesley, J., 1033
West, D. J., 588
West, G., 912
West, G. P., 129, 131, 132, 654
West, M., 483
Westendorf, W., 241, 244
Wester, J., 654
Westwood, T., 54, 58
Wethered, H. N., 415, 684
Wettley, A., 782, 928
Wettstein, R. von, 968
Weyer, J., 788
Weyl, T., 1031
Weymouth, A., 801
Wharton, T., 780
Wheeler, F. J., 946
Wheeler, L. R., 152, 157
Wheeler, W. M., 1008
Wheelwright, E. G., 665
Whetman, E. H., 698, 701
Whetzel, H. H., 690
Whipple, A. O., 448, 767, 815
Whipple, G. H., 77
White, A. D., 27
White, G., 560, 1033, 1034
White, J. G. Department of
  folklore, Cleveland Public
  Library, see Catalog of
  folklore
White, K. D., 386, 387, 388,
  389
White, S., 767
White, T. H., 497, 499
Whitehead, A. N., 19
Whitehead, P. J. P., 900
Whitehouse, H. L. K., 906
Whitman, C. O., 596
Whitlock, R., 698, 701, 703,
  704
Whitney, E., 708
Whitrow, G. J., 158
Whitteridge, G., 952
Whittle, T., 685
Whyte, L. L., 595
Whytt, R., 795
Wichler, G., 912
Wichmann, J. E. W., 744
Wichtermann, R., 641
Wickersheimer, E., 508, 511,
  516, 546, 742
Widal, F., 742
Widdess, J. D. H., 751
Widdra, K., 381
Wiecko, E., 706
Wiedemann, A., 233
Wiedemann, E., 461, 462, 463,

464, 478, 483
Wiener, N., 580
Wier, J., 26
Wiesner, J., 666, 964
Wight, R., 943
Wightman, W. P. D., 28
Wilcocks, C., 831
Wilcox, J., 444
Wildhaber, R., 40
Wiley, H. W., 708
Wilhelm, R., 967
Wilke, G., 215
Wilkie, J. S., 906
Wilkins, M., 629
Wilkinson, K. D., 1035
Willerding, U., 695
Willey, G. R., 581
William de Brescia, 513
William the Clerc, 496, 558
William de Congenis, 504, 510,
  513
William the Falconer, 498, 499
William Gratarolus, see
  Gratarolo, G.
William of Ockham, 11
William of Saliceto, 476, 513,
  514, 515, 536, 543, 558, 781
Williams, B., 855, 924
Williams, R. C., 831
Williams, R. R., 799
Williams, T. I., 79
Williamson, G. C., 79
Willier, B. H., 605
Willis, J. C., 118, 570, 599, 603
Willis, R., 950, 953
Willis, T., 780, 1034
Willius, F. A., 567, 575, 579
Wills, G., 318
Willstätter, R., 1034, 1035
Willughby, F., 81, 649
Wilms, H., 525
Wilpert, P., 546
Wilsdorf, H., 865
Wilson, A., 79
Wilson, E. B., 605, 984
Wilson, H. F., 647
Wilson, J. A., 161, 235
Wilson, J. V. Kinnier, see
  Kinnier Wilson, J. V.
Wilson, J. W., 10
Wilson, L. G., 607
Wilson, M. L., 965
Wilson, R. H. L., 812, 814
Wimmer-Aeschlimann, U., 948
Winburne, J. N., 123
Winchell, C. M., 100
Winckler, E., 666
Winckler, L., 857
Windisch, W., 56, 58, 59
Windler, E., 527
Wingate, S. D., 500
Winick, C., 110, 962
Winney, J., 888
Winogradski, S. N., 615, 616,
  1035
Winslow, C. E. A., 834, 835

Winspear, A. D., 409
Winstedt, R. O., 232
Winter, H. J. J., 28
Winter, I., 730
Winter, J., 396
Winters, R. K., 714
Wirth, D., 129
Wirth, W., 587
Wirz, P., 232
Wirzen, J. E. A., 667
Wisberg, H. A., 947
Wissler, C., 224
Wissowa, G., 331
Wit, C. de, 239
Wit, H. C. D. de, 1009
Wither, G., 331, 410
Withering, W., 736, 853, 1035
Withers, S., 79
Withington, E. T., 351, 365,
  736
Witt, F. H., 776
Wittop Koning, D. A., 898
Wittstein, G. C., 116
Woelderen, C. A. van, 381
Woenig, F., 238, 239
Woglom, W. H., 736
Woillez, E., 73
Wolf-Heidegger, G., 598, 603
Wolf, A., 28, 29
Wolf, K. L., 939
Wolfe, L. S., 128
Wolff, C. F., 601, 618, 627,
  640, 980, 1036
Wolff, E., 878
Wolff, G., 800
Wolff, J., 809
Wolff, K. F., 152
Wolff, R. L., 9
Wolfson, H. A., 312
Wollaston, W. H., 809
Wolska, W., 427
Wolstenholme, G., 745
Wong, K. Chimin, 303, 310
Wong, M., 283, 284, 302, 310
Wood, A., 1036
Wood, C. A., 59, 60, 466, 528,
  533
Wood, E. S., see Wood, C. A.
Wood, J. G., 316, 317, 381
Woodcock, G., 872
Woodcock, P. G., 334
Woodger, J. H., 150
Woodham-Smith, C., 988
Woods, R. S., 110, 615
Woodward, J., 837
Woodward, M., 937
Woodworth, R. S., 587
Wootton, A. C., 850
World geography of forest
  resources
World List of scientific
  periodicals, see Brown, P.
World medical periodicals, see
  Unesco list of world medical
  periodicals
Worlidge, J., 699

1070

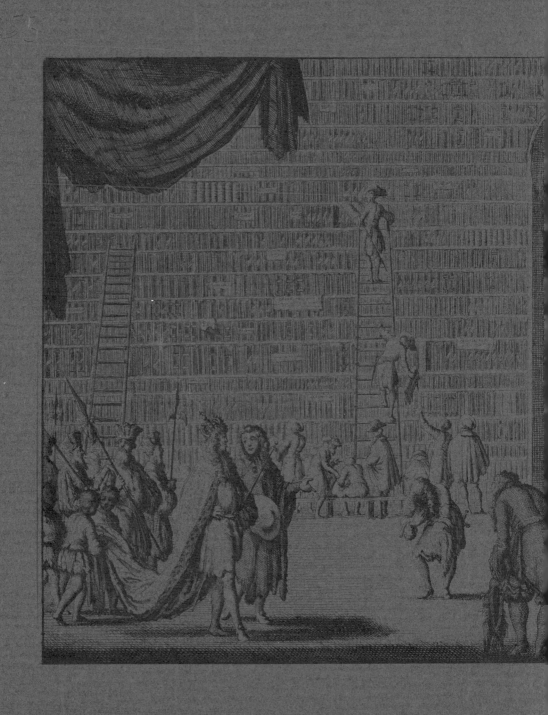